AMBULATORY OBSTETRICS

Third Edition

WINIFRED L. STAR, RNC, NP, MS

MAUREEN T. SHANNON, CNM, FNP, MS

LISA L. LOMMEL, FNP, MS, MPH

YOLANDA M. GUTIERREZ, PhD, RD

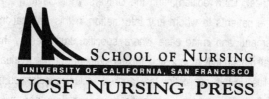

SCHOOL OF NURSING
UNIVERSITY OF CALIFORNIA, SAN FRANCISCO

UCSF NURSING PRESS

Copyright 1999 by The Regents, University of California

Senior Publications Coordinator: Kathleen McClung
Design/Production: Patricia Walsh Design, Claire Keaveney
Editor: Sara Shopkow
Proofreader: Lisa Carlson
Index: ALTA Indexing Service

For information, contact:

UCSF Nursing Press
School of Nursing
University of California, San Francisco
521 Parnassus Avenue, Room N535C
San Francisco, CA 94143-0608 U.S.A.
Phone: (415) 476-4992
Fax: (415) 476-6042
Internet: http://nurseweb.ucsf.edu/www/books.htm

ISBN # 0-943671-18-3

First Printing, 1999
Printed in U.S.A.

DISCLAIMER

The authors of Ambulatory Obstetrics (Third edition), and the University of California, San Francisco disavow any responsibility for the outcomes of the patients to whom any information in this publication is applied, including general assessment and treatment/management, and in the case where specific drug therapy has been delineated. It is the individual practicing clinician who shall remain fully responsible for the outcome of the evaluation and management of the patients to whom any clinical guidelines in this publication are applied, including instances in which specific drug therapy has been set forth. For additional information concerning specific drugs and drug therapy, health care providers should consult the drug package insert, the Physicians' Desk Reference, and/or a clinical pharmacist.

DEDICATION

To Judy Carlson, my mentor and friend—a wonderfully unique person who provided me with a sound and practical foundation in the advanced nursing practice of clinical obstetrics, and who, as an internationally working nurse-midwife, has improved maternal-child health care in many developing nations of the world. And to all of my loving friends, family members, patients, and colleagues who helped me face the challenges of 1998 with strength, dignity, and courage.

WLS

To my patients who continue to teach me my most valuable clinical lessons; and to the members of the Shannon-Pantell Family Circus (Matthew, Gregory, Megan, and Bob) who continue to keep me smiling.

MTS

To Michael, for always believing in my dreams and not letting me forget them. And to Liam and Tess for teaching me not to take anything too seriously.

LLL

To my husband Adolfo, and Richard and Nancy for their constant support, love, and encouragement.

YG

ACKNOWLEDGMENTS

The publication of the third edition of *Ambulatory Obstetrics* would not have been possible without the participation and support of a number of people.

A special thanks to our research assistant, Ann-Marie McNamara, for her dedication and good spirit, and for enduring a multitude of hours of literature retrieval. We thank Kristina Keilman, MS, for her expert review of the hemoglobinopathy chapters and the section on preconceptional health, and for being so graciously indulgent of all our many questions. For taking the time to read and improve the travel during pregnancy chapter, we are grateful to Jerome Greenbaum, MD. Thanks also to Lee Wilkinson, MD for reviewing the anemia tables. We extend thanks to Phyllis Acosta, DrPH, RD, for providing valuable information regarding nutritional support for persons with PKU; to Merry-K. Moos, FNP, MPH and Robert Cefalo, MD, PhD, for their excellent publication on preconceptional health care; and, to Perinatal Health, Inc., for sharing their written materials on preconceptional health matters. And, to Barbara Murphy, RN, MSN, Donald Coustan, MD, Robin Field, MD, and David Sacks, MD, we thank you for the discussions regarding gestational diabetes mellitus and providing us with information on screening, diagnosis, and guidelines for care of pregnant women with this condition. To Tony Cesnik and Vince Lagano, many thanks for your assistance with online literature searches and the timely acquisition of a great number of journal articles. And, thanks to Ethel Gamboa for her graciousness and skillful technical assistance in creating many of the figures and tables in the book.

The contributing authors also wish to thank a number of individuals. Kristina Keilman would like to thank Bruce Blumberg, MD, Cody Cotulla, Christine Hartlove, MS, Tamara Treisman, MS and Amy Vance, MS, for their ideas and encouragement. Susan Adams wishes to thank and acknowledge Ronald J. Ruggiero, PharmD, for his comments and suggestions about substance abuse in pregnant women. He has been an invaluable resource. Fritzi Drosten thanks her younger children, Allyson and Emma, for their patience and understanding, her older son, Leben, who taught her how to use a word processor, and Rebecca Matthews for her assistance and encouragement.

For our medical editors, Dr.'s Susan Schaefer, Robin Henson, Tracy Flanagan, Karen Beckerman, and Robert Pantell—thank you for the expert review of the manuscripts and for your astute comments and practical suggestions for clarification and augmentation of the material.

For his professional guidance and continuing support of the book, we are grateful to William Holzemer, PhD, at the University of California, San Francisco. To Kathleen McClung, senior publications coordinator of the UCSF Nursing Press, thank you for your assistance in organizing the many administrative details of the book's publication. A very special thanks to our extremely good-natured and insightful editor, Sara Shopkow, for all her hard work and diligence in getting this manual to become a readable, finished product. And, to Theo Crawford and Claire Keaveney, many thanks for performing the painstaking task of input and formatting of the publication.

Finally, as always, we thank our mentors, colleagues and students for sharing their insights an experiences with us; and, our patients, for making the practice of obstetrics so rewarding.

PRINCIPAL AUTHORS

Winifred L. Star, RNC, NP, MS
Women's Health Nurse Practitioner
Coordinator, Young Mother's Clinic
Department of Obstetrics and Gynecology
Kaiser Permanente Medical Center
San Francisco, California

Associate Clinical Professor
Department of Family Health Care Nursing
University of California, San Francisco
San Francisco, California

Maureen T. Shannon, CNM, FNP, MS
Associate Clinical Professor
Department of Family Health Care Nursing
University of California, San Francisco
San Francisco, California

Perinatal Study Coordinator
Bay Area Perinatal AIDS Center
San Francisco General Hospital
San Francisco, California

Lisa L. Lommel, FNP, MS, MPH
Associate Clinical Professor
Co-Director, Family and Women's Primary Care Nurse Practitioner Program
Department of Family Health Care Nursing
University of California, San Francisco
San Francisco, California

Family and Women's Health Nurse Practitioner
Director, Young Women's Clinic
University of California, San Francisco/Mt. Zion Medical Center
San Francisco, California

Yolanda M. Gutierrez, PhD, RD
Associate Clinical Professor
Department of Family Health Care Nursing
University of California, San Francisco
San Francisco, California

Regional Perinatal Nutrition Consultant
Stanford University School of Medicine
Mid-Coastal California Perinatal Outreach Program
Palo Alto, California

CONTRIBUTING AUTHORS

Susan L. Adams, RNC, NP, PhD
Women's Health Nurse Practitioner
Obstetrics and Gynecology Continuity Practice
Ambulatory Care Center
University of California, San Francisco
San Francisco, California

Assistant Clinical Professor
Department of Family Health Care Nursing
University of California, San Francisco
San Francisco, California

Pilar Bernal de Pheils, RNC, MS, FNP
Associate Clinical Professor
Family and Women's Primary Care Nurse
    Practitioner Program
Department of Family Health Care Nursing
University of California, San Francisco
San Francisco, California

Family and Women's Health Nurse Practitioner
Young Women's Clinic
Department of Obstetrics
University of California, San Francisco
San Francisco, California

Mission Neighborhood Health Center
San Francisco, California

Barbara J. Burgel, RN, MS, ANP, COHN-S
Clinical Professor
Occupational Health Nursing Program
Department of Community Health Systems
University of California, San Francisco
San Francisco, California

Fritzi Drosten, RN, IBCLC
Lactation Consultant
Kaiser Foundation Hospital
Oakland, California

Visiting Nurse Association
Emeryville, California

Kristina Keilman, MS
Genetic Counselor
Clinical Services Manager
Department of Genetics
Kaiser Permanente Medical Center
San Francisco, California

Ann-Marie McNamara, RNC, NP, MS
Women's Health Nurse Practitioner
Sacred Circle of Birth
Perinatal Department
Native American Health Center
Oakland, California

Joan R. Murphy, RNC, MS, NP, CNS
Women's Health Nurse Practitioner
Perinatal Clinical Specialist
Department of Obstetrics and Gynecology
Kaiser Permanente Medical Center
San Francisco, California

Hoff Medical Group
Redwood City, California

Lucy Newmark Sammons, RNC, NP, ACCE, DNS
Assistant Clinical Professor
Department of Family Health Care Nursing
University of California, San Francisco
San Francisco, California

Ellen M. Scarr, RNC, MS, FNP, WHNP
Associate Clinical Professor
Family and Women's Primary Care Nurse
    Practitioner Program
University of California, San Francisco
San Francisco, California

Family and Women's Health Nurse Practitioner
Young Women's Clinic
Department of Obstetrics
University of California, San Francisco
San Francisco, California

Women's Clinic
City College of San Francisco
San Francisco, California

Maxine Hall Health Center
Department of Public Health
San Francisco, California

PREFACE TO THE THIRD EDITION

The authors are pleased to introduce the third edition of *Ambulatory Obstetrics*. This edition brings a reorganization of the book with new depth and breadth to the material contained in prior publications. Several new sections and chapters have also been included with the collaboration of contributing authors from a variety of backgrounds, who have brought new expertise to this edition. We hope you will find this expanded version useful.

The publication is meant to be a "working manual" for use in the clinical setting—as a source of information on common obstetrical conditions, as well a framework from which to formulate site-specific guidelines for practice. As before, the Subjective-Objective-Assessment-Plan (SOAP) format is used for ease of reading the clinical guidelines sections of the book. For more in-depth information on selected conditions the reader is directed to the reference section contained within each chapter or current textbooks in the field of obstetrics.

The reader may have noticed the change in the book's title. It is our hope that this edition will target a broader audience of clinicians: *all* of the health professionals who provide ambulatory obstetrical services. We would like to mention that the "sister book" to this publication, entitled *Women's Primary Health Care: Protocols for Practice** is a comprehensive primary care guide that will complement *Ambulatory Obstetrics* and enhance the reader's library on women's health publications.

We welcome your comments and suggestions. Please address correspondence to

UCSF Nursing Press
School of Nursing, Room N-535-C
521 Parnassus Avenue, Box 0608
San Francisco, CA 94143-0608.

*Star, W. L., Lommel, L. L., and Shannon, M. T. (1995). *Women's primary health care: Protocols for practice.* Washington, D. C.: American Nurses' Publishing. 1-800-637-0323.

TABLE OF CONTENTS

(continued)

(continued)

(continued)

SECTION 1

PRECONCEPTION HEALTH CARE—AN OVERVIEW

Section 1

PRECONCEPTION HEALTH CARE—AN OVERVIEW

Winifred L. Star

In the 1990 U.S. Public Health Service document, *Healthy People 2000: National Health Promotion and Disease Prevention Objectives*, one of the stated national objectives for improvement in the area of maternal/child health was to "increase to at least 60 percent the proportion of primary care providers who provide age-appropriate preconception care and counseling" (U.S. Department of Health and Human Services, 1990, p. 99). Indeed, throughout this country, an increasing number of programs have been developed to provide preconception care, with the ultimate goal to improve reproductive outcomes.

Preconception health care focuses on identifying and reducing reproductive risks for women and couples before conception. Components of care include 1) risk assessment, 2) health promotion, and 3) medical and psychosocial intervention, including education, counseling, referral, and follow-up (Jack & Culpepper, 1991). Care can be provided in a variety of settings, such as a primary care setting in private practice or a health maintenance organization, a sexually transmitted disease (STD) or family planning clinic, a substance abuse treatment center, a school health education program, or a community or occupational health center. Often, a multidisciplinary team of health care providers is involved.

Preconception health education and counseling includes such topics as effects of lifestyle choices on reproduction, the interplay of genetics, workplace and environmental hazards, the impact of nutrition, and the effects of medication and specific disease states on maternal/fetal health (Frede, 1993). According to Cefalo & Moos (1995), the overriding goal of preconception counseling should be to provide each client and, if desired, her partner with adequate information to make informed decisions about reproduction. The information can empower clients to accept risks or modify them, to forego their childbearing potential or choose other reproductive options (such as donor insemination, oocyte donation, surrogacy, or adoption) (Cefalo & Moos, 1995; Holtzman, 1990).

Strategies for implementing preconception health care will vary from site to site depending on the capabilities and constraints of the system; however, programs of preconception health promotion should include three basic components: 1) systematic and comprehensive identification of individual risks, 2) provision of personalized, nonjudgmental education, and 3) availability of complementary services (e.g., genetics, nutritional counseling, behavioral modification programs) (Cefalo & Moos, 1995). Since comprehensive preconception counseling encompasses a vast area of knowledge, the clinician may need to increase his/her skills in this area through in-service education or specialty training.

The information contained in this section is intended to provide an overview of preconception health care in a primary care setting and is structured to provide basic information to aid the clinician in counseling a client or couple. Complete information on all medical diagnoses affecting pregnancy is beyond the scope of this text. Additional information from other chapters in this book and/or a current textbook will be an essential supplement to the information here. The publication by Cefalo and Moos (1995) is a valuable resource. See also Patient Education Materials and Referral Resources, Appendix 1b.

Database

Subjective

- Individual client assessment requires an extended time frame, and the counselor's schedule must allow for this. Follow-up visits may be necessary.

- A complete health history is imperative. See Table 1.1, Risk Assessment. Use a preprinted preconception risk assessment questionnaire to expedite the process of evaluation. The form may be mailed to the client prior to the initial visit. See Appendix 1a, Preconceptional Health Assessment—Client History Form, for an example of a preprinted questionnaire.

- Encourage the client or couple to bring to the preconception counseling session a list of specific questions and concerns; this further individualizes care.

- See Intervention/Management and Patient Education in this chapter for further discussion.

Objective

- Physical examination parameters will vary depending on the setting, the time frame of the visit, and the client's health history. Components may include

  - ▶ Height, weight, calculation of desirable body weight (DBW)

  - ▶ Vital signs (blood pressure, pulse)

  - ▶ Complete or screening physical examination, including the following, as indicated: skin, HEENT, thyroid, heart, lungs, breasts, abdomen, genitalia, rectum, lymph nodes, pulses, reflexes, other musculoskeletal and neurological components

  - ▶ Dental examination (provide referral if needed)

  - ▶ Additional specific physical examination components will depend on the client's medical history and identified risk factors. See Intervention/Management and Patient Education below.

- Review laboratory and other test results. See Diagnostic Tests in this chapter.

Assessment

- Identify risk factors, including

  - ▶ Age

  - ▶ Current medical diagnoses

  - ▶ Past medical, STD, infectious disease or reproductive history that may have an impact on future reproduction

  - ▶ Genetic risk factors: client, partner, and family members

  - ▶ Medications that pose a risk to reproduction

  - ▶ Lifestyle risks—including use of drugs, alcohol, tobacco; STD risk factors; and exercise and hyperthermia risks

  - ▶ Environmental hazard exposures at work and home

► Nutritional risk factors

► Psychosocial risk factors

► Partner issues that may impact reproductive health

Plan

Diagnostic Tests

● Order routine laboratory tests based on current primary care screening recommendations (e.g., U.S. Preventive Services Task Force, 1996) and/or site-specific practices and policies. See Table 1.2, Laboratory Tests for the Preconception Period.

● Additional laboratory evaluation will depend on the specific disease state or risk involved. See Intervention/Management and Patient Education.

Intervention/Management and Patient Education

The provider's goals and objectives of preconception counseling for the client or couple may include identification, modification or elimination of risk behaviors, improvement or correction of underlying problems, or understanding of risks when risk factors cannot be modified. In cases where modification of risk may not be feasible (e.g., unalterable medication regimen that may have harmful fetal effects), inform the client/couple regarding alternative reproductive options (Kuller & Laifer, 1994).

● Include the following in education, counseling, and/or intervention activities:

► Health-promoting behaviors—advice on good nutrition and exercise; recommendations for avoidance of smoking, alcohol, illicit drugs, unnecessary over-the-counter medicines and teratogens; good dental hygiene

► Vaccination: provision or referrals

► Pregnancy prevention, spacing, and planning; provision of contraception

► Potential risks of lifestyle factors on early embryological development, discussion about the importance of early and consistent prenatal care, and education toward realistic expectations concerning pregnancy outcome

► Education regarding primary prevention of infectious disease and STD; information on safer sex guidelines

► Identification of medical and lifestyle risk factors that may have an impact on reproduction and pregnancy, treatment of identified medical problems, and modification of chronic disease medication regimens, as indicated

► Alternative reproductive options

► Environmental hazards

► Referral to treatment programs to reduce psychosocial risks

► Referrals to appropriate agencies for medical and social support, including social services, nutrition services, public health nursing, community mental health, housing, medical, financial and/or vocational assistance programs and shelters (Cefalo & Moos, 1995; Jack &

Culpepper, 1991; Moos, 1989; U.S. Public Health Service Expert Panel on the Content of Prenatal Care, 1989)

- Counseling/intervention regarding specific identified risks may be undertaken within a multidisciplinary framework; thus, referral to several specialists may be necessary depending upon the client profile. Several visits may be required to complete the process. Ideally, counseling occurs within the context of the client's or couple's cultural, economic, and sociopolitical belief systems. Foreign language interpreters should be utilized as indicated and available. (Please note that reference to the "couple" may include the biological parent, a same-sex partner, or a nonpaternal partner and should be interpreted as applicable.)

- Specific information regarding lifestyle risks, medical risks, infectious disease/STD risks, genetic/reproductive risk factors, and male factors is discussed in separate sections to follow. The reader is also directed to other chapters in this book and the references for further information.

Lifestyle Risks

Nutritional and Weight Factors

The provider's goals and objectives are to gather data on the client's food intake, evaluate her diet for adequacy of nutrients to identify malnutrition, identify overweight or underweight status individuals, identify women with eating disorders, and educate regarding the value of adequate nutrition in enhancing health and reducing the potential for reproductive problems/poor pregnancy outcomes (Cefalo & Moos, 1995).

- Take a nutritionally oriented history using a 24-hour dietary recall format. Ask about vitamin/mineral supplements. Evaluate eating disorders (bulimia, anorexia) and idiosyncratic eating habits (pica). Assess signs and symptoms of diabetes and hypertension in overweight women.

- Ascertain height and weight; perform DBW calculations.

- Laboratory tests may include complete blood count (CBC), serum iron, serum ferritin, transferrin saturation, folate, B_{12}, glucose, and urinalysis as indicated by subjective and objective data.

- Refer individuals with identified nutritional risk factors or those with special dietary needs (vegetarians, over- or underweight) to a nutritionist for further counseling and intervention.

  ▶ Women who are overweight should be encouraged to lose weight, then maintain a desirable weight for 2 to 3 months prior to conception (*Before Pregnancy Planning Guide*, 1994; Scioscia, 1991).

  ▶ Vegetarians, especially those who exclude animal proteins, may be at risk for deficiencies in iron, vitamin B_{12}, essential amino acids, and calories (Scioscia, 1991). Supplementation with vitamins/minerals, calcium, and/or iron may be indicated based on identified nutritional deficiencies.

- As indicated, refer the client to a weight loss or eating disorders support group.

- Include the following information in education about nutritional factors and weight:

  ▶ Preconception risk reduction

► Role nutrition plays in a healthy pregnancy

► Potential risks of being underweight for poor pregnancy outcomes (e.g., spontaneous abortion, low-birthweight infants, intrauterine growth restriction, congenital anomalies [particularly of the central nervous system], increased perinatal mortality)

► Risks of being overweight/obese (e.g., hypertension, diabetes, thromboembolic complications, postpartum infections; macrosomic infants); potential undernourishment in obesity due to intake of high calorie foods that are low in essential nutrients

► Encouragement for healthy eating habits based on the recommended dietary allowance (RDA) for nutrients, vitamins, and minerals

NOTE: Show the Food Pyramid to the client. The graphic displays the following food groups with suggested numbers of servings: bread, cereal, rice, and pasta (6–11); fruits (2–4); vegetables(3–5); milk, yogurt, and cheese (2–3); meat, poultry, fish, dry beans, eggs, and nuts (2–3); fats, oils, and sweets (use sparingly) (U.S. Department of Agriculture Human Nutrition Information Service, 1992).

► Encouragement to achieve and/or maintain ideal body weight in the preconceptional period (ideally weight should stabilize 2 to 3 months before conception) (Cefalo & Moos, 1995)

► Recommendations for a regular exercise routine (see Exercise section below)

► Discussion about excesses and deficiencies of vitamins and minerals and their effects on reproduction and pregnancy

► Specific instruction regarding the need to avoid excess amounts of vitamin A, which confers risk of fetal teratogenicity

NOTE: A recent case report suggests the teratogenic dose of vitamin A may be as little as 10,000 IU. The malformations among some infants resembled those associated with isotretinoin exposure, that is, craniofacial, central nervous system, cardiac, and thymic abnormalities. The RDA for vitamin A for females (and during pregnancy) is 800 µg RE (retinol equivalents) per day (Food and Nutrition Board, 1989). This RDA is equivalent to 2700 IU of supplemental vitamin A as retinol or 4800 µg beta carotene. Supplementation of 5000 IU/day vitamin A (as retinol or retinyl esters) should be the maximum intake prior to or during pregnancy (American College of Obstetricians and Gynecologists [ACOG], 1995b). Beta carotene, (found in fruits and vegetables) has not been associated with vitamin A toxicity and should be the main source of vitamin A (Teratology Society Position Paper, 1987).

► Advice regarding the U.S. Public Health Service recommendations for all women of childbearing potential to consume 0.4 mg of folic acid daily prior to conception to reduce the incidence of neural tube defects (NTDs)

  – Women who have had a child with an NTD should begin consuming 4 mg folic acid daily at least one month prior to conception and continue through the first three months of pregnancy (CDC, 1991, 1992).

  – For women without a history of an offspring with an NTD, folate intake should be less than 1 mg/day in order not to mask the diagnosis of vitamin B_{12} deficiency (CDC, 1991, 1992).

NOTE: Adequate amounts of folic acid can be attained via dietary intake or by the use of over-the-counter (OTC) supplements. When supplementation is required it should be in the form of a folic acid supplement rather than multiple doses of vitamins containing folic acid. Doses of 1 mg or more per day require a prescription.

- Refer to Section 18, *Nutrition,* and the phenylketonuria (PKU) section following later for further information.

Exercise

The provider's goals and objectives are to educate the client about the effects of a safe, regular exercise program on enhancement of overall health and well-being and the potential exercise-related risks to reproduction and general health.

- Review the menstrual cycle history. Ask about past and present exercise routines and exercise-induced injuries. Evaluate the client's interest in starting a preconceptional exercise program.

- Unless contraindicated, encourage an inactive person to start a regular exercise program at least 3 months before pregnancy. Fast walking, swimming, aerobic dance, and bicycling are all good forms of aerobic exercise (March of Dimes, 1995). A 20 to 30 minute jog or 45 to 60 minute walk three to four times a week will accomplish aerobic fitness for almost any person (ACOG,1992).

- Advise persons with underlying medical conditions to discuss plans for an exercise program with their primary health care provider.

- Include the following information in education about exercise:

  ▶ Preconceptional benefits of exercise

  ▶ Guidelines for aerobic exercise, strengthening, and stretching. See Table 1.3, Exercise Safety Guidelines.

    NOTE: Target heart rate formula
    * 220 - age x 60% = lower limit
    * 220 - age x 80% = upper limit

  ▶ Benefits of exercise, such as improved cardiovascular and respiratory health, protection against osteoporosis, stress reduction, weight management, and a sense of well-being (*Before Pregnancy Planning Guide*, 1994)

  ▶ Effects of exercise on the menstrual cycle and reproduction

    NOTE: Intensive exercise has been associated with menstrual irregularities (e.g., short luteal phase, oligomenorrhea, secondary amenorrhea) and may interfere with conception. In addition, exercise-associated menstrual dysfunction is associated with osteoporosis (Constantini & Warren, 1994; Scioscia, 1991).

  ▶ Guidelines for safe exercise during pregnancy (walking and swimming are good choices); contraindications to exercise during pregnancy; effects of pregnancy on the musculoskeletal system

▶ Effects of hyperthermia

NOTE: Women attempting pregnancy should not exercise in hot, humid climates and should avoid saunas and hot tubs. Maternal core temperatures >38.9°C (102°F) during the first trimester of pregnancy have been associated with neural tube defects (Olsen, 1994; Milunsky, Ulcickas, & Rothman, 1991)

▶ Suggestions for a healthy diet

● Refer to Chapter 4.4, *Exercise During Pregnancy*, for additional information.

Environmental Factors

The provider's goals and objectives are to identify environmental exposure risks, educate about the hazards in the environment and workplace and their potential effects on reproduction, and encourage limitation of exposure to potentially harmful substances in order to maximize a healthy pregnancy (Cefalo & Moos, 1995).

● Obtain a thorough history of environmental and worksite exposures for both client and partner; assess reproductive history for problems that may have been due to environmental hazards. "Right-to-know" laws have made it possible for employees to obtain information about worksite exposures: encourage client or partner to ask employers for Material Safety Data Sheets.

● Laboratory evaluation may include blood test for lead level (should be less than 25 µg/dL).

● Use more than one resource for information about the effects of environmental exposure on pregnancy and recommended precautions at home and work. Clinicians should have an overall working knowledge of potentially hazardous substances and be able to use on-line databases, such as REPROTOX (part of Micromedex Computerized Clinical Information System), for specific information. Other resources include a state's teratogen hotline, local March of Dimes, or the Occupational Health and Safety Administration (OSHA). Consult with an occupational health expert or industrial medicine specialist to aid in tailoring counseling and care. Refer clients to a specialist or a genetic counselor as indicated. (See also Appendix 1b, Patient Education Materials and Referral Resources, and Table 1.4, Teratogenic Agents.

● Based on the subjective and objective information obtained and the known effects of specific substances, tailor the counseling to the individual circumstances. In some instances it may be necessary to advise work modifications or precautions. Rarely, an individual may be advised to discontinue a certain type of work if it involves harmful exposure (Cefalo & Moos, 1995).

● Include the following information in education about environmental exposures:

▶ Preconception risk reduction

▶ Potentially hazardous environmental or worksite exposures—specifically the known effects of the substance on reproductive health

NOTE: Substances that are known to be harmful include metals (lead, mercury), solvents (trichloroethylene, chloroform, benzene, carbon disulfide), vinyl monomers (vinyl chloride), pollutants (polychlorinated biphenyl [PCB], polybrominated biphenyl [PBB]), pesticides, 2,4,5-T and 2,4-D organophosphates (e.g., malathion), gases (carbon monoxide, anesthetic gases), radiation (x-rays), and antineoplastic drugs (Cefalo & Moos, 1995).

 ▶ Ways to minimize toxic exposures (e.g., adequate ventilation; wearing gloves, aprons, and other barriers; proper handwashing; avoiding eating, drinking or smoking in the exposed environment) (*Before Pregnancy Planning Guide*, 1994)

 ▶ Biologic effects of ionizing radiation

 ▶ Statements regarding the relative safety of electromagnetic fields based on available data (Schnorr, et al., 1991)

• Refer to Section 15, *Pregnancy and Occupational Health*, Chapter 6.14, *Ionizing Radiation Exposure*, and Section 2, *Genetic Counseling*, for further information.

Stress

The provider's goals and objectives are to assist in identifying stressors, educate the client regarding the potential effects of prolonged stress on physical and psychological health, and facilitate stress management.

• Ask client to identify factors that are sources of stress.

• Explore psychosocial variables; review past medical, psychological, medication, and habits history. Evaluate somatic symptom complex as indicated. Assess coping style.

• On physical examination, pay attention to those systems that may receive target organ damage from prolonged stress or may be the cause of stress-related symptoms (Kelber, 1995).

• Laboratory evaluation may include thyroid function tests, CBC, and/or fasting blood glucose, as appropriate (Kelber, 1995).

• Make recommendations for stress management. Various approaches include assertiveness or time management training, cognitive restructuring techniques, relaxation techniques, massage therapy (Kelber, 1995). Suggest "time-out" for pleasurable activities.

• Refer the client to a support group, stress management class, or mental health counselor as indicated.

• Include the following information in education about stress:

 ▶ Preconception stress reduction

 ▶ Effects of prolonged stress and its potential effects on pregnancy (e.g., low birth weight due to premature deliveries, poor fetal growth)

 ▶ Strategies to avoid, prevent, and counteract the effects of stress

  NOTE: It may be warranted for client to delay conception until significant stress is reduced to a manageable level.

 ▶ Recommendations for proper nutrition, adequate rest and exercise

 ▶ Advice regarding limitation of alcohol and caffeine (Kelber, 1995)

Drug and Other Substance Risks

OTC Drugs and Prescriptive Medication

The provider's goals and objectives are to identify use of OTC or prescriptive substances and to advise reduction or elimination of products known to be addictive or harmful to reproduction.

- Have client list all OTC and prescriptive substances she is currently taking. Consult with the prescribing health care provider to determine the absolute necessity for certain medications used during the preconceptional period.

- Specific substances that have the potential to be harmful to pregnancy include aspirin, nonsteroidal anti-inflammatory drugs (NSAIDs), angiotensin-converting enzyme (ACE) inhibitors, antineoplastic drugs, aminopterin, methotrexate, carbamezine, warfarin, etretinate, daunorubicin, lithium, methyl mercury, gold, lead, thalidomide, phenytoin, propylthiouracil, methimazole, quinolones, isotretinoin, retinoic acid, tetracycline, trimethadione, valproic acid, folic acid antagonists, excess vitamin A (Dacus, Meyer, & Sibai, 1995; Jack & Culpepper, 1991; Summers & Price, 1993).

  NOTE: This list may not identify *all* potentially harmful substances. See Table 1.4 for additional information.

- Refer the client/couple to a genetic counselor if there has been exposure to known teratogen(s) in the preconceptional period.

- Include the following information in education about OTC and prescriptive medication:

  ▶ Preconception risk reduction

  ▶ Recommendations for avoiding of OTC medication when possible

  ▶ Known effects of specific OTCs and prescriptive substances on the preconceptional period and pregnancy (client should be aware of the dosage and timing of medication[s] taken)

  ▶ Recommendations for client to check with her health care provider regarding medication usage

  ▶ Advice about not taking other people's medications

- Refer to the Illicit Drugs and Controlled Substances section below and Section 2, *Genetic Counseling,* for additional information.

Caffeine

The provider's goals and objectives are to discuss the potential effects of caffeine consumption on general health and its potential risks to pregnancy.

- Assess average intake. Recommend client consume only moderate amounts of caffeine— this degree of intake has not been found harmful to the average healthy adult (moderate is defined as less than 300 mg caffeine/day or approximately three cups of coffee).

  NOTE: Studies are conflicting with respect to adverse effects on pregnancy related to caffeine; however, the U.S. Food and Drug Administration (FDA) has cautioned pregnant women to limit caffeine intake.

- Include the following information in education about caffeine:

  ▶ Preconception lowering of intake if excessive

  ▶ General physical effects of excessive caffeine intake (e.g., potential for anxiety, restlessness, sleep disturbances, palpitations) (Cefalo & Moos, 1995)

  ▶ Amount of caffeine in certain beverages:
  80–200 mg per 6 oz cup of coffee
  2–6 mg per 6 oz cup decaffeinated coffee
  10–20 mg per cup cocoa
  25–70 mg per cup tea (depending on brew)
  30–70 mg per 12 oz soft drink (*Before Pregnancy Planning Guide*, 1994)

  ▶ Potential effects of caffeine on pregnancy (e.g., spontaneous abortion, premature delivery, intrauterine growth restriction, low birth weight infants)

  NOTE: There is no conclusive scientific evidence that caffeine causes birth defects in humans (*Before Pregnancy Planning Guide,* 1994).

Alcohol

The provider's goals and objectives are to assess alcohol consumption, assess medical complications of alcohol abuse, provide information on the potential effects of alcohol on the fetus, and support the alcohol-dependent woman in achieving a decision to discontinue drinking.

- Use one of the standard tools to determine alcohol intake (e.g., Ten-Question Drinking History [TQDH], Michigan Alcohol Screening Test [MAST], the CAGE questionnaire, the T-ACE questionnaire). Inquire about her partner's alcohol intake.

- Observe objective signs and indicators for alcohol abuse. See Chapter 6.31, *Substance Abuse*.

- Laboratory evaluation may include blood alcohol level, toxicology screen, ALT, AST, uric acid, CBC (to assess MCH, MCV), albumin, total protein, serum magnesium, potassium, folate, and B_{12} (Jessup, 1995).

- Demonstrate concern about her drinking to the client. Refer her to a specific alcohol counselor or Alcohol Anonymous meeting. Additional resources may be indicated, for example, alcohol treatment centers, various residential programs.

  NOTE: Use of Antabuse® is contraindicated preconceptionally and during pregnancy (Cefalo & Moos, 1995).

- Maintain continuing interest in and contact with the client. Ask about on-going alcohol use. Consult with the client's 12-step program sponsor as needed. Utilize social services.

- Include the following information in education about alcohol:

  ▶ Preconception risk reduction

  ▶ Recommendations to reduce alcohol intake prior to conception

  ▶ Effects of alcohol on pregnancy (in particular, fetal alcohol syndrome) and the possible physical effects to self

▶ The uncertainty of determining a safe level of alcohol consumption in pregnancy but with reassurance that the occasional drink when pregnancy was unsuspected is unlikely to cause harm

▶ Impact of continued drinking on the client's emotional, financial, spiritual, and psychological realms (Jessup, 1995)

▶ Importance of proper nutrition

● Refer to Table 1.4, Teratogenic Agents, and Chapter 6.31, *Substance Abuse,* for further information.

Tobacco

The provider's goals and objectives are to educate regarding general health risks of tobacco use and the effects of smoking on reproduction (Cefalo & Moos, 1995).

● Obtain a smoking history. Ask about prior attempts to quit.

● Assess medical history for cardiorespiratory system illness, cancers, and obstetrical and gynecological problems. Explore psychosocial history. Inquire about partner's smoking habits.

● Observe for physical indicators of tobacco use (skin changes, periodontal findings/disease, chest and peripheral vascular findings).

● Encourage client to stop smoking (tapering off is also beneficial) and avoid second-hand smoke when possible. Assist client in picking a "quit date." Provide referrals for a smoking cessation program and utilize appropriate Patient Education and self-help materials. Continue to be available as a support person for client's endeavors to quit (Cefalo & Moos, 1995; Sheehan, 1995).

NOTE: Nicotine gum/patch is contraindicated during pregnancy but may be utilized preconceptionally if there are no health risks which would prohibit its use (e.g., cardiovascular disease, hypertension).

● Include the following information in education about tobacco:

▶ Preconception risk reduction

▶ Risks that tobacco use may have on general health, reproduction, and pregnancy (e.g., tobacco-related illnesses [lung cancer, chronic obstructive pulmonary disease (COPD)]; lower fecundity; ovulatory and tubal disorders; delayed conception; increase in incidence of ectopic pregnancy, spontaneous abortion, intrauterine growth restriction, premature rupture of membranes, preterm delivery, low birth weight infants, placental/bleeding complications, and fetal/neonatal death) (ACOG, 1995a; Cefalo & Moos, 1995; Dacus, Meyer, & Sibai, 1995; REPROTOX, 1995a; Teratogen Information System [TERIS], 1995, on-line).

NOTE: There is no consistent evidence that smoking causes an increase in the incidence of congenital malformations (REPROTOX, 1995a; TERIS, 1995, on-line).

▶ Importance of fresh air, exercise, and proper nutrition (Sheehan, 1995).

Illicit Drugs and Controlled Substances

The provider's goals and objectives are to identify history of past or present drug use, determine the specific substance and route of administration, and educate regarding the potential effects on maternal and fetal health.

- Drug use patterns may be elicited with the aid of specific assessment tools. See Chapter 6.31, *Substance Abuse.*

- Observe objective signs and indicators for substance abuse. See Chapter 6.31, *Substance Abuse.*

- Laboratory tests may include toxicology screen, hepatitis B surface antigen (HBsAg), hepatitis C antibody, human immunodeficiency virus (HIV) antibody screen and STD testing. Tuberculosis skin testing may also be offered. Offer partner screening, if indicated.

- Counsel the substance user individually or refer her to group education or a substance abuse treatment program (residential or out-patient). Offer substance-addicted women a structured and supervised withdrawal program, which may include medicated withdrawal management (e.g., methadone). Other medically managed withdrawals will depend on the substance used and site-specific practices. Consult with a drug counselor or addiction expert to aid in tailoring care.

- Include the following information in education about illicit drugs and controlled substances:

  ▶ Preconception risk reduction, with emphasis on the risks for exposure to HIV and hepatitis B and C

  ▶ Specific information regarding the effects of the particular substance on general health and well-being and on maternal/fetal health

  ▶ Importance of proper nutrition

- Refer to Table 1.4, Teratogenic Agents, and Chapter 6.31, *Substance Abuse,* for further information.

Medical Risk Factors

Age

The provider's goals and objectives are to evaluate physiological and psychological variables related to age to provide appropriate preconceptional risk assessment and counseling, to offer information on age-related fertility factors, to provide data on specific age-related risks to pregnancy, to inform about the incidence of chromosomal abnormalities associated with aging, and facilitate discussion and communication between partners regarding parenthood (Cefalo & Moos, 1995; March of Dimes, 1995).

- Explore client's/couple's psychological readiness and desire for pregnancy.

- Assess psychosocial variables: employment, education, career plans and goals, financial arrangements, and social support network.

- Identify medical problems that may impact pregnancy. In general, women over age 35 should be evaluated for signs and symptoms of hypertension, diabetes, and renal disease. Adolescents are at higher risk for STDs. A health habits history is important in all age groups.

- Provide an overview of prenatal screening and genetic assessment modalities.

- Provide referrals to specialty services as indicated (e.g., reproductive endocrinologist, infertility nurse-specialist, genetic counselor and/or geneticist).

- Laboratory evaluation will be driven by the client profile and specific underlying medical history. See Table 1.2, Laboratory Tests for the Preconception Period, for routine tests that may be ordered.

- Include the following information in education and counseling about age-related factors:

  ▶ Preconception risk reduction; safer sex practice guidelines for high-risk individuals

  ▶ Sensitive, appropriate counseling regarding decision-making for pregnancy and parenting, important at any age

  ▶ Age-related risks to reproduction: fertility, medical conditions associated with aging and their impact on pregnancy, and the incidence of chromosomal abnormalities.

    – Counsel women of advancing years that there is no time to waste in attempting to achieve pregnancy because fertility declines with age. About one-third of women who defer pregnancy until the mid-to late-30s and at least half of women over age 40 will have an infertility problem) (Speroff, Glass, & Kase, 1994).

    – Discuss the research regarding obstetrical complications and pregnancy outcomes for women 35 years and older.

      * Data from various studies suggest that women of advanced maternal age are at increased risk for placenta previa, abruptio placentae, placental infarcts, preterm birth, increased perinatal mortality, small-for-gestational-age and low birth weight infants, prolonged labor, and increased cesarean section rates.

      * Other studies, however, indicate that older women are at no higher risk for adverse outcomes when preexisting medical disorders or reproductive problems are controlled for (Berkowitz, Skovron, Lapinski, & Berkowitz, 1990).

    – Discuss the incidence of fetal chromosomal abnormalities associated with aging:

      * 1/200 live-born infants of women aged 35 years and 1/65 for women aged 40 years (Hook, Cross, & Schreinemachers, 1983).

      * Trisomy 21 (Down syndrome, which accounts for about one-half of chromosomal abnormalities) affects 1/384 live-born infants of women age 35 and 1/112 infants of woman age 40 (Cuckle, Wald, & Thompson, 1987).

      * In addition, spontaneous abortion rates increase with age largely as a result of fetal chromosomal abnormalities.

- Refer to Section 2, *Genetic Counseling,* and the following section for additional information.

Genetic and Reproductive Factors

The provider's goals and objectives are to identify familial factors that may express themselves through Mendelian or alternative inheritance patterns; identify women with poor reproductive or pregnancy outcomes and investigate factors contributing to these outcomes; provide counseling regarding the genetic effects associated with advanced maternal/paternal age; provide counseling regarding specific autosomal recessive, autosomal dominant and x-linked disorders; provide unbiased, objective information to allow prospective parents to make informed decisions regarding planning, preventing or terminating a pregnancy; and provide emotional and grief support (Cefalo & Moos, 1995).

- A thorough medical, OB/GYN, and habits history is imperative. Ask about
  - ▶ Diethylstilbestrol (DES) exposure (given from the 1940s to early 1970s)
  - ▶ Exposure to environmental toxins
  - ▶ Partner history
  - ▶ Family history (for both client and partner); in particular, ask about family history of known genetic diseases, birth defects, stillbirths, early unexplained deaths, childhood surgeries, early adult deaths, mental retardation, disability, and involuntary infertility (Simpson, 1995)

- Review the medical records of an affected family member; this may be useful in some cases because medical information is often passed on inaccurately within families.

- Perform a hormonal evaluation if the client presents with infertility. Tests may include follicle-stimulating hormone (FSH), luteinizing hormone (LH) and prolactin on day 2 to 3 of the menstrual cycle, and midluteal phase progesterone level. Semen analysis may be ordered for the prospective father. Additional infertility evaluation may include thyroid stimulating hormone (TSH), testosterone, dehydroepiandrosterone sulfate (DHEAS), screening for STDs, post-coital test, endometrial biopsy, hysterosalpingogram, and endoscopy. Refer client to an infertility specialist as indicated.

- Clients exposed to DES in utero may require evaluation of the uterus to rule out anomalies (especially if there is a history of pregnancy loss). Consult with physician.

- Counsel women who are 35 years or older about the genetic risks associated with advanced maternal age. (When a client in this age group is pregnant, antenatal genetic testing for chromosomal abnormalities will be offered.)

- Refer any woman with personal or family histories of congenital anomalies, known genetic condition, or mental retardation to a genetic counselor. Also evaluate the prospective father's history for familial disorders, as noted above. An evaluation by a medical geneticist may be needed to establish a diagnosis.

- Refer women who have given birth to a child with a congenital anomaly, known genetic condition, or mental retardation to a genetic counselor.

- Offer carrier testing for Tay-Sachs disease to Askenazi Jewish and French Canadian couples.

- Offer preconception testing for thalassemia and sickle-cell traits to people of African, African-American, Asian, Middle Eastern, and Mediterranean descent. Laboratory evaluation should include, at a minimum, CBC and hemoglobin electrophoresis. See individual hemoglobinopathy protocols for additional tests that may be ordered.

- Offer screening to individuals with a family history of cystic fibrosis and refer them to a genetic counselor.

- Refer the couple to a genetic counselor in instances where both client and prospective father have known hemoglobinopathies or hemoglobin traits, or both are known carriers for Tay-Sachs.

- Offer genetic counseling to women with histories of poor pregnancy outcomes (e.g., spontaneous abortion [three or more, or more than two after age 35] or stillbirth).

  ▶ Preconception testing may include evaluation for anatomic and/or genetic factors with a karyotype, ultrasound, hysterosalpingogram and/or hysteroscopy. Infectious disease factors should be considered as well.

  ▶ Carefully review previous medical records, including the autopsy report, of clients with histories of perinatal death.

  ▶ Consult with a physician as indicated.

- Testing for antiphospholipid antibodies (lupus anticoagulant, anticardiolipin) may be in order to screen for systemic lupus erythematosus (SLE) or the antiphospholipid syndrome in women with a history of recurrent pregnancy loss or poor obstetrical outcomes (Carson, 1995).

- Evaluate for and treat luteal phase deficiency in women with early recurrent pregnancy loss, if indicated. Refer client to an infertility specialist as indicated.

- Note and discuss with the client previous pregnancy complications such as preterm labor/delivery, low birth weight infant, and intrauterine growth restriction. Prevention strategies should be discussed as appropriate to the history. Education regarding preterm birth prevention is a routine part of prenatal care.

- Make education specific to the age of the client and the client/couple/family history. Involve a genetic counselor, if necessary. Topical areas include

  ▶ Preconception risk reduction

  ▶ Age-related chromosomal disorders

  ▶ Genetic causes of recurrent spontaneous abortion

  ▶ Risk-estimates for inherited diseases of the offspring as indicated by personal, family, and partner history

  ▶ Potential impact on reproduction and pregnancy of known genetic disorders in client/partner/family

  ▶ Screening for hemoglobin disorders

  ▶ Strategies to prevent pregnancy complications

  ▶ Preconceptional testing for anatomic, infectious disease, autoimmune, or endocrine disorders as indicated by reproductive/obstetrical history

  ▶ Reproductive options

  ▶ Emotional/psychological responses to genetic disorders

- Refer to Section 2, *Genetic Counseling,* and other associated chapters for further information.

Diabetes

The provider's goals and objectives are to educate the client about the maternal, fetal, neonatal risks of diabetes; reduce occurrence of obstetric and diabetic complications; and decrease the incidence of congenital anomalies (Cefalo & Moos, 1995).

- A thorough medical evaluation should be undertaken. Meticulous preconceptional metabolic control should be achieved to reduce the risk of congenital malformations (i.e., caudal regression, neural tube defects, congenital heart defects, and renal anomalies) and spontaneous abortion (Kuller & Laifer, 1994; Moore, 1994). Assess carefully for the presence of end-organ system disease (Scioscia, 1991). Diabetic women should be managed by a physician or co-managed in consultation with a perinatologist, internist, and other specialists as indicated. Referral to a registered dietitian is advisable. Additional referrals may include ophthalmology, podiatry, and nephrology as indicated.

- Preconceptional evaluation may include the following tests (Cefalo & Moos, 1995; Moore, 1994):

  ▶ Fasting and postprandial plasma glucose; HbA$_1$c

    NOTE: Normal glucose values are 80–100 mg/dL (fasting) and <120 mg/dL (2-hour postprandial). Pregnancy should be avoided until HbA$_1$c is in the normal, nonpregnant range (4–8 percent; may vary by laboratory) (Moore, 1994).

  ▶ Electrocardiogram (ECG) (if diabetes present for more than 10 years)

  ▶ Cardiac, renal evaluation

  ▶ Thyroid function studies; antithyroid antibodies

  ▶ 24-hour urine for protein, creatinine clearance

  ▶ Lipid profile

  ▶ Ophthalmologic examination

  ▶ Baseline neurologic examination

- Include the following information in education about diabetes:

  ▶ Preconception risk reduction and the importance of tight control of the disease

  ▶ Contraception

  ▶ Medical, fetal, obstetrical, and neonatal risks associated with diabetes

  ▶ Routine obstetrical surveillance

  ▶ Glucose monitoring/control

  ▶ Symptoms of hypoglycemia

  ▶ Nutrition (ideally, provided by a nutritionist)

  ▶ Importance of family and social support

  ▶ Economic considerations (Moore, 1994)

- Refer to Chapter 6.11, *Gestational Diabetes Mellitus,* for further information.

Cardiovascular Disease

The provider's goals and objectives are to assess cardiac status and inform the client about risks specific to her underlying heart condition (Cefalo & Moos, 1995).

- Refer the patient to a perinatologist and manage her care in close consultation with a cardiologist. Determine the nature of the underlying disease before preconception recommendations can be made (Cefalo & Moos, 1995). Referral to a registered dietitian may also be appropriate.

- The work-up may include an ECG, chest x-ray, or cardiac catheterization if not already performed. Diagnostic and therapeutic modalities should be determined by the physician in charge of the patient's care.

- Encourage patients on anticoagulants for recent deep vein thrombosis or pulmonary emboli to avoid pregnancy while still on medication (Scioscia, 1991).

Hypertension

The provider's goals and objectives are to achieve and maintain blood pressure within a range compatible with good maternal and fetal outcomes and educate the mother about the effects of medication and the risks of uncontrolled hypertension (Cefalo & Moos, 1995).

- The client may be managed in consultation with a physician or referred to a specialist. Referral to a registered dietitian may also be appropriate.

- Perform a careful physical examination, including a fundoscopic examination, auscultation for renal artery stenosis, and assessment of femoral pulses (Scioscia, 1991).

- Laboratory tests may include blood urea nitrogen (BUN), creatinine, 24-hour urine for protein, creatinine clearance. Additional testing may include an ECG and a chest x-ray.

- Medication may require adjustment preconceptionally. ACE-inhibitors are contraindicated. Drugs that are relatively safe during pregnancy include methyldopa, atenolol, clonidine, and hydralazine (Cefalo & Moos, 1995). Some clients may not require medication. Consult with a physician.

- Include the following information in education about hypertension:

  ▶ Preconception risk reduction and the importance of hypertension control

  ▶ Drug regimen, if utilized, and drug side effects

  ▶ Possible obstetrical complications

  ▶ Increased rest during pregnancy and possible work restrictions

- Refer to Table 1.4, Teratogenic Agents, and Chapter 6.13, *Hypertensive Disorders of Pregnancy,* for further information

Kidney Disease

The provider's goals and objectives are to assess degree of renal impairment and to provide individualized maternal and fetal risk assessment (Cefalo & Moos, 1995).

- The client may be co-managed with a physician or referred to a perinatologist. Consultation with a nephrologist is advisable. Referral to a registered dietitian may also be appropriate.

- Laboratory evaluation may include complete urinalysis; serum creatinine, and BUN; 24-hour urine for protein and creatinine clearance. Ongoing monitoring of renal function and assessment for urinary tract infection during pregnancy will be necessary (Cefalo & Moos, 1995).

- Include the following information in education about renal disease:

  ▶ Preconception risk reduction and the importance of disease stability

  ▶ Specific maternal and fetal risks, depending on the degree of renal impairment and the underlying form of renal disease.

  NOTE: Advice and preconceptional education should be undertaken in consultation with the physician responsible for the client's care.

Epilepsy

The provider's goals and objectives are to review nature of the seizure disorder and the history of treatment, educate about the risk of congenital malformations with epilepsy and the use of antiepileptic drugs (AEDs), and, ideally, promote a seizure-free state and decrease the incidence of malformations in offspring (Cefalo & Moos, 1995; Delgado-Escueta & Janz, 1992; Scioscia, 1991).

- Practitioners may wish to consult the Guidelines for the Care of Epileptic Women of Childbearing Age (1989) developed by the Commission on Genetics, Pregnancy, and the Child for the International League Against Epilepsy (ILAE).

- Co-management with an obstetrician is indicated. Consult with a neurologist to discuss appropriate drug regimens and the appropriateness of weaning client from AEDs.

- Preconceptional evaluation may include skull x-rays, an electroencephalogram (EEG), or a computed tomography (CT) scan per order of the physician.

- A complete diet, medication, and alcohol history is important.

- Refer the client to a genetic counselor if a genetic disease or syndrome is the basis for the seizure disorder (Scioscia, 1991).

- Include the following information in education about epilepsy:

  ▶ Preconception risk reduction and the importance of well-controlled seizure disorder

  ▶ Comprehensive counseling regarding the possible effects of epilepsy on pregnancy

    – Teratogenicity of specific seizure medications and those that are contraindicated during pregnancy

    – Increased risks of congenital malformation

NOTE: Women with epilepsy who are treated with AEDs have a two- to three-fold increased risk for producing offspring with birth defects (especially congenital heart defects and cleft lip with or without cleft palate) (Delgado-Escueta & Janz, 1992; Friis, 1989; McCormick, 1987; Scioscia, 1991). In addition, offspring of mothers with epilepsy (treated or not) tend to have slightly more minor anomalies than do offspring of epileptic fathers or nonepileptic parents (Delgado-Escueta & Janz, 1992).

▶ Statistics about AED treatment and pregnancy outcome (the vast majority of women with epilepsy—at least 90 percent—who are treated with AEDs have normal children) (McCormick, 1987)

▶ Anticipatory guidance regarding seizure frequency during pregnancy and the potential for certain complications of pregnancy

▶ Advice about dietary folate in the preconceptional period to reduce risk for NTDs

- Refer to Table 1.4, Teratogenic Agents, Section 2, *Genetic Counseling,* Chapter 6.28, *Seizures,* and Section 18, *Nutrition,* for further information.

Asthma

The provider's goals and objectives are to educate the client about the effect that pregnancy may have on asthma and to stabilize disease with least amount of effective medication (Cefalo & Moos, 1995).

- The client may require co-management with an internist or pulmonologist, and obstetrician.

- The client should make an effort to have asthma stabilized through lifestyle modification and medication (Scioscia, 1991).

- Review drug regimens and tailor them to the status of the client's asthma. Most asthma medications are safe during the preconceptional period and during pregnancy. Ideally, steroid use should be kept to a minimum. Iodine preparations should not be used during pregnancy (Scioscia, 1991).

- Influenza vaccine may be advisable. Consult with physician.

- Include the following information in education about asthma:

  ▶ Preconception risk reduction and the importance of well-controlled asthma

  ▶ Review of medication regimens and discussion of drug side effects as necessary

  ▶ Advice regarding avoidance of environmental conditions that may act as precipitants to attacks

  ▶ Recommendations for prompt evaluation of symptoms of respiratory infection

  ▶ Anticipatory guidance regarding the influence that pregnancy may have on the disease (i.e., minimal change, improvement, or worsening)

- Refer to Chapter 11.1, *Asthma,* for further information.

Thyroid Disorders

The provider's goals and objectives are to educate the client about the effects of thyroid dysfunction on pregnancy and to achieve and maintain thyroid function within normal range with the least amount of medication (Cefalo & Moos, 1995).

- The client may be managed in consultation with a physician or referred. Review her thyroid medication regimen with the physician.

- Laboratory tests may include T_3, T_4, TSH, and antithyroid antibodies.

- Include the following information in education about thyroid disease:

  ▶ Preconception risk reduction and the importance of disease stability

  ▶ Avoiding pregnancy for one year after treatment with radioactive iodine

  ▶ Importance of continuing medication during pregnancy

  ▶ Maternal and fetal risks and surveillance during pregnancy (Cefalo & Moos, 1995)

- Refer to Section 12, *Thyroid Conditions,* for further information.

Cancer

The provider's goals and objectives are to educate the woman about the effects of cancer on pregnancy, the overall prognosis during pregnancy, and the potential fetal complications of cancer therapy (Cefalo & Moos, 1995).

- Cancer patients should be managed by a physician. Preconceptional counseling should be tailored to the specific form of cancer and undertaken in consultation with the physician responsible for the patient's care. All patients should receive general counseling on overall preconception risk reduction.

- Assess the family history of cancer(s)

Multiple Sclerosis

The provider's goals and objectives are to review the client's history of disease relapse and progression and to educate her about the effect of pregnancy on the disease.

- The client may require co-management with a physician.

- Assess the degree of disability present. Review medication use to assess safety during preconception and pregnancy.

- Refer the client to a genetic counselor for education about risk to the offspring (generally small, about 3 percent) (Scioscia, 1991).

- Include the following information in education about multiple sclerosis:

  ▶ Preconception risk reduction and the importance of disease stability

  ▶ Effects that pregnancy may have on the disease state

NOTE: Pregnancy does not appear to increase the frequency of relapse or progression; however, disease may be exacerbated in the postpartum period (Scioscia, 1991).

Systemic Lupus Erythematosus (SLE)

The provider's goals and objectives are to assess the current activity and complications of disease and to provide counseling about maternal/fetal risks and course of the disease in pregnancy.

- Manage the client in consultation with specialists in nephrology, rheumatology, etc.

- Assess the past disease course and review medications. Evaluate for presence of renal or central nervous system disease.

- Laboratory evaluation may include CBC, platelet count, glucose, BUN, creatinine, creatinine clearance, partial thromboplastin time (PTT), antiphospholipid antibodies, anti-Ro (SS-A) antibodies, urinalysis.

- Advise patients to delay pregnancy until a state of remission has been entered and sustained. In women with active disease at conception, relapses, exacerbations, and fetal complications are more common.

NOTE: Women with lupus anticoagulant or anticardiolipin antibodies are at significant risk of poor pregnancy outcomes, specifically, pregnancy wastage (Scioscia, 1991).

- Clients with the following history should be screened for lupus anticoagulant and anticardiolipin antibodies: recurrent spontaneous abortion or fetal death, SLE, false-positive VDRL (or RPR), thrombotic episodes, Coombs + hemolytic anemia, and presence of anti-Ro (SS-A) antibodies. If results are positive, prepregnancy treatment with aspirin/glucocorticoid therapy may be indicated (Cefalo & Moos, 1995). Consult with physician.

- Include the following information in education about SLE:

  ▶ Preconception risk reduction and the importance of disease stability

  ▶ Contraceptive options to be employed until patient is in remission

  ▶ Effects of pregnancy on the disease, medication effects, and maternal/fetal risks, including

  – Variability of the disease course (in absence of multisystem disease pregnancy may not worsen SLE)

  – The incidence of preterm delivery, fetal wastage, and small-for-gestational age infants (increases to 30 to 50 percent in women who have chronic renal disease or creatinine greater than 1.6 mg/dL)

  – Fetal survival with inactive disease at conception (about 85%; with active disease it is 50-75%)

  – Corticosteroids and azathioprine have not been associated with congenital anomalies in humans; these drugs should be continued in the pre- and postconception period (other chemotherapeutic agents should be evaluated for safety)

  – The permanent or transient effect of placental transfer of maternal antibodies (discoid lupus rash, hemolytic anemia, cardiac conduction system impairment, or complete heart block) (Cefalo & Moos, 1995)

- See Chapter 6.2, *Antiphospholipid Syndrome.*

Phenylketonuria (PKU)

The provider's goals and objectives are to identify women with hyperphenylalaninemia and initiate diet therapy, educate the mother regarding the effects of PKU on pregnancy, and optimize the chances for a healthy mother and baby (Cefalo & Moos, 1995).

- Do a preconceptional screening to disclose PKU in undiagnosed women if the following history exists: born before 1967; immigrated to the U.S.; intellectually "slow"; has seizures or poor coordination of unknown etiology; has a "mousy" or "barnlike" odor; or has a poor reproductive history, including spontaneous abortion(s), or a neonate with congenital anomalies, mental retardation, microcephaly, or who was stillborn (Acosta & Wright, 1992). Also, inquire whether the client had "special feeding" in infancy.

- Laboratory testing may include serum levels of phenylalanine (PHE), tyrosine, or other plasma amino acids. Refer women with PHE concentrations of 4 mg/dL or more on screening for diagnostic workup for PKU (Acosta & Wright, 1992).

- A multidisciplinary team consisting of a women's primary care nurse practitioner, obstetrician or perinatologist, medical geneticist, and metabolic nutritionist will usually be needed to manage the client. The client's cooperation with a center in the Collaborative Study of Maternal Phenylketonuria may be in her best interest (Koch, Acosta, & Williams, 1995).

- The Medical Research Council has provided preconceptional guidelines for women with PKU (Cockburn et al., 1993). Lab determinations, as above, should be made prior to staring the PHE-restricted diet.

  NOTE: Blood PHE concentration most likely to yield the best reproductive outcomes is unknown; a PHE-restricted diet that maintains blood PHE concentrations between 60 and 180 μmol/L has been suggested (Acosta, 1995; Smith, Glossup, & Beasley, 1990).

- The client should be on an individualized PHE-restricted diet for at least 3 months before a planned pregnancy and continue through the pregnancy. Preconceptional and prenatal vitamin supplementation is not recommended (Acosta et al., 1982; Acosta & Wright, 1992; Cefalo & Moos, 1995). A protocol is available to plan and evaluate nutrition support during pregnancy. (See Acosta & Yannicelli, 1993.) Refer woman to metabolic nutritionist for dietary instruction/management.

  ▶ A PHE-free medical food is prescribed.

  ▶ Access to medical food is necessary. Four medical foods are available in the United States: Phenex®-2 Amino Acid Modified Medical Food (Ross Products Division, Abbott Laboratories); XP Maxamum® (Scientific Hospital Supplies, Inc., Gaithersburg, MD); Phenyl-Free® and PKU-3 (Mead Johnson Nutritionals, Evansville, IN) (Acosta, 1995).

- Include the following information in education about PKU:

  ▶ Preconception risk reduction and the importance of strict dietary control

► Contraceptive options to be employed until the client is in good control of her PKU (fetal risk reduction is substantial when treatment and control is achieved prior to pregnancy) (Scioscia, 1991)

► Specific fetal hazards associated with elevated maternal phenylalanine levels (i.e., risk for spontaneous abortion, congenital malformations, mental retardation, microcephaly, congenital heart defects, and intrauterine growth restriction) (Dacus, Meyer, & Sibai, 1995; Taysi, 1988)

► Absolute importance of a strict diet preconceptionally and during pregnancy to lower the risk of birth defects, cost of the diet (approximately $4500 for one year), and the importance of self-motivation and social support to maintain it (programs such as Women, Infants, Children [WIC], state and federal programs, or client's health insurance may help with costs)

► Genetic information, including the carrier rate in the general population of about 1/50 (combined U.S. ethnic groups), and information regarding risk to offspring

NOTE: A 1/50 carrier rate × a 1/2 risk that a carrier father will pass on his PKU gene yields an approximately 1/100 chance that a woman with PKU will produce an offspring with PKU (Scriver, Beaudet, Sly, & Valle, 1995).

► Multidisciplinary team management as ideal to improved outcomes during pregnancy, frequency of labs (may be twice weekly) and serial ultrasound during pregnancy, and frequent changes in individualized diet prescription (Acosta, 1995).

Infectious Disease and STD

The provider's goals and objectives are to assess history of naturally occurring childhood diseases; advise the client/couple regarding the potential effects of a variety of infectious diseases and STDs on the course and outcome of pregnancy; provide strategies for primary prevention of infectious disease and STD; assist the client/couple with lifestyle choices that promote health; identify and treat STDs prior to pregnancy; and offer appropriate immunizations as indicated.

• Infectious diseases and STDs that may affect pregnancy include (but are not limited to) viral hepatitis, rubella, varicella, toxoplasmosis, group B streptococcal infection, cytomegalovirus infection, herpesvirus infection, chlamydia, gonorrhea, syphilis, human papillomavirus infection, human immunodeficiency virus (HIV) infection. Inquire about signs and symptoms that may be related to these infections.

• Administer vaccinations, if necessary, well in advance of a planned pregnancy (e.g., measles, mumps, rubella, and varicella vaccine should be given at least 3 months prior to conception). All women of childrearing age should be immune to measles, mumps, rubella, tetanus, diphtheria, and poliomyelitis. Persons born prior to 1957 are likely to have been naturally infected with measles and mumps and can be considered immune. Poliomyelitis risk in the United States is very small and most adults are immune; thus, routine vaccination of adults who have not received a primary series is not necessary. Advise the preconceptional woman to keep up-to-date on booster doses of tetanus and diphtheria (ACOG, 1991).

• Assess rubella and varicella with appropriate laboratory tests as indicated.

NOTE: Persons with a positive clinical history of varicella do not require screening; serologic confirmation of rubella immunity is essential unless the individual has a documented history of rubella vaccination at 12 months of age or older. Offer rubella and varicella immunization preconceptionally to nonimmune women. Caution against pregnancy for 3 months after administration of these vaccines (ACOG, 1991). Advise preconceptional, nonimmune individuals who are not candidates for vaccination to avoid contact with people exhibiting rashes (especially school-age children). See also Chapter 4.5, *Travel During Pregnancy,* Chapter 10.5, *Measles (Rubeola)*, Chapter 10.8, *Rubella*, Chapter 10.11, *Varicella Zoster Virus*, and the inserts found in vaccine package for additional information. Refer also to the recommendations of the Advisory Committee on Immunization Practices, the American Academy of Pediatrics, and the American Academy of Family Physicians (American Academy of Pediatrics, 1997).

- Additional laboratory assessment may include HBsAg (with liver function studies and hepatitis E antigen [HBeAg] if positive), HIV antibody tests, serologic test for syphilis, screening for gonorrhea, chlamydia and herpes simplex virus. Pap smears should be individualized.

- Routine preconceptional screening for *Toxoplasma gondii* or cytomegalovirus is not recommended (Cefalo & Moos, 1995).

- Hepatitis B vaccine may be indicated for some women. See Chapter 10.2, *Hepatitis A, B, C, D, and E.*

- Advise preconceptional clients with syphilis to defer pregnancy until treatment has been completed. Careful, close follow-up for resolution of the disease is mandatory. See Chapter 14.6, *Syphilis.*

- Risk reduction for acquisition of HIV is of utmost importance. Primary prevention is the key message. Women with HIV infection and their partners will require intensive preconceptional counseling. The possible effects of HIV on the pregnancy and neonate should be clearly understood by the client/couple. Additional laboratory tests will usually be indicated. Refer to Chapter 14.5, *Human Immunodeficiency Virus,* for further information.

- Include the following information in education about infectious disease and STD:
  - ▶ Preconception risk reduction
  - ▶ Review of immunization schedule
  - ▶ Prevention of specific infectious disease and STD and their potential effects on pregnancy
  - ▶ Instruction to client that she inform her prenatal care provider regarding history of infectious disease and/or STD in herself and/or her sexual partner

- Refer to Table 1.4, Teratogenic Agents, and to the individual infectious disease and STD chapters for further information.

Psychiatric Illness

The provider's goals and objectives are to determine the psychiatric diagnosis and medication(s) being used, to evaluate the safety of the medication(s) during the preconception period and during pregnancy, to observe for deterioration in mental health, and to educate the client regarding the possible effects that pregnancy may have on psychopathology.

- Review medical/psychological history and current psychiatric diagnosis. Ask about prescriptive medications and substance use. Consultation with the client's mental health care provider is advisable; client should be followed closely.

  NOTE: Regarding antidepressants, antipsychotic drugs, and tranquilizers:

  ▶ There has been concern that tricyclic antidepressants may cause congenital malformations with specific attention on limb bud reduction defects. Retrospective studies of large populations have failed to show significant increases of congenital limb defects, however (REPROTOX, 1995b).

  ▶ According to Jones (1994), "No study has been performed from which it can be concluded that benzodiazepines are teratogenic in humans." (p. 171).

  ▶ "Three human studies of diazepam exposure during the first trimester have reported an increased relative risk of oral clefts." (Jones, 1994, p. 171).

  ▶ Data suggest that meprobamate and chlordiazepoxide are not human teratogens (Jones, 1994).

  ▶ Phenothiazides are probably not teratogenic in humans (Jones, 1994). However, neonatal withdrawal effects have been reported following third-trimester exposure (McElhatton, 1992).

  ▶ Prenatal exposure to lithium is associated with an increased risk for Ebstein's anomaly (tricuspid valve malformation) (Jones, 1994); true magnitude of risk is currently controversial.

  NOTE: The preconceptional counselor should review the most current literature regarding the use of these drugs. The teratogen registry, or *Physicians' Desk Reference* can be utilized for specific information. A clinical pharmacist can also be consulted.

- Sensitive questioning about the client's motivation and desire for pregnancy and parenting is in order.

- Assess coping skills; ask about past history of suicidal gestures. Consider psychosocial support systems.

- Individualize the physical examination and laboratory tests based on the client's presenting psychological profile.

- Referral to a perinatal support group may be indicated.

- Include the following information in education about psychiatric illness:

  ▶ Preconception risk reduction

  ▶ Common emotional and psychological reactions to pregnancy (Aminoff, 1994)

  ▶ Anticipatory guidance on common discomforts of pregnancy

  ▶ Reassurance regarding natural fears about childbirth and pregnancy outcome

  ▶ Recommendations for perinatal education or a support group

  ▶ Postpartum adjustment to parenting

Male Issues

The provider's goals and objectives are to assess the risk factors of the prospective father that may impact reproduction, present information regarding male effects on reproductive risk, evaluate partner's influence on lifestyle choices for the woman, support and encourage participation of the partner in pregnancy decision-making, and advise as to the importance of the partner as source of social support for the woman during the preconceptional period and pregnancy.

- Ascertain race and ethnic background.

- Obtain a medical, reproductive, genetic, habits/lifestyle, occupational/environmental exposure, and family history of the father, with emphasis on factors that could adversely affect reproduction or pregnancy outcome. Evaluate paternal drug and chemical exposures carefully in couples with repeated pregnancy loss. See Table 15.5 in Section 15, *Pregnancy and Occupational Health,* for information on exposures associated with male reproductive dysfunction.

- Order laboratory tests as indicated (e.g., STD screen, HIV testing, semen analysis for infertility clients, CBC and hemoglobin electrophoresis to rule out hemoglobinopathies, and Tay-Sachs screen).

- As indicated, refer partner (or client and partner) to support groups to assist with lifestyle alterations that promote health (e.g., 12-step program, smoking cessation program).

- Include the following information in education about male issues:

  ▶ Preconception risk reduction

  ▶ Specific STD risk-reduction, especially if the partner is nonmonogamous, bisexual, or an intravenous drug user

  ▶ Importance of the partner in social support of the woman during the preconceptional period and pregnancy

  ▶ Statements such as "no strong, consistent human evidence exists that male-mediated factors affect the occurrence of congenital anomalies" (Cefalo & Moos, 1995, p. 235). To date there have been no human congenital abnormalities attributable to drug- or disease-altered sperm (REPROTOX, 1995c).

  ▶ The following additional information may be conveyed:

    – Genetic disease can be attributed to increased frequencies of male gene mutations and advanced paternal age (more than 40 to 50 years) has been associated with an increased risk for single gene mutations.

    NOTE: Autosomal dominant mutations in which association with paternal age has been confirmed include achondroplasia, Marfan's syndrome, and neurofibromatosis, although the absolute risk is small for a given family (Hook, 1986; Scioscia, 1991).

    – Tobacco smoking may affect male fertility by impairing erectile function and altering spermatogenesis, sperm motility, and sperm morphology; secondary smoke may affect birth weight of an infant and increase risk of respiratory infections.

    – Paternal epilepsy does not appear to increase the risk of congenital birth defects, however, the data are inconclusive (Friis, 1989).

- Germ cell loss due to radiation exposure and after treatment with antineoplastic drugs results in male infertility.

  NOTE: After treatment with platinum-containing chemotherapy for testicular cancer spermatogenesis may be recovered in a substantial proportion of men (REPROTOX, 1995c).

- Certain chemical exposures could affect male germinal tissue and increase the frequency of spontaneous abortion rates. Substances may include lead, vinyl chloride, benzene, anesthetic gases, chloroprine, and others (Cefalo & Moos, 1995). Due to lack of consistency in the findings of epidemiological studies that report paternal occupational/workplace exposures and abnormal pregnancy outcomes, no firm conclusions regarding possible risks to offspring can be made at this time (REPROTOX, 1995c).

Consultation

- A multidisciplinary approach to preconceptional health care may be indicated. The team can include (but is not limited to) a primary care provider, nutritionist, obstetrician and/or perinatologist, internist, cardiologist, nephrologist, pulmonologist, genetic counselor and/or geneticist, infertility nurse-specialist and/or reproductive endocrinologist, substance abuse counselor, mental health counselor and/or psychiatrist, and clinical pharmacist.

- See the Intervention/Management and Patient Education section above.

Follow-up

- Individualize follow-up according to case presentation.

- Use primary care and family planning visits to discuss preconceptional health promotion and reproductive risk reduction.

- Encourage clients to review their health care insurance to determine what services are covered in the pre-pregnancy and perinatal periods. Assist the client/couple in decision making regarding the setting(s) in which they would like to receive prenatal and postpartum care (Summers & Price, 1993).

- Document all important diagnoses and risk factors in the problem list. Progress notes should be thorough and include summaries provided by the consultants.

Table 1.1

Risk Assessment

- Complete medical history, including
  - Age
  - Childhood illnesses
  - Adulthood illness (acute and chronic; incl. STD/infectious disease)
  - Immunization history
  - Surgical history
  - Injuries
  - Hospitalizations
  - Psychiatric illness
  - Allergies
  - Medications
  - Transfusions
- Menstrual, OB/GYN, contraceptive, and sexual history
- Race and ethnic background of client and partner*
- Genetic disease risk factors, client and partner*
- Family history, client and partner*
- Lifestyle risk factors, including:
  - Nutritional history; use of vitamin/mineral supplements
  - STD risk factors
  - Drug, alcohol, tobacco, caffeinated beverage use
  - Exercise patterns
  - Environmental exposures/hazards, home and work
  - Cat exposure
- Partner* history
  - Infectious disease and STD history
  - History of chemotherapy, radiation
  - Substance use
- Psychosocial history
  - Marital status
  - Identified stressors; coping mechanisms
  - Social support
  - Mental status
  - Housing, finances, etc.
  - Education
  - History of physical, emotional abuse
  - Pregnancy readiness
  - Barriers to health care

* Assumes prospective father of the baby

Table 1.2

Laboratory Tests for the Preconception Period

- Hemoglobin, hematocrit or complete blood count (CBC)

- Hemoglobin electrophoresis*

- Iron studies*

- Rh factor

- Rubella titer

- Varicella titer*

- Urinalysis

- Papanicolaou smear

- Tests for cervical infection with gonorrhea, chlamydia*

- Genital cultures for herpes simplex virus*

- Serological test for syphilis

- Hepatitis B surface antigen

- HIV antibody (with informed consent)

- Tuberculosis screen*

- Toxoplasmosis screen*

- Cytomegalovirus screen*

- Toxicology screen (offered)*

- Tay-Sachs screen*

- Antiphospholipid antibodies (lupus anticoagulant, anticardiolipin)*

- Parental karyotype*

- Mammogram*

*As indicated

Source: Adapted from U.S. Public Health Service Expert Panel on the Content of Prenatal Care. (1989). *Caring for our future: The content of prenatal care.* Washington, DC: U.S. Department of Health and Human Services. U.S. Government Printing Office.

Table 1.3

Exercise Safety Guidelines

GUIDELINES FOR AEROBIC EXERCISE

1. For impact activities, it is recommended that exercise routines involving repeated foot impacts be limited to 30 minutes in duration at intensities not exceeding 75% of maximal heart rate. There should be a day of rest between such sessions.

2. A resilient floor should be selected for exercise that involves repeated foot impacts. If such a surface is not available, the exercise routines should be modified to ensure that the feet remain close to the floor throughout the program.

3. Aerobic exercise should be preceded by a gentle warm-up routine that utilizes the full range of motion of the joints. This increases the elasticity of the muscles and will help prevent potentially injurious movements.

4. Muscles that are used repeatedly during aerobic exercise must be carefully stretched before and afterward.

5. To reduce the severity of impact shock on the lower extremities, repetitive jumping on the same foot should not exceed four consecutive jumps.

6. Extremes of joint flexion and extension (such as deep knee bends and ballistic hyperextension of the knee) should be avoided.

7. The feet should be moved repeatedly to prevent cramping in the intrinsic muscles of the foot.

8. Trunk rotation should be avoided while on the feet with hips or lower spine flexed. Rotational activity in this position subjects the intervertebral disks to very high mechanical stress.

9. Intense physical activity should always be followed by a cool-down period of at least 10 minutes of lighter activity to prevent pooling of blood in the extremities. Hot showers and baths should be avoided immediately after intense physical activity.

10. Participants should be given a specific means of assessing physical status and progress. Working heart rate should be measured during peak levels of exercise to ensure that the intensity of activity is within the desired range. Regular measurement of the recovery heart rate will motivate participants by documenting their progress. Failure to progress as measured by this method may indicate the need for more intense activity during the aerobic phase or may signal the presence of other problems.

GUIDELINES FOR STRENGTHENING EXERCISES

1. Strengthening exercises should not be performed on the same muscles on consecutive days.

2. A general warm-up routine should be performed before muscles are made to work against resistance.

3. Muscle-strengthening exercises should be preceded and followed by stretching exercises that are specific for the muscles that are made to work against resistance.

4. All strengthening exercises should be performed in a slow and controlled manner. Ballistic (rapid or jerky) movements increase the risk of injury.

5. The most efficient way to improve strength is to allow brief rest periods between bouts of vigorous exercise. Repetitions should be limited to short sets (10 or fewer) that are repeated later.

6. When the strength of one muscle or muscle group is disproportionate to that of the antagonist(s) for that muscle or group, the weaker muscle should be strengthened to restore balance around the joint.

7. The breath should not be held during strength-training exercises. Exhalation should take place during the exertion phase of each repetition.

GUIDELINES FOR STRETCHING EXERCISES

1. Stretching exercises may be performed as often as desired, preferably at least once a day.

2. A general warm-up routine should be performed before muscles are stretched.

3. Stretching routines should be performed statically, without holding the breath. Rapid, jerky movements should be avoided.

4. Each stretch should be held long enough so that relaxation will occur sufficiently to achieve the maximum benefit of the stretch. This can vary from as little as 6 seconds in some individuals to 20 seconds in others.

5. Muscles should be stretched only to the point of tension. Pain should be regarded as a signal that a stretch has gone too far.

Source: American College of Obstetricians and Gynecologists. (1992). *Women and exercise*. Technical Bulletin No. 173. Washington, DC.: ACOG. © 1992. Reprinted with permission.

Table 1.4 Teratogenic Agents

Agent	Effects	Comments
Drugs and chemicals		
Alcohol	Growth restriction before and after birth, mental retardation, microcephaly, midfacial hypoplasia producing atypical facial appearance, renal and cardiac defects, various other major and minor malformations	Nutritional deficiency, smoking, and multiple drug use confound data. Risk due to ingestion of one to two drinks per day is not well defined but may cause a small reduction in average birth weight. Fetuses of women who ingest six drinks per day are at a 40% risk of developing some features of the fetal alcohol syndrome.
Androgens and testosterone derivatives (eg, danazol)	Virilization of female, advanced genital development in males	Effects are dose dependent and related to the stage of embryonic development at the time of exposure. Given before 9 weeks of gestation, labioscrotal fusion can be produced; clitoromegaly can occur with exposure at any gestational age. Risk related to incidental brief androgenic exposure is minimal.
Angiotesin-converting enzyme (ACE) inhibitors (eg, enalapril, captopril)	Fetal renal tubular dysplasia, oligohydramnios, neonatal renal failure, lack of cranial ossification, intrauterine growth restriction	Incidence of fetal morbidity is 30%. The risk increases with second- and third-trimester use, leading to in utero fetal hypotension, decreased renal blood flow, and renal failure.
Coumarin derivatives (eg, warfarin)	Nasal hypoplasia and stippled bone epiphyses are most common; other effects include broad short hands with shortened phalanges, ophthalmologic abnormalities, intrauterine growth restriction, developmental delay, anomalies of neck and central nervous system	Risk for a seriously affected child is considered to be 15–20% when anticoagulants that inhibit vitamin K are used in the first trimester, especially during 6–9 weeks of gestation. Later drug exposure may be associated with spontaneous abortion, stillbirths, central nervous system abnormalities, abruptio placentae, and fetal or neonatal hemorrhage.
Carbamazepine	Neural tube defects, minor craniofacial defects, fingernail hypoplasia, microcephaly, developmental delay, intrauterine growth restriction	Risk of neural tube defect, mostly lumbosacral, is 1–2% when used alone during first trimester and increased when used with other antiepileptic agents.
Folic acid antagonists (methotrexate and aminopterin)	Increased risk for spontaneous abortions, various anomalies	These drugs are contraindicated for the treatment of psoriasis in pregnancy and must be used with extreme caution in the treatment of malignancy. Cytotoxic drugs are potentially teratogenic. Effects of aminopterin are well documented. Folic acid antagonists used during the first trimester produce a malformation rate of up to 30% in fetuses that survive.
Cocaine	Bowel atresias; congenital malformations of the heart, limbs, face, and genitourinary tract; microcephaly; intrauterine growth restriction; cerebral infarctions	Risks may be affected by other factors and concurrent abuse of multiple substances. Maternal and pregnancy complications include sudden death and placental abruption.
Diethylstilbestrol	Clear-cell adenocarcinoma of the vagina or cervix, vaginal adenosis, abnormalities of cervix and uterus, abnormalities of the testes, possible infertility in males and females	Vaginal adenosis is detected in more than 50% of women whose mothers took these drugs before 9 weeks of gestation. Risk for vaginal adenocarcinoma is low. Males exposed in utero may have a 25% incidence of epididymal cysts, hypotrophic testes, abnormal spermatozoa, and induration of the testes.
Lead	Increased abortion rate, stillbirths	Fetal central nervous system development may be adversely affected. Determining preconceptional lead levels for those at risk may be useful.
Lithium	Congenital heart disease, in particular Ebstein anomaly	Risk of heart malformations due to first-trimester exposure is low. The effect is not as significant as reported in earlier studies. Exposure in the last month of gestation may produce toxic effects of the thyroid, kidneys and neuromuscular systems.

(Continued)

Preconception Health Care—An Overview

Table 1.4 Teratogenic Agents (continued)

Agent	Effects	Comments
Drugs and chemicals (continued)		
Organic mercury	Cerebral atropy, microcephaly, mental retardation, spasticity, seizures, blindness	Cerebral palsy can occur even when exposure is in the third trimester. Exposed individuals include consumers of fish and grain contaminated with methyl mercury.
Phenytoin	Intrauterine growth restriction, mental retardation, microcephaly, dysmorphic craniofacial features, cardiac defects, hypoplastic nails and distal phalanges	The full syndrome is seen in less than 10% of children exposed in utero, but up to 30% have some manifestations. Mild- to-moderate mental retardation is found in some children who have severe physical stigmata. The effect may depend on whether the fetus inherits a mutant gene that decreases production of epoxide hydrolase, an enzyme necessary to decrease the teratogen phenytoin epoxide.
Streptomycin and kanamycin	Hearing loss, eighth-nerve damage	No ototoxicity in the fetus has been reported from use of gentamicin or vancomycin.
Tetracycline	Hypoplasia of tooth enamel, incorporation of tetracycline into bone and teeth, permanent yellow-brown discoloration of deciduous teeth	Drug has no known effect unless exposure occurs in second or third trimester.
Thalidomide	Bilateral limb deficiencies, anotia and microtia, cardiac and gastrointestinal anomalies	Of children whose mothers used thalidomide between 35 and 50 days of gestation, 20% show the effect.
Trimethadione and paramethadione	Cleft lip or cleft palate; cardiac defect; growth deficiency; microcephaly; mental retardation; characteristic facial appearance; ophthalmologic, limb and genitourinary tract abnormalities	Risk for defects or spontaneous abortion is 60–80% with first-trimester exposure. A syndrome including V-shaped eyebrows, low-set ears, high arched palate, and irregular dentition has been identified. These drugs are no longer used during pregnancy due to the availability of more effective, less toxic agents.
Valproic acid	Neural tube defects, especially spina bifida; minor facial defects	Exposure must occur prior to normal closure off neural tube during first trimester to produce open defect (incidence of approximately 1%).
Vitamin A and its derivatives (eg, isotretinoin, etretinate, and retinoids)	Increased abortion rate, microtia, central nervous system defects, thymic agenesis, cardiovascular effects, craniofacial dysmorphism, microphthalmia, cleft lip and palate, mental retardation.	Isotretinoin exposure before pregnancy is not a risk because the drug is not stored in tissue. Etretinate has a long half-life and effects occur long after drug is discontinued. Topical application does not have a known risk.
Infections		
Cytomegalovirus	Hydrocephaly, microcephaly, chorioretinitis, cerebral calcifications, symmetric intrauterine growth restriction, microphthalmos, brain damage, mental retardation, hearing loss	Most common congenital infection. Congenital infection rate is 40% after primary infection and 14% after recurrent infection. Of infected infants, physical effects as listed are present in 20% after primary infection and 8% after secondary infection. No effective therapy exists.
Rubella	Microcephaly, mental retardation, cataracts, deafness, congenital heart disease; all organs may be affected	Malformation rate is 50% if the mother is infected during first trimester. Rate of severe permanent organ damage decreases to 6% by midpregnancy. Immunization of children and nonpregnant adults is necessary for prevention. Immunization is not recommended during pregnancy, but the live attenuated vaccine virus has not been shown to cause the malformations of congenital rubella syndrome.
Syphilis	If severe infection, fetal demise with hydrops; if mild, detectable abnormalities of skin, teeth, and bones	Penicillin treatment is effective for *Treponema pallidum* eradication to prevent progression of damage. Severity of fetal damage depends on duration of fetal progression of damage. Severity of fetal damage depends on duration of fetal infection; damage is worse if infection is greater than 20 weeks. Prevalence is increasing; need to rule out other sexually transmitted diseases.

(Continued)

Table 1.4 Teratogenic Agents (continued)

Agent	Effects	Comments
Infections (continued)		
Toxoplasmosis	Possible effects on all systems but particularly central nervous system: microcephaly, hydrocephaly, cerebral calcifications. Chorioretinitis is most common. Severity of manifestations depends on duration of disease.	Low prevalence during pregnancy (0.1–0.5%); initial maternal infection must occur during pregnancy to place fetus at risk. *Toxoplasma gondii* is transmitted to humans by raw meat or exposure to infected cat feces. In the first trimester, the incidence of fetal infection is as low as 9% and increased to approximately 59% in the third trimester. The severity of congenital infection is greater in the first trimester than at the end of gestation. Treat with pyrimethamine, sulfadiazine, or spiramycin.
Varicella	Possible effects on all organs, including skin scarring, chorioretinitis, cataracts, microcephaly, hypoplasia of the hands and feet, and muscle atrophy	Risk of congenital varicella is low, approximately 2–3% and occurs between 7 and 21 weeks of gestation. Varicella-zoster immune globulin is available regionally for newborns exposed in utero during last 4–7 days of gestation. No effect from herpes zoster.
Radiation	Microcephaly, mental retardation	Medical diagnostic radiation delivering less than 0.05 Gy* to the fetus has no teratogenic risk. Estimated fetal exposure of common radiologic procedures is 0.01 Gy or less (eg, intravenous pyelography, 0.0041 Gy).

* 1 gray = 100 rad

Source: American College of Obstetricians and Gynecologists. (1997). *Teratology.* Educational Bulletin No. 236. Washington, DC. © ACOG, April 1997. Reprinted by permission.

NOTE: This table only includes agents for which the preponderance of evidence suggests a significant teratogenic risk. The reader should consult additional sources for information regarding other possible teratogens. See Appendix 1.B, Patient Education Materials and Additional Resources.

Appendix 1a

PRECONCEPTIONAL HEALTH ASSESSMENT
Client History Form

What is your main interest in seeking preconceptional counseling?

So that we can address your specific interests and concerns, we ask that you complete the following questionnaire.

Instructions: Place an X next to any item that applies to you.

SOCIAL HISTORY

Are you

___ 35 years of age or older?

Do you

___ Drink beer, wine, or hard liquor?

___ Smoke cigarettes or use any other tobacco products?

___ Use marijuana, cocaine, or any other recreational drugs?

___ Use lead or chemicals at home or at work? If yes, please list the specific chemicals.

___ Work with radiation?

___ Participate in an exercise program?

NUTRITION HISTORY

On the back of this sheet, please write down everything you ate or drank for the last 24 hours, including the approximate amount.

Do you

___ Practice vegetarianism?

___ Have an intolerance for milk or other dairy products?

___ Eat things like laundry starch, clay, refrigerator frost?

___ Have a history of bulimia or anorexia?

___ Follow a special diet? If yes, describe:

___ Supplement your diet with vitamins? If yes, list vitamins and dosages:

MEDICAL HISTORY

Do you now have or have you ever had

___ Diabetes?

___ Thyroid disease?

___ PKU?

___ Asthma?

___ Heart disease?

___ High blood pressure?

___ Blood clots?

___ Lupus?

___ Epilepsy?

___ Sickle cell disease?

___ Cancer?

___ Other health problems that require medical or surgical care? If yes, describe:

INFECTIOUS DISEASE HISTORY

Do you or your partner have a history of

___ Recurrent genital infection?

___ Herpes simplex?

___ Chlamydia?

___ Warts?

___ Syphilis?

___ Gonorrhea?

___ Viral hepatitis?

___ HIV infection?

___ AIDS?

___ Occupational exposure to blood or body fluids?

___ Blood transfusion(s)?

___ Intravenous street drug use?

___ Intimate bisexual/homosexual contact?

___ Multiple sexual partners?

Do you

___ Own or work with cats?

___ Have documented immunity to rubella (German measles)?

___ Have documented immunity to varicella?

MEDICATION HISTORY

Do you

___ Routinely or occasionally take prescribed medication? If yes, list names and dosages:

___ Routinely or occasionally take over-the-counter medications? If yes, list names and dosages:

REPRODUCTIVE HISTORY

Do you have a history of

___ Uterine or cervical abnormalities?

___ Two or more pregnancies that ended in first-trimester miscarriages?

___ One or more pregnancies that ended between 14 and 28 weeks of gestation?

___ One or more fetal deaths?

___ One or more infants who were admitted to a neonatal intensive care unit?

___ One or more infants with a birth defect?

FAMILY HISTORY

Do you, your partner, or members of either of your families, including children, have

___ Hemophilia?

___ Thalassemia?

___ Tay-Sachs disease?

___ Sickle cell trait or disease?

___ PKU?

___ Cystic fibrosis?

___ A birth defect?

___ Mental retardation (such as Down syndrome, fragile X syndrome)?

___ Blindness?

___ Deafness?

___ Neurological condition (such as muscular dystrophy, Huntington's disease)?

___ Spina bifida?

___ An inherited disease?

___ Are you and your partner related?

What is your race and ethnic background? _____

What is your partner's race and ethnic background? _____

Source: Cefalo, R. C., & Moos, M.-K. (1995). *Preconceptional health care* (2nd ed., pp. 243-248). St. Louis: Mosby. Adapted with permission.

Appendix 1b

Patient Education Materials and Referral Resources

<u>Organizations</u>

Phenylketonuria

Maternal PKU Collaborative Study
Coordinating Center
PKU Program - #73
Division of Medical Genetics
4650 Sunset Blvd.
Los Angeles, CA 90027

Smoking

American Lung Association
1740 Broadway
New York, New York 10019
(212) 315-8700
        or
1-(800) LUNG-USA (1-800/586-4872)

American Cancer Society
1599 Clifton Road, NE
Atlanta, Georgia 30329
(404) 320-3333

National Cancer Institute
1-(800) 4-CANCER (1-800/422-6237)

Nicotine Anonymous World Services
3410 Geary Boulevard
San Francisco, California 94117
(415) 750-0328

Drugs and alcohol

Alcohol Help/Referral Hotline
1-(800) ALCOHOL (1-800/252-6465)

National Council on Alcoholism and Drug Dependence
1-(800) NCA-CALL (1-800/622-2255)

Cocaine
1-(800) COCAINE (1-800/262-2463) or 1-(800) HELP

Occupational Safety and Health

Agency for Toxic Substances and Disease Registry (ATSDR-Chamblee)
1600 Clifton Road, NE
Atlanta, GA   30333

Environmental Protection Agency (EPA)
Public Information Center
PM-211B
401 M Street, SW
Washington, DC 20460

Occupational Safety and Health Administration (OSHA)
U.S. Department of Labor
200 Constitution Avenue, NW
Washington, DC 20212

National Institute for Occupational Safety and Health (NIOSH)
1600 Clifton Road, NE
Atlanta, GA   30333

Preconceptional Health

Perinatal Health, Inc. (Preconceptional risk assessment and education service)
7777 Greenback Lane, Suite 205
Citrus Heights, CA 95610

Reproductive Risks

California Teratogen Registry
(619) 543-2131 or 1-(800) 532-3749

Environmental Protection Agency Pesticide Hotline
1-(800) 858-7378

Pregnancy Riskline *(western United States)*
(801) 328-2229

Reproductive Toxicology Center (REPROTOX)
202-293-5137

REPRORISK
1-(800) 525-9083

Shepard's Catalog of Teratogenic Agents
(206) 543-3373

Teratogen Information System (TERIS)
(206) 543-2465

Toxic Information Center

On-line Services

Micromedex Computerized Clinical Information System, including
    REPRORISK (Reproductive reviews of chemicals, drugs, physical agents, and nutritional
        status)
    REPROTEXT
    REPROTOX
    Shepard's Catalog of Teratogenic Agents
    TERIS (Teratogen Information System)

Pamphlets

Smart Move! A Stop Smoking Guide
American Cancer Society.
88-900M-Rev.8/89-No. 2515-LE
1-(800) ACS-2345 (1-800/227-2345)

Weight Control Guidance in Smoking Cessation
American Heart Association.
7320 Greenville Avenue
Dallas, Texas 75231

Think Ahead! Is There a Baby in Your Future? March of Dimes (1995)
ISBN# 1-56066-471-1/36173.
Obtain from Mosby-Great Performance
14964 NW Greenbrier Parkway
Beaverton, OR 97006
(503) 222-9434

Clearing the air: How to Quit Smoking...and Quit for Keeps
Publication No. 87-1647
U.S. Department of Health and Human Services (USDHHS), Public Health Service, National
Institutes of Health.

Textbooks/Manuals

Acosta, P.B., & Yannicelli, S. (1993). *Nutrition support protocols*. Columbus, OH: Ross Laboratories. (May be obtained by writing to Ross Laboratories, PO. Box 1317, Columbus, OH 43216-1317)

Barlow, S.M., & Sullivan, F.M. (1982). *Reproductive hazards of industrial chemicals*. London: Academic Press.

Briggs, G.G., Freeman, R. K., & Yaffe, S.J. (1994). *Drugs in pregnancy and lactation* (4th ed.). Baltimore: Williams & Wilkins.

LaDou, J. (1990). *Occupational Medicine*. Norwalk, CT: Appleton & Lange.

Physicians' Desk Reference. Montvale, NJ: Medical Economics.

Schardein, J. L. (1993). *Chemical induced birth defects* (2nd ed.). New York: Marcel Dekker. Shepard, T.H. (1995) *Catalog of teratogenic agents* (8th ed.). Baltimore, MD: Johns Hopkins University Press.

References

Acosta, P.B. (1995). Nutritional support of maternal phenylketonuria. *Seminars in Perinatology, 19*(3), 182–190.

Acosta, P.B., Blaskovics, Cloud, H., Lis, E., Stroud, H., & Wenz, E. (1982). Nutrition in pregnancy of women with hyperphenylalaninemia. *Research, 80*, 443–450.

Acosta, P.B., & Wright, L. (1992). Nurses' role in preventing birth defects in offspring of women with phenylketonuria. *Journal of Obstetric, Gynecologic, and Neonatal Nursing, 21*(4), 270–276.

Acosta, P.B., & Yannicelli, S. (1993). *Nutrition support protocols.* Columbus, OH: Ross Laboratories (P.O. Box 1317, Columbus, OH 43216-1317).

Advisory Committee on Immunization Practices (ACIP). (1994). General recommendations on immunizations. *Morbidity and Mortality Weekly Report, 43*(RR–1), 1–38.

American Academy of Pediatrics, Committee on Infectious Diseases (1997). Recommended childhood immunization schedule—United States, January–December 1997. *Pediatrics. 99*(1), 136–137.

American College of Obstetricians and Gynecologists (ACOG). (1991). *Immunization during pregnancy.* Technical Bulletin No. 160. Washington, DC: Author.

American College of Obstetricians and Gynecologists (ACOG). (1992). *Women and exercise.* Technical Bulletin No. 173. Washington, DC: Author.

American College of Obstetricians and Gynecologists (ACOG). (1995a). *Smoking and reproductive health.* Technical Bulletin No. 180. Washington, DC: Author.

American College of Obstetricians and Gynecologists (ACOG). (1998). *Vitamin A supplementation during pregnancy.* Committee Opinion No. 197. Washington, DC: Author.

American College of Obstetricians and Gynecologists (ACOG). (1997). *Teratology.* ACOG Educational Bulletin No. 233. Washington, DC: Author.

Aminoff, M.J. (1994). Neurologic disorders. In R.K. Creasy & R. Resnik (Eds.), *Maternal-fetal medicine. Principles and practice* (3rd ed.), pp. 1071–1100). Philadelphia: W.B. Saunders.

Before Pregnancy Planning Guide. (1994). Perinatal Health, Inc. Preconceptional Risk Assessment and Education Service. Citrus Heights, CA: Comprehensive Informatics for Perinatal Health, Inc.

Berkowitz, G.S., Skovron, M.L., Lapinski, R.H., & Berkowitz, R.L. (1990). Delayed childbearing and the outcome of pregnancy. *The New England Journal of Medicine, 322*(10), 659–664.

Brachen, M.B., Eshenazi, B., Sachse, K., McSharry, J.E., et al. (1990). Association of cocaine use with sperm concentration, motility and morphology. *Fertility and Sterility, 53*, 315–322.

Briggs, G.G., Freeman, R.F., & Yaffe, S.J. (1994). *Drugs in pregnancy and lactation* (4th ed.). Baltimore: Williams & Wilkins.

Brent, R.L., & Beckman, D.A. (1991). Angiotensin-converting enzyme inhibitors, an embryopathic class of drugs with unique properties: Information for clinical teratology counselors. *Teratology, 43*, 543–546.

Carson, S. (1995). Fetal wastage when genetics is not involved. *Contemporary OB/GYN, 40*(6), 77–84.

Cefalo, R.C., & Moos, M-K. (1995). *Preconceptional health care* (2nd ed.). St. Louis: Mosby.

Centers for Disease Control and Prevention. (1991). Use of folic acid for prevention of spina bifida and other neural tube defects 1983–1991. *Morbidity and Mortality Weekly Report, 40*, 513–516.

Centers for Disease Control and Prevention. (1992). Recommendations for the use of folic acid to reduce the number of cases of spina bifida. *Mortality and Morbidity Weekly Report, 41*(No. RR-14), 1–5.

Chan, K.W., & Ng, W.L. (1985). Gentamycin nephropathy in a neonate. *Pathology, 17*, 514–515.

Cockburn, F. Barnwell, B.E., Brenton, D.P., et al. (1993). Recommendations on the dietary management of phenylketonuria. *Archives of Disease in Childhood, 63*, 432–430.

Constantini, N.W., & Warren, M.P. (1994). Special problems of the female athlete. *Baillière's Clinical Rheumatology, 8*(1), 199–219.

Cuckle, H.A., Wald, N.J., & Thompson, S.C. (1987). Estimating a woman's risk of having a pregnancy associated with Down's syndrome using her age and alfa-fetoprotein level. *British Journal of Obstetrics and Gynaecology, 94*, 387.

Dacus, J.V., Meyer, N.L. & Sibai, B.M. (1995). How preconception counseling improves pregnancy outcome. *Contemporary OB/GYN, 40*(6), 111–126.

Delgado-Escueta, A.V., & Janz, D. (1992). Consensus guidelines: Preconception counseling, management, and care of the pregnant woman with epilepsy. *Neurology, 42*(5), 149–160.

Drogari, E., Beasley, M., Smith, I., & Lloyd, J.K. (1987). Timing of strict diet in relation to fetal damage in maternal phenylketonuria. *Lancet, 2*, 927–930.

Food and Nutrition Board. National Academy of Sciences, National Research Council. (1989). *Recommended dietary allowances* (10th ed.). Washington, DC: National Academy Press.

Frede, D.J. (1993). Preconceptional education. *AWHONN's Clinical Issues, 4*(1), 60–65.

Friis, M.L. (1989). Facial clefts and congenital heart defects in children of parents with epilepsy: Genetic and environmental etiologic factors. *Acta Neurol Scand, 79*, 433–459.

Guidelines for the care of epileptic women of childbearing age. (1989). *Epilepsia, 30*, 409–410.

Holtzman, N.A. (1990). Prenatal screening: When and for whom? *Journal of General Internal Medicine, 5*(September/October Supplement), S42–S46.

Hook, E.B. (1986). Paternal age and genetic outcome: Implications for genetic counseling. In I.H. Porter, N.H. Hatcher, & A.M. Wiley (Eds.), *Perinatal genetics: Diagnosis and treatment* (pp. 243–274). New York: Academic Press.

Hook, E.B., Cross, P.K., & Schreinemachers, D.M. (1983). Chromosomal abnormality rates at amniocentesis and in liveborn infants. *Journal of the American Medical Association, 249*(15), 2034–2038.

Jack, B.W., & Culpepper, L. (1991). Preconception care. *The Journal of Family Practice, 32*(3), 306–315.

Jessup, M. (1995). Alcoholism and other drug dependencies. In W.L. Star, L.L. Lommel, & M.T. Shannon (Eds.), *Women's primary health care: Protocols for practice.* Washington, DC: American Nurses Publishing.

Jones, K.L. (1994). Effects of therapeutic, diagnostic, and environmental agents. In R.K. Creasy & R. Resnik (Eds.), *Maternal-fetal medicine. Principles and practice* (3rd ed., pp. 171–181). Philadelphia, PA: W.B. Saunders.

Kelber, C.M. (1995). Stress management. In W.L. Star, L.L. Lommel, & M.T. Shannon (Eds.), *Women's primary health care: Protocols for practice.* Washington, DC: American Nurses Publishing.

Koch, R., Acosta, P.B., & Williams, J.C. (1995). Nutritional therapy for pregnant women with a metabolic disorder. *Clinics in Perinatology, 22*(1), 1–14.

Koch, R., Friedman, E.G., Levy, H., Matalon, R., Rouse, B., de la Cruz, F., Aezn, C., Gross, E., & Friedman, N. (1990). A preliminary report of the collaborative study of maternal phenylketonuria in the United States and Canada. *Journal of Inherited Metabolic Disease, 13,* 541–650.

Koch, R., Levy, H.L., Matalon, R., Rouse, B., Hanley, W., & Azen, C. (1993). The North American Collaborative Study of Maternal Phenylketonuria. *American Journal of Diseases of Children, 147,* 1224–1230.

Kuller, J.A., & Laifer, S.A. (1994). Preconceptional counseling and intervention. *Archives of Internal Medicine, 154,* 2273–2280.

Lian, Z.H., Zack, M.M., & Erickson, J.D. (1986). Paternal age and the occurrence of birth defects. *American Journal of Human Genetics, 39,* 648.

March of Dimes. (1995). *Think ahead! Is there a baby in your future?* Beaverton, OR: Mosby-Great Performance.

McCormick, K.B. (1987). Pregnancy and epilepsy: Nursing implications. *Journal of Neuroscience Nursing, 19*(2), 66–76.

McElhatton, P.R. (1992). The use of phenothiazines during pregnancy and lactation. *Reproductive Toxicology , 6,* 475–490.

Medical Research Council Working Party on Phenylketonuria. (1993). *Archives of Disease in Childhood, 68*(3), 426–427.

Milunsky, A., Ulcickas, M., & Rothman, K.J. (1991). Maternal heat exposure and neural tube defects. *Journal of the American Medical Association, 268,* 882–885.

Moore, T.R. (1994). Diabetes in pregnancy. In R.K. Creasy & R. Resnik (Eds.), *Maternal-fetal medicine. Principles and practice* (3rd ed., pp. 934–978). Philadelphia: W.B. Saunders.

Moos, M-K. (1989). Preconceptional health promotion: A health education opportunity for all women. *Women and Health, 15*(3), 55–68.

Olsen, M.E. (1994). Preconception evaluation and intervention. *Southern Medical Journal, 87*(6), 639–645.

REPROTOX. (1995a). *Cigarette smoking.* The REPROTOX System. 1975–1995 Micromedex, Inc. Vol. 86, pp. 1–5. (On-line).

REPROTOX. (1995b). *Desiparimine.* The REPROTOX System. 1975–1995 Micromedex, Inc. Vol. 86, pp. 1–3. (On-line).

REPROTOX. (1995c). *Paternal exposures.* The REPROTOX System. 1975–1995 Micromedex, Inc. Vol. 86, pp. 1–4. (On-line).

Schnorr, T.M., Grajewski, B.A., Hornung, R.W., Thun, M.J., Egeland, G.M., Murray, M.S., Conover, D.L., & Halperin, W.E. (1991). Video display terminals and the risk of spontaneous abortion. *The New England Journal of Medicine, 324*(11), 727–733.

Scioscia, A.L. (1991). Preconceptional counseling. *Current Problems in Obstetrics, Gynecology, and Fertility, 14,* 45–66.

Scriver, C.R., Beaudet, A.L., Sly, W.S., & Valle, D. (1995). *The metabolic and molecular basis of inherited diseases* (7th ed.). New York: McGraw-Hill.

Sheehan, K. (1995). Smoking cessation. In W. L. Star, L. L. Lommel, & M. T. Shannon (Eds.), *Women's primary health care: Protocols for practice.* Washington, DC: American Nurses Publishing.

Simpson, J.L. (1995). Genetic evaluation for spontaneous abortion. *Contemporary OB/GYN, 40*(6), 86–90.

Smith, I., Glossop, J., & Beasley, M. (1990). Fetal damage due to maternal phenylketonuria: Effects of dietary treatment and maternal phenylalanine concentration around the time of conception. *Journal of Inherited Metabolic Diseases, 13,* 651–657.

Speroff, L., Glass, R.H., & Kase, N.G. (1994). *Clinical gynecologic endocrinology and infertility.* (5th ed., pp. 809–839). Baltimore: Williams & Wilkins.

Streissguth, A.P., Barr, H.M., & Sampson, P.D. (1990). Moderate prenatal alcohol exposure: Effects on child IQ and learning problems at age 7½ years. *Alcohol Clinical Exposure Research, 14,* 662–669.

Summers, L. & Price, R.A. (1993). Preconception health care. An opportunity to maximize health in pregnancy. *Journal of Nurse-Midwifery, 38*(4), 188–198.

Taysi, K. (1988). Preconceptional counseling. *Obstetrics and Gynecology Clinics of North America, 15*(2), 1667–178.

Teratology Society Position Paper. (1987). Recommendations for vitamin A use during pregnancy. *Teratology, 35,* 269–275.

Teratogen Information System (TERIS) (1995). *Cigarette smoking (Tobacco).* University of Washington. Vol. 86, pp. 1–9. (On-line).

U.S. Department of Agriculture Human Nutrition Information Service. (1992). *The food guide pyramid.* Hyattsville, MD: Author.

U.S. Department of Health and Human Services. (1990). *Healthy people 2000: National health promotion and disease prevention objectives.* (DHHS pub. no. 91-50213). Washington, DC: USDHHS.

U.S. Preventive Services Task Force. (1996). *Guide to clinical preventive services* (2nd ed.). Baltimore: Williams & Wilkins.

U.S. Public Health Service Expert Panel on the Content of Prenatal Care. (1989). *Caring for our future. The content of prenatal care.* Washington, DC: U.S. Department of Health and Human Services. U.S. Government Printing Office.

SECTION 2
GENETIC COUNSELING

Section 2

GENETIC COUNSELING

Kristina Keilman

Women and their partners receive much of the screening and provision of basic information about genetic conditions from their primary obstetrical care providers (Robinson & Linden, 1993). However, with the rapid pace of gene identification through the Human Genome Project, this area of prenatal care is becoming increasingly complex, and consultation with genetics professionals (master's level genetic counselors, M.D. geneticists, genetic nurses, and genetic social workers) is becoming more common. The purpose of this section is to familiarize primary obstetrical care providers with the components of the genetic counseling process, to review indications for genetic counseling referrals, and to augment the knowledge base of primary providers about the content of genetic counseling sessions for the most common of these indications.

Genetic counseling is defined as

> . . . a communication process which deals with the human problems associated with the occurrence, or the risk of occurrence, of a genetic disorder in a family. This process involves an attempt by one or more appropriately trained persons to help the individual or family to (1) comprehend the medical facts, including the diagnosis, probable course of the disorder, and the available management; (2) appreciate the way heredity contributes to the disorder, and the risk of recurrence in specified relatives; (3) understand the alternatives for dealing with the risk of recurrence; (4) choose the course of action which seems to them appropriate in view of their risk, their family goals, and their ethical and religious standards, and to act in accordance with that decision; and (5) to make the best possible adjustment to the disorder in an affected family member and/or to the risk of recurrence of that disorder (Ad Hoc Committee on Genetic Counseling, 1975, pp. 240–241).

Components of Genetic Counseling

- The timing of a genetics referral primarily depends on when the client presents for care and her particular needs.

  ▶ When possible, preconceptional counseling is beneficial because it allows the couple to consider the options for managing the risk in advance and to explore the psychological impact of the decisions they may make (Cefalo & Moos, 1995).

  ▶ If a client may be at significant risk to have a child with a genetic disorder and does not present preconceptionally, refer her as early in pregnancy as possible to allow her and her partner time to understand the implications of the risk and to maximize the testing and management options available to them.

  ▶ In many cases, referral prior to the discovery of an abnormality in the baby is not possible, such as when an anomaly or fetal demise is identified through prenatal ultrasound. Genetics evaluation is useful in these circumstances, also.

NOTE: The cause of late pregnancy loss may be detectable in up to 80 percent of cases (Curry, 1992). The identification of a specific diagnosis helps with the long-term emotional adjustment of couples who have experienced a fetal loss or have had a child with abnormalities (Frets, Duivenvoorden, Verhage, & Niermeijer, 1992).

- After a referral is made, genetic counseling is most often a multistage process involving assessment, informational counseling, supportive counseling, and follow-up (Robinson & Linden, 1993).

Assessment

The genetic counselor's goal in the assessment phase is to develop an understanding of the client's concerns and history.

- A genetics evaluation begins with the gathering of the following information:
  - ▶ Client's presenting concerns and questions, which are often different from the counselor's expectations (Kessler, 1992)
  - ▶ Pregnancy history
  - ▶ Medications, including dosage, frequency, and gestational age at exposure
  - ▶ Detailed family history and pedigree construction (see Bennett et al., 1995, for pedigree standards)
  - ▶ Medical history for affected family members, which may include a review of medical records or photographs
  - ▶ In some cases, physical examination and diagnostic evaluation of the client, the father of the baby, or a previous child may be necessary (particularly when a specific diagnosis or etiology has not been established)
  - ▶ The family's psychological adjustment to the condition
  - ▶ Sources of psychosocial support

Counseling

The genetic counselor's goals are to provide information to clients, to help clients reach their own decisions after exploring the options, and to support clients emotionally throughout the process. The counseling approach in genetics is nondirective (National Institutes of Health [NIH], 1992).

- Informational counseling
  - ▶ The genetic counselor discusses the same basic types of information, whether the referral is for maternal age or a more complex condition such as cystic fibrosis.
    - – Description of the condition
      - * Prevalence
      - * Underlying defect, if known

        *   Natural history

        *   Prognosis

        *   How often the condition is genetic

        *   Pattern of inheritance (autosomal dominant, autosomal recessive, X-linked, mitochondrial, imprinting, multifactorial, chromosomal)

   –   Risks for the current pregnancy and the couple's future offspring

        *   Basis for risk calculation (by pattern of inheritance or by empiric data)

        *   Risk of 2 to 4 percent for birth defects in the general population

   –   Implications of the diagnosis for other family members

   –   Diagnostic, treatment, and management options

   –   Future reproductive options, which may include

        *   Pursuing pregnancy

        *   Remaining child free

        *   Prenatal diagnosis

        *   Adoption

        *   Oocyte or sperm donation

        *   Experimental technologies such as preimplantation diagnosis

- Supportive counseling

  ▶ The majority of couples who discover they are at risk to have a child with a genetic condition are able to come to a decision about current and future reproduction even with short-term genetic counseling (Van Spijker, 1991). Critical factors in the decision-making process are (D'Amico, Jacopini, Vivona, & Frontali, 1992; Frets et al., 1992; Van Spijker, 1991).

    –   Recurrence risks

    –   Availability of prenatal diagnosis

    –   Burden of the disorder (including age of onset of symptoms, severity of disorder, life expectancy, physical versus mental disabilities, quality of life)

    –   Reactions of family members

    –   Couple's resources

    –   Demands of caring for a previously affected child

    –   Desire to have (more) children

  ▶ Couples who discover their offspring may be at risk for abnormalities experience a variety of emotional responses including fear, guilt, disbelief, sadness, and shame (Chapple, May, & Campion, 1995; Kessler, 1979). Parents of children with disabilities express a strong preference for being afforded the opportunity to talk, particularly about their feelings, when given the diagnosis (Sharp, Strauss, & Lorch, 1992). The emotional component of supportive counseling may involve

- Telling the story (it can be therapeutic to relate the history of a previous pregnancy loss, child with birth defects, or loss of a family member [Suslak, Scherer, & Rodriguez, 1995])

- Exploring the psychological, social, and financial impact of the condition for the client, the couple, and their families

- Discussing the couple's responses to the information provided

- Exploring strategies for coping with ambiguity, particularly when a specific diagnosis is not available

- Providing referrals to support groups, other parents, and appropriate local service agencies (see appendix 2.1b, Counseling Resources for National Referral Agencies)

Follow-up

The genetic counselor's goals in the follow-up are to evaluate clients' current needs for information and psychosocial support, to offer ongoing assistance, and to help clients identify which studies or referrals might be helpful to them.

- Follow-up telephone calls or appointments may provide an opportunity to assess the couple's current level of understanding of the condition and their adjustment to the decisions they have made.

  ▶ The genetic counselor discusses additional evaluations if a specific diagnosis is not found.

  ▶ Written materials about the condition are given when available, because it can be difficult for couples to take in the volume of information discussed in a genetic counseling session, particularly because of the psychological implications (Chapple et al., 1995; Kessler, 1979).

- Psychotherapy referrals may be indicated. Some couples experience long-term psychological sequelae following the diagnosis of a genetic disorder (Elder & Laurence, 1991; Frets et al., 1992; Heimler, 1990; Van Spijker, 1991).

- Depending on the reason for genetic consultation and the couple's needs, genetic counseling may continue through the pregnancy and after delivery.

Genetic Counseling After Diagnosis of a Fetal Abnormality

The components of genetic counseling outlined above are employed if a referral is made prior to conception, during pregnancy, or after delivery. Counseling issues that arise at the time of discovery of a fetal abnormality merit specific exploration. Whether the fetus is found to have a chromosome problem, an apparently isolated physical birth defect, or a genetic condition, the detection of a fetal abnormality is a crisis situation for a pregnant woman and her partner. In this emotional state the couple receives a mass of complex information that they must rapidly assimilate to make decisions about the pregnancy. It can be particularly difficult for couples to cope when a specific diagnosis is not available or the fetal prognosis is uncertain. In such situations, it is useful for the genetic counselor and primary obstetrical care provider to work together to provide support and anticipate both short- and long-term needs for the couple, who are frequently too overwhelmed to consider questions they may have in the future when contemplating another pregnancy.

Informational Counseling

- If possible, discuss in advance how results will be given (by telephone or in person).

- Decide who will give the results (primary obstetrical care provider or genetic counselor). Most couples prefer to talk with someone who can answer their questions as soon as possible.

- Informational counseling may include

  ▶ Option to continue or terminate the pregnancy

    – Information about foster care and adoption placement may be helpful since some couples are unaware of these options.

    – Specific information about the abortion procedures that are available is reported to be of particular value to couples considering termination (Suslak et al., 1995).

      NOTE: Couples who would choose to continue the pregnancy upon discovery of a fetal abnormality often decline prenatal testing.

  ▶ Accuracy of the testing

    – A common reason for persistent ambivalent feelings about terminating the pregnancy is uncertainty about the accuracy of the diagnosis (White-van Mourik, Connor, & Ferguson-Smith, 1992).

  ▶ The specific diagnosis and prognosis

    – The prognosis for the fetus is a primary factor in decision making for clients who elect to have prenatal testing and is more critical than the age of the fetus or personal characteristics of the couple (Hassed et al., 1993; Pryde et al., 1992).

    – Most couples choose to abort the pregnancy when an autosomal chromosome abnormality like Down syndrome is detected, but are less likely to chose termination with milder conditions such as sex chromosome abnormalities (Verp, Bombard, Simpson, & Elias, 1988).

    – Many couples elect to continue the pregnancy when the fetus is diagnosed with a lethal anomaly, the prognosis for the fetus is uncertain, or detection of the fetal abnormality occurs too late in pregnancy for abortion to be an option (Fonda Allen & Mulhauser, 1995; Hassed et al, 1993).

  ▶ Availability of additional studies

    – Additional studies may identify a specific diagnosis, which is of benefit because couples experience more long-term distress when a diagnosis is not available (Frets et al., 1992).

- Further evaluations may clarify the prognosis for the fetus even when a specific diagnosis is known (e.g., echocardiography for a fetus with Down syndrome may identify an atrioventricular canal).

- Additional studies may include

  * Ultrasound

  * Echocardiography

  * Chromosome studies

  * Biochemical studies

  * DNA analysis

  * Autopsy

  * Physical exam of fetus or newborn by the geneticist

  NOTE: If desired by the client, autopsy following termination of pregnancy or perinatal death can be particularly useful with isolated ultrasound abnormalities because additional anomalies are detected in 50 percent of cases; discovery of these additional anomalies can impact diagnosis, recurrence risks, and future pregnancy management (Julian-Reynier et al., 1994; Weston, Porter, Andrews, & Berry, 1993).

▶ Availability of referrals to other medical specialists (e.g., perinatologists, pediatric specialists), especially when the pregnancy is continued

▶ Discussion of recurrence risks and testing options for future pregnancies

Supportive Counseling

● The genetic counselor's goals in supportive counseling are to

  ▶ Provide written materials about the specific condition, the stages of grief, and decision making

  ▶ Discuss strategies to facilitate decision making, especially when the diagnosis or prognosis remain uncertain

  ▶ Explore feelings, including grief, guilt, and disbelief

  - Families report this to be one of the most helpful parts of genetic counseling after the discovery of a fetal abnormality (Elder & Laurence, 1991).

  - Discuss whether the couple would find it helpful to create memories (e.g., photographs, memorial service) following an abortion, stillbirth, or neonatal death.

  ▶ Discuss social supports and what the couple plans to tell family members and friends

  - Offer referrals to local and national support groups for specific diagnoses (see Appendix 2.1b, Counseling Resources).

- Offer referrals to groups which provide peer support after genetic termination of pregnancy.

- Discuss the availability of social work and psychotherapeutic services.

Follow-up

- Offer follow-up genetic counseling, in person or by telephone.

  ▶ Women who miscarry or terminate a pregnancy because of a fetal abnormality report that the people in their lives expect them to recover from the experience much sooner than they do.

    - Grief can remain unresolved as long as 18 months after the pregnancy loss for some couples (White-van Mourik et al., 1992).

    - Prolonged grief is less common for couples who undergo counseling or have other supports (Elder & Laurence, 1991).

  ▶ Clients who continue the pregnancy also face emotional challenges as they try to balance the need to cope with the loss of the normal child they hoped for with the need to bond with their child with disabilities or chronic health concerns (Fonda Allen & Mulhauser, 1995).

- With clients who discontinue the pregnancy, the genetic counselor discusses

  ▶ Ability of each partner to return to regular activities

  ▶ Impact of the experience on the relationship as a couple

    - Marital and sexual disruption is frequently reported by couples following termination of pregnancy for a fetal abnormality (Elder & Lawrence, 1991; White-van Mourick et al., 1992).

    - The grief period is often shorter for fathers (Suslak et al., 1995; White-van Mourik et al., 1992).

  ▶ Reactions of family members and friends

  ▶ Use of social support, including peer referrals or formal support groups

  ▶ Results of follow-up or confirmation studies

  ▶ Decisions about future pregnancies

    - Review of the risks of having another affected child

    - Prevention strategies (e.g., folate supplementation for neural tube defects)

    - Reproductive options, which may include oocyte or sperm donation, adoption, surrogacy, or remaining child free

    - Testing options, including ultrasound, chorionic villus sampling (CVS), amniocentesis, or experimental technologies such as preimplantation diagnosis

- With clients who continue the pregnancy after diagnosis of a fetal anomaly, the genetic counselor explores

  ▶ Ability of each partner to return to regular activities

▶ Impact of the experience on the relationship as a couple

▶ Reactions of family members and friends

▶ Use of social support, including peer referrals, formal support groups, and community agencies for individuals with disabilities

▶ Plans for contact with adoption professionals if placement is planned

▶ Plans for meeting the medical and developmental needs of the child

▶ Fears and hopes for the child's future

▶ Ability to bond with the baby

▶ Decisions about future pregnancies

   – Review of the risks of having another affected child

   – Prevention strategies (e.g., folate supplementation for neural tube defects)

   – Reproductive options, which may include oocyte or sperm donation, adoption, surrogacy, or remaining child free

   – Testing options, including ultrasound, CVS, amniocentesis, or experimental technologies such as preimplantation diagnosis

Genetic Counseling Indications

History

• Obtain a detailed history to determine the usefulness of a genetic counseling referral for an individual patient.

   ▶ Collect information about pregnancy losses, birth defects, mental retardation, chronic health conditions, or genetic disorders in the client, previous children, and her extended family members.

   ▶ Obtain the same information about the father of the baby, any children he has from previous relationships, and his extended family.

   ▶ Ask about the couple's ethnic background and any consanguinity (blood relationship).

   NOTE: Harper (1993) and Robinson & Linden (1993) are useful resources for guidance about family history taking for genetic assessment.

• Psychological, social, cultural, and economic factors can influence a client's ability and willingness to provide genetic information.

   ▶ Genetic information is often kept secret in families and may not be shared with members known to be at risk to have affected children (Varekamp, Suurmeijer, Brocker-Vriends, & Rosendaal, 1992).

   ▶ Client-provider communication about genetic disorders may also be limited, due to the client's fear of insurance discrimination if a family history of genetic conditions is divulged (Lynch et al., 1997).

Genetics and Environment

- The evaluation of individuals with birth defects or mental retardation frequently involves sorting out genetic and environmental influences.

  ▶ Therefore, genetic consultation is not limited to conditions with straightforward autosomal dominant, recessive, or X-linked inheritance.

  NOTE: For a review of the basics of inheritance patterns, see Harper (1993), Robinson & Linden (1993), or Thompson, McInnes, & Willard (1991) listed in Appendix 2.1a, General Book Resources.

  ▶ Genetics consultation is also useful for conditions (e.g., hypercholesterolemia) or birth defects (e.g., spina bifida) that are known to cluster in families as a result of the interaction of environment and genetics (multifactorial inheritance).

  ▶ Genetic counseling also may be offered when there is potential for harm to the developing baby as a result of environmental exposures.

Indications for Genetics Referral

- Standard indications for genetics referral or consultation include but are not limited to (American Academy of Pediatrics Committee on Genetics, 1994; D'Alton & DeCherney, 1993; D'Alton, Craigo, & Bianchi, 1994; Harper, 1993; Robinson & Linden, 1993)

  ▶ Maternal age 35 years or older at estimated date of confinement (EDC)

  ▶ Abnormal alpha-fetoprotein (AFP) or triple marker (AFP, human chorionic gonadotropin [hCG], unconjugated estriol [μE_3]) screen

  ▶ Positive results for both parents through carrier screening programs for hemoglobinopathies, Tay-Sachs disease, Canavan disease, or cystic fibrosis

  ▶ Teratogen exposure

  ▶ Ultrasound identification of fetal abnormalities

  ▶ Personal or family history of

    - Mental retardation, especially Down syndrome or fragile X syndrome

    - Chromosome abnormalities, including both numerical abnormalities (e.g., trisomies) and structural rearrangements (e.g., translocations, inversions)

    - Congenital malformations (e.g., neural tube defect, cleft lip, polydactyly)

    - Neurologic conditions (e.g., muscular dystrophy, Huntington's disease, epilepsy)

    - Metabolic diseases (e.g., phenylketonuria [PKU], Gaucher disease, Hurler syndrome)

    - Hereditary blood disorders (e.g., sickle cell disease, thalassemia, hemophilia, immune deficiency)

    - Connective tissue disorders (e.g., Marfan syndrome, Ehlers-Danlos syndrome, osteogenesis imperfecta)

    - Hereditary skin disorders (e.g., neurofibromatosis, tuberous sclerosis)

- Any condition known to be genetic (e.g., cystic fibrosis, polycystic kidney disease)
- Multiple congenital anomalies
- Dysmorphic appearance
- Dwarfism
- Deafness or blindness
- Consanguinity
- Two or more miscarriages

Common Genetic Consultations

- The most common indications for genetic counseling are explored in more detail below.

- See the Components of Genetic Counseling discussion earlier in this section for general guidelines used in genetic counseling.

Maternal Age

- The risk for numerical chromosome abnormalities in the fetus increases as maternal age increases, and the current standard of care in the United States is to offer prenatal diagnosis via CVS or amniocentesis when maternal age will be 35 years or greater at delivery (Centers for Disease Control and Prevention [CDC], 1994).

  NOTE: A shift away from the use of maternal age alone to the use of maternal age plus triple marker screening to determine which women should be offered prenatal diagnosis has been suggested (Haddow et al., 1994), but this approach remains controversial (D'Alton et al., 1994).

- Paternal age is not associated with an increased risk for fetal chromosome abnormalities, so although there may be an increased risk for autosomal dominant disorders in the offspring of older men, prenatal diagnosis is not offered for advanced paternal age (Friedman, 1981; Hook, 1986).

- Specific information about triple marker screening, amniocentesis, and CVS is provided in Triple Marker Screening below and in Section 3, *Prenatal Diagnosis and Surveillance Techniques*.

- It can be a challenge for patients to sort through the testing options, so one of the genetic counselor's primary goals is to facilitate decision making about testing.

  ▶ Some women decline all testing for the fetus.

  ▶ If testing is desired, clients choose between a screening test (triple marker) and a diagnostic test (CVS or amniocentesis).

- Factors that have an impact on clients' choice of tests include (Cefalo & Moos, 1995; CDC, 1994; D'Alton et al., 1994)

  ▶ Risks of procedure

- Between 1 in 400 and 1 in 200 women will experience a miscarriage due to amniocentesis (CDC, 1994).

- With CVS, 1 in 200 to 1 in 100 women will miscarry due to the procedure. Transverse limb deficiencies have been reported in approximately 1 in 3,000 to 1 in 1,000 births following CVS (CDC, 1994).

▶ Stage of pregnancy when results are available

▶ Client's perception of accuracy of testing

- Triple marker provides screening for chromosome abnormalities but is not diagnostic.

- The screen-positive rate for triple marker increases dramatically after age 40 (Haddow & Palomaki, 1993), rendering triple marker a less useful screening tool for these patients.

- A mosaic result, in which the sample includes both chromosomally normal cells and chromosomally abnormal cells, is more common with CVS than with amniocentesis (Fryburg, 1993).

▶ Client's perception of comprehensiveness of testing

- Triple marker screens only for select chromosome abnormalities (i.e., Down syndrome and trisomy 18).

- Although amniocentesis tests for chromosome abnormalities and screens for neural tube defects, CVS provides testing for chromosome abnormalities only.

▶ Client's perception of risk for fetal chromosome abnormalities as high or low

▶ Fear of procedures (especially needles)

▶ Client's anticipated plan for her course of action if fetus is found to have an abnormality

- When an abnormality is found, most couples do elect to terminate the pregnancy (Verp et al., 1988).

- Some patients elect to have prenatal diagnosis, with the knowledge that they will continue the pregnancy if an abnormality is detected, because they feel the information will be useful to them in psychologically preparing for the birth of an affected child (Fonda Allen & Mulhauser, 1995).

● See Genetic Counseling after Diagnosis of a Fetal Abnormality above for guidelines about genetic counseling following discovery of fetal anomalies through CVS or amniocentesis.

Triple Marker Screening

● The triple marker screen is considered to be positive when the risk for Down syndrome, trisomy 18, or neural tube defects is above a specified threshold.

▶ Maternal age and maternal serum levels of AFP, hCG, and μE3 are taken into account when calculating the risk for these abnormalities.

● Offer consultation with a genetic counselor when the triple marker screen is positive.

▶ Women referred for genetic counseling because of a positive triple marker screen describe feelings of anxiety upon being informed of the result (Statham & Green, 1993).

▶ As with women referred for advanced age, psychosocial support and assistance with the process of decision making about prenatal diagnosis are primary goals of the genetic counselor.

• Triple marker screening is covered in detail in Chapter 3.3, *Triple Marker Prenatal Screening*.

Screen Positive for Down Syndrome

• Offer genetic counseling referral.

• The triple marker screen is positive when the combination of maternal age and levels of serum markers indicates a risk for Down syndrome above a specified threshold.

▶ The most common pattern with a screen positive for Down syndrome is decreased AFP, decreased μE_3, and increased hCG levels.

▶ In the California program, the triple marker screen is positive when the risk for Down syndrome is greater than 1 in 190 pregnancies (at the time of the second trimester).

▶ Triple marker screening laboratories provide a risk assessment that is individualized for the client.

▶ Because a threshold is used, the screen can be positive in selected cases even when the risk for Down syndrome is lower with the triple marker screen than it would have been based on age alone. For example, in the California program a 40-year-old woman would have a positive triple marker screen if her risk to have a fetus with Down syndrome was calculated to be 1 in 150, even though this is lower than the 1 in 110 risk based on her age alone.

• The genetic counselor will offer

▶ Detailed ultrasound

– Dating changes may result in reinterpretation of the risk.

– Most fetuses with Down syndrome have no detectable abnormality on ultrasound (Garmel & D'Alton, 1993).

▶ Amniocentesis

– Risk for birth defects is not increased if the fetal karyotype is found to be normal.

• The risk for complications (e.g., fetal growth restriction, preterm delivery, low birth weight) may be increased with hCG elevations above 2.0 multiples of the median (MOM) (Gonen et al., 1992; Lieppman et al., 1993).

Screen Positive for Trisomy 18

• Offer genetic counseling referral.

• The triple marker screen is positive when the combination of maternal age and levels of serum markers indicates a risk for trisomy 18 above a specified threshold.

▶ The most common pattern with a screen positive for trisomy 18 is decreased levels of all three metabolites (AFP, hCG, and μE3).

▶ In the California program, the triple marker screen is positive when the risk for trisomy 18 is greater than 1 in 100 pregnancies (at the time of the second trimester).

▶ Many, but not all, triple marker screening laboratories provide a risk assessment that is individualized for the client.

- The genetic counselor may offer the client

  ▶ Detailed ultrasound

  - Dating changes do not usually lead to reinterpretation of the risk for trisomy 18.

  - Some features of trisomy 18 may be detectable, but ultrasound is not diagnostic.

  ▶ Amniocentesis

  - Risk for birth defects is not increased if the fetal karyotype is found to be normal.

Screen Positive for Neural Tube Defects

- Offer genetic counseling referral

- A triple marker screen is positive for neural tube defects when the level of AFP in maternal serum is above a specified multiple of the median (MOM) level, usually set at 2.0 or 2.5.

  ▶ Risks for neural tube defects do not depend on maternal age or levels of hCG or μE3.

  ▶ Most triple marker screening laboratories do not provide an individualized risk assessment for neural tube defects.

- The genetic counselor may offer the following testing options:

  ▶ Detailed ultrasound

  - At least 90 percent of neural tube defects are detectable by ultrasound (Platt et al., 1992).

  - Other abnormalities such as abdominal wall defects, renal abnormalities, or placental anomalies may be associated with an elevation of the AFP (Milunsky et al., 1989).

  - Genetic counseling issues for fetal neural tube or abdominal wall defects are discussed in Ultrasound Abnormalities below.

  ▶ Amniocentesis

  - Testing of amniotic fluid for acetylcholinesterase and AFP levels may increase detection rate for neural tube defects (Platt et al., 1992).

  - Chromosome abnormalities may be found in up to 1 percent of cases (Feuchtbaum et al., 1995).

- See Chapter 3.3, *Triple Marker Prenatal Screening,* for discussion of the risks for pregnancy complications when follow-up studies are normal and the elevation of maternal serum AFP remains unexplained.

Carrier Screening

- Carrier testing is most frequently offered when there is a previous family history of a specific genetic disorder; however, there are genetic screening programs designed to identify at-risk couples in the general population who were previously unaware of the risk to their offspring.

  ▶ Screening is usually offered to individuals known to be at increased risk to carry a gene for a specified genetic disorder, most often based on ethnic background.

  ▶ Clients' decisions about screening depend on factors such as the severity of the genetic disorder, treatment options, ethnocultural background, and religious beliefs (D'Alton et al., 1994).

  NOTE: Knowledge of carrier status appears to have an impact on self-image, anxiety levels, reproductive behavior, and social image (Evers-Kiebooms, Denayer, Welkenhuysen, Cassiman, & Van den Berghe, 1994; Marteau, 1992), so screening is ideally offered on a voluntary basis (Elias, Annas, & Simpson, 1991).

- Standard programs provide prenatal carrier screening for cystic fibrosis, sickle cell, thalassemia, Tay-Sachs, and Canavan diseases.

  ▶ Offer genetic counseling

  - Because Tay-Sachs disease, Canavan disease, cystic fibrosis, and hemoglobinopathies are inherited in an autosomal recessive pattern, there is a risk for disease in the child only if both the client and her partner are carriers.

  - Prenatal diagnosis and/or newborn screening is possible for most families at risk to have children with these disorders.

  - Guidelines for genetic counseling are outlined above in the Components of Genetic Counseling section.

  ▶ Cystic fibrosis carrier screening

  - Carrier frequencies vary by ethnic background as follows (NIH, 1997).

    * 1 per 29 individuals of Caucasian descent

    * 1 per 29 individuals of Ashkenazi (Eastern European) Jewish descent

    * 1 per 32 individuals of Native American descent

    * 1 per 46 individuals of Latino descent

    * 1 per 60 individuals of African-American descent

    * 1 per 90 individuals of Asian descent

  - Carrier screening consists of DNA analysis for the most common mutations in the cystic fibrosis gene.

  - Sensitivity in the detection of carriers is (NIH, 1997)

    * 90 percent in individuals of Caucasian descent

    * 97 percent in individuals of Ashkenazi (Eastern European) Jewish descent

* 94 percent in individuals of Native American descent

* 57 percent in individuals of Latino descent

* 75 percent in individuals of African-American descent

* 30 percent in individuals of Asian descent

► Sickle cell trait screening

– Carrier frequency is approximately 1 in 14 for individuals of African-American descent (Lorey, Arnopp, & Cunningham, 1996).

– Carrier screening can be accomplished with hemoglobin electrophoresis, isoelectric focusing, or high-performance liquid chromatography, with greater than 99 percent sensitivity in the detection of sickle cell trait (Lorey, Cunningham, Shafer, Lubin, & Vichinsky, 1994). See the hemoglobinopathy chapters for details about hemoglobin screening.

► Thalassemia trait screening

– Carriers are most often of African-American, Mediterranean, Middle Eastern, or Asian descent. Carrier frequencies vary significantly depending on the country of origin (Lorey et al., 1996) and will therefore not be reviewed here.

– Laboratory analysis for thalassemia trait screening is described in detail in the hemoglobinopathy chapters.

► Tay-Sachs disease carrier screening

– Carrier frequency is 1 in 30 for individuals of Ashkenazi Jewish or French Canadian descent (Kaback et al., 1993).

– Screening is accomplished by measuring levels of hexosaminidase A, with greater that 99 percent sensitivity in the detection of carriers. Pregnancy alters serum hexosaminidase levels, so prenatal carrier screening should be performed on white blood cells rather than serum (Kaback et al., 1993).

► Canavan disease carrier screening

– Carrier frequency is 1 in 40 for individuals of Ashkenazi Jewish descent (Matalon, Michals, & Kaul, 1995).

– Carrier screening consists of DNA analysis for the most common mutations, with 97 percent sensitivity in the detection of carriers of Ashkenazi Jewish descent (Matalon et al., 1995).

Teratogens

● Background

► A teratogen is a drug, chemical, infectious agent, or environmental exposure that has deleterious effects on the developing fetus (Conover, 1994; Juchau, 1993).

▶ Table 2.1 lists several agents that are known teratogens. This listing is not exhaustive and is likely to expand in the future.

▶ When there is a question about the teratogenic potential of an exposure, patients find it useful to be provided with a specific numerical risk for birth defects in the fetus (Ludowese, Marini, Laxova, & Pauli, 1993).

    – Although most exposures during pregnancy are not teratogenic, patients perceive medications and environmental exposures to be a major cause of birth defects and consistently overestimate the magnitude of the risks of their own exposures (Friedman et al., 1990; Koren, Bologa, Long, Feldman, & Shear, 1989).

    – The press plays a role in establishing these misperceptions; one study assessing 15 popular magazines found that articles about exposures in pregnancy were misleading or inaccurate 55 percent of the time (Gunderson-Warner et al., 1990).

    – Women revise their estimates of the teratogenic potential of exposures as a result of genetic counseling, with fewer electing to terminate the pregnancy after discovering that the fetal risks were lower than anticipated (Koren et al., 1989; Ludowese et al., 1993).

    – Preconception counseling may be especially helpful as it allows a woman who will continue the exposure to make choices about alternative medications, strategies for minimizing her exposures at work, or methods to improve control of maternal disease such as diabetes or maternal phenylketonuria (PKU). See Section 1, *Preconception Heath Care–An Overview,* and Section 15, *Pregnancy and Occupational Health*, for additional information.

▶ Standard medical sources can be difficult to use to assess exposures in pregnancy.

    – For example, the *Physicians' Desk Reference* focuses primarily on whether or not a medication should be prescribed during pregnancy rather than on the risks to the fetus when a pregnant woman has already taken the medication, which is the more common question (Friedman et al., 1990).

    – Other sources that specifically address the teratogenic potential of exposures such as books, on-line data bases, or regional teratogen information phone lines may be more useful in counseling (see Appendix 2.1c, Resources for Assessing Teratogens and Table 2.1, Established Teratogens).

● Risk assessment

  ▶ The teratogenic potential of an agent is dependent on several factors (Conover, 1994).

    – Dosage

    – Timing of the exposure

      * First trimester exposures are of specific concern.

      * Exposure at other times in pregnancy may pose some risk to the fetus, depending on the specific agent.

    – Duration of the exposure

    – Interaction effects with concurrent drugs or exposures

- Susceptibility of the fetus

  * For example, genetic differences may account for the development of fetal hydantoin syndrome in some but not all fetuses exposed to antiepileptic drugs (Buehler, Delimont, van Waes, & Finnel, 1990).

- Maternal disease

  * A normal diet, not restricted for phenylalanine intake, is teratogenic for the offspring of women with phenylketonuria, for example (Koch et al., 1993).

▶ Studies that evaluate the teratogenic potential of exposures during pregnancy focus on two primary questions:

- Does this agent lead to an increase in the risk for birth defects above the background risk of 2 to 4 percent in any pregnancy?

- Is there a specific pattern of birth defects associated with in utero exposure to this agent?

▶ In most instances, counseling about exposures during pregnancy can provide reassurance that the specific agent of concern is not known to increase the risk for birth defects.

- The majority (>90 percent) of the most commonly prescribed medications have not been found to be teratogenic (Friedman et al., 1990).

- Women who report exposures limited to the all-or-nothing time period through 4 weeks after the last menstrual period can be reassured that the risk to the fetus is not increased (Conover, 1994).

- Most paternal exposures are not associated with a risk to the fetus (Conover, 1994).

  NOTE: Of course, patients should be advised of the 2 to 4 percent general population risk for birth defects even in these situations.

The most commonly encountered teratogens are discussed below. These and other potential teratogens (e.g., radiation exposure, maternal disease) are addressed in specific chapters, also.

Antiepileptic Drugs

● Offer genetic counseling

● Risks

▶ The offspring of women using antiepileptic drugs during pregnancy are at a 6 to 8 percent risk for birth defects, which is increased above the rate in the general population of 2 to 4 percent (Delgado-Escueta & Janz, 1992).

- The increased risk is probably not entirely due to the use of antiepileptic drugs, however, because some studies have reported increased rates for birth defects in the offspring of women with epilepsy who *did not* take antiepileptic drugs during pregnancy (Delgado-Escueta & Janz, 1992; Koch et al., 1992; McCormick, 1987).

- Congenital heart defects and cleft lip with or without cleft palate are specifically seen at higher rates than in the general population, particularly with polydrug therapy (Delgado-Escueta & Janz, 1992).

- Valproate or carbamazepine use confers an increased risk for spina bifida, which has been reported in approximately 1 percent of exposed fetuses (Lindhout, Omtzigt, & Cornel, 1992; Rosa, 1991).

- Some infants prenatally exposed to antiepileptic medications have fetal anticonvulsant syndrome, characterized by dysmorphic facial features, hypoplastic nails, and developmental and growth delay (Delgado-Escueta & Janz, 1992; Jones, Lacro, Johnson, & Adams, 1989).

  NOTE: It has been suggested that this syndrome occurs primarily in fetuses with a genetic defect in the epoxide hydrolase enzyme (Buehler et al., 1990), but this finding has not been replicated by other investigators.

▶ Some studies suggest an increased risk for developmental problems with anticonvulsant use even in the absence of visible birth defects (Scolnik et al., 1994), but whether this constitutes a real risk following in utero exposure to antiepileptic drugs remains unresolved.

▶ When the cause for the mother's epilepsy is unknown, the risk for her offspring to develop epilepsy is 5 to 10 percent, but it can be as high as 50 percent because epilepsy follows an autosomal dominant pattern in some families (Gardiner, 1990).

- Evaluations and options
    ▶ Neurology consultation

    - The most commonly used antiepileptic drugs (carbamazepine, valproate, phenytoin, and phenobarbital) all have some teratogenic potential.

    - A change in dosage or specific antiepileptic regimen may be recommended during pregnancy.

    ▶ Obstetrics or perinatology consultation

    - There is an increased risk for neonatal hemorrhage due to deficiency of vitamin K clotting factors in exposed infants (Delgado-Escueta & Janz, 1992).

    - See Chapter 6.28, *Seizures,* for further information.

    ▶ Folate supplementation

    - The utility of supplementation has not been specifically documented in the offspring of women on antiepileptic medications as yet, but supplementation may help prevent neural tube defects when used preconceptionally and through the first trimester (Delgado-Escueta & Janz, 1992). See *Preconception Health Care—An Overview,* for dosing information.

    ▶ Detailed ultrasound in the second trimester

    - Sonography can screen for facial clefting, congenital heart defects, and neural tube defects, but many of the effects of prenatal antiepileptic drug exposure are not detectable (Garmel & D'Alton, 1993).

    - See Ultrasound Abnormalities below for a discussion of neural tube defects.

▶ Alpha-fetoprotein screening via maternal serum or amniocentesis for women on valproate or carbamazepine

   – Although more cases of neural tube defects can be detected by amniocentesis than by serum screening, amniocentesis is associated with a risk for miscarriage.

   – See Triple Marker Prenatal Screening in Chapter 3.3 and the appropriate chapters in Section 3, *Prenatal Diagnosis and Surveillance Techniques* for more information.

▶ Option to terminate or continue the pregnancy

▶ Neonatal evaluation by a dysmorphologist or geneticist for infants suspected to have fetal anticonvulsant syndrome

● Specific psychosocial issues

▶ General supportive counseling (see Components of Genetic Counseling above)

▶ Balancing concerns about maternal and fetal health

▶ Strategies for coping with uncertainty regarding fetal prognosis

Alcohol

● Offer genetic counseling

● Risks

▶ The risk for fetal alcohol syndrome may be as high as 40 percent in the offspring of women who consume six or more drinks per day (Coles, 1993). Fetal alcohol syndrome affects an estimated 1 to 2 per 1,000 infants born in the United States (Levy & Koren, 1990).

   – Fetal alcohol syndrome is characterized by growth delay, mental retardation, and dysmorphic facial features, including short palpebral fissures, hypoplastic philtrum, and low set ears. Some individuals with fetal alcohol syndrome also have congenital heart defects, genitourinary abnormalities, hearing loss, or behavioral problems (Coles, 1993).

▶ Fetal alcohol effects such as neurobehavioral abnormalities have been reported even with moderate alcohol exposure (two to three drinks per day), and consumption limited to binge drinking also has been associated with developmental problems (Coles, 1993; Levy & Koren, 1990).

▶ Complications such as placental abruption and pregnancy loss are reported more frequently for women who use alcohol (Levy & Koren, 1990).

▶ See Section 1, *Preconception Health Care—An Overview*, and Chapter 6.31, *Substance Abuse,* for additional information.

● Evaluation and options

▶ Detailed ultrasound

   – Growth restriction may be found, but most of the effects of in utero alcohol exposure are not detectable by sonography (Garmel & D'Alton, 1993).

▶ Option to continue or terminate the pregnancy

- ▶ Neonatal evaluation by a dysmorphologist or geneticist for infants at risk for fetal alcohol syndrome
- ● Specific psychological issues
  - ▶ General supportive counseling (see Components of Genetic Counseling above)
  - ▶ Referral to local alcohol treatment programs
  - ▶ Impact of addiction
    - – Guilt feelings can interfere with the patient's ability to seek prenatal care and treatment programs.
    - – Many women with alcohol problems use other substances as well, which may increase the risks to the fetus (Levy & Koren, 1990).
  - ▶ Strategies for coping with uncertainty about fetal prognosis

Cocaine

- ● Offer genetic counseling
- ● Risks
  - ▶ Physicians *and* patients perceive cocaine to be a potent teratogen and significantly over-estimate the magnitude of the risk for birth defects in exposed pregnancies. The specific magnitude of the risk for birth defects following in utero cocaine exposure is not well delineated, but it is not as high as with chronic alcohol exposure. (Koren, Gladstone, Robeson, & Robieux, 1992).
    - – Established risks of cocaine use in pregnancy include fetal intracranial hemorrhage, cerebral infarction, genitourinary anomalies, intrauterine growth restriction, premature delivery, and placental problems (Plessinger & Woods, 1993; Volpe, 1992).
    - – Some studies have suggested a risk for limb reductions and congenital heart defects (Plessinger & Woods, 1993).
    - – There may also be a risk of fetal cocaine syndrome, characterized by developmental delay and dysmorphic features such as a midline lip pit, diagonally split eyebrows, and periorbital edema (Fries et al., 1993).
  - ▶ Studies assessing the neurobehavioral effects have been contradictory (Volpe, 1992).
  - ▶ See Section 1, *Preconception Health Care—An Overview*, and Chapter 6.3, *Substance Abuse,* for additional information.
- ● Evaluation and options
  - ▶ Detailed ultrasound
    - – Sonography may detect growth restriction, placental abnormalities, and some fetal malformations such as limb reductions or renal agenesis/dysplasia, but most of the effects of in utero cocaine exposure are not detectable by ultrasound (Garmel & D'Alton, 1993).
  - ▶ Option to continue or terminate the pregnancy

- ▶ Neonatal evaluation by a dysmorphologist or geneticist for infants suspected to have fetal cocaine syndrome
- Specific psychological issues
  - ▶ General supportive counseling (See Components of Genetic Counseling above)
  - ▶ Referral to local substance abuse treatment programs
  - ▶ Impact of addiction
    - – Guilt feelings can interfere with the patient's ability to seek prenatal care and treatment programs.
    - – Polydrug or concurrent alcohol use is common in women who use cocaine, which may increase the risks to the fetus (Levy & Koren, 1990).
  - ▶ Strategies for coping with uncertainty about fetal prognosis

Retinoids

Drugs in this class are most commonly used in the treatment of skin disorders.

- Offer genetic counseling
- Risks
  - ▶ Isotretinoin
    - – Exposure in the first trimester has been associated with a risk as high as 20 percent for mental retardation and a specific pattern of birth defects, including microcephaly, hydrocephalus, retinal abnormalities, microtia, clefting, thymus abnormalities, and conotruncal congenital heart defects (Lammer et al., 1985).
    - – Advise clients to cease using isotretinoin at least one month before attempting pregnancy (Oakley & Erickson, 1995; Teratology Society, 1987).
  - ▶ Vitamin A supplements, either in the form of retinol (a true retinoid) or as beta carotene (a retinol precursor)
    - – Some studies suggest an increased risk for birth defects with consumption of over 10,0000 IU of vitamin A supplements in the form of retinol (Rothman et al., 1995). However, it is not clear if large doses of retinol are truly teratogenic, and if they are, at what level of exposure they become so (Mitchell, 1992).

      NOTE: The U.S. RDA for retinol is 800 µg, equivalent to approximately 2,700 IU.

    - – Large doses of beta carotene have not been associated with teratogenic effects (Teratology Society, 1987).

      NOTE: The average American diet generally provides adequate amounts of vitamin A, so supplementation during pregnancy may not be necessary and should not exceed 5,000 IU if it is used (American College of Obstetricians and Gynecologists [ACOG] Committee on Obstetric Practice, 1995).

  - ▶ See Section 1, *Preconception Health Care—An Overview,* for additional information.

- Evaluation and options
  - ▶ Detailed ultrasound
    - – Many of the features of retinoic acid embryopathy can potentially be detected by sonography.
  - ▶ Option to continue or terminate the pregnancy
  - ▶ Neonatal evaluation by a dysmorphologist or geneticist for infants suspected to have retinoic acid embryopathy
- Specific psychological issues
  - ▶ General supportive counseling (see Components of Genetic Counseling above)
  - ▶ Strategies for coping with uncertainty about fetal prognosis

Rubella

Although immunization programs have decreased the overall rate of rubella infection, 5 to 20 percent of women of reproductive age living in developed countries are still seronegative (CDC, 1990; Cooper, Preblud, & Alford, 1995). Recent clusters of congenital rubella syndrome in Los Angeles and among the Amish in Pennsylvania demonstrate that rubella infection remains an obstetric concern (CDC, 1991a; CDC, 1992).

- Offer genetic counseling
- Risks
  - ▶ Rubella vaccination
    - – Vaccination is not recommended during pregnancy. Advise women to avoid becoming pregnant for a 3-month period after inoculation because the vaccine uses a live, attenuated form (CDC, 1990).
    - – However, reassure women who have been inadvertently vaccinated that there have been no reported cases of congenital rubella syndrome with vaccination immediately prior to conception or during the critical first trimester of pregnancy (CDC, 1989).
  - ▶ Rubella infection
    - – Maternal rubella infection is associated with significant risks for miscarriage, stillbirth, and congenital rubella syndrome (Cooper et al., 1995). The classic features of congenital rubella syndrome are congenital cataracts, heart defects (patent ductus arteriosus or pulmonic stenosis), and deafness. The condition can also be associated with mental retardation, microcephaly, growth delay, long bone radiolucency, glaucoma, and pigmentary retinopathy along with later onset problems such as diabetes mellitus, hypothyroidism, and hypertension (Cooper et al., 1995; Givens, Lee, Jones, & Ilstrup, 1993; Peckham, 1985).

      NOTE: It is difficult to accurately assess the magnitude of the risk for congenital rubella syndrome after maternal infection because many of the features of the condition are not apparent at birth.

* The period of greatest risk for classic congenital rubella syndrome is with maternal infection in the first trimester. Estimates vary widely, but the risk may be as high as 60 to 70 percent at this time in pregnancy (Cooper et al., 1995; Miller, Crodock-Watson, & Pollock, 1982; Peckham, 1985).

* Maternal infection in the second trimester still poses a risk to the fetus in the range of 10 to 25 percent, with some affected infants presenting with isolated hearing loss or developmental delay (Cooper et al., 1995; Miller et al., 1982; Peckham, 1985).

* Maternal infection after 20 weeks of pregnancy does not appear to be associated with a significant risk for congenital rubella syndrome, but growth restriction has been reported with maternal rubella infection in the third trimester (Miller et al., 1982).

   – Referral to a genetic counselor may be helpful for women with documented rubella infection in the first or second trimester of pregnancy.

▶ See Chapter 10.8, *Rubella,* for detailed information about the evaluation and management of women who report exposure to rubella or have rubella infection during pregnancy.

● Evaluation and options

   ▶ Option to terminate or continue the pregnancy

   ▶ Prenatal diagnosis

      – Prenatal diagnosis is not readily available (Cooper et al., 1995).

      * Other than growth restriction, the primary defects associated with fetal rubella infection are not detectable with ultrasound.

      * Amniocentesis and fetal umbilical blood sampling for measurement of specific immunoglobulin M or for viral culture have been tried on a research basis (Hwa et al., 1994; Skvorc-Ranko et al., 1991). Interpretation of these tests is problematic because of the potential for false negative results and because such testing provides indirect information (i.e., about fetal infection) rather than direct information about fetal abnormalities.

   ▶ Obstetrics or perinatology consultation

   ▶ Pediatric infectious disease consultation

      – Couples who elect to continue the pregnancy may benefit from having the opportunity to psychologically prepare for the evaluation and management of the infant at risk for congenital rubella syndrome.

   ▶ Neonatal evaluation by a dysmorphologist or geneticist for infants suspected to have congenital rubella syndrome

● Specific psychological issues

   ▶ General supportive counseling (see Components of Genetic Counseling above)

   ▶ Strategies for coping with uncertainty about fetal prognosis

Varicella

The potential impact of the newly available varicella vaccine on infection rates in pregnant women is unknown. Prior to introduction of the vaccine, less that 10 percent of women of reproductive age were seronegative for varicella (CDC, 1996), and approximately 1 per 2,000 women in the U.S. contracted varicella during pregnancy (Gilbert, 1993).

- Risks

  ▶ Varicella vaccination

  - Vaccination during pregnancy is not recommended. Advise women to avoid pregnancy for one month after each dose of vaccine (CDC, 1996).

  - Encourage women who have been inadvertently vaccinated immediately prior to conception or early in pregnancy to contact the CDC Registry at 1-800-986-8999. The risk of fetal varicella syndrome is expected to be low following periconceptional vaccination, but the vaccine has not been in use for a sufficient period of time for adequate assessment of in utero exposure (CDC, 1996; White, 1997).

  ▶ Varicella infection

  - Recent studies suggest the risk for fetal varicella syndrome is 1 to 2 percent in infants whose mothers are infected during the critical period of exposure between 8 and 20 weeks after the last menstrual period (CDC, 1996; Jones, Johnson, & Chambers, 1994; Pastuszak et al., 1994). Features of fetal varicella syndrome may include neurologic abnormalities (hydrocephalus, microcephaly, developmental delay), eye anomalies (cataracts, microphthalmia, chorioretinitis), limb hypoplasia due to cicatricial lesions, and growth retardation (Gilbert, 1993).

  - Reassure clients that there is a risk for fetal varicella syndrome only when the mother has a varicella infection, not simply because she has been exposed to someone with varicella.

  - Maternal varicella near delivery *is* associated with a risk for neonatal varicella infection.

  - Referral to a genetic counselor may be helpful for women with documented varicella infection in the first or second trimester of pregnancy.

  ▶ For further details about varicella in pregnancy, see Chapter 10.11, *Varicella Zoster Virus*.

- Evaluation and options

  ▶ Detailed ultrasound

  - Although hydrocephalus, microcephaly, growth restriction, or limb hypoplasia may be detected, other features of fetal varicella syndrome are not detectable by sonography.

  ▶ Option to terminate or continue the pregnancy

  - Some patients will elect to terminate a pregnancy with a 1 to 2 percent risk for fetal varicella syndrome (Pastuszak et al., 1994).

  ▶ Obstetrics or perinatology consultation

▶ Pediatric infectious disease consultation

▶ Neonatal evaluation by a dysmorphologist or geneticist for infants suspected to have congenital varicella syndrome

● Specific psychological issues

▶ General supportive counseling (see Components of Genetic Counseling above)

▶ Strategies for coping with uncertainty about fetal prognosis

Ultrasound Abnormalities

● The use of ultrasound for routine prenatal screening remains controversial.

▶ Some studies demonstrate benefits such as decreased perinatal mortality while others have not found improved perinatal outcomes (Chitty, 1995; Garmel & D'Alton, 1993). Differences between studies in rates of detection and rates of abortion for fetal abnormalities may in part account for this discrepancy (Chitty, 1995).

▶ In spite of the controversy, ultrasound evaluation during pregnancy is common, with fetal abnormalities found in up to 1 percent of routine scans (Saari-Kemppainen, Karjalainen, Ylostalo, & Heinonen, 1990).

● The timing for prenatal sonography has also generated some debate.

▶ Early ultrasound allows improved accuracy of pregnancy dating.

– Accurate dating is crucial for correct interpretation of triple marker screening (Wald, Cuckle, Densem, Kennard, & Smith, 1992).

▶ Ultrasound in the latter part of the second trimester (approximately 18 to 22 weeks after the last menstrual period) permits more thorough anatomic visualization of the fetus (Constantine & McCormack, 1991).

– Detection rates for fetal abnormalities are higher in *targeted scans,* performed in pregnancies known to be at increased risk of specific abnormalities, than in routine scans (Chitty, 1995; Garmel & D'Alton, 1993).

– When fetal abnormalities are detected in the second trimester, couples usually have time to consider options, such as amniocentesis and termination of pregnancy, although the timing of legal abortion varies from state to state.

▶ When determining the appropriate timing for ultrasound, balance the individual client's concerns against pregnancy management needs.

● The expectations of clients who undergo prenatal sonography vary.

▶ Some clients are not aware that many birth defects cannot be detected by ultrasound. They assume that a normal scan provides a guarantee for a normal pregnancy outcome.

▶ Most clients do not consider in advance the possibility that an abnormality might be discovered via ultrasound, so the detection of a fetal abnormality is experienced as an unanticipated crisis.

- Many couples find it difficult to make decisions in such a complicated and emotionally charged situation, especially because of the limited time window in which prenatal diagnosis and abortion are available.

- Genetics consultation can be helpful in the decision-making process after ultrasound detection of a fetal abnormality.

  NOTE: It can be particularly challenging for patients to understand the difference between structural abnormalities, such as spina bifida, and abnormalities that are most often normal variants, such as choroid plexus cysts or hyperechogenic bowel. These variants may be associated with an increased risk for disorders in the fetus but are usually associated with a normal outcome. When a true structural abnormality is identified in the fetus, follow-up testing frequently reveals additional abnormalities which impact pregnancy management and recurrence risks for future pregnancies (Julian-Reynier et al., 1994; Weston, 1993).

It is beyond the scope of this chapter to review fetal abnormalities detected by ultrasound in detail. The most frequently encountered anomalies are discussed below. General counseling guidelines are provided above in Counseling After Diagnosis of a Fetal Abnormality in this chapter. For information about the use of ultrasound, see Chapter 3.4, *Ultrasound.* Texts providing more detailed information about prenatal ultrasound and fetal anomalies are listed in General Resources.

Choroid Plexus Cysts

- Offer genetic counseling

- Risks

  ▶ In most pregnancies a fetal choroid plexus cyst represents a normal variant.

  ▶ Choroid plexus cysts have been reported in 1 to 2 percent of second-trimester fetal ultrasounds (Garmel & D'Alton, 1993).

  ▶ Several studies have found an increased risk for chromosome abnormalities

    - Estimates of the risk range from 0.5 percent to as high as 9.5 percent, with trisomy 18 specifically over-represented (Nadel, Bromley, Frigoletto, Estroff, & Benacerraf, 1992; Porto, Murata, Warneke, & Keegan, 1993).

    - Small sample sizes in the studies and variability in the background incidence of choroid plexus cysts between the studies make the actual magnitude of the risk unclear, but it has been estimated to be approximately 1 percent when choroid plexus cysts are an isolated finding (Achiron, Barkai, Katznelson, & Masahiach, 1991; Garmel & D'Alton, 1993).

  ▶ Choroid plexus cysts have not been associated with an increased risk for mental retardation or birth defects in the absence of chromosome abnormalities (Achiron et al., 1991).

- Evaluation and options

  ▶ Detailed ultrasound

- In fetuses with trisomy 18, other anomalies are usually seen on ultrasound (Gabrielli et al., 1989; Nadel et al. 1992), although the cysts are the only anomaly detected in some cases (Perpignano et al., 1992).

- Cysts usually disappear by 28 weeks of pregnancy regardless of the karyotype of the fetus, so serial ultrasound does not provide additional information (Nadel et al., 1992).

▶ Amniocentesis for fetal karyotype

- There is debate about whether or not to offer amniocentesis when choroid plexus cysts are an isolated finding (Nadel et al., 1992; Perpignano et al., 1992).

- If fetal karyotype is normal, the risk for adverse fetal outcome is not increased (Achiron et at., 1991).

● Specific psychological issues

▶ General supportive counseling (see Components of Genetic Counseling and Genetic Counseling after Diagnosis of a Fetal Abnormality above)

▶ Methods of coping during waiting period for prenatal diagnosis results or birth of baby if testing is declined

● Implications for future pregnancies

▶ No known specific risk if fetal chromosomes are normal

Hyperechogenic Bowel

● Offer genetic counseling

● Risks

▶ Hyperechogenic bowel has been reported in approximately 1 percent of fetal ultrasounds (Bromley et al., 1994; Hill, Fries, Hecker, & Grzybek, 1994).

▶ Hyperechogenic bowel in the fetus has been associated with problems such as chromosome abnormalities, cystic fibrosis, intrauterine infection, and gastrointestinal malformations (Bahado-Singh, Morotti, Copel, & Mahoney, 1994).

▶ Quantifying the risk for fetal abnormalities is quite difficult, because estimates vary widely among studies, and investigators have not been consistent in the system used to rate the severity of the echogenicity (Bahado-Singh et al., 1994; Slotnick & Abuhamad, 1996).

- Risks are highest when

* The bowel is severely echogenic (usually defined as being as echogenic as bone)

* Other abnormalities such as intrauterine growth restriction are present

- Normal outcomes have been reported in 20 to 60 percent of pregnancies with severe hyperechogenic bowel and in approximately 80 percent of milder cases (Bromley et al., 1994; Hill et al., 1994; Muller et al., 1995; Nyberg et al., 1993).

▶ There may be some risk for adverse pregnancy outcomes such as intrauterine growth restriction, fetal demise, or premature delivery with severe echogenic bowel (Bahado-Singh et al., 1994; Bromley et al., 1994; Muller et al., 1995; Nyberg et al., 1993).

- Evaluation and options

  ▶ Detailed ultrasound to rule out other abnormalities and to determine the severity of echogenicity in the bowel

  ▶ Amniocentesis for fetal karyotype

  ▶ Screening for cystic fibrosis mutations

    – There are two testing options: carrier screening for the couple or fetal testing through amniocentesis.

      * Normal results reduce the probability but do not eliminate the possibility that the fetus has cystic fibrosis.

      * The utility is limited in some populations, such as Asians, in which cystic fibrosis is rare (NIH, 1990).

  ▶ Testing for intrauterine infection (see the chapters in Section 10, *Infectious Diseases.*)

  ▶ Obstetrics or perinatology consultation, especially with severe hyperchogenic bowel

- Specific psychological issues

  ▶ General supportive counseling (see Components of Genetic Counseling and Genetic Counseling after Diagnosis of a Fetal Abnormality above)

  ▶ Methods of coping during waiting period for prenatal diagnosis results or birth of baby if testing is declined

  ▶ Strategies for dealing with uncertainty about fetal prognosis

- Implications for future pregnancies

  ▶ Recurrence risks and testing options depend on the evaluation results

Nuchal Cystic Hygroma

A cystic hygroma is a collection of lymphatic fluid, most often found at the posterior and lateral neck of the fetus.

- Offer genetic counseling

- Risks

  ▶ Fetal cystic hygroma is detected in approximately 1 per 600 routine prenatal ultrasounds (Edwards & Graham, 1990).

    – Chromosome abnormalities are diagnosed in 60 to 80 percent of fetuses with nuchal cystic hygroma. Turner syndrome (45,X) is most often seen in cases diagnosed in the second trimester and Down syndrome in cases presenting in the first trimester (Edwards & Graham, 1990; Johnson et al., 1993).

    – Genetic disorders such as Noonan syndrome or multiple pterygium syndrome may also be associated with nuchal cystic hygroma in the fetus.

▶ The prognosis for cases of cystic hygroma detected in the second trimester is poor regardless of the fetal karyotype, with the majority developing hydrops fetalis (Edwards & Graham, 1990).

    – Outcomes may be better for fetuses diagnosed with nuchal cystic hygroma in the first trimester; in one series, only 11 percent of the chromosomally normal pregnancies miscarried (Trauffer et al., 1994).

● Evaluation and options

  ▶ Detailed ultrasound to examine the fetus for other anomalies

    – Repeat ultrasound if pregnancy is continued

    – Fetal echocardiography

  ▶ Chorionic villus sampling or amniocentesis to test for fetal chromosome abnormalities

  ▶ Genetics evaluation of the parents in some cases when the fetal karyotype is normal

  ▶ Obstetrics or perinatology consultation

  ▶ Option to continue or terminate the pregnancy

● Specific psychological issues

  ▶ General supportive counseling (see Components of Genetic Counseling and Genetic Counseling after Diagnosis of a Fetal Abnormality above)

  ▶ Methods of coping during waiting period for prenatal diagnosis results or birth of baby if testing is declined

  ▶ Strategies for dealing with uncertainty about fetal prognosis

  ▶ Grief over loss of idealized normal fetus

● Implications for future pregnancies

  ▶ Recurrence risks and testing options depend on evaluation results

Neural Tube Defects

The neural tube closes at 4 weeks gestation, and defective closure can result in anencephaly (absence of cerebral hemispheres and cranial vault), encephalocele (bony defect in the cranium with herniation of brain), or spina bifida (exposure of spinal neural tissue).

● Offer genetic counseling

● Risks

  ▶ Nationwide, neural tube defects are seen in approximately 1 per 1,000 births, but rates vary geographically with higher rates in the east and lower rates in the west (Shaw, Jensvold, Wasserman, & Lammer, 1994; Yen et al., 1992).

  ▶ Known risk factors include maternal use of the anticonvulsants valproic acid and carbamazepine, a family history of neural tube defects, and maternal *diabetes mellitus* (Lindhout et al., 1992; Main & Mennuti, 1986).

- – Periconceptional supplementation with folic acid has been found to reduce the incidence of neural tube defects (Czeizel & Dudas, 1992).

- – When a neural tube defect occurs, however, it is usually in the absence of any known risk factor (Main & Mennuti, 1986).

▶ In over 80 percent of cases of spina bifida or anencephaly, the neural tube defect is an isolated anomaly.

- – However, 10 to 15 percent of affected fetuses are found to have chromosome abnormalities (Harmon, Hiett, Palmer, & Golichowski, 1995; Luthy et al., 1991; Shaw et al., 1994).

- – Neural tube defects, especially encephaloceles, can be seen in association with genetic syndromes, such as Meckel syndrome (encephalocele, polycystic kidneys, facial clefting, and polydactyly).

• Evaluation and options

▶ Detailed ultrasound to examine the fetus for other anomalies

- – Serial ultrasounds are indicated when a client continues a pregnancy in which the fetus has spina bifida, because of the risk for hydrocephalus (Budorick, Pretorius, & Nelson, 1995).

▶ Amniocentesis to rule out fetal chromosome abnormalities

▶ Option to continue or terminate the pregnancy

▶ Obstetrics or perinatology consultation

- – Cesarean section prior to the onset of labor has been found to improve motor function in infants prenatally diagnosed with spina bifida (Luthy et al., 1991).

▶ Pediatric surgery consultation

- – Couples who elect to continue the pregnancy may benefit from having the opportunity to psychologically prepare for surgery in the neonatal period.

- – A tour of the newborn intensive care unit may also be helpful.

• Specific psychological issues

▶ General supportive counseling (see Components of Genetic Counseling and Genetic Counseling after Diagnosis of a Fetal Abnormality above)

▶ Methods of coping during waiting period for prenatal diagnosis results or birth of baby if testing is declined

▶ Strategies for dealing with uncertainty about fetal prognosis

▶ Grief over loss of idealized normal fetus

• Implications for future pregnancies

▶ Recurrence risks

- – Recurrence risk is 2 to 3 percent when the neural tube defect is determined to be an isolated anomaly (Main & Mennuti, 1986).

- Risks may be higher if the fetus is diagnosed with a syndrome (e.g., Meckel syndrome).

▶ Folate supplementation

- Women who have had a fetus or child with a neural tube defect are advised of the CDC (1991b) recommendation to take 4 mg folic acid daily from one month preconceptionally through the first 3 months of pregnancy to help reduce the chance for recurrence.

▶ Testing options, including maternal serum alpha-fetoprotein screening, ultrasound, and amniocentesis

Abdominal Wall Defects

There are two distinct types of abdominal wall defects, gastroschisis and omphalocele (Torfs, Curry, & Roeper, 1990). Omphalocele is characterized by a protrusion of intestines and sometimes other organs such as liver or bowel through a membrane-covered opening at the umbilicus. Gastroschisis is characterized by right-sided protrusion of the intestines without a membranous covering and is usually smaller in size than an omphalocele.

- Offer genetic counseling

- Risks

  ▶ Because of inconsistencies in classification of cases in the past, estimates of the incidence of gastroschisis and omphalocele have varied widely. Recent studies suggest abdominal wall defects occur in approximately 1 in 4,000 births (Calzolari et al., 1993; Torfs et al., 1990).

  ▶ Omphalocele

   - Other fetal anomalies, such as heart defects, neural tube defects, or genitourinary tract anomalies, are found in 30 to 75 percent of infants with omphalocele (Calzolari et al., 1993; Torfs et al., 1990).

   - Syndromes such as trisomy 13, trisomy 18, or Beckwith-Wiedemann syndrome may be associated with omphalocele (Calzolari et al., 1993; Torfs et al., 1990).

  ▶ Gastroschisis

   - Gastroschisis is most often an isolated defect, but it can be seen with other anomalies in up to 20 percent of cases (Torfs et al., 1990).

   - The rate of gastroschisis is increased in the offspring of young, socially disadvantaged women with a history of substance abuse (Torfs, Velie, Oechsli, Bateson, & Curry, 1994).

- Evaluation and options

  ▶ Detailed ultrasound to confirm the type of abdominal wall defect and to examine the fetus for other abnormalities

   - Serial ultrasounds may be offered when pregnancies are continued because of the risk for complications such as intrauterine growth restriction (Calzolari et al., 1993).

   - Fetal echocardiography may help in the assessment of syndromic causes of omphalocele.

▶ Amniocentesis to test for fetal chromosome abnormalities, particularly with omphalocele

▶ Option to continue or terminate the pregnancy

▶ Perinatology consultation

    – There is conflicting evidence about the benefits of cesarean section (Novotny, Klein, & Boeckman, 1993; Sakala, Erhard, & White, 1993).

▶ Pediatric surgery consultation

    – Couples who elect to continue the pregnancy may benefit from having the opportunity to psychologically prepare for treatment and surgery in the neonatal period.

    – A tour of the newborn intensive care unit may also be helpful.

● Specific psychological issues

▶ General supportive counseling (see Components of Genetic Counseling and Genetic Counseling after Diagnosis of a Fetal Abnormality above)

▶ Methods of coping during waiting period for prenatal diagnosis results or birth of baby if testing is declined

▶ Strategies for dealing with uncertainty about fetal prognosis

▶ Grief over loss of idealized normal fetus

● Implications for future pregnancies

▶ Recurrence risks are dependent on the specific diagnosis

▶ Testing options, including maternal serum alpha-fetoprotein screening, ultrasound, and amniocentesis

Table 2.1

Established Teratogens

Medications/Drugs

Alcohol
Aminoglycosides
Angiotensin-converting enzyme inhibitors
Anticonvulsants
Antithyroid agents
Cocaine
Coumarin derivatives
Folic acid antagonists
Hormonal agents
Lithium salts
Penicillamine
Purine/pyrimidine analogs
Retinoids/arotinoids
Tetracyclines
Thalidomide

Environmental Agents

Lead/lead salts
Organic mercurials
Organic solvents
Polychlorinated biphenyls
Radiation (high doses)

Maternal Conditions

Cytomegalovirus
Diabetes mellitus
Phenylketonuria
Rubella
Seizure disorder
Toxoplasmosis
Varicella

Source: Juchau, M. R. (1993). Chemical teratogenesis. *Progress in Drug Research, 41*, 9-50. Adapted with permission.

Appendix 2.1a

General Book Resources

General

Harper, P. S. (1993). *Practical genetic counselling* (4th ed.). Oxford, England: Butterworth-Heinemann.

King, R. A., Rotter, J. L., & Motulsky, A. G. (Eds.). (1992). *The genetic basis of common diseases.* New York: Oxford University Press.

Robinson, A., & Linden, M. G. (1993). *Clinical genetics handbook* (2nd ed.). Boston: Blackwell Scientific Publications.

Stevenson, R. E., Hall, J. G., & Goodman, R. M. (1993). *Human malformations and related anomalies.* New York: Oxford University Press.

Thompson, M. W., McInnes, R. R., & Willard, H. F. (1991). *Thompson & Thompson: Genetics in medicine* (5th ed.). Philadelphia: W.B. Saunders.

Genetic Syndromes

Jones, K. L. (1997). *Smith's recognizable patterns of human malformation* (5th ed.). Philadelphia: W. B.. Saunders.

McKusick, V. A. (1994). *Mendelian inheritance in man* (11th ed.). Baltimore: The Johns Hopkins University Press.

Prenatal Diagnosis

Callen, P. W. (Ed.). (1994) *Ultrasonography in obstetrics and gynecology* (3rd ed.). Philadelphia: W. B.. Saunders.

Filkins, K., & Russo, J. F. (Eds.). (1990). *Human prenatal diagnosis* (2nd ed.). New York: Marcel Dekker.

Harrison, M. R., Golbus, M. S., & Filly, R. A. (Eds.). (1991). *The unborn patient: Prenatal diagnosis and treatment.* Philadelphia: W. B. Saunders.

Hegge, F. N. (1992). *A practical guide to ultrasound of fetal anomalies.* New York: Raven Press.

Milunsky, A. (Ed.). (1992). *Genetic disorders and the fetus: Diagnosis, prevention, and treatment* (3rd ed.). Baltimore: The Johns Hopkins University Press.

Simpson, J. L., & Golbus, M. S. (1992). *Genetics in obstetrics & gynecology* (2nd ed.). Philadelphia: W. B. Saunders.

Appendix 2.1b

Counseling Resources

Newsletters

A Heartbreaking Choice (after genetic termination)
(517)224-1881

Support Groups

To locate a support group for a specific disorder, contact

Alliance of Genetic Support Groups
1-(800)336-GENE (800/336-4363)

National Organization for Rare Disorders
(203)746-6518

Professional Societies in Genetics

To locate genetics services in the local area, contact

American Society of Human Genetics
(301)571-1825

International Society of Nurses in Genetics
(703)876-3896

National Society of Genetic Counselors
(610)872-7608

Appendix 2.1c

Resources For Assessing Teratogens

<u>Texts</u>

Briggs, E.G., Freeman, R.K., & Yaffe, S.J. (1994). *Drugs in pregnancy and lactation: A reference guide to fetal and neonatal risks* (4th ed.). Baltimore: Williams & Wilkins.

Friedman, J.M., & Polifka, J.E. (1994). *Teratogenic effects of drugs: A resource for clinicians (TERIS).* Baltimore: The Johns Hopkins University Press.

Paul, M. (1992). *Occupational and environmental reproductive hazards: A guide for clinicians.* Baltimore: Williams & Wilkins.

Schardein, J.L. (1993). *Chemical induced birth defects* (2nd ed.). New York: Marcel Dekker.

Scialli, A.R., Lione, A., & Padgett, G.K.B. (1995). *Reproductive effects of chemical, physical, and biologic agents (REPROTOX®).* Baltimore: The Johns Hopkins University Press.

Shepard, T.H. (1995). *Catalog of teratogenic agents* (8th ed.). Baltimore: The Johns Hopkins University Press.

<u>Hotline Services</u>

Hotlines are operated in several states but each hotline provides services to clients in a specified geographic region only. To locate the nearest service, call:

East of the Mississippi
      Massachusetts Teratogen Information
      Service, National Birth Defects Center
      (781)466-8474

West of the Mississippi
      Utah Pregnancy RiskLine
      (801) 328-2229

<u>On-line Services</u>

REPROTOX® (Reproductive reviews of
chemicals, drugs, physical agents,
and nutritional status)
(202) 293-5137

TERIS (Teratogen Information System)
(206) 543-2465

References

Achiron, R., Barkai, G., Katznelson, B-M., & Masahiach, S. (1991). Fetal lateral ventricle choroid plexus cysts: The dilemma of amniocentesis. *Obstetrics and Gynecology, 78,* 815–818.

Ad Hoc Committee on Genetic Counseling.(1975). Genetic counseling. *American Journal of Human Genetics, 27,* 240–242.

American Academy of Pediatrics Committee on Genetics. (1994). Prenatal genetic diagnosis for pediatricians. *Pediatrics, 93,* 1010–1015.

American College of Obstetricians and Gynecologists (ACOG) Committee on Obstetric Practice. (1995). *Vitamin A supplementation during pregnancy.* Technical Bulletin No. 157. Washington, DC: ACOG.

Bahado-Singh, R., Morotti, R., Copel, J.A., & Mahoney, M.J. (1994). Hyperechoic fetal bowel: The perinatal consequences. *Prenatal Diagnosis, 14,* 981–987.

Bennett, R.L., Steinhaus, K.A., Uhrich, S.B., O'Sullivan, C.K., Resta, R.G., Lochner-Doyle, D., Markel, D.S., Vincent, V., & Hamanishi, J. (1995). Recommendations for standardized human pedigree nomenclature. *American Journal of Human Genetics, 56,* 745–752.

Bromley, B., Doubilet, P., Frigoletto, F.D., Jr., Krauss, C., Estroff, J.A., & Benacerraf, B.R. (1994). Is fetal hyperechoic bowel on second-trimester sonogram an indication for amniocentesis? *Obstetrics and Gynecology, 83,* 647–651.

Budorick, N.E., Pretorius, D.H., & Nelson, T.R. (1995). Sonography of the fetal spine: Technique, imaging findings, and clinical implications. *American Journal of Radiology, 164,* 421–428.

Buehler, B.A., Delimont, D., van Waes, M., & Finnel, R.H. (1990). Prenatal prediction of risk of the fetal hydantoin syndrome. *New England Journal of Medicine, 322,* 1567–1572.

Calzolari, E., Volpato, S., Bianchi, F., Cianciulli, D., Tenconi, R., Clementi, M., Calabro, A., Lungarotti, S., Mastroiacovo, P.P., Botto, L., Spagnolo, A., & Milan, M. (1993). Omphalocele and gastroschisis: A collaborative study of five Italian congenital malformation registries. *Teratology, 47,* 47–55.

Cefalo, R.C., & Moos, M.K. (1995). *Preconceptional health care: A practical guide* (2nd ed.). St. Louis, MO: Mosby-Year Book.

Centers for Disease Control and Prevention (CDC). (1989). Rubella vaccination during pregnancy—United States, 1971–1988. *Morbidity and Mortality Weekly Report, 38,* 289–292.

Centers for Disease Control and Prevention (CDC). (1990). Rubella prevention. Recommendations of the Immunization Practices Advisory Committee (ACIP). *Morbidity and Mortality Weekly Report, 39(RR–15),* 1–18.

Centers for Disease Control and Prevention (CDC). (1991a). Increase in rubella and congenital rubella syndrome—United States, 1988–1990. *Morbidity and Mortality Weekly Report, 40,* 93–99.

Centers for Disease Control and Prevention (CDC). (1991b). Use of folic acid for prevention of spina bifida and other neural tube defects, 1983–1991. *Morbidity and Mortality Weekly Report, 40,* 513–516.

Centers for Disease Control and Prevention (CDC). (1992). Congenital rubella syndrome among the Amish - Pennsylvania, 1991–1992. *Morbidity and Mortality Weekly Report, 41,* 468–469, 475–476.

Centers for Disease Control and Prevention (CDC). (1994). Chorionic villus sampling and amniocentesis: Recommendations for prenatal counseling. *Morbidity and Mortality Weekly Report, 44*(RR–9), 1–12.

Centers for Disease Control and Prevention (CDC). (1996). Prevention of varicella: Recommendations of the Advisory Committee on Immunization Practices (ACIP). *Morbidity and Mortality Weekly Report, 45 (*RR–11), 1–36.

Chapple, A., May, C., & Campion, P. (1995). Lay understanding of genetic diseases: A British study of families attending a genetic counseling service. *Journal of Genetic Counseling, 4,* 281–300.

Chitty, L.S. (1995). Ultrasound screening for fetal abnormalities. *Prenatal Diagnosis, 15,* 1241–1257.

Coles, C.D. (1993). Impact of prenatal alcohol exposure on the newborn and the child. *Clinical Obstetrics and Gynecology, 36,* 255–266.

Conover, E. (1994). Hazardous exposures during pregnancy. *The Journal of Obstetric, Gynecologic, and Neonatal Nursing, 23,* 524–532.

Constantine, G., & McCormack, J. (1991). Comparative audit of booking and mid-trimester ultrasound scans in the prenatal diagnos of congenital anomalies. *Prenatal Diagnosis, 11,* 905–914.

Cooper, L.Z., Preblud, S.R., & Alford, C.A. (1995). Rubella. In J.S. Remington & J.O. Klein (Eds.), *Infectious diseases of the fetus and newborn infant* (pp. 268–311). Philadelphia, PA: W.B. Saunders.

Curry, C.J. (1992). Pregnancy loss, stillbirth, and neonatal death: A guide for the pediatrician. *Pediatric Clinics of North America, 39,* 157–192.

Czeizel, A.E., & Dudas, I. (1992). Prevention of the first occurrence of neural-tube defects by periconceptional vitamin supplementation. *New England Journal of Medicine, 327,* 1832–1835.

D'Alton, M.E., & DeCherney, A.H. (1993). Prenatal diagnosis. *New England Journal of Medicine, 28,* 114–120.

D'Alton, M.E., Craigo, S., & Bianchi, D.W. (1994). Prenatal diagnosis. *Current Problems in Obstetrics, Gynecology and Fertility, 17,* 48–78.

D'Amico, R., Jacopini, G., Vivona, G., & Frontali, M. (1992). Reproductive choices in couples at risk for genetic disease: A qualitative and quantitative analysis. *Birth Defects: Original Article Series, 28,* 41–46.

Delgado-Escueta, A.V., & Janz, D. (1992). Consensus guidelines: Preconception counseling, management, and care of the pregnant woman with epilepsy. *Neurology, 42*(Suppl. 5), 149–160.

Edwards, M.J., & Graham, J.M., Jr. (1990). Posterior nuchal cystic hygroma. *Clinics in Perinatology, 17,* 611–640.

Elder, S.H., & Laurence, K.M. (1991). The impact of supportive intervention after second trimester termination of pregnancy for fetal abnormality. *Prenatal Diagnosis, 11,* 47–54.

Elias, S., Annas, G.J., & Simpson, J.L. (1991). Carrier screening for cystic fibrosis: Implications for obstetric and gynecologic practice. *American Journal of Obstetrics and Gynecology, 164,* 1077–1083.

Evers-Kiebooms, G., Denayer, L., Welkenhuysen, M., Cassiman, J.J., & Van den Berghe, H. (1994). A stigmatizing effect of the carrier status for cystic fibrosis? *Clinical Genetics, 46,* 336–343.

Feuchtbaum, L.B., Cunningham, G., Waller, D.K., Lustig, L.S., Tompkinson, D.G., & Hook, E.B. (1995). Fetal karyotyping for chromosome abnormalities after an unexplained elevated maternal serum alpha-fetoprotein sccreening. *Obstetrics and Gynecology, 86,* 248–254.

Fonda Allen, J.S., & Mulhauser, L.C. (1995). Genetic counseling after abnormal prenatal diagnosis: Facilitating coping in families who continue their pregnancies. *Journal of Genetic Counseling, 4,* 251–265.

Frets, P.G., Duivenvoorden, H.J., Verhage, F., & Niermeijer, M.F. (1992). The reproductive decision-making process after genetic counseling: Psychosocial aspects. *Birth Defects: Original Article Series, 28,* 21–28.

Friedman, J.M. (1981). Genetic disease in the offspring of older fathers. *Obstetrics and Gynecology, 57,* 745–749.

Friedman, J.M., Little, B.B., Brent, R.L., Cordero, J.F., Hanson, J.W., & Shepard, T.H. (1990). Potential human teratogenicity of frequently prescribed drugs. *Obstetrics and Gynecology, 75,* 594–599.

Fries, M.H., Kuller, J.A., Norton, M.E., Yankowitz, J., Kobori, J., Good, W.V., Ferriero, D., Cox, V., Donlin, S.S., & Golabi, M. (1993). Facial features of infants exposed prenatally to cocaine. *Teratology, 48,* 413–420.

Fryburg, J.S. (1993). Mosaicism in chorionic villus sampling. *Obstetrics and Gynecology Clinics of North America, 20,* 523–532.

Gabrielli, S., Reece, A., Pilo, G., Perolo, A., Rizzo, N., Bovicelli, L., & Hobbins, J.C. (1989). The clinical significance of prenatally diagnosed choroid plexus cysts. *American Journal of Obstetrics and Gynecology, 160,* 1207–1210.

Gardiner, R.M. (1990). Genes and epilepsy. *Journal of Medical Genetics, 27,* 537–544.

Garmel, S.H., & D'Alton, M.E. (1993). Fetal ultrasonography. *Western Journal of Medicine, 159,* 273–285.

Gilbert, G.L. (1993). Chickenpox during pregnancy. *British Medical Journal, 306,* 1079–1080.

Givens, K.T., Lee, D.A., Jones, T., & Ilstrup, D.M. (1993). Congenital rubella syndrome: Ophthalmic manifestations and associated systemic disorders. *British Journal of Ophthalmology, 77,* 358–363.

Gonen, R., Perez, R., David, M., Dar, H., Merksamer, R., & Sharf, M. (1992). The association between unexplained second-trimester maternal serum hCG elevation and pregnancy complications. *Obstetrics & Gynecology, 80,* 83–86.

Gunderson-Warner, S., Martinez, L.P., Martinez, I.P., Carey, J.C., Kochenour, N.K., & Emery, M.G. (1990). Critical review of articles regarding pregnancy exposures in popular magazines. *Teratology, 42,* 469–472.

Haddow, J.E., & Palomaki, G.E. (1993). Prenatal screening for Down syndrome. In J.L. Simpson & S. Elias (Eds.), *Essentials of prenatal diagnosis* (pp. 185–220). New York: Churchill Livingstone.

Haddow, J.E., Palomaki, G.E., Knight, G.J., Cunningham, G.C., Lustig, L.S., & Boyd, P.A. (1994). Reducing the need for amniocentesis in women 35 years of age or older with serum markers for screening. *New England Journal of Medicine, 330,* 1114–1118.

Harmon, J.P., Hiett, A.K., Palmer, C.G., & Golichowski, A.M. (1995). Prenatal ultrasound detection of isolated neural tube defects: Is cytogenetic evaluation warranted? *Obstetrics and Gynecology, 86,* 595–599.

Harper, P.S. (1993). *Practical genetic counseling* (4th ed.). Oxford, England: Butterworth-Heinemann.

Hassed, S.J., Miller, C.H., Pope, S.K., Murphy, P., Quirk, J.G., Jr., & Cunniff, C. (1993). Perinatal lethal conditions: The effect of diagnosis on decision making. *Obstetrics and Gynecology, 82,* 37–42.

Heimler, A. (1990). Group counseling for couples who have terminated a pregnancy following prenatal diagnosis. *Birth Defects: Original Article Series, 28,* 161–167.

Hill, L.M., Fries, J., Hecker, J., & Grzybek, P. (1994). Second-trimester echogenic small bowel: An increased risk for adverse perinatal outcome. *Prenatal Diagnosis, 14,* 845–850.

Hook, E.B. (1986). Paternal age and genetic outcome: Implications for genetic counseling. In I.H. Porter, N.H. Hatcher & A.M. Wiley (Eds.), *Perinatal genetics: Diagnosis and treatment* (pp. 243–274). New York: Academic Press.

Hwa, H-L., Shyu, M-K., Lee, C-N., Wu, C-C., Kao, C-L., & Hsieh, F-J. (1994). Prenatal diagnosis of congenital rubella infection from maternal rubella in Taiwan. *Obstetrics and Gynecology, 84,* 415–419.

Johnson, M.P., Johnson, A., Holzgreve, W., Isada, N.B., Wapner, R.J., Treadwell, M.C., Heeger, S., & Evans, M.I. (1993). First-trimester simple hygroma: Cause and outcome. *American Journal of Obstetrics and Gynecology, 168,* 156–161.

Jones, K.L., Johnson, K.A., & Chambers, C.D. (1994). Offspring of women infected with varicella during pregnancy: A prospective study. *Teratology, 49,* 29–32.

Jones, K.L., Lacro, R.V., Johnson, K.A., & Adams, J. (1989). Pattern of malformations in the children of women treated with carbamazepine during pregnancy. *New England Journal of Medicine, 320,* 1661–1666.

Juchau, M.R. (1993). Chemical teratogenesis. *Progress in Drug Research, 41,* 9–50.

Julian-Reynier, C., Macquart-Moulin, G., Philip, N., Scheiner, C., Potier, A., Gambarelli, D., & Ayme, S. (1994). Fetal abnormalities detected by sonography in low-risk pregnancies: Discrepancies between pre- and post-termination findings. *Fetal Diagnosis and Therapy, 9,* 310–320.

Kaback, M., Lim-Steele, J., Dabholkar, D., Brown, D., Levy, N., & Zeiger, K. (1993). Tay-Sachs disease-Carrier screening, prenatal diagnosis, and the molecular era: An international perspective, 1970 to 1993. *Journal of the American Medical Association, 270,* 2307–2315.

Kessler, S. (1979). The psychological foundations of genetic counseling. In S. Kessler (Ed.), *Genetic counseling: Psychological dimensions* (pp. 17–33). New York: Academic Press.

Kessler, S. (1992). Process issues in genetic counseling. *Birth Defects: Original Article Series, 28,* 1–10.

Koch, R., Levy, H. L., Matalon, R., Rouse, B., Hanley, W., & Azen, C. (1993). The North American collaborative study of maternal phenylketonuria. Status report 1993. *American Journal of Diseases in Children, 147,* 1224–1230.

Koch, S., Losche, G., Jager-Roman, E., Jakob, S., Rating, D., Deichl, A., & Helge, H. (1992). Major and minor birth malformations and antiepileptic drugs. *Neurology, 42*(Suppl. 5), 83–88.

Koren, G., Bologa, M., Long, D., Feldman, Y., & Shear, N.H. (1989). Perception of teratogenic risk by pregnant women exposed to drugs and chemicals during the first trimester. *American Journal of Obstetrics and Gynecology, 160,* 190–194.

Koren, G., Gladstone, D., Robeson, C., & Robieux, I. (1992). The perception of teratogenic risk of cocaine. *Teratology, 46,* 567–571.

Lammer, E.J., Chen, D.T., Hoar, R.M., Agnish, N.D., Benke, P.J., Braun, J.T., Curry, C.J., Fernhoff, P.M., Grix, A.W., Lott, I.T., Richard, J.M., & Sun, S.C. (1985). Retinoic acid embryopathy. *New England Journal of Medicine, 313,* 837–841.

Levy, M., & Koren, G. (1990). Obstetric and neonatal effects of drugs of abuse. *Emergency Medicine Clinics of North America, 8,* 633–652.

Lieppman, R.E., Williams, M.A., Cheng, E.Y., Resta, R., Zingheim, R., Hickok, D.E., & Luthy, D.A. (1993). An association between elevated levels of human chorionic gonadotropin in the midtrimester and adverse pregnancy outcome. *American Journal of Obstetrics and Gynecology, 168,* 1852–1857.

Lindhout, D., Omtzigt, J.G.C., & Cornel, M.C. (1992). Spectrum of neural-tube defects in 34 infants prenatally exposed to antiepileptic drugs. *Neurology, 42*(Suppl. 5), 111–118.

Lorey, F.W., Arnopp, J., & Cunningham, G.C. (1996). Distribution of hemoglobinopathy variants by ethnicity in a multiethnic state. *Genetic Epidemiology, 13,* 501–512.

Lorey, F., Cunningham, G., Shafer, F., Lubin, B., & Vichinsky, E. (1994). Universal screening for hemoglobinopathies using high-performance liquid chromatography: Clinical results of 2.2 million screens. *European Journal of Human Genetics, 2,* 262–271.

Ludowese, C.J., Marini, T., Laxova, R., & Pauli, R.M. (1993). Evaluation of the effectiveness of a teratogen information service: A survey of patient and professional satisfaction. *Teratology, 48,* 233–245.

Luthy, D.A., Wardinsky, T., Shurtleff, D.B., Hollenbach, K.A., Hickok, D.E., Nyberg, D.A., & Benedetti, T.J. (1991). Cesarean section before the onset of labor and subsequent motor function in infants with meningomyelocele diagnosed antenatally. *New England Journal of Medicine, 324,* 662–666.

Lynch, H.T., Lemon, S.J., Durham, C., Tinley, S.T., Connolly, C., Lynch, J.F., Surdham, J., Orinion, E., Slominski-Caster, S., Watson, P., Lerman, C., Tonin, P., Lenoir, G., Serova, O., & Narod, S. (1997). A descriptive study of BRCA1 testing and reactions to disclosure of test results. *Cancer, 79,* 2219–2228.

Main, D.M., & Mennuti, M.T. (1986). Neural tube defects: Issues in prenatal diagnosis and counseling. *Obstetrics and Gynecology, 67,* 1–16.

Marteau, T.M. (1992). Psychological implications of genetic screening. *Birth Defects: Original Article Series, 28,* 185–190.

Matalon, R., Michals, K., & Kaul, R. (1995). Canavan disease: From spongy degeneration to molecular analysis. *The Journal of Pediatrics, 127,* 511–517.

McCormick, K.B. (1987). Pregnancy and epilepsy: Nursing implications. *Journal of Neuroscience Nursing, 19,* 66–76.

Miller, E., Cradock-Watson, J.E., & Pollock, T.M. (1982). Consequences of confirmed maternal rubella at successive stages of pregnancy. *Lancet, 2,* 781–784.

Milunsky, A., Jick, S.S., Bruell, C.L., MacLaughlin, D.S., Tsung, Y.-K., Jick, H., Rothman, K.J., & Willett, W. (1989). Predictive values, relative risks, and overall benefits of high and low maternal serum alpha-fetoprotein screening in singleton pregnancies: New epidemiological data. *American Journal of Obstetrics and Gynecology, 161,* 291–297.

Mitchell, A.A. (1992). Oral retinoids: What should the prescriber know about their teratogenic hazards among women of child-bearing potential? *Drug Safety, 7,* 79–85.

Muller, F., Dommergues, M., Aubry, M.-C., Simon-Bouy, B., Gautier, E., Oury, J.F., & Narcy, F. (1995). Hyperechogenic fetal bowel: An ultrasonographic marker for adverse fetal and neonatal outcome. *American Journal of Obstetrics and Gynecology, 173,* 508–513.

Nadel, A.S., Bromley, B.S., Frigoletto, F.D., Jr., Estroff, J.A., & Benacerraf, B.R. (1992). Isolated choroid plexus cysts in the second-trimester fetus: Is amniocentesis really indicated? *Radiology, 185,* 545–548.

National Institutes of Health (NIH). (1990). Statement from the National Institutes of Health workshop on population screening for the cystic fibrosis gene. *New England Journal of Medicine, 323,* 70–71.

National Institutes of Health (NIH). (1992). National Institutes of Health workshop statement. Reproductive genetic testing: Impact on women. *American Journal of Human Genetics, 51,* 1161–1163.

National Institutes of Health (NIH). (1997, April 14–16). Genetic testing for cystic fibrosis. *NIH Consensus Statement Online. 15*(4): in press.

Novotny, D.A., Klein, R.L., & Boeckman, C.R. (1993). Gastroschisis: An 18-year review. *Journal of Pediatric Surgery, 28,* 650–652.

Nyberg, D.A., Dubinsky, T., Resta, R.G., Mahony, B.S., Hickok, D.E., & Luthy, D.A. (1993). Echogenic fetal bowel during the second trimester: Clinical importance. *Radiology, 188,* 527–531.

Oakley, G.P., & Erickson J.D. (1995). Vitamin A and birth defects. Continuing caution is needed. *New England Journal of Medicine, 333,* 1414–1415.

Pastuszak, A.L., Levy, M., Schick, B., Zuber, C., Feldkamp, M., Gladstone, J., Bar-Levy, F., Jackson, E., Donnenfeld, A., Meschino, W., & Koren, G. (1994). Outcome after maternal varicella infection in the first 20 weeks of pregnancy. *New England Journal of Medicine, 330,* 901–905.

Peckham, C. (1985). Congenital rubella in the United Kingdom before 1970: The prevaccine era. *Reviews of Infectious Diseases, 7*(Suppl. 1), S11–S16.

Perpignano, M.C., Cohen, H.L., Klein, V.R., Mandel, F.S., Streltzoff, J., Chervenak, F.A., & Goldman, M.A. (1992). Fetal choroid plexus cysts: Beware the smaller cyst. *Radiology, 182,* 715–717.

Platt, L.D., Feuchtbaum, L., Filly, R., Lustig, L., Simon, M., & Cunningham, G.C. (1992). The California maternal serum alpha-fetoprotein screening program: The role of ultrasonography in the detection of spina bifida. *American Journal of Obstetrics and Gynecology, 166,* 1328–1329.

Plessinger, M.A., & Woods, J.R. (1993). Maternal, placental, and fetal pathophysiology of cocaine exposure during pregnancy. *Clinical Obstetrics and Gynecology, 36,* 267–278.

Porto, M., Murata, Y., Warneke, L.A., & Keegan, K.A. (1993). Fetal choroid plexus cysts: An independent risk factor for chromosomal anomalies. *Journal of Clinical Ultrasound, 21,* 103–108.

Pryde, P.G., Isada, N.B., Hallak, M., Johnson, M.P., Odgers, A.E., & Evans, M.I. (1992). Determinants of parental decision to abort or continue after non-aneuploid ultrasound-detected fetal abnormalities. *Obstetrics and Gynecology, 80,* 52–56.

Robinson, A, & Linden, M.G. (1993). *Clinical genetics handbook* (2nd ed.). Boston: Blackwell Scientific Publications.

Rosa, F.W. (1991). Spina bifida in infants of women treated with carbamazepine during pregnancy. *New England Journal of Medicine, 324,* 674–677.

Rothman, K.J., Moore, L.L., Singer, M.R., Nguyen, U.-S.D.T., Mannino, S., & Milunsky, A. (1995). Teratogenicity of high vitamin A intake. *New England Journal of Medicine, 333,* 1369–1373.

Saari-Kemppainen, A., Karjalainen, O., Ylostalo, P., & Heinonen, O.P. (1990). Ultrasound screening and perinatal mortality: Controlled trial of systematic one-stage screening in pregnancy. *Lancet, 336,* 387–391.

Sakala, E.P., Erhard, L.N., & White, J.J. (1993). Elective cesarean section improves outcomes of neonates with gastroschisis. *American Journal of Obstetrics and Gynecology, 169,* 1050–1053.

Scolnik, D., Nulman, I., Rovet, J., Gladstone, D., Czuchta, D., Gardner, A., Gladstone, R., Ashby, P., Weksberg, R., Einarson, T., & Koren, G. (1994). Neurodevelopment of children exposed in utero to phenytoin and carbamazepine monotherapy. *Journal of the American Medical Association, 271,* 767–770.

Sharp, M.C., Strauss, R.P., & Lorch, S.C. (1992). Communicating medical bad news: Parents' experiences and preferences. *Journal of Pediatrics, 121,* 539–546.

Shaw, G.M., Jensvold, N.G., Wasserman, C.R., & Lammer, E.J. (1994). Epidemiologic characteristics of phenotypically distinct neural tube defects among 0.7 million California births, 1983–87. *Teratology, 49,* 143–149.

Skvorc-Ranko, R., Lavoie, H., St-Denis, P., Villeneuve, R., Gagnon, M., Chicoine, R., Boucher, M., Guimond, J., & Dontigny, Y. (1991). Intrauterine diagnosis of cytomegalovirus and rubella infections by amniocentesis. *Canadian Medical Association Journal, 145,* 649–654.

Slotnick, R.N., & Abuhamad, A.Z. (1996). Prognostic implications of fetal echogenic bowel. *Lancet, 347,* 85–87.

Statham, H., & Green, J. (1993). Serum screening for Down's syndrome: Some women's experiences. *British Medical Journal, 307,* 174–176.

Suslak, L., Scherer, A., & Rodriguez, G. (1995). A support group for couples who have terminated a pregnancy after prenatal diagnosis: Recurrent themes and observations. *Journal of Genetic Counseling, 4,* 169–178.

Teratology Society. (1987). Teratology Society position paper: Recommendations for vitamin A use during pregnancy. *Teratology, 35,* 269–275.

Torfs, C., Curry, C., & Roeper, P. (1990). Gastroschisis. *The Journal of Pediatrics, 116,* 1–6.

Torfs, C.P., Velie, E.M., Oechsli, F.W., Bateson, T.F., & Curry, C.J.R. (1994). A population-based study of gastroschisis: Demographic, pregnancy, and lifestyle risk factors. *Teratology, 50,* 44–53.

Trauffer, P.M.L., Anderson, C.E., Johnson, A., Heeger, S., Morgan, P., & Wapner, R.J. (1994). The natural history of euploid pregnancies with first-trimester cystic hygromas. *American Journal of Obstetrics and Gynecology, 170,* 1279–1284.

Van Spijker, H.G. (1991). Support in decision making processes in the post-counseling period. *Birth Defects: Original Article Series, 28,* 29–35.

Varekamp, I., Suurmeijer, T., Brocker-Vriends, A., & Rosendaal, F.R. (1992) Hemophilia and the use of genetic counseling and carrier testing within family networks. *Birth Defects: Original Article Series, 28,* 139–148.

Verp, M.S., Bombard, A.T., Simpson, J.L., & Elias, S. (1988). Parental decision following prenatal diagnosis of fetal chromosome abnormality. *American Journal of Medical Genetics, 29,* 613–622.

Volpe, J.J. (1992). Effect of cocaine use on the fetus. *New England Journal of Medicine, 327,* 399–405.

Wald, N.J., Cuckle, H.S., Densem, J.W., Kennard, A., & Smith, D. (1992). Maternal serum screening for Down's syndrome: the effect of routine ultrasound scan determination of gestational age and adjustment for maternal weight. *British Journal of Obstetrics and Gynaecology, 99,* 144–149.

Weston, M.J., Porter, H.J., Andrews, H.S., & Berry, P.J. (1993). Correlation of antenatal ultrasonography and pathological examinations in 153 malformed fetuses. *Journal of Clinical Ultrasound, 21,* 387–392.

White, C.J.(1997). Varicella-zoster virus vaccine. *Clinical Infectious Diseases, 24,* 753–763.

White-van Mourik, M.C.A., Connor, J.M., & Ferguson-Smith, M.A. (1992). The psychosocial sequelae of a second-trimester termination of pregnancy for a fetal abnormality. *Prenatal Diagnosis, 12,* 189–204.

Yen, I.H., Khoury, M.J., Erickson, D., James, L.M., Waters, G.D., & Berry, R.J. (1992). The changing epidemiology of neural tube defects: United States, 1968–1989. *American Journal of Diseases of Children, 146,* 857–861.

SECTION 3
PRENATAL DIAGNOSIS AND SURVEILLANCE TECHNIQUES

Chapter 1

AMNIOCENTESIS

Lisa L. Lommel

Amniocentesis is the removal of a sample of amniotic fluid from the amniotic sac. There are a variety of indications for amniocentesis including

- Assessment of fluid for presence of bilirubin secondary to erythroblastosis fetalis

- Assessment of lecithin and sphingomyelin (L/S) ratio indicating level of fetal lung maturity

- Analysis of fluid for genetic fetal abnormalities

Depending upon the indication, amniocentesis may be completed at varying times during the pregnancy. Amniocentesis for genetic diagnosis may be completed between 12 and 14 weeks' gestation (early amniocentesis) or 15 and 20 weeks (traditional amniocentesis) both of which are 99 percent accurate in detecting trisomy 21 (Down Syndrome) and other chromosomal defects (California Department of Health Services, 1995).

The amniocentesis protocol includes an ultrasound, performed immediately prior to the procedure to determine fetal age, position of the placenta, location of amniotic fluid, fetal cardiac movement, and number of fetuses. Ultrasound is also used during the amniocentesis to help avoid puncturing the placenta, fetus, and umbilical cord. After the patient has emptied her bladder, a 19 to 22 gauge needle is passed through the lower abdomen into the uterus and amniotic sac. In traditional amniocentis, approximately 15 to 30 mL of fluid is aspirated. In early amniocentesis, approximately 1 mL of fluid per gestational week is obtained.

Amniotic cells that originate from fetal skin, the amnion, and fetal mucous membranes are grown in culture for analysis. Cells obtained from amniotic fluid undergo cytogenic, enzymatic, and DNA analysis. In addition, levels of alpha-fetoprotein (AFP) and acetylcholinesterase (ACHE) can be measured to diagnose neural tube and other anterior wall defects. With early amniocentesis, there is a slightly increased risk of obtaining an inadequate sample because of the lower fluid volume. Karyotype results are usually available within 10 days to 3.5 weeks depending upon cell development and the laboratory.

The overall risk for pregnancy loss following traditional amniocentesis is 0.25 to 0.50 percent (1/400–1/200) when the procedure is done by an experienced clinician (Centers for Disease Control, 1995). The risk of pregnancy loss after early amniocentesis is approximately 1 percent, which is slightly greater than the risk of traditional amniocentesis (Wright, 1994). These rates are related to the amniocentesis procedure alone and do not include the background rate of miscarriage.

Maternal complications associated with amniocentesis include puncture of the bladder or intestine, amnionitis, vaginal bleeding, amniotic fluid leakage, and Rh sensitization. Maternal organ puncture is very rare and can be avoided by an experienced clinician using concurrent ultrasound visualization. Symptomatic amnionitis occurs very rarely. Transient vaginal bleeding occurs more often and usually is not associated with fetal complications. Amniotic fluid leakage occurs in approximately 1 to 2 percent of patients after amniocentesis (Schemmer & Johnson, 1993). Most cases of fluid leakage are transient; only a few continue until delivery and require hospitalization. The rate of Rh sensitization after second trimester genetic amniocentesis is between 2.1 and 5.4 percent. Although routine administration of Rh immune globulin is controversial, most centers recommend prophylactic treatment in the Rh-negative, antibody screen negative patient (Schemmer & Johnson, 1993).

Fetal complications associated with amniocentesis are rare. Only a small number of cases of damage to the fetus and placenta by needle injury have been reported. The preterm birth rate, stillbirth rate, perinatal mortality rate, and physical growth and neurological development of the infant have not been affected by genetic amniocentesis (Schemmer & Johnson, 1993). The major disadvantage of early amniocentesis compared to traditional amniocentesis is the decreased detection rate of neural tube birth defects through AFP analysis below 16 to 18 weeks' gestation. AChE analysis can be combined with AFP analysis from 11 to 15 weeks to improve detection rates to 90 percent at 13 to 15 weeks' gestation (Wright, 1994).

Second trimester amniocentesis has several major advantages and disadvantages when compared to chorionic villus sampling (see Chapter 3.2, *Chorionic Villus Sampling*). Advantages include the ability to detect neural tube defects through alpha-fetoprotein analysis, visualization of fetal anatomy and function via the second trimester ultrasound, and well-established maternal-fetal risks and laboratory analysis.

Disadvantages relate to the timing of the procedure. Since most amniocenteses are completed at 15 to 18 weeks' gestation, the results are usually not available until approximately 17 to 21 weeks' gestation. An elected termination at that time poses a greater risk to the mother than an earlier termination done after chorionic villus sampling. Studies show that maternal anxiety is maintained and "maternal attachment to the fetus" is delayed in patients who undergo amniocentesis due to the later availability of results (Robinson et al., 1988; Sjögren & Uddenberg, 1989; Spencer & Cox, 1988).

Database

Subjective

- Common indications for amniocentesis include (Cunningham, MacDonald, Gant, Leveno & Gilstrap, 1993):

  ▶ Advanced maternal age (Standard practice is to offer prenatal diagnosis to women who will be 35 or older when their infant is born. These women have an increased risk for chromosomal problems in the fetus because of misdivision of the ovum during meiosis.)

  ▶ Flexibility is recommended when women under 35 years of age request prenatal diagnosis; see Table 3.1, Chromosomal Abnormalities in Liveborns

  ▶ Previous child with chromosomal abnormality

  ▶ A previous infant with multiple major malformations in whom no cytogenic study was performed

  ▶ Parental chromosomal abnormality (balanced translocations, inversion, aneuploidy, mosaicism)

  ▶ A previous child or parent with a neural tube defect or abnormally low or high level of maternal serum alpha-fetoprotein. See Chapter 3.3, *Triple Marker Prenatal Screening*

▶ Down syndrome or other chromosomal abnormality in a close family member

▶ Fetal sex determination in pregnancies at risk of a serious X-linked disease for which specific prenatal diagnosis is not available

▶ Increased risk for mendelian disorders detectable by molecular biologic techniques (i.e., sickle cell anemia, cystic fibrosis)

▶ Increased risk for mendelian disorders detectable by enzyme assays (Tay-Sachs)

▶ History of three or more successive spontaneous abortions

▶ Abnormal fetus identified by sonographic examination

● The most common difficulties associated with performing an amniocentesis include

▶ Maternal obesity

▶ Anteriorly-placed placenta

▶ Needle placement in early amniocentesis (a large anterior fibroid or severely retroverted uterus may also make needle placement difficult)

▶ Multiple gestation (early amniocentesis would not be possible because of too little amniotic fluid to obtain a safe sample)

● Common effects related to the procedure include

▶ Local discomfort described as a "stick" on the surface

▶ Deep pelvic pressure during needle insertion

▶ A push-pull feeling when the fluid sample is withdrawn

▶ Cramping (sometimes experienced immediately following the procedure, usually self-limited)

Objective

● Data review for accurate dating of pregnancy

● Data review for RH status and irregular antibodies

● Ultrasound confirming viable pregnancy at 15 to 21 weeks' gestation and documentation of placental position, location of amniotic fluid, and number of fetuses

● Karyotype result possibilities

▶ Normal 46 XX chromosomes

▶ Normal 46 XY chromosomes

▶ Abnormal chromosomes

- Alpha-fetoprotein result possibilities
  - ▶ Elevated for gestational age
  - ▶ Normal for gestational age
  - ▶ Low for gestational age

  NOTE: Bloody amniotic fluid is aspirated in 2 percent of amniocenteses. It is often maternal in origin and does not adversely affect cell growth. Brown, dark-red, or wine-colored amniotic fluid is associated with an increased likelihood of adverse pregnancy outcome. Greenish amniotic fluid has not been associated with adverse pregnancy outcome (American College of Obstetrican and Gynecologists [ACOG], 1987).

Assessment

- Abnormal chromosome with diagnosed condition (indications for amniocentesis)
- Family, maternal, or paternal risk for chromosomal abnormality or genetic disorder
- Increased fetal risk for physical abnormality or mental retardation
  - ▶ Maternal disease
  - ▶ Maternal drug use or chemical exposure
- Abnormal alpha-fetoprotein level

Plan

Diagnostic Tests

- Amniocentesis performed by a physician trained in the procedure
- Ultrasound to confirm viable fetus, location of placenta, location of amniotic fluid, and number of fetuses
- Amniotic fluid analysis (type ordered depends on diagnosis to be ruled out)
  - ▶ Chromosome
  - ▶ DNA
  - ▶ Biochemical
  - ▶ In situ hybridization on amniotic fluid

Treatment/Management

- Continue routine prenatal care for the client whose fetus has a normal karyotype and alpha-fetoprotein level.
- A client whose fetus has an abnormal karyotype and/or abnormal alpha-fetoprotein level should be referred to a physician.

- Administer 300 μg of Rh immune globulin to Rh-negative, antibody screen negative women after the procedure.

Consultation

- A client who is at risk for delivering an infant with a genetic disorder should be referred to a geneticist or genetic counselor as early as possible in their pregnancy. See Section 2, *Genetic Counseling*.

- Clients who desire amniocentesis should be referred to a physician for the procedure.

- A client whose fetus has an abnormal karyotype and/or abnormal alpha-fetoprotein level should be referred to a physician.

Patient Education

- Provide a thorough explanation of the procedure.

- Discuss the common discomforts associated with the procedure.

- Advise the woman to call her provider for persistent uterine cramping, vaginal bleeding, or leakage of amniotic fluid.

- Teach the common signs of infection including temperature elevation, flu-like symptoms, and/or change in vaginal discharge.

- Advise the client to refrain from strenuous activity and intercourse for the remainder of the day following the procedure.

- Discuss avoidance of heavy lifting (more than 20 pounds) for several days.

- Discuss avoidance of bending at the waist.

- Encourage the client to take the rest of the day off following the procedure, if possible.

- Advise resting for a couple of hours after the procedure.

- Provide emotional support to the client and her partner. This is most important after the procedure while waiting for the results, a time of increased anxiety for the client and her family.

- Genetic counseling should be completed by a geneticist and should include the woman's risk of delivering an infant with a genetic disorder.

Follow-up

- Provide emotional support to the client and her family when an abnormal result is obtained.

- Refer women with abnormal results to social workers or counselors, as appropriate.

- Document risks and indications for chromosomal/genetic disorder and karyotype result in progress notes and problem list.

References

American College of Obstetricians and Gynecologists (ACOG) (1987). *Antenatal diagnosis of genetic disorders* (Technical Bulletin No. 108). Washington, DC: Author.

California Department of Health Services, Genetic Disease Branch (1995). *Summary of prenatal testing choices.* Berkeley, CA: Author.

Centers for Disease Control and Prevention (1995). Chorionic villus sampling and amniocentesis: Recommendations for prenatal counseling. *Morbidity and Mortality Weekly Report, 44,* No. RR-9, 1–12.

Cunningham, F.G., MacDonald, D.C., Gant, N.F., Leveno, K.J., & Gilstrap, L.C. (1993). Prenatal diagnosis and invasive techniques to monitor the fetus. In *Williams Obstetrics* (19th Ed.) (pp. 945–954) Norwalk, CT: Appleton & Lange.

Robinson, G.E., Garner, D.M., Olmstead, M.P., Shime, J., Hutton, E.M., & Crawford, B.M. (1988). Anxiety reduction after chorionic villus sampling and genetic amniocentesis. *American Journal of Obstetrics and Gynecology, 159*(4), 953–956.

Schemmer, G. & Johnson, A. (1993). Genetic amniocentesis and chorionic villus sampling. *Obstetric and Gynecology Clinics of North America, 20* (3), 497–521.

Sjögren, B., & Uddenberg, N. (1989). Prenatal diagnosis and psychological distress: Amniocentesis or chorionic villus biopsy? *Prenatal Diagnosis, 9,* 477–487.

Spencer, J.W., & Cox, D.V. (1988). A comparison of chorionic villi sampling and amniocentesis: Acceptability of procedure and maternal attachment to pregnancy. *Obstetrics and Gynecology, 72*(5), 714–718.

Wright, L. (1994). Prenatal diagnosis in the 1990s. *Journal of Obstetric, Gynecologic and Neonatal Nursing, 23* (6), 506–519.

Chapter 2

CHORIONIC VILLUS SAMPLING

Lisa L. Lommel

Chorionic villus sampling (CVS) removes a small sample of chorionic (placental) tissue for prenatal genetic diagnosis. The overall accuracy rate for trisomy 21 (Down syndrome) and other chromosomal defects is 98 percent (California Department of Health Services, 1995).

The two most common methods of CVS are the transcervical and transabdominal techniques. The selection of an appropriate approach is based on placental location, although certain other conditions may preclude a particular approach, (e.g. presence of uterine myoma or active cervical/vaginal herpes). Both techniques are completed at 9 to 12 weeks' gestation when the chorionic villi are abundant enough to be easily sampled while avoiding the gestational sac. The transcervical method is the most widely used. Under ultrasound guidance, and with the woman's bladder full, a catheter is passed through the vagina and cervix into the uterine cavity (transcervical technique). The transabdominal technique usually requires an empty bladder while the catheter is passed through the abdominal wall into the uterine cavity under ultrasound guidance. When the chorionic villi is located and visualized, approximately 5 to 30 mg of villi are removed by applying suction to the end of the catheter with a syringe. Karyotype results can be available within 3 to 4 days when using the direct method of tissue analysis. It is recommended that a tissue culture also be completed on the same sample to confirm the results (available in 2 to 3 weeks in most laboratories).

The overall risk of miscarriage from CVS is 0.5 percent to 1.0 percent (1/200–1/100) (Centers for Disease Control and Prevention [CDC], 1995). Additional complications associated with CVS include bleeding, infection, and RH isoimmunization. Vaginal spotting or light bleeding is rare following transabdominal CVS but has a 10 to 25 percent incidence rate after the transcervical method. Vaginal spotting due to CVS usually resolves in 10 to 14 days and does not persist or recur later in pregnancy. Heavy vaginal bleeding is infrequent and rarely presents serious complications.

Intrauterine infection poses a threat to the woman and her fetus. It is believed that the risk of infection using the transcervical method is higher than the transabdominal method. Risk of infection has been found to be 0.2 percent for the transcervical method. Many providers require negative *Neisseria gonorrhoeae* testing before the procedure. Careful client education regarding signs and symptoms of infection is important in reducing the risk of serious sequelae.

Rh sensitization has been of concern following CVS because of a reported rise in maternal serum alpha-fetoprotein following 50 percent of the procedures, implying a fetal maternal hemorrhage. Prophylactic use of 50 μg of Rh immune globulin is recommended in Rh negative patients who have a negative antibody screen.

Fetal complications sometimes result from the CVS procedure, particularly certain congenital defects of the extremities known as limb deficiencies or limb reduction defects. The majority of limb deficiencies are transverse terminal defects, which involve the absence of parts of one or more fingers or toes. Rarely, oromandibular-limb hypogenesis (the absence or hypoplasia of the tongue and lower jaw) occurs. The theory is that these defects occur as a result of vascular disruption (from the CVS procedure) during the formation of embryonic limbs or in already formed fetal limbs. The gestational age of the fetus appears to be closely linked with the risk and severity of the defect. The risk of defect from CVS done at less than 10 weeks gestation (0.20 percent) is higher than the risk of defect from CVS at 10 weeks' gestation or later (0.07 percent). Because of these reports, it is recommended that CVS be performed at 9 to 12 weeks' gestation. Recent data indicate an overall risk of transverse limb deficiency from CVS to be 0.03 to 0.10 percent (CDC, 1995).

Chorionic villi sampling has some major advantages and disadvantages when compared to second trimester amniocentesis for genetic diagnosis. The primary advantage is the availability of results early in the pregnancy. Because of early availability of results, studies have shown that maternal anxiety is reduced and maternal attachment to the fetus is enhanced in patients who undergo CVS (Robinson et al., 1988; Sjögren & Uddenberg, 1989; Spencer & Cox, 1988). Additionally, if termination was elected by the patient, the termination procedure would pose less risk at 11 to 14 weeks' gestation compared to that of 20 to 22 weeks. Disadvantages to CVS include a higher total pregnancy loss rate of 0.5 percent when compared to amniocentesis (CDC, 1995), the inability to screen for neural tube defects with amniotic fluid alpha-fetoprotein analysis, the inability to visualize fetal anatomy via ultrasound at the earlier weeks of gestation, and the increased frequency of chromosomal mosaicism (1–2 percent), which is usually confined to the placenta (the majority of fetuses do not manifest mosaicism) (Fryberg, 1993; Bramboti, 1995; Schemmer & Johnson, 1993).

Database

Subjective

- Common indications for CVS include (Cunningham, MacDonald, Gant, Leveno & Gilstrap, 1993):

  ▶ Advanced maternal age

    – Standard practice is to offer prenatal diagnosis to women who will be 35 or older when their infant is born. These woman have an increased risk for chromosomal problems in the fetus because of misdivision of the ovum during meiosis

    – Flexibility is recommended when women under 35 years of age request prenatal diagnosis. See Table 3.1, Chromosomal Abnormalities in Liveborns.

  ▶ Previous child with chromosomal abnormality

  ▶ A previous infant with multiple major malformations in whom no cytogenic study was performed

  ▶ Parental chromosomal abnormality (balanced translocations, inversions, aneuploidy, mosaicism)

  ▶ Down syndrome or other chromosomal abnormality in a close family member

  ▶ Fetal sex determination in pregnancies at risk for serious X-linked diseases for which specific prenatal diagnosis is not available

  ▶ Increased risk for mendelian disorders detectable by molecular biologic technique (i.e. sickle cell anemia, cystic fibrosis)

  ▶ History of three or more successive spontaneous abortions

  ▶ Abnormal fetus identified by sonographic examination

- Relative contraindication for CVS include
  - ▶ Alpha-fetoprotein analysis for neural tube and abdominal wall defects can be conducted using amniotic fluid only. Patients at increased risk for these abnormalities are not candidates for CVS.

- Absolute contraindications for CVS
  - ▶ Presence of intrauterine device
  - ▶ Active bleeding
  - ▶ Cervical stenosis (transabdominal technique may be utilized)
  - ▶ Untreated endocervicitis or pelvic inflammatory disease
  - ▶ Positive *N. gonorrhoeae* testing of the cervix
  - ▶ Active genital herpes simplex viral infection

- Common effects related to the procedure
  - ▶ Discomfort attributed to a full bladder
  - ▶ Cramping associated with placement of the tenaculum and insertion and removal of the catheter.

Objective

- Data review for accurate dating of pregnancy
- Data review for Rh status and irregular antibodies
- Pre-procedure ultrasound confirming viable pregnancy at 9 to 12 weeks' gestation and absence of uterine anomalies
- Karyotype result:
  - ▶ Normal 46 XX chromosomes or
  - ▶ Normal 46 XY chromosomes or
  - ▶ Abnormal chromosomes
- *N. gonorrhea* testing negative

Assessment

- Abnormal chromosomes with diagnosed condition (see the Subjective section for indications for CVS)
  - ▶ Family, maternal or paternal risk for chromosomal abnormality or genetic disorder
  - ▶ Maternal disease or drug or chemical exposure increasing fetal risk for physical abnormality or mental retardation

Plan

Diagnostic Tests

- Chorionic villus sampling (done by a physician who is trained in this procedure)

- Cervical testing for *N. gonorrhoeae*

- Culture for herpes simplex if suspicious lesion is present or if the patient has a history of herpes simplex lesion within previous 6 months

- Ultrasound to confirm viability of fetus and date pregnancy between 9 and 12 weeks

- Ultrasound to rule out uterine abnormalities, presence of intrauterine device, and presence of multiple gestation (CVS *can* be accomplished in a twin gestation with an experienced clinician)

Treatment/Management

- Continue routine prenatal care for patients whose fetus has a normal karyotype.

- Patients whose fetuses have an abnormal karyotype should be referred to a physician.

- Administer 50 µg of Rh immune globulin to Rh-negative, antibody screen negative patients after CVS procedure has been performed.

Consultation

- Refer clients who are at risk of delivering an infant with a genetic disorder to a geneticist as early as possible in their pregnancy.

- Refer clients who desire CVS to a physician for the procedure.

- Refer clients whose fetuses have an abnormal karyotype to a physician.

Patient Education

- Genetic counseling should be completed by a geneticist or genetic counselor and should include the woman's risks of delivering an infant with a genetic disorder. See Section 2, *Genetic Counseling*.

- Explain that CVS cannot evaluate for neural tube defects. Women should be offered maternal serum alpha-fetoprotein (MSAFP) screening at 16–18 weeks' gestation. See Chapter 3.3, *Antepartum Fetal Surveillance*.

- Provide explanation of the procedure.

- Discuss the common discomforts that are associated with the procedure.

- Explain that spotting is common after the procedure but should subside within 3 days. Advise woman to contact her care provider if bleeding persists or increases in amount.

- Teach the client common signs of infection including temperature elevation, flu-like symptoms, or change in vaginal discharge. Advise the woman to contact her care provider if any of the symptoms are present.

- Advise the client to refrain from strenuous activity for the remainder of the day following the procedure. For women who have experienced vaginal spotting, advise avoiding intercourse until one week after vaginal spotting has stopped.

- Provide emotional support to the client and her partner. This will be most important after the procedure while waiting for the results. This is a time of increased anxiety for the client and her family.

- Provide emotional support to the patient and her family when an abnormal result is obtained.

Follow-up

- Offer maternal serum alpha-fetoprotein screening for neural tube defects at 16 to 18 weeks gestation.

- Many CVS programs recommend a second-trimester ultrasound to evaluate the fetus for malformations and organ function.

- Refer women with an abnormal result to a social worker or counselor, as appropriate.

- Document risk, indication for chromosomal/genetic disorder, and karyotype result in progress notes and problem list.

Table 3.1

Chromosomal Abnormalities in Liveborns*

Maternal Age	Risk for Down Syndrome	Total Risk for Chromosomal Abnormalities**
20	1/1,667	1/526
21	1/1,667	1/526
22	1/1,429	1/500
23	1/1,429	1/500
24	1/1,250	1/476
25	1/1,250	1/476
26	1/1,176	1/476
27	1/1,111	1/455
28	1/1,053	1/435
29	1/1,000	1/417
30	1/952	1/385
31	1/909	1/385
32	1/769	1/322
33	1/602	1/286
34	1/485	1/238
35	1/378	1/192
36	1/289	1/156
37	1/224	1/127
38	1/173	1/102
39	1/136	1/83
40	1/106	1/66
41	1/82	1/53
42	1/63	1/42
43	1/49	1/33
44	1/38	1/26
45	1/30	1/21
46	1/23	1/16
47	1/18	1/13
48	1/14	1/10
49	1/11	1/8

* Because sample size for some intervals is relatively small, 95% confidence limits are sometimes relatively large. Nonetheless, these figures are suitable for genetic counseling.

** 47 XXX excluded for ages 20-32 (data not available)

Source: American College of Obstetricians and Gynecologists (1987). *Antenatal diagnosis of genetic disorders* (Technical Bulletin No. 108). Washington, DC: Author. Reprinted with permission.

References

Centers for Disease Control and Prevention (1995). Chorionic villus sampling and amniocentesis: Recommendations for prenatal counseling. *Morbidity and Mortality Weekly Report, 44,* No. RR-9, 1–12.

California Department of Health Services, Genetic Disease Branch (1995). Summary of prenatal testing choices. Berkeley, CA: Author.

American College of Obstetricians and Gynecologists (1987). *Antenatal diagnosis of genetic disorders* (Technical Bulletin No. 108). Washington, DC: Author.

Bramboti, B. (1995) Chorionic villus sampling. *Current Opinion in Obstetrics and Gynecology, 7,* 109–114.

Cunningham, F.G., MacDonald, D.C., Gant, N.F., Leveno, K.J. & Gilstrap, L.C. (1993). *Williams Obstetrics* (19th Ed.) (pp. 945–954). Norwalk, CT : Appleton & Lange.

Freyburg, J.S. (1993). Mosaicism in chorionic villus sampling. *Obstetrics and Gynecology Clinics of North American 20*(3), 523–532.

Robinson, G.E., Garner, D.M., Olmstead, M.P., Shime, J., Hutton, E.M., & Crawford, B.M. (1988). Anxiety reduction after chorionic villus sampling and genetic amniocentesis. *American Journal of Obstetrics and Gynecology, 159*(4), 953–956.

Schemmer, G. & Johnson, A. (1993). Genetic amniocentesis and chorionic villus sampling. *Obstetric and Gynecology Clinics of North America, 20*(3), 497–521.

Shulman, L.P. & Elias, S. (1993) Amniocentesis and chorionic villus sampling. *The Western Journal of Medicine, 159*(3) 260–268.

Sjögren, B., & Uddenberg, N. (1989). Prenatal diagnosis and psychological distress: Amniocentesis or chorionic villus biopsy? *Prenatal Diagnosis, 9,* 477–487.

Spencer, J.W., & Cox, D.V. (1988). A comparison of chorionic villi sampling and amniocentesis: Acceptability of procedure and maternal attachment to pregnancy. *Obstetrics and Gynecology, 72*(5), 714–718.

Chapter 3

Triple Marker Prenatal Screening

Maureen T. Shannon

The first referrals of women for prenatal counseling and diagnosis were based on a family history of a genetic abnormality, or maternal age greater than or equal to 35 years of age, which is associated with increased risk of fetal aneuploidy (Hook, 1981). However, 95 percent of pregnant women with fetuses affected by neural tube defects (NTDs) are without an associated identified risk factor (California Department of Health Services, 1994). In addition, 80 percent of children with Down syndrome are born to women less than 35 years of age (Phillips et al., 1992). During the past two decades, advances in biochemical analysis of maternal serum have provided an opportunity to screen large populations of pregnant women for these and, to a limited extent, other fetal chromosomal and congenital abnormalities. Studies have demonstrated that an analysis of a combination of one or more maternal serum biochemical substances (i.e., analytes), in addition to maternal age, is more sensitive and specific than using maternal age alone in detecting risk (Cheng et al., 1993; Kellner et al., 1995; Phillips, et al., 1992; Rose, Palomake, Haddow, Goodman, & Mennuti, 1994). In addition to the identification of maternal serum analytes, a statistical model estimates a woman's individual risk for a particular chromosomal or congential abnormality using maternal age and a combination of the levels of these maternal serum analytes (Wald et al., 1988).

In response to these advances, various prenatal screening programs were developed to afford access to maternal prenatal testing for large populations of pregnant women. A study of laboratories responsible for processing prenatal screening tests revealed that in the United States between 1988 to 1992 maternal serum screening for Down syndrome (using either one, or a combination of two or three maternal analytes) almost doubled (Palomaki, Knight, McCarthy, Haddow, & Eckfeldt, 1993). As a result of such programs, a considerable reduction in the prevalence of some birth defects and chromosomal abnormalities has been observed (Centers for Disease Control and Prevention [CDC], 1995).

Currently, there are three maternal serum analytes used for prenatal diagnostic screening for risk of NTDs, abdominal wall defects, Down syndrome, and trisomy 18.

- Alpha-fetoprotein (AFP): a protein produced in the fetal yolk sac during the first trimester and later in pregnancy by the fetal liver.

  > In pregnant women AFP is found in both the amniotic fluid and maternal serum in significantly lower concentrations than is found in fetal serum. The highest concentration of AFP in fetal serum and amniotic fluid occurs at approximately the 13th gestational week, after which time these levels decrease rapidly. In maternal serum, the AFP concentration remains at low levels, but does exhibit a gradual increase in concentration until 30 -32 weeks gestation.

  > Abnormally elevated levels of AFP alone (either from amniotic fluid or maternal serum samples) have been associated with several fetal disorders including open NTDs, abdominal wall defects, congenital nephrosis, and other birth defects. Elevated AFP levels are also noted in multiple gestations. (Women with abnormally elevated maternal serum AFP (MSAFP) levels during the second trimester but normal fetal evaluations are at an increased risk of preterm delivery, low birth weight infants, and fetal death [California Department of Health Services, 1994; Waller, Lustig, Cuningham, Golbus, & Hook, 1991].)

> Abnormally low AFP levels are associated with an increased risk of Down Syndrome (Knight, Palomaki, & Haddow, 1988) and other chromosomal abnormalities (Drugan et al., 1989).

- Human chorionic gonadotropin (hCG): a hormone produced and secreted by the placenta.

  > During early normal pregnancy, the level of this hormone rises rapidly and then begins to decline between the 10th to the 20th week of gestation.

  > In Down syndrome, the level of hCG during the second trimester is, on the average, higher than expected (Bogart, Pandian, & Jones, 1987; California Department of Health Services, 1994; Chard, Lowings, & Kitau, 1984; Wald et al., 1988).

- Unconjugated estriol (μE_3): a hormone that is produced by the placenta, and by the fetal adrenal glands and liver.

  > The level of this hormone rises as normal pregnancy progresses.

  > In pregnancies with fetal Down syndrome, the levels of mE_3 are, on the average, lower than unaffected pregnancies (California Department of Health Services, 1994; Canick et al., 1988; Heyl, Miller, & Canick, 1990; McDonald, Wagner, & Slotnick, 1991; Norgaard-Pedersen, Larsen, Arends, Svenstrup, & Tabor, 1990; Wald et al., 1988).

Prenatal testing programs offering triple marker screening to women during the second trimester analyze all three of these analytes. To ascertain an individual woman's risk, the level of each analyte and the pattern that is derived from their individual levels are analyzed. The result is reported as multiples of the median (MoMs) for the woman's gestational age at the time her blood sample was drawn, reflecting a level that may be normal, high, or low in relation to this median value. In addition, the possibility of a pregnancy being affected by Down syndrome is reported in relation to a particular cutoff value for a population based on demographic and ethnic statistics (e.g., a positive screen for Down syndrome in California is reported as a risk greater than or equal to 1 in 250) (California Department of Health Services, 1994).

When a sample for triple marker screening (or for prenatal serum screening for any of the analytes) is ordered, a woman must have her blood sample drawn between the 15th and 20th gestational weeks (ideally between 112 and 126 gestational days), for these tests to be accurate (see Table 3.3, Time Window for Expanded AFP Blood Collection) (California Department of Health Services, 1994). Other factors that can affect the accuracy of these tests include

- incorrect pregnancy dating (the median level of each analyte changes daily during pregnancy).

- improper laboratory collection of the maternal specimen.

- maternal weight (heavier women have lower median values).

- race (there are different median values for some races).

- number of fetuses (multiple gestation is associated with an increase in some values).

- diabetic status (insulin dependent diabetics, *not* gestational diabetics, usually have lower MSAFP values) (California Department of Health Services, 1994). Maternal medical and family history is also important.

- A family history of neural tube defects (NTDs) (i.e., in mother, father, or sibling of the fetus) or maternal ingestion of carbamazepine or valproic acid prior to or during the first few weeks of pregnancy is associated with an increased risk of NTDs in the present fetus.

Once a positive result is reported, women are usually referred to prenatal diagnostic centers (PDCs) for further evaluation (usually an ultrasound and possibly an amniocentesis) (California Department of Health Services, 1994).

For pregnant women who will be 35 years of age or older at the time of their estimated date of confinement (EDC), the current recommendation for the detection of chromosomal abnormalities remains amniocentesis or chorionic villus sampling (CVS) (American College of Obstetricians and Gynecologists [ACOG], 1993). Women who choose to have an early amniocentesis (i.e., 12 to 14 gestational weeks) or CVS (10 to 12 gestational weeks) should have MSAFP testing done, since AFP levels cannot be determined using specimens obtained during this time (see Table 3.4, Summary of Prenatal Testing Choices). Some women may decline MSAFP testing on the basis of the 1 percent fetal loss rate associated with the procedure or for other personal reasons. Studies investigating the efficacy of using triple marker screening (i.e., MSAFP, hCG, μE_3) plus maternal age to calculate the risk of specific fetal chromosomal abnormalities and congenital defects compared to amniocentesis in pregnant women older than 35 years of age have demonstrated that using a combination of maternal age and one or more of the three analytes is better than using maternal age alone (Haddow et al., 1994; Kellner et al., 1995; Rose et al., 1994). Nevertheless, there remains a decreased sensitivity of detecting risks of Down syndrome or other chromosomal abnormalities when compared to amniocentesis in this age group (Rose et al., 1994). For women in this age category electing to have triple marker screening instead of amniocentesis, this difference needs to be clearly presented as part of their counseling.

Database

Subjective

The woman may report one or more of the following risk factors:

- A family history positive for NTD, abdominal wall defect, or chromosomal abnormality (e.g., Down syndrome)

- A history of vaginal bleeding during the first trimester (Bernstein, Barth, Miller, & Capeless, 1992)

- Ingestion of valproic acid or carbamazepine

- Insulin-dependent diabetes (prior to pregnancy)

- Age of 35 years or older at the time of her EDD (estimated date of delivery)

Objective

- The woman undergoing triple marker prenatal screening, in general, does not exhibit abnormal clinical manifestations.

Assessment

- A positive result for any of the triple marker analytes *is not* diagnostic, since this is only a screening test. Therefore, the assessment is simply a "positive" or "negative" screen.

Plan

Diagnostic Tests

- Initial triple marker screening must be done between 15 and 20 weeks' gestational age (105 to 140th day from the last menstrual period [LMP]). The ideal time for sample collection is between 112 to 126 days (California Department of Health Services, 1994).

- When filling out the forms accompanying the sample, only one method of determining the gestational age should be designated (e.g., LMP, first trimester pelvic examination, or ultrasound results) with the most reliable method of determining gestation cited. The most reliable method of determining gestational age for the purposes of obtaining accurate results from this prenatal screening test is ultrasound dating (California Department of Health Services, 1996).

- Once the sample is obtained, mail it to the specified laboratory within 24 hours to ensure accuracy of results (California Department of Health Services, 1996).

NOTE: Invalid test results occur if the wrong specimen collection tube is used, or if there is contamination of the specimen by EDTA. Therefore, when obtaining several laboratory specimens in addition to the triple marker screen, the triple marker screen specimen should be drawn first and should be collected in a serum separator tube (California Department of Health Services, 1996).

- A negative triple marker screen result indicates a *low risk* of Down syndrome, trisomy 18, open NTDs, and abdominal wall defects. It does not eliminate the possibility of these or other fetal conditions.

  - Under some circumstances, a woman with a negative screen result may be referred to the PDC for additional services (i.e., counseling, other testing). Women who are usually included in this group are those with a family history of NTDs or who have taken carbamazepine or valproic acid just prior to or during the first few weeks of pregnancy.

- A positive triple marker screen result may be reported as follows:

  - A positive screen for an increased risk of open NTDs or abdominal wall defects occurs when the AFP value is elevated at 2.5 MoM or more for a single fetus and 4.5 MoM or more for multiple gestations. The AFP value is the only analyte used since hCG and μE_3 are not useful indicators of NTDs (California Department of Health Services, 1994).

    NOTE: A positive screen may be reported as a result of underestimation of gestational age, multiple gestation, fetal renal abnormalities, fetomaternal hemorrhage, or fetal demise. In some normal pregnancies with a positive screen, there have been increased incidences of low birth weight, preterm delivery, and fetal demise.

  - A positive screen for an increased risk for Down syndrome is reported when the combined measurements of the three analytes demonstrates the following pattern: a decreased level of AFP and μE_3 with an increased level of hCG. A woman is classified as being at an increased risk for a fetus with this condition when the above results produce a calculated risk greater than the cutoff risk for the particular population or geographic region.

NOTE: A positive screen may be reported because of an overestimation of gestational weeks, or presence of triploidy or Turner syndrome (California Department of Health Services, 1994).

- A positive screen for an increased risk for trisomy 18 occurs when there are low levels of all three analytes.

- When a woman is referred to a state-funded PDC she usually receives genetic counseling and a high-resolution ultrasound to confirm or eliminate evidence of a fetal abnormality. If there is no evidence of a fetal abnormality demonstrated by ultrasonography, further testing is indicated (e.g., amniocentesis).

Treatment/Management

- Continue routine prenatal care for a woman with normal triple marker screen results.

- Refer a woman who has been diagnosed with a fetus with an open NTD, abdominal wall defect, Down syndrome, trisomy 18, or other fetal abnormality to the consulting physician for care.

- Comanage the care of a woman with a "low" MSAFP level, without evidence of a fetal abnormality, with an MD secondary to a possible increased incidence of adverse pregnancy outcomes.

- Comanage the care of a woman with an elevated MSAFP level and no evidence of fetal abnormalities with the consulting physician because of an increased risk of IUGR, preterm labor, and fetal demise.

Consultation

- Refer all women with a positive triple marker screen to the regional PDC for further counseling and diagnostic testing. Base follow-up on the results of these evaluations.

- Consult with a physician for a woman with either a low or elevated MSAFP result and no evidence of an abnormal fetal condition secondary to the increased rates of adverse perinatal outcomes associated with these results.

Patient Education

- Educate the woman about the triple marker screening test

  ▶ What fetal conditions it screens for

  ▶ Information about the limitations of the test (e.g., MSAFP screening will not help in the prenatal diagnosis of *closed* neural tube defects, which constitutes about 10 percent of all NTDs)

- For a woman with a positive screen result, reinforce the fact that this test *does not* diagnose a fetal abnormality but indicates an increased possibility of a problem. Discuss the need for referral to a PDC for further counseling and evaluation.

- For a woman who will be 35 years of age or older at the time of her EDD who declines amniocentesis, discuss the triple marker screening test, including the limitations of the test for a woman in her age category.

Follow-up

- See Treatment/Management.
- Document triple marker screening results in laboratory section of chart.
- Document abnormal triple marker screening results in the problem list.

Table 3.3

Time Window for Expanded AFP Blood Collection

Based on the 1st day of the Last Menstrual Period (LMP)

"Time Window" is from 105th through 140th day (between 15 and 20 weeks). For use during 365-day year.

LMP Date	Draw Blood From	Through	LMP Date	Draw Blood From	Through	LMP Date	Draw Blood From	Through	LMP Date	Draw Blood From	Through
Jan 01	Apr 16	May 21	Feb 01	May 17	Jun 21	Mar 04	Jun 17	Jul 22	Apr 04	Jul 18	Aug 22
Jan 02	Apr 17	May 22	Feb 02	May 18	Jun 22	Mar 05	Jun 18	Jul 23	Apr 05	Jul 19	Aug 23
Jan 03	Apr 18	May 23	Feb 03	May 19	Jun 23	Mar 06	Jun 19	Jul 24	Apr 06	Jul 20	Aug 24
Jan 04	Apr 19	May 24	Feb 04	May 20	Jun 24	Mar 07	Jun 20	Jul 25	Apr 07	Jul 21	Aug 25
Jan 05	Apr 20	May 25	Feb 05	May 21	Jun 25	Mar 08	Jun 21	Jul 26	Apr 08	Jul 22	Aug 26
Jan 06	Apr 21	May 26	Feb 06	May 22	Jun 26	Mar 09	Jun 22	Jul 27	Apr 09	Jul 23	Aug 27
Jan 07	Apr 22	May 27	Feb 07	May 23	Jun 27	Mar 10	Jun 23	Jul 28	Apr 10	Jul 24	Aug 28
Jan 08	Apr 23	May 28	Feb 08	May 24	Jun 28	Mar 11	Jun 24	Jul 29	Apr 11	Jul 25	Aug 29
Jan 09	Apr 24	May 29	Feb 09	May 25	Jun 29	Mar 12	Jun 25	Jul 30	Apr 12	Jul 26	Aug 30
Jan 10	Apr 25	May 30	Feb 10	May 26	Jun 30	Mar 13	Jun 26	Jul 31	Apr 13	Jul 27	Aug 31
Jan 11	Apr 26	May 31	Feb 11	May 27	Jul 01	Mar 14	Jun 27	Aug 01	Apr 14	Jul 28	Sep 01
Jan 12	Apr 27	Jun 01	Feb 12	May 28	Jul 02	Mar 15	Jun 28	Aug 02	Apr 15	Jul 29	Sep 02
Jan 13	Apr 28	Jun 02	Feb 13	May 29	Jul 03	Mar 16	Jun 29	Aug 03	Apr 16	Jul 30	Sep 03
Jan 14	Apr 29	Jun 03	Feb 14	May 30	Jul 04	Mar 17	Jun 30	Aug 04	Apr 17	Jul 31	Sep 04
Jan 15	Apr 30	Jun 04	Feb 15	May 31	Jul 05	Mar 18	Jul 01	Aug 05	Apr 18	Aug 01	Sep 05
Jan 16	May 01	Jun 05	Feb 16	Jun 01	Jul 06	Mar 19	Jul 02	Aug 06	Apr 19	Aug 02	Sep 06
Jan 17	May 02	Jun 06	Feb 17	Jun 02	Jul 07	Mar 20	Jul 03	Aug 07	Apr 20	Aug 03	Sep 07
Jan 18	May 03	Jun 07	Feb 18	Jun 03	Jul 08	Mar 21	Jul 04	Aug 08	Apr 21	Aug 04	Sep 08
Jan 19	May 04	Jun 08	Feb 19	Jun 04	Jul 09	Mar 22	Jul 05	Aug 09	Apr 22	Aug 05	Sep 09
Jan 20	May 05	Jun 09	Feb 20	Jun 05	Jul 10	Mar 23	Jul 06	Aug 10	Apr 23	Aug 06	Sep 10
Jan 21	May 06	Jun 10	Feb 21	Jun 06	Jul 11	Mar 24	Jul 07	Aug 11	Apr 24	Aug 07	Sep 11
Jan 22	May 07	Jun 11	Feb 22	Jun 07	Jul 12	Mar 25	Jul 08	Aug 12	Apr 25	Aug 08	Sep 12
Jan 23	May 08	Jun 12	Feb 23	Jun 08	Jul 13	Mar 26	Jul 09	Aug 13	Apr 26	Aug 09	Sep 13
Jan 24	May 09	Jun 13	Feb 24	Jun 09	Jul 14	Mar 27	Jul 10	Aug 14	Apr 27	Aug 10	Sep 14
Jan 25	May 10	Jun 14	Feb 25	Jun 10	Jul 15	Mar 28	Jul 11	Aug 15	Apr 28	Aug 11	Sep 15
Jan 26	May 11	Jun 15	Feb 26	Jun 11	Jul 16	Mar 29	Jul 12	Aug 16	Apr 29	Aug 12	Sep 16
Jan 27	May 12	Jun 16	Feb 27	Jun 12	Jul 17	Mar 30	Jul 13	Aug 17	Apr 30	Aug 13	Sep 17
Jan 28	May 13	Jun 17	Feb 28	Jun 13	Jul 18	Mar 31	Jul 14	Aug 18	May 01	Aug 14	Sep 18
Jan 29	May 14	Jun 18	Mar 01	Jun 14	Jul 19	Apr 01	Jul 15	Aug 19	May 02	Aug 15	Sep 19
Jan 30	May 15	Jun 19	Mar 02	Jun 15	Jul 20	Apr 02	Jul 16	Aug 20	May 03	Aug 16	Sep 20
Jan 31	May 16	Jun 20	Mar 03	Jun 16	Jul 21	Apr 03	Jul 17	Aug 21	May 04	Aug 17	Sep 21

Table 3.3 (cont.)

Time Window for Expanded AFP Blood Collection

Based on the 1st day of the Last Menstrual Period (LMP)

"Time Window" is from 105th through 140th day (between 15 and 20 weeks). For use during 365-day year

LMP Date	Draw Blood From	Through	LMP Date	Draw Blood From	Through	LMP Date	Draw Blood From	Through	LMP Date	Draw Blood From	Through
05 May	18 Aug	22 Sep	05 Jun	18 Sep	23 Oct	06 Jul	19 Oct	23 Nov	06 Aug	19 Nov	24 Dec
06 May	19 Aug	23 Sep	06 Jun	19 Sep	24 Oct	07 Jul	20 Oct	24 Nov	07 Aug	20 Nov	25 Dec
07 May	20 Aug	24 Sep	07 Jun	20 Sep	25 Oct	08 Jul	21 Oct	25 Nov	08 Aug	21 Nov	26 Dec
08 May	21 Aug	25 Sep	08 Jun	21 Sep	26 Oct	09 Jul	22 Oct	26 Nov	09 Aug	22 Nov	27 Dec
09 May	22 Aug	26 Sep	09 Jun	22 Sep	27 Oct	10 Jul	23 Oct	27 Nov	10 Aug	23 Nov	28 Dec
10 May	23 Aug	27 Sep	10 Jun	23 Sep	28 Oct	11 Jul	24 Oct	28 Nov	11 Aug	24 Nov	29 Dec
11 May	24 Aug	28 Sep	11 Jun	24 Sep	29 Oct	12 Jul	25 Oct	29 Nov	12 Aug	25 Nov	30 Dec
12 May	25 Aug	29 Sep	12 Jun	25 Sep	30 Oct	13 Jul	26 Oct	30 Nov	13 Aug	26 Nov	31 Dec
13 May	26 Aug	30 Sep	13 Jun	26 Sep	31 Oct	14 Jul	27 Oct	01 Dec	14 Aug	27 Nov	01 Jan
14 May	27 Aug	01 Oct	14 Jun	27 Sep	01 Nov	15 Jul	28 Oct	02 Dec	15 Aug	28 Nov	02 Jan
15 May	28 Aug	02 Oct	15 Jun	28 Sep	02 Nov	16 Jul	29 Oct	03 Dec	16 Aug	29 Nov	03 Jan
16 May	29 Aug	03 Oct	16 Jun	29 Sep	03 Nov	17 Jul	30 Oct	04 Dec	17 Aug	30 Nov	04 Jan
17 May	30 Aug	04 Oct	17 Jun	30 Sep	04 Nov	18 Jul	31 Oct	05 Dec	18 Aug	01 Dec	05 Jan
18 May	31 Aug	05 Oct	18 Jun	01 Oct	05 Nov	19 Jul	01 Nov	06 Dec	19 Aug	02 Dec	06 Jan
19 May	01 Sep	06 Oct	19 Jun	02 Oct	06 Nov	20 Jul	02 Nov	07 Dec	20 Aug	03 Dec	07 Jan
20 May	02 Sep	07 Oct	20 Jun	03 Oct	07 Nov	21 Jul	03 Nov	08 Dec	21 Aug	04 Dec	08 Jan
21 May	03 Sep	08 Oct	21 Jun	04 Oct	08 Nov	22 Jul	04 Nov	09 Dec	22 Aug	05 Dec	09 Jan
22 May	04 Sep	09 Oct	22 Jun	05 Oct	09 Nov	23 Jul	05 Nov	10 Dec	23 Aug	06 Dec	10 Jan
23 May	05 Sep	10 Oct	23 Jun	06 Oct	10 Nov	24 Jul	06 Nov	11 Dec	24 Aug	07 Dec	11 Jan
24 May	06 Sep	11 Oct	24 Jun	07 Oct	11 Nov	25 Jul	07 Nov	12 Dec	25 Aug	08 Dec	12 Jan
25 May	07 Sep	12 Oct	25 Jun	08 Oct	12 Nov	26 Jul	08 Nov	13 Dec	26 Aug	09 Dec	13 Jan
26 May	08 Sep	13 Oct	26 Jun	09 Oct	13 Nov	27 Jul	09 Nov	14 Dec	27 Aug	10 Dec	14 Jan
27 May	09 Sep	14 Oct	27 Jun	10 Oct	14 Nov	28 Jul	10 Nov	15 Dec	28 Aug	11 Dec	15 Jan
28 May	10 Sep	15 Oct	28 Jun	11 Oct	15 Nov	29 Jul	11 Nov	16 Dec	29 Aug	12 Dec	16 Jan
29 May	11 Sep	16 Oct	29 Jun	12 Oct	16 Nov	30 Jul	12 Nov	17 Dec	30 Aug	13 Dec	17 Jan
30 May	12 Sep	17 Oct	30 Jun	13 Oct	17 Nov	31 Jul	13 Nov	18 Dec	31 Aug	14 Dec	18 Jan
31 May	13 Sep	18 Oct	01 Jul	14 Oct	18 Nov	01 Aug	14 Nov	19 Dec	01 Sep	15 Dec	19 Jan
01 Jun	14 Sep	19 Oct	02 Jul	15 Oct	19 Nov	02 Aug	15 Nov	20 Dec	02 Sep	16 Dec	20 Jan
02 Jun	15 Sep	20 Oct	03 Jul	16 Oct	20 Nov	03 Aug	16 Nov	21 Dec	03 Sep	17 Dec	21 Jan
03 Jun	16 Sep	21 Oct	04 Jul	17 Oct	21 Nov	04 Aug	17 Nov	22 Dec	04 Sep	18 Dec	22 Jan
04 Jun	17 Sep	22 Oct	05 Jul	18 Oct	22 Nov	05 Aug	18 Nov	23 Dec			

Table 3.3 (cont.)

Time Window for Expanded AFP Blood Collection

Based on the 1st day of the Last Menstrual Period (LMP)

"Time Window" is from 105th through 140th day (between 15 and 20 weeks). For use during 365-day year

LMP Date	Draw Blood From	Through
Sep 05	Dec 19	Jan 23
Sep 06	Dec 20	Jan 24
Sep 07	Dec 21	Jan 25
Sep 08	Dec 22	Jan 26
Sep 09	Dec 23	Jan 27
Sep 10	Dec 24	Jan 28
Sep 11	Dec 25	Jan 29
Sep 12	Dec 26	Jan 30
Sep 13	Dec 27	Jan 31
Sep 14	Dec 28	Feb 01
Sep 15	Dec 29	Feb 02
Sep 16	Dec 30	Feb 03
Sep 17	Dec 31	Feb 04
Sep 18	Jan 01	Feb 05
Sep 19	Jan 02	Feb 06
Sep 20	Jan 03	Feb 07
Sep 21	Jan 04	Feb 08
Sep 22	Jan 05	Feb 09
Sep 23	Jan 06	Feb 10
Sep 24	Jan 07	Feb 11
Sep 25	Jan 08	Feb 12
Sep 26	Jan 09	Feb 13
Sep 27	Jan 10	Feb 14
Sep 28	Jan 11	Feb 15
Sep 29	Jan 12	Feb 16
Sep 30	Jan 13	Feb 17
Oct 01	Jan 14	Feb 18
Oct 02	Jan 15	Feb 19
Oct 03	Jan 16	Feb 20
Oct 04	Jan 17	Feb 21

LMP Date	Draw Blood From	Through
Oct 05	Jan 18	Feb 22
Oct 06	Jan 19	Feb 23
Oct 07	Jan 20	Feb 24
Oct 08	Jan 21	Feb 25
Oct 09	Jan 22	Feb 26
Oct 10	Jan 23	Feb 27
Oct 11	Jan 24	Feb 28
Oct 12	Jan 25	Mar 01
Oct 13	Jan 26	Mar 02
Oct 14	Jan 27	Mar 03
Oct 15	Jan 28	Mar 04
Oct 16	Jan 29	Mar 05
Oct 17	Jan 30	Mar 06
Oct 18	Jan 31	Mar 07
Oct 19	Feb 01	Mar 08
Oct 20	Feb 02	Mar 09
Oct 21	Feb 03	Mar 10
Oct 22	Feb 04	Mar 11
Oct 23	Feb 05	Mar 12
Oct 24	Feb 06	Mar 13
Oct 25	Feb 07	Mar 14
Oct 26	Feb 08	Mar 15
Oct 27	Feb 09	Mar 16
Oct 28	Feb 10	Mar 17
Oct 29	Feb 11	Mar 18
Oct 30	Feb 12	Mar 19
Oct 31	Feb 13	Mar 20
Nov 01	Feb 14	Mar 21
Nov 02	Feb 15	Mar 22
Nov 03	Feb 16	Mar 23

LMP Date	Draw Blood From	Through
Nov 04	Feb 17	Mar 24
Nov 05	Feb 18	Mar 25
Nov 06	Feb 19	Mar 26
Nov 07	Feb 20	Mar 27
Nov 08	Feb 21	Mar 28
Nov 09	Feb 22	Mar 29
Nov 10	Feb 23	Mar 30
Nov 11	Feb 24	Mar 31
Nov 12	Feb 25	Apr 01
Nov 13	Feb 26	Apr 02
Nov 14	Feb 27	Apr 03
Nov 15	Feb 28	Apr 04
Nov 16	Mar 01	Apr 05
Nov 17	Mar 02	Apr 06
Nov 18	Mar 03	Apr 07
Nov 19	Mar 04	Apr 08
Nov 20	Mar 05	Apr 09
Nov 21	Mar 06	Apr 10
Nov 22	Mar 07	Apr 11
Nov 23	Mar 08	Apr 12
Nov 24	Mar 09	Apr 13
Nov 25	Mar 10	Apr 14
Nov 26	Mar 11	Apr 15
Nov 27	Mar 12	Apr 16
Nov 28	Mar 13	Apr 17
Nov 29	Mar 14	Apr 18
Nov 30	Mar 15	Apr 19
Dec 01	Mar 16	Apr 20
Dec 02	Mar 17	Apr 21
Dec 03	Mar 18	Apr 22

LMP Date	Draw Blood From	Through
Dec 04	Mar 19	Apr 23
Dec 05	Mar 20	Apr 24
Dec 06	Mar 21	Apr 25
Dec 07	Mar 22	Apr 26
Dec 08	Mar 23	Apr 27
Dec 09	Mar 24	Apr 28
Dec 10	Mar 25	Apr 29
Dec 11	Mar 26	Apr 30
Dec 12	Mar 27	May 01
Dec 13	Mar 28	May 02
Dec 14	Mar 29	May 03
Dec 15	Mar 30	May 04
Dec 16	Mar 31	May 05
Dec 17	Apr 01	May 06
Dec 18	Apr 02	May 07
Dec 19	Apr 03	May 08
Dec 20	Apr 04	May 09
Dec 21	Apr 05	May 10
Dec 22	Apr 06	May 11
Dec 23	Apr 07	May 12
Dec 24	Apr 08	May 13
Dec 25	Apr 09	May 14
Dec 26	Apr 10	May 15
Dec 27	Apr 11	May 16
Dec 28	Apr 12	May 17
Dec 29	Apr 13	May 18
Dec 30	Apr 14	May 19
Dec 31	Apr 15	May 20

Source: Reprinted with permission from California Department of Health Services, Genetic Disease Branch. *The California expanded alpha-fetoprotein screening program: Prenatal care provider handbook.* (pp. 29-30). Berkeley, CA: Author.

Table 3.4

Summary of Prenatal Testing Choices

A diagnostic test tells whether or not the fetus actually has a certain birth defect.

A screening test estimates the chances (risk) of the fetus having a certain birth defect. If the risk is high, a woman is referred for diagnostic tests.

Diagnostic Tests Available to Pregnant Women of All Ages				
CVS	10–12 weeks of pregnancy	• Diagnoses 98% of Down syndrome and other chromosomal defects • Not a test for neural tube defects, so an AFP blood test is recommended at 15–20 weeks • Chance of miscarriage is about 1 to 3%	Approx. $1200 to $1800 plus $57 for AFP blood test	
Early Amniocentesis	12–14 weeks of pregnancy	• Diagnoses 99% of Down syndrome and other chromosomal defects • May not diagnose neural tube defects, so an AFP blood test is recommended at 15–20 weeks • Chance of miscarriage is about 1%	Approx $1000 to $1500 plus $57 for AFP blood test	
Amniocentesis	15–20 weeks of pregnancy	• Diagnoses 99% of Down syndrome and other chromosomal defects • Also diagnoses most neural tube defects abdominal wall defects, and some other birth defects • Chance of miscarriage is less than 1%	Approx $1000 to $1500	

Screening Test Available to Women at High Risk for Birth Defects or Women Who Are 35 Years or Older				
Expanded AFP Screening Program (blood tests)	15–20 weeks of pregnancy	• Estimates a woman's chance of having a fetus with Down syndrome or trisomy 18 • Also detects most neural tube defects and abdominal wall defects • If the result is positive, the Program pays for amniocentesis at a State-approved Prenatal Diagnosis Center. • Accurately predicts 70% to 90% of fetuses with Down syndrome in women 35 and older. Will miss detecting some Down syndrome and other chromosomal defects.	$115	

References

American College of Obstetricians and Gynecologists (ACOG). (1991). Alpha-fetoprotein. *(Technical Bulletin No. 154)*. Washington, DC: Author.

Bernstein, I.M., Barth, R.A., Miller, R., & Capeless, E.L. (1992). Elevated maternal serum alpha-fetoprotein: Association with placental sonolucencies, fetomaternal hemorrhage, vaginal bleeding, and pregnancy outcome in the absence of fetal anomalies. *Obstetrics and Gynecology, 79*(1), 71–74.

Bogart, M.H., Pandian, M.A., & Jones, D.W. (1987). Abnormal maternal serum chorionic gonadotropin levels in pregnancies with fetal chromosome abnormalities. *Prenatal Diagnosis, 7*(9), 623–638.

California Department of Health Services, Genetic Disease Branch (1994). *The California expanded Alpha-fetoprotein Screening Program. Prenatal care provider handbook.* Berkeley, CA: Author.

California Department of Health Services, Genetic Disease Branch (1996). *Expanded Alpha-fetoprotein Screening Program update.* Berkeley, CA: Author.

Canick, J.A., Knight, G.J., Palomaki, G.E., Haddow, J.E., Cuckle, H.S., & Wald, N.J. (1988). Low second-trimester maternal serum unconjugated oestriol in pregnancies with Down's syndome. *British Journal of Obstetrics and Gynaecology, 95*(4), 330–333.

Centers for Disease Control and Prevention (CDC). (1995). Surveillance for anencephaly and spina bifida and the impact of prenatal diagnosis—United States, 1985–1994. *Morbidity and Mortality Weekly Report, 44*(SS-4), 1–13.

Chard, T., Lowings, C., & Kitau, M.J. (1984). Alpha-fetoprotein and chorionic gonadotropin levels in relation to Down's syndrome. *Lancet, 2*(8485), 758.

Cheng, E.Y., Luthy, D.A., Zebelman, A.M., Williams, M.A., Lieppman, R.E., & Hickok, D.E. (1992). A prospective evaluation of a second-trimester screening test for fetal Down syndrome using maternal serum alpha-fetoprotein, hCG, and unconjugated estriol. *Obstetrics and Gynecology, 81*(1), 72–77.

Drugan, A., Dvorin, E., Koppitch, F.C., Greb, A., Krivchenia, E.L., & Evans, M.I. (1989). Counseling for low maternal serum alpha-fetoprotein should emphasize all chromosome anomalies, not just Down's syndrome! *Clinical Obstetrics and Gynecology, 73*(2), 271 –274.

Evans, M.I., Chik, L., O'Brien, J.E., Chin, B., Dvorin, E., Ayoub, M., Krivchenia, E.L., Ager, J.W., Johnson, M.P., & Sokol, R.J. (1995). MOMs (multiples of the median) and DADs (discriminant aneuploidy detection): Improved specificity and cost-effectiveness of biochemical screening for aneuploidy with DADs. *American Journal of Obstetrics and Gynecology, 172*(4), 1138–1149.

Haddow, J.E., Palomaki, G.E., Knight, G.J., Cunningham, G.C., Lustig, L.S., & Boyd, P.A. (1994). Reducing the need for amniocentesis in women 35 years of age or older with serum markers for screening. *New England Journal of Medicine, 330*(16), 1114–1118.

Heyl, P.S., Miller, W., & Canick, J.A. (1990). Maternal serum screening for aneuploid pregnancy by alpha-fetoprotein, hCG, and unconjugated estriol. *Obstetrics and Gynecology, 76*(6), 1825–1831.

Hook, E.B. (1981). Rates of chromosome abnormalities at different maternal ages. *Obsetrics and Gynecology, 58*(3), 282–285.

Kellner, L.H., Weiss, R.R., Weiner, Z., Neuer, M., Martin, G.M., Schulman, H., & Lipper, S. (1995). The advantages of using triple-marker screening for chromosomal abnormalities. *American Journal of Obstetrics and Gynecology, 172*(3), 831–836.

Knight, G.J., Palomake, G.E., & Haddow, J.E. (1988). Use of maternal serum alpha-fetoprotein measurements to screen for Down's syndrome. *Clinical Obstetrics and Gynecology, 31*(2), 306–327.

MacDonald, M.L., Wagner, R.M., & Slotnick, R.N. (1991). Sensitivity and specificity of screening for Down syndrome with alpha-fetoprotein, hCG, unconjugated estriol, and maternal age. *Obstetrics and Gynecology, 77*(1), 63–68.

Norgaard-Pedersen, B., Larsen, S.D., Arends, J., Svenstrup, B., & Tabor, A. (1990). Maternal serum markers in screening for Down syndrome. *Clinical Genetics, 37*(1), 35–43.

Palomaki, G.E., Knight, G.J., McCarthy, J., Haddow, J.E., & Eckfeldt, J.H. (1993). Maternal serum screening for fetal Down syndrome in the United States: A 1992 survey. *Obstetrics and Gynecology, 169*(6), 1558–1562.

Phillips, O.P., Elias, S., Shulman, L.P., Andersen, R.N., Morgan, C.D., & Simpson, J.L. (1992). Maternal serum screening for fetal Down syndrome in women less than 35 years of age using alpha-fetoprotein, hCG, and unconjugated estriol: A prospective 2-year study. *Obstetrics and Gynecology,80*(3), 353–358.

Rose, N.C., Palomaki, G.E., Haddow, J.E., Goodman, D.B.P., & Mennuti, M.T. (1994). Maternal serum alpha-fetoprotein screening for chromosomal abnormalities: A prospective study in women aged 35 and older. *American Journal of Obstetrics and Gynecology, 170*(4), 1073–1080.

Wald, N.J., Cuckle, H.S., Densem, J.W., Nanchahal, K., Rayston, P., Chard, T., Haddow, J.E., Knight, G.J., Palomaki, G.E., & Canick, J.A. (1988). Maternal serum screening for Down's syndrome in early pregnancy. *British Medical Journal, 297*(6653), 883–887.

Waller, D.K., Lustig, L.S., Cunningham, G.C., Golbus, M.S., & Hook, E.B. (1991). Second-trimester maternal serum alpha-fetoprotein levels and the risk of subsequent fetal death. *New England Journal of Medicine, 325*(1), 6–10.

Chapter 4

Obstetric Ultrasound

Pilar Bernal de Pheils

Obstetric ultrasound is a safe and noninvasive procedure that obtains information about the fetus and mother to aid in diagnosis and patient management. It also is used in the performance of high-risk perinatal procedures and antenatal fetal surveillance described elsewhere in the book. This technique has replaced X-ray as the primary method of fetal imaging during pregnancy.

Ultrasound is any sound with a frequency of greater than 20,000 hertz (Hz) (undetectable by the human ear). In obstetrical examinations, a frequency of 3 to 5 megahertz (MHz) (3 to 5 million cycles per second) is most commonly used with abdominal transducers, while 5 to 7 MHz is used with transvaginal transducers (American College of Obstetricians and Gynecologists [ACOG], 1993). The two basic types of ultrasound equipment are static and real time. Static scanners produce a "frozen" image from several different points of the examining field. Real-time scanners detect fetal movement, heart activity, and breathing movement, which allows evaluation of structural and functional characteristics of the fetus (ACOG, 1993).

Obstetric ultrasound instrumentation emits sound waves into the abdomen. The sound waves reflect when they collide with tissue or structures with varying densities. The analysis of the reflected sound waves' frequency, length, speed, amplitude, and intensity produces a visible image. The safety level of ultrasound exposure has been defined as less than 100 mW/cm^2. Most obstetric instruments use energy well below this level. There are no studies, to date, that have detected or reported adverse biologic effects of fetal exposure to diagnostic ultrasound (ACOG, 1995; Gabbe, 1994; Grisso et al., 1994; Salvensen, Bakketeig, EiK-Nes, Undheim & Oakland, 1992).

There are two techniques for ultrasound imaging in obstetrics: the transabdominal and the transvaginal procedures. The transabdominal procedure usually requires the client to drink three 8-ounce glasses of clear fluid (no milk) 1 hour prior to the exam to fill the bladder. A full bladder is necessary to elevate the uterus into the abdomen of a client who is not pregnant or who is in her first trimester, permitting optimal visualization of the fetus. The client is instructed not to urinate and that the exam will take between 30 minutes to an hour. In the second or third trimester, a full bladder may not be necessary because the fetus is out of the pelvis. The ultrasound probe, covered with coupling gel, is placed on the abdomen and slowly passed over all four quadrants. The only discomfort may be from the full bladder.

The transvaginal procedure is performed by inserting the probe, covered with a condom and coupling gel, into the vagina. Insertion may be performed by the ultrasonographer or the client. The transvaginal technique, enhanced by a higher sound frequency and by the fact that the sound waves travel to a depth of only 1 to 2 cm before reaching the area to be examined, produces an image with greater resolution than the transabdominal technique. The ability to identify a gestational sac as early as 5 weeks' gestation, thus aiding in the diagnosis of ectopic pregnancies, is the primary advantage of the transvaginal ultrasound. Transvaginal ultrasound also facilitates the diagnosis of cervical incompetence and ovarian lesions, as well as the diagnosis of pregnancy in obese clients (Bromley, Frioletto, & Benacerraf, 1993). The disadvantage of the technique is that insertion of the probe into the vagina makes many women uncomfortable.

First-trimester ultrasound is indicated in the presence of vaginal bleeding; when there is a need to diagnose fetal viability, a multiple pregnancy, or a pelvic mass; and to identify an intrauterine gestational sac (to rule out ectopic pregnancy). Ultrasound can also be used to determine gestational age as early as 6-10 menstrual weeks (with an accuracy to within 3 to 5 days in 95 percent of cases), using crown-rump measurements.

Second-trimester ultrasound is most commonly performed to determine gestational age, particularly when the last menstrual period (LMP) is not exact or unknown, or when there is a discrepancy of more than 3 weeks between the fundal height and LMP. The measurements that best estimate gestational age are the fetal biparietal diameter (BPD), head circumference, and femur length and the mother's abdominal circumference (Nazarian & Kurtz, 1993). BPD measurements up to week 24 are accurate to within 5 to 7 days (Nazarian & Kurtz, 1993). Ultrasonography alone in the first half of pregnancy (less than 24 weeks) has been found to predict delivery date better than calculation from LMP, even when LMP is certain (Mongelli, Wilcox, & Gardosi, 1996). Postponing obstetric ultrasound for the purposes of gestational age determination until 18 to 20 weeks' gestation is beneficial because it also allows for assessment of fetal anatomical malformations (ACOG, 1993).

Third-trimester ultrasound is not as accurate for gestational age calculation because there are large variations in individual fetal growth. The accuracy of the BPD decreases after 30 weeks' gestation to $\pm$ 2 weeks and may approach $\pm$ 4 weeks by term (ACOG, 1993). However, it is possible to estimate fetal growth and weight when measurements of the head, abdomen, and femur can be obtained. If there is concern about fetal growth, serial ultrasounds may be performed as early as 28 weeks' gestation, but not more often than every 2 weeks (ACOG, 1993). Measurement of fetal abdominal circumference in the third trimester of pregnancy (after 34 weeks) is the most accurate test to predict birth weight that will be less than the tenth percentile (Harding, Evans, & Newnham, 1995). Ultrasound in the third trimester is also indicated in the presence of vaginal bleeding to localize the placenta.

The use of routine ultrasound is still under debate (ACOG, 1993). Routine ultrasound at 19 weeks' gestation performed by trained, experienced ultrasonographers has been shown to have a high level of accuracy in the diagnosis of fetal anomalies in an unselected population (Chitty, Hunt, Moore, & Lobb, 1991; Luck, 1992) as well as in high-risk populations (Ott, Arias, Sheldon, Sunderji, & Taysi, 1995). Early identification of fetal anomalies gives health care providers the ability to inform and prepare parents for the child's future needs.

The argument for using ultrasound routinely is supported by the accuracy of dating in the first half of pregnancy. The percentage of incorrectly diagnosed post-term pregnancies is reduced from 11.5 to 3.5 percent (Mongelli et al., 1996). This increase in accuracy could result in financial savings because further precision may reduce induction rates, hospital length-of-stays, and need for medical and surgical intervention. On the other hand, the majority of randomized control trials have not demonstrated evidence of improved maternal or perinatal outcome because fetal structural and growth anomalies, multiple pregnancies or gestational age measurements were more accurately determined (Ewigman, et al., 1993; LeFevre, et al., 1993). The argument against routine ultrasound in these studies is viewed from the perspective of cost versus benefit. The increase in costs of routinely screening all pregnancies has not shown a positive cost-benefit and, in fact, may diminish the availability of resources for other interventions that demonstrate positive impact on maternal-fetal health.

Although routine use of ultrasound during pregnancy is not recommended in the United States as of this writing (ACOG, 1993; Cunningham, MacDonald, Gant, Leven, & Gilstrap, 1993), this diagnostic modality is commonly used in many institutions (Ott et al., 1995). Skupski, Chervenak, and McCullough (1994) argue strongly that use of routine ultrasound is supported by the principles of beneficence and respect of autonomy. These are defined as "an ethical principle that requires the physician to act in a way that produces no harm for the patient," and "an ethical principle that requires the physician to acknowledge the integrity of the patient's values and beliefs, to elicit her preferences, and to carry out those performances," respectively (Chervenak & McCullough 1993).

Database

Subjective

- Indications for use of ultrasound during pregnancy may include the following (ACOG, 1993):

  ▶ Estimation of gestational age for clients with

    – Uncertain dates

    – History of irregular menstrual cycles

    – History of oral contraceptive or fertility drug use with last menstrual cycle

  ▶ Verification of dates for clients who are to undergo scheduled, elective repeat cesarean delivery; induction of labor; or elective termination of pregnancy

  ▶ Evaluation of fetal growth when intrauterine growth restriction is suspected or if there is a history of small-for-gestational-age baby

  ▶ Evaluation of fetal condition for late registrants for prenatal care

  ▶ Vaginal bleeding of unknown origin

  ▶ Suspected ectopic pregnancy

  ▶ Suspected hydatidiform mole

  ▶ Possible abruptio placenta or previa

  ▶ Follow-up for evaluation of placental localization of identified placenta previa

  ▶ Pelvic mass

  ▶ Suspected uterine anomaly

  ▶ Suspected fetal demise

  ▶ Abnormal maternal serum alpha-fetoprotein value

  ▶ Determination of fetal presentation

  ▶ Suspected polyhydramnios or oligohydramnios

  ▶ Significant uterine size/date discrepancy (at least 3 weeks discrepancy)

  ▶ Suspected multiple gestation

  ▶ Estimation of fetal weight and/or presentation in premature rupture of membranes and/or premature labor

▶ History of previous congenital anomaly

▶ Follow-up observation of identified fetal anomaly

▶ Observation of intrapartum events

▶ Antenatal maternal conditions known to affect fetal growth (diabetes mellitus, preexisting hypertension, renal disease)

- Obstetric ultrasound is also used as an adjunct to special procedures.

   ▶ Cervical cerclage

   ▶ Suspected cervical incompetence

   ▶ External version

   ▶ Manual removal of placenta

   ▶ Intrauterine transfusion

   ▶ Percutaneous umbilical blood sampling

   ▶ Amniocentesis

   ▶ Chorionic villus sampling (CVS)

   ▶ In vitro fertilization

   ▶ IUD localization

   ▶ Ovarian follicle surveillance

   ▶ Biophysical profile

Objective

- Basic ultrasound should provide the following information (ACOG, 1993; Cunningham, MacDonald, Grant, Leveno, & Gilstrap, 1993)

   ▶ First trimester

      - Gestational sac location

      - Embryo identification

      - Crown-rump length

      - Fetal heart motion

      - Fetal number

      - Uterus and adnexal evaluation

   ▶ Second and third trimesters

      - Fetal number

      - Fetal presentation

      - Documentation of fetal life

      - Placental location

- – Assessment of amniotic fluid volume
- – Assessment of gestational age/estimation of fetal weight
- – Survey for gross malformations
- – Evaluation for maternal pelvic masses

- Second and third trimester examinations should provide information regarding abnormal findings in the survey of the following fetal anatomical structures (ACOG, 1993):

  ▶ Cerebral ventricles

  ▶ Four chambers of the heart and the heart's position within the thorax

  ▶ Spine

  ▶ Stomach

  ▶ Urinary bladder

  ▶ Umbilical cord insertion site on the anterior abdominal wall

  ▶ Kidneys

- Comprehensive fetal anatomical surveys may not be possible in the presence of oligohydramnios, hyperflexed fetus, engaged fetal heat, compression of fetal body parts, or maternal obesity.

- A *limited* obstetric ultrasound (avoiding survey for gross malformations) may be indicated for the following reasons:

  ▶ Assessment of amniotic fluid volume

  ▶ Biophysical profile

  ▶ Determination of fetal lie or presentation

  ▶ Confirmation of fetal life or death

  ▶ Special procedures, such as amniocentesis or external cephalic version

  ▶ A client who has had a previous basic ultrasound or comprehensive anatomical survey examination in the second trimester

  ▶ Determination of multiple gestation

  ▶ Estimation of gestational age and weight in an emergency situation

  ▶ For urgent evaluation of antepartal or intrapartal problems (e.g., hemorrhage)

Assessment

- IUP at _____ weeks by obstetric ultrasound
- Identification of abnormal conditions of the fetus, placenta, umbilical cord, amniotic fluid, pelvic structures, etc.

Plan

Diagnostic Tests

Basic ultrasound should be performed by a trained provider (Seeds, 1992).

- Basic ultrasound is indicated for the following:
  - ▶ Documentation of fetal life
  - ▶ Fetal number and presentation
  - ▶ Evaluation of gestational age, amniotic fluid, and maternal pelvic masses
  - ▶ Placental localization
  - ▶ Fetal survey, when performed beyond 18 weeks' gestational age
- Comprehensive ultrasound examination is indicated for the evaluation of specific suspected fetal malformations and should be performed by an operator experienced in this type of sophisticated scanning.
- Limited ultrasound examination is employed when a previous basic ultrasound has been performed to obtain specific limited information
  - ▶ For urgent evaluation of antenatal or intrapartal problems (e.g., hemorrhage)
  - ▶ For use with a biophysical profile

Treatment/Management

- Continue routine prenatal care for women whose obstetric ultrasound is within normal limits.
- Manage clients with identified abnormal fetal or maternal conditions according to the recommendations for the specific condition. See specific chapters for specific conditions.

Consultation

- Consult with and refer to a physician clients with abnormal obstetrical ultrasound findings.

Patient Education

- Discuss the limitations of ultrasound in detecting all fetal anomalies (Chervanak & McCullough, 1993).
- Advise client not to empty her bladder at least 1 hour before the procedure. Some institutions advise ingestion of up to three 8-ounce glasses of water 1 hour prior to the procedure if abdominal ultrasound is performed before the second or third trimester.
- Discuss results with client based on the findings and concern of the woman.

Follow-up

- Provide emotional support to the woman and her family when an abnormal obstetric ultrasound result is obtained.

- Refer women with structural fetal malformations to a social worker or counselor, as appropriate.

- Document any abnormality or problem reported in the obstetric ultrasound on the problem list and in the progress notes.

References

American College of Obstetrics and Gynecologists (ACOG). (1993, December). Ultrasonography in pregnancy. (Technical Bulletin No. 187). *International Journal of Gynecology & Obstetrics, 44,* 173–183.

American College of Obstetrics and Gynecologists (ACOG). (1995, September). *Guidelines for Diagnostic Imaging during Pregnancy.* (Committee Opinion No. 158). Washington DC: Author.

Bromley, B., Frigoletto, F.D., & Benacerraf, B.R. (1993). Pitfalls and opportunities in fetal sonography. *Contemporary OB/GYN, 38,* 22–37.

Chervenak, F.A., & McCullough, L.B. (1993). The importance of ethics to the practice of obstetric ultrasound. *Annals of Medicine, 25,* 271–273.

Chitty, L.S., Hunt, G.H., Moore, J., & Lobb, M.O. (1991). Effectiveness of routine ultrasonography in detecting fetal structrual abnormalities in a low-risk population. *British Medical Journal. 303*(6811), 1165–1169.

Cunningham, F.G., MacDonald, P.C., Gant, N.F., Leveno, K.L., & Gilstrap, K.L. (1993). Ultrasound in obstetrics. *Williams Obstetrics* (19th ed., pp. 1045–1063). Norwalk, CT: Appleton & Lange.

Ewigman, B., Crane, J.P., Frigoletto, F.D., LeFevre, M.L., Bain, R.P., & McNellis, D. (1993). A randomized trial of prenatal ultrasound screening: Impact on perinatal outcome. *New England Journal of Medicine, 329,* 821–827.

Gabbe, S.G. (1994). Routine versus indicated scans. In R.E. Sabbagha (Ed.), *Diagnostic ultrasound applied to obstetrics and gynecology* (3rd ed.). Philadelphia, PA: J.B. Lippincott.

Grisso, J.A., Strom, B.L., Cosmatos, I., Tolsa, J., Main, D., & Carson, J. (1994). Diagnostic ultrasound in pregnancy and low birth weight. *American Journal of Perinatology, 11*(4), 297–301.

Harding, K., Evans, S., & Newnham, N. (1995). Screening for the small fetus: A study of the relative efficacies of ultrasound biometry and symphysiofundal height. *Australian and New Zealand Journal of Obstetrics and Gynecology, 35*(2), 160–164.

LeFevre, M.L., Bain, R.P., Ewigman, B.G., Frigoletto, F.D., Crane, J.P., McNellis, D., & the Routine Antenatal Diagnostic Imaging with Ultrasound (RADIUS) Study Group. (1993). A randomized trial of prenatal ultrasonographic screening: Impact on maternal management and outcome. *American Journal of Obstetrics and Gynecology, 169*(3), 483489.

Luck, C.A. (1992). Value of routine ultrasound scanning at 19 weeks: A four-year study of 8,849 deliveries. *British Medical Journal, 304,* 1474–1478.

Mongelli, M., Wilcox, M., & Gardosi, J. (1996). Estimating the date of confinement: Ultrasonographic biometry versus certain menstrual dates. *American Journal of Obstetrics and Gynecology, 174,* 278–281.

Nazarian, L.V., & Kurtz, A.B. (1993). Routine ultrasound of the pregnant uterus. *Seminars in Ultrasound, CT, and MRI, 14*(1), 3–22.

Ott, W.J., Arias, F., Sheldon, G., Sunderji, S., & Taysi, K. (1995). Comprehensive ultrasound evaluation in a private practice. *American Journal of Perinatology, 12*(6), 385–391.

Salvensen, K.A., Bakketeig, L.S., Eik-Nes, S.H., Undheim, J.O., & Oakland, O. (1992). Routine ultrasonography in utero and school performance at age 8–9 years. *Lancet, 339,* 85–89.

Seeds, J.W. (1992). Commentary: Who should perform sonograms? Those with the skills and experience to provide complete and accurate service. *Birth, 19*(2), 101–102.

Skupski, D.W., Chevernak, F.A., & McCullough, L.B. (1994). Is routine ultrasound screening for all patients? *Clinics in Perinatology, 21*(4), 707–722.

Chapter 5

ANTEPARTUM FETAL SURVEILLANCE

Lisa L. Lommel

Pilar Bernal de Pheils

Fetal surveillance evaluates fetal well-being in high-risk populations. Its major goal is to reduce fetal demise in those populations at high risk for this complication (American College of Obstetricians and Gynecologists [ACOG], 1994). Fetal heart rate monitoring, ultrasonography, and fetal movement assessment are the most commonly utilized surveillance techniques for the evaluation of fetal well-being. The previously used indirect biochemical tests, the human placental lactogen levels and serial estriol levels, have been replaced by direct biophysical testing of the fetus. Doppler flow assessment is the most recent technique introduced for the evaluation of fetal well-being and has been shown to correlate well with antenatal fetal compromise. This assessment may involve additional resources without an added benefit, however, (Johnstone, et al., 1993), and hence remains an investigational technique (ACOG, 1994).

The primary indication for surveillance testing of fetal well-being is the high-risk pregnancy. There are a variety of conditions that require testing by a trained health care provider. They include (ACOG, 1994; University of California, San Francisco (UCSF), 1994):

- Hypertensive disorders (except for chronic hypertension without superimposed pre-eclampsia and normal fetal growth)

- Diabetes mellitus (insulin dependent)

- Suspected oligohydramnios

- Intrauterine growth retardation (< 10th percentile)

- Prolonged pregnancy (≥ 42 weeks)— some centers begin surveillance at 41 to 41.5 weeks

- Isoimmunization (moderate to severe)

- Chronic renal disease

- Maternal cyanotic heart disease

- Hemoglobinopathies (e.g., SC, S-Thal)

- Multiple gestation with significant discordant growth (greater than 20 percent discrepancy)

- Previous unexplained fetal demise

- Decreased fetal movement (maternal perception)

- Preterm premature rupture of membranes

- Vaginal bleeding

- Systemic lupus erythematous or antiphospholipid syndrome

- Severe polyhydramnios

- Cholestasis of pregnancy with objective evidence

- Increase maternal serum alpha fetoprotein (MSAFP) with normal amniocentesis

- Hyperthyroidism

- Active drug/alcohol abuse

The choice of surveillance test to evaluate fetal well-being will vary, but there are important points that should be considered when choosing the most appropriate test. These include the availability of the test client compliance, early predictability of fetal compromise, and the rate of the test's false-positive results and false-negative results.

The initiation of testing depends upon the prognosis for neonatal survival (cumulative risk of fetal death and gestational week specific probability of fetal death) and the specificity of the test (Rouse, Owen, Goldberger, & Cliver, 1995). The frequency of testing depends upon the severity, timing, and number of clinical conditions. Generally, with multiple or severe high-risk conditions, testing may begin as early as 26 to 28 weeks when there is a possibility of extrauterine survival. In these cases, the criteria for interpretation of the contraction stress test and the biophysical profile (see below) appear to be valid (ACOG, 1994). In most high-risk pregnancies, testing usually begins at 32 to 34 weeks gestation or when evidence of fetoplacental compromise is found. The frequency of repeat testing is every 7 days unless the previous test was abnormal or specific conditions necessitate more frequent surveillance (i.e., post date pregnancy, insulin-dependent diabetes, or intrauterine growth restriction) (ACOG, 1994). Refer to protocols of specific conditions for fetal surveillance manage-ment recommendations.

Pregnancies monitored by surveillance tests should be co-managed by a physician. For specific conditions, such as insulin-dependent diabetes, management may be provided primarily by the physician. Management of abnormal tests requires further evaluation or delivery as appropriate. In the absence of obstetric contraindications, delivery of a fetus with an abnormal test is usually attempted by induction of labor. Cesarean delivery may be indicated for obstetric complications or with abnormal fetal heart rates. Descriptions of each of the common antepartum fetal surveillance tests follow below.

Fetal Movement Counts

Although fetal activity has been recognized with ultrasound as early as 6 weeks gestational age (American Institute of Ultrasound in Medicine [AIUM], 1991), the majority of women feel fetal movements between 16 to 20 weeks' gestational age. Early fetal movements are weak, infrequent, and sometimes difficult to distinguish from abdominal movements of the intestines. Fetal activity increases in strength and is most frequent between 20 and 39 weeks of gestation. A decline in the number of fetal movements is expected to occur within weeks of delivery but maternally perceived fetal movement does not significantly change in the healthy fetus (Rayburn,

1990). The average number of recorded daily fetal movements varies between 4 and 1,440. Most women perceive a certain number of movements daily that stay fairly constant throughout the pregnancy (Sadovsky & Polishuk, 1977). Fetal movement is greatest during the late night hours (between 9:00 PM and 1:00 AM), when compared to the rest of the day (Patrick, Campbell, Carmichael, & Probert, 1982).

Fetal movements may be altered by maternal ingestion of medications and cigarette smoke. Sedatives such as barbiturates, benzodiazepines, narcotics, methadone, and alcohol cross the placenta, causing a reduction in the number and duration of fetal movements. Nicotine has a depressant effect on the fetal nervous systems causing a temporary reduction in fetal gross body movement and breathing (Goodman, Visser, & Dawes, 1984). Altered fetal body movement will usually reverse after drug clearance (Rayburn, 1990). A transitory reduction or cessation of fetal movements has been observed with the administration of steroids for the enhancement of fetal lung maturity (Katz, et al., 1988).

Maternally perceived fetal activity is used as an indicator of fetal well-being. Maternal recording of fetal activity near term correlates with approximately 85 percent of motions recorded by ultrasound (Cunningham, MacDonald, Gant, Leveno, Gilstrap, 1993). A drop or decrease in fetal activity is associated with fetal distress, especially when chronic uteroplacental insufficiency is present (Rayburn, 1990). If the fetal distress is severe enough to cause intrauterine fetal demise, fetal movements may rapidly diminish and stop 12 to 48 hours before death (Pearson & Weaver, 1976).

Fetal movement monitoring is used as a generally acceptable, noninvasive, cost-effective method of fetal surveillance in high- and low-risk pregnancies. Because a large proportion of stillbirths occur at term in pregnancies that were not classified as high risk, monitoring should be done on all pregnant women starting at 28 weeks' gestation (Moore & Piacquadio, 1989; Neldman, 1980). The specificity of fetal movement counting is considered high (90 to 95 percent) with only a moderate sensitivity of 50 to 70 percent (Newton, 1989). Given the high rate of false-positive testing, it is recommended that an abnormal fetal movement count be followed by additional evaluation (e.g., electronic fetal monitoring or biophysical profile).

Several techniques and methods of quantification for evaluating fetal movements have been proposed; however, no one technique has been shown to improve compliance or acceptability over another (Comeford, Freda et al., 1993). Furthermore, the ideal number of kicks recorded by the mother, as well as the time interval for movement count, has not been defined. What is considered to be most important is the maternal perception of decreased activity level compared with a perception of previous fetal movements (ACOG, 1994). One of the most commonly used methods is the count-to-ten method, which has been well accepted by pregnant women (Smith, Davis, & Rayburn, 1992). It proposes that less than ten fetal movements in 2 hours is inadequate and should be followed by additional fetal surveillance (Moore & Piacquadio, 1989). Education includes advising all patients beginning at 28 weeks' gestation to record daily the time it takes to count ten fetal movements (rolling, stretching, kicking, jabbing, punching, hiccuping, or flutters). In the healthy fetus, ten movements are usually felt within 10 to 60 minutes. Advise the client to monitor movements at the same time every day, preferably after eating a meal. Teach her to rest in the lateral recumbent position with her hands extending over the abdomen. External stimuli should be reduced so she can concentrate on the movements. The client should call her health care provider if 10 movements have not been felt within a two-hour period. See Table 3.5, Example of Kick Count Record.

Nonstress Test

It has been well established and accepted that fetal heart rate increases during periods of fetal movement. The premise for the nonstress test (NST) is that the normal fetus demonstrates movement at varying intervals and that the fetal central nervous system and myocardium responds to this movement in a reflex action by demonstrating fetal heart-rate accelerations. An increase in fetal heart rate during movement is accepted as a sign of fetal well-being. A fetus that fails to show fetal heart rate accelerations may be at risk for or suffering from hypoxemia.

Interpretation of criteria for reactivity of the NST vary widely. The most commonly accepted criteria are as follows (Ware & Devoe, 1994):

- Reactive pattern (normal NST) is defined as the presence of two accelerations, lasting 15 seconds or more and reaching a zenith 15 beats or more per minute (bpm) within a 20-minute period.

- Nonreactive pattern (abnormal NST) fails to meet any one criterion over a 40-minute period.

Nonreactive tests should be followed immediately by a contraction stress test or biophysical profile. Reactive NSTs are usually repeated in 7 days and twice weekly in patients with insulin-dependent diabetes with poor control, prolonged pregnancy, or intrauterine growth retardation (Keegan, 1987). NST criteria for evaluating fetuses less than 32 to 34 weeks' gestational age should be analyzed with caution and multiple parameter biophysical testing should be performed when there is an abnormal NST tracing at very early gestations (28 to 32 weeks) (Ware & Devoe, 1994). Low-risk patients with a perception of decreased fetal movements and a reactive NST do not require further testing unless there is further complaint of decreased fetal movement (Whitty, Garfield, & Divon, 1991).

The NST is the most commonly used antepartum fetal surveillance test. It is currently recommended in most high-risk obstetric conditions in combination with amniotic fluid volume evaluation (Ware & Devoe, 1994). When compared to other test techniques, the NST has many advantages:

- Less time consuming

- Less costly

- No contraindications

- Easier to interpret

- Does not require frequent repeat testing for suspicious or hyperstimulation test results

- Can be employed in an outpatient setting

- Is reassuring when it is reactive (less than 1 percent chance of fetal death within one week of reactive NST) (Field, 1989).

The major disadvantage of the NST is its high false-positive rate (nonreactive NST with a normal outcome). The false-positive rate averages 58 percent, test specificity averages 45 percent, and false-negative rates generally are less than 10 percent (Devoe, 1990). The major reason for high false-positive rates is the nonuniformity of what is interpreted as normal fetal reactivity. Other factors that increase the false-positive rates include gestational age of less than 30 weeks, relative sleep-wake cycles of the fetus, and maternal ingestion of depressant drugs including alcohol and nicotine.

The NST is performed with the woman in the semi-Fowler's position. The patient should be nonfasting and have not smoked recently. The fetal heart rate is monitored with an ultrasound transducer for approximately 20 minutes. If no accelerations occur within 20 minutes, the monitoring is continued for 40 minutes to account for fetal sleep-wake cycles. Various techniques have been used to stimulate the fetus to achieve reactivity. Fetal vibroacoustic stimulation (FVAS) has been the only technique to show a meaningful impact on the outcome of the non-stress test (Smith, 1994). The FVAS technique includes the application of a vibratory device on the maternal abdomen overlying the fetus. Sound and vibration are used to startle the fetus, thereby accelerating its heart rate. It has been shown to elicit fetal heart rate accelerations, thus decreasing the high false-positive rate of the NST (Zimmer & Divon, 1993). There is some evidence that the FVAS technique causes pain and stress in the fetus (Visser, Mulder, Mulder, Wit, & Prechtl, 1989; Zimmer, Chao, Guy, Marks, & Fifer, 1992), and despite the fact that it has been found to have had no effect in four-year-old children when measured by neurologic development or hearing loss (Nyman, Barr & Westgren, 1992), its safety is still under investigation (Zimmer & Divon, 1993). When FVAS is used, its application is recommended after 10 minutes of a nonreactive pattern, initially stimulating the fetus for 1 second and then waiting for 1 minute. If the fetus is still nonreactive, the fetus can be stimulated up to two more times for a 2-second duration, with an interval of 1 minute. Failure to become reactive requires further evaluation (UCSF, 1994).

Contraction Stress Test

The contraction stress test (CST) is based on the observation of fetal heart rate response to uterine contractions. The premise for the test is that the fetus that is beginning to develop marginal basal oxygenation with the ordinary hypoxic stresses of normal uterine contractions will manifest decelerations (Huddleston & Quinland, 1987). Recurrent late decelerations indicate that the fetus has suboptimal oxygenation of its blood. The absence of late decelerations is considered to be a sign of fetal well-being.

The CST is performed with the patient in the semi-Fowler's or lateral tilt position to prevent maternal hypotension and decrease of uterine blood flow (ACOG, 1994). The fetal heart rate is obtained with an ultrasound transducer, and contraction activity is monitored with a tocodynamo-meter. A baseline tracing is obtained for 15 to 20 minutes. No uterine stimulation is needed if adequate uterine contractions are present spontaneously. Adequate contractions are defined as at least three contractions of 40 seconds duration within a 10-minute period of time. If fewer than three contractions of at least 40 seconds duration are observed, uterine stimulation can be produced by oxytocin infusion (oxytocin challenge test, [OCT]) or manual nipple massage (breast self-stimulation test, [BSST]). Breast self-stimulation is generally more acceptable than OCT because of the increased discomfort and cost associated with the OCT. If the BSST is inadequate in producing the desired contractions, an intravenous oxytocin infusion is given at a rate 0.5 milliunits/minute and doubled every 15 to 20 minutes until adequate contractions are achieved. The BSST is accomplished by instructing the patient to rub one nipple, through her clothing, in a to-and-fro motion with the palmar surface of her fingers, rapidly but gently for 2 minutes or until contractions begin. Stimulation is then stopped for 5 minutes to evaluate uterine activity. If three 40- to 60-second contractions do not occur within 10 minutes, another cycle of 2 minutes of stimulation and 5 minutes of rest is started. Stimulation should be discontinued if contractions begin. It takes approximately

40 minutes to complete BSST including a baseline tracing of 15 to 20 minutes.   The success rate of adequate uterine activity with the BSST is 80 to 100 percent (Huddleston, Sutliff, & Robinson, 1984), with the added benefit of reduced cost and shortened testing times (Cunningham, et al., 1993).

Interpretation and management of the CST is as follows (ACOG, 1994), (Cunningham, et al., 1993):

- Negative CST (normal): There are no late decelerations.   Repeat test in one week.

- Positive CST (abnormal): Late decelerations are seen with 50 percent or more contractions. Requires further evaluation or delivery.

- Suspicious or equivocal CST: Late decelerations are seen with less than 50 percent of all contractions.   Requires further evaluation *and* repeat CST within 24 hours.   Repeat suspicious tests are most often negative.   Only 10 to 15 percent become positive in repeated testing (Huddleston & Quinlan, 1987).

- Hyperstimulated CST: There are late decelerations and the uterine contractions are closer together than every 2 minutes or last longer than 90 seconds.   No late decelerations with excessive contractions is considered negative.   Repeat test within 24 hours.

- Unsatisfactory CST: The quality of tracing is inadequate for accurate interpretation or adequate uterine activity cannot be achieved.

Most institutions have replaced the CST with the NST and amniotic fluid volume evaluation as the primary screening tool for uteroplacental insufficiency (Miller, Rabello & Paul, 1996; Smoleniec & James, 1992).

The major advantages of the CST are

- Low false-negative rate of 1 percent (Huddleston & Quinlan, 1987)

- False-positive rate of 50 percent, which is lower than that of the NST

- False-positive rate that does not increase at gestational ages less than 33 weeks (Gabbe, Freeman & Goebelsman, 1978)

- Negative CST, which is associated with a lower antepartum fetal death rate within 1 week after testing compared to the NST (Freeman, 1987)

- The CST appears to be a more sensitive indicator of fetal hypoxia and acidosis making it a better long-range predictor of uteroplacental deterioration (Freeman, 1987).

Contraindications to the CST include clinical conditions that would preclude stimulating uterine contractions

- Known placenta previa

- Previous uterine scar (classical scar)

- Conditions for which risk of preterm delivery is increased (i.e., premature rupture of the membranes, multiple gestation, incompetent cervix, hydramnios, previous preterm delivery) (McCaul & Morrison, 1990)

Additional disadvantages of the CST include

- Need for I.V. infusion if OCT is performed
- Need for hospital-based setting in which to perform the test
- Increased cost compared to the NST
- Large number of equivocal results (10 to 25 percent) (Porto, 1987)
- Difficulty in interpreting the results
- Length of time required to complete the test

The OCT can take 1 to 2 hours, while the BSST has a shorter test time, which reduces the cost of testing.

Biophysical Profile

The Biophysical Profile (BPP) has evolved with the introduction of real-time ultrasonography, allowing the evaluation of multiple biophysical activity other than the fetal heart rate. The components of the BPP include the non-stress test (NST) and four ultrasound parameters: Fetal Breathing Movements (FBM), Body Movement (FM), Tone (FT), and Amniotic Fluid Volume (AFV) (ACOG, 1994). The NST is performed and interpreted according to the criteria outlined in the section for NST. Real-time ultrasound is used to evaluate the remaining variables. Ultrasound observation is continued until the variable becomes normal or when 30 minutes have elapsed.

There are currently two types of scoring systems

- Each variable is either normal (score=2) or abnormal (score=0) (Table 3.6, Technique of Biophysical Profile Scoring)
- Each variable receives a score of 0, 1, or 2 (Table, 3.7, Criteria for Scoring Biophysical Variables). Placental grading has been introduced as a sixth variable in the BPP because of the association of placental grade 3 with abnormal heart rate patterns and abruption during labor. Since the incidence of fetal distress and perinatal death has remained the same, this variable has not been found to be a significant prognostic test (Finberg, Kurtz, Johnson, & Wapner, 1990).

The pathophysiological explanation of the biophysical variables is based on the "gradual hypoxia concept" (Vintzileos, Campbell & Rodis, 1994). The components of the BPP combine acute and chronic markers. Fetal heart rate, fetal breathing movements, fetal movements, and fetal tone are considered to be acute markers. Amniotic fluid and placental grading are considered to be chronic markers. Of the acute markers, fetal heart rate reactivity and fetal breathing movements are the first biophysical variables to become compromised during uterine hypoxia and acidosis (mild hypoxemia). Cessation of fetal movements and, finally, loss of fetal tone are associated with progressively more profound hypoxemia. Consider the gradual hypoxia concept when interpreting the biophysical parameters because of the different degrees of sensitivity to acidemia.

- The nonreactive NST and absence of fetal breathing indicates early stage fetal acidemia.
- The absence of fetal movements and tone are late manifestations of fetal asphyxia.

- The normal findings of all biophysical parameters rule out fetal hypoxia. However, the absence of biophysical activity is not always the result of fetal hypoxia and acidosis. In such cases, it is necessary to rule out factors such as normal periodicity and maternal depressant medication, such as sedatives, before attributing the effect to fetal hypoxia (Vintzileos et al., 1994).

Guidelines for obstetric management based on the BPP score have been developed. It is recommended to use this protocol as a guide and to individualize management according to the patient and her presenting condition. See Table 3.8, Biophysical Profile Scoring: Management Protocol, for the BPP management protocol.

The major advantage of the BPP is a lower false-positive rate when compared to the single variable tests. The single variable tests (NST, CST) are accurate predictors of normal fetal condition (false-negative rate of less than 1 percent and up to 2.7 percent) but are relatively inaccurate in predicting the fetus at risk for poor outcome (high false-positive rates of 50 percent to more than 75 percent), (Vintzileos et. al., 1994). Using a combination of variables, the BPP has a greater ability to accurately identify the sick fetus. The BPP provides other useful information with regard to fetal number and position, placental location and grading, risks of intrauterine growth restriction (IUGR) where oligohydramnios is common, and identification of major congenital anomalies (Brar, Platt, & DeVore, 1987). The BPP may be used as a confirmatory test for the fetus with an abnormal NST and amniotic fluid index (Nageotte, Towers, Asrat, & Freeman, 1994), which may prevent unnecessary intervention when well-being is assured. When performed by trained personnel, the BPP can be completed in as little as 20 minutes.

Limitations of the BPP include

- Lack of knowledge regarding the sequelae of fetuses with low scores
- How the duration and frequency of hypoxia will affect the fetus
- The relative weight of each of the scoring criteria (i.e., whether the absence of fetal movement or amniotic fluid volume has the same significance as the absence of fetal breathing movements and a non-reactive NST) (Manning, Morrison, Lange, & Harman, 1982).

A major disadvantage of the BPP is that it requires sonographic skills for interpretation and it may be more costly and time consuming than the single variable tests. These factors may make it too cumbersome for use as a primary mode of fetal surveillance in some settings. The modified BPP (NST and amniotic fluid assessment) has been shown to be quicker and at least as effective as a full BPP or a CST (Miller et al., 1996). With the modified BPP, assessment of fetal breathing, body movement, and tone are reserved for cases when the NST is nonreactive (Vintzileos, Campbell, Nochimson, & Weinbaum, 1987).

Amniotic Fluid Volume and the Modified Biophysical Profile

Amniotic Fluid Volume

The evaluation of amniotic fluid is another important tool in the assessment of fetal well-being and fetal surveillance. Poor pregnancy outcome, such as intrauterine growth restriction, post-term pregnancy and fetal distress in labor, have been associated with abnormalities of amniotic fluid volume (Berg & Devoe, 1994). Fetal urine output and fetal swallowing are the major determinants of amniotic fluid volume. It has been hypothesized that oligohydramnios may be the result of diminished urinary fetal output caused by fetal hypoxemia (Nicolaides et al., 1990) and that placental insufficiency may cause hypoxemia and hence oligohydramnios (Campbell, Wladimiroff & Dewhurst, 1973). Therefore, assessment of long-term uteroplacental function may be performed by evaluating amniotic fluid volume (ACOG, 1994).

With the introduction of ultrasound, the evaluation of the amniotic fluid volume has moved away from invasive techniques to indirect measurements that provide an estimate of the amniotic fluid volume. The techniques most recognized are the subjective assessment, the maximum vertical pocket, and the amniotic fluid index (Williams, 1993).

The subjective assessment of amniotic fluid volume is widely used by ultrasonographers in the evaluation of the fetal compartment. The clinician observes the fluid in the gestational sac of the entire uterus with real-time ultrasound. An overall sense of overcrowding of the fetus, the obvious lack of amniotic fluid, and/or the inability to identify any significant pocket of fluid in any sector of the uterus is assessed subjectively as decreased amniotic fluid. Excessive fluid assessment is subjectively defined when there is an obvious excess of fluid and when the fetal trunk can be placed comfortably in a fluid pocket of a transverse ultrasound, performed at various levels of the uterine cavity (Williams, 1993). The fluid is subjectively classified as normal, high, or low for gestational age. When the subjective evaluation of the amniotic fluid volume is either increased or decreased, it is suggested an amniotic fluid index (see below) be performed for confirmation of the subjective impression (Hallack, Kirshon, Smith, Evans, & Cotton, 1993). The advantage of this method is that it is fast and efficient and takes into account the amniotic fluid volume variations related to gestational age. Disadvantages include unreliability if the operator is inexperienced and difficulty in documenting the findings of fluid (i.e., low, normal or high), such as in cases when the operator does not make the final report or when the fluid is followed over repeated scans (Doubilet & Benson, 1994).

Assessment of the maximum vertical pocket is done by identifying the largest pocket of amniotic fluid. A measurement of the depth of a pocket is done at right angles to the uterine contour. A maximum vertical pocket of less than 2 centimeters indicates oligohydramnios; greater than 8 centimeters indicates polyhydramnios (see Chapter 6.21, *Oligohydramnios,* and Chapter 6.22, *Polyhydraminios*) (Williams,1993).

The disadvantages of this method include

- The difficulty in accurately calculating amniotic fluid volume with a single measurement in such a highly irregular shape as that occupied by the amniotic fluid

- Variation of this measurement if the fetus changes position

- Variation of the fluid with gestational age

- Measurements of deep but thin pockets alongside the fetus or between the fetal legs, which may yield a normal value in the presence of severe oligohydramnios (Doubliet & Benson, 1994).

Assessment of the amniotic fluid index (AFI) is determined by dividing the maternal abdomen into four quadrants by sagittal and transverse lines through the umbilicus. A linear ultrasound transducer is placed along the longitudinal axis of the mother and perpendicular to the floor. Vertical dimensions of the deepest pocket that are not occupied by more than 50 percent of the umbilical cord or fetal extremities are measured in milliliters in each quadrant. The AFI is the sum of each four measurements. Mean values of the AFI has been described based on longitudinal and cross-sectional measurements from the second trimester of pregnancy (Berg & Devoe, 1994; Nwosu,

Welch, Manasse & Walkinshaw, 1993), and although it varies slightly with gestational age the normal range is considered to be between 5.1 cm to 24 cm.

The UCSF Guidelines for Fetal Surveillance (1994) AFI results are defined as follows:

≤ 5 cm	Oligohydramnios
5.1 to 8 cm	Low Normal
8.1 to 24 cm	Normal
> 24 cm	Polyhydramnios

When the AFI is normal (8.1 to 24 cm), repeat the test every 7 days. For women 41 weeks' gestational age or more, the test should be repeated twice a week (the risk of oligohydramnios is very low). If the measurement is low normal (5.1 to 8) a scheme of twice weekly is recommended (Wing, Fishman, Gonzalez, & Paul, 1996). An AFI of ≤ 5 requires further evaluation (BPP or CST) or delivery. Maternal hydration has been demonstrated to increase AFI in women with decreased amniotic fluid index (Kilpatrick et al., 1991).

There are conflicting studies on the superiority of semiquantitative evaluations of the amniotic fluid (i.e., maximum vertical pocket vs. amniotic fluid index), and further studies are needed to determine the superiority of one test over the other (Croom et al., 1992; Magann et al., 1994). Nonstress test, with acoustic fetal stimulation when needed, along with AFI has been recommended as an integral part of antepartum fetal surveillance in high-risk pregnancies. The predictive value of the NST alone is increased from 83 to 99 percent when combined with the AFI (Anandakumar, et al., 1993).

The Modified Biophysical Profile

The Modified Biophysical Profile is a combination of the NST, as an immediate indicator of fetal well-being, and the amniotic fluid index, which reflects long-term uteroplacental function, and is now a commonly used test as a primary mode of fetal surveillance (ACOG, 1994). The false-negative rate of the modified biophysical profile has been found to be lower than that of the NST and has been compared favorably with the false-negative rates of the CST and the complete biophysical profile (Miller et al., 1996).

Doppler Flow Studies

Doppler ultrasound measures the speed of blood through the vessels or chambers. It has been used in the adult and pediatric populations for assessment of blood vessels and the myocardium. Recently, Doppler ultrasound has been found to be an important tool for fetal assessment.

Doppler ultrasound is performed by applying a transducer to the maternal abdomen and directing an ultrasound beam at a maternal or fetal blood vessel. The beam is reflected from the red cells moving within the vessel which causes a change in frequency of the ultrasound beam. These changes in frequency are proportional to the velocity of the reflecting red cells moving at various rates within the vascular channels (Watson, Young, & Hegge, 1987).

There are three types of Doppler ultrasound: continuous-wave, pulsed-wave, and color-flow imaging. Continuous-wave ultrasound emits a continuous beam that records the velocity of blood cells moving in its path. This form of Doppler is used for fetal heart rate monitoring and determination of fetal heart rate via the pocket Doppler system. The disadvantages of the continuous-wave Doppler is that there is no real-time imaging of the vessels. Parameters of flow velocity and total blood flow cannot be determined.

The pulsed-wave Doppler uses real-time ultrasound to locate and measure a specific vessel or specific area of the fetal heart. The pulsed-wave Doppler system is more expensive and more difficult to operate, although it allows for precise velocity and flow determinations.

Doppler color-flow imaging is a new technology in which a sample of an entire image is taken instead of a selected area. The image is color coded so that it looks like an angiogram of blood flow with velocity superimposed upon a real-time image (Platt, DeVore, Schulman, & Wladimiroff, 1989).

Doppler flow has a variety of clinical uses for fetal assessment. Early in the first trimester, the continuous-wave system is used to detect a fetal heart beat. Color-flow imaging is used to investigate maternal-fetal circulation in early pregnancy and to differentiate pathological conditions of endometrial origin during this period (such as gestational trophoblastic disease or post-abortal uterus) (Kurjak, Kupesic, & Zudenigo, 1994). Color-flow imaging also enhances early detection of abnormal cord insertion, which is associated with adverse pregnancy outcome, particularly fetal growth restriction. In the presence of fetal growth restriction, umbilical cord insertion examination is recommended (Heinonem, Ryynänen, Kirkinen, Saarikoski, 1996).

During the second half of pregnancy, Doppler velocimetry has been used to evaluate the fetus at risk for intrauterine compromise or fetal death by assessing blood flow changes in the fetal heart, aorta, kidney, cerebrum, and maternal and umbilical arteries (Maulik, 1991). Doppler studies also help assess umbilical artery velocity waveforms and identify discordant fetal growth in multiple gestations with a specificity of 95.8 percent and a sensitivity of 77.8 percent (Huch, Kurmanovicius, Hebisch, & Huch, 1994).

Currently, Doppler flow studies are being used as an adjunct technique in pregnancies at risk for growth restriction and preeclampsia (Ålmström, et al., 1992; Bower, Schuchter, & Campbell, 1993). An extremely abnormal flow study within the context of abnormal fetal surveillance test may be considered in formulating a management plan; however, at the present time doppler ultrasound is not recommended as a routine method for antenatal surveillance (ACOG, 1994). This technique remains in an investigational arena until there is proof of effectiveness (Johnstone et al., 1993). There is no evidence to date that shows Doppler ultrasound to be harmful to the fetus (Watson et. al., 1987).

Percutaneous Umbilical Blood Sampling

Percutaneous umbilical blood sampling (PUBS) or cordocentesis is an invasive procedure that allows vascular access to the fetus and has opened up new possibilities for the diagnosis and treatment of the high-risk perinatal conditions affecting the fetus. Due to its complexity, it is limited to regional referral centers where an adequate number of procedures are performed with the necessary technical equipment and by a skilled practitioner (Westgren, Stangenberg, & Lingman, 1995). This procedure is most commonly performed beginning at a gestational age of 18 weeks. PUBS as early as 12 weeks gestational age has been performed but with a higher rate of fetal loss. Pregnancy loss rate is influenced by the procedure itself and by the condition for which this procedure is indicated (Wilson, Farquharson, Wittmann, & Shaw, 1994). Procedural fetal loss rate varies from 3.5 percent (chromosomal indication), 1.25 percent (nonchromosomal indications), and 2.75 percent (in the total population). Overall, fetal loss in chromosomal risk populations is 47 percent (procedural and nonprocedural). Discussion of this risk should be included in the counseling of women undergoing this procedure.

Percutaneous umbilical blood sampling is primarily used for rapid fetal karyotyping and in the evaluation and treatment of fetuses affected by isoimmune hemolytic disease. Other indications for PUBS include evaluation of

- Intrauterine infection
- Nonimmune hydrops fetalis
- Intrauterine growth restriction/fetal acid-bace status
- Twin to twin transfusion
- Fetal alloimmune thrombocytopenia
- Idiopathic thrombocytopenia purpura of pregnancy
- Immunological deficiencies
- Coagulation factor deficiencies
- Hemoglobinopathies
- Fetal thyroid disease
- Fetal drug therapy (Bell & Weiner, 1993; Megerian & Ludomirsky, 1994).

The advantage of PUBS over amniocentesis for karyotyping is the rapidity of the results, allowing the modification of care in the second and third trimester and the option of termination in the presence of aneuploidy before fetal viability. Percutaneous umbilical blood sampling has improved perinatal outcome and dramatically altered the diagnosis and treatment of fetal red blood-cell immunization. PUBS is preferred to intraperitoneal transfusion in the management of erythrocyte isoimmunization because it can be performed 4 to 5 weeks earlier and because the red cells are transfused directly into the fetal circulation. In the diagnosis of the pregnancy at risk for adverse outcome in the immunized mother, the justification of PUBS over simpler tests, such as maternal serologic studies, amniocentesis, and ultrasound remains unclear (Bell & Weiner, 1993). Platelets can also be transfused into a fetus with severe thrombocytopenia. Transfusion therapy can be started as early as 19 weeks' gestation or when PUBS reveals a Coomb's-positive fetus to have a hematocrit of less than 30 percent (Ludomirski & Weiner, 1988). PUBS has contributed to the diagnosis and treatment of congenital toxoplasmosis, cytomegalovirus, and the hydropic fetus infected with human parvovirus (Bell & Weiner, 1993)

PUBS is performed by inserting a 10 to 16 cm, 20 to 22 gauge needle through the maternal abdomen into the umbilical vessel under the guidance of a high image resolution ultrasound.   The umbilical cord is punctured 1 to 2 cm from its placental insertion where it is more stable. Cord insertion near the placenta may be difficult when the placenta is posterior, when obstructed by fetal parts, or in the presence of oligohydramnios. In such cases, the risk of needle displacement is increased.   Insertion directed to a free umbilical cord loop or directly into the fetus may be necessary to avoid injury to a vessel wall or the fetus (Sonek & Nicolaides, 1994). An artery or vein can be sampled. A vein is used most frequently because it has a larger diameter and is easily punctured, although an artery has greater advantage for fetal transfusion. A sample of 0.5 to 3 cc of blood is removed and assayed by a Kleinhauer-Betke test to evaluate sample purity. Maternal blood contamination is more common when samples are taken closer to the placenta. When testing for acid-base parameters, the practitioner must recognize the type of vessel punctured because there is a significant difference in normal values between the veins and arteries.

NOTE: There can be other technical difficultites with PUBS related to maternal obesity, size or thickness of the umbilical cord, gestational age, and fetal movements.

Complications from the PUBS procedure include

- Cord laceration and/or hematoma

- Fetal bradycardia, which is relatively common at blood transfusion

- Vessel constriction

- Thrombosis, thromboembolism or air embolism

- Transient fetal arrhythmias

- Placental abruption

- Fetal-maternal hemorrhage

Delayed consequences of the procedure are premature labor, premature rupture of membranes, and chorioamnionitis (Sonek & Nicolaides, 1994). Chorioamnionitis is a common complication, particularly when multiple punctures are involved.   To reduce the incidence of chorioamnionitis, a broad spectrum antibiotic can be administered after the procedure. Cord bleeding is commonly observed; 10 percent bleed more than a minute but almost all bleeding subsides within 3 minutes (Westgren et al., 1995).

A nonstress test is usually performed immediately after the PUBS procedure. An ultrasound 1 hour after the procedure is also performed to ensure that there is no further bleeding or hematoma formation.   Postprocedure education should include premature labor precautions and the signs and symptoms of infection.

Table 3.5

Example of Kick Count Record

An easy way to check the health of your baby is once each day to count the number of times the baby kicks. At the same time every day, after you have eaten, record the amount of time it takes for your baby to kick 10 times.

For example, on Monday, you begin to count your baby's kicks at 7:00 PM. By 7:30 PM your baby has kicked 10 times. You fill in the chart as in the example below.

Remember that every baby is an individual. It has times when it sleeps and times when it is active. If you start counting and the baby is not kicking, stop, walk around for 5 minutes, and then count again. (Helpful hint: count baby's kicks after you have eaten). If, at the end of two hours, your baby has not kicked 10 times, call this number_____

Kicks = movements, twists, turns.

EXAMPLE

DATE:

40th Week		M	T	W	T	F	S	S
MINUTES	10							
	20							
	30	X						
	40							
	50							
HOURS	1							
	1.5							
	2							

DATE:

		28th WEEK								29th WEEK								30th WEEK							
		M	T	W	T	F	S	S	M	T	W	T	F	S	S	M	T	W	T	F	S	S		
Minutes	10																							
	20																							
	30																							
	40																							
	50																							
Hours	1																							
	1.5																							
	2																							

(Charting would continue through end of pregnancy)

Source: Adapted from UCSF Department of Obstetrics (1988).

Table 3.6

Technique of Biophysical Profile Scoring

Biophysical Variable	Normal (Score = 2)	Abnormal (Score = 0)
Fetal breathing movements	At least 1 episode of at least 30 seconds' duration in 30 minutes' observation	Absent or no episode of $\geq$ 30 seconds in 30 minutes
Gross body movements	At least 3 discrete body/limb movements in 30 minutes (episodes of active continuous movement considered as a single movement)	Two or fewer episodes of body/limb movements in 30 minutes
Fetal tone	At least 1 episode of active extension with return to flexion of fetal limb(s) or trunk. Opening and closing of hand considered normal tone	Either slow extension with return to partial flexion, or movement of limb in full extension, or absent fetal movement
Reactive fetal heart rate	At least 2 episodes of acceleration of $\geq$ 15 bpm and at least 15 seconds' duration associated with fetal movement in 30 minutes	Less than two accelerations or acceleration < 15 bpm in 30 minutes
Qualitative amniotic fluid volume	At least 1 pocket of amniotic fluid that measures at least 2 cm* in two perpendicular planes	Either no amniotic fluid pockets or a pocket < 1 cm in two perpendicular planes

Sources:

Manning, F.A., Morrison, I., Lange, J.R., & Harman, C. (1982). Antepartum determination of fetal health: Composite biophysical profile scoring. *Clinics in Perinatology, 9(2)*, 285–396. Reprinted with permission.

*Chamberlain, P.F., Manning, F.A., Morrison, J., Harman, C.R., & Lange, J.R. (1984). Ultrasound evaluation of amniotic fluid volumes. I. The relationship of marginal and decreased amniotic fluid to perinatal outcome. *American Journal of Obstetrics & Gynecology, 150*(3), 245–249.

Table 3.7

Criteria for Scoring Biophysical Variables

Nonstress Test

Score 2 (NST 2): $\geq$ 5 FHR accelerations of at least 15 bpm in amplitude and at least 15 seconds duration associated with fetal movements in a 20-minute period.

Score 1 (NST 1): 2-4 acceleration of at least 15 bpm in amplitude and at least 15 seconds duration associated with fetal movements in a 20-minute period.

Score 0 (NST 0): $\leq$ 1 acceleration in a 20-minute period.

Fetal Movements

Score 2 (FM 2): $\geq$ 3 gross (trunk and limbs) episodes of fetal movements within 30 minutes. Simultaneous limb and trunk movements counted as a single movement.

Score 1 (FM 1): 1-2 fetal movements within 30 minutes.

Score 0 (FM 0): Absence of fetal movements within 30 minutes.

Fetal breathing movements

Score 2 (FBM 2): $\geq$ 1 episode of fetal breathing of at least 60 seconds duration within a 30-minute observation period.

Score 1 (FBM 1): $\geq$ 1 episode of fetal breathing lasting 30-60 seconds within 30 minutes.

Score 0 (FBM 0): Absence of fetal breathing or breathing lasting < 30 seconds within 30 minutes.

Fetal Tone

Score 2 (FT 2): $\geq$ 1 episode of extension of extremities with return to position of flexion and 1 episode of extension of spine with return to position of flexion.

Score 1 (FT 1): $\geq$ 1 episode of extension of extremities with return to position of flexion or 1 episode of extension of spine with return to position of flexion.

Score 0 (FT 0): Extremities in extension. Fetal movements not followed by return to flexion. Open hand.

Amniotic fluid volume

Score 2 (AF 2): Fluid evident throughout the uterine cavity. A pocket that measures $\geq$ 2 cm in vertical diameter.

Score 1 (AF 1): A pocket that measures < 2 cm but > 1 cm in vertical diameter.

Score 0 (AF 0): Crowding of fetal small parts. Largest pocket < 1 cm in vertical diameter.

Placenta grading

Score 2 (PL 2): Placental grading of 0, 1, or 2.

Score 1 (PL 1): Placenta posterior difficult to evaluate.

Score 0 (PL 0): Placental grading 3.

Source:

Vintzileos, A.M., Campbell, W.A., Ingardia, C.J., & Nochimsom, D.J. (1983). The fetal biophysical profile and its predictive value. *Obstetrics and Gynecology, 62(3)*, 271–278. Reprinted with permission.

Table 3.8

Biophysical Profile Scoring: Management Protocol

Score	Interpretation	Recommended management
10	Normal infant, low risk for chronic asphyxia	Repeat testing at weekly intervals. Repeat twice weekly in insulin dependent diabetic patient and patients $\geq$ 42 wk.
8	Normal infant, low risk for chronic asphyxia	Repeat testing at weekly intervals. Repeat twice weekly in insulin dependent diabetic patient and patients $\geq$ 42 wk. Indication for delivery = oligohydramnios.
6	Suspected chronic asphyxia	Repeat testing within 24 hr. Indication for delivery = oligohydramnios or repeat score remaining at $\leq$ 6.
4	Suspected chronic asphyxia	Indication for delivery = $\geq$ 36 week and favorable cervix. If < 36 wk and lecithin/sphingomyelin ratio < 2.0, repeat test in 24 hr. Indication for delivery = repeat score $\leq$ 6 or oligohydramnios.
0 –2	Strong suspicion of chronic asphyxia	Extend testing time to 120 min. Indication for delivery = persistent score $\leq$ 4, regardless of gestational age.

Source:

Adapted from: Manning, F.A., Morrison, I., Lange, J.R., Harman, C. R., & Chamberlain, P.F. (1985). Fetal assessment based on fetal biophysical profile scoring: Experience in 12,620 referred high-risk pregnancies. *American Journal of Obstetrics and Gynecology, 151*(3), 343–350. Reprinted with permission.

References

Ålmström, H., Axelsson, O., Cnattingius, S., Ekman, G., Maesel, A., Ulmsten, U., Årström, K., & Marsál., K. (1992). Comparison of umbilical-artery velocimetry and cardiotacography for surveillance of small-for-gestational-age fetuses. *Lancet, 340*, 936–940.

American College of Obstetricians & Gynecologists (ACOG). (1994). *Antepartum fetal surveillance* (Technical Bulletin, Number 188). Washington, DC. Author.

American Institute of Ultrasound in Medicine (AIUM). (1991). *Guidelines for the performance of the antepartum obstetrical ultrasound examination.* Rockville, MD: Author.

Andakumar, C., Biwas, A., Arulkumaran, S., Wong, Y.C., Malarvishy, G., & Ratnam, S.S. (1993). Should assessment of amniotic fluid volume form an integral part of antenatal fetal surveillance of high risk pregnancy? *Australian and New Zealand Journal of Obstetrics and Gynaecology, 33*(3), 272–275.

Bell, J.G., & Weiner S. (1993). Has percutaneous umbilical blood sampling improved the outcome of high-risk pregnancies? *Clinics in Perinatology, 20*(1), 61–80.

Berg, T.G., & Devoe, L.D. (1994). Amniotic fluid assessment methods and role in fetal assessment. *Clinics in Perinatology, 21*(4), 809–822.

Bower, S., Schuchter, K. & Campbell, S. (1993). Doppler ultrasound screening as part of routine antenatal scanning: Prediction of preeclampsia and intrauterine growth retardation. *British Journal of Obstetrics and Gynaecology, 100*, 989–994.

Brar, H.S., Platt, L.D., & Devoe, G.R. (1987). The biophysical profile. *Clinical Obstetrics and Gynecology, 30*(4), 936–947.

Campbell, S., Wladimiroff, J.W., & Dewhurst, C.J. (1973). The antenatal measurement of fetal urine production. *British Journal of Obstetrics and Gynaecology, 80*, 680–686.

Chamberlain, P.F., Manning, F.A., Morrison, J., Harman, C.R., & Lange, J.R. (1984). Ultrasound evaluation of amniotic fluid volumes. I. The relationship of marginal and decreased amniotic fluid to perinatal outcome. *American Journal of Obstetrics & Gynecology, 150*(3), 245–249.

Comeford Freda, M., Mikhail, M., Mazloom, E., Polizzotto, K.D., Damus, K. & Merkatz, I. (1993). Fetal movement counting: Which method? *Maternal Child Nursing, 18*, 314–321.

Croom, C.S., Banias, B.B., Ramos-Santos, E., Devoe, L.D., Bezhadian, A., & Hiett, A.K. (1992). Do semi-quantitative fluid index reflect actual volume? *American Journal of Obstetrics & Gynecology, 107*, 995–999.

Cunningham, F.G., MacDonald, P.C., Gant, N.F., Leveno, K.L., & Gilstrap, L.C. (1993). Techniques used to assess fetal health. *Williams Obstetrics* (19th ed, pp. 1031–1044). Norwalk, CT: Appleton & Lange.

Devoe, L.D. (1990). Assessment and care of the fetus: physiological, clinical, and medicolegal principles. In F. Boehm & R. Eden (Eds.), *Care of the Fetus* (pp. 365–383). Norwalk, CT: Appleton and Lange.

Doubilet, P.M., & Benson, C.L. (1994). Ultrasound evaluation of amniotic fluid. In W. Peter Callen (Ed.), *Ultrasonography in obstetrics and gynecology* (3rd ed.) (pp. 475–486). Philadelphia: W.B Saunders.

Field, D.R. (1989). Changing patterns in antepartum surveillance. In J.T. Parer (Ed.), *Antepartum and intrapartum management* (pp.85–99). Philadelphia: Lea and Febinger.

Finberg, H.J., Kurtz, A.B., Johnson, R.L., & Wapner, R.J. (1990). The biophysical profile: A literature review and reassessment of its usefulness in the evaluation of fetal well-being. *Journal of Ultrasound Medicine, 9*, 583–591.

Freeman, R.K. (1987). Antepartum case management. *Clinical Obstetrics and Gynecology, 30*(4),1007–1014.

Gabbe, S.G., Freeman, R.K., & Goebelsman, U.W.E. (1978). Evaluation of the contraction stress test before 33 weeks' gestation. *Obstetrics and Gynecology, 52*(6), 649–652.

Goodman, L.D., Visser, F.G., & Dawes, G.S. (1984). Effects of maternal smoking on fetal trunk movements, fetal breathing movements and fetal heart rate. *British Journal of Obstetrics and Gynaecology, 91*(70), 657–661.

Hallack, M., Kirshon, B., Smith, E.M., Evans, M.I., & Cotton, D.B. (1993). Subjective ultrasonographic assessment of amniotic fluid depth: Comparison with the amniotic fluid index. *Fetal Diagnostic Therapy, 8*, 256–260.

Heinonen, S. Ryynänen, M., Kirkinen, P., & Saarikoski, S. (1996). Perinatal diagnostic evaluation of velamentous umbilical cord insertion: Clinical, Doppler, and ultrasonic findings. *Obstetrics & Gynecology, 87*(1), 112–117.

Huch, R., Kurmanovicius, J., Hebisch, G., & Huch, A. (1994). Doppler ultrasound in twins. In H.P. van Geijn and F.J.A. Copray (Eds.), *A critical appraisal of fetal surveillance,* (p. 483–492). Amsterdam: Excerpta Medica.

Huddleston, J.F., & Quinlan, R.W. (1987). Clinical utility of the contraction stress test. *Clinical Obstetrics & Gynecology, 30* (4), 912–920.

Huddleston, J.F., Sutliff, J.B., & Robinson, D. (1984). Contraction stress test by intermittent nipple stimulation. *Obstetrics and Gynecology, 63*(5), 669–673.

Johnstone, F.D., Prescott, R., Hoskins, P., Greer, I.A., McGlew, T., & Comptom, M. (1993). The effect of introduction of umbilical doppler recordings to obstetric practice. *British Journal of Obstetrics and Gynaecology, 100*, 733–741.

Katz, M., Meizner, I., Holcberg, G., Mazor, M., Hagay, Z.J., & Insler, V. (1988). Reduction or cessation of fetal movements after administration of steroids for enhancement of lung maturation: I. Clinical evaluation. *Israel Journal of Medical Sciences, 24*, 5–9.

Keegan, K.A. (1987). The nonstress test. *Clinical obstetrics and Gynecology, 30*(4), 921–935.

Kilpatrick, S.J., Safford, K.L., Pomeroy, T., Hoedt, L., Sheerer, L., & Laros, R.K. (1991). Maternal hydration increases amniotic fluid index. *Obstetrics & Gynecology, 78*, 1098–1102.

Kurjak, A., Kupesic, S., & Zudenigo, D. (1994). Doppler ultrasound in all three trimesters of pregnancy. *Current Opinion in Obstetrics & Gynecology, 6*, 472–478.

Ludomirski, A., & Weiner, S. (1988). Percutaneous fetal umbilical blood sampling. *Clinical Obstetrics and Gynecology, 31*(1), 19–26.

Magann, E.F., Morton, M.L., Nolan, T.E.. Martin, J.N., Whitworth, N.S., & Morrison, J.C. (1994). Comparative efficacy of two sonographic measurements for the detection of aberrations in the amniotic fluid volume and the effect of amniotic fluid volume on pregnancy outcome. *Obstetrics and Gynecology, 83(60),* 959–962.

Manning, F.A., Morrison, I., Lange, I.R., & Harman, C. R. (1982). Antepartum determination of fetal health: Composite biophysical profile scoring. *Clinics in Perinatology, 9(2),* 285–296.

Manning, F.A., Morrison, I., Lange, J.R., Harman, C.R., & Chamberlain, P.F. (1985). Fetal assessment based on fetal biophysical profile scoring: Experience in 12,620 referred high-risk pregnancies. *American Journal of Obstetrics and Gynecology, 151*(3), 343–350.

Maulik, D. (1991). Doppler for clinical management: what is its place? *Obstetrics and Gynecology Clinics of North America, 18*(4), 853–874.

McCaul, J.F., & Morrison, J.C. (1990). Antenatal fetal assessment: An overview. *Obstetrics and Gynecology Clinics of North America, 17*(1), 1–16.

Megerian, G., & Ludomirsky, A. (1994). Role of cordocentesis in perinatal medicine. *Current Opinion in Obstetrics and Gynecology, 6*(1), 30–35.

Miller, D.A., Rabello, Y.A., & Paul, R.H. (1996). The modified biophysical profile: Antepartum testing in the 1990s. *American Journal of Obstetrics and Gynecology, 174*(3), 812–817.

Moore, T.R., & Piacquadio, K. (1989). A prospective evaluation of fetal movement screening to reduce the incidence of antepartum fetal death. *American Journal of Obstetrics and Gynecology, 160*(5), 1075–1080.

Nageotte, M.P., Towers, C.V., Asrat, T., & Freeman, R.K. (1994). Perinatal outcome with the modified biophysical profile. *American Journal of Obstetrics and Gynecology, 170*(6), 1672–1676.

Neldman, S. (1980). Fetal movements as an indicator of fetal wellbeing. *The Lancet, 1* (8180), 1222–1224.

Newton, E.R. (1989). The fetus as a patient. *Medical Clinics of North America, 73*(30), 517–539.

Nicolaides, K.H., Peters, M.T., Vyas, S., Rabinowitz, R., Rosen, D.J.D., & Campbell, S. (1990). Relation of rate of urine production to oxygen tension in small for gestational age fetus. *American Journal of Obstetrics and Gynecology, 162,* 387–391.

Nwosu, E.C., Welch, C.R., Manasse, P.R., & Walkinshaw, S.A. (1993). Longitudinal assessment of amniotic fluid index. *British Journal of Obstetrics and Gynaecology, 100,* 816–819.

Nyman, M., Barr, M., & Westgren, M. (1992). A four-year follow-up of hearing and development in children exposed in utero to vibroacoustic stimulation. *British Journal of Obstetrics and Gynaecology, 81*(3), 451–457.

Patrick, J., Campbell, K., Carmichael, L., & Probert, C. (1982). Influence of maternal heart rate and gross body movements on the daily pattern of fetal heart rate near term. *American Journal of Obstetrics and Gynecology, 144*(5), 533–538.

Pearson, J.F., & Weaver, J.B. (1976). Fetal activity and fetal well-being: An evaluation. *British Medical Journal, 1(6020),* 1305–1307.

Platt, L.C., DeVore, G.R., Schulman, H. & Wladimiroff, J. (1989). Assessing the fetus with Doppler ultrasound. *Contemporary Ob/Gyn, 33*(1), 168–199.

Porto, M. (1987). Comparing and contrasting methods of fetal surveillance. *Clinical Obstetrics and Gynecology, 30*(4), 956–967.

Rayburn, W.F. (1990). Fetal body movement monitoring. *Obstetrics and Gynecology Clinics of North America, 17*(1), 95–110.

Rouse, D.J., Owen, J., Goldberger, R.L., & Cliver, Z.P. (1995). Determinants of the optimal time in gestation to initiate antenatal fetal testing: A decision-analytic approach. *American Journal of Obstetrics and Gynecology, 173*(5), 1357–1363.

Rutherford, S.E., Phelan, J.P., Smith, C.V., & Jacobs, N. (1987). The four quadrant assessment of amniotic fluid: An adjunct to antepartum fetal heart rate testing. *Obstetric and Gynecology, 70,* 249–251.

Sadovsky, E., & Polishuk, W. (1977). Fetal movements in utero. *Obstetrics and Gynecology, 50*(1), 49–55.

Smith, C.V. (1994). Vibroacoustic stimulation for risk assessment. *Clinics in Perinatology, 21*(4) 797.

Smith, C.V., Davis, S.A., & Rayburn, W.F. (1992). Patients' acceptance of fetal monitoring movement: A randomized comparison of charting techniques. *Journal of Reproductive Medicine, 37*(2), 144–146.

Smoleniec, J.S., & James, D.K. (1992). The unreactive fetal heart rate. *Arch Disease Child, 67,* 1237.

Sonek, J., & Nicolaides, K. (1994). The role of cordocentesis in the diagnosis of fetal well-being. *Clinics in Perinatology, 21*(4), 743–764.

University of California, San Francisco. (1994). *Guidelines for Fetal Surveillance.* Department of Obstetrics and Gynecology.

Vintzileos, A.M., Campbell, W.A., Ingardia, C.J., & Nochimsom, D.J. (1983). The fetal biophysical profile and its predictive value. *Obstetrics and Gynecology, 62*(3), 271–278. Reprinted with permission.

Vintzileos, A.M., Campbell, W.A., Nochimson, D.J., & Weinbaum, P.J. (1987). The use and misuse of the fetal biophysical profile. *American Journal of Obstetrics and Gynecology, 156*(3), 527–533.

Vintzileos, A.M., Campbell, W.A., & Rodis, J.F. (1994). Antepartum fetal assessment by ultrasonography: The fetal biophysical profile. In P. W Callen (Ed.), *Ultrasonography in Obstetrics and Gynecology* (p. 487–501), Philadelphia: W.B. Saunders.

Visser, G.H.A., Mulder H.H., Wit H.P., Mulder, E.J.H., & Prechtl, H.F.R. (1989). Vibro-acoustic stimulation of the human fetus: Effect on behavioral state organization. *Early Human Development, 19,* 285–96.

Ware, J.D. & Devoe, L.D. (1994). The non-stress test: Reassessment of the gold standard. *Clinics in Perinatology, 21*(4), 779–796.

Watson, P.T., Young, W.P., & Hegge, F.N. (1987). Doppler measurement of maternal and fetal blood flow. *Clinical Obstetrics and Gynecology, 30*(4), 948–955.

Westgren, M., Stangenberg, M., & Lingman, G. (1995). Cordocentesis. *Gynecologic and Obstetric Investigation, 40*(4), 227–230.

Whitty, J.E., Garfield, D.A., & Divon, M.Y. (1991). Maternal perception of decreased fetal movement as an indication for antepartum testing in a low-risk population. *American Journal of Obstetrics and Gynecology, 165*, 1084–1088.

Williams, K. (1993). Amniotic fluid assessment. *Obstetrics & Gynecology Survey, 48*(12), 795–800.

Wilson, D.R., Farquharson, D.F., Wittmann,B.K., & Shaw, D. (1994) Cordocentesis: Overall pregnancy loss rate as important as procedure loss rate. *Fetal Diagnosis and Therapy, 9*(3), 142–148.

Wing, D.A., Fishman, A., Gonzalez, C., & Paul, R.H. (1996). How frequently should the amniotic fluid index be performed during the course of antepartum testing? *America Journal of Obstetrics and Gynecology, 174*(1), 33–36.

Zimmer, E.Z., & Divon, M.Y. (1993). Fetal vibroacoustic stimulation *Obstetrics and Gynecology, 81*(3), 451–457.

Zimmer, E.Z., Chao, C.R., Guy, G.P., Marks, F., & Fifer, W.P. (1992). Vibratory acoustic stimulation stimulates human fetal voiding. *America Journal of Obstetrics and Gynecology, 166*, 417.

SECTION 4

ROUTINE PRENATAL AND POSTPARTUM CARE

Chapter 1

INITIAL PRENATAL VISIT

Maureen T. Shannon

Prenatal care is the ongoing assessment and clinical care of a pregnant woman, her fetus, and her family. According to the report by the U. S. Public Health Services Expert Panel on the Content of Prenatal Care (U.S. Department of Health and Human Services [DHHS], 1989), the objectives of prenatal care for the pregnant woman, her fetus, and her family are as follows:

The objectives of prenatal care *for the woman* are

- to increase her well-being before, during, and after pregnancy and to improve her self-image and self-care;

- to reduce maternal mortality and morbidity, fetal loss, and unnecessary pregnancy interventions;

- to reduce the risks to her health prior to subsequent pregnancies and beyond childbearing years; and

- to promote the development of parenting skills.

The objectives of prenatal care for *the fetus and infant* are

- to increase well-being;

- to reduce preterm birth, intrauterine growth retardation, congenital anomalies, and failure to thrive;

- to promote healthy growth and development, immunization, and health supervision;

- to reduce neurologic, developmental, and other morbidities; and

- to reduce child abuse and neglect, injuries, preventable acute and chronic illness, and the need for extended hospitalization after birth.

The objectives of prenatal care for *the family* during pregnancy and the first year of the infant's life are

- to promote family development, and positive parent-infant interaction;

- to reduce unintended pregnancies; and

- to identify and treat behavior disorders leading to child neglect and family violence (U.S. Department of Health and Human Services, 1989, p. 5).

Public agencies currently seek a national health goal to have a minimum of 90 percent of pregnant women initiate prenatal care during their first trimester by the year 2000 (U.S. Public Health Service, 1991). However, in the United States only 76 percent of pregnant women receive prenatal care (National Center for Health Statistics, 1992). To successfully accomplish the majority, if not all, of the objectives of prenatal care listed above, obstetric care providers need to educate pregnant women and women considering pregnancy about the importance of early and ongoing prenatal evaluations. Women considering pregnancy, especially those women with known medical or gynecologic conditions, should have a preconception evaluation by a qualified clinician to assess and improve her health status before conception (see Section 1, *Preconceptional Health Care—An Overview*). Women who suspect or know they are pregnant should have immediate access to perinatal services early in gestation. Guidelines for perinatal care (prenatal, intrapartum, postpartum, and infancy) have been developed by professional organizations (i.e., American College of Obstetricians and Gynecologists [ACOG], American Academy of Pediatrics [AAP]) to assist clinicians with the provision of these services.

The initial prenatal assessment should be as comprehensive as possible. In clinical settings where time constraints prevent the completion of all of the components of this evaluation, the most important aspects of the evaluation should be completed (e.g., determining gestational age) with a subsequent visit scheduled as soon as possible to complete the remainder of the assessment. If a woman is unlikely to return in a timely manner to continue the initial evaluation, all of the components of the initial prenatal assessment should be completed during the first visit (U. S. Department of Health and Human Services, 1989).

Database

Subjective

The provider should obtain a comprehensive history that includes the following information (AAP & ACOG, 1997; U.S. Department of Health and Human Services, 1989):

Menstrual History

- Past menstrual history including
  - ▶ Age at menarche
  - ▶ Characteristics of cycle (i.e., cycle interval, length of flow, amount of flow)
  - ▶ Abnormal bleeding (i.e., intermenstrual bleeding, metrorrhagia)
  - ▶ Associated symptoms (i.e., dysmenorrhea, premenstrual syndrome)
- Date of last normal menstrual period (LNMP)—including characteristics—and previous normal menstrual period (PNMP)
- Date of ovulation (if known)
- Date of conception (if known)
- Contraceptive use prior to LNMP and possibly during conception (e.g., oral contraceptives)

Obstetrical History

- Pregnancies
  - ▶ Current pregnancy, whether planned, unplanned, or assisted reproduction
  - ▶ Total number of pregnancies
  - ▶ Date(s) of births
  - ▶ Length of gestation (for each pregnancy)

> ► Abortions: spontaneous (SAB) and therapeutic (TAB); if TAB, type of termination procedure and any complications

> ► Type of delivery for each birth, sex and birthweight of child(ren), length of labor(s), anesthesia received, postpartum complications

> ► Neonatal complications, number of living children, and general health of child(ren)

- Past obstetrical complications (e.g., pregnancy-induced hypertension [PIH], gestational diabetes, intrauterine growth restriction [IUGR], preterm labor [PTL], preterm birth [PTB], etc.)

Gynecologic History

- Pap smear

> ► Date of most recent smear and result

> ► History of any abnormal Pap smear result(s), date, result, treatment, and follow-up

- Sexual history

> ► Age when first sexually active and whether consensual or nonconsensual

> ► Current number of sexual partners; average number of partners per year

> ► Sexual orientation (i.e., heterosexual, bisexual, lesbian)

> ► Safer sex methods used; frequency of use

- Contraceptive history

> ► Type of contraceptive most recently used; consistency of use

> ► Previous methods used; reason(s) for discontinuing use

- Infertility

- Sexually transmitted diseases (e.g., herpes simplex virus [HSV] infection, human papillomavirus [HPV] infection, gonorrhea, chlamydia, syphilis, human immunodeficiency virus [HIV] infection, pelvic inflammatory disease [PID])

> ► Date(s) of diagnosis, treatment(s), hospitalization

> ► Date(s) of follow-up test(s) and result(s)

> ► Complications

> ► Partner(s) notification and whether treated

- DES exposure

- History of sexual assault

> ► Date

> ► Forensic evaluation

> ► Treatment(s) (e.g., postcoital contraception, STD)

> ► Counseling

> ► Any sequelae

- Other genitourinary conditions (e.g., vaginitis, urinary tract infection, pyelonephritis, myoma, ovarian cyst, breast masses/biopsy, etc.)

General Medical History

- Current medications and medications taken just prior to pregnancy (including over-the-counter [OTC] preparations)
  - ▶ Date of administration
  - ▶ Type of medication
  - ▶ Reason for use
- Significant illnesses
  - ▶ Chronic diseases (e.g., anemia, asthma, diabetes mellitus, cardiovascular conditions [i.e., hypertension, mitral valve prolapse], blood clotting or bleeding disorders, collagen vascular disease, tuberculosis, renal/bladder disease, seizure disorder, musculoskeletal problems, gastrointestinal disorders, cancer, thyroid disease)
  - ▶ Infectious diseases (e.g., hepatitis B or C, tuberculosis, HIV)
  - ▶ Accidents with date, treatment required, complications
  - ▶ Surgical procedures with date, procedure, complications
- Transfusions with dates and reasons for transfusion
- Allergies with type and reaction
- Immunizations
  - ▶ Documented or estimated dates for completion of polio, measles, mumps, rubella, diptheria, tetanus, pertussis, hepatitis B vaccination series
  - ▶ Other immunizations (e.g., pneumococcus, influenza, *Calmette-Guerin bacillus* [BCG])
  - ▶ Date of last diptheria/tetanus toxoid (dT) immunization
- Tuberculosis testing with date of last TB skin test and result
- Exposure to environmental or occupational toxins or pollutants
- Personal habits
  - ▶ Exercise
  - ▶ Sleeping patterns
  - ▶ Stress reduction
  - ▶ Use of tobacco, cannabis, alcohol, caffeine, social or street drugs (i.e., cocaine, crack, heroin, methamphetamine, etc.), OTC preparations, herbal preparations
- Review of systems

Family History

- Alcoholism or other substance abuse
- Allergies
- Cardiovascular disease
- Cancer
- Congenital anomalies
- Endocrine disorders
- Ethnic and/or racial extraction
- Gastrointestinal disorders
- Genetic or chromosomal disorders
- Hematologic disorders
- Lung disease
- Mental retardation
- Multiple gestations
- Neurological problems
- Psychiatric illness
- Renal disease
- Family dysfunction (child abuse or neglect, sexual assault or incest, domestic violence)

Social History

- Current living situation
- Educational level
- Occupation
- Primary language
- Age and occupation of spouse/father of the baby
- Relationship with father of the baby
- Previous and current support systems

Nutritional History

- Height
- Pregravid weight
- Weight gain to date
- Adequacy of intake of four food groups
- See Section 18, *Nutrition,* for further information or if specific problems are encountered

Problems with Current Pregnancy

- Common discomforts of pregnancy (e.g., nausea, vomiting, breast tenderness, etc.)

- Illnesses, injuries, accidents, surgeries since conception

- Bleeding

Objective

The provider should perform a complete physical examination that includes the following including (AAP and ACOG, 1997; U.S. Department of Health and Human Services, 1989):

- Height, weight, blood pressure

- General, including observation of affect, mood

- Skin examination noting presence of chloasma, striae gravidarum, spider angiomas, linea nigra, increased pigmentation of areola, pallor, jaundice, scars, lesions, or pigmented nevi

- Head examination noting presence of any edema, lesions, deformities, lymphadenopathy, or sinus tenderness

- Hair examination noting consistency, or alopecia

- Eyes

  ▶ Determine the woman's reading ability.

  ▶ Check EOMs and pupils.

  ▶ Test for lid lag.

  ▶ Perform ophthalmoscopic examination and note presence of A-V nicking, papilledema or exudates.

- Ears

  ▶ Test for hearing ability (e.g., normal conversation; ability to repeat words whispered from behind her).

  ▶ Perform otoscopic exam and note presence of serous otitis, otitis media, scarred tympanic membrane, or excessive cerumen.

- Nose examination noting pallor, edema, hyperemia, ulcerations, perforation of septum

- Lip examination noting pallor, cyanosis, presence of lesions, inflammation

- Gum examination noting gingivitis, epulis, or bleeding

- Oral mucosa/palate examination noting erythema, lesions or ulcerations

- Tongue examination noting lesions, thrush or, hairy leukoplakia

- Teeth examination noting decay, missing teeth, condition of dental repairs, and quality of hygiene

- Posterior pharynx examination noting presence of tonsils, hyperemia, edema, exudate

- Neck examination noting position of trachea, lymphadenopathy, tenderness

- Thyroid examination noting size, consistency, and presence of masses or nodules

- Thorax and lung examination noting respiratory rate, dullness to percussion, decreased or absent breath sounds; presence of wheezes, rhonchi, crackles, or friction rubs

- Heart examination noting heart rate and rhythm, presence of murmurs, clicks, rubs, extrasystoles

- Breast examination noting size, symmetry, masses, puckering, retraction, dimpling, areolar pigment changes, striae, presence of supernumerary nipples; whether nipples are everted, flat, or inverted; lymphadenopathy of axilla or supraclavicular region

- Back examination noting costovertebral angle tenderness (CVAT), scoliosis, kyphosis, lordosis

- Abdomen
  - ▶ Note presence of bowel sounds, striae, diastasis recti, rashes, lesions, masses, organomegaly, and inguinal lymphadenopathy.
  - ▶ Measure uterine fundus (if appropriate).
  - ▶ Auscultate fetal heart tones (if appropriate).
  - ▶ Determine fetal presentation (if appropriate).

- Musculoskeletal examination noting any limitation of movement, abnormal gait, or swollen or tender joints

- Extremities examination noting edema, or varicosities

- Neurological examination noting orientation and deep tendon reflexes (DTRs); presence of clonus, tics, or tremors; evaluation of cranial nerves, sensorimotor, and proprioception (if indicated)

- Pelvic examination
  - ▶ External genitalia/perineum with note made of lesions, varicosities, episiotomy scar, edema, erythema, discharge
  - ▶ Vagina with note made of rugae, discharge, lesions, hyperemia, masses, quality of muscle tone
  - ▶ Cervix with note made of color, position, consistency, patency, status of os, symmetry, surface characteristics, length, mobility, tenderness, lesions, masses, discharge
  - ▶ Uterus with note made of shape, size, consistency, position, masses, mobility, tenderness
  - ▶ Adnexa with note made of size, mobility, tenderness, presence of masses (if palpated)

- Clinical pelvimetry with assessment of splay of sidewalls, ischial spines, sacrosciatic notch, curve and length of the sacrum, mobility of coccyx, diagonal conjugate measurement, suprapubic angle, bituberous diameter

- Rectal or rectovaginal examination
  - ▶ Confirm uterine examination.
  - ▶ Note hemorrhoids, masses, or lesions.

Assessment

- IUP at an estimation of weeks by LMP
- Uterine size is equal to, less than, or greater than dates
- Weight gain adequate, inadequate, or excessive
- Problems identified from history or physical examination

Plan

Diagnostic Tests

The following tests should be considered for a woman initiating prenatal care and be ordered according to institution specific guidelines or protocols (AAP & ACOG, 1997; U.S. Preventative Services Task Force, 1996):

- Complete blood count (CBC)
- Blood type, Rh, and antibody screen
- Hemoglobin electrophoresis with quantitative A$_2$ and F for all black women
- Syphilis serology (e.g., VDRL, RPR)
- Rubella titer
- Hepatitis B virus screening (i.e., hepatitis B surface antigen and surface antibody)
- Tuberculin skin test (i.e., PPD)
- Counsel and offer triple marker screening if between 15 to 20 weeks of pregnancy are completed.
- Counsel and offer amniocentesis or chorionic villus sampling if the client's age is advanced or there is a history of chromosomal abnormalities or hereditary diseases.
- Urine culture
- Cervical cytology
- Wet prep of cervicovaginal secretions (as indicated)
- *Neisseria gonorrhoeae* culture
- *Chlamydia trachomatis* testing
- Offer an HIV antibody test to all pregnant woman after appropriate counseling and after obtaining specific consent from the woman for this test (Centers for Disease Control and Prevention [CDC], 1995).
- Offer an illicit drug screen (urine toxicology) (as indicated) to a woman but send only after obtaining consent from the client (AAP & ACOG, 1997).
- Provide obstetrical ultrasound if indicated (see Chapter 6.29, *Size/Dates Discrepancy*, and Chapter 6.4, *First Trimester Bleeding*). Some practices routinely offer an obstetrical ultrasound between 18 to 22 weeks gestation.
- Other lab tests as indicated (e.g., 1-hour glucose screen; hemoglobin A1C, etc.)

Treatment/Management

- During the first trimester the woman should receive 0.4 to 0.8 mg of folic acid a day to reduce the development of neural tube defects.

  ▶ Ideally, this daily dose of folic acid should begin at least one month prior to conception.

  ▶ Women with prior pregnancies affected by a neural tube defect should receive 4.0 mg folic acid daily beginning 1 to 3 months prior to conception and continuing through the first trimester of pregnancy (U.S. Preventative Services Task Force, 1996).

- Routine multivitamin supplementation is not necessary if the woman is maintaining a balanced diet that results in appropriate maternal weight gain (see Section 18, *Nutrition*, for dietary requirements during pregnancy and indications for multivitamin and mineral supplementation).

- Prescribe other medications as indicated by history and physical exam findings.

- If the woman has completed her primary immunization series for diptheria-tetanus (dT) and has not had a dT booster for 10 years, she should receive a booster after the first trimester (ACOG, 1991a). Other immunizations may be indicated for her (e.g., hepatitis B, influenza, pneumococcus) based on coexistant medical conditions, but should be administered after consultation with a physician (see Table 4.1, Immunizations During Pregnancy).

- Make appropriate referrals as indicated by the results of the woman's history and physical examination findings (e.g., genetics counselor, social worker, nutritionist, perinatologist).

- If available, refer the woman to pregnancy education classes.

Consultation

- Physician referral is indicated for a woman who is considered high-risk either because of her medical/family history or because of abnormal findings found during her physical examinations (See Table 4.2, Guidelines for Medical Consultation).

- Consultation with a genetic counselor is indicated for a woman who is at an increased risk for a pregnancy affected by a neural tube defect, chromosomal abnormality, or hereditary disorder.

- Social worker referral is indicated for a woman with complex psychosocial issues (See Table 4.3, Guidelines for Social Service Consultation).

Patient Education

- Educate the woman about her estimated date of delivery (EDD), the plan of care for her pregnancy, normal fetal growth and development, signs and symptoms of possible complications, and emergency contacts.

- Educate the woman about avoidance of potentially hazardous substances (i.e., tobacco, alcohol, etc.). If the woman has a chemical dependency problem, discuss with her the treatment options available and refer her to an appropriate program.

- Educate the woman about the importance of folic acid 0.4 to 0.8 mg daily intake during the first trimester.

- Educate the woman about the nutritional requirements for pregnancy and the importance of maintaining adequate nutrition (see Section 18, *Nutrition*).

- Advise the woman not to take any OTC or prescription medications unless recommended by a clinician. Emphasize the importance of informing other clinicians she may be seeing for care (e.g., dentist, dermatologist, emergency room clinicians) that she is pregnant.

- Educate the woman about treatments for common discomforts of pregnancy (see specific protocols for recommended self-help remedies).

- Reinforce the use of automobile passenger restraints. Educate the woman about the proper placement of the restraint during pregnancy. Specifically, advise her to place the lap belt portion of lap-shoulder belts under her abdomen (when it is enlarging) and across her upper thighs. The shoulder restraint should be applied in the usual manner. Both the lap and shoulder belts should be comfortably snug (ACOG, 1991b).

- Educate/review safer sex methods. Present information relevant to the specific situation(s).

- Educate the woman about domestic violence and the increased incidence noted during pregnancy. Discuss the need to have a plan to reach a safe place if she is verbally threatened or physically abused. Also present information about available local resources (e.g., police departments, legal services, women's and children's shelters, support groups).

- Educate the woman about ways to decrease the possibility of toxoplasmosis infection during pregnancy. Specifically, advise her to make sure that meat is thoroughly cooked. If she has a cat, she should have someone else in the household change the litter; if she is not able to arrange this she should be instructed to wear gloves and a mask when changing the litter and thoroughly wash her hands after completing this task (see Chapter 10.9, *Toxoplasmosis*, for additional information).

- Teach/review cancer prevention strategies including monthly self-breast examination (BSE), cervical/pelvic screening, and other assessments (e.g., skin, oral) based on her age and personal/family history of cancer.

- Address any specific concerns the client has.

- Discuss with the woman being referred for physician consultation why this evaluation is indicated.

Follow-up

- If no problems are identified that require consultation with a physician, the woman should return to see the clinician at screening intervals recommended by institution specific guidelines (see Chapter 4.2, *Return Prenatal Visits*, for the recommended schedule for routine prenatal visits).

- Refer for physician evaluation those women who are in high-risk categories.

- Document any significant historical, chronic, or acute problem in the progress notes and on the problem list.

Table 4.1

Immunizations During Pregnancy*

Diptheria-Tetanus (dT) Toxoid	Recommended: Booster every 10 years for adults who have completed primary series. Dose: 0.5 mL IM (preferably in the deltoid muscle) If primary series never received, administer series of 3 immunizations (0.5 mL per dose) with the second and third injections given at 4 - 8 weeks and 6 - 12 months, respectively, after the first dose. Note: A primary series may be completed without restarting the entire series regardless of elapsed time between vaccinations.
Hepatitis B (Recombivax HB®; Engerix-B®)	Recommended: In adolescents, young adults, and other adults considered "high risk" for hepatitis B exposure/infection (see Hepatitis protocol). Dose: Series of 3 injections in deltoid muscle. Note: Women > 19 years: 1.0 mL IM (either preparation); second and third injections given at 1 and 6 months after the first dose. Women $\leq$ 19 years (same schedule as above): 0.5 mL (5µg) per dose of Recombivax HB® or 1.0 mL (20 µg) per dose of Engerix-B®. Requires documentation of negative hepatitis B surface antigen and surface antibody status.
Influenza	Recommended: Annual administration prior to influenza season (usually mid-October to mid-December) for pregnant women > 14 weeks gestation (see Chapter 11.3, Influenza). Dose: 0.5 mL IM Note: If needed, may be given at same time (but at different site) as pneumococcus vaccine.
Pneumococcus	Recommended: Every ten years for individuals at high risk for pneumococcal infection (see Pneumonia protocol). Dose: 0.5 mL subcutaneously or IM Note: If needed, may be given at the same time (but at different site) as influenza vaccine.
Rubella Measles, Rubella (MR) Mumps, Measles, Rubella (MMR)	Recommended: **Contraindicated during pregnancy.** May administer postpartum to women lacking immunity. Dose: 0.5 mL subcutaneously (type of preparation to administer depends upon woman's immunization history, natural disease history, and possible side effects associated with immunization). Note: Reliable method of contraception should be employed for at least 3 months after receiving vaccine. Immunization may be given to women who received Rh(D) immunoglobulin during the third trimester and postpartum.

* Whenever possible administration of a vaccine should be postponed until after the first trimester of pregnancy.

Sources:

American College of Obstetricians & Gynecologists (ACOG). Immunizations during pregnancy. *Technical bulletin 160.* 1991. Washington, DC: Author.

U.S. Department of Health & Human Services, Public Health Service. *Clinicians handbook of preventive services. Put prevention into practice.* 1994. Washington, DC: Author.

American Academy of Pediatrics. *1997 Red Book.* Report of the Committee on Infectious Diseases (24th ed.). Elk Grove Village, IL.

Table 4.2

Guidelines for Medical Consultation

Women who present with or develop a specific high risk condition should be referred for an evaluation by a physician.*

Specific high-risk categories include but are not limited to the following:

- Preeclampsia
- Diabetes mellitus and glucose intolerance of pregnancy
- Third trimester bleeding
- Previous fetal wastage: greater than 16 weeks gestation
- Habitual abortions: 3 or more serial abortions under 16 weeks gestation
- Known drug abuse
- Rhesus sensitization or other IgG antibody sensitization
- Post-maturity: all women at 41 weeks or more by reliable menstrual dating or early obstetrical ultrasound
- Hemoglobinopathies
- Anemias: hemoglobin less than 10 gm/dl or hematocrit less than 30%, unresponsive to iron therapy
- Multiple gestation
- Premature rupture of membranes
- Suspicion of intrauterine growth restriction
- High-risk score on preterm labor assessment
- Polyhydramnios or oligohydramnios
- Severe maternal malnourishment
- Maternal cardiac disease
- Maternal hypertensive disease
- Maternal renal disease, or repeated urinary tract infections
- Maternal collagen disease
- Abnormal maternal triple marker screen
- Fetal malpresentation after 35 weeks gestation
- Family or personal history of severe congenital anomalies or chromosomal abnormalities
- Psychiatric illness
- Positive human immunodeficiency virus (HIV) test result
- Miscellaneous maternal gynecological, endocrine, neuromuscular, pulmonary, gastrointestinal, or infectious disease(s).

* In some instances, the physician may review the pertinent data and make recommendations for management without the need for a consultation visit. In other situations, a consultation visit may be all that is necessary, with the woman being referred back to the primary obstetrical care provider after this evaluation.

Table 4.3

Guidelines for Social Service Consultation

- Family/marital problems
- Difficulty in planning for the care of the baby
- History of being abused as a child or being a child abuser
- History of being a victim of domestic violence/sexual assault
- History of psychiatric disease
- Financial problems
- Need for other community resources (e.g., placement for adoption, special schools if a pregnant adolescent, etc.)

References

American Academy of Pediatrics (AAP) *1997 Redbook*. Report of the Committee on Infectious Diseases (24th ed.). Elk Grove Village, IL: Author.

American Academy of Pediatrics (AAP) & American College of Obstetricians and Gynecologists (ACOG). (1997). *Guidelines for perinatal care* (4th ed.). Elk Grove Village, IL: Author.

American College of Obstetricians and Gynecologists (ACOG). (1991a). *Immunization during pregnancy. Technical bulletin no.160*. Washington, DC: Author.

American College of Obstetricians and Gynecologists (ACOG). (1991b). *Automobile passenger restraints for children and pregnant women*. (Technical bulletin no.151). Washington, DC: Author.

Centers for Disease Control and Prevention (CDC). (1995). U.S. Public Health Service recommendations for human immunodeficiency virus counseling and voluntary testing for pregnant women. *Morbidity and Mortality Weekly Report, 44*(RR–7), 1–15.

National Institutes of Health. (1992). *Report of the National Institutes of Health: Opportunities for research on women's health*. Bethesda, MD: Author.

U.S. Preventative Services Task Force. (1996). *Guide to clinical preventative services* (2nd ed.). Alexandria, VA: International Medical Publishing.

U.S. Public Health Service. (1991). *Healthy people 2000: National health promotion and disease prevention objectives—full report, with commentary*. DHHS publication no. (PHS) 91–50212. Washington, DC: U.S. Government Printing Office.

U.S. Department of Health and Human Services. (1989). *Caring for our future: The content of prenatal care. A report of the Public Health Service Expert Panel on the Content of Prenatal Care*. Washington, DC: Author.

U.S. Department of Health and Human Services. (1994). *Clinicians handbook of preventive services: Put prevention into practice*. Washington, DC: U.S. Government Printing Office.

Chapter 2

RETURN PRENATAL VISIT

Maureen T. Shannon

The purposes of return prenatal visits are 1) to evaluate the progress of the woman's pregnancy, 2) to provide the woman and her partner with information and support appropriate to their needs, and 3) to make appropriate referrals to other health care workers or community resources as indicated. These visits allow the provider to detect deviations from the expected clinical parameters of pregnancy. In addition, the provider can implement and evaluate ongoing psychosocial and health education assessments and interventions.

After the initial pregnancy evaluation has been completed, routine follow-up visits for low-risk women are usually scheduled every 4 weeks until 28 weeks, then every 2 weeks until 36 weeks, with weekly visits thereafter until delivery (American Academy of Pediatrics [AAP] & American College of Obstetricians and Gynecologists [ACOG], 1997; ACOG, 1990). However, in 1989 the U.S. Public Health Service Expert Panel on the Content of Prenatal Care recommended a schedule of return prenatal visits with fewer appointments for low-risk women (U.S. Department of Health and Human Services, 1989). A recent study investigated the incidence of adverse perinatal outcomes (i.e., preterm delivery, preeclampsia, low birth weight, and cesarean section delivery) and patient satisfaction in a group of low-risk pregnant women who were randomly assigned to either the ACOG-recommended routine schedule of visits (a total of 14 visits) or the U.S. Public Health Service schedule with fewer visits (a total of 9 visits). The results of this study demonstrated no significant differences in the perinatal complications between the groups and patient satisfaction was maintained in both groups (McDuffie, Beck, Bischoff, Cross, & Orleans, 1996). The experimental group of women in this study using the USPHS guidelines were scheduled for routine prenatal visits at 8, 12, 16, 24, 28, 32, 36, 38, and 40 weeks. For parous women, a telephone call at 12 weeks was scheduled instead of an office appointment. The investigators limited the generalizeability of their findings to populations of low-risk, white pregnant women. Similar studies investigating this schedule of visits and the impact on low-risk pregnant women of different ethnicity are needed to determine the validity of these findings in other populations.

Database

Subjective

- Symptoms associated with pregnancy (e.g., quickening)

- Problems or complaints since last visit

- Follow-up of problems identified on preceding visit(s)

- Woman (and her partner) discuss preparation for pregnancy, childbirth, and parenting (within cultural context).

Objective

- May include, but are not limited to the following examinations and assessments

  ▶ Weight

  ▶ Blood pressure

▶ Dipstick check of clean catch midstream urine for glucose, protein and ketones

▶ General affect noting of increased stress, anxiety, depression

▶ Abdominal examination

- palpation of uterine fundus including McDonald's measurement and Leopold maneuvers when appropriate

- presence or absence of fetal heart tones and how auscultated

  * by Doppler beginning at 12 weeks

  * by fetoscope or stethoscope when 20 weeks by dates or when fundus at umbilicus

● Extremities: assess for the presence of edema, varicosities

● Other physical examination components as indicated by the woman's complaints and concerns

● Review laboratory reports

Assessment

● IUP at _____ weeks

● Identify any size or dates discrepancies

● Identify any abnormal physical or laboratory findings

● Determine whether weight gain or nutritional status are appropriate/inappropriate

● Evaluate the woman's (and partner's) level of acceptance of pregnancy

● Identify social problems and support system

Plan

Diagnostic Tests (AAP & ACOG, 1997)

● Women 35 years of age or older and women with a family history of chromosomal abnormalities—counsel and offer chorionic villus sampling (CVS) between 10 and 12 weeks' gestation, or amniocentesis between 15 and 18 weeks' gestation (see Section 2, *Genetic Counseling*, Chapter 3.3, *Amniocentesis*, and Chapter 3.2, *Chorionic Villus Sampling*).

● Between 15 to 20 weeks' gestation—provide counseling. Offer triple marker screening (see Section 2, *Genetic Counseling* and Chapter 3.3, *Triple Marker Prenatal Screening*).

● Between 24 and 28 weeks gestation

  ▶ Order a gestational diabetes screen (i.e., 50 gram one-hour glucose test).

  NOTE: If the results of this screen are abnormal, a three-hour glucose tolerance test should be ordered (see Chapter 6.11, *Gestational Diabetes Mellitus*).

  ▶ Repeat hemoglobin (Hgb)/hematocrit (Hct) or complete blood count (CBC).

  ▶ Repeat antibody test for unsensitized Rh-negative women, unless the father of the baby is also known to be Rh-negative. (See Chapter 9.10, *Rh Isoimmunization,* for diagnostic evaluation and treatment of sensitized Rh-negative women.)

- During latter part of third trimester:

  ▶ Screen for sexually transmitted diseases (STDs), as indicated—gonorrhea and chlamydia tests, syphilis serology, HIV testing (if not already done or if woman is at risk for seroconversion during the previous 6 months; testing requires counseling and informed consent) (see STD protocols)

  ▶ Repeat Hgb/Hct or CBC as indicated

- Tests ordered as indicated by office- or institution-specific protocols

- Obstetrical ultrasound, if indicated by physical examination findings

- Other laboratory tests as indicated by history or physical examination findings

Treatment/Management

- Begin therapy for iron deficiency anemia if indicated. See Chapter 9.3, *Anemia—Iron, Folate, and Vitamin B12 Deficiency.*

- Review the woman's weight gain and dietary intake, and discuss indicated changes in her nutritional intake.

  NOTE: Multivitamin and calcium supplement should be recommended if inadequate dietary intake of nutrients or calcium is evident (see Section 18, *Nutrition*).

- Treat specific problems as indicated (e.g., urinary tract infection, vaginitis, etc.).

- Follow-up on any prior abnormal laboratory results.

- Give women who are Rh-negative and antibody-screen negative Rh (D) immune globulin 300 μg I. M. at 28 weeks. This intervention is not indicated if the father of the baby is proven to be Rh-negative.

- Women who are hepatitis surface antigen negative and antibody negative may begin or continue the hepatitis B immunization series after the first trimester. See Chapter 10.2, *Hepatitis A, B, C, D, and E.*

- Evaluate any woman manifesting signs or symptoms of psychosocial stress and refer her (as indicated) to the appropriate health care clinicians (e.g., licensed clinical social worker, psychologist, psychiatrist) for therapeutic interventions to reduce stress and improve functioning.

Consultation

- Refer to or consult with a physician if problems specified in Table 4.2, Guidelines for Medical Consultation, are documented.

Patient Education

- Review results from recent laboratory tests with the client.

- Address the woman and her partner's specific concerns and questions.

- Inform the woman about the gestational age of her fetus and provide information regarding fetal growth and development, discomfort signs and symptoms (e.g., round ligament syndrome), and signs and symptoms of complications (e.g., preterm birth).

- Educate the woman who is Rh-negative and antibody-screen negative about the need for Rh (D) immune globulin administration at 28 weeks gestation and within 72 hours after birth (unless the father of the baby is proven to be Rh-negative).

- Offer formal childbirth education programs appropriate to stage of pregnancy and needs of the woman (e.g., early pregnancy classes, childbirth preparation, breastfeeding, child care, contraception).

- Discuss contraceptive options with the woman (usually during the third trimester).

- Review and reinforce safer sex methods as indicated.

- During the third trimester, discuss and/or refer the client to a pediatric clinician for discussion of pediatric care.

Follow-up

- Repeat routine laboratory studies as indicated under Diagnostic Tests section.

- Schedule routine follow-up visits for pregnant women at low risk for complications according to current clinical practice or institution protocols.

- Make sure woman referred to a physician for consultation attends follow-up visits per the consulting physician's recommendation.

- Arrange routine physician visits per institution-specific policies and protocols.

- Document ongoing problem(s) in progress notes and problem list.

References

American Academy of Pediatrics (AAP) & American College of Obstetricians and Gynecologists (ACOG) (1997). *Guidelines for perinatal care* (3rd ed.). Elk Grove Village, IL: Author.

American College of Obstetricians and Gynecologists (ACOG) (1990). *Scope of services for uncomplicated obstetric care* (Committee Opinion No. 79). Washington, DC: Author.

McDuffie, R.S., Beck, A., Bischoff, K., Cross, J., & Orleans, M. (1996). Effect of frequency of prenatal care visits on perinatal outcome among low-risk women. A randomized controlled trial. *Journal of American Medical Association, 275*(11), 847–851.

U.S. Department of Health and Human Services (1989). *Caring for our future: The content of prenatal care. A report of the Public Health Service Expert Panel on the content of prenatal care.* Washington, DC: Author.

Chapter 3

THE POSTPARTUM VISIT

Maureen T. Shannon

Lucy Newmark Sammons

The postpartum period can be divided arbitrarily into three segments. The immediate puerperium is the first 24 hours after delivery, during which time dramatic physiologic changes take place. The early puerperium extends from the second day to the end of the first postpartal week. The remote puerperium is usually considered to be the time from the end of the first postpartal week to the end of the sixth week, the amount of time generally required for healing and restoration of the reproductive organs (Novy, 1994).

Following delivery, the scheduling of maternal postpartum office visits depends upon a number of factors, including: the length of the hospital or birth center stay, availability and use of home nurse visits, telephone follow-up procedures, complications during delivery, and limitations of the provider and family resources for multiple visits. This chapter addresses the nursing assessment, problem-solving, and management aspects of care that should be accomplished by the end of the remote puerperium, regardless of the number and structure of health care contacts.

Database

Subjective

- Review antenatal record for problems identified prenatally.
- Review the medical record and the labor and delivery summary for intrapartum description.
  - ▶ Type of labor and delivery
  - ▶ Anesthesia
  - ▶ Episiotomy or laceration
  - ▶ Infant weight
  - ▶ Maternal and/or infant complications
  - ▶ Medications required/given during hospitalization
  - ▶ Discharge orders
- Elicit interval maternal history since hospital discharge
  - ▶ Any hospital readmissions, calls/visits to providers or emergency care, additional medications, and any episodic or acute illness/fever/pain/procedures
  - ▶ Abdominal pain

    NOTE: Afterpains caused by uterine contractions, especially in multigravidas and during infant suckling, normally are quite mild after 3 days postpartum (Novy, 1994). If significant abdominal pain is experienced later during the puerperium, consider other causes such as endometritis. See Chapter 6.9, *Endometritis.*

▶ Headache pain

NOTE: Headaches occur in 30 to 40 percent of women during the first week postpartum and are usually responsive to minor analgesics (Reik, 1988). A headache that persists after the use of an analgesic or is accompanied by other symptoms (e.g., fever, nausea, visual problems, etc.) requires further evaluation.

▶ Breastfeeding assessment

   – Symptoms of mastitis

   – Condition of nipples

   – Nursing pattern

   – Woman's perception of success and ease of breastfeeding

▶ Bottlefeeding

   – Clarify method and ease of lactation suppression

   – Address problems preparing formula

   – Note bottlefeeding pattern

▶ Bowels assessment

   – Pattern of elimination and comparison to normal for woman

   – Presence of discomfort associated with defecation

   – Use of medications/aids

▶ Expected puerperal changes predisposing for postpartum constipation include

   – Normal to mild ileus

   – Perineal or rectal discomfort, postpartum fluid loss

   – If problematic, see Chapter 5.2, *Constipation*

▶ Hemorrhoids assessment

   – Discomfort

   – Presence of bleeding

   – Use of medications/sitz baths

   – See Chapter 5.9, *Hemorrhoids*

▶ Episiotomy assessment

   – Discomfort

   – Perineal hygiene

   – Symptomatic treatment, including sitz baths or medications

▶ Bladder

   – Voiding pattern

   – History of urinary tract infection (UTI) during pregnancy

- Catheterization during peripartum/postpartum period
- Symptoms of UTI
- Ability to stop flow with Kegel's maneuver

NOTE: Urinary frequency and high volume due to diuresis are normal during postpartal days 2 to 5; however, urinary frequency thereafter may indicate the presence of a UTI. See Chapter 13.2, *Cystitis*.

▶ Bleeding assessment

- Amount
- Color
- Change with time or activity
- The normal pattern for lochial flow is a continual decrease in amount and change in color/consistency as follows (Baxley, 1996; Novy, 1994):

  * Lochia rubra: red discharge (similar to a heavy menstrual flow) during postpartum days 1 to 3
  * Lochia serosa: paler color (usually serosanguinous) during postpartum days 4 to 10
  * Lochia alba: white to yellowish white color with thick, mucoid consistency during postpartum days 10 to 28/through 35

- Variation in lochia amount may occur and is considered normal when associated with postural changes (some increase in amount or clots may be noted when rising) and with increased activity.
- Reddish color beyond 2 weeks suggests retained placental parts or subinvolution—see Chapter 6.30, *Subinvolution*.
- Foul smelling lochia suggests infection—see Chapter 6.9, *Endometritis,* and Chapter 14.7, *Vaginitis*.
- Resumption of menses usually occurs within 6 to 8 weeks for most non-nursing women. Women who nurse their infants have a return of menses that varies between 2 to 18 months, and often depends on the length of nursing.The first menses that occurs postpartum is usually heavier than a woman's previous menstrual periods, is often anovulatory, and is noted earlier in multiparous women compared to primiparous women.

▶ Intercourse assessment

- Pattern
- Libido
- Associated discomfort
- New partner(s)
- Contraception used or anticipated
- Satisfaction with method
- Incorporation of safer sex (as indicated)

- Elicit information about the woman's general adaptation including (Killeen & Osborn, 1996)
  - ▶ Activity and exercise type and amount
  - ▶ Rest and sleep patterns
    - – Amount
    - – Hindrances
    - – Sleeping aids (e.g., medications, bedtime routine)
  - ▶ Nutrition Assessment should be specific to the needs of the woman (e.g., lactation, anemia)
    - – Appetite
    - – Supply of food
    - – WIC enrollment (as indicated)
  - ▶ Progress with future plans
    - – Plans for returning to work if woman is employed outside home
    - – Child care arrangements
    - – Social services support
    - – Moving
    - – Continued education if attending school
- Elicit maternal and family behavioral and psychological responses to childbearing and childrearing (Killeen & Osborn, 1996; Novy, 1994)
  - ▶ Global response to birthing experience
  - ▶ Note infant's name
  - ▶ Responses of the woman, significant others, and siblings to infant's personality/temperament
  - ▶ Identify the woman's greatest strengths and her most important need for continued assistance.
  - ▶ Maternal experience of "postpartum blues," crying spells, or depression.

    NOTE: Up to 50 percent of women may experience postpartum blues during the first 1 to 2 weeks after delivery; however, 10 percent of women may develop significant clinical depression. Women reporting prolonged symptoms or significant manifestations of depression require further evaluation by a qualified clinician. See Chapter 6.23, *Postpartum Depression*.

  - ▶ Maternal sense of self, worthiness, social isolation versus connectedness
  - ▶ Extent of maternal return of functional ability (resumption of household, social, community and occupational activities)

    NOTE: In one study, the majority of low-risk women interviewed after delivery (both primiparas and multiparas) reported substantial fatigue during the postpartum period which they perceived delayed their ability to return to the level of functioning they were capable of prior to delivery (Ruchala & Halstead, 1994).

▶ Family accommodation to household tasks while client is recuperating and getting acquainted with her new infant

Objective

● Observe the woman's mood, affect, level of distress, and note any alterations or disturbances.

● Vital signs are usually within normal limits (WNL); however, the following may be observed (Baxley, 1996; Novy, 1994; Stover & Marnejon, 1995):

▶ Temperature elevations associated with breast engorgement are normally observed during the first 2 to 3 days postpartum and usually do not exceed 38°C (101°F). Temperature elevations greater than this should be evaluated to rule out the possibility of infection.

▶ During the immediate postpartum period there are major hemodynamic changes including a decrease in maternal heart rate by 4 to 17 beats per minute (bpm) with within 12 to 24 hours after delivery (Poole, 1993). The pulse rate should be WNL at the time of a woman's routine postpartum office visit.

▶ Compare current blood pressure to the range observed during pregnancy.

NOTE: During the first 5 days after delivery an elevated blood pressure may be observed in normal women as a result of the effects of increased uterine vascular resistance and a transient increase in plasma volume. An elevated blood pressure after this period may indicate chronic hypertension, late preeclampsia, improper use of a prescription medication, or use of an illicit drug (e.g., crack, cocaine, methamphetamine).

▶ Compare to the woman's prepregnant weight and weight at delivery. The pattern of weight loss after delivery is influenced by a number of factors; however, the following findings may be observed (Crowell, 1995):

- The greatest weight loss is observed during the first 3 months postpartum, with the majority of loss occuring during the first week postpartum. From 3 to 6 months postpartum, a steady more gradual decline in weight loss is usually observed.

- A prenatal weight gain of more than 15.7 kg/35 lb is often associated with significant weight retention at 6 months postpartum. Additional factors reportedly associated with an increased weight retention by 6 months postpartum include smoking cessation, increased parity, education less than 12 years, lower socioeconomic status, unmarried status, and a high prepregnancy body mass index. (Crowell, 1995)

- Women who have low prepregnant weights are reported to have a more rapid return to prepregnant weight during the puerperium.

- Women who breastfeed exclusively do not demonstrate a significantly different weight loss by 6 months postpartum compared to women who bottlefeed or combine bottle and breastfeeding.

● Note size, consistency, and presence of nodules/masses or tenderness to palpation of thyroid.

NOTE: There is a 6 percent incidence of transient thyroiditis or hypothyroidism after delivery. See Chapter 12.4, *Postpartum Transient Thyroid Dysfunction* (postpartum thyroiditis).

● Assess costovertebral angle tenderness (CVAT), and/or pain and tenderness along paraspinous muscles of the back.

- Note size, shape, consistency, masses, galactorrhea, and nipple condition of the breasts; lactation status; and presence of axillary and supra-clavicular nodes.

  NOTE: Distension, firmness, tenderness, and warmth are normal with engorgement days 3 to 4 postpartum; beyond that consider the possibility of mastitis—see mastitis chapter. Presence of dimpling, retraction, bloody nipple discharge, and/or a discrete mass may indicate a tumor. See Chapter 6.6, *Breast Mass*.

- Examine the abdomen.

  ▶ Ausculate bowel sounds (should be WNL).

  ▶ Palpate and assess diastasis in fingerbreadths, tenderness, masses, cesarean section incision (women who have had a cesarean secion are often evaluated at 2 weeks and 6 weeks postpartum), striae, and inguinal lymph nodes. Abdominal musculature involution may require 6 to 7 weeks.

    NOTE: The uterine fundus usually involutes as follows (Novy, 1994):

    – First postpartum day—at the umbilicus

    – Fifth postpartum day—between the umbilicus and symphysis pubis

    – Tenth postpartum day—at the symphysis pubis

    – Thereafter—no longer palpable by abdominal examination

- Conduct a pelvic examination.

  ▶ Perineum/external genitalia

    – Check episiotomy healing for edema, inflammation, hematoma, suppuration, wound dehiscence, and ecchymosis.

    – If lochia present, check appearance and odor.

    NOTE: Red, brawny, swollen, gaping opposing episiotomy edges, with serous, serosanguinous, or purulent exudate indicates a localized infection of the episiotomy.

  ▶ Vagina

    – Assess presence and healing of lacerations; evaluate rugae, coloration, dryness, inflammation, leukorrhea, and odor.

    – Assess pelvic muscle tone by requesting the woman do a Kegel's maneuver during the digital exam.

    – Palpate episiotomy scar on posterior vaginal septum for tenderness and integrity.

    NOTE: The vaginal epithelium appears thin and smooth until ovaries function to produce estrogen; lactation extends hypoestrogenic condition. Rugae reappear by third week postpartum (Novy, 1994).

  ▶ Cervix

    – Check for lacerations, healing, normal changes of parity with vaginal delivery, discharge, and presence of foul odor.

    – During bimanual examination note the presence of cervical motion tenderness.

NOTE: The cervical canal is reformed by 10 to13 days postpartum. The external os is converted to a transverse slit after a vaginal birth (Novy, 1994).

▶ Bimanual examination of the uterus

   – Note position, size, shape, tenderness, consistency, and mobility.

NOTE: Uterine size by bimanual examination is as follows:

   – 1 week postpartum—approximately 12-week gestation size

   – 6 weeks postpartum—near complete involution

▶ Palpation of the adnexa: Note size, shape, tenderness, masses, consistency

▶ Rectum

   – Assess sphincter tone.

   – Check rectovaginal septum for episiotomy scar/integrity of repair.

   – Palpate sacrospinous ligaments.

   – Assess masses, fistulas, external or internal hemorrhoids, and presence/absence of stool.

NOTE: A rectovaginal examination should be performed on all women who have delivered vaginally to adequately assess the integrity of the rectovaginal septum.

▶ General muscle tone

   – Check for cystocele or rectocele.

● Assess extremities for edema, varicosities, calf tenderness, increased warmth, erythema, nodularity, and Homan's sign

Assessment

● Normal _____ week postpartum exam

● Nonlactating, nonproblematic suppression or breastfeeding, lactation well established

● Episiotomy or cesarean section incision well healed

● Maternal-infant interactions appropriate with progressing social and emotional adaptations

● Family adjustment normal or abnormal

● Contraception method in use or planned

● Nutritional status adequate/inadequate; weight appropriate/high/low

● Identified problems, e.g., episiotomy or cesarean section incision problems, dyspareunia, pyelonephritis, postpartum depression or maternal maladaptation, unstable social situation, hemorrhoids, history of recurrent asymptomatic bacteriuria, cystitis, gestational diabetes, anemia, thyroid dysfunction, domestic violence, substance use (see pertinent chapters).

Plan

Diagnostic Tests

Check the woman's previous laboratory results (e.g., prenatal and postpartum hematocrit [Hct]/hemoglobin [Hgb], Rubella titer, Rh factor, Pap smear and sexually transmitted disease [STD] screening tests) and obtain the following tests as indicated:

- Pap smear

- Gonorrhea and chlamydia tests

- Wet prep of cervicovaginal secretions

- Complete blood count or hematocrit/hemoglobin ordered (if there is a history of anemia or significant blood loss during the delivery)

- Clean catch midstream urine for dipstick

  NOTE: If the woman has a history of bacteriuria during pregnancy, has sickle cell trait/anemia, is reporting symptoms that are associated with cystitis, or has evidence of a possible UTI on her urine dipstick, obtain a urine culture. See Chapter 13.2, *Cystitis*.

- If no documentation of the offering of human immunodeficiency virus (HIV) counseling and testing during the antepartum or intrapartum period, or the woman has declined this in the past, review this option with her.

Treatment/Management

- Provide the contraceptive method the woman has chosen if there are no contraindications to its use.

- Continue adequate nutrition and vitamin or mineral supplementation as indicated (see Section 18, *Nutrition*).

- Provide/continue iron supplementation if the woman is anemic.

- Provide/continue calcium supplement if dietary sources are inadequate.

- Review the woman's immunization status.

  ▶ If the woman has an inadequate immunization history (e.g., no evidence of diptheria/ tetanus (dT) toxoid vaccination in 10 years, lack of rubella immunity and no evidence of postpartum Rubella vaccine administration), administer appropriate immunization(s) after discussing the indications for vaccination.

  ▶ See Chapter 4.1, *Inital Prenatal Visit*, Section 10, *Infectious Diseases*, and Chapter 11.3, *Influenza*.

- Initiate specific treatment(s) for identified problem(s). See the specific protocols

- See the Patient Education section.

Consultation

- Medical consultation for the following variations from normal:

  ▶ Infection or abnormal healing of surgical site

▶ Abnormal vaginal bleeding

▶ Suspected breast abscess or mass

▶ Suspected pelvic infection

▶ Episiotomy breakdown

▶ Uterine subinvolution

▶ Late preeclampsia

▶ Postpartum depression

▶ Postpartum thyroid dysfunction.

● Nutritional consultation if nutritional status severely compromised

● Social services, public health nursing services, or child protective service referrals as needed

● Lactation consultant (if available) for a comprehensive evaluation and intervention for a woman with significant breastfeeding difficulties. See Section 16, *Lactation*.

Patient Education

● Sleep/rest

▶ Provide practical, concrete suggestions to enhance maternal rest and recuperation, sensitive to the client's lifestyle and cultural milieu.

● Contraception/sexual adaptation

▶ Provide specific guidelines about when to resume intercourse if the woman has not yet become sexually active since delivery.

▶ Provide anticipatory guidance regarding postpartal differences in sensation, lubrication, elasticity, arousal, and strategies for increasing satisfaction (e.g., suggestions for lubricants such as Astroglide®).

▶ Assist the woman in selecting and implementing contraceptive measures best suited to her lifestyle.

▶ Review/reinforce safer sex methods as indicated.

● Nutritional counseling

▶ Review nutritional recommendations for lactation and/or recuperative diet with attention to any special problems. See Section 18, *Nutrition,* for specific recommendations.

▶ Refer the woman to WIC if she is eligible for this service.

● Lactation support

▶ Provide anticipatory guidance, helpful suggestions, and recommend readings, as indicated.

▶ Refer women with significant breastfeeding difficulties to a lactation consultant (if available) for further evaluation. See Section 18, *Nutrition,* for lactation diet.

● Exercise/activity/weight guidance

▶ Describe the average weight loss pattern after delivery and assist the woman in determining realistic, healthy short- and long-term goals for weight loss.

▶ Provide postpartum exercise instructions.

– Emphasize the gradual return of muscle tone and weight

– Focus on the need for recuperation during the early postpartum period before beginning moderate or strenuous exercise regimens (this usually requires 3 to 4 weeks of recovery after delivery) (Novy, 1994; Stover & Marnejon, 1995). See also Chapter 4.4, *Exercise During Pregnancy*.

▶ Teach/reinforce Kegel's exercise.

● Parenting

▶ Support realistic expectations for parenting and parent-infant interaction.

▶ If the infant is present, identify positive characteristics of the infant and reinforce the woman's strengths in dealing with infant.

▶ Educate the woman about parents' groups and support services available to her and the father of the infant. See Appendix 4.3a for organizations and reading material resources.

● Infant care concerns

▶ Discuss the normal activity level, behaviors, feeding patterns, and elimination patterns of infants.

▶ Review the usual schedule for pediatric visits and immunizations, infant safety (e.g., car seat use, CPR classes), and signs/symptoms of possible problems (e.g., fever, diarrhea, change in behavior). See Section 17, *Infant Health Supervision*.

● Health maintenance

▶ Instruct the woman in self-breast examination techniques.

▶ Provide anticipatory guidance regarding continued postpartal recuperation (e.g., timing of return of menses).

▶ Encourage regular gynecologic care/Pap smears and primary care visits per current national guidelines/institution specific protocols.

▶ Advise about the individual need for specific immunizations (e.g., hepatitis B) and tuberculosis screening, as indicated (see Chapter 10.10, *Tuberculosis*).

▶ Discuss the woman's (and her partner's) past and current coping strategies, especially review these of the current and future demands of their family. Review current sources for psychosocial support, including family, friends, and community agencies.

● Immunization update

▶ Address questions about rubella immunization as needed.

▶ Women at risk for inadequate measles (rubeola) and/or mumps protection, in addition to lack of rubella immunity, should be immunized with a vaccine combining measles-rubella (MR) or measles-mumps-rubella (MMR). See Chapter 10.5, *Measles (Rubeola)*, Chapter 10.6, *Mumps*, and Chapter 10.8, *Rubella*

▶ Diptheria-tetanus (dT) toxoid boosters should be administered to women if they have not received a booster in ten years.

▶ Other immunizations (e.g., hepatitis B, pneumococcal, influenza) should be administered to the woman as indicated by her individual situation and at appropriate intervals. See Chapter 10.2, *Hepatitis A, B, C, D and E*, Chapter 11.3, *Influenza*, and Chapter 11.4, *Pneumonia*;

● Explain findings

▶ Review laboratory results as needed.

▶ Clarify questions about Rho(D) Immune Globulin (RhIG) given postpartally.

▶ Discuss findings from postpartum examination.

● Additional problems

▶ Discuss comfort/recuperative measures for any identified problems. See also particular chapters.

Follow-up

● Encourage continued health maintenance: primary care, Pap smear, and gynecologic examinations every 1 to 3 years as indicated by institution specific protocols and current national guidelines.

● Suggest that infant to be followed by a primary care provider at intervals suggested by current national guidelines and institution specific protocols.

● Encourage woman to return for specific contraceptive method as needed.

● Make referrals to special interest groups: La Leche League, single mothers, parent-infant classes, play groups, etc.

● Make a referral to lactation specialist as indicated for nursing problems.

● For identified problems as necessary, document in progress notes and problem list.

APPENDIX 4.3a
Resources

Some resources for new parents include the following organizations and reading materials (Stover & Marnejon, 1995). See Section 16, *Lactation*, and Section 17, *Neonatal Care*, for other resources specific to these topics.

Organizations

Postpartum Support International
927 North Kellogg Avenue
Santa Barbara, CA 93111
(805) 967-7636

An international support group that provides information about the emotional changes women experience during pregnancy and after birth.

National Association of Mothers' Centers
336 Fulton Avenue
Hempstead, NY 11550
(800) 645-3828 or (516) 486-6614

An organization with groups in most states that provides support and education on a variety of topics (including postpartum depression).

Books

A. Dunnewold & D. G. Sanford. (1994). *Postpartum survival guide.* Oakland, CA: New Harbinger Publications, 1994.
Presents several aspects of postpartum adjustment.

K. R. Kleinman & V. D. Raskin. (1994). *This isn't what I expected: recognizing and recovering from depression and anxiety after childbirth.* New York: Bantam Books.
Primarily focuses on postpartum depression. Comprehensive and easy to use parent's guide to care of infant/children.

S. Placksin. (1994). *Mothering the new mother: your postpartum resource companion.* New York: Newmarket Press.

References

Baxley, E. (1996). Postpartum biomedical concerns. In S.D. Ratcliffe, J.E. Byrd, & E.L. Sakornbut (Eds.), *Handbook of pregnancy and prenatal care in family practice. Science and practice* (pp. 430–446). Philadelphia: Hanley & Belfus.

Crowell, D.T. (1995). Weight change in the postpartum period. A review of the literature. *Journal of Nurse-Midwifery, 40*(5), 418–423.

Killeen, I., & Osborn, C. (1996). Postpartum care: Psychosocial concerns. In S.D. Ratcliffe, J.E. Byrd, & E.L. Sakornbut (Eds.), *Handbook of pregnancy and prenatal care in family practice. Science and practice* (pp. 447–458). Philadelphia: Hanley & Belfus.

Novy, M. J. (1994). The normal puerperium. In A.H. DeCherney & M.L. Pernoll (Eds.), *Current obstetric and gynecologic diagnosis and treatment* (8th ed., pp. 240–274). Norwalk, CT: Appleton & Lange.

Poole, J. (1993). HELLP syndrome and coagulopathies of pregnancy. *Critical Care Nursing Clinics of North America, 5*(3), 475–487.

Reik, L. (1988). Headaches in pregnancy. *Seminars in Neurology, 8*(3), 187–192.

Ruchala, P.L., & Halstead, L. (1994). The postpartum experience of low-risk women: A time of adjustment and change. *Maternal-Child Nursing Journal, 22*(3), 83–89.

Stover, A. M., & Marnejon, J.G. (1995). Postpartum care. *American Family Physician, 52*(5), 1465–1472.

Chapter 4

EXERCISE DURING PREGNANCY

Winifred L. Star

Many women today enjoy the health benefits of exercise and wish to continue their physical fitness programs during pregnancy. In years past, traditional advice has been for a pregnant woman to rest throughout gestation; however, it is now generally accepted that pregnancy should not result in a sedentary lifestyle, unless indicated by the presence of obstetrical or medical conditions (Artal, 1992; Wolfe, Brenner, & Mottola, 1994). Moreover, pregnancy can be a time for a healthy woman engaging in moderate levels of physical activity to maintain cardiorespiratory and muscular fitness (American College of Obstetricians and Gynecologists [ACOG], 1994). Additional benefits of exercise may include positive effects on self-image and psychological state, improved bowel function, better weight management, and improved joint flexibility (Fishbein & Phillips, 1989).

A wealth of research and narrative literature exists on the topic of exercise during pregnancy, examining both maternal and fetal responses. See Table 4.4, Summary and Conclusions of the Effects of Exercise on Maternal and Fetal Health. The prenatal care provider should be knowledgeable regarding the maternal/fetal risks and benefits of exercise, however, an extensive review of the subject matter is beyond the scope of this chapter. The reader is directed to the bibliography for additional information.

Database

Subjective

- Comprehensive medical and obstetrical history
- Social, recreational and lifestyle history
  - ▶ Employment status
  - ▶ Drug, alcohol and tobacco use
  - ▶ Family commitments and social support
- Current level of physical activity and exercise
- History of past exercise type and pattern
- History of musculoskeletal problems and/or sports trauma
- Patient's desire and motivation to exercise, especially if sedentary
- Nutritional history and history of eating disorders

Objective

- Routine prenatal physical examination at initial obstetrical visit
- Desirable body weight calculations (see Section 18, *Nutrition*)

- 24-hour diet recall to assess nutritional status
- Attention to routine prenatal laboratory indices
- Ongoing routine prenatal evaluation
  - ▶ Weight
  - ▶ Blood pressure
  - ▶ Urine dipstick for protein/glucose/ketones
  - ▶ Serial measures of fundal height
- Additional specific physical assessment modalities as indicated by maternal obstetrical complaints (e.g., serial cervical examination and tokodynamometry to assess preterm labor symptoms; fetal heart rate monitoring to evaluate maternal concerns regarding fetal movement)
- Additional specific physical examination components related to cardiorespiratory or musculoskeletal systems as indicated by patient history and/or complaints related to exercise

Assessment

- Current level of physical activity
- Interest/motivation for exercise program during pregnancy
- R/O obstetrical and medical conditions that would contraindicate exercise

Plan

Diagnostic Tests

- Routine initial and follow-up prenatal laboratory tests
- Additional laboratory evaluation as indicated by pregnancy course
- Ultrasound evaluation and additional fetal surveillance modalities as indicated
- Physical examination specific to maternal complaints (see Objective section)

Treatment/Management

- Rule out obstetrical and/or medical complications that may contraindicate exercise during pregnancy and the postpartum period.
  - ▶ See Table 4.5, Contraindications to Exercise. Consult with a physician as indicated.
  - ▶ Any number of medical/obstetrical conditions may warrant modifications in an exercise program; thus, recommendations should be tailored accordingly.
- Assess the individual's current level of physical activity in order to assist with development of a sensible training program for pregnancy; goals may be to maintain or improve functional capacity and fitness (Clapp III, 1994).

NOTE: Exercise for weight reduction should be discouraged during pregnancy.

- Unless conditions exist to the contrary, women who have been exercising prior to pregnancy may cautiously continue their customary regimen unless the specific activity is risky (see below). The competitive athlete should be monitored frequently; overtraining should be avoided (Clapp III, 1994; Revelli et al., 1992).

- Women without complications that would contraindicate exercise and who have been previously inactive may be encouraged to undertake an exercise program at the beginning of the second trimester. Safe activities include nonweight-bearing exercise such as swimming and stationary cycling (which minimize risk of soft-tissue injury) and weight-bearing modalities such as walking or low-impact aerobics (which involve minimal vertical displacement of the center of gravity) (Wolfe & Mottola, 1993).

  NOTE: A woman with a history of an extremely sedentary lifestyle should not begin strenuous exercise in pregnancy. Consult with physician.

- It is prudent to set limitations on certain activities in pregnancy.

  ▶ Avoid hyperthermia during the first weeks of gestation (Artal, 1992).

    NOTE: An increased risk of neural tube defects among offspring of women exposed to heat in the form of hot tub, sauna, or fever during early pregnancy has been reported (Milunsky et al., 1992). A possible maternal threshold for human teratogenesis is 39.2°C (102.6°F). (ACOG, 1994).

  ▶ Approach sports requiring rapid changes in direction, balance, and muscular strength cautiously (Artal, 1992; Clapp III, 1994).

  ▶ Avoid the performance of certain activities that present risks for blunt trauma (e.g., contact sports, [hockey, soccer, basketball], downhill skiing, waterskiing, ice skating, hang gliding) (Clapp III, 1994; Revelli, Durando, & Massobrio, 1992; Wolfe & Mottola, 1993). (Tennis, racquetball, and squash are considered fairly safe sports [Artal & Buckenmeyer, 1995]).

  ▶ Do not initiate jogging after the pregnancy has begun because it increases risk for musculoskeletal injuries (Artal & Buckenmeyer, 1995).

    – Experienced joggers are advised to reduce mileage to less than 2 miles per day to prevent hyperthermia and dehydration (Artal & Buckenmeyer, 1995; Wolfe & Mottola, 1993).

    – An alternative to jogging is a brisk-walking program (Artal & Buckenmeyer, 1995).

  ▶ Avoid exercise in the supine position.

  ▶ Limit lifting of heavy weight, rowing exercises, and squatting-type exercises to prevent injury to the lower back (Artal, 1992); heavy resistance on weight machines and heavy free-weights also should be avoided (Artal & Buckenmeyer, 1995).

  ▶ Avoid deep flexion or hyperextension of joints and avoid stretching muscles to the point of maximum resistance (Artal & Buckenmeyer, 1995).

  ▶ Avoid scuba diving and hiking at high altitudes during pregnancy (Clapp III, 1994; Wolfe & Mottola, 1993).

Consultation

- Consult with an obstetrician/perinatologist as indicated regarding advisability of a prenatal exercise program.

- Women with risk factors that could compromise physiological adaptation to exercise (e.g., obesity, anemia, diabetes, extreme sedentary lifestyle) or that may lead to adverse maternal/fetal outcomes should be evaluated by a physician prior to establishing a prenatal exercise program (Fishbein & Phillips, 1990).

- Consult with a physician when a client has had significant adverse symptoms while exercising.

- Refer clients to a community pre- and post-natal exercise program run by certified leaders.

- If the patient sustains an exercise-related injury, refer her to a sports medicine specialist or orthopedist if required.

- Refer the obese or underweight client to a registered dietician for nutritional counseling. Clients with an underlying history of an eating disorder should also be referred.

- Counsel professional athletes before conception regarding the potential effects of competitive exercise on pregnancy. Close obstetrical surveillance should be maintained.

  NOTE: Information on this topic will not be covered in depth in this chapter.

Patient Education

- Discuss the benefits of exercise on maternal health.

  ▶ Advise that a healthy pregnant woman may begin or maintain a sensible, regular exercise program during pregnancy which can be beneficial to health and should not adversely affect the course and outcome of the pregnancy (Artal, 1992; Clapp III, 1994; Clapp & Capeless, 1991; Jarrett II & Spellacy, 1983; Pivarnik et al., 1993).

  ▶ Ideally, fitness should be achieved prior to becoming pregnant. See Section 1, *Preconception Health Care—An Overview.*

- Include the following information in education about exercise during pregnancy:

  ▶ Specifics of an exercise program

  ▶ Prevention of injury

  ▶ Danger signs

  ▶ Contraindications for exercise during pregnancy

  ▶ See Table 4.6, Summary of Recommendations for Exercise in Pregnancy/Postpartum, and Table 4.5, Contraindications to Exercise. See also Table 1.3, Exercise Safety Guidelines, in Section 1, *Preconception Health Care — An Overview* (most of the guidelines in Section 1 also apply to exercise *during* pregnancy).

- In addition to the guidelines listed in Table 4.6, the following information may be discussed with the patient regarding exercise:

  ▶ Proper clothing that encourages heat loss

  ▶ Supportive bras

  ▶ Appropriate footwear

  ▶ Exercise on terrain that provides sure footing (Artal & Buckenmeyer, 1995; Fishbein & Phillips, 1990)

  ▶ Lower abdominal support is often helpful to alleviate abdominal/pelvic discomfort associated with exercise and advancing pregnancy (Clapp III, 1994)

  ▶ Proper intake (liberal amounts) of fluid before and after exercise to prevent dehydration and hyperthermia (Artal & Buckenmeyer, 1995)

  ▶ Ensurance of adequate carbohydrate intake (Artal & Buckenmeyer, 1995)

  ▶ Proper convective heat loss during exercise on stationary equipment (e.g., using electric fans) (Wolfe & Mottola, 1993)

  ▶ Proper breathing (i.e., avoid breath holding or Valsalva maneuver) during weight lifting or isometrics

  ▶ Adequate "spotting" during lifting of free weights

  NOTE: Very light weights (2 to 5 kg) are recommended as pregnancy progresses (Artal & Buckenmeyer, 1995; Clapp III, 1994).

  ▶ Monitoring of exercise intensity

    – Suggested target heart rate zones (Wolfe & Mottola, 1993):

      * Under age 20: 140–155 beats per minute (bpm)
      * Ages 20–29: 135–150 bpm
      * Ages 30–39: 130–145 bpm
      * Over age 40: 124–140 bpm

    NOTE: Ideally, target heart rates should be established on an individual basis. Most healthy pregnant women can safely exercise at heart rates up to 150 bpm (Wolfe & Mottola, 1993).

    – Alternatively, the 6- through 20-point *Borg Scale Rating of Perceived Exertion* (RPE) may be used to guide exercise intensity:

      * No exertion = 6
      * Extremely light exertion = 7–8
      * Very light exertion = 9–10
      * Light exertion = 11–12
      * Somewhat hard exertion = 13–14
      * Hard exertion = 15–16
      * Very hard exertion = 17–18

    *   Extremely hard exertion = 19
    *   Maximal exertion = 20

NOTE: An RPE level of 12 to 14 has been suggested as appropriate for most pregnant women (Artal & Buckenmeyer, 1995; Wolfe & Mottola, 1993). Overexertion should be avoided. Exercise is to be adjusted to accommodate nausea, fatigue, and/or musculoskeletal pain (Jarski & Trippett, 1990). Use of the "talk test" is a way to prevent overexertion (i.e., if a pregnant woman can not comfortably carry on a conversation while exercising she should reduce her exercise effort) (Fitness Canada, 1982).

▶ Immediate cessation of exercise if any of the following signs or symptoms occur:

   – Vaginal bleeding or fluid loss

   – Abdominal pain

   – Uterine contractions

   – Severe tachycardia, palpitations

   – Chest, back, or pubic pain

   – Severe shortness of breath

   – Headache

   – Loss of muscle control, difficulty walking

   – Dizziness, faintness

   – Nausea, vomiting

   – Absence of fetal movement once established

▶ Discuss nutritional recommendations, healthy eating patterns, and weight gain trends. Recommend consultation with a nutritionist for the underweight or overweight woman.

▶ See the Treatment/Management section in this chapter. See also Section 18, *Nutrition*.

Follow-up

● Carefully monitor obstetrical parameters and the client's individual progress. Pay special attention to weight trends and fundal height measurements, which should remain within normal limits.

● Use diet recalls to assess an individual's intake to offer advice regarding a problem with weight gain or loss. Refer the client to a nutritionist to discuss healthy eating patterns, as indicated.

● Evaluate clients who experience musculoskeletal injuries related to exercise; the client may need to be referred to an orthopedic or sports medicine specialist.

● The client can monitor her own responses to her exercise program: e.g., caloric intake, weight, color of urine, overall strength and fitness, musculoskeletal comfort, rest cycles, etc. (Clapp III, 1994).

NOTE: It is common for pregnant women who partake of weight-bearing exercise to note a progressive decline in performance beginning in early pregnancy. Nonweight-bearing exercisers may be able to maintain a moderate-duration regimen through the third trimester (ACOG, 1994).

- Make sure client reports significant weight loss or danger signs (see above) to the provider.

- Evaluate symptoms of preterm labor promptly.

- Modify the exercise program as indicated based on the clinical status of the patient.

- Postpartum resumption of exercise will depend on the woman's physical capability.

  ▶ Joints and ligaments may take up to 3 months to return to their prepregnancy state (Artal & Buckenmeyer, 1995).

  ▶ Education may include instruction on Kegel exercises.

  ▶ After cesarean section, it is usually recommended that a patient not begin exercise (other than walking) until 4 to 6 weeks postpartum.

  NOTE: A minimum of 21 days is required for the scar to become maximally strong (Warren, 1991).

- Document exercise-related injuries or other significant problems associated with exercise in the problem list and in the progress notes. Document in the problem list "professional athlete" status, as appropriate.

Table 4.4

Summary and Conclusions of the Effects of Exercise on
Maternal and Fetal Health

MATERNAL EFFECTS

- Uterine blood flow decreases during acute strenuous exercise with magnitude of reduction directly correlated with exercise intensity and duration.

  ▶ The reduced blood flow may be compensated by redistribution of blood flow favoring the cotyledons, exercise-induced hemoconcentration, and increased fetal arteriovenous oxygen extraction.

  ▶ The magnitude of splanchnic shunting may be reduced by increased maternal blood volume and cardiac output and reduction in systemic vascular resistance.

- Exercise posture appears to be an important determinant of uterine blood flow (and pregnancy complications) during exercise.

  ▶ Exercise in the supine position is not recommended due to relative obstruction of venous return and decrease in cardiac output (which may lead to the supine hypotensive syndrome).

- Decreased oxygen is available for the performance of aerobic exercise during pregnancy because of the increased resting oxygen requirements and the increased respiratory work secondary to the physical effects of the uterus on the diaphragm. This does not appear to change the acid-base balance in some fit women during exercise in pregnancy.

- Caloric requirements are increased in regularly-exercising pregnant women.

  ▶ Maternal hypoglycemia may occur in response to strenuous aerobic exercise in late gestation.

  ▶ Adequate carbohydrate intake is essential for the exercising pregnant woman.

- Hormonal influences during pregnancy may result in increased joint laxity, predisposing a woman to mechanical trauma or sprains, especially of the metacarpophalangeal joints.

- Elevations in core temperature in response to strenuous exercise in pregnancy appear to attenuate as a result of increased sweating and augmented skin blood flow.

  ▶ Fit individuals thermoregulate core temperature more efficiently.

  ▶ There have been no demonstrated increases in neural tube defects in women who exercise (even vigorously) during pregnancy.

  NOTE: Hot tub use in early pregnancy has been associated with increases in congenital anomalies.

- Without additional risk factors for preterm labor, the majority of healthy, exercising pregnant women do not have increases in baseline uterine activity or increased incidences of preterm labor/delivery.

FETAL EFFECTS

- The most common fetal heart rate (FHR) response to vigorous maternal exercise is an increase of about 5 to 25 beats/minute with a gradual return to baseline in the postexercise recovery period.

  ▶ Degree of elevation depends on gestational age as well as intensity, modality, and duration of maternal exercise.

  ▶ Brief periods of fetal bradycardia have been occasionally noted during (usually maximal) maternal aerobic exercise, most commonly in the postexercise period; this FHR deceleration is most likely a transient reflex vagal response to acute hypoxia and is not associated with significant perinatal morbidity or mortality.

- Several studies have demonstrated slight reductions in gestational length and decreased birth weights (averages of 300–350 g) among infants of recreational athletes who exercised at high intensities throughout pregnancy.

  ▶ Moderate aerobic conditioning of healthy well-nourished pregnant women can improve physical fitness and does not appear to increase the risk of fetal growth retardation.

Sources: American College of Obstetricians and Gynecologists. (1994). *Exercise during pregnancy and the postpartum period.* Technical Bulletin No. 189. Washington, D.C.: ACOG. Used with permission.

Wolfe, L.A., Brenner, I.K., & Mottola, M.F. (1994). Maternal exercise, fetal well-being and pregnancy. *Exercise and Sports Sciences Reviews, 22,* 145–194.

Table 4.5

Contraindications to Exercise

- Pregnancy-induced hypertension

- Preterm rupture of membranes

- Preterm labor during the prior or current pregnancy or both

- Incompetent cervix/cerclage

- Persistent second- or third-trimester bleeding

- Intrauterine growth retardation

- Other medical or obstetrical conditions (chronic hypertension, active thyroid disease, cardiac/vascular/pulmonary disease should be evaluated carefully to determine whether an exercise program is appropriate)

- Any additional risk factors for adverse maternal or perinatal outcome

Source: American College of Obstetricians and Gynecologists. (1994). *Exercise during pregnancy and the postpartum period.* Technical bulletin No. 189. Washington, D.C.: ACOG. Used with permission.

Table 4.6

Summary of Recommendations for Exercise in Pregnancy/Postpartum

● **During pregnancy**

▶ Women can continue to exercise and derive health benefits from even mild-moderate exercise routines.

▶ Modify and individualize exercise programs to meet specific physical and mental needs.

▶ Regular exercise at least 3 times/week is preferable to intermittent activity.

▶ Warm-up and cool-down periods of 5-10 minutes should precede and follow exercise sessions.

▶ Intensity of exercise should be maintained at "light to somewhat hard." Heart rates of up to approximately 150 beats/minute are safe for most healthy pregnant women.*

▶ Moderately intense aerobic activities can be safely conducted for up to 30-minute periods. Lower-intensity activities should not exceed 45 minutes in duration.

▶ Transition from weight-bearing to non-weight-bearing activities is recommended during pregnancy. Nonweight-bearing exercises (stationary cycling, swimming) will minimize the risk of injury and facilitate the continuation of exercise.

▶ Avoid deep flexion or hyperextension of joints. Stretching should not be taken to the point of maximal resistance.

▶ Limit or avoid jumping/jarring motions or rapid direction changes.

▶ Avoid heavy free-weights and heavy resistance on weight machines. Resistance training with low weights and moderate repetitions is advisable.*

▶ Pregnant women who exercise should augment heat dissipation by ensuring adequate hydration, appropriate clothing, and optimal environmental surroundings during exercise. They should refrain from exercising in hot, humid weather. Women who are febrile should not exercise.*

▶ Avoid exercise in the supine position after the first trimester because this position is associated with decreased cardiac output in most pregnant women.

▶ Avoid prolonged periods of motionless standing.

▶ Pregnant women should stop exercising when fatigued or if danger signs develop and should not exercise to exhaustion.*

▶ Avoid exercise that has the potential to cause physical trauma or expose the woman to hyperbaric, hypothermic, hyperthermic or hypoxic environmental conditions, and/or awkward positions.*

▶ Pregnancy requires an additional 300 kcal/day (without additional exercise) to maintain metabolic homeostasis. Thus, women who exercise during pregnancy should be particularly careful to ensure an adequate diet.

● **Postpartum**

▶ Many of the physiologic and morphologic changes of pregnancy persist 4 to 6 weeks postpartum and joints and ligaments may require up to 3 months to reconfigure. Thus, prepregnancy exercise routines should be resumed gradually based on a woman's physical capability.

* See chapter for additional discussion.

Sources: American College of Obstetricians and Gynecologists. (1994). *Exercise during pregnancy and the postpartum period.* Technical bulletin # 189. Washington, D.C.: ACOG. Used with permission.

Artal, R., & Buckenmeyer, P. J. (1995). Exercise during pregnancy and postpartum. *Contemporary OB/GYN, 40(5),* 62-90.

Wolfe, L. A., & Mottola, M. F. (1993). Aerobic exercise in pregnancy: An update. *Canadian Journal of Applied Physiology, 18(2),* 116-147.

References

American College of Obstetricians and Gynecologists (ACOG). (1994). *Exercise during pregnancy and the postpartum period.* Technical bulletin No. 189. Washington, D.C.: Author.

Artal, R. (1992). Exercise and pregnancy. *Clinics in Sports Medicine, 11(2),* 363–377.

Artal, R., & Buckenmeyer, P. J. (1995). Exercise during pregnancy and postpartum. *Contemporary OB/GYN, 40(5),* 62–90.

Clapp, J. F. III. (1994). A clinical approach to exercise during pregnancy. *Clinics in Sports Medicine, 13(2),* 443–458.

Clapp, J. F., & Capeless, E. (1991). The VO_{2max} of recreational athletes before and after pregnancy. *Medicine and Science in Sports and Exercise, 23,* 1128–1133.

Fishbein, E. G., & Phillips, M. (1989). How safe is exercise during pregnancy? *Journal of Obstetric, Gynecologic, and Neonatal Nursing, 19(1),* 45–49.

Fitness Canada. (1982). Fitness and pregnancy: A leader's manual. Ottowa: Fitness and Amateur Sport Canada.

Jarski, R. W., & Trippett, D. L. (1990). The risks and benefits of exercise during pregnancy. *The Journal of Family Practice, 30(2),* 185–189.

Jarrett, J. C. II, & Spellacy, W. N. (1983). Jogging during pregnancy: An improved outcome? *Obstetrics & Gynecology, 61(6),* 705–709.

Milunsky, A., Ulcickas, M., Rothman, K. J., Willett, W., Jick, S. S., & Jick, H. (1992). Maternal heat exposure and neural tube defects. *Journal of the American Medical Association, 268(7),* 882–885.

Pivarnik, J. M., Ayres, N. A., Maure, M. B., Cotton, D. B., Kirshon, B., & Dildy, G. A. (1993). Effects of maternal aerobic fitness on cardiorespiratory responses to exercise. *Medicine and Science in Sports and Exercise, 25,* 993–998.

Revelli, A., Durando, A., & Massobrio, M. (1992). Exercise and pregnancy: A review of maternal and fetal effects. *Obstetrical and Gynecological Survey, 47(6),* 355–367.

Warren, M. P. (1991). Exercise in women. Effects on reproductive system and pregnancy. *Clinics in Sports Medicine, 10(1),* 131–139.

Wolfe, L. A., & Mottola, M. F. (1993). Aerobic exercise in pregnancy: An update. *Canadian Journal of Applied Physiology, 18(2),* 116–147.

Wolfe, L. A., Brenner, I. K., & Mottola, M. F. (1994). Maternal exercise, fetal well-being and pregnancy outcome. *Exercise and Sport Sciences Reviews, 22,* 145–194.

Chapter 5

TRAVEL DURING PREGNANCY

Winifred L. Star

Travel during pregnancy may be planned or unexpected and may include a wide range of itineraries. The stresses of traveling during pregnancy vary depending upon the reason for the trip, length of the trip, destination, itinerary, and planned activity while away. Travel for vacation purposes should be enjoyable, rather than stressful, and the health care provider can provide information to reduce potential hazards. Recommendations for the traveling pregnant woman encompass general health and safety guidelines as well as strategies for disease prevention. Of course, international travel poses different risks than travel within the United States, and predeparture considerations may include certain vaccinations.

The underlying health status of the mother is an important consideration for determining the safety and impact of travel on the pregnancy. Women with medical complications are at increased risk for adverse pregnancy outcomes; the effects of long-distance travel may further compromise the pregnancy. On the other hand, a healthy pregnant woman may have little difficulty traveling and derive much pleasure from the experience. Many of the recommendations for the pregnant traveler are common sense guidelines to optimize a healthy pregnancy and avoid discomforts and potential complications.

Women with cardiovascular conditions made worse by pregnancy or with congenital/acquired heart disease may need to avoid travel during pregnancy. Multiple gestation after 20–22 weeks and incompetent cervix are also contraindications to travel. Strong relative contraindications to long-distance travel include threatened abortion or vaginal bleeding, known placenta previa in the third trimester, history of preterm labor or premature rupture of membranes, and/or a history of other pregnancy complications (e.g., placental abruption, pregnancy induced hypertension, gestational diabetes). Pregnant diabetics will require careful monitoring of blood sugar and insulin dosing during long-distance/duration travel (Barry & Bia, 1989; Lee, 1989).

General Information

Vehicle of Travel

The vehicle of travel may pose inherent risks to the pregnant traveler. Air travel in modern commercial aircraft is generally felt to be safe during pregnancy provided additional risk factors are excluded (Huch et al., 1986). When placental function is uncompromised, the fetus should be unaffected during flights in pressurized aircraft (Cameron, 1973; Parer, 1982; Sholten, 1976); however, certain medical complications of pregnancy may be significant enough to preclude air travel altogether or to warrant supplemental oxygen (see the Treatment/Management section). Prolonged periods of sitting during air travel increase the possibility of venous stasis.

The major risk to the woman during air travel is incidental trauma (e.g., from turbulence). It has been proposed that sudden, severe deceleration forces encountered during flight or landing may precipitate placental abruption in late pregnancy; however, this phenomenon requires further study (Matzkel, Lurie, Elchalal, & Blickstein, 1991).

Pregnant crew members or frequent flyers who fly high-altitude, high-latitude flights of long duration may be exposed to radiation that exceeds the maximum permissible fetal dose (5 mSv) during the gestation period (Barish, 1990; Friedberg, Faulkner, Snyder, Darden, & O'Brien, 1989). The Federal Aviation Administration (FAA) has indicated that pregnant crew members who fly these high-altitude, high-latitude, and long-duration flights should be given the opportunity to make an informed decision whether or not to transfer to short-distance flights in the contiguous United States (FAA, 1986 as cited in Barish, 1990).

Cruise ship travel may pose a risk for gastrointestinal (GI) disease if sanitation standards are not well-maintained. Vessels with foreign itineraries are subject to twice yearly inspections, with reinspections as necessary. The Centers for Disease Control and Prevention (CDC) has established specific criteria for the insurance of a clean and healthy environment aboard ship.

Motor vehicle accidents are the leading cause of disability and death worldwide. Pregnant travelers should be diligent about the use of seat belts. Airbags and antilock brakes are other vehicular features that may prevent serious injury.

Additional information on health, safety, and comfort measures are covered in the Treatment/ Management and Patient Education sections and Tables 4.7 through 4.10.

International Travel

The risk of acquiring illness during international travel depends upon the areas to be visited and length of stay. Travel to developing countries poses a greater risk. In most developed countries (i.e., Canada, Australia, New Zealand, Japan, and western Europe) the traveler's general health risk will be no greater than that incurred while traveling in the United States, except for, possibly, a higher risk of measles, mumps, and rubella (MMR) (CDC, 1997a). Women of childbearing age should be immune to MMR before leaving the United States.

In many areas of the world, living conditions and standards of sanitation and hygiene vary considerably and immunization coverage levels may be low. The risk of acquiring disease in these areas can vary greatly (CDC, 1997a). The majority of American international travelers will not require additional immunizations or prophylaxis if their routine immunization status is up-to-date according to the U.S. current standards (American Academy of Pediatrics, 1997; CDC, 1997a). (Childhood vaccinations in the United States include diphtheria, tetanus, pertussis, measles, mumps, rubella, polio, *H. influenza* type b, hepatitis B, and varicella zoster virus.)

During pregnancy, the decision whether or not to vaccinate against a particular disease will depend on the degree of risk, safety of the vaccine and the prior immunization status of the woman. For travelers, selective vaccination against specific diseases (e.g., yellow fever, cholera, typhoid, polio, hepatitis A) is recommended based upon known/perceived disease-specific risks in the areas to be visited, plus the type/duration of travel (Advisory Committee on Immunization Practices [ACIP], 1991). Risk from vaccination during pregnancy is largely theoretical; benefits of vaccination usually outweigh potential risks when a) the risk for disease exposure is high, b) the infection poses a special risk to mother or fetus, or c) the vaccine is unlikely to cause harm (CDC, 1997a). See Table 4.7, Vaccination During Pregnancy.

Live-virus vaccines should not be given during pregnancy or to a woman who may become pregnant within three months of the vaccination. (Note that despite the theoretical hazards of administration of live virus vaccine during pregnancy, no specific complication of pregnancy has been linked to their use. Women who are inadvertently vaccinated with live virus vaccine during pregnancy should be appropriately counseled and be generally reassured [K. P. Beckerman, personal communication, October 8, 1996]). Vaccines (live or killed) do not affect the safety of breastfeeding for women or their infants (CDC, 1997a).

Specific Diseases

Hepatitis A

Hepatitis A is an enterically transmitted viral infection, highly endemic throughout the developing world but of low endemicity in the United States and other developed countries. Risk of transmission is increased with duration of travel and risk is highest in rural areas of developing countries and in settings with poor sanitation. Transmission occurs via direct person-to-person contact or from contaminated water, ice, fruit, vegetables or other uncooked foods, or from shellfish contaminated by sewage water. Foods may be also be contaminated after cooking via improper handling processes.

Symptoms, which usually appear 2 to 6 weeks after exposure, consist of malaise, nausea, anorexia, vomiting, abdominal pain, myalgia, fever, and jaundice. Avoidance of potentially contaminated food or water is the key to prevention. Hepatitis A vaccine or immune globulin (IG) is recommended for susceptible persons traveling to areas of intermediate-high endemicity of infection (CDC, 1996a, CDC, 1997a; Greenbaum, 1996).

Hepatitis B

Hepatitis B virus (HBV) infection risk for international travel is generally low, except for certain travelers to countries with high HBV endemicity. Refer to the *Yellow Book* for geographic distribution of hepatitis B.

Symptoms are similar to those of hepatitis A infection. Transmission is through breaks in the skin, via mucous membranes or blood, and through parenteral or perinatal exposure. Vaccination is available for prevention and is recommended for certain groups. Pregnancy/lactation is not a contraindication for the vaccine (CDC, 1997a; Lommel, 1995).

Hepatitis E

Hepatitis E viral infection is spread by sewage-contaminated food or water or close personal contact. In recent years, it has been reported in several areas of Asia, North America, and rural areas of central Mexico.

Symptoms of disease are similar to hepatitis A. Epidemics generally affect adults, and pregnant women may have an unusually high mortality rate. Unfortunately, immune globulin has not been effective in preventing disease during hepatitis E outbreaks and no vaccine is available. As with hepatitis A and other enteric infections, prevention is key and is accomplished by avoiding potentially contaminated food and water (CDC, 1997a).

Travelers' Diarrhea

Travelers' diarrhea (TD) may be acquired anywhere in the world. High-risk destinations include most developing countries in Latin America, Africa, the Middle East, and Asia (CDC, 1997a). Bacterial enteropathogens cause approximately 80 percent of TD (DuPont & Ericsson, 1994). The predominant organisms, acquired through fecally contaminated food and/or water, include enterotoxigenic *Escherichia coli* (ETEC), salmonella species, shigella species, and *Campylobacter jejuni*. Less common bacterial pathogens include *E. coli*, *Yersinia enterocolitica*, *Vibrio cholerae* O1, 0139 and other non-01, and *Vibrio fluvialis*. *Vibrio parahaemolyticus*, acquired via ingestion of raw or undercooked seafood, has caused TD in passengers on Caribbean cruise ships and in Japanese people traveling in Asia. Parasitic enteric pathogens include *Giardia lamblia*, *Entamoeba histolytica*, and occasionally *Cryptosporidium* (Buckley, 1995; CDC, 1997a; DuPont & Ericsson, 1993). Infrequent causes of TD are viral enteric pathogens including rotaviruses and Norwalk-like viruses. Twenty to fifty percent of TD cases remain without identified etiologies (CDC, 1997a).

The TD syndrome is characterized by a twofold or greater increase in the frequency of unformed bowel movements. Other associated symptoms include abdominal cramps, nausea, vomiting, bloating, fecal urgency, tenesmus, fever, malaise, or the passage of bloody or mucoid stools. Onset is usually within the first week of travel but may occur at any time, even after returning home. Most episodes resolve in a few days and can be treated with medication (CDC, 1997a; DuPont & Ericsson, 1993).

Malaria

Worldwide, parasitic infection during pregnancy is very common (Tietze & Jones, 1991). Of special significance is malarial infection. Travelers to malaria-endemic areas should be provided with an appropriate prophylactic drug regimen and advised about personal protection measures to prevent disease (CDC, 1997a). Ideally, travel to areas of highly endemic disease should be postponed until after pregnancy.

Malaria is caused by one of four protozoan species of *Plasmodium*: *P. falciparum* (most significant), *P. vivax*, *P. ovale*, and *P. malariae*. All are transmitted by the bite of an infected female *Anopheles* mosquito. Places in the world where malaria exists include large areas of Central and South America, Hispaniola, sub-Saharan Africa, the Indian subcontinent, Southeast Asia, the Middle East, and Oceania. The risk of acquiring malaria varies markedly, however, from area to area. Infection may occasionally be spread by blood transfusion, or congenitally from mother to fetus. Malaria infection may be more severe during pregnancy and may increase the risk for adverse outcomes (e.g., prematurity, abortion, stillbirth); thus, pregnant women should avoid travel to malarious areas.

Symptoms of the disease include fever, chills, headache, myalgia, and malaise, which may occur intermittently. These symptoms can develop as early as eight days after initial exposure to as late as several months after departure from a malarious area, after chemoprophylaxis has been terminated. Anemia and jaundice may also occur. *P. falciparum* infections may cause kidney failure, coma, and death. Antimalarial drugs such as chloroquine or mefloquine are appropriate during pregnancy and neither has a harmful effect on the fetus (CDC, 1996b, CDC, 1996c; CDC, 1997a).

Yellow Fever

Yellow fever, a viral disease transmitted by the bite of the female *Aedes aegypti* mosquito (among other species), occurs only in parts of Africa and South America. It is rare among travelers but significant due to its high mortality rate. Most countries have regulations and require yellow fever vaccination.

Illness severity ranges from a flu-like syndrome to severe hepatitis and hemorrhagic fever. Vaccination during pregnancy is generally contraindicated, however, and pregnant women may obtain a waiver. No definitive treatment measures exist. Precautions against exposure to mosquito bites are of utmost importance (CDC, 1997a).

Cholera

Cholera is an acute intestinal infection caused by *Vibrio cholerae* O-group 1 or O-group 139 and spread by contaminated food and water. The disease is common in the Indian subcontinent, sub-Saharan Africa, and South America, predominantly in areas of poor sanitation. The bacteria may also live in brackish rivers and coastal waters. A few cases have been contracted by eating raw or undercooked shellfish from the Gulf of Mexico. In epidemics, contamination sources are usually the feces of an infected person. Rapid spread of disease is common in areas of inadequate sewage and water treatment. Casual contact with infected persons is not a risk for disease. The disease is very rare in industrialized countries and travelers are at little risk if staying in international tourist accommodations.

Symptoms are usually mild but one in 20 infected persons may have severe disease characterized by profuse watery diarrhea, vomiting, and leg cramps. Dehydration, shock, and death may ensue within hours. Attention to food and water precautions will prevent illness. Treatment consists of fluid replacement and antibiotics (CDC, 1996d; Pust, Campos-Outcalt, & Cordes, 1991). A vaccine is available for prevention, but should be avoided during pregnancy on theoretical grounds.

Typhoid Fever

Typhoid fever is prevalent in developing countries of Africa, Asia, and Latin America. The disease is caused by a particular species of salmonella bacteria, *Salmonella typhi*, which is transmitted by contaminated food/beverages and water. Infected persons carry bacteria in their bloodstream and intestinal tract; carriers can recover from the acute illness but continue to carry *S. typhi* which can be shed in the stool.

Symptoms include chills, high fever, headache, weakness, myalgia, anorexia, abdominal pain, and diarrhea (may be bloody) or constipation. A macular, rose-colored rash may appear on the chest and abdomen. Treatment consists of antibiotics and supportive therapy. Untreated individuals may have fever for weeks to months; as many as 20 percent die of complications. Information on vaccine safety during pregnancy is not available, thus the CDC feels it is prudent to avoid vaccinating pregnant women (CDC, 1996e; CDC, 1997a; Greenbaum, 1996).

Dengue Fever

Dengue fever is a viral disease transmitted by *Aedes* mosquitoes (usually *Aedes aegypti*, a daytime feeder). There are four immunologically related dengue viruses. However, they do not provide cross-protective immunity. The illness is rapidly expanding worldwide in tropical areas (urban as well as resort and rural areas). Risk is greatest in the Indian subcontinent, Southeast Asia, Southern China, Central and South America, the Caribbean, Mexico, and Africa. Epidemics have become more frequent and larger, and increased transmission in all tropical locales is anticipated. Unless an epidemic is occurring, however, risk to an international traveler is small.

Symptoms of dengue fever include sudden onset of high fever, severe frontal headache, joint/muscle pain, nausea, vomiting, and rash (which appears 3 to 5 days after fever onset and may spread from torso to arms, legs, or face). Although the disease is usually benign and self-limited, convalescence can be prolonged (2 to 4 weeks). Treatment consists of supportive care including rest, fluid replacement, and analgesics. No vaccine is available, thus prevention, by avoidance of mosquito bites, is key. A severe, fatal form of the disease known as dengue hemorrhagic fever (DHF) exists. Symptoms include syncope, shock, and generalized bleeding. Other infectious illnesses (e.g., influenza, measles, malaria, typhoid/scarlet fever) can be confused with dengue fever (CDC, 1996f; CDC, 1997a; Greenbaum, 1996).

Meningococcal disease

Meningococcal disease is caused by a bacterium, *Neisseria meningitidis*. Epidemics of serogroup A or C meningococcal disease occur frequently during the dry season (December through June) in sub-Saharan Africa. However, disease among Americans traveling to these areas is rare (CDC, 1997a).

Affected individuals present with symptoms/signs of fever, vomiting, severe headache, nuchal rigidity, confusion, or lethargy. Treatment consists of antibiotic and supportive therapy. Vaccine is available but recommended only for certain travelers. During pregnancy, however, vaccination should be avoided unless there is substantial risk of infection (CDC, 1997a; Greenbaum, 1996).

Japanese encephalitis

Japanese encephalitis is a mosquito-borne viral encephalitis infection, transmitted by the bite of the *Culex* species. The host may include man, domestic animals, and birds. Areas supporting the transmission cycle of the virus are primarily rural, agricultural zones of Asia (mostly during the months of June through September). Risk to short-term urban travelers is low. Only 1 in 50 to 1 in 1,000 persons infected by a mosquito bite will develop illness, and symptoms are generally mild or absent.

Early symptoms include headache, fever, GI symptoms, confusion, and behavioral changes. The disease can progress to encephalitis, which in one third of cases is fatal. In survivors, serious neurological sequelae may persist. Infection during the first and second trimester of pregnancy has been associated with spontaneous abortion. Mosquito bite prevention measures are important because after infection sets in, only supportive treatment is available. Vaccine is available but recommended only for selected persons. During pregnancy the risk/benefit ratio of vaccination must be weighed, but generally it should be avoided (CDC, 1996g; CDC, 1997a).

Plague

Plague is an acute bacterial disease caused by *Yersinia pestis*, which is transmitted from animal-to-animal or animal-to-human by the bites of infected fleas. Rodents, domestic cats and dogs, and other animals also serve as sources of infection. Most human cases result from the bites of infected fleas, but infection may also occur as a result of direct contact with the tissues or body fluids of plague-infected animals. Primary plague pneumonia may result from the inhalation of infectious droplets exhaled from persons or animals with pneumonic plague. Wild rodent plague exists in the western third of the United

States and many areas of Africa, Asia, South America, the Middle East, and eastern European countries. Risk to urban travelers is small; rural agricultural areas are the predominant places where disease is found.

The incubation period is 2 to 6 days. Illness features include fever, headache, malaise, and extreme exhaustion followed by painful, swollen regional lymph nodes (buboes). Disease can progress rapidly to plague septicemia and plague pneumonia. Mortality in plague pneumonia is over 50 percent. Treatment consists of antibiotic and supportive therapy. Vaccination is rarely indicated for travelers, especially if they are only frequenting urban areas (CDC, 1992a; CDC, 1994a, 1994b; CDC, 1997a).

Rabies

Rabies is a viral illness transmitted by animal bites and scratches and, occasionally, by nonbite exposures that introduce virus into open cuts or mucus membranes. Dogs are the main reservoir for disease. However, all animal bites warrant evaluation. Internationally, the highest risk for rabies is in Mexico, Central and South America, the Indian subcontinent, Africa and Southeast Asia. In the United States, rabies is found in all states except Hawaii.

Signs of rabies in an animal include nervousness, aggressiveness, excessive drooling or foaming at the mouth, and abnormal behavior. The population at large rarely requires preexposure vaccination (CDC, 1992b; CDC, 1996h; CDC, 1997a).

Schistosomiasis

Schistosomiasis, caused by flukes, with fresh water snails as the intermediate hosts, is a risk for travelers to endemic areas of the Caribbean, South America, Africa, and Asia. The larvae of the infected snail can penetrate unbroken skin of the human host, and even brief encounters in contaminated waters can lead to infection. Wading, swimming, or bathing in fresh water in rural areas with poor sanitation presents the greatest risk.

Symptoms of acute infection, which may occur 2 to 3 weeks after exposure to infected waters, include fever, anorexia, weight loss, abdominal pain, weakness, headache, joint/muscle pain, nausea, diarrhea, and cough; most infections, however are asymptomatic. The central nervous system can be involved (rarely) to produce seizures or transverse myelitis. A chronic infection can cause disease of the lung, liver, intestines and/or bladder (CDC, 1996i; CDC, 1997a). Chemoprophylaxis is not available, but treatment with effective oral medication exists.

Tuberculosis

Tuberculosis (TB) is an increasingly serious public health problem caused by *Mycobacterium tuberculosis*. The organism is transmitted through droplets in the air (although unpasteurized milk or milk products can also spread disease); prolonged exposure in a closed environment with an infected, coughing person is usually required for disease acquisition.

Persons who become infected with *Mycobacterium tuberculosis* can be treated to prevent active disease. Multiple medication therapy is indicated for the treatment of tuberculosis (CDC, 1997a). See Chapter 10.10, *Tuberculosis*, for additional information.

Human Immunodeficiency Virus

Human immunodeficiency virus (HIV) infection and acquired immunodeficiency syndrome (AIDS) are worldwide. The incubation period for AIDS is long and variable, ranging from months to years. Currently a vaccine is not available for prevention. The World Health Organization estimates that 18 million people are infected with HIV (CDC, 1997a). Travelers are at risk for HIV acquisition if they a) have heterosexual or homosexual intercourse with an HIV-infected person; b) use or allow the use of contaminated, unsterilized syringes, or needles for any injections or other skin-piercing procedures (including acupuncture, use of illicit drugs, steroid/vitamin injections, medical/dental procedures, ear/body piercing, or tattooing); and/or c) receive infected blood, blood components, or clotting factor concentrates (CDC, 1996k; CDC, 1997a). If an individual is HIV-infected, travel, especially to developing countries, carries significant risks for exposure to opportunistic pathogens and food and waterborne diseases (CDC, 1996). Precautions for the prevention of these infections is imperative (see chapter 14.5, *Human Immunodeficiency Virus*, for additional information).

Additional Diseases

Additional diseases that may pose risk to international travelers, beside the ones mentioned above, include American trypanosomiasis (Chagas' disease), African trypanosomiasis (sleeping sickness), cryptosporidiosis, cyclospora, diphtheria, tetanus, measles, rubella, giardiasis, tick-borne encephalitis, leishmaniasis, filariasis, onchocerciasis (river blindness), bartonellosis (Oroya fever), relapsing fever, Chikungunya fever, Oropouche virus disease, Ross River virus (epidemic polyarthritis), Congo-Crimean hemorrhagic fever, and typhus. Rift Valley fever, Lassa fever, Ebola, and Marborg disease are severe, often fatal viral illnesses that occur in rural areas of Africa, but are not a significant health problem to travelers (CDC, 1996m). Discussion of the above entities is beyond the scope of this chapter. The reader is directed to a current journal or textbook for information.

In the sections to follow, considerations regarding travel during pregnancy are approached on three levels: a) details about general safety and comfort guidelines, b) current recommendations regarding immunizations for international travel, and c) general treatment, management, and follow-up recommendations of commonly encountered international diseases. This chapter is not intended to take the place of a current textbook or the resources of governmental health agencies and experts in the area of travel medicine. These sources of information should be utilized for the most current information on international disease patterns and vaccination requirements and additional specific treatment recommendations.

Database

Subjective

- Obtain a complete medical, obstetrical, and social history.

- Obtain an immunization history.

- Ascertain planned travel itinerary during pregnancy to determine risk for infectious and environmental disease. Important considerations include destination and locale (urban, rural), season of travel, place of stay (hotel, other), duration of stay, planned activities, type of vehicle(s) to be used to transport traveler.

- See introductory section for information on specific diseases.

Objective

- Perform physical and/or laboratory examination, as indicated, based on specific travel plans and health status.

- Document all pertinent medical history and plans for international travel during pregnancy on the problem list.

- Certain countries may require an International Certificate of Vaccination against Yellow Fever; this must be given at an official Yellow Fever Vaccination center as designated by a state's health department. The certificate must be validated by the center administering the vaccine and signed by a licensed physician (or physician-designee). See Treatment/Management section and Table 4.7 for further information regarding vaccination during pregnancy.

- See introductory and Diagnostic Tests sections for additional information.

Assessment

- Document specific travel itinerary.
- Document immunization status.
- Assess underlying health status and lifestyle risks.
- R/O health conditions which may pose a risk to travel.

Plan

Diagnostic Tests

- Determine routine prenatal laboratory evidence of rubella immunity, hepatitis B surface antigen status, HIV antibody status.

- Screen for hepatitis A antibodies (anti-HAV) to determine susceptibility of frequent travelers to hepatitis A viral infection. (An antibody-positive screen precludes need for hepatitis A vaccination or passive immunization with immune globulin [CDC, 1996a; CDC, 1997a; Pust et al., 1991].)

- Perform tuberculin skin testing.

  NOTE: HIV-infected persons may have an impaired response to the skin test and may require anergy testing (CDC, 1996k).

- Cultures may be indicated for assessment of disease status:

  ▶ Stool cultures (and microscopy) for diarrheal episodes

  ▶ Blood, stool, and urine cultures for febrile travelers

- Women with symptoms of malaria should have thick and thin blood smears as soon as possible; if negative, should be repeated every 6–12 hours for 36–48 hours if the provider has a strong suspicion of malaria (Yung & Ruff, 1994).

- Dengue fever may be diagnosed by special blood tests for the presence of the virus or its antibodies. (Check with a local laboratory for availability.)

- Diagnostic tests to rule out plague include chest X-ray and laboratory examination of blood, bubo aspirate, exudates, purulent drainage and sputum if appropriate.

  ▶ Acute and convalescent serum studies are required to confirm the diagnosis if microorganisms are not isolated initially (CDC, 1992a).

  ▶ Contact local laboratory for further information.

  NOTE: Wound drainage, blood, and body fluids are all potentially hazardous to laboratory/medical personnel.

- Perform stool and urine microscopic examinations for schistosome eggs 6 to 8 weeks after exposure; serologic studies are also available.

- Additional specific laboratory tests (e.g., complete blood count [CBC], erythrocyte sedimentation rate [ESR], liver function tests) may be indicated to assist with diagnosis of parasitic, viral and/or bacterial infections.

- See Follow-up section.

Treatment/Management

<u>General Information and Recommendations</u>

- The International Air Transport Association (IATA) policy adopted by most airlines allows unrestricted travel on domestic flights up to 36 weeks of gestation, and up to 35 weeks of gestation on international flights. (Policies may vary with individual airlines.) If the pregnancy is more advanced or complications exist, medical clearance by the client's provider and the airline's medical department is required. After 38 weeks of gestation the airline usually does not permit travel unless there is demonstrable and acceptable need to make the journey. The client should be provided with sufficient obstetrical records as appropriate/indicated. Mothers and newborns should avoid air travel within the several days after birth (Breen, Gregori, & Neilson, 1986; Lee, 1989; Matzkel et al., 1991).

- Travel in pressurized aircraft poses little risk to a pregnant woman.

  ▶ Conditions that are exceptions and for which supplemental oxygen is indicated are severe anemia, hemoglobinopathies, cardiopulmonary conditions causing hypoxia, intrauterine growth restriction, compromised placental function, preeclampsia, and premature labor (Lee, 1989).

    – Arrangements for oxygen should be made with the airline at least 24 hours in advance.

    – The airline's medical department may need to be contacted regarding the patient's suitability for travel.

  NOTE: Generally a patient with a complicated pregnancy should not be permitted to fly except in extremely unusual circumstances (Breen et al., 1986). Consultation with a physician is mandatory for a pregnant traveler prior to embarking if there is a history of an obstetrical complication or medical problem. If the health and well-being of the mother and fetus is at serious risk, nonessential travel should be postponed.

  ▶ During flight, if depressurization should occur, a pregnant woman should receive oxygen and pay attention to fetal kick counts; medical evaluation should be sought as soon as possible if there is persistent reduction in or absence of fetal movement (Lee, 1989).

▶ Frequent flyers or pregnant flight crew may wish to consult with an occupational health specialist or contact the Environmental Protection Agency (EPA) and FAA for guidance regarding flight safety during pregnancy.

- Individuals susceptible to motion sickness can be protected by the use of anti–motion-sickness medication or antihistamines as indicated. Refer to the *Physicians' Desk Reference (PDR)* regarding side effects and use in pregnancy.

- See also the introductory and Patient Education sections.

International Travel

- Review the patient's immunization status and travel itinerary with a travel medicine specialist to determine need for malaria prophylaxis and vaccination against specific diseases. Allow ample time to review the particulars prior to patient's departure (at least 6 weeks).

- Obtain from the CDC the following publications:

  ▶ Latest edition of *Health Information for International Travel* (the *Yellow Book*), a compendium of information and recommendations for international travelers; also contains information regarding yellow fever vaccination requirements by country

  ▶ The *Summary of Health Information for International Travel* (the *Blue Sheet*), a biweekly update to the *Yellow Book,* which lists where cholera and yellow fever are being reported and official changes in individual country's vaccination requirements (see References and Appendix 4.5a for details on obtaining these publications)

- Use information from the CDC's 24-hour Hotline, the International Travelers Hotline, the Fax Information Service, the Drug Information Service, and the Internet. (See Appendix 4.5a for further information.)

- Ideally, immunizations such as tetanus, diphtheria, polio, and MMR will be up-to-date prior to pregnancy.

  ▶ For administration of certain vaccines, weigh the risk/benefit ratio. Some immunizations require sufficient time to complete the series (e.g., hepatitis B vaccine, 6 months).

  ▶ MMR is contraindicated during pregnancy or if pregnancy is planned in the next 3 months.

  ▶ Consult with a travel medicine specialist as needed and refer to the CDC's *Morbidity and Mortality Weekly Report* for updates on adult immunization.

  ▶ Refer to package inserts of specific vaccines for dosage and administration information.

  ▶ See also Table 4.7.

NOTE: Clinicians should be aware of the potential side effects and adverse effects of vaccines and toxoids. These are discussed in ACIP statements found in selected issues of the *Morbidity and Mortality Weekly Report* and in *Health Information for International Travel.* Although adverse events (i.e., events usually requiring recipient to seek medical attention) are rare, health care providers are required by law to report problems associated with DTP, DT, Td, MMR, MR, measles, OPV, or IPV vaccine administration (CDC, 1997a). Reports should be called to the Vaccine Adverse Event Reporting System (VAERS) (800-822-7967).

Specific Diseases

Hepatitis A

- Discuss prevention measures. Avoidance of potentially contaminated food and water is the key to prevention. See Table 4.8 for food and water precautions. See also Chapter 10.2, *Hepatitis A, B, C, D, and E.*

- Hepatitis A vaccine or immune globulin (IG) prophylaxis is recommended for susceptible travelers to all areas except Japan, Australia, New Zealand, Northern and Western Europe, and North America (excluding Mexico) (CDC, 1996a; CDC, 1997b; Greenbaum, 1996).

  NOTE: If an individual is shown to be antibody positive, prophylaxis is not indicated. See Diagnostic Tests section.

  ▶ Vaccination is preferred for persons who plan to travel repeatedly or reside for long periods in countries with intermediate or high endemicity of infection (CDC, 1996a; CDC, 1997a).

    – Two hepatitis A vaccines are currently available: HAVRIX® and VAQTA®. Refer to the drug package inserts for dosage information, contraindications, and side effects.

    – Travelers are protected 4 weeks after receiving the initial dose. Persons traveling to intermediate- or high-risk areas less than 4 weeks after the initial dose of vaccine should receive immune globulin 0.02 mL/kg of body weight at a different injection site (CDC, 1996a; CDC, 1997a).

  NOTE: The safety of hepatitis A vaccines during pregnancy has not been determined, however, theoretical risk is expected to be low. Risk/benefit ratio should be weighted prior to administration.

  ▶ Immune globulin (IG) is recommended for persons desiring only short-term protection or those who elect not to be vaccinated:

    – For travel up to 3 months: single IG dose of 0.02 mL/kg.

    – For travel longer than 3 months: IG dose is 0.06 mL/kg; repeated every 5 months (CDC, 1996a; CDC, 1997a).

  NOTE: IG may be given simultaneously at different sites with inactivated vaccines (e.g., DPT, hepatitis A, etc.). IG does not interfere with OPV or yellow fever vaccines but diminishes the effectiveness of live virus vaccines (e.g., MMR) when given simultaneously (CDC, 1997b).

Hepatitis B

- Prevention measures should be discussed. See Chapter 10.2, *Hepatitis A, B, C, D, and E,* for further information.

- Vaccination is recommended for health care workers who come into contact with blood and body fluids and individuals who will reside for 6 months or longer in areas of intermediate to high HBV endemicity where they may engage in activities that will place them at risk for HBV transmission. These activities may include

  ▶ Sexual or close physical contact with locals

  ▶ Receipt of medical/dental/other treatment in local facilities

- Hepatitis B vaccination is not contraindicated during pregnancy or lactation but is not indicated for routine travel unless high-risk conditions exist (see above information and the introductory section).

- Short-term travelers to areas of moderate to high endemicity who are likely to be in direct contact to blood or body fluids of local residents should also be vaccinated.

- Two types of hepatitis B vaccines exist: Recombivax HB® and Energix-B® (see package inserts for information on dosage and administration, side effects, and contraindications).

Hepatitis E

- Discuss prevention measures. With hepatitis E, prevention is key.

  ▶ Immune globulin is not effective in preventing disease.

  ▶ No vaccine is currently available.

  ▶ See Table 4.8 for food and water precautions.

Travelers' Diarrhea (TD)

- Prevention includes information on food and beverage consumption (see Table 4.8).

- The CDC does not recommend routine use of prophylactic antibiotics (CDC, 1997a). Advise client that she should, ideally, consult a health care provider rather than attempt self-medication (CDC, 1996n).

- Treatment of TD may include the following (CDC, 1997a; Greenbaum, 1996):

  ▶ Dietary measures

    - Soup (lightly salted rice or noodle), broth, toast, salted crackers

    - The "BRAT" diet is well tolerated: bananas, rice, applesauce, toast

    - Oral rehydration solution (ORS) for severe dehydration, available at stores or pharmacies in developing countries

    Note: Simple home-made solutions can be made by mixing any of the following:

    a) One teaspoon salt and 2 to 3 tablespoons sugar or honey to one liter clean water

    b) One 8-ounce cup of orange juice (or other fruit juice) and one teaspoon salt to 3 cups clean water

    c) Half teaspoon table salt, $1/4$ teaspoon salt substitute (KCL), $1/2$ teaspoon baking soda and 2 to 3 tablespoons of sugar or 2 tablespoons of honey or Karo syrup to one liter clean water

  NOTE: Dairy products, iced drinks, and noncarbonated bottled beverages that contain water of questionable quality should be avoided (CDC, 1996n). Fruit juices, soft drinks, Gatorade®, and Jell-O® should not be ingested unless heavily diluted (Greenbaum, 1996).

▶ Nonspecific agents

- Kaolin and pectin

    * Over-the-counter (OTC): follow directions on bottle

    * Widely used but not too effective

- Bismuth subsalicylate

    * OTC: 2 tablespoons liquid (one dose cup, 1 oz) or two, 262.5 mg tablets p.o. Every 30 minutes to one hour for a maximum of eight doses in a 24-hour period

    * Treatment limited to 48 hours (CDC, 1996n)

    * Use with caution during gestation, restrict to the first half of pregnancy, and do not exceed recommended doses

    * Avoid during lactation (Briggs, Freeman, & Yaffe, 1994)

    NOTE: Reduces number of unformed stools and shortens duration of diarrhea but has no antibacterial or anti-inflammatory action (DuPont & Ericsson, 1993). Medication may cause temporary darkening of tongue and/or stool (stool darkening not to be confused with melena). Refer to the *PDR* or a clinical pharmacist for further information.

▶ Antimotility agents (synthetic agents)

- Loperamide

    * Initial dose 4 mg (two capsules) p.o., followed by 2 mg (one capsule) p.o. after each unformed stool until diarrhea controlled, after which dose should be reduced to meet individual requirements

    * Daily dose not to exceed 16 mg (eight capsules) (*PDR*, 1995); an OTC liquid formulation is available

    NOTE: Use of this drug has not been linked to congenital defects and is compatible with breast feeding (Briggs et al., 1994).

- Diphenoxylate

    * Two tablets p.o. four times daily or 10 ml liquid (2 teaspoons) p.o. four times daily.

    * Dosage may be reduced to meet individual requirements after initial diarrhea control achieved (*PDR*, 1995).

    NOTE: Diphenoxylate is a narcotic related to meperidine, available only in combination with atropine. Data does not support an association between the drug and congenital birth defects; should be used with caution during breastfeeding as the drug is probably excreted into breast milk (Briggs et al., 1994). Refer to the *PDR* for further information.

NOTE: Antimotility agents should not be used if there is blood in the stool or fever is present. If diarrhea does not resolve within 48 hours drug should be discontinued. Refer to the *PDR* or a clinical pharmacist for further information. Discuss with client side effects of all drugs used.

▶ Antimicrobials

    – Trimethoprim/sulfamethoxazole (160 mg/800 mg, double-strength [DS] tablet)

        * One DS tablet p.o. twice daily for 3 days (although 2 days or less may be sufficient) (CDC, 1997a; Greenbaum, 1996).

        NOTE: Use with caution during pregnancy; avoid in first trimester (trimethoprim is a folate acid antagonist); sulfonamides should be avoided close to delivery; compatible with breast feeding of healthy, full-term neonate (Briggs et al., 1994).

    – Ciprofloxacin is also used in the treatment of TD but is *contraindicated during pregnancy and lactation.*

NOTE: Patients should consult a physician rather than attempting self-treatment if diarrhea is severe or contains blood and/or mucus, or if there is fever/chills, dehydration or persistent diarrhea (CDC, 1997a). Drugs should be prescribed with caution, weighing the risk/benefit ratio. Discuss with client side effects of all drugs used. Nausea and vomiting without diarrhea should not be treated with antimicrobials (CDC, 1997a).

● See also the HIV/STD section in this chapter for additional information about TD.

Malaria

● Pregnant women should avoid travel to malarious areas.

● If travel to these places is unavoidable, offer prophylaxis.

● Consult with a travel medicine specialist. Detailed recommendations for the prevention of malaria are available 24-hours-a-day by phone by calling the CDC International Travelers Hotline at (404) 332-4559.

● Personal protection measures for malaria prevention are listed in Table 4.9. Infants (both bottle and breast-fed) and children will require prophylaxis if traveling with their mothers to malaria-endemic areas—consult with a pediatrician, a travel medicine specialist, or the CDC regarding regimens.

NOTE: If febrile illness occurs during travel in malaria-endemic areas, professional medical evaluation is imperative! Treatment of malaria during pregnancy will not be covered in this chapter.

● Prophylactic regimens

    ▶ Chloroquine phosphate alone is used in areas where the malarial strain is sensitive to the drug.

    – Dosage is 300 mg base (500 mg salt) p.o. once a week.

        * Medication should be taken 1 to 2 weeks prior to entering a malarious area, weekly while there, and weekly for 4 weeks after leaving malarious area (CDC, 1996b, CDC, 1996c, CDC, 1997a).

        * If intolerable side effects occur (see below), the dose may be taken with meals or in twice weekly, divided doses.

        NOTE: Alternatively, hydroxychloroquine sulfate 310 mg base (400 mg salt) p.o. once a week may be better tolerated (CDC, 1997a).

- Side effects/adverse reactions can be GI upset, headache, dizziness, blurred vision, pruritus (all rare), or exacerbation of psoriasis.

- Chloroquine and hydroxychloroquine are not contraindicated during pregnancy.

▶ Mefloquine alone is recommended in areas with chloroquine-resistant *P. falciparum*.

- Dosage is 228 mg base (250 mg salt) p.o. once a week

   * Medication should be taken 1 to 2 weeks prior to entering malarious area, weekly while there, and for 4 weeks after leaving malarious area (CDC, 1996b; CDC, 1996c; CDC, 1997a).

- Side effects/adverse reactions can be GI disturbances and dizziness (tend to be mild, temporary), psychoses (rarely), convulsions.

- Contraindications are known hypersensitivity or history of epilepsy, psychiatric disorders, and cardiac conduction abnormalities.

- "Mefloquine may be considered for use by health care providers for prophylaxis in women who are pregnant or likely to become so, when exposure to chloroquine-resistant *P. falciparum* is unavoidable" (CDC, 1997a, p. 136).

NOTE: Information on use of the drug in the first trimester is limited; if use is elected during this time, women or their health care providers are asked to report the exposure to the Malaria Section, CDC, telephone 770-488-7760 for inclusion in a registry to assess pregnancy outcomes (CDC, 1997a). Adverse reactions to the drug should also be reported to this number.

NOTE: Self-treatment regimens and alternatives to mefloquine for travelers to areas with drug resistant *P. falciparum* should be discussed with a travel medicine specialist or the CDC.

Yellow fever

- Yellow fever prevention is accomplished by avoidance of mosquito bites. See Table 4.9.

- Some countries require an International Certificate of Vaccination Against Yellow Fever as a condition for entry. Vaccination must be given at an approved Yellow Fever Vaccination Center and the vaccination certificate must be validated with the center's official stamp. The certificate is valid for 10 years. Yellow fever vaccination requirements and recommendations are listed in the *Yellow Book* and the *Blue Sheet* as well as in the CDC's fax documents.

- Yellow fever vaccine virus can potentially infect the fetus. Risk of adverse events associated with congenital infection is unknown, however. Pregnant women should be advised to postpone travel to epidemic areas until after delivery (CDC, 1997a).

  ▶ If a pregnant woman must travel to areas in which the risk of yellow fever is high, she should be vaccinated.

  ▶ If the travel itinerary poses no substantial risk of exposure and international travel regulations constitute the only reason for vaccination, a waiver should be provided for the client.

  NOTE: Contraindications to vaccination may be indicated on the designated section of the vaccination card and waiver letter written on physician's (or physician-designee's) letterhead stationery (CDC, 1995; CDC, 1997a).

- Prophalaxis

  ▶ Vaccine dosage is 0.5 mL for individuals over 9 months of age; one dose every 10 years.

  ▶ Side effects may include mild headache, myalgia, low-grade fever, other minor symptoms 5 to 10 days after vaccination.

  ▶ Contraindications are egg hypersensitivity and immunosuppression.

  NOTE: Persons with asymptomatic HIV infection who cannot avoid potential exposure should be offered the vaccine (CDC, 1996L; CDC, 1997a).

  NOTE: Clinicians should be knowledgeable regarding the precautions, contraindications, reactions, and information about simultaneous administration of other drugs and vaccines if yellow fever vaccine is used.

Cholera

- Disease is easily prevented by proper food and water precautions (see Table 4.8).

- Cases generally respond to simple fluid/electrolyte replacement via an ORS (see section on Travelers' Diarrhea). Antibiotics may also be indicated. Persons with severe diarrhea and vomiting should seek medical attention promptly.

- Vaccination is not routinely recommended for travelers; on theoretical grounds, cholera vaccination should be avoided during pregnancy (CDC, 1996d, CDC, 1997a).

Typhoid

- Discuss prevention measures. See Table 4.8, Water and Food Precautions.

- Vaccination is not required for international travel. Information is unavailable regarding safety of the vaccines during pregnancy, therefore, on theoretical grounds the CDC advises against vaccinating pregnant women (CDC, 1996e; CDC, 1997a).

- If typhoid fever is suspected medical care should be sought immediately.

- Antibiotics used in treatment include ampicillin, trimethoprimsulfamethoxazole, and ciprofloxacin (cipro is contraindicated in pregnancy).

  NOTE: Persons who have had typhoid fever may need medical clearance prior to returning to a food handling job or a job caring for small children.

Dengue Fever

- Treatment consists of supportive care, including rest, fluid replacement, and analgesics (e.g., acetaminophen) (Greenbaum, 1996).

- No vaccine is available, thus prevention, by avoidance of mosquito bites, is key—see Table 4.9.

Meningococcal Disease

- Travelers with symptoms of meningococcal disease should seek medical help immediately.

- Vaccination is indicated for travelers to areas with recognized epidemic meningococcal disease due to vaccine-preventable serogroups A, C, Y, and W135.

  ▶ Areas include the "meningitis belt" of sub-Saharan Africa, and certain areas outside of the "meningitis belt" in Kenya, Tanzania, Burundi, or Mongolia. Vaccination is required for pilgrims traveling to Mecca, Saudi Arabia for the annual hajj.

  ▶ In the U.S. one formulation of meningococcal polysaccharide vaccine is currently available.

  ▶ Unless there is a substantial risk of infection, pregnant women should not be vaccinated (CDC, 1997a).

Japanese encephalitis

- Mosquito-biting prevention measures are important. See Table 4.9.

- Travelers with symptoms of this infection should seek medical help immediately.

- Vaccination recommendations are as follows:

  ▶ Vaccination should be avoided during pregnancy unless the risk of acquiring the disease clearly outweighs the theoretical risk of vaccination (i.e., there is high risk of infection during travel in Asia [trips into rural, farming areas]).

  ▶ Short-term travel (less than 30 days) to urban areas does not require vaccination (CDC, 1996g; CDC, 1997a). Consult the *Yellow Book* for information on risk of infection by country, region, and season.

  ▶ Dosage is 1.0 mL for persons over 3 years of age on days 0, 7, and 30.

    – Protection is conferred 10 days after last dose

    – Booster after 3 years if the traveler is still at risk for infection (CDC 1996g; CDC, 1997a).

    – Side effects/adverse reactions: fever, headache, myalgia; redness, swelling, pain in injection site; generalized urticaria, angioedema, respiratory distress, and anaphylaxis.

      NOTE: Serious reactions can occur within the range of minutes to up to 1 week after administration. **Observe vaccinees for 30 minutes after injection and warn them about delayed reactions.** Close medical supervision should be available for at least 48 hours after vaccination (CDC, 1996g; CDC, 1997a).

    – Contraindications are a known hypersensitivity to vaccine components or a history of multiple allergies.

Plague

- Travel to plague-infected areas should be avoided by pregnant women.

- If travel to an endemic area is imperative, DEET-containing insect repellent should be applied to the skin of the legs and ankles.

  ▶ Also apply insecticides and repellents to clothes and outer bedding. Permethrin sprays are effective for fleas (see Table 4.9, Personal Protection Measures Against Insect Bites).

- Sick, dead, stray or wild animals should not be handled.

- Antibiotic prophylaxis may be considered in the event of exposure to wild rodent or flea bites during a plague outbreak, or when coming into contact with the tissues of a plague infected animal or close exposure to a human or pet with suspected plague pneumonia (CDC, 1992a; CDC, 1994a, 1994b; CDC, 1997a). Consult the CDC or a travel medicine specialist.

- Plague vaccination is indicated for persons at high risk due to research activities or field work in epizootic areas.

  ▶ Selective vaccination of other at-risk groups may be considered.

  ▶ Vaccination is rarely indicated for travelers, especially if they are only frequenting urban ares.

- Vaccination during pregnancy should be evaluated on a case-by-case basis (CDC, 1994a, 1994b, 1994c; CDC, 1997a).

- Individuals with plague should be hospitalized, placed in isolation, and managed by a physician.

  NOTE: In the United States, local and state health departments must be notified of plague diagnosis (CDC, 1992a).

Rabies

- Domestic or wild animals (especially skunks, raccoons, and bats) should be avoided.

  ▶ Pet owners should ensure their animals are vaccinated.

  ▶ Animal bite wounds and scratches should be immediately well-cleansed with soap and water.

  ▶ Exposed persons should contact local health authorities immediately and their primary care provider or state health department as soon as possible thereafter (CDC, 1997a).

- Preexposure immunization is not indicated for the population-at-large.

- Consult with a travel medicine specialist or the CDC regarding preexposure prophylaxis of pregnant women whose activities may place them at higher risk of rabies exposure. Postexposure prophylaxis may be given to pregnant women.

- Prophalaxis

  ▶ Persons not previously immunized should receive

    – One dose of rabies immune globulin (RIG) 20 I.U./kg body weight, one-half infiltrated at bite site (if possible), the remainder IM,

  PLUS

    – 5 doses of human diploid cell rabies vaccine (HDCV) **or** rabies vaccine adsorbed (RVA), 0.1 mL IM (deltoid area), one injection on days 0, 3, 7, 14, and 28 (CDC, 1997a).

  ▶ Side effects: local reactions (e.g., pain, erythema, swelling, itching), mild systemic reactions (e.g., headache, nausea, abdominal pain, myalgia, dizziness).

    NOTE: Once initiated, postexposure prophylaxis should not be discontinued or interrupted due to mild local/systemic reactions.

Schistosomiasis

- Wading, swimming, or bathing in fresh water in rural areas with poor sanitation should be avoided. (Swimming or wading in salt water or chlorinated pools does not present a risk.)
- Travelers with symptoms of schistosomiasis should seek medical attention as soon as possible.
  - ▶ Medications are available for treatment. Consult the CDC or a travel medicine specialist.
  - ▶ Refer to Table 4.10 for information on prevention measures. Also see the Diagnostic Tests and Follow-up sections.

Tuberculosis

- Pregnant travelers who anticipate prolonged exposure to TB should have a tuberculin skin test prior to departure and, if negative, a repeat test upon returning. HIV-infected individuals may require anergy testing.
- Persons with infectious tuberculosis should travel by private transportation rather than commercial carrier (CDC, 1996j).
- Refer to Chapter 10.10, *Tuberculosis,* for further treatment information.

HIV/Sexually Transmitted Disease (STD)

- Address HIV and STD prevention. See Chapter 14.5, *Human Immunodeficiency Virus*, and Table 14.1, *Safer Sex Recommendations.*
- HIV-infected pregnant women should consult with a physician or travel medicine specialist prior to embarking.
  - ▶ Recommendations
    - − Carry an antibiotic along for treatment of travelers' diarrhea, to be taken empirically should diarrhea develop.
    - − Use malaria chemoprophylaxis as appropriate for anticipated exposure.
    - − Avoid live virus vaccines (see section on yellow fever in this chapter).
    - − Killed vaccines (e.g., diphtheria-tetanus, rabies) may be used, as for non-HIV infected persons as indicated.
    - − Cholera vaccine is not recommended (CDC, 1996L).
- Contact the CDC for information regarding blood transfusion guidelines for international travelers. (This information is also contained in the *Yellow Book.*)

Consultation

- Consult with or refer the client to a travel medicine specialist or the traveler's clinic of the local health department when caring for a pregnant woman planning international travel.
  - ▶ Specific up-to-date information regarding health information for international travel may also be sought from the CDC: Information regarding appropriateness of vaccination during pregnancy is

contained in CDC publications (see also Treatment/Management section, Table 4.7, and References.)

- Consult with a physician if patient has a medical or obstetrical problem that may pose a risk for traveling.

- Consult with or refer client to an occupational health specialist regarding health risks from radiation exposure when caring for a pregnant flight crew member or business frequent flyer. The client should understand airline policy regarding flying during pregnancy.

- Persons with travel-related illness who are severely ill should be hospitalized and managed by a physician. See Appendix 4.5a, Additional Resources, at the end of the chapter.

- For treatment/management guidelines of infections not covered in this chapter the reader should consult a textbook or current journal, or discuss the case with a travel medicine specialist.

Patient Education

General Information and Recommendations

- The pregnant traveler should contact her insurance company regarding health care coverage while traveling.

- Client should carry a synopsis of her medical/prenatal records and a lay language compendium of travel advice (Pust et al., 1991).

- Client should carry a back-up supply of prescriptive medication and the written prescription(s) should be available. Extra eyeglasses, contact lenses and the vision correction prescription should be carried along (Greenbaum, 1996).

- If client requires routine/frequent injections (e.g., insulin-dependent diabetics), she should carry a sufficient supply of syringes, needles, and alcohol wipes.

- Take along OTC analgesics (i.e., acetaminophen), antimotility drugs, antimotion-sickness medication, decongestants, stool softener (or glycerine suppositories), sunscreen, antibacterial soap, and insect repellent along with a small first-aid kit (Greenbaum, 1996).

- Advise client regarding issues related to general health, safety, and comfort measures. See Table 4.10, General Health, Safety, and Comfort Measures for Traveling While Pregnant.

- Discuss the general effects of travel, such as disturbed sleep/wakefulness cycle, disruption of usual eating and drinking habits, etc.

  ▶ Advise the patient that it is common to experience fatigue, nausea, indigestion, constipation, or insomnia due to the effects/stress of traveling.

  ▶ Discuss strategies for reducing jet lag (Greenbaum, 1996)

    – Plan trip to arrive at the new destination in early evening; go to bed on local time.

    – Reset watch to new destination time upon boarding airplane; adjust eating and sleeping accordingly.

    – Sleep on a night flight if scheduled to arrive in the morning; stay awake during flight that will arrive in the evening.

    – Force the body to adjust to new local time as soon as possible with activity, exercise, and mealtime adjustments; exposure to bright daylight may help to readjust the body's timeclock.

- Drink plenty of water; do not drink alcohol, and minimize coffee and other caffeinated beverages.

- Advise that air travel late in pregnancy may precipitate labor (CDC, 1997a).

- Advise that magnetometers at airport security checkpoints are not harmful to the fetus (Barry & Bia, 1989).

International Travel

- See General Information/Recommendations above.

- Have the client obtain (or provide for her) the various CDC fax documents from the International Travel Directory (404-332-4565).

NOTE: These documents contain very valuable information on many facets of international travel, i.e., reference information, disease risk and prevention information, disease outbreak bulletins, and other additional information.

- Obtain information on cruise ship sanitation from the *Summary of Sanitation Inspections of International Cruise Ships* (the "Green Sheet"). See Appendix 4.5a. for particulars.

- Recommend postponing nonessential travel to high-risk areas (DuPont & Ericsson, 1993).

- Address specific questions about health problems in various countries to the embassy or local consulate general's office of the particular country.

- Discuss safety and efficacy of immunizations and prophylactic medications if utilized.

  ▶ Advise that vaccines (killed or live) do not affect the safety of breastfeeding for mothers or infants.

  ▶ Breastfeeding is not a contraindication for any vaccine (CDC, 1997a).

- Mothers traveling with infants or children should ensure that the immunization status of their offspring is up-to-date. Consultation with a travel medicine specialist regarding pediatric vaccination and prophylaxis is advisable prior to departure.

- Food and water precautions and insect-biting protection measures are essential to preventing a variety of diseases; discuss these with client. See Tables 4.8 and 4.9 and Treatment/Management section for further information.

- Discuss travelers' diarrhea prevention and treatment measures. See Table 4.8 and the Treatment/Management section.

  ▶ Advise the client that she must seek medical attention if experiencing more than a few days of diarrhea, associated fever or chills, blood/mucus in the stool or dehydration with persistent diarrhea (CDC, 1997a).

  ▶ Good hand washing is important after using the toilet and before preparing food.

- Inform client regarding the risk of malaria infection.

  ▶ Discuss signs and symptoms of infection, prophylaxis, and side effects of medication given.

  ▶ Stress the importance of early treatment in the event of an infection (delay of therapy can have serious/fatal consequences).

> ▶ Refer to the CDC for information on malaria-endemic areas and the presence of drug resistant *P. falciparum* in certain areas.

> ▶ See Treatment/Management section and Table 4.9.

- Advise client regarding the potential of a carrier state for *S. typhi*.

> ▶ Good hygiene is essential during treatment.

> ▶ Individuals should not prepare or serve food to others during treatment.

- Address HIV/STD prevention and management.

> ▶ See Table14.1, Safer Sex Recommendations.

> ▶ HIV-infected individuals should be counseled that travel to certain areas poses risk for opportunistic infection and food and waterborne disease.The use of public conveyances (i.e., airplanes, automobiles, boats, buses, trains) by persons with HIV or AIDS does not pose a risk of infection to travelers.

> ▶ International travelers should be aware that some countries serologically screen incoming travelers for HIV infection (primarily persons with extended visits); they may be denied entry to certain countries (CDC, 1996k). Obtain further information on these policies from the consular officials of specific nations (CDC, 1996k).

- International travelers should be aware that some countries require the spraying (i.e., disinfection) of aircraft passenger compartments while the passengers are on board to prevent the importation of insects, such as mosquitos.

> ▶ Though determined safe by the World Health Organization, the disinfection procedures may aggravate certain health conditions such as allergies.

> ▶ Countries that may spray are located in Latin America, the Caribbean, Australia, and the South Pacific regions (CDC, 1996o).

> ▶ Travelers may contact the airline for further information.

- The U.S. embassy or consulate in the destination country may be contacted for information regarding hospitals, physicians, or emergency medical services.

- The International SOS, and the U.S. State Department, Overseas Emergency Center can be of assistance to travelers in medical or legal difficulties (Buckley, 1995). See Appendix 4.5a, Additional Resources.

- See also the introduction to the chapter and the Treatment/Management section, for additional particulars on specific diseases.

Follow-up

- Review the itinerary upon client's return and inquire as to health/illness status of the client during her travels. Explore the psychosocial impact of the trip with her.

- Malaria prophylaxis, if used, should be continued for 4 weeks after traveler leaves a malarious area.

- Advise client to report *any* illness which occurs after her return.

  ▶ Most individuals who acquire viral, bacterial, or parasitic infection abroad become ill within 6 weeks of returning home (exception is malaria which may not manifest for 6 months to 1 year) (CDC, 1997a).

  ▶ The most common complaints of returning travelers are diarrhea, upper respiratory infections, fever, rash, abdominal pain, or malaise.

  ▶ The most common diagnoses are STDs, giardia, hepatitis A, and malaria (Pust et al., 1991).

- Clinical consultation with a travel medicine specialist may be indicated because more than one infection may exist. CDC physician consultation is available via the CDC International Travelers Hotline at (404) 639-2572.

- Expectant and conservative management is appropriate for returning travelers with mild, nonprogressive diarrhea without fever, weight loss, or rectal bleeding (Yung & Ruff, 1994). See Travelers' Diarrhea under Treatment/Management.

- Diarrhea persisting for more than 3 weeks may require fecal examinations (x 3), CBC, ESR, liver function tests, amoebic and *Strongyloides* serology. Additional tests that may be indicated include enterotest (string test), sigmoidoscopy and rectal biopsy, fecal fat collection, and colonoscopy (Yung & Ruff, 1994).

- Fever in returning travelers most commonly is due to malaria, hepatitis A, typhoid or dengue fever.

  ▶ Important considerations include

    – The possible etiologies based on the client's itinerary

    – The possible diagnoses based on the clinical presentation

    – Which diseases require urgent intervention

  ▶ **Every fever in a returning traveler should be regarded as malaria until proven otherwise** (Yung & Ruff, 1994). See Diagnostic Tests section.

  ▶ Client should be managed in consultation with a travel medicine specialist.

- Hemorrhagic fevers are potentially lethal, although rare in travelers.

  ▶ Client should be managed by a travel medicine specialist.

  ▶ Suspected cases should be reported to the CDC immediately.

- Neurological symptoms (e.g., headache, mental status changes) may be the result of a wide variety of meningitis or encephalitis etiologies. Consult with/refer client to physician.

- Respiratory infections may be acute or have latency periods (months to years, as in TB).

  ▶ New-onset asthma symptoms after tropical-country travel is suspicious for helminthic infection (i.e., ascaris, hookworm, strongyloides) (Yung & Ruff, 1994).

- Jaundice is most likely due to viral hepatitis, but may be due to a variety of other causes.

  ▶ Serological diagnosis is important.

  ▶ Abdominal ultrasound is indicated if the laboratory picture is atypical (Yung & Ruff, 1994).

▶ Offer Hepatitis B vaccine to susceptible household members and sexual partners of patients with hepatitis B.

▶ See Chapter 10.2, *Hepatitis A, B, C, D, and E,* for further information.

● Physical findings of hepatosplenomegaly, lymphadenopathy, and/or rash in an asymptomatic returning traveler suggest infection and should be worked up appropriately. Consult with specialist.

● STDs should be treated appropriately. See chapters in Section 14, Vaginitis and Sexually Transmitted Disease.

▶ Serologic tests for syphilis, hepatitis B, and HIV should be performed 6 weeks after exposure to an STD.

▶ HIV testing may be repeated in 3 to 6 months.

● Stool examinations for ova and parasites may be obtained 8 weeks after client's return from international travel to rule out asymptomatic parasitic infestation. Consult with a travel medicine specialist regarding treatment during pregnancy, as indicated.

● Stool cultures for *S. typhi* should be performed in individuals treated for typhoid fever to rule out a carrier state.

● Tuberculin skin testing may be performed 6 to 8 weeks after client's return from international travel, as indicated.

● If exposure to possible schistosome-infected water occurred during travel, client should undergo screening tests on returning (e.g., serologic studies; microscopic examination of urine and stool for schistosome eggs—6 to 8 weeks after exposure) (CDC, 1997a). Consult with travel medicine specialist regarding treatment.

● Health care providers should report suspected/confirmed cases of dengue fever to the state health department. In addition, certain STDs are reportable to the local health department.

● See also Treatment/Management and Consultation sections.

● Document client's itinerary and any illness acquired during travel in the progress notes and problem list.

Table 4.7

Vaccination During Pregnancy

Type of Vaccine	Indications for Vaccination During Pregnancy
Live virus vaccines	
Measles	Contraindicated
Mumps	
Rubella	
Yellow fever	Contraindicated except if exposure to yellow fever virus is unavoidable.
Poliomyelitus (OPV)	Persons at substantial risk of exposure to polio.
Inactivated virus vaccines	
Hepatitis A	Safety undetermined. Weigh risk/benefit.
Hepatitis B	Pregnancy is not a contraindication.
Influenza	Usually recommended only for patients with serious underlying disease. Consult health authorities for current recommendations.
Japanese encephalitis	Avoid; should reflect actual risks of disease and probable benefits of vaccine.
Poliomyelitis (IPV)	OPV preferred when immediate protection of pregnant females is needed; however, IPV is alternative if complete vaccination series can be administered before exposure.
Rabies	Substantial risk of exposure; not contraindicated for postexposure prophylaxis.
Live bacterial vaccines	
Typhoid	Avoid; should reflect actual risks of disease and probable benefits of vaccine.
Inactivated bacterial vaccines	
Cholera	Avoid; should reflect actual risks of disease and probable benefits of vaccine.
Typhoid	
Plague	Selective vaccination of exposed persons.
Meningococcal	Only in unusual outbreak situations.
Pneumococcal	Only for high-risk persons.
Haemophilus b conjugate	Only for high-risk persons.
Toxoids	
Tetanus-diphtheria (Td)	Lack of primary series, or no booster within past 10 years.
Immune globulins, pooled or hyperimmune	Exposure or anticipated unavoidable exposure to measles, hepatitis A, hepatitis B, rabies, or tetanus.

Source: Centers for Disease Control and Prevention. (1997). *Health information for international travel 1996-97* (Table 6, p. 94). Atlanta: Department of Health and Human Services.

Table 4.8

Water and Food Precautions

WATER
- Usage
  - ▶ The following beverages may be safe to drink in areas with poor sanitation:
    - Boiled water.
    - Hot beverages, such as coffee or tea made with boiled water.
    - Canned or bottled carbonated beverages.
  - ▶ Avoid ice, flavored ices, and popsickles because they may be made with unsafe water.
  - ▶ It is safer to drink from a canned or bottled beverage than from a container not known to be clean and dry. Wipe clean and dry the area of a can or bottle that touches the mouth. Avoid beverages from street vendors.
  - ▶ No brushing teeth with tap water in areas where water is known to be contaminated.
- Treatment
  - ▶ Boiling is the most reliable method.
    - Bring water to a vigorous boil, boil for 1 minute, allow to cool, *do not* add ice.
    - At very high altitudes, boil for several minutes longer.
  - ▶ To improve taste, add a pinch of salt or pour from one clean container to another.
  - ▶ Strain cloudy water through a clean cloth into a clean container then treat by boiling or chemical means.
  - ▶ To chemically disinfect water use either iodine or chlorine
    - Iodine provides greater disinfection in wider circumstances.
    - Tincture of iodine or iodine tablets (e.g., Globaline® Portable-Aqua®) may be used.
      - * For tablets, follow manufacturer's instructions, double number of tablets if water cloudy; if water extremely cold, warm it or allow increased contact time.
      - * For tincture of iodine 2% - use 5 drops/quart or liter of *clear* water, 10 drops/quart or liter of *cloudy* or *cold* water and let stand for 30 minutes; if water very cloudy or cold may require prolonged contact time, let stand up to several hours prior to use.

FOOD
- Source
  - ▶ Select with care!
  - ▶ Avoid raw food because it could be contaminated. Of particular concern: salads, uncooked vegetables, salsa, fruits and juices, flavored ices, unpasteurized milk/milk products, raw or undercooked eggs, meat, fish or shellfish.
  - ▶ Highest risk areas for poisonous biotoxins from fish are tropical insular areas of the West Indies, Pacific and Indian oceans. Cholera has occurred among persons who ate crab brought back from Latin America by travelers; thus, travelers should *not* bring perishable seafood (or other food items) back with them.
  - ▶ Eat only food that has been thoroughly cooked and is still hot and steaming, or fruit/vegetables that have been peeled by the traveler after thorough hand washing. Peels should not be eaten.
  - ▶ Avoid buffet food that's been handled frequently and served repeatedly.
    - If eating in a private home make sure food is cooked and served hot.
    - Avoid foods from street vendors.
  - ▶ Certain fish, even when cooked, may not be safe.
    - Of particular concern: tropical reef fish, red snapper, amberjack, grouper, and sea bass if caught on tropical reefs rather than open ocean; barracuda should *not* be eaten.
    - Raw fish or uncooked shellfish should *not* be eaten.

Sources: Centers for Disease Control and Prevention. (1997a). *Health information for international travel 1996–97.* Atlanta: Department of Health and Human Services.

Greenbaum, J.J. (1996). *Travel companion.* Copyright 1996, Kaiser Permanente Medical Group. Adapted with with permission.

Table 4.9
Personal Protection Measures Against Insect Bites

- Reduce contact with *Anopheles* mosquitos, especially between dusk and dawn. Remain in well-screened areas as much as possible, especially during these hours.

- Inspect self and clothing frequently for insects or ticks and remove promptly.

- Wear clothing that covers most of the body.

  - ▶ Shirts should be tucked into pants, and pants tucked into socks and boots.

  - ▶ Wear a hat.

  - ▶ Boots or shoes should be worn, sandals avoided. Avoid bright or dark-colored clothing.

  - ▶ Avoid using or applying substances with strong scents (e.g., deodorants, perfumes, lotions, soaps).

- Use insect repellent that contains 30% DEET (N,N diethylmethyltoluamide).[*]

  - ▶ Apply sparingly to exposed areas of the skin and on clothing. An application will last about 4 to 12 hours depending on the brand; saturation does not increase efficacy.

  - ▶ Avoid eyes; do not inhale or ingest.

  - ▶ Do not use on wounds or inflamed/irritated skin.

  - ▶ Wash repellent-treated areas of skin after returning indoors.

  - ▶ If a reaction develops, wash treated skin and see a physician (bring the container).

- Permethrin[*] cloth-impregnating solutions may be applied to clothing, shoes, and camping gear (not utensils) to kill and repel ticks, mosquitos, and other insects (effect lasts for several weeks, and is retained after repeated laundering).

- Permethrin-containing shampoo or cream may be effective as an insect repellent when applied to hair or skin.

- Reduce insect access to living quarters and sleeping areas.

  - ▶ Use mosquito netting impregnated with permethrin to afford protection while maintaining airflow. (Bednets are more effective if treated with insecticide.)

  - ▶ Use a pyrethroid-containing flying-insect spray in living and sleeping areas during evening and nighttime hours.

  - ▶ Before retiring, check bedding for insects.

- Use mosquito coils, especially in nonscreened rooms (some contain DDT so use with caution). *Minimize use if pregnant or breastfeeding.*

- **Minimize use of repellents if pregnant or breastfeeding.**

[*] May be purchased in hardware or backpacking stores. Use according to label directions.

Sources: Centers for Disease Control and Prevention. (1997). *Health information for international travel 1996-97.* Atlanta: Department of Health and Human Services.

Greenbaum, J. J. (1996). *Travel companion.* Copyright 1996, Kaiser Permanente Medical Group. Adapted with permission.

Table 4.10
General Health, Safety, and Comfort Measures for Traveling While Pregnant

Exercise
- Avoid prolonged immobilization.
- Walking about every 1–2 hours and exercising the legs periodically (calf/Achilles tendon stretches) will decrease dependent edema, lower back/symphysis pubis discomfort, and leg cramps.
- Physical fitness should be maintained during the travel period.

Clothing/Garments/Luggage
- Wearing of loose, comfortable clothing appropriate to the climate; cold-weather travel requires more adequate dress.
- Support hose may be utilized if a woman has varicosities or history of lower limb thrombosis (Skjenna, Evans, Moore, Thibeault, & Tucker, 1991).
- Avoid bringing heavy luggage. Baggage should be relatively easy to maneuver and never left unattended.

Diet
- Avoid
  ▶ Alcohol
  ▶ Caffeinated beverages
  ▶ Heavy, fatty foods
- Drink liberal fluids to prevent dehydration
- Avoid gas-producing foods prior to flight

Health and Hygiene
- Avoid overdistention of the bladder, both for comfort and to prevent uterine contractions.
- Wash hands thoroughly with soap and water before meals and after using public restrooms or changing a child's diaper.
- For susceptibility to symptoms produced by low humidity during air travel, use artificial tears if needed.
  ▶ Contact lens wearers should avoid prolonged wearing time.
  ▶ Patients with skin conditions aggravated by dryness should carry a moisturizing cream (Skjenna et al., 1991).
- To prevent upper respiratory tract illness, avoid breathing or swallowing dust from travel on unpaved roads or in arid areas.
- High-altitude trekking may cause acute altitude sickness; extreme care should be taken during pregnancy (ideally should be avoided) (Barry & Bia, 1989).
- To prevent/relieve airsickness, take night flights, place the seat in the reclining position, select a seat near the wing base, and take antimotion-sickness medication (Kusumi, 1981).
- Use sunscreen (SPF 15), protective eyewear and hats (Buckley, 1995).
- Avoid over-the-counter medications unless familiar with ingredients that are known to be safe during pregnancy.
- Seek medical attention for insect bites which cause redness, swelling, bruising or persistent pain, and for snake bites which break the skin. See also Table 4.9, Personal Protection Measures Against Insect Bites.
- Avoid wading, swimming or bathing in freshwater streams, canals, and lakes liable to be infested with the snail hosts of schistosomiasis or contaminated with urine from animals infected with *Leptospira* (vigorous towel-drying after accidental water exposure may remove snail larvae). Heating bathing water to 50°C (122°F) for 5 minutes or treating it with iodine or chlorine will destroy snail larvae.
- Apply STD/HIV prevention measures and safer sex guidelines.

Vehicular Travel
- Use vehicles in good working order and equipped with airbags and antilock brakes; wear helmet while cycling.
- Avoid nonessential night driving or riding with persons under the influence of drugs or alcohol; drive only when alert and well-rested.
- Wear seat belts during air and motor vehicle travel—lap portion of belt should be worn low around the pelvic girdle rather than higher up around the soft mid-abdomen.

Environment
- Awareness of fire safety measures/devices and fire escape routes in hotels/buildings.
- Avoid high-risk areas for violence (assault, terrorist attack).
  ▶ Local residents and the U.S. Embassy or Consul may be consulted.
  ▶ Avoid going out at night and when alone.
- Avoid domestic or wild animals in areas where endemic rabies exists; avoid all snakes.
- Avoid beaches and waters contaminated with sewage or animal waste. Wear shoes and protective clothing and use towels where fecal contamination of sand/soil is likely. Swallowing of water should be avoided while swimming. For safety's sake, never swim alone.

NOTE: Many of the above recommendations derive from the CDC publication, *Health Information for International Travel 1996–97*.

Appendix 4.5a

Additional Resources

Literature

Health Information for International Travel (the *Yellow Book*)

This publication may be obtained for a fee from the Superintendent of Documents, U.S. Government Printing Office, Washington, D.C. (202-512-1800); it is also available free of charge to health care providers from the CDC by calling (404) 639-2572.

Summary of Health Information for International Travel (the *Blue Sheet*)

A biweekly update to the *Yellow Book* which lists where cholera and yellow fever are being reported and official changes in individual country's vaccination requirements. This publication is free of charge to health care providers and can be obtained from the CDC by calling the fax information service at (404) 332-4565 and requesting document # 220022. The *Blue Sheet* is also available via the Internet at http://www.cdc.gov (choose "Travelers' Health" and look for first document in references titled "Biweekly HIIT Summary")

The Summary of Sanitation Inspections of International Cruise Ships (the *Green Sheet*)

Vessel Sanitation Program, National Center for Environmental Health
Centers for Disease Control and Prevention
1015 North America Way, Room 107
Miami, Florida 33132

For cruise ship sanitation information for an individual vessel; published every 2 weeks. Summaries may also be obtained from a travel agent, via the CDC fax information service at (404) 332-4565 (request document # 510051), or via Internet at FTP.CDC.GOV/PUB/SHIP_INSPECTIONS/ SHIPSCORE.TXT

Centers for Disease Control and Prevention

24-hour Hotline

Recorded information from the 24-hour CDC Hotline may be utilized by calling (404) 332-4555 or the CDC International Travelers' Hotline at (404) 639-2572.

Fax Information Service

Materials from the automated CDC Fax Information service can be obtained by calling (404) 332-4565. The International Travel Directory is document # 00005.

Drug Service

The CDC Drug Service at (404) 639-3670 provides phone consultation on unusual parasitic diseases and provides pharmaceuticals which may not be available commercially.

Internet Address

The CDC's Internet address on the World Wide Web Server is: http://www.cdc.gov or the File Transfer Protocol server at ftp.cdc.gov.

Emergency Assistance

Overseas Citizens Services
Room 4811 A
Department of State
Washington, DC 20520
(202) 647-5225
Assistance to travelers in medical and legal difficulty and advisories on countries with political unrest or high levels of violence-related injuries to travelers

The International Association for Medical Assistance to Travelers (IAMAT).
417 Center Street
Lewiston, New York
(716) 754-4883
Travel advisors for many countries with addresses and telephone numbers for English-speaking travel physicians in major cities.

International SOS Assistance
P.O. Box 11568
Philadelphia, PA 19616
(215) 245-4707
Emergency medical evacuation and travelers' insurance

Disabled Traveler Information

The U.S. Architectural and Transportation Barriers Compliance Board (ATBCB)
Access Board, Suite 1000
1331 F Street, NW
Washington, D.C. 20004-1111
1(800) USA-ABLE (voice/TTY)
Distributes publications at no cost

Access Travel: Airports (booklet)
Consumer Information Center
Pueblo, CO 81009
List of accessibility features at over 500 airports worldwide

Sources: Centers for Disease Control and Prevention. (1997). *Health information for international travel 1996–97.* Atlanta: CDC.

Buckley, G. E. (1995). Traveling healthy: A guide for counseling the international traveler. *The Nurse Practitioner, 20*(10), 38–50.

References

Advisory Committee on Immunization Practices (ACIP). (1991). Update on adult immunization: Recommendations of the Immunization Practices Advisory Committee (ACIP). *Mortality and Morbidity Weekly Report, 40*(No. RR–12), 1–94.

American Academy of Pediatrics Committee on Infectious Diseases. (1997). Recommended childhood immunization schedule - United States, January-December 1997. *Pediatrics, 99*(1), 136–137.

Barish, R.J. (1990). Health physics concerns in commercial aviation. *Health Physics, 59*(2), 199–204.

Barry, M., & Bia, F. (1989). Pregnancy and travel. *Journal of the American Medical Association 261*(5), 728–731.

Breen, J.L., Gregori, C.A., & Neilson, R.N. (1986). Travel by airplane during pregnancy. *New Jersey Medicine, 83*(5), 297–299.

Briggs, G.G., Freeman, R.K., & Yaffe, S.J. (1994) Drugs in pregnancy and lactation (4th ed.) Balitmore: Williams & Wilkins.

Buckley, G.E. (1995). Traveling healthy: A guide for counseling the international traveler. *The Nurse Practitioner, 20*(10), 38–50.

Cameron, R.G. (1973). Should air hostesses continue flight duty during the first trimester of pregnancy? *Aerospace Medicine, 44*, 552–556.

Centers for Disease Control and Prevention. (1992a). *Plague information. Health worker information.* Fax document # 351510. Atlanta: CDC.

Centers for Disease Control and Prevention. (1992b). *Rabies.* Fax document # 361501. Atlanta: CDC.

Centers for Disease Control and Prevention. (1994a). *Plague.* Fax document # 351500. Atlanta: CDC.

Centers for Disease Control and Prevention. (1994b). *Plague information. Vaccine information.* Fax document # 351511. Atlanta: CDC.

Centers for Disease Control and Prevention. (1994c). *Plague information - Drug guidelines: Plague.* Fax document # 351513. Atlanta: CDC.

Centers for Disease Control and Prevention. (1995). *Comprehensive yellow fever vaccination requirements.* Fax document # 220005. Atlanta: CDC.

Centers for Disease Control and Prevention. (1996a). *Hepatitis A vaccine and immune globulin (IG): Disease and vaccine information.* Fax document # 221100. Atlanta: CDC.

Centers for Disease Control and Prevention. (1996b). *Malaria information: Pregnancy and children.* Fax document # 221012. Atlanta: CDC.

.Centers for Disease Control and Prevention. (1996c). *Prescription drugs for malaria.* Fax document # 221010. Atlanta: CDC.

Centers for Disease Control and Prevention. (1996d). *Cholera information.* Fax document # 221120. Atlanta: CDC.

Centers for Disease Control and Prevention. (1996e). *Preventing typhoid fever: A guide for travelers.* Fax document # 221061. Atlanta: CDC.

Centers for Disease Control and Prevention. (1996f). *Dengue fever.* Fax document # 221030. Atlanta: CDC.

Centers for Disease Control and Prevention. (1996g). *Japanese encephalitis.* Fax document # 351601. Atlanta: CDC.

Centers for Disease Control and Prevention. (1996h). *Rabies information: International traveler rabies immunization recommendations.* Fax document # 351502. Atlanta: CDC.

Centers for Disease Control and Prevention. (1996i). *Schistosomiasis.* Fax document # 578004. Atlanta: CDC.

Centers for Disease Control and Prevention. (1996j). *Tuberculosis risk on aircraft.* Fax document # 221090. Atlanta: CDC.

Centers for Disease Control and Prevention. (1996k). *HIV/AIDS prevention. International travelers health information.* Fax document # 221070. Atlanta: CDC.

Centers for Disease Control and Prevention. (1996l). *HIV infected traveler precautions.* Fax document # 221071. Atlanta: CDC.

Centers for Disease Control and Prevention. (1996m). *Other insect diseases.* Fax document # 221050. Atlanta: CDC.

Centers for Disease Control and Prevention. (1996n). *Food and water and traveler's diarrhea.* Fax document # 220004. Atlanta: CDC.

Centers for Disease Control and Prevention. (1996o). *Spraying of aircraft for insects.* Fax document # 221080. Atlanta: CDC.

Centers for Disease Control and Prevention. (1997a). *Health information for international travel 1996–97.* Atlanta: Department of Health and Human Services.

Centers for Disease Control and Prevention. (1997b). *Vaccine recommendations for travelers 2 years of age and older.* Fax document # 220002. Atlanta: CDC.

DuPont, H.L. & Ericsson, C.D. (1993). Prevention and treatment of traveler's diarrhea. *The New England Journal of Medicine, 328*(25), 1821–1827.

Federal Aviation Administration (1986). Regulatory docket no. 24016 - "Denial of petition." Washington, D.C.: FAA.

Friedberg, W., Faulkner, D.N., Snyder, L., Darden, E.B., Jr., & O'Brien, K. (1989). Galactic cosmic radiation exposure and associated risks for air carrier crewmembers. *Aviation Space Environmental Medicine, 60,* 1104–1108.

Furesz, J., Scheifele, D., & Palkonyay, L. Safety and effectiveness of the new inactivated hepatitis A virus vaccine. *Canadian Medical Association Journal, 152,* 343–348.

Goldman, M. (1982). Ionizing radiation and its risks. *Western Journal of Medicine, 137*(6), 540–547.

Greenbaum, J.J. (1996). *Travel companion.* USA: Kaiser Permanente Medical Group.

Huch, R,, Baumann, H., Fallenstein, F., Schneider, KT., Holdener, F., & Huch, A. (1986). Physiologic changes in pregnant women and their fetuses during jet air travel. *American Journal of Obstetrics and Gynecology, 154*, 996.

Kusumi, R. (1981, June). Medical aspects of air travel. *American Family Physician*, 125–129.

Lee, R.V. (1989). The pregnant traveller. *Travel Medicine, 7*, 51–58.

Lommel, L.L. (1995). Hepatitis - viral. In W. L. Star, L.L. Lommel, & M.T. Shannon (Eds.), *Women's primary health care: Protocols for practice* (pp. 11–15 - 11–24). Washington, D.C.: American Nurses Publishing.

Matzkel, A., Lurie, S., Elchalal, U., & Blickstein, I. (1991). Placental abruption associated with air travel. A case report and overview on safety of air travel in pregnant women. *Journal of Perinatal Medicine, 19*, 317–320.

Parer, J.T. (1982). Effects of hypoxia on the mother and fetus with emphasis on maternal air transport. *American Journal of Obstetrics and Gynecology, 142*, 957.

Pust, R.E., Campos-Outcalt, D., & Cordes, D.H. (1991). International travel. Preparing your patient. *Primary Care, 18*(1), 213–240.

Pust, R.E., Peate, W.F., & Cordes, D.H. (1986). Comprehensive care of travelers. *Journal of Family Practice, 23*(6), 572–579.

Sholten, P. (1976). Pregnant stewardess - should she fly? *Aviation Space and Environmental Medicine, 47*, 77–81

Skjenna, O.W., Evans, J.F., Moore, M.S., Thibeault, C., & Tucker, A. G. (1991). Helping patients travel by air. *Canadian Medical Association, 144*(3), 287–293.

Tietze, P.E., & Jones, J.E. (1991). Parasites during pregnancy. *Primary Care, 18*(1), 75–98.

Yung, A.P., & Ruff, T.A. (1994). Tropical health: Travel medicine. 2. Upon return. *The Medical Journal of Australia, 160*(21), 206–212.

SECTION 5

COMMON DISCOMFORTS OF PREGNANCY

Chapter 1

BACKACHE

Winifred L. Star

Ellen M. Scarr

Back pain in pregnancy is a common occurrence, affecting 50 to 90 percent of pregnancies (Heckman, 1990; Orvieto, Achiron, Ben-Rafael, Gelernter & Achiron, 1994; Ostgaard, Andersson, Schultz & Miller, 1993; Rungee, 1993). Normal lumbar lordosis (anterior convexity of the spine) becomes exaggerated during pregnancy as the enlarging uterus shifts the woman's center of gravity forward and upward. Lack of support from lax abdominal muscles may contribute to this compensatory lordosis. The increased lordosis creates stress on the posterior lumbosacral spine, with resulting pain, commonly in the fifth to seventh month of pregnancy.

The hormone relaxin, secreted during pregnancy, promotes softening of the sacroiliac (SI) joints and symphysis pubis to facilitate delivery. This resulting joint instability promotes increased movement in both the spine and the SI joint, normally a minimally moving articulation. This may result in inflammation and pain of the SI joint (sacroilitis), the most common cause of low back pain in pregnancy, which can begin as early as the first trimester (Rungee, 1993). Sacroiliac subluxation is also a result of this joint instability and commonly causes severe low back pain in the second trimester (Daly, Frame, & Rapoza, 1991). Vascular compromise contributes to nocturnal back pain, a frequent occurrence 1 to 2 hours after the woman lies down. Dependent edema, which accumulates during the day returns to the intravascular space, which in turn increases venous return. Pressure on the inferior vena cava from the fetus, coupled with the increase in venous return, compromises pelvic blood flow and results in neural hypoxia, causing pain and occasionally radicular symptoms (Hainline, 1994).

Pain in the cervicothoracic, as well as sternocostal and costovertebral areas, may result from the increased weight of the breasts during pregnancy. Lumbosacral pain with radicular symptoms may result from direct pressure of the gravid uterus on the lumbosacral nerve root (Orvieto et al., 1994). Other factors that may precipitate backache in pregnancy include excessive weight gain, repetitive lifting and bending, inadequate rest and mechanical strain from improper body mechanics. Pathologic causes of back pain, such as sprain due to trauma, intervertebral disc herniation, vertebral fractures, and pyelonephritis, should be evaluated as indicated. Obstetric causes of backache such as preterm labor should be ruled out.

Database

Subjective

- Client may report history of
  - ▶ Back problems/injury/surgery
  - ▶ Recent trauma
  - ▶ Excessive exercise, bending, lifting, twisting, sitting, or walking
  - ▶ Obesity

▶ Excessive weight gain in pregnancy

▶ Wearing high-heeled or improperly fitting shoes

▶ Improper use of body mechanics

▶ Fatigue

- Client may report

   ▶ Pain (unilateral or bilateral), aching, tightness, or spasm in upper or lower back; pain may be aggravated by coughing, sneezing, laughing, standing, walking

   ▶ Numbness, tingling, weakness in back, buttocks, or extremities

   ▶ Audible popping or "catching" of joints

   ▶ Associated bowel or bladder incontinence

   ▶ Signs and symptoms of premature labor. See Chapter 6.25, *Preterm Labor.*

   ▶ Signs and symptoms of urinary tract infection. See Chapter 13.2, *Cystitis,* and Chapter 13.3, *Pyelonephritis.*

Objective

- Lax abdominal musculature

- Lordotic curve

- Abnormal gait

- May have tenderness/spasm over SI joint

- May have tenderness/spasm along paraspinous muscles

- May have decreased, uneven, or absent patellar, ankle or plantar deep tendon reflexes may be decreased, uneven or absent (indicates neurological deficit)

- Straight leg raising may cause or increase pain in back, buttocks, or legs (indicates disc/neurological involvement, sacroiliac joint involvement)

- Decreased sensation along lower extremity nerve root may be present

- Asymmetry of the anterior or posterior superior iliac spines may be present (indicates sacroiliac subluxation)

- May have pain in sacral area with downward pressure on anterior superior iliac spines (pelvic compression test, indicating sacroiliac subluxation)

- Abdominal exam may reveal tenderness or decreased bowel sounds

- Costovertebral angle tenderness may be present

- Vaginal exam may reveal abnormal lesions/discharge

- If in labor, uterine contractions may be palpable by examiner.

Assessment

- Physiologic backache
  - ▶ R/O lumbar, cervicothoracic, sternocostal, or costovertebral muscle strain/sprain
  - ▶ R/O sciatica
  - ▶ R/O intervertebral disc herniation
  - ▶ R/O vertebral tumor/fracture
  - ▶ R/O pyelonephritis
  - ▶ R/O gastrointestinal disorder/disease
  - ▶ R/O pelvic infection (sexually transmitted infection, chorioamnionitis)
  - ▶ R/O premature labor

Plan

Diagnostic Tests

- If symptoms and examination are suggestive of physiologic backache, no diagnostic testing needed.
- X-rays are to be avoided in pregnancy except per physician recommendation.
- Laboratory tests may include complete blood count (CBC), urinalysis with culture and sensitivities, cervical cultures, as indicated.

Treatment/Management

- Physiologic Causes or Strain
  - ▶ Ice to affected area(s) for first 24 hours after an acute injury, or if spasm is present. (Application may be for 10 to 20 minutes at a time, 20 minutes/hour, or as indicated.)
  - ▶ Local, moist heat with proper padding or toweling to affected area(s) if there is no acute injury or if pain is due to physiologic cause. (Dry heat [i.e., heating pad] is nonpenetrating and does not reach the deep muscles of the back.)
  - ▶ Warm (not hot) tub baths not to exceed 30 minutes
  - ▶ Bed rest on firm supportive surface; a bed board may be necessary
  - ▶ Massage and relaxation
  - ▶ Supportive brassiere
  - ▶ Low-heeled, supportive, and comfortable shoes
  - ▶ Support stockings to decrease dependent edema
  - ▶ Pelvic rocking exercise—about 10 to12 times a day (see Patient Education)
  - ▶ Proper body mechanics; avoidance of heavy lifting

    ▶ Abdominal muscle strengthening exercises

    ▶ Corset or trochanteric belt for lumbosacral spine support (decreases SI joint movement, supports abdomen, decreases symphysis pubis movement)

    ▶ Maternity girdle—especially useful in obese women, multiparas, or women with extreme lordosis

    ▶ Analgesics, such as acetaminophen 325 mg, one to two tablets every 4 hours as needed for pain. Long-term use of analgesics may indicate more serious pathology and would require physician evaluation.

    ▶ General fitness exercise three to four times a week for at least 30 minutes (e.g., stretching, walking, swimming, prenatal exercise class)

    ▶ Physical therapy as indicated

- See Patient Education.

- Pathologic Causes

    ▶ Refer to either an orthopedic specialist, neurologist, or internal medicine physician for significant pathologic back pain, or if physical exam findings are indicative of pathology.

    ▶ Refer to physical therapy, as indicated.

    ▶ Treat genitourinary infections as indicated. See Section 13.

    ▶ See also Chapter 6.25, *Preterm Labor.*

Consultation

- Consultation is not required for cases of physiologic back pain, but should be sought when pain is secondary to acute strain/sprain or other pathologic causes.

- Discuss with physician the appropriateness of referrals to alternative sources of care such as chiropractic, acupuncture, or acupressure.

Patient Education

- See Treatment/Management.

- Stress avoidance of sitting, standing, or walking for long periods of time; encourage patient to wear low-heeled, comfortable shoes.

- Advise use of firm, straight back chair when sitting, with one foot elevated on small stool to relax back muscles. A cushion can provide support for the lower back.

- Discuss need for adequate rest periods and avoidance of fatigue and excess stress.

- Encourage proper body mechanics (bend both knees when lifting, hold object close to body, lift with leg muscles, avoid heavy lifting).

- Encourage daily abdominal/back exercises (Hainline, 1994; Heckman, 1990; Jacobson, 1991)

    ▶ Pelvic tilt (lie supine with hips/knees flexed, feet flat on floor; press lower back into floor by contracting abdominal/gluteal muscles; hold for 5 seconds, then relax; repeat 10 times)

- ▶ Pelvic rocking (do pelvic tilt; raise buttocks off floor; rock pelvis slowly 10 times)

- ▶ Straight leg lift (lie flat, feet on floor, knees bent; straighten and lift one leg 10 inches off floor, hold for 10 seconds, slowly relax; repeat with other leg; repeat sequence 5 times)

- ▶ Curl-ups (do pelvic tilt, bend chin to chest, slowly reach to knees, lift head and shoulders off floor; slowly lower to floor; repeat 10 times)

- ▶ Hip flexion (do pelvic tilt; lift one knee slowly to chest, then relax; repeat with other knee, relax; repeat with both knees, relax; repeat 10 times)

- Recommend against excessive weight gain during pregnancy.

- Encourage general fitness; suggest formal prenatal exercise class or nonimpact aerobic exercise three to four times/week for at least 30 minutes (stretching, walking, swimming).

- Suggest that a friend or partner give the client a back massage.

- Suggest incorporation of relaxation techniques into daily living.

- Give hints for supporting lower back area while resting/sleeping (e.g., use of pillows under knees and between legs).

  NOTE: Sleeping on left side with pillow to elevate protuberent abdomen will avoid nocturnal backache.

- Offer suggestions for reading materials related to relaxation, exercise in pregnancy, massage, etc.

- Encourage maintenance of well-balanced diet and give suggestions for meal planning if on bed rest. See Section 18, *Nutrition*.

Follow-up

- Refer to physician all patients with significant pathologic causes of back pain, or those whose pain is not responding to routine conservative therapies.

- Provide referrals for prenatal exercise class in facility or community.

- Encourage client compliance with suggested treatment modalities.

- Evaluate response to therapy as indicated; may need to see client more frequently for return visits.

- If the client is on restrictive bed rest, refer her to social services for assistance with child care arrangements as indicated.

- Document a significant ongoing problem with backache in problem list and progress notes.

References

Daly, J.M., Frame, P.S., & Rapoza, P.A. (1991). Sacroiliac subluxation: A common, treatable cause of low back pain in pregnancy. *Family Practice Research Journal, 11*(2), 149–159.

Hainline, B. (1994). Low–back pain in pregnancy. *Advances in Neurology, 64*, 65–76.

Heckman, J.D. (1990). Managing musculoskeletal problems in pregnant patients. Part 1: Back and leg pain are not inevitable. *Journal of Musculoskeletal Medicine, 7*(8), 29–41.

Jacobson, H. (1991). Protecting the back during pregnancy. *AAOHN Journal, 39*(6), 286–291.

Orvieto, R., Achiron, A., Ben–Rafael, Z., Gelernter, I., & Achiron, R. (1994). Low–back pain of pregnancy. *Acta Obstetricia et Gynecologica Scandinavica, 73*(3), 209–214.

Ostgaard, H., Andersson, G., Schultz, A., & Miller, J. (1993). Influence of some biomechanical factors on low–back pain in pregnancy. *Spine, 18*(1), 61–65.

Rungee, J. (1993). Low back pain during pregnancy. *Orthopedics, 16*(12), 1339–1344.

Chapter 2

CONSTIPATION

Ellen M. Scarr

Lucy Newmark Sammons

Constipation is the infrequent or difficult evacuation of hard stools, accompanied by straining (West, Warren & Cutts, 1992). It affects up to one-third of pregnant women, most often in the second and third trimesters. Constipation may be caused by

- Decreased gastrointestinal motility due to increased levels of progesterone (a smooth muscle relaxant) and decreased levels of motilin (a gastrointestinal stimulating hormone)

- Pressure from the gravid uterus on abdominal and back muscles and the rectum

- Increased fluid absorption from the large intestine

- The presence of hemorrhoids or other painful rectal lesions

- Weakened abdominal and pelvic floor muscles (especially levator ani) from prior pregnancies

- The constipating effect of iron supplementation

- Changes in dietary habits, activity or exercise patterns

- Tension and anxiety (Baron, Ramirez & Richter (1993).

Database

Subjective

- Client reports decreased frequency of defecation and/or increased hardness of stool with difficulty emptying bowels

- Client may also report

  ▶ History of irregular/difficult bowel movements (obtain prepregnant bowel history)

  ▶ History of laxative habit

  ▶ Diet lacking adequate roughage and fluids; high in refined carbohydrates

  ▶ Sedentary activity level or bedrest

  ▶ Use of drugs that increase constipation

    – Antacids with aluminum hydroxide, or calcium

    – Iron supplements

    – Anticholinergics

    – Tricyclic antidepressants

    – Codeine analgesics or cough syrup

- Client may report
  - ▶ Feeling of incomplete evacuation of stool
  - ▶ Abdominal discomfort (distention, bloating, cramping)
  - ▶ Increased flatus
  - ▶ Anorexia
  - ▶ Hemorrhoids or other rectal lesions contributing to suppression of defecation
  - ▶ Emotional tension, inability to relax
- Patient denies severe abdominal pain or passing of blood, pus, or mucus per rectum.

Objective

- Abdominal examination may reveal palpable fullness in the large intestine (left lower quadrant)
- Rectal examination may reveal unevacuated stool in vault
- Anoscopic examination may reveal hemorrhoids, rectal fissure, hard stool in rectum

Assessment

- Constipation
  - ▶ R/O pathologic causes of abdominal pain if warranted by data base (e.g., appendicitis, irritable colon)
  - ▶ R/O alternative causes of abdominal cramping (e.g., labor, Braxton-Hicks contractions)
  - ▶ R/O alternative causes of constipation (e.g., intestinal obstruction, pseudo-obstruction of the colon, fecal impaction, irritable bowel syndrome, hypothyroidism)

Plan

Diagnostic Tests

- No further diagnostic tests indicated in absence of other suspected pathology

Treatment/Management (Gilstrap & Little, 1992)

- See Patient Education for modifications of diet, activity, and lifestyle.
- If symptoms warrant additional intervention
  - ▶ Bulk laxative
    - – Psyllium hydrophilic mucilloid: one rounded teaspoon in 8 oz liquid p.o. qd to t.i.d. for 2 to 3 days as needed, followed by additional 8 oz liquid (higher dosages may be considered).
  - ▶ Stool softener may be useful, especially if client on iron supplementation
    - – Docusate sodium 50–100 mg p.o. per day

▶ If necessary in severe cases

- Magnesium hydroxide (milk of magnesia): 2 to 4 tablespoons p.o., followed by glass of water

- Glycerin suppository 3 gm per rectum one time

- Bisacodyl 10 mg p.o. one time

▶ In extreme cases, may consider senna concentrate natural laxative: one to two tablets p.o. at bedtime as needed.

NOTE: Caution is necessary because senna may stimulate gravid uterus and produce abdominal discomfort/cramping.

● Correct any perianal problems interfering with bowel evacuation.

● If administering iron supplement, client to take with prune juice or consider interrupting use until severe constipation resolves. Re-evaluate use of other constipating medications.

Consultation

● Consult with a physician if client has an impaction or fails to respond to conservative treatment.

Patient Education

● Explain the multiple causes of constipation in pregnancy and rationale for treatment approaches.

● Explore a variety of treatment approaches (modification of diet and activities), maintaining sensitivity to the lifestyle and habits of the woman.

▶ Advise modification of dietary intake to include sufficient roughage (e.g., bran—3 tablespoons daily; fruits and vegetables; whole grain products).

▶ Recommend avoidance or reduction of constipating foods (e.g., cheese, refined carbohydrates).

▶ Advise improving hydration by drinking 6 to 8 glasses of water daily in addition to mealtime beverages.

▶ Recommend drinking warm beverages upon rising.

▶ Tell client to establish regular time for bowel evacuation and not to ignore the urge to defecate.

- Reliance on laxatives and enemas should be avoided.

- Prolonged attempts to empty bowels with exertion, which predisposes to hemorrhoids, should be avoided. When defecating, feet may be supported on stool or box to reduce straining.

▶ Encourage regular pelvic floor exercises (i.e., Kegel's have been found to reduce constipation, when used with biofeedback [West, Abell & Cutts, 1992]).

▶ Encourage walking or other exercise to improve abdominal muscle tone.

▶ Stress maintenance of good posture.

Follow-up

- Reassess bowel activity and related lifestyle habits in subsequent visits.
- Document a significant ongoing problem with constipation in progress notes and problem list.

References

Baron, T., Ramirez, B., & Richter, J. (1993). Gastrointestinal motility disorders during pregnancy. *Annals of Internal Medicine, 118*(5), 366–375.

Gilstrap, L., & Little, B. (1992). *Drugs and pregnancy,* (pp.277–291). New York: Elsevier Science.

West, L., Abell, T., & Cutts, T. (1992). Longterm results of pelvic floor muscle rehabilitation in the treatment of constipation. *Gastroenterology, 102*(4, part 2), A533.

West, L., Warren, J., & Cutts, T. (1992). Diagnosis and management of irritable bowel syndrome, constipation and diarrhea in pregnancy. *Gastroenterology Clinics of North America, 21*(4), 793–802.

Chapter 3

DIZZINESS AND VERTIGO

Ellen M. Scarr

Lucy Newmark Sammons

Dizziness may be described as lightheadedness (or a sense of unsteadiness), or actual vertigo, which refers to a sensation that either one's internal or external environment is moving or revolving in space (Goroll, 1995). Neither condition involves a loss of consciousness (syncope), although a syncopal episode may be preceded by vertigo.

Dizziness and vertigo have many causes (Goroll, 1995)

- Vestibular disorders
    - > Ménière's disease
    - > Acute labyrinthitis
    - > Acoustic neuroma
- Neurologic disease
    - > Neoplasms
    - > Migraine headaches
    - > Seizure disorders
    - > Multiple sclerosis
- Cardiovascular disease
    - > Arrhythmias
    - > Aortic stenosis
    - > Cardiac insufficiency
- Anemia
- Psychiatric illness
- Metabolic disturbances
    - > Hypoglycemia
- Ocular disease
- Substance toxicity
- Hyperventilation
- Emotional distress

Common in the first trimester of pregnancy, dizziness is usually caused by orthostatic hypotension, vasomotor instability, or hypoglycemia (Andolsek, 1990). Blood pools in the lower extremities, splanchnic, and pelvic areas because of hormonally mediated vasomotor instability, which decreases venous return to the heart and leads to orthostatic hypotension. Dizziness results when quickly rising from a lying or sitting position (Zeldis, 1992). Hypoglycemia may result from inadequate nutrient intake, possibly from nausea and vomiting in early pregnancy.

Dizziness may persist throughout the pregnancy. Increasing venous pressure in the lower extremities and the subsequent venous stasis contributes to orthostatic hypotension. Supine hypotensive syndrome, a common cause of third trimester dizziness, is caused by compression of the vena cava by the gravid uterus in the recumbent position (Ikeda, Ohbuchi, Ikenoue & Mori, 1992).

Database

Subjective

- Client reports occasional lightheadedness, especially upon changing to upright or standing position; onset during pregnancy.

- History negative for use of possible toxic agents (e.g., alcohol or drugs, such as antihypertensives, anti-epileptic drugs, diuretics, antidepressants).

- History negative for middle ear or central nervous system disease, visual problems, endocrine disorders, seizure disorders, or migraine headaches.

- Client may report erratic food intake patterns.

Objective

- Differential between lying and standing BP (≥ 20 percent) and pulse rate may be observed (Guarnieri, 1996).

- Eye, ear, thyroid, cardiac and neurologic examination within normal limits (WNL).

Assessment

- Dizziness/lightheadedness—benign
    - ▶ R/O orthostatic hypotension/systemic hypotension/vena caval syndrome
    - ▶ R/O vestibular disease
        - Ménieré's disease
        - Labyrinthitis
        - Acoustic neuroma
    - ▶ R/O neurologic disease
        - Neoplasm
        - Migraine headache
        - Seizure disorder
        - Multiple sclerosis

- ▶ R/O cardiovascular disease
  - – Arrhythmia
  - – Aortic stenosis
  - – Cardiac insufficiency
- ▶ R/O anemia
- ▶ R/O anxiety/psychological disturbance
- ▶ R/O metabolic disturbances (e.g., hypoglycemia)
- ▶ R/O ocular strain/refractive error
- ▶ R/O substance toxicity

Plan

Diagnostic Tests

- No specific laboratory test is diagnostic for benign dizziness.
- If obtained, hemoglobin/hematocrit are within normal limits (WNL).

Treatment/Management

See Patient Education.

Consultation

- Consult with a physician for severe symptoms nonresponsive to palliative treatment or if underlying pathologic condition is suspected.

Patient Education

- Explain that vascular changes are usually responsible for dizziness in pregnancy when no underlying pathology exists.
- Suggest use of elastic stockings or vigorous pumping leg motions to reduce pooling of blood in lower extremities.
- Advise avoiding prolonged periods of standing or sitting.
- Recommend slow change of positions (i.e., from lying/sitting to rising).
- Suggest that the client structure activities so that loss of balance would be of minimal danger (e.g., no climbing of ladders).
- Identify anxiety-provoking situations and counsel in relation to these, if the psychological component is apparent.
- Advise client to avoid prolonged periods with no food intake; recommend five to six small meals a day if needed; increase fluid intake, if low.

- To avoid compression of vena cava, advise the client to rest on her left side rather than her back when recumbent.

Follow-up

- Reevaluate the number and circumstances of dizzy episodes on subsequent visits.

- Evaluate and consult further if dizziness is not responsive to therapeutic measures and is interfering with patient safety or activities of daily living.

- Document a significant ongoing problem with dizziness in progress notes and problem list.

References

Andolsek, K.M. (1990). *Obstetric care: Standards of prenatal, intrapartum, and postpartum management* (pp. 8–18). Philadelphia, PA: Lea & Febiger.

Goroll, A. (1995). Evaluation of dizziness. In A. Goroll, L. May, & A. Mulley (Eds.), *Primary care medicine* (3rd ed., pp. 829–8335). Philadelphia, PA: J.B. Lippincott.

Guarnieri, T. (1996). Syncope and cardiac arrhythmias. In J. Stobo, D. Hellman, P. Ladenson, B. Petty & T. Traill (Eds.), *The principles and practice of medicine* (23rd ed., pp. 71– 82). Stamford, CT: Appleton & Lange.

Ikeda, T., Ohbuchi, H., Ikenoue, T., & Mori, N. (1992). Maternal cerebral hemodynamics in the supine hypotensive syndrome. *Obstetrics and Gynecology, 79*(1), 27–31.

Zeldis, S. (1992). Dyspnea during pregnancy: Distinguishing cardiac from pulmonary causes. *Clinics in Chest Medicine, 13*(4), 567–585.

Chapter 4

DYSPNEA

Ellen M. Scarr

Maureen T. Shannon

Dyspnea, the sensation of an increase in the work of breathing, is a common complaint in pregnancy, occurring in 50 to 75 percent of women with no prior history of cardiopulmonary disease (Elkus & Popovich, 1992; Zeldis, 1992). Normal hormonal and anatomic changes of pregnancy, particularly those involving the respiratory system, lead to a mild respiratory alkalosis, resulting in dyspnea, a heightened awareness of the act of breathing, and a perceived decrease in exercise tolerance (Hume & Killam, 1990). Physiologic dyspnea occurs in the first and second trimesters and does not progress, and remains stable or improves near term. While bothersome, physiologic dyspnea usually does not interfere with normal daily activity; dyspnea at rest is rare. The nonprogressive nature of physiologic dyspnea suggests that the growing uterus does not contribute to the development of dyspnea; third trimester studies indicate the gravid uterus does not hinder diaphragmatic excursion (Field, Bell, Cenaiko & Whitelaw, 1991).

While dyspnea is a common occurrence in pregnancy, the physical demands of pregnancy may exacerbate underlying respiratory and cardiac disease. Cardiac dyspnea typically begins in the second half of pregnancy and peaks in the seventh month, when fluid overload is maximal. It is important to rule out the possibility of underlying pathology as the cause of dyspnea (Zeldis, 1992).

Database

Subjective

- Nonpathologic Dyspnea

    ▶ Increased awareness of the need to breathe—may or may not be associated with exercise

    ▶ Dizziness

    ▶ Lightheadedness

    ▶ May need an extra pillow at night during the third trimester

- Pathologic Dyspnea

    ▶ Acute, severe, or progressive

    ▶ Paroxysmal nocturnal dyspnea, frequently 1 to 2 hours after lying down

    ▶ Progressive orthopnea

    ▶ Dyspnea at rest or at a level of activity not expected to cause dyspnea

    ▶ Chest pain

    ▶ Palpitations

    ▶ Acute, extreme anxiety

    ▶ Severe fatigue

▶ Audible wheezing

▶ Signs and symptoms of an upper respiratory tract infection (URI)

   – Rhinorrhea

   – Sneezing

   – Sore throat

   – Headache

   – Fever

   – Coughing (productive or nonproductive)

▶ Signs and symptoms of lower respiratory infection

   – Fever

   – Chills

   – Cough (productive or nonproductive)

   – Pleuritic chest pain

▶ Hemoptysis

▶ Dry, irritating non-productive cough that worsens at night (may indicate pulmonary hypertension)

▶ History of cardiac problems, asthma, or other respiratory problems

▶ Smoker

Objective

● Nonpathologic

  ▶ Vital signs are normal

  ▶ No clinical signs found when client examined

● Pathologic

  ▶ May appear anxious

  ▶ Vital signs

    – May have elevated temperature, increased or irregular pulse, rapid respirations

    – Blood pressure may be elevated, decreased or normal

  ▶ Auscultation of the lungs and heart may reveal

    – Presence of rhonchi, wheezes or crackles that do not clear after two to three deep breaths or coughs

    – Cardiac arrhythmias

    – Systolic murmur, intensity greater than grade III/VI

    – Diastolic or continuous murmur

- Unequivocal cardiac enlargement
- Cardiac rub

► Examination of the neck and chest may reveal
- Prominent jugular vein distention
- Intercostal retractions

► Examination of the extremities may reveal
- Cyanosis
- Clubbing

Assessment

● Dyspnea secondary to anatomic/physiologic changes of pregnancy

► R/O URI (e.g., common cold, bronchitis)

► R/O lower respiratory infection (e.g., pneumonia, pleurisy)

► R/O pulmonary diseases (e.g., reactive airway disease, pulmonary edema, pulmonary hypertension, pulmonary embolism)

► R/O cardiac disorders (e.g., rheumatic heart disease, congenital heart disease, ischemic heart disease, arrhythmias, cardiomyopathy)

► R/O anxiety

Plan

Diagnostic Tests

● Nonpathologic dyspnea: No further diagnostic tests needed

● Pathologic dyspnea: Some of the following tests may be ordered after consultation with a physician:

► Transcutaneous O_2 saturation

► Arterial blood gas (ABG)

► Pulmonary function tests (PFTs)

► Electrocardiogram (ECG)

► Echocardiogram

► Chest X-ray

► Sputum cultures

Treatment/Management

- Nonpathologic dyspnea
  - ▶ Symptomatic treatment
  - ▶ See Patient Education section
- Pathologic dyspnea
  - ▶ Treatment of underlying condition after consultation with physician and appropriate referrals (e.g., pulmonologist, cardiologist, cardiac surgeon)

Consultation

- Consultation is required for suspected pathologic causes of dyspnea with referral to physician care if long-term follow-up is necessary (e.g., cardiac disease)

Patient Education

- Nonpathologic dyspnea
  - ▶ Educate client about anatomic and physiologic changes that contribute to dyspnea.
  - ▶ Advise client to sit and stand correctly.
  - ▶ Advise client not to overexert herself and to rest after exercise.
  - ▶ Encourage client to avoid restrictive clothing.
  - ▶ Advise client to turn onto her side if dyspnea occurs when resting on her back.
  - ▶ Suggest using an additional pillow for the head and upper torso when sleeping.
- Pathologic dyspnea
  - ▶ Educate client about the need for consultation and possible follow-up by physician.
  - ▶ Educate client about tests that will be ordered.

Follow-up

- Nonpathologic dyspnea
  - ▶ No specific follow-up indicated; continue routine prenatal care.
  - ▶ Document a significant on-going problem with dypsnea in problem list and progress notes.
- Pathologic dyspnea
  - ▶ Have physician follow up until problem resolves.

References

Elkus, R., & Popovich, J. (1992). Respiratory physiology in pregnancy. *Clinics in Chest Medicine, 13*(4), 555–565.

Field, S., Bell, S., Cenaiko, D., & Whitelaw, W. (1991). Relationship between inspiratory effort and breathlessness in pregnancy. *Journal of Applied Physiology, 71*(5), 1897–1902.

Hume, R., & Killam, A. (1990). Maternal physiology. In J. Scott, P. DiSaia, C. Hammond, & W. Spellacy (Eds.), *Danforth's obstetrics and gynecology*, (6th ed., pp. 93–100). Philadelphia, PA: JB Lippincott.

Zeldis, S. (1992). Dyspnea during pregnancy: Distinguishing cardiac from pulmonary causes. *Clinics in Chest Medicine, 13*(4), 567–585.

Chapter 5

EDEMA—PHYSIOLOGIC

Ellen M. Scarr

Lucy Newmark Sammons

Edema is defined as an increase in the extravascular or interstitial fluid volume. During normal pregnancy, plasma volume increases an average of 50 percent over nonpregnant levels (Iams, 1990; Moore, 1994). As a consequence, cardiac output, renal blood flow, glomerular filtration rate, and levels of renin and angiotensin II also increase during pregnancy. Angiotensin II stimulates secretion of aldosterone, which, along with antidiuretic hormone (ADH), promotes retention of water and salt. Estrogen increases vascular capacity by causing vasodilation. There is normally no increase in blood pressure because the usual response to elevated levels of angiotensin II is blunted during pregnancy (Moore, 1994).

Eighty percent of healthy pregnant women demonstrate clinical edema (Malee, 1993). In pregnancy, peripheral edema is caused by alteration of the near-equilibrium (Starling equilibrium) maintained at the capillary membrane, where fluid filtered outward through arterial capillaries no longer approximates the amount reabsorbed at the venous end of the capillaries. Concentrations of several plasma proteins, particularly albumin, are decreased in pregnancy; this decrease in proteins contributes to edema by lowering colloidal osmotic pressure of the plasma (Goroll, 1995; Malee, 1993).

Venous pressure in the upper extremities remains unchanged in pregnancy but increases in the lower extremities as pregnancy progresses. Uterine pressure on the inferior vena cava and pressure from the fetal head on the common iliac veins impedes venous return to the heart from the lower extremities, contributing to dependent edema late in pregnancy (Pernoll & Taylor, 1994). However, generalized edema seen in the hands and face requires further evaluation, as it may be a sign of preeclampsia/eclampsia.

Database

Subjective

- Client reports swelling in lower extremities, particularly after periods of standing or sitting; symptons are present in mid- to third trimester of pregnancy

- Client denies presence of symptoms related to preeclampsia (see Chapter 6.13, *Hypertensive Disorders of Pregnancy*)

- Client may report:

  ▶ Low protein intake, high intake of salty foods

  ▶ Recent greater than expected weight gain

  ▶ Exposure to warm/hot weather

Objective

- Edema of the lower extremities

    ▶ Extent of the edema may be quantified by gently pressing the affected area (e.g., pretibial area) with examiner's thumb for 5 seconds. If a depression persists, edema is described as pitting and may be ranked (Jarvis, 1996):

        – 1+: slight indentation, no visible swelling

        – 2+: pitting is moderate but resolves quickly, minimal swelling may be evident

        – 3+: deeper pit of several seconds duration, obvious swelling

        – 4+: deeper pit possibly lasting minutes, frank swelling

- Mild swelling in hands and fingers may be present

- Absence of signs suggestive of preeclampsia:

    ▶ No significant increase in BP

    ▶ Trace to 1+ proteinuria (see Chapter 6.27, *Proteinuria*)

    ▶ No increase in deep tendon reflex (DTR) tonicity

    ▶ Absence of periorbital or generalized edema

- Greater-than-expected weight gain may be exhibited

Assessment

- Edema of pregnancy—physiologic

    ▶ R/O preeclampsia/eclampsia and related disorders

    ▶ R/O renal disease

    ▶ R/O localized inflammatory response, trauma

    ▶ R/O varicosities

    ▶ R/O thrombophlebitis

    ▶ R/O carpal tunnel syndrome

Plan

Diagnostic Tests

- No laboratory tests indicated for diagnosis
- Urine dipstick for protein

Treatment/Management

See Patient Education.

Consultation

Seek medical and nutritional consultation if client fails to respond to conservative therapeutics and she is in significant discomfort.

Patient Education

- Explain basis of edema and distinction between dependent and generalized edema.

- Advise elevation of affected extremities above the level of the heart for 1 to 2 hours 1 to 2 times per day, as needed, using left lateral recumbent position when possible.

- Advise client to avoid prolonged standing or sitting.

- Include the following instructions in nutritional counseling:

  ▶ Avoid excessive sodium intake, but do not overly restrict.

  ▶ Limit added salt and processed foods.

  ▶ Avoid excessive carbohydrate intake.

  ▶ Maintain a high protein diet.

  ▶ Maintain a high fluid intake: 8 glasses/day, especially water.

  NOTE: It may be necessary to explain that increased water intake will decrease edema, especially in warmer weather.

- Explain the danger of diuretics and the need to avoid them.

- Recommend avoidance of constricting garters, socks, etc.; supportive hose (with adequate abdominal room) may be helpful.

- Explain increased susceptibility of swollen tissues to injury and the need to prevent trauma. Advise of need to wear protective foot covering, even though difficult because of enlarged size.

- Review signs and symptoms of preeclampsia.

Follow-up

- Reevaluate edema in 1 to 2 weeks.

- Request that client contact the provider if she gains 2 or more pounds in 1 week (Dickason, Schult & Silverman, 1990)

- Document a significant ongoing problem with edema in progress notes and problem list.

References

Goroll, A. (1995). Evaluation of leg edema. In A. Goroll, L. May, & A. Mulley (Eds.), *Primary care medicine* (3rd ed., pp. 105–108). Philadelphia, PA: JB Lippincott.

Iams, J. (1990). Physiologic changes in pregnancy. In J. Iams & F. Zuspan (Eds.), *Zuspan and Quilligan's manual of obstetrics and gynecology,* (2nd ed., pp. 31–38). St. Louis, MO: Mosby.

Jarvis, C. (1996). *Physical examination and health assessment* (pp. 569–598). Philadelphia, PA: W.B. Saunders.

Malee, M. (1993). Physiology of pregnancy. In J. Brown & N. Crombleholm (Eds.), *Handbook of gynecology and obstetrics* (pp. 301–311). Norwalk, CT: Appleton & Lange.

May, K., & Mahlmeister, L. (1994). *Maternal and neonatal nursing: Family centered care* (3rd ed., pp. 275–301). Philadelphia, PA: JB Lippincott.

Moore, P. (1994). Maternal physiology during pregnancy. In A. DeCherney & M. Pernoll (Eds.), *Current obstetric and gynecologic diagnosis and treatment,* (8th ed., pp. 146–154). Norwalk, CT: Appleton & Lange.

Pernoll, M., & Taylor, C. (1994). Normal pregnancy and prenatal care. In A. DeCherney & M. Pernoll (Eds.), *Current obstetric and gynecologic diagnosis and treatment,* (8th ed., pp. 183– 201). Norwalk, CT: Appleton & Lange.

Chapter 6

EPISTAXIS

Ellen M. Scarr

Lucy Newmark Sammons

Epistaxis, or nasal bleeding, originates most often from Kiesselbach's plexus, the rich network of veins on the antero-inferior portion of the nasal septum. Posteriorly, bleeding often occurs at the back third of the inferior meatus. Because of the highly vascular nature of the nasal turbinates and mucosa, bleeding may be profuse.

Factors that contribute to nosebleeds are

- Local infections, such as sinusitis
- Systemic infections
- Drying of nasal mucous membranes
- Local trauma
- Arteriosclerotic changes
- Hypertension
- Bleeding disorders
- Ulcerative disease or malignancy
- Overheating
- Cocaine use

During pregnancy, nosebleeds are more common because of the vasodilating effects of estrogen on mucous membranes, relaxing effects of progesterone on venous walls, engorgement of the blood vessels of the nasal passages, and increased nasal secretions (Hume & Killam, 1990).

Database

Subjective

- Description of nosebleeding incident(s), which may include
  - ▶ History of nosebleeds prior to pregnancy
  - ▶ Precipitating event, such as nose picking, overexertion
- Ability to control nosebleeds within 10 to 15 minutes
- History negative for other local or systemic disease, or trauma

Objective

- Vital signs within normal limits (WNL)
- Physical examination otherwise normal; no evidence of local or systemic disease
- Nasal mucosa pink or dull red
  - ▶ May see residual clotted blood
  - ▶ May see superficial vessels, particularly in triangular area on antero-inferior nasal septum of affected side
- Absence of visible nasal growths or polyps

Assessment

- Epistaxis of pregnancy, uncomplicated
  - ▶ R/O acute or chronic local infections, such as rhinitis, sinusitis, vestibulitis
  - ▶ R/O systemic infections, such as scarlet fever, infectious mononucleosis, influenza, measles
  - ▶ R/O elevated blood pressure
  - ▶ R/O anemias and bleeding disorders
  - ▶ R/O local ulcerative disease, malignant polyp
  - ▶ R/O cocaine abuse

Plan

Diagnostic Tests

- No diagnostic test(s) indicated
- Complete blood count WNL, if obtained, unless underlying pathology exists (e.g., bleeding disorder)

Treatment/Management

- Immediate care
  - ▶ Loosen clothing around neck.
  - ▶ Sit with head tilted forward or lie with head and shoulders elevated, and use mouth breathing.
  - ▶ Apply pressure by pinching nostrils for 10 to 15 minutes.
  - ▶ Apply ice packs or cold compresses across nose.
  - ▶ Pack affected nostril with small sterile pad (optional).
- Continued care
  - ▶ Treat any concomitant local infections as indicated.

- ▶ Apply a topical antibiotic ointment t.i.d.
    - – May combat local inflammation, if needed
    - – Moisturizes mucous membranes
- ▶ Increase moisture to dry mucous membranes by using a humidifier or aerosol moisturizer or by topical application of petroleum jelly.
- ▶ See also Patient Education.

Consultation

- Consult a physician if the bleeding is not relieved by above measures, or if there is a suspicion of underlying related pathology.

Patient Education

- Explain that, in the absence of identified pathology, nosebleeds may be considered normal in pregnancy.

- Explain the physiologic basis for nosebleeds in pregnancy and the rationale and techniques of management described above. Have the client contact her health care provider immediately for nosebleeds not responsive to described treatment approaches.

- Advise client to avoid trauma to nasal mucosa.

    - ▶ Avoid nose picking.

    - ▶ Avoid forceful nose blowing or sneezing.

    - ▶ Avoid coughing.

- Advise client to avoid overheating or excessive exertion, which may precipitate nosebleed.

- Advise woman who is prone to nosebleeds that they may occur with change in atmospheric pressure (e.g., when flying).

Follow-up

- The client should contact provider if nosebleeds not responsive to described treatments.

- Reevaluate pattern and management of nosebleeds at next regularly scheduled appointment.

- Document a significant ongoing problem with epistaxis in progress notes and problem list.

Reference

Hume, R., & Killam, A. (1990). Maternal physiology. In J. Scott, P. DiSaia, C. Hammond, & W. Spellacy (Eds.), *Danforth's obstetrics and gynecology* (6th ed., pp. 93–100). Philadelphia, PA: J.B. Lippincott.

Chapter 7

FATIGUE AND INSOMNIA

Ellen M. Scarr

Lucy Newmark Sammons

Fatigue, defined for the purposes of this book as feelings of tiredness or weariness, is a common complaint in pregnancy, noted by up to 90 percent of women (Reeves, Potempa & Gallo, 1991). Usually beginning early in pregnancy and continuing on throughout the pregnancy, fatigue has an often significant impact on the life of the pregnant woman.

The normative fatigue of pregnancy may be caused by increased levels of progesterone, a hormone known to have sedative effects. Other factors contributing to fatigue include

- Normal physiologic changes (cardiovascular, respiratory, urinary, metabolic)
- Physical factors (anemia, inadequate nutrition, inadequate rest)
- Environmental factors (employment, lifestyle, lack of social support)
- Psychological factors (anxiety, depression)

Late in pregnancy, fatigue may be increased by additional weight gain, physical discomforts because of the growing fetus, increased metabolic demands, and difficulty falling asleep or staying asleep (Pugh & Milligan, 1993; van Lier, Manteuffel, Dilorio, & Stalcup, 1993).

Insomnia, the difficulty in initiating or maintaining sleep, may have multiple causes in pregnancy

- Disturbance from fetal movement
- Inability to assume a position of comfort because of the enlarging abdomen
- Interruption by the need to urinate
- Discomfort from gastric reflux or other gastrointestinal changes
- Feelings of shortness of breath
- Psychological concerns and thoughts

Database

Subjective

- Complaints of tiredness
- Reports of difficulty sleeping that may be aggravated by fetal movement or nocturia
- Perceptions of fatigue, often increased during the first and third trimesters
- Reports of adequate (or inadequate) nutritional intake

- Reports difficulty concentrating or completing tasks
- Negative history of circulatory, respiratory, endocrine, infectious, or emotional problems

Objective

- Lethargic, inattentive, yawning
- May have poor posture
- Respiratory impairment (refer to Chapter 5.4, *Dyspnea*)
- Vital signs are within normal limits (WNL).

Assessment

- Fatigue—physiologic fatigue of pregnancy
  - ▶ R/O respiratory disorder
  - ▶ R/O circulatory/hematologic disorder
  - ▶ R/O preeclampsia
  - ▶ R/O inadequate nutritional intake
  - ▶ R/O depression, anxiety, or stress
  - ▶ R/O infectious process
  - ▶ R/O hypothyroidism

Plan

Diagnostic Tests

- Consider complete blood count (CBC) if warranted by database; will WNL.
- No further diagnostic tests are indicated.

Treatment/Management

- See Patient Education.

Consultation

- Consultation is not required without evidence of pathology.

Patient Education

- Explain that in the absence of identified pathology, feelings of fatigue are a normal part of the pregnancy experience.

- Encourage adequate periods for sleep, which may extend to 8 to 12 hours.

- Encourage periods for napping/resting during the day as work/school/child care arrangements permit.

- For difficulty sleeping at night:
  - ▶ Explore comfort measures (pillows, bladder emptying in late evening, relaxation techniques)
  - ▶ Suggest toleration of awakening at night while maintaining physical rest.

- Suggest sleep-inducing aids (warm milk, outdoor exercise, music, reading, love-making, shower) if there is difficulty falling asleep.

- Reinforce adequate nutritional intake.

- Instruct in relaxation techniques or refer to resource.

- Advise good posture to relieve fatigue.

- Explore possible sources of anxiety or emotional discomfort that may be increasing fatigue and counsel appropriately; refer to psychological health care provider if indicated by emotional status.

- Advise client that daily schedule may need modification to accommodate fatigue while pregnant.
  - ▶ Decrease number of hours worked.
  - ▶ Devise flexible scheduling of work hours.
  - ▶ Work at home.
  - ▶ Decrease social activities.

- Encourage spouse and children to assume more responsibility for household tasks.

- Discourage the use of sleeping medications.

- Discourage consumption of central nervous system stimulants or heavy meals in late evening.

Follow-up

- Reevaluate degree of fatigue and effectiveness of therapeutics on following visit.

- Document a significant ongoing problem with fatigue/insomnia in progress notes and problem list.

References

Pugh, L., & Milligan, R. (1993). A framework for the study of childbearing fatigue. *Advances in Nursing Science, 15*(4), 60–70.

Reeves, N., Potempa, K., & Gallo, A. (1991). Fatigue in early pregnancy: An exploratory study. *Journal of Nurse–Midwifery, 36*(5), 303–309.

van Lier, D., Manteuffel, B., DiIorio, C., & Stalcup, M. (1993). Nausea and fatigue during early pregnancy. *Birth, 20*(4), 193–197.

Chapter 8

HEADACHE

Ellen M. Scarr

Lucy Newmark Sammons

Headache is the most common neurological symptom in both pregnant and nonpregnant women (Cartlidge, 1995; Feller & Franko-Filipasic, 1993; Fox, Harms, & Davis, 1990), with vascular-type and muscle tension headaches occurring most frequently. Characteristics of preexisting headaches may change during pregnancy, or benign headaches may occur for the first time. While the etiology of most headaches is unclear, it has been postulated that low levels of the neurotransmitter serotonin result in swelling of cerebral blood vessels, contributing to vascular-type headaches. Fluctuations in sex hormones, particularly estrogen, have also been linked to vascular-type headaches. Muscle tension headaches result from tightening and/or spasm of neck and back muscles (Feller & Franko-Filipasic, 1993).

Migraine headaches, the most common vascular headache, occur in 20 percent of women (Fox et al., 1990). Migraine headaches peak in the reproductive years, likely influenced by estrogen and progesterone (Silberstein & Merriam, 1993). Although preexisting migraines usually worsen in the first trimester of pregnancy, up to 80 percent of women note near or complete resolution of migraines in the second and third trimesters, possibly due to sustained levels of estrogen (Cartlidge, 1995; Chan & Leviton, 1994). While headaches generally pose no risk to the pregnant woman or her fetus, women with migraines have been reported to have an increased incidence of preeclampsia and perinatal mortality (Fox et al., 1990). Muscle tension headaches are the most common type of headache occurring in pregnancy (Feller & Franko-Filipasic, 1993); they are less likely than migraines to improve.

Benign headaches often develop for the first time in pregnancy. Of these, migraines are the most typical, usually beginning in the first trimester (Fox et al., 1990). The other commonly developing benign headache of pregnancy is nonmigrainous vascular headache of early pregnancy, which usually occurs in the first trimester and spontaneously resolves after several days to weeks. Physiologic changes of pregnancy may increase the occurrence of other types of benign headaches. Vasodilation of the sinus passages may contribute to sinusitis and resultant headache. Ocular changes of pregnancy may lead to headaches caused by eye strain or refractive changes.

Serious conditions that may also cause headaches during pregnancy include the following (Feller & Franko-Filipasic, 1993; Fox et al., 1990):

- Preeclampsia/eclampsia
- Pseudotumor cerebri
- Subarachnoid hemorrhage from an aneurysm or arteriovenous malformation
- A rapidly growing solid brain lesion
- Thrombosis of the cortical vein
- Listeria meningitis

Database

Subjective

- Client complains of mild to moderate diffuse pain in the head; may report visual changes or difficulty using glasses.

- Obtain detailed history of symptoms, using descriptors (i.e., onset, frequency, precipitating factors, location, radiation, quality, associated symptoms, aggravating or alleviating measures) to allow for categorization of headache

  ► Tension headache

  - Often begins in the morning, lasting all day, worsening in the evening

  - Dull, not throbbing, steady, of low persistent intensity

  - Usually occipital, suboccipital, and bilateral, like a constrictive band or tightness of the scalp

  - May radiate to neck and upper back, with local soreness of muscles

  - Constant or persisting several days

  ► Migraine headache

  - Severe, throbbing, or boring

  - Common migraine usually unilateral in frontotemporal or supraorbital region

  - May last 4 hours to several days

  NOTE: Classic migraines are preceded by aura and prodrome (e.g., flashing lights, colors, wavy lines, photophobia, vomiting), occur unilaterally, lasting 2 to 8 days.

  ► Sinus headache

  - Pain over involved sinuses (maxillary, ethmoid, or frontal)

  ► Benign vascular headache of pregnancy

  - Mild, throbbing, bifrontal

  - Usually limited to first trimester, occurring daily for days to weeks

  - Spontaneously resolves

- Personal or family history may be positive for migraines or other headache categories

- General health history otherwise unremarkable. In particular, history negative for

  ► Recent trauma to head

  ► Symptoms suggesting disease or trauma to paranasal sinuses, teeth, eye, ear, nose, or throat

  ► Exposure to toxic chemicals or agents

Objective

- Blood pressure, ophthalmic examination, weight pattern, fluid retention, urine laboratory values are within normal limits (WNL)
- Afebrile, free of signs of infection
- Fundoscopic examination WNL
- Ear, nose, throat examination WNL
- Nasal sinuses nontender, no nasal drainage
- Neck
  - ▶ Full range of motion
  - ▶ Nontender without spasm
  - ▶ No signs of meningeal irritation
- Nonfocal neurologic examination
  - ▶ Cranial nerves
  - ▶ Cerebellar function

Assessment

- Headache—physiologic vascular headache of early pregnancy, benign
- Migraine headache, classic or common
- Tension headache
  - ▶ R/O muscle tension, trapezius muscle spasm
  - ▶ R/O temporomandibular joint (TMJ) dysfunction or bruxism (teeth grinding)
  - ▶ R/O stress or psychological tension
- Sinus headache
  - ▶ R/O sinusitis
  - ▶ R/O allergies
- R/O preeclampsia/eclampsia
- R/O eye strain/refractive changes
- R/O infectious disease (e.g., meningitis)
- R/O cerebrovascular disease (e.g., cortical thrombosis, arteriovenous malformation [AVM])
- R/O space-occupying lesion (e.g., cerebral tumor)

Plan

Diagnostic Tests

- No diagnostic tests indicated in absence of neurologic abnormalities and if signs and symptoms conform to standard headache syndromes.

Treatment/Management (Cartlidge, 1995; Fox et al., 1990; Gilstrap & Little, 1992; Peleg & Niebyl, 1997; Silberstein, 1993)

- Vascular headache of early pregnancy
  - ▶ Rest and reassurance about absence of serious neurologic problem
  - ▶ Acetaminophen 325 mg p.o. one to two tablets every 4 hours as needed
  - ▶ Consider caffeinated beverage if severe.
- Migraine
  - ▶ Acute episode
    - – Analgesicss (e.g., acetaminophen 325 mg p.o., one to two tablets every 4 hours as needed, acetaminophen with codeine one tablet p.o. every 4 hours as needed.)

      NOTE: Tolerance to codeine can develop with continued use. Drug should be used with caution. Warn client about side effects.
    - – Antiemetics
    - – Meclizine 12.5 to 25 mg p.o. every 6 hours as needed
    - – Doxylamine 12.5 mg p.o. b.i.d. and 25 mg p.o. at bedtime as needed
    - – Metoclopramide 10 mg p.o. one hour before meals and at bedtime as needed
    - – Prochlorperazine 5 to 10 mg p.o. t.i.d. to q.i.d. as needed
  - ▶ If severe, may need intravenous fluids, parenteral narcotics

    NOTE: The usual agent, ergotamine, is contraindicated in pregnancy.
  - ▶ Preventive therapy
    - – Avoid triggers, if known (see Patient Education)
    - – May be able to await improvement in later pregnancy
    - – Consider prophylactic medication if needed
      - * Beta-blockers (propranolol, atenolol)
      - * Calcium channel blocker (verapamil)
      - * Amitriptyline if needed
    - – Consult with physician
- Tension headache

- ▶ Acetaminophen
- ▶ Rest, ice packs to neck and shoulders
- ▶ Relaxation techniques, new coping skills
- ▶ Consider biofeedback, physical therapy, exercise
- Treat contributing disorders as needed.
- See also Patient Education.

Consultation

- Consult for prescription medication(s) as needed.
- Obtain medical consultation for
  - ▶ Headaches accompanied by neurologic abnormalities or not conforming to standard headache syndromes
  - ▶ Headaches not relieved by treatment approaches within scope of practice
  - ▶ Suspicion of underlying pathology
- Refer to eye care specialist as needed for relief of headache caused by visual strain/difficulty
- Refer to psychologic health care provider, as needed, for stress and anxiety management.

Patient Education

- Explain the physiologic basis of headaches during pregnancy and the rationale for the treatment approaches selected.
- Explain that, in the absence of identified pathology, mild, transient headaches may be considered normal in pregnancy.
- Explore tension reduction techniques with client (e.g., progressive relaxation, use of imagery, meditation, exercise).
- Suggest massage, moist heat, or cold application to neck muscles, which may relax muscles in spasm.
- Advise client to avoid aspirin and nonsteroidal anti-inflammatory drugs (NSAIDs).
- Advise client to eliminate foods and beverages from diet if strongly associated with symptom occurrence. Contributing foods may include
  - ▶ Those with nitrites/nitrates (e.g., hot dogs, bacon)
  - ▶ Tyramines (e.g., chocolate, cheese, red wine)
  - ▶ Monosodium glutamate
- Recommend that client eat at regular intervals.
  - ▶ Skipping meals leads to hypoglycemia.
  - ▶ Overeating carbohydrates at one time leads to hyperglycemia and also should be avoided.

- Ask client to explore and identify environmental factors that precipitate headaches.
  - ▶ Structure activities to avoid these stimuli when possible. Examples are
    - Bright lights
    - Loud noises
    - Intense odors
    - Cigarette smoke
    - Stuffy rooms
    - Alterations in sleep.
- Suggest plenty of rest and sleep.
- A headache calendar can help identify headache triggers. Have the client note the time of onset, severity, duration, associated activity and/or food intake, emotional state, relief measures.

Follow-up

- Patient to contact provider if headache not relieved with rest and analgesic in 24 hours, or if marked increase in severity of headache.

- If good relief obtained, no additional follow-up is required.

- Document a significant ongoing problem with headaches in progress notes and problem list.

References

Cartlidge, N. (1995). Neurologic disorders. In W. Barron & M. Lindheimer (Eds.), *Medical disorders during pregnancy* (2nd ed., pp. 430–450). St. Louis, MO: Mosby.

Chan, T., & Leviton, A. (1994). Headache recurrence in pregnant women with migraine. *Headache*, *34*(2), 107–110.

Feller, C., & Franko-Filipasic, K. (1993). Headaches during pregnancy: Diagnosis and management. *Journal of Perinatal and Neonatal Nursing*, *7*(1), 1–10.

Fox, M., Harms, R., & Davis, D. (1990). Selected neurologic complications of pregnancy. *Mayo Clinic Proceedings*, *65*(12), 1595–1618.

Gilstrap, L., & Little, B. (1992). *Drugs and pregnancy* (pp. 111–132). New York: Elsevier Science.

Peleg, D. & Niebyl, J. (1997). Prescribing antiemetic therapy during pregnancy. *Contemporary OB/GYN*, *42*(6), 164–171.

Silberstein, S. (1993). Headaches and women: Treatment of the pregnant and lactating migraineur. *Headache*, *33*(10), 533–540.

Silberstein, S., & Merriam, G. (1993). Sex hormones and headache. *Journal of Pain and Symptom Management*, *8*(2), 98–114.

Chapter 9

HEMORRHOIDS

Ellen M. Scarr

Lucy Newmark Sammons

Hemorrhoids are anorectal protrusions that may result from increased venous pressure and dilation of the anorectal vascular network, arteriovenous communications in rectal tissue, and/or collapse of the anal canal cushions (Goroll, 1995; Medich & Fazio, 1995). Internal hemorrhoids involve the superior hemorrhoidal plexus above the dentate margin, the border separating pink mucosa from the modified squamous-lined anoderm. External hemorrhoids lie distal to the dentate margin, arise from the inferior hemorrhoidal plexus and are covered with pain-sensitive anal skin (Goroll, 1995). Hemorrhoids may be classified clinically from first degree to fourth degree, determined by increasing protrusion of the mucosa (Medich & Fazio, 1995).

Hemorrhoids become clinically significant when they cause symptoms. Symptoms are produced by protrusion of the vascular submucosa through an increasingly congested anal canal. Common complications are bleeding, seen with either internal or external hemorrhoids, and thrombosis (painful clot formation within the hemorrhoid, usually external).

Other entities associated with hemorrhoids include anal fissures, perianal hematomas, skin tags, and mucosal prolapse. However, cause and effect relationships are difficult to establish.

Hemorrhoids are the most common anorectal problem in both men and women, and are associated with diets low in fiber and high in fat. Also common in the second and third trimester of pregnancy (up to one-third of pregnant women develop hemorrhoids), the factors which promote the development of hemorrhoids include

- Constipation, due to the effect of progesterone on the intestinal smooth muscle and the pressure of the gravid uterus

- Straining at stool

- Vascular engorgement and decreased venous return from pressure of the gravid uterus

- Venous dilation from the increase in circulating blood volume. Heredity, parity, obesity and increasing age may also be contributing factors (Baron, Ramirez & Richter, 1993; Saleeby et al, 1991; Wijayanegara, Mose, Achmad, Sobarna & Permadi, 1992).

Database

Subjective

- History may include
  - ▶ Family history of symptomatic hemorrhoids
  - ▶ Personal history of symptomatic hemorrhoids
  - ▶ Multiparity

- ▶ Increased age
- ▶ Obesity
- ▶ Constipation or straining during defecation
- ▶ Sitting for prolonged periods of time
- Complaints of perianal prolapse or "lump," pruritus, discomfort, pain, swelling, or discharge
  - ▶ More severe rectal pain most often associated with thrombosis or rectal fissure
- Client may describe perianal bleeding
  - ▶ Painless, bright red bleeding on surface of stool at time of defecation (suggests internal hemorrhoids)
  - ▶ Spontaneous bleeding (suggests large internal and external hemorrhoids)

Objective

- External hemorrhoids are visible on examination, at rest, or when bearing down.
- Internal hemorrhoids may be palpable on digital examination of anal canal, visible externally when prolapsed, or visible with anoscopy.
- Thrombosis (shiny blue or purple masses; subcutaneous clots adjacent to anus) or infection (inflamed appearance) may be evident.
- Fecal soiling may be noted where swelling of the external component makes hygiene difficult.

Assessment

- Hemorrhoids
  - ▶ R/O anal fissures, skin tags
  - ▶ R/O condylomata acuminata
  - ▶ R/O perirectal abscess
  - ▶ R/O idiopathic pruritus ani
  - ▶ R/O cancerous lesions
  - ▶ R/O inflammatory bowel disease

Plan

Diagnostic Tests

- Obtain hemoglobin/hematocrit if bleeding has been substantial and continued.

Treatment/Management

- Attempt to reduce hemorrhoids with gentle digital pressure.
- Topical anesthetic: Hemorrhoidal suppositories and ointment with or without hydrocortisone
  - ► Suppositories—insert one per rectum as needed, three to five per day, especially every morning, at bedtime, and after every bowel movement
  - ► Ointment—apply freely and gently rub into anal area, three to five times per day, especially every morning, at bedtime and after every bowel movement
- Sitz baths (warm or cool) for 15 to 20 minutes as needed for comfort, when bleeding absent
- Ice pack or cold compress; epsom salt bath to aid reduction
- Astringent compresses: witch hazel pads, as needed, to alleviate discomfort
- Petroleum jelly or glycerin suppository per rectum to ease defecation, as needed
- Stool softeners/laxatives, as needed (see Chapter 5.2, *Constipation*)
- See Patient Education.

Consultation

- For extremely painful, large, strangulated, or thrombosed hemorrhoids or continued bleeding, refer the client to a surgical consultant for evaluation and intervention.

Patient Education

- Explain the cause and treatment approaches for hemorrhoids in pregnancy.
- Advise client to correct and avoid constipation. See Chapter 5.2, *Constipation,* for education and therapeutics (includes high-fiber diet and adequate hydration).
- Teach digital replacement, if possible.
- Advise regarding careful anal hygiene.
- Recommend elevation of hips while sidelying to reduce discomfort; elevate foot of bed if tolerated.

Follow-up

- Client to call provider if pain becomes severe, bleeding continues, or no relief is obtained from therapeutic measures in one week. Otherwise reassess at next regular appointment.
- Document a significant ongoing problem with hemorrhoids in progress notes and problem list.

References

Baron, T., Ramirez, B., & Richter, J. (1993). Gastrointestinal motility disorders during pregnancy. *Annals of Internal Medicine, 118*(5), 366–375.

Goroll, A. (1995). Approach to the patient with anorectal complaints. In A. Goroll, L. May, & A. Mulley (Eds.), *Primary care medicine*, (3rd ed., pp. 372–379). Philadelphia, PA: JB Lippincott.

Medich, D., & Fazio, V. (1995). Hemorrhoids, anal fissure and carcinoma of the colon, rectum and anus during pregnancy. *Surgical Clinics of North America, 75*(1), 77–88.

Saleeby, R., Rosen, L., Stasik, J., Riether, R., Sheets, J., & Khubchandani, I. (1991). Hemorrhoidectomy during pregnancy: Risk or relief. *Diseases of the Colon and Rectum, 34*(3), 260–261.

Wijayanegara, H., Mose, J., Achmad, L., Sobarna, R., & Permadi, W. (1992). A clinical trial of hydroxyethylrutosides in the treatment of haemorrhoids in pregnancy. *Journal of International Medical Research, 20*(1), 54–60.

Chapter 10

LEG CRAMPS

Ellen M. Scarr

Lucy Newmark Sammons

Leg cramps are spasmodic, usually painful, contractions of leg muscles, most often affecting the gastrocnemius, but they may also involve the gluteal, thigh, or foot muscles (Cartlidge, 1995; Maldonado & Barger, 1995). Common in pregnancy, the etiology is not completely understood and is probably multifactorial. Reduced serum calcium levels and/or elevated serum phosphorus levels may contribute to the development of leg cramps, with pressure by the gravid uterus on lower extremity vessels and nerves as a contributing factor (Pernoll & Taylor, 1994). Leg cramps usually occur in the first few hours of sleep and disrupt sleep patterns, or may occur upon awakening, when muscle activity increases (Maldonado & Barger, 1995; Walton & Kolb, 1991).

Database

Subjective

- Client complains of painful cramping in calf, buttock, thigh, or foot
- Client may report
  - ▶ Previous history of muscle cramping
  - ▶ Fatigue in extremities
  - ▶ Diet may be very high or very low in calcium sources

Objective

- No evidence of
  - ▶ Dehydration
  - ▶ Hyperthyroidism
  - ▶ Hypothyroidism
  - ▶ Hypomagnesemia
  - ▶ Salt depletion
  - ▶ Uremia
  - ▶ Nerve root compression
- Absence of local warmth, redness, or positive Homan's sign

Assessment

- Leg cramps, physiologic
  - ▶ R/O varicose veins
  - ▶ R/O thrombophlebitis

Plan

Diagnostic Tests

- No diagnostic test is indicated.

Treatment/Management

- Immediate relief measures include
  - ▶ Extension of calf muscle by dorsiflexion of the foot
  - ▶ Compression of calf muscle
  - ▶ Attempt at ambulation
  - ▶ Application of heat
  - ▶ Massage
- Many providers recommend increasing calcium intake (without phosphorus), although the efficacy of the treatment is questionable (Institute of Medicine, 1990).
  - ▶ Calcium carbonate 1200 to 1500 mg/day p.o. in divided doses with meals, not with iron supplements

    NOTE: Chewable calcium carbonate tablets improve absorption of calcium because of increased surface area. Calcium carbonate contains 40 percent elemental calcium; 1500 mg provides 600 mg calcium.
  - ▶ Trial of reduction of phosphate intake
    - – Reduce milk
    - – Reduce excessive sources of phosphates (e.g., sodas, processed snacks)
    - – Reduce nutritional supplements containing calcium phosphate

Consultation

- No consultation necessary if symptoms mild and responsive to treatment

Patient Education

- Explain causes of leg cramps and rationale for therapeutics.
- Discuss dietary modifications as indicated above.

- Teach patient prophylactic measures:
  - ▶ Shake legs for 30 seconds before bedtime to improve circulation.
  - ▶ Avoid pointing toes when stretching or walking, which may trigger a cramp.
  - ▶ Avoid fatigue in legs.
  - ▶ Keep legs warm (with knee socks or leg warmers) and use leg massage if helpful.
  - ▶ Use relief measures above (dorsiflexion, compression, massage, warmth) as needed.
  - ▶ Maintain good circulation through exercise, posture, and positioning.

Follow-up

- Reevaluate symptoms and calcium/phosphate intake on next prenatal visit, or sooner if symptoms severe or nonresponsive to treatment.
- Document a significant ongoing problem with leg cramps in progress notes and problem list.

References

Cartlidge, N. (1995). Neurologic disorders. In W. Barron & M. Lindheimer (Eds.), *Medical disorders during pregnancy* (2nd ed., pp. 430–450). St. Louis, MO: Mosby.

Institute of Medicine. (1990). *Nutrition during pregnancy*. Washington, DC: National Academy Press.

Maldonado, A., & Barger, M. (1995). Primary care for women: Comprehensive assessment of common musculoskeletal disorders. *Journal of Nurse–Midwifery, 40*(2), 202–215.

Pernoll, M., & Taylor, C. (1994). Normal pregnancy and prenatal care. In A. DeCherney & M. Pernoll (Eds.), *Current obstetric and gynecologic diagnosis and treatment*, (8th ed., pp. 183– 201). Norwalk, CT: Appleton & Lange.

Walton, T., & Kolb, K. (1991). Treatment of nocturnal leg cramps and restless leg syndrome. *Clinical Pharmacology, 10*(6), 427– 428.

Chapter 11

LEUKORRHEA—PHYSIOLOGIC

Winifred L. Star

Ellen M. Scarr

Physiologic leukorrhea is an increased amount of normal vaginal and cervical discharge, consisting of epithelial cells and cervical mucus (Pernoll & Taylor, 1994). A result of hormonal stimulation, the amount and duration of leukorrhea varies from woman to woman and, in the same woman, from pregnancy to pregnancy. There should be no concomitant signs or symptoms of infection. The presence of coexisting vaginitis or cervicitis or other cervical pathology should be ruled out.

Database

Subjective

- Client may complain of increased amount of vaginal discharge or sensation of increased wetness in vulvar area without symptoms of vulvar or vaginal itching, irritation, burning, or odor.

Objective

- Pelvic examination is within normal limits (WNL)
  - ▶ Presence of increased amount of moderately thick, white vaginal discharge.
  - ▶ Note color and amount
- Wet mounts
  - ▶ Saline preparation (NaCl)
    - Normal amount of lactobacilli present
    - Normal squamous epithelium
    - Lack of white blood cells (WBCs)
    - No clue cells or trichomonads

    NOTE: With marked ectropion, there may be WBCs.
  - ▶ Potassium hydroxide (KOH)
    - No yeast
    - Negative amine odor
    - pH between 3.5 and 4.5 (acidic)

Assessment

- Physiologic leukorrhea
  - ▶ R/O rupture of membranes

▶ R/O onset of labor/preterm labor

▶ R/O vaginitis/cervicitis

▶ R/O condylomata acuminata

▶ R/O squamous intraepithelial lesion (SIL)

Plan

Diagnostic tests

- Pap smear as indicated by history and physical examination
- Wet mounts to be performed to rule out infection
- Testing for *Chlamydia trachomatis* and *Neisseria gonorrhoeae* as indicated by history and/or physical examination
- Testing for rupture of membranes as indicated (see Chapter 6.24, *Premature Rupture of Membranes*).
- Other tests, as indicated (e.g., herpes simplex viral culture)

Treatment

- Symptomatic relief; see Patient Education section in Chapter 14.7, *Vaginitis.*
- Advise client to avoid overtreatment with over-the-counter (OTC) preparations.
- If vulvar, vaginal, and/or cervical pathology identified, treat accordingly.

Consultation

- Consultation is not required.

Patient Education

- Educate about normal vaginal discharge.
- Advise against overtreatment of physiologic leukorrhea.
- See Chapter 14.7, *Vaginitis.*

Follow-up

- As necessary for signs/symptoms of infection, and as indicated by results of diagnostic testing.
- Refer patients with SIL for colposcopy.
- Document a significant ongoing problem with leukorrhea in progress notes and problem list.

References

Pernoll, M., & Taylor, C. (1994). Normal pregnancy and prenatal care. In A. DeCherney & M. Pernoll (Eds.), *Current obstetric and gynecologic diagnosis and treatment*, (8th ed., pp. 183– 201). Norwalk, CT: Appleton & Lange.

Chapter 12

NAUSEA AND VOMITING

Ellen M. Scarr

Lucy Newmark Sammons

Nausea and vomiting of pregnancy (NVP) are among the most common complaints of pregnancy, occurring in 50 to 90 percent of women (Baron, Ramirez & Richter, 1993; Belluomini, Litt, Lee & Katz, 1994; DiIorio, van Lier & Manteuffel, 1994). While often dismissed as a normal discomfort of pregnancy, NVP often has a substantial impact on the daily lives of pregnant women, 25 percent of whom take time off from work and an additional 50 percent feel their job performance is impacted by their symptoms (O'Brien & Naber, 1992). NVP is categorized as mild (nausea alone), moderate (nausea and vomiting), or severe (intractable vomiting with fluid and electrolyte disturbances) (Deuchar, 1995). NVP is most common in Western cultures, in younger women and in obese women (Baron et al., 1993).

Mild-moderate NVP usually begins by 4 to 6 weeks' gestation, peaks in severity by the third month, and usually resolves by 14 to 16 weeks of gestation (Hume & Killam, 1990). Symptoms are often worse in the early morning, and usually diminish as the day progresses. The etiology of NVP is unknown, despite numerous studies, and is likely multifactorial. All of the following have been postulated:

- Elevated hormone levels (serum hCG, progesterone or estradiol)
- Decreased gastric acidity and resulting gastric hypofunction
- Alterations in gastrointestinal motility due to increased progesterone and decreased motilin
- Vitamin B_6 deficiency
- Psychiatric/genetic/cultural factors

Mild-moderate NVP occurring in or persisting into the second or third trimester may be precipitated by the enlarging uterine fundus compressing the diaphragm and pyloric sphincter (Baron et al., 1993; Deuchar, 1995; Stainton & Neff, 1994). Mild-moderate NVP poses no threat to the fetus; in fact, early NVP has been reported to be a favorable risk factor for pregnancy outcome (Behrman, Hedigar, Scholl, & Arkangel, 1990; Peleg & Niebyl, 1997).

Severe NVP, also known as hyperemesis gravidarum, results in dehydration, electrolyte imbalance and weight loss. While hyperemesis gravidarum usually resolves by the third month, frequent relapses are not uncommon, and up to 20 percent of women suffer intractable nausea and vomiting throughout the pregnancy (Baron et al., 1993; Best & Hill, 1995). The cause of hyperemesis gravidarum remains poorly understood. High levels of serum hCG and serum estradiol have been implicated, as hyperemesis gravidarum is more common in pregnancies with higher hormonal levels, such as multiple gestation or molar pregnancies. Adrenal dysfunction, thyroid disease, reflux esophagitis and psychosocial factors have also been studied. The incidence of hyperemesis gravidarum is 0.5 to 2 percent of pregnancies, and occurs more frequently in Caucasians, primiparas, obese, unmarried and younger women (Best & Hill, 1995). While the prognosis for women with hyperemesis gravidarum is usually considered good, severe persistent symptoms have been associated with as high as a 40 percent pregnancy loss risk, intrauterine growth restriction, and low birth weight babies (Abbott, 1994; Deuchar, 1995; Mabie, 1992). Nausea and vomiting that initially presents in the second or third trimesters may be due to liver disease, eclampsia, or occult infection, and warrants further investigation (Abbott, 1994).

Database

Subjective

- Client complaints
  - ▶ Loss of appetite
  - ▶ Sensations of nausea
  - ▶ Aversion to sight, smell or thought of food
  - ▶ "Queasy stomach"
  - ▶ Retching and/or vomiting
- Symptoms may be limited to the morning or persist throughout the day, particularly increasing with fatigue.
- Symptoms most frequent during weeks 4 to 14 of pregnancy.
- Client may report history of nausea when using oral contraceptives.
- Data inconclusive to support any greater risk for NVP due to parity, maternal age, fetal gender, racial or ethnic group, intendedness of pregnancy, or socioeconomic status.
- Remainder of history unremarkable; particularly noting absence of abdominal pain, diarrhea, or fever.

Objective

- Mild-moderate NVP
  - ▶ Vital signs within normal limits (WNL)
  - ▶ Weight may show increase, stability, or decrease, depending on severity of symptoms
  - ▶ Mucous membranes, skin turgor, and urine specific gravity indicate absence of dehydration
  - ▶ Mucosal surfaces free of bleeding, indicating absence of severe vitamin C and B complex deficiency or hypoprothrombinemia
  - ▶ Fundoscopic exam WNL, indicating absence of retinal hemorrhage
  - ▶ Abdominal exam elicits no pain or tenderness, no organomegaly
  - ▶ Fetal heart tones audible at appropriate gestation, indicating fetal well-being and absence of molar pregnancy (in almost all cases)
  - ▶ Uterine size appropriate for dates

▶ Urine multi-dipstick/urinalysis negative for ketones, indicating absence of ketosis; negative or trace proteinuria

NOTE: If patient has ketonuria see Chapter 6.16, *Ketonuria*.

▶ Serum electrolytes, if obtained, WNL, indicating absence of severe dehydration or acidosis

▶ Complete blood count (CBC), if done, WNL, indicating absence of severe hemoconcentration

▶ Ultrasound shows normal intrauterine pregnancy, indicating absence of molar or multiple gestation

• Severe NVP

▶ Patient may appear anxious, fatigued

▶ Vital signs

   − Heart rate may be elevated

   − Blood pressure may be low

   − Respiratory rate may be elevated

   − Evidence of postural changes

▶ Weight usually is decreased

▶ Mucous membranes and skin turgor show evidence of dehydration and bleeding

▶ Fundoscopic exam may show retinal hemorrhage

▶ Fetal heart tones may be absent (molar pregnancy) or multiple (multiple gestation)

▶ Uterine size may be small for dates (from maternal weight loss) or enlarged from molar or multiple pregnancy

▶ Urine dipstick positive for protein (>1+) and/or ketones; specific gravity elevated

▶ Serum electrolytes abnormal (hypokalemia, hyponatremia, hypochloremia, elevated BUN and creatinine), indicating severe dehydration and metabolic alkalosis

▶ CBC shows evidence of hemoconcentration (i.e., elevated red blood count, hemoglobin, hematocrit)

▶ Ultrasound may show evidence of molar pregnancy, multiple gestation or intrauterine growth restriction (IUGR)

Assessment

• Nausea/vomiting of pregnancy

▶ R/O hyperemesis gravidarum

▶ R/O multiple gestation

▶ R/O molar pregnancy

▶ R/O gastrointestinal influenza

▶ R/O acute infection (e.g., appendicitis, pancreatitis, or urinary tract infection/pyelonephritis)

▶ R/O hiatal hernia, peptic ulcer, gastric carcinoma, or other disorders of the alimentary tract, biliary system, pancreas and peritoneum

▶ R/O eating disorders (anorexia, bulimia)

▶ R/O pica

▶ R/O food poisoning

▶ R/O migraine headache

▶ R/O preeclampsia/eclampsia

▶ R/O anemia

▶ R/O diabetic ketosis

▶ R/O hyperthyroidism

Plan

Diagnostic Tests

- Mild-moderate NVP

  ▶ Urine dipstick for protein and ketones to rule out proteinuria and ketosis

- Severe NVP

  ▶ Urine dipstick for protein, specific gravity, and ketones to assess level of proteinuria, dehydration, and ketosis

  ▶ Serum electrolytes to assess level of dehydration and alkalosis

  ▶ CBC to assess level of hemoconcentration

  ▶ Ultrasound to determine presence of multiple gestation, molar pregnancy or IUGR

Treatment/Management

- Mild NVP

  ▶ Obtain an accurate dietary history to assess quality, quantity, and pattern of food intake and food loss by vomiting.

  ▶ Administer iron and vitamin supplementation after meals, rather than on an empty stomach—If iron and/or vitamins still cause distress, the client may defer supplementation until symptoms resolve.

  NOTE: While vitamins may be an irritant for some women, one study showed a decrease in first trimester NVP with multivitamin use (Czeizel et al., 1992).

  ▶ It is best to avoid medication in the first 10 weeks of pregnancy (because of organogenesis) (Kousen, 1993); may use pyridoxine HCL (vitamin B_6) 25 to 50 mg p.o., t.i.d. to q.i.d., not to exceed 200 mg q.d.

NOTE: More than 200 to 300 mg/day vitamin B_6 can cause toxic neuropathies (Ditmars, 1993; Hunt & Osterman, 1994; Newman, Fullerton & Anderson, 1993). Recent studies show B_6 may decrease or eliminate NVP (Sahakian, Rouse, Sipes, Rose & Niebyl, 1991; Vutyavanich, Wongtra-ngan & Ruangsri, 1995).

▶ Consider Emetrol® 15 to 30 ml p.o. on arising, repeated every 3 hours as needed for nausea or every 15 minutes for a maximum of five doses for vomiting. Emetrol, a hyperosmolar carbohydrate solution with phosphoric acid, acts locally on the gastrointestinal (GI) tract to reduce smooth muscle contraction and delay gastric emptying time (Silberstein, 1993).

- Moderate NVP

  ▶ Consider an upper GI tract stimulant (e.g., metoclopramide hydrochloride, 10 mg p.o. 1 hour before meals and at bedtime).

  ▶ Consider an antihistamine (e.g., hydroxyzine 50 mg p.o., one-half hour before meals and at bedtime [Briggs, 1997]; or doxylamine succinate 25 mg p.o., given at bedtime with pyridoxine 25 mg p.o. [Kousen, 1993]).

  NOTE: A combination of doxylamine and vitamin B_6 reproduces the effective elements of Bendectin®, which is no longer available because of earlier concerns of fetal safety. Bendectin is *not* associated with an increased risk of congenital malformations (Gilstrap & Little, 1992; Silberstein, 1993). Client and provider may discuss implications of relevant litigation and controversy.

  ▶ Consider "resting" the GI tract with a clear liquid diet only for 24 hours, then advance to full liquid, then add complex carbohydrates. Avoid dairy products and fats for 48 hours.

  ▶ If moderate NVP is unresponsive to conservative measures, treat with antiemetics, either oral or rectal suppository with physician consultation as needed (Gilstrap & Little, 1992; Peleg & Neibyl, 1997):

    – Promethazine 5 to10 mg p.o., t.i.d. to q.i.d., as needed, or 25 mg rectal suppository every 4 hours, as needed

    – Prochlorperazine 5 to10 mg p.o., t.i.d. to q.i.d., as needed, or 5 to 10 mg rectal suppository b.i.d. to t.i.d., as needed

    – Chlorpromazine 10 to 25 mg p.o., every 4 hours, as needed, or 50 to 100 mg rectal suppository every 8 hours, as needed

  ▶ See also Patient Education.

- Severe NVP

  ▶ Medical referral required for

    – Documented weight loss of 4 or more pounds or 5 percent of body weight

    – 1+ or greater ketonuria

    – Electrolyte imbalance

    – Signs of dehydration

    – Suspected underlying pathology

▶ Patients are likely to require intravenous fluids, parenteral nutrition, antiemetics and possibly enteral feeding via nasogastric tube.

NOTE: Reports of both IV and enteral home therapy for hyperemesis gravidarum have shown that patients can successfully be managed outside of the hospital (Boyce, 1992; Naef et al., 1995).

▶ Refer to mental health professional as indicated for extreme anxiety, psychological disturbance or evidence of eating disorder.

Consultation

● See Treatment/Management section.

● Consult with physician for use of antiemetics, as indicated.

● Nutritional consultation may be indicated where strong food preferences, food allergies, or other dietary restrictions compound the problem of maintaining adequate intake.

Patient Education

● Explain possible causes of nausea and vomiting in pregnancy, the therapeutic plan, and signs or symptoms requiring return contact with provider.

● Provide reassurance that mild symptoms do not appear to have negative effects on fetal growth and development.

● Encourage additional rest, sleep, and relaxation. See Chapter 5.7, *Fatigue and Insomnia*.

NOTE: Lying down and resting during pregnancy has been found to be the most frequently used relief measure for nausea (DiIorio et al., 1994).

● Considering patient's lifestyle and preferences, explore alterations in solid and liquid nutritional intake patterns, food preparation techniques, and activity patterns that may be helpful in relieving NVP.

▶ Although rigorous evidence of their effectiveness has not been established in all cases, the following self-help measures may provide relief (Baron et al., 1993; Deuchar, 1995; DiIorio et al., 1994):

– Eat a small amount of a dry, complex carbohydrate in the morning before rising (e.g., crackers, toast, or cereal).

– Avoid letting the stomach become overly full or empty for too long; try small, frequent meals that are high in carbohydrate, low in fat.

– Try snacks of high protein foods (yogurt, nuts).

– Try taking fluids between meals instead of with meals.

– Sip carbonated beverages or clear juices.

– Drink milk, or eat apples or potatoes to neutralize gastric acid.

– Avoid brushing teeth within 1 to 2 hours after meals; may also need to avoid brushing teeth upon arising in the morning if this aggravates NVP.

- Maintain good ventilation while sleeping.

- Avoid foods/substances that irritate the stomach (e.g., coffee, alcohol, and cigarettes; iron; fried foods and spices).

- Avoid food preparation if it aggravates nausea; avoid offensive odors; maintain good ventilation when preparing foods.

• Acupressure at the P6 (Neiguan) acupuncture point near the wrist crease (either with digital pressure or the wearing of SeaBands®) has been shown to decrease nausea and vomiting (Belluomini et al., 1994; Stainton & Neff, 1994).

• Alternative remedies, which may be helpful but lack rigorous medical testing

  ▶ Herbal/spice teas: spearmint, peppermint, chamomile, ginger root, fennel, anise, raspberry leaf, and cinnamon (Dilorio et al., 1994; Peleg & Niebyl, 1997)

  ▶ Ginger capsules 250 mg p.o. four times a day (Peleg & Niebyl, 1997)

  ▶ Hypnosis (Stanford, 1994)

  ▶ Cold compresses to forehead or throat

  ▶ Hard candies

  ▶ Regular exercise

• If woman is employed, consider degree of disability and responsibilities of the job. Discuss alternative strategies for coping.

• Advise avoidance of constrictive clothing around abdomen.

• Advise avoidance of reclining immediately after eating, when the relaxed cardiac sphincter may more readily allow reflux regurgitation.

• Consider maintaining a diary to monitor food intake, identify precipitating factors, and evaluate effectiveness of relief measures.

Follow-up

• Client to contact provider if unable to retain minimum of liquids for 12 hours or more or for continued weight loss after identification of problem.

• If client able to maintain weight, recheck weekly (weight, urine ketones, signs and symptoms of dehydration) until symptoms subside.

• If symptoms are mild and respond well to therapeutics, and the weight gain pattern is appropriate, recheck at routine intervals.

• Document a significant ongoing problem with nausea/vomiting in progress notes and problem list.

References

Abbott, J. (1994). Medical disorders during pregnancy. *Emergency Medicine Clinics of North America, 12*(1), 115–128.

Baron, T., Ramirez, B., & Richter, J. (1993). Gastrointestinal motility disorders during pregnancy. *Annals of Internal Medicine, 118*(5), 366–375.

Behrman, C., Hediger, M., Scholl, T., & Arkangel, C. (1990). Nausea and vomiting during teenage pregnancy: Effects on birth weight. *Journal of Adolescent Health Care, 11*(5), 418–422.

Belluomini, J., Litt, R., Lee, K., & Katz, M. (1994). Acupressure for nausea and vomiting of pregnancy: A randomized, blinded study. *Obstetrics and Gynecology, 84*(2), 245–248.

Best, C., & Hill, J. (1995). Early pregnancy disorders: Hyperemesis and vaginal bleeding. In K. Carlson & S. Eisenstat (Eds.), *Primary care of women*, (pp. 321–326). St. Louis, MO: Mosby.

Boyce, R. (1992). Enteral nutrition in hyperemesis gravidarum: A new development. *Journal of the American Dietetic Association, 92*(6), 733–736.

Briggs, G. (1997). A guideline for treating hyperemesis gravidarum. *Contemporary OB-GYN, 42*(6), 70–79.

Czeizel, A., Dudas, I., Fritz, G., Tecsoi, A., Hanck, A., & Kunovits, G. (1992). The effect of periconceptional multivitamin–mineral supplementation on vertigo, nausea and vomiting in the first trimester of pregnancy. *Archives of Gynecology and Obstetrics, 251*(4), 181–185.

Deuchar, N. (1995). Nausea and vomiting in pregnancy: A review of the problem with particular regard to psychological and social aspects. *British Journal of Obstetrics and Gynaecology, 102*(1), 6–8.

Dilorio, C., van Lier, D., & Manteuffel, B. (1994). Recommendations by clinicians for nausea and vomiting of pregnancy. *Clinical Nursing Research, 3*(3), 209–227.

Ditmars, D. (1993). Patterns of carpal tunnel syndrome. *Hand Clinics, 9*(2), 241–252.

Gilstrap, L., & Little, B. (1992). *Drugs and pregnancy*, (pp. 269–275). New York: Elsevier Science.

Hume, R., & Killam, A. (1990). Maternal physiology. In J. Scott, P. DiSaia, C. Hammond, & W. Spellacy (Eds.), *Danforth's obstetrics and gynecology*, (6th ed., pp. 93–100). Philadelphia, PA: JB Lippincott.

Hunt, T., & Osterman, A. (1994). Complications of the treatment of carpal tunnel syndrome. *Hand Clinics, 10*(1), 63–71.

Kousen, M. (1993). Treatment of nausea and vomiting in pregnancy. *American Family Physician, 48*(7), 1279–1283.

Mabie, W. (1992). Obstetric management of gastroenterologic complications of pregnancy. *Gastroenterology Clinics of North America, 21*(4), 923–935.

Naef, R., Chauhan, S., Roach, H., Roberts, W., Travis, K., & Morrison, J. (1995). Treatment for hyperemesis gravidarum in the home: An alternative to hospitalization. *Journal of Perinatology, 15*(4), 289–292.

Newman, V., Fullerton, J., & Anderson, P. (1993). Clinical advances in the management of severe nausea and vomiting during pregnancy. *Journal of Obstetrics, Gynecologic and Neonatal Nursing, 22*(6), 483–490.

O'Brien, B. & Naber, S. (1992). Nausea and vomiting during pregnancy: Effects on the quality of women's lives. *Birth, 19*(3), 138–143.

Peleg, D. & Niebyl, J. (1997). Prescribing antiemetic therapy during pregnancy. *Contemporary OB-GYN, 42*(6), 164–171.

Sahakian, V., Rouse, D., Sipes, S., Rose, N., & Niebyl, J. (1991). Vitamin B6 is effective therapy for nausea and vomiting of pregnancy: A randomized, double-blind placebo-controlled study. *Obstetrics and Gynecology, 78*(1), 33–36.

Silberstein, S. (1993). Headaches and women: Treatment of the pregnant and lactating migraineur. *Headache, 33*(10), 533–540.

Stainton, M., & Neff, E. (1994). The efficacy of SeaBands for the control of nausea and vomiting in pregnancy. *Health Care for Women International, 15*(6), 563–575.

Stanford, J. (1994). Hypnosis for nausea and vomiting in pregnancy. *American Family Physician, 49*(8), 1733, 1736.

Vutyavanich, T., Wongtra–ngan, S., & Ruangsri, R. (1995). Pyridoxine for nausea and vomiting of pregnancy: A randomized, double-blind, placebo-controlled trial. *American Journal of Obstetrics and Gynecology, 173*(3), 881–884.

Chapter 13

PICA

Ellen M. Scarr

Lucy Newmark Sammons

Pica (cissa) refers to the abnormal craving for, and regular ingestion of, foods and nonfood substances with no nutritive value. The most common substances ingested are dirt or clay (geophagia), laundry starch or cornstarch (amylophagia) and ice or frost scraped from a refrigerator (pagophagia). Pica has also been reported with hair, stone/plaster, burnt matches, ashes, lead, wood, coffee grounds, uncooked rice, mothballs and powdered bricks.

The prevalence of pica is unknown, but it is estimated to occur in 20 to 75 percent of various pregnant populations. In the United States it is most common in poor, African-American women living in the rural Southeast or inner cities (Horner, Lackey, Kolasa & Warren, 1991; Lacey, 1990). Other risk factors that have been proposed include maternal age, nutrient and nutritional status, and a childhood or family history of pica, although studies are controversial (Horner et al., 1991).

There are multiple theories of the etiology of pica (Lacey, 1990). The homeostatic theory supports an attempt to restore minerals that are lacking in the diet. Physiologic disorder theories are based on the hypothesis that there is neurotransmitter substance malfunction or damage to the lateral or ventral medial areas of the hypothalamus. Some picas may have psychological origins based in reinforced behaviors of learning theory, modeling, compulsive disorders, or addictive behaviors. Strong cultural components are recognized. Certain picas are associated with protective beliefs for the welfare and comfort of the mother and baby.

Numerous medical complications are associated with pica, although study results have been variable and inconclusive (Horner et al., 1991; Lacey, 1990). Gastrointestinal problems include nausea, vomiting, obstruction, perforation, intussusception, parotid enlargement and constipation. Obesity or weight loss depend on the caloric value of the substance ingested. Hypercalcemia, lead poisoning in the woman and fetus, and fetal hemolytic anemia (from mothballs or air freshener) are potential complications. Although the cause-and-effect relationship between pica and commonly co-existing iron and zinc deficiencies and the related anemias remains unclear, it is known that ingestion of starch and clay interferes with maternal absorption of iron (Mitus, 1995).

Database

Subjective

- Client reports cravings for/ingestion of nonfood items such as starch, clay, ashes, plaster, antacids, ice, coffee grounds, or paraffin.

- Client states nonfood items (e.g., clay, cornstarch, flour) relieve discomforts of pregnancy and delivery or promote well-being of infant, while denial of such items affects the fetus (e.g., causes birthmarks).

- Client may have history of having eaten clay or dirt as a child.

- Client may also complain of
  - ► Fatigue, dyspnea on exertion, or other symptoms of anemia
  - ► Constipation, fecal impaction, persistent vomiting, or anorexia
  - ► Ptyalism

Objective

- Client may demonstrate any of the following:
  - ► Low serum iron values and iron deficiency anemia
  - ► Maternal weight gain below ideal, equal to ideal, or in excess of ideal
  - ► Severe abrasion to teeth
- Blood pressure and urine protein/ketones within normal limits (WNL)
- Fetal growth parameters WNL

Assessment

- Pica
  - ► R/O nutritional deficiency
  - ► R/O anemia
  - ► R/O ketonuria
  - ► R/O parasitic infection
  - ► R/O maternal intestinal and pyloric obstruction or chronic constipation
  - ► R/O preeclampsia
  - ► R/O emotional problems
  - ► R/O hypercalcemia
  - ► R/O lead intoxication

Plan

Diagnostic Tests

- Obtain ferritin or serum iron/TIBC to rule out concomitant iron deficiency anemia, as indicated. See Chapter 9.3, *Anemia—Iron, Folate, and Vitamin B_{12} Deficiency*.

Treatment/Management

- Thoroughly evaluate
  - ▶ Nutritional status
  - ▶ Maternal weight gain pattern
  - ▶ Fetal status
- See also Patient Education.

Consultation

- Nutritional consultation may be needed if food intake is markedly distorted.
- Medical consultation is needed if pathology from malnutrition or complications of pica develop.
- Social services referral is needed if warranted by socioeconomic situation.

Patient Education

- Explain need for well-balanced, adequate nutritional intake during pregnancy, with sensitivity to the beliefs of the client. Reinforce nutritional counseling.
- Demonstrate tolerance towards cravings if nutrition is otherwise adequate and ingested substances are not harmful.
- Provide additional education for related problems (e.g., constipation, obesity) as needed.

Follow-up

- Reassess food and nonfood intake patterns at subsequent visits.
  - ▶ If nutritional deficiencies are minimal, progress of pregnancy and fetal growth is unremarkable, and there are no signs of complications of pica, routine scheduling is adequate.
- Document a significant ongoing problem with pica in progress notes and problem list.

References

Horner, R., Lackey, C., Kolasa, K., & Warren, K. (1991). Pica practices of pregnant women. *Journal of the American Dietetic Association, 91*(1), 34–38.

Lacey, E. (1990). Broadening the perspective of pica: Literature review. *Public Health Reports, 105*(1), 29–35.

Mitus, A. (1995). Blood disorders. In K. Carlson & S. Eisenstat (Eds.), *Primary care of women* (pp. 98–105). St. Louis, MO: Mosby.

Chapter 14

URINARY FREQUENCY—PHYSIOLOGIC

Ellen M. Scarr

Lucy Newmark Sammons

Hormonal effects on the urinary system begin in the first trimester and, together with vascular engorgement, result in marked dilation of the urinary collecting system (calyces, pelves, and ureters), an increase in glomerular filtration rate, and increased diuresis (Davison, 1992). Mechanical obstruction by the growing uterus also promotes urinary tract dilation and decreases bladder capacity, contributing to urinary frequency later in pregnancy. Additionally, as the uterus enlarges, urinary control diminishes (Hume & Killam, 1990).

Database

Subjective

- Complaints of increased frequency of urination coinciding with onset of pregnancy, particularly in first and third trimesters, *without* symptoms of urinary tract infection (UTI)
- Client denies dysuria, urgency, hematuria, foul odor to urine, suprapubic discomfort, flank pain, or fever
- May complain of loss of urine when coughing or laughing
- Client not taking diuretic medication

Objective

- Afebrile
- Absent costovertebral angle tenderness (CVAT)
- Lower abdominal exam and genitourinary exam within normal limits (WNL)
- Urinalysis (dipstick/microscopic) WNL
  - ▶ Negative leukocyte esterase or nitrite
  - ▶ Negative pyuria, bacteriuria, or hematuria
- Urine culture, if obtained, WNL

Assessment

- Urinary frequency—physiologic
  - ▶ R/O urinary tract infection (UTI)
  - ▶ R/O asymptomatic bacteriuria
  - ▶ R/O diabetes mellitus

▶ R/O hypercalcemia

▶ R/O hypokalemia

▶ R/O psychogenic origin, particularly if nocturia is absent (Goodson, 1995)

Plan

Diagnostic Tests

- See Objective section.

Treatment/Management

- See Patient Education.

Consultation

- No consultation is required.

Patient Education

- Explain multiple causes of changed bladder function during pregnancy and expected return to previous function after delivery.

- Teach pelvic floor muscle exercises (i.e., Kegel's) to increase control over voluntary muscles.

- Instruct the client she should maintain good hydration but reduce excessive fluid intake, especially late in evening, if nocturia is interfering with sleep.

- Advise client to reduce excessive intake of foods and beverages containing alcohol and caffeine (e.g., coffee, tea, cocoa, chocolate, and soft drinks; alcohol should be avoided in pregnancy).

- Suggest the use of a panty liner if occasional incontinence is a problem.

- Advise client to empty bladder frequently and fully to deter urinary stasis and infection.

- Explain the signs and symptoms of UTI that require further attention.

Follow-up

- Monitor degree of discomfort and effect of therapeutics at next regular prenatal visit.

- Document a significant ongoing problem with urinary frequency in progress notes and problem list.

References

Davison, J. (1992). Renal disorders. In A. Calder & W. Dunlop (Eds.), *High risk pregnancy* (pp. 165–209). Oxford, England: Butterworth–Heineman.

Goodson, J. (1995). Approach to incontinence and other forms of lower urinary tract dysfunction. In A. Goroll, L. May, & A. Mulley (Eds.), *Primary care medicine* (3rd ed., pp. 687– 694). Philadelphia, PA: J.B. Lippincott.

Hume, R., & Killam, A. (1990). Maternal physiology. In J. Scott, P. DiSaia, C. Hammond, & W. Spellacy (Eds.), *Danforth's obstetrics and gynecology* (6th ed., pp. 93–100). Philadelphia, PA: J.B. Lippincott.

Chapter 15

VARICOSITIES

Ellen M. Scarr

Lucy Newmark Sammons

Varicosities are superficial veins that are enlarged, swollen, knotted or twisted. They are the most common vascular condition, occurring in 10 to 20 percent of the population (Brewster, 1995; Kontos, 1996). Pregnancy can aggravate preexisting varicosities, or promote the development of new varicosities in the legs, feet, vulva, or anal area. Proximal obstruction to venous return by the gravid uterus, increased venous stasis, congenital and acquired weakness of the vascular walls, constipation, obesity and decreased smooth muscle tone from hormonal effects or inactivity contribute to the development or worsening of varicosities in pregnancy.

Database

Subjective

- Client describes prominent, enlarged blood vessels, which may feel painful, achy, or cause a feeling of heaviness, in the legs, feet, vulva, or anal area.

- Occurrence increases with following risk factors:

  ▶ Family history of varicosities

  ▶ Increased age

  ▶ Greater gravidity

  ▶ Obesity

  ▶ Occupations requiring prolonged standing

Objective

- Pattern of purple or blue vessels, varying from flat and thin to raised and wide, visible superficially

- The following signs of thrombophlebitis are *absent:*

  ▶ Inflammation (i.e., overlying skin is red and hot)

  ▶ Involved superficial veins feel firm, cordlike

  ▶ Veins on dorsa of foot remain distended after elevation to 45 degrees

  ▶ Dependent cyanosis

  ▶ Deep tenderness elicited on palpation of vein or calf

  ▶ Positive Homan's sign (i.e., pain on abrupt ankle dorsiflexion)

> ▶ Louvel's sign (i.e., pain in calf upon sneezing or coughing, which disappears on digital compression proximal to obstruction)

> ▶ Restlessness, fever, tachycardia

- Edema may be present
- Peripheral pulses present and adequate

Assessment

- Varicosities (state site)
  - ▶ R/O thrombophlebitis
  - ▶ R/O edema
  - ▶ R/O hemorrhoids

Plan

Diagnostic Tests

- No tests indicated.

Treatment/Management

- See Patient Education.

Consultation

- Medical consultation for severe or thrombosed varicosities

Patient Education

- Explain causes of varicosities and rationale for treatment approach.
- Advise modification of activities to allow rest and elevation of extremities.
  - ▶ Elevate legs at least 30 minutes twice a day.
  - ▶ Avoid prolonged standing.
  - ▶ Avoid sitting for more than 1 hour at a time without walking around.
- Advise use of supportive elastic stockings (preferably full-length, pantyhose type, rather than calf or thigh length); place prior to rising from bed.

  NOTE: Elastic stockings for use in pregnancy are made by Jobst®, a national company. Their customer service line (800/537-1063) can give the name(s) of local dealer(s).

- Explain that a vulvar pad held snugly by belt or binder may give relief for vulvar varicosities; advise client to elevate hips with pillow when resting.

- Advise client to wear loose, nonconstrictive clothing, to avoid further impediment of circulation.

  ▶ Avoid clothing such as knee-high socks or pants with constrictive bands.

- Avoid crossing legs at the knee.

- Control weight gain and lose excess weight postpartally, as needed.

- Alert client to possible complications and their prevention

  ▶ Orthostatic hypotension and faintness on standing

    – Arise slowly from sitting or lying positions.

    – Maintain hydration.

  ▶ Predisposition to superficial thrombophlebitis, muscle aching, edema, or skin ulcers

    – Elastic stockings may prevent muscle aching, superficial thrombophlebitis, or edema of legs and feet.

    – Advise client to check skin frequently for breakdown or ulcerations.

- Reassure women that visible veins are normal and require no treatment

  ▶ Early or primary varicose veins are benign and best dealt with conservatively with compression stockings, or by compression sclerotherapy.

  ▶ If surgery or injection therapy is required, it is usually considered after all childbearing is completed.

Follow-up

- Reevaluate discomfort/extent of varicosities and success of therapeutics on next regularly scheduled visit. If symptoms increase or are not responsive to treatment, or if complications arise, see sooner.

- Document a significant ongoing problem with varicosities in progress notes and problem list.

References

Brewster, D. (1995). Management of peripheral venous disease. In A. Gorroll, L. May, & A. Mulley (Eds.), *Primary care medicine* (3rd ed., pp. 206–211). Philadelphia, PA: J.B. Lippincott.

Kontos, H. (1996). Vascular diseases of the limbs. In J. Bennett & F. Plum (Eds.), *Cecil textbook of medicine* (20th ed., pp. 346–357). Philadelphia, PA: W.B. Saunders.

SECTION 6

PERINATAL CONDITIONS

Chapter 1

ABNORMAL CERVICAL CYTOLOGY

Maureen T. Shannon

Papanicolaou (Pap) smear testing is a screening mechanism that detects early cellular changes associated with the development of cervical neoplasia or carcinoma. The identification of abnormal cervical findings in such a manner allows intervention early in the disease process. As a result of routine Pap smear testing of women, a decline in the incidence of invasive cervical cancer during the past several decades has been documented. However, during recent years an increase in cervical neoplasia and cancer rates has been observed (Devesa et al., 1987). One significant factor associated with this increase is the higher rate of human papillomavirus (HPV) infection reported in sexually active women during this time. Specific types of HPV (i.e., types 16, 18, 45, 56) have been correlated with a later development of cervical neoplasia and carcinoma in numerous investigations (Durst, Gissmann, Ikenberg, & zur Hausen, 1983; Lorincz, Temple, Kurman, Jenson, & Lancaster, 1987). Other factors reportedly associated with an increased risk for cervical neoplasia include: early age of first coital episode; use of tobacco, alcohol, or drugs; multiple sexual partners; in-utero diethylstilbestrol (DES) exposure; and immunosuppression (e.g., human immunodeficiency virus [HIV] infection, iatrogenic immunosuppression) (Cuzick, Singer, De Stavola, & Chomet, 1990; Maiman et al., 1990).

Currently the classification system used to report Pap smear results is the Bethesda system (TBS), which replaced the numerical system (i.e., Class I through V) previously used for this purpose. The Bethesda system gives a detailed analysis of Pap smear findings so that clinicians will have more comprehensive information regarding the results and the possible need for further evaluation. TBS attempts to provide the following information for the clinician:

- Determines whether the specimen is adequate for interpretation; if it is not, gives specific reasons for the unsatisfactory nature of the specimen

- Determines whether the specimen is within normal limits

- Provides a detailed descriptive diagnosis of any pathology that is identified (e.g., infections, reactive and reparative changes, epithelial cell abnormalities, nonepithelial malignant neoplasms) (see Table 6.1, The Bethesda System for Reporting Cervical/Vaginal Cytologic Diagnosis) (American College of Obstetricians and Gynecologists [ACOG], 1993; National Cancer Institute Workshop, 1989).

The Bethesda system uses different terminology than the previous numerical classification system to describe the various cytopathologic findings. The term "squamous intraepithelial lesion" (SIL) is used to describe the cervical changes that were previously classified as cervical intraepithelial neoplasia (CIN). According to the Bethesda system, low-grade SIL (LGSIL) findings encompass cellular changes associated with HPV and CIN I, while high-grade SIL (HGSIL) describes lesions encompassing changes seen in CIN II through CIN III (carcinoma in situ). These results also include a detailed description of the actual cell analysis (see Table 6.1, The Bethesda System for Reporting Cervical/Vaginal Cytologic Diagnosis).

In addition to the new classification of cytology results, the use of colposcopy and directed biopsies allows clinicians with specialized training in these procedures to further rule out the presence of pre-invasive and invasive lesions in the genital tract (e.g., cervix, vagina, vulva, and perianal regions). The colposcope magnifies suspicious lesions, and directed biopsy of these areas provides specimens for histologic evaluation. In some instances, the directed biopsy completely excises the abnormal tissue and no further treatment may be necessary. As part of the colposcopic evaluation, the squamocolumnar junction (SCJ) must be visualized, since this is the area where the majority of cervical abnormalities (e.g., neoplasia) will be found (Beckmann et al., 1995; Goodman & Hill, 1994). The SCJ may be located on the portio cervix or within the endocervical canal. The location of the SCJ will influence treatment strategies. When the SCJ is not adequately visualized, the colposcopy is classified as inadequate. In nonpregnant women, an endocervical curettage (ECC) is usually performed to obtain endocervical tissue for histologic evaluation to rule out any abnormalities in this location. In pregnant women ECC is usually *not* performed because of the possibility of iatrogenic rupture of membranes or stimulating labor (Beckmann et al., 1995; Sakornbut & Baxley, 1996). In addition to the detection and diagnosis of cervical neoplasia and cancer, the thorough evaluation of a woman's vaginal, vulvar, and perianal regions during the examination is essential to assess clinical evidence of multifocal genital tract lesions (e.g., vaginal intraepithelial neoplasia [VAIN], or vulvar intraepithelial neoplasia [VIN]).

Once an abnormal lesion is diagnosed, management is based upon several factors, including the severity of the lesion, extent of the lesion (i.e., single lesion, multifocal lesion), the woman's history (e.g., previous abnormal lesions), and the health status of the woman (e.g., immunocompetent or immunocompromised). The management of abnormal lesions may include the following methods:

- Expectant management

  ▶ Approximately 30 percent of LGSIL spontaneously regresses (Goodman & Hill, 1994).

  ▶ In some patient populations (e.g., reliable, immunocompetent), close monitoring of such lesions through repeat Pap smear and/or colposcopic evaluations at specific intervals (e.g., every 3 to 6 months) to observe regression or changes in the lesion(s) may be considered (Cruickshank & Kitchener, 1996; Goodman & Hill, 1994).

- Directed biopsy

  ▶ This is usually done to obtain a histologic sample to determine the severity of a suspicious lesion. It can be an effective treatment if complete excision of the abnormal tissue occurs during the biopsy.

- Cryotherapy

  ▶ Using nitrous oxide or carbon dioxide as the refrigerant, a cryoprobe (a stainless-steel probe varying in size) is used to freeze the lesion(s). Directed freezing must include the abnormal lesion and extend beyond the lesion's margins to include at least 5 mm of normal tissue.

    – Cervical stenosis may result; and follow-up colposcopic evaluations may be inadequate because visualization of the SCJ may not be possible (Beckmann et al., 1995; Goodman & Hill, 1994).

- Laser

  ▶ A carbon dioxide laser may be used to ablate abnormal tissue, including the lesions of the vulva, vagina, cervix, perineum. A carbon dioxide laser also may be used as a method of performing a cone biopsy for diagnosis and treatment of CIN in the cervical canal.

  NOTE: It is considered to be more effective than cryotherapy, and is less likely to cause cervical stenosis (Goodman & Hill, 1994; Kawada, 1994).

- Loop electrosurgical excision procedure (LEEP)

▶ A small wire loop is connected to an electrosurgical generator which emits low-voltage, high-frequency alternating currents resulting in thermal destruction of tissue.

▶ LEEP is frequently used for excision of vulvar and cervical lesions and may be used to perform a cone biopsy (i.e., large loop excision of the transformation zone or "LEETZ" procedure) (Goodman & Hill, 1994; Kawada, 1994).

- Cone biopsy

  ▶ Cervical cone biopsy is a minor surgical procedure that can be performed under local or general anesthesia using a scalpel (i.e., cold knife conization), a laser, or LEETZ procedure.

  ▶ The procedure removes a cone-shaped specimen that encompasses all of the lesions of the exocervix, the SCJ, and a portion of the endocervical canal (Beckmann et al., 1995; Goodman & Hill, 1994).

  ▶ Analysis of this specimen determines the severity and extent of cervical disease, and the type of treatment indicated.

  ▶ The procedure may also be therapeutic if the margins of the specimen are without evidence of abnormal cells (i.e., depth of endocervical canal invasion is determined to be less than 1 mm).

  NOTE: Cervical incompetence may result if the internal os is compromised as a result of this procedure (Beckmann et al., 1995).

- Hysterectomy, pelvic lymphadenectomy, and/or pelvic irradiation

  ▶ Surgical interventions are indicated in the treatment of invasive cervical carcinoma.

  ▶ The type of treatment is based upon the stage of the cervical cancer diagnosed. (A detailed discussion of the treatment of invasive cervical cancer is beyond the scope of this book.)

Overall, the incidence of abnormal cervical cytology during pregnancy is approximately 3 percent (Beckmann et al., 1995). An investigation of risk factors associated with the development of cervical neoplasia and carcinoma in pregnant women has not demonstrated a statistically significant increase in their incidence during pregnancy (Kemp, Hakenewerth, Laurent, Gravitt, & Stoerker, 1992). Furthermore, the majority of pregnant women diagnosed with varying degrees of cervical neoplasia respond to conservative management strategies similar to those recommended for nonpregnant women (ACOG, 1993; Economos, Veridiano, Delke, Collado, & Tancer, 1993; Giuntoli et al., 1991; Ueki et al., 1995). The successful outcome observed with conservative management during pregnancy is correlated with routine cervical cytology as a part of prenatal care, detection and further diagnosis of abnormalities (i.e., through the use of colposcopy and directed biopsies by experienced clinicians), and appropriate treatment and follow-up (ACOG, 1993).

Database

Subjective

- The woman may be asymptomatic or report one or more of the following:

  ▶ Epidemiologic factors associated with an increased incidence of cervical neoplasia or carcinoma

    – History of HPV infection or exposure to a partner with HPV

    – Multiple sexual partners

- Early age at first coitus
- Use of tobacco, alcohol, or drugs
- In utero DES exposure
- Immunosuppression (e.g., disease [HIV] or therapeutic interventions [cancer treatments])

▶ Previously abnormal Pap smear

▶ History of infrequent Pap smears

▶ Painless spotting or bleeding after coitus

▶ History of intermenstrual bleeding prior to pregnancy

▶ Thin, watery vaginal discharge.

▶ Complaints associated with cervicitis

▶ Weight loss and painful vaginal bleeding (the latter stages of cervical carcinoma)

Objective

- Physical examination may reveal one or more of the following findings:

  ▶ Vital signs within normal limits (WNL)

  ▶ External genitalia and perianal areas may appear normal or may have

    - Evidence of verruciform lesions (condylomata acuminata)
    - Areas of pallor or abnormal white epithelium (AWE)

  ▶ Speculum examination may reveal

    - Vaginal mucosa may appear normal or may have verruciform lesions, areas of pallor
    - Cervix may appear normal, or may be erythematous, friable, ulcerated; colposcopic evaluation may reveal evidence of mosaicism, punctation and/or abnormal blood vessels

    - Failure of abnormal epithelium to stain with iodine (Schiller's test)
    - Evidence of leukoplakia when suspicious areas on the vulva, perineum, vagina, and cervix have 3 to 5 percent acetic acid solution applied to them.

  ▶ Bimanual palpation of cervix (a hard, enlarged mass may be revealed in latter stages of carcinoma of cervix).

- No effect on clinical parameters of pregnancy is usually evident unless the woman is in latter stages of carcinoma at which time she may demonstrate weight loss with subsequent intrauterine growth restriction (i.e., fundal height less than gestational age).

Assessment

- Adequate or inadequate cervical cytology specimen

- Abnormal cervical cytology result (the specific Bethesda system classification should be included [e.g., ASCUS, LGSIL, HGSIL, squamous cell carcinoma])

  ▶ R/O condylomata acuminata

▶ R/O cervicitis/sexually transmitted diseases (STDs)

▶ R/O vaginitis

• Reactive changes (e.g., inflammation, infection)

▶ R/O coexistent vulvar, vaginal, or perianal neoplasia

▶ R/O HIV infection

• Colposcopic evaluation (if performed) adequate or inadequate (i.e., SCJ location completely or not completely visualized)

• Colposcopic lesion(s)— location, extent, characteristics

▶ R/O intrauterine growth restriction (IUGR)

Plan

Diagnostic Tests

• The false negative rate of Pap smear cytology is usually due to sampling error. The proper technique to obtain and fix a Pap smear specimen is as follows (ACOG, 1993; Hanson, 1995):

▶ Specimens should be obtained prior to the bimanual examination.

– Lubricant contaminates specimens and any contact with this should be avoided.

NOTE: Warm water can be used instead of lubricant to reduce friction.

– If sexually transmitted disease (STD) testing is to be done, the Pap smear should be obtained first.

– If large amounts of vaginal discharge are present, carefully remove this prior to obtaining the Pap smear.

▶ Visualize the entire portio to provide optimum sampling. Reposition the speculum if necessary for better visualization of the cervix.

▶ Obtain the sample from the portio that includes the entire transformation zone first by gently rotating the spatula 360 degrees.

▶ Obtain the endocervical sample by gently rotating the endocervical brush or cotton-tipped swab 180 degrees.

NOTE: Preliminary evidence indicates that the endocervical brush can be used during pregnancy (Foster & Smith, 1996; Orr, Barrett, Orr, Holloway, Holimon, 1992).

▶ Once the specimens are obtained apply them evenly to either a single slide or a slide for the portio and another for the endocervical sample. The slide(s) should then be fixed to prevent air drying.

NOTE: When using spray fixatives, the spray should be held at least 10 inches away from the slide to prevent destruction of the cells by the propellant.

▶ Obtaining a four-quadrant sample from the upper two thirds of the vagina should be considered for women with a history of in utero DES exposure. This sample should be placed on a separate slide from the cervical specimens, and labeled as a vaginal sample.

- Obtain colposcopic evaluation on women with abnormal cervical cytology, as indicated (see Treatment/Management section).

  NOTE: Colposcopy should be performed by an *experienced* clinician, especially in pregnant women because of the increased vascularity of the cervix as a result of pregnancy. This may make adequate visualization and assessment difficult and possibly result in the overinterpretation (i.e., HGSIL) of cervical vascular patterns. In addition, there is an increased risk of bleeding from punch biopsies performed during pregnancy. Therefore, the clinician performing the colposcopic evaluation should be prepared to intervene in a timely and appropriate manner if this occurs (Sakornbut & Baxley, 1996).

- Obtain a directed biopsy of a suspicious lesion or area (e.g., AWE) during colposcopy, if indicated.

- Endocervical curettage *is not* done during pregnancy.

- Wet prep of cervico-vaginal discharge may reveal evidence of vaginitis or cervicitis (see Section 14, *Vaginitis and Sexually Transmitted Diseases*).

- Obtain additional STD testing (e.g., gonorrhea testing, chlamydia testing, syphilis serology, HIV antibody testing), as indicated.

  NOTE: HIV antibody testing should be done only after adequate pretest counseling and voluntary consent of the woman has been obtained (see Chapter 14.5, *Human Immunodeficiency Virus*).

Treatment/Management

- A normal Pap smear result and without a history of any abnormal cervical cytologic result or other risk factors associated with the rapid development of cervical or genital neoplasias (e.g., HIV infection)

  ▶ Woman may have her Pap smear repeated every 1 to 3 years at the discretion of the clinician and preference of the woman (ACOG, 1993; U.S. Preventative Services Task Force, 1996).

- Pap smear result that is benign but without evidence of endocervical cells

  ▶ In general, this finding does not require a repeat Pap smear be obtained earlier than routinely recommended (i.e., every 1 to 3 years) unless

    – The woman is immunocompromised

    – Woman has a history of abnormal Pap smear results (El Sadr et al., 1994; Hanson, 1995).

- Atypical squamous cells of undetermined significance (ASCUS)

  ▶ The management depends upon the clinical circumstances specific to the woman (e.g., immunocompromised) and whether the diagnosis of ASCUS was qualified (see Table 6.1, The Bethesda System for Reporting Cervical/Vaginal Cytological Diagnosis). Several management options are possible (Beckmann et al., 1995; Hanson, 1995):

    – Repeat Pap smear every 6 months for up to 2 years until there are three consecutive smears that are WNL.

      * If a repeat Pap smear result reveals ASCUS or higher grade lesion, colposcopic evaluation is indicated.

    – A Pap smear with ASCUS qualified with severe inflammation requires evaluation of the woman to determine the etiology of the inflammation (e.g., vaginitis). A repeat Pap smear should be obtained 2 to 3 months after treatment of any identified infection. If this result is WNL, then another Pap smear should be obtained in 6 to 12 months. If this is normal, follow-up Pap smears can be obtained at the discretion of the clinician or per institution specific policies and protocols.

- – A woman considered to be at risk for the development of SIL (e.g., an immunosuppressed woman) who has a single Pap smear with ASCUS reported should obtain a colposcopic evaluation.

- – A report of ASCUS qualified by a statement favoring a premalignant or malignant condition indicates the need for colposcopic evaluation of the woman.

- A woman with evidence of LGSIL should be referred for colposcopic evaluation and treatment (as indicated).

- A woman with HGSIL or evidence of cancer should be referred for colposcopic evaluation and appropriate treatment.

- Evidence of early stromal invasion or microinvasion based on Pap smear findings may require excision of the area to rule out invasive carcinoma. If a pregnant woman does not have evidence of invasive carcinoma based on the histologic evaluation of this specimen, treatment may be postponed until after delivery (ACOG, 1993; Beckmann et al., 1995). However, repeat cytologic samples should be obtained and colposcopic evaluations performed during the pregnancy at intervals determined by the physician responsible for her care (Sakornbut & Baxley, 1996).

- Obstetrical ultrasound: in a woman with suspected IUGR as a result of advanced stages of invasive cervical cancer. Serial ultrasound testing every 3 to 4 weeks should be ordered for women with a diagnosis of IUGR (see IUGR protocol).

- Antepartum fetal surveillance (e.g., nonstress tests [NST], amniotic fluid index [AFI]): may be indicated in women with advanced cervical or metastatic disease if coexistent IUGR.

Consultation

- Consultation may be necessary for an immunocompetent woman with premalignant findings reported on cervical cytology.

- Consultation is indicated for an immunosuppressed woman with a cervical cytology result indicating ASCUS or higher grade lesion.

- Refer a woman with a cervical cytologic abnormality of HGSIL or carcinoma to a physician.

Patient Education

- Explain the Pap smear and other laboratory tests and interpret the results for the woman.

  ▶ Discuss the importance of having follow-up testing (as indicated).

- Reassure the woman that in general, the abnormal cervical cytology will not adversely effect the infant. However, in the situation where invasive cervical cancer has been diagnosed, the illness could result in poor/adverse maternal and/or fetal outcome. Information about the possible complications associated with invasive cervical cancer should be presented to the woman (and her partner) by the physician managing her care.

- Explain to the woman who is being referred to the consulting physician the reason(s) for the referral/transfer of care.

- A woman diagnosed with an STD should be educated about the condition, the indicated treatment, the treatment option(s) for her and her partner(s), and the recommended follow-up tests to evaluate the success of the treatment. Discuss with the woman safer sex methods (see STD Chapter).

Follow-up

Follow-up depends on the result of the cytologic evaluation, additional diagnostic tests (e.g., biopsy results), and site-specific guidelines. Generally, every woman should have a Pap smear during her 6-week postpartum examination with subsequent Pap smears obtained, as indicated, based upon her history. The following guidelines have been proposed but may vary depending upon site-specific protocols (see also Treatment/Management section for suggested schedules based on clinical and cytologic findings) (Beckmann et al., 1995):

- Benign Pap result

  ▶ Repeat Pap smear test every 1 to 3 years in women without a history of immunocompromise or previous abnormal cervical cytology/diagnosis.

  ▶ Women with immunocompromise or a history of abnormal cervical cytology/diagnosis should have Pap smears repeated at intervals recommended for their specific clinical/cytologic/ histologic findings.

- ASCUS result

  ▶ Pap smear every 6 months for up to 2 years until three consecutive negative results, then every 1 to 3 years based upon the clinician's discretion and/or institution specific policies and procedures.

  ▶ If a second Pap smear result indicates ASCUS or higher grade lesion, perform or refer for colposcopy with follow-up based upon results of colposcopy/cytology/histology findings.

- Treatment for LGSIL/HGSIL

  ▶ Pap smear every 3 months for a year (after a complete colposcopic evaluation), then every 6 months for 2 years.

  ▶ If all Pap smear results are normal, the woman may begin annual Pap smear evaluations beginning the third year.

- Treatment for cervical carcinoma

  ▶ Pap smear every 3 months for 2 years, then every 6 months for 3 years.

  NOTE: Women who have been treated for cervical carcinoma should receive follow-up evaluations per the recommendations of their gynecologist and/or oncologist.

- Guidelines for Pap smear evaluations of woman with immunosuppression (specifically HIV infection) vary. However, the following schedules have been proposed for HIV-infected women (El Sadr et al., 1994):

  ▶ A woman with early HIV infection and without a history or evidence of any abnormal cervical cytology should have two Pap smears obtained 6 months apart. If both of these are adequate specimens and benign, then Pap smears may be obtained annually.

  ▶ A woman should have a repeat Pap smear if there is no evidence of endocervical cells on the smear or after treatment for an identified cause of underlying inflammation (e.g., vaginitis).

▶ A woman who has had a colposcopic evaluation for ASCUS, LGSIL, or higher-grade lesion should have follow-up Pap smears obtained and/or colposcopic evaluations performed per recommendation of the clinician responsible for her care.

▶ A woman without a history of abnormal cervical cytology who has symptomatic HIV disease or a CD4 count less than 500 should have a Pap smear every 6 months.

● Follow-up evaluation intervals for a woman who is referred for colposcopy are determined by the colposcopist/consulting physician.

● Document Pap results in laboratory section of chart. If abnormal, then record specific diagnosis and treatment thereof in progress notes and on problem list.

Table 6.1

The Bethesda System for Reporting Cervical/Vaginal Cytologic Diagnosis

Format of the Report
       a. A statement on adequacy of the specimen
       b. A general categorization which may be used to assist with clerical triage (optional)
       c. The descriptive diagnosis

Adequacy of the Specimen
       Satisfactory for evaluation
       Satisfactory for evaluation but limited by. . . (specify reason)
       Unsatisfactory for evaluation . . . (specify reason)

General Categorization (Optional)
       Within normal limits
       Benign cellular changes: See descriptive diagnoses
       Epithelial cell abnormality: See descriptive diagnoses

Descriptive Diagnoses
Benign cellular changes
       Infection
              Trichomonas vaginalis
              Fungal organisms morphologically consistent with *Candida* species
              Predominance of coccobacilli consistent with shift in vaginal flora
              Bacteria morphologically consistent with *Actinomyces* species
              Cellular changes associated with herpes simplex virus
              Other
Reactive changes
       Reactive cellular changes associated with
               Inflammation (includes typical repair)
              Atrophy with inflammation ("atrophic vaginitis")
              Radiation
              Intrauterine contraceptive device (IUD)
       Other
Epithelial Cell Abnormalities
       Squamous cell
              Atypical squamous cells of undetermined significance: Qualify[†]
              Low-grade squamous intraepithelial lesion encompassing:
                     HPV[‡]
                     Mild dysplasia/CIN 1
              High-grade squamous intraepithelial lesion encompassing:
                     Moderate and severe dysplasia
                     CIS/CIN 2 and CIN 3
              Squamous cell carcinoma
       Glandular cell
              Endometrial cells, cytologically benign, in a postmenopausal woman
              Atypical glandular cells of undetermined significance: Qualify[†]
              Endocervical adenocarcinoma
              Endometrial adenocarcinoma
              Extrauterine adenocarcinoma
              Adenocarcinoma, not otherwise specified (NOS)
Other malignant neoplasms: Specify
Hormonal evaluation (applied to vaginal smears only)
       Hormonal pattern compatible with age and history
       Hormonal pattern incompatible with age and history: Specify
       Hormonal evaluation not possible due to . . .Specify

[†] Atypical squamous or glandular cells of undetermined significance should be further qualified as to whether a reactive or premalignant/malignant process is favored.

[‡] Cellular changes of human papillomavirus (HPV)—previously termed koilocytosis atypia, or condylomatous atypia—are included in the category of low-grade squamous intraepithelial lesion.

Source: Reprinted with permission from American College of Obstetricians and Gynecologists. (1993). *Cervical cytology: Evaluation and management of abnormalities.* (Technical bulletin no. 183, p. 3). Washington, DC: Author.

References

American College of Obstetricians and Gynecologists (ACOG). (1993). *Cervical cytology: Evaluation and management of abnormalities.* (Technical bulletin no. 183). Washington, DC: Author.

Beckmann, C.R.B., Ling, F.W., Barzansky, B.M., Bates, G.W., Herbert, W.N.P. Laube, D.W., & Smith, R.P. (1995). *Obstetrics and gynecology* (2nd ed., pp. 413–438). Baltimore, MD: Williams & Wilkins.

Cruickshank, M.E., & Kitchener, H.C. (1996). The problem with low-grade Pap smears. *Contemporary OB/GYN, 41*(8), 80–93.

Cuzick, J., Singer, A., De Stavola, B.L., & Chomet, J. (1990). Case-control study of risk factors for cervical intraepithelial neoplasia in young women. *European Journal of Cancer, 26*(6), 684–690.

Devesa, S.S., Silverman, D.T., Young, Jr., J.L., Pollack, E.S., Brown, C.C., Horm, J.W., Percy, C.L., Myers, M. ., McKay, F.W., & Fraumeni, Jr., J.F. (1987). Cancer incidence and mortality trends among whites in the United States, 1947–1984. *Journal of the National Cancer Institute, 79*, 701–770.

Durst, M., Gissmann, L., Ikenberg, H., & zur Hausen, H. (1983). A papillomavirus DNA from cervical carcinoma and its prevalence in cancer biopsies from different geographic regions. *Proceedings from the National Academy of Sciences USA, 80*, 3812–3817.

Economos, K., Veridiano, N.P., Delke, I., Collado, M.L., & Tancer, M.L. (1993). Abnormal cervical cytology in pregnancy: A 17 year experience. *Obstetrics and Gynecology, 81*(6), 915–918.

El-Sadr, W., Oleske, J.M., Agins, B. D., Bauman, K., Brosgart, C., et al. (1994). *Evaluation and management of early HIV infection.* Clinical practice guideline No. 7, AHCPR Publication No. 94-0572. Rockville, MD: Agency for Health Care Policy and Research, Public Health Service, U.S. Department of Health and Human Services.

Foster, J.C., & Smith, H.L. (1996). Use of a cytobrush for Papanicolaou smear screens in pregnant women. *Journal of Nurse-Midwifery, 41*(3), 211–217.

Giuntoli, R., Yeh, I.T., Bhuett, N., Chu, W., Van Leewen, K., & Van Der Lans, P. (1991). Case report. Conservative management of cervical intraepithelial neoplasia during pregnancy. *Gynecologic Oncology, 42*, 68–73.

Goodman A., & Hill, E.C. (1994). Premalignant and malignant disorders of the uterine cervix. In A. H. DeCherney & M. L. Pernoll (Eds.), *Current obstetric & gynecologic diagnosis & treatment* (8th ed., pp. 920–936). East Norwalk, CT Appleton & Lange.

Hanson, L. N. (1995). Abnormal cervical cytology. In W.L. Star, L.L. Lommel, & M.T. Shannon (Eds.), *Women's primary health care: Protocols for practice* (pp. 12–3, 12–12). Washington, DC: American Nurses Publishing.

Kawada, C.Y. (1994). Gynecologic history, examination & diagnostic procedures. In A.H. DeCherney & M.L. Pernoll (Eds.), *Current obstetrics & gynecologic diagnosis & treatment* (8th ed., pp. 612–632). East Norwalk, CT: Williams & Wilkins.

Kemp, E.A., Hakenewerth, A.M., Laurent, S.L., Gravitt, P.E., & Stoerker, J. (1992). Human papillomavirus prevalence in pregnancy. *Obstetrics and Gynecology, 79*(5), 649–656.

Lorincz, A.T., Temple, G.F., Kurman, R.J., Jenson, A.B., & Lancaster, W.D. (1987). Oncogenic association of specific human papillomavirus types with cervical neoplasia. *Journal of the National Cancer Institute, 79*, 671–677.

Maiman, M., Fruchter, R.G., Serur, E., Remy, J.C., Feuer, G., & Boyce, J. (1990). Human immunodeficiency virus infection and cervical neoplasia. *Gynecologic Oncology, 38*, 377 – 382.

National Cancer Institute Workshop. (1989). The 1988 Bethesda system of reporting cervical/vaginal cytological diagnoses. *Journal of the American Medical Association, 262*(7), 931–934.

Orr, Jr., J.W., Barrett, J.M., Orr, P.F., Holloway, R.W., & Holimon, J.L. (1992). The efficacy and safety of the cytobrush during pregnancy. *Gynecologic Oncology, 44*, 260–262.

Sakornbut, E., & Baxley, E. (1996). Commonly encountered medical problems in pregnancy. In S.D. Ratcliffe, J. E. Byrd, & E. L. Sakornbut (Eds.), *Handbook of pregnancy and perinatal care in family practice* (pp. 168–205). Philadelphia, PA: Hanley & Belfus.

Ueki, M., Ueda, M., Kumagai, K., Okamoto, Y., Noda, S., & Matsuoka, M. (1995). Cervical cytology and conservative management of cervical neoplasias during pregnancy. *International Journal of Gynecological Pathology, 14*(1), 63–69.

United States Preventative Services Task Force. (1996). *Guide to clinical preventative services* (2nd ed., pp. 105–116). Alexandria, VA: International Medical Publishing.

Chapter 2

Antiphospholipid Syndrome

Joan R. Murphy

Antiphospholipid syndrome (APS) is an autoimmune disorder characterized by the presence of maternal autoantibodies, specifically lupus anticoagulant (LA), anticardiolipin antibody (aCL), and the antibody responsible for the false-positive serologic test for syphilis (FP-STS), in combination with one or more clinical sequelae (Atterbury, Munn, Groome, & Yarnell, 1997; Branch, 1991; Silver & Branch, 1994). The primary clinical features associated with the APS are venous or arterial thrombosis (including stroke), recurrent spontaneous abortion or fetal death, and thrombocytopenia (American College of Obstetricians & Gynecologists [ACOG], 1998; Bowles, 1990; Branch, 1991; Ordi-Ros, Perez-Peman, & Monasterio, 1994; Silver & Branch, 1994). Fetal death, especially late in the first trimester or in the second trimester, appears to be the type of pregnancy loss most specific for APS (Dizon-Townson, & Branch, 1998; Patton, 1993).

Antiphospholipid antibodies occur in a variety of medical and obstetrical conditions (including other autoimmune disorders, neoplastic disorders, and infectious diseases), in association with certain drugs, and in otherwise healthy individuals (Ordi-Ros, et al., 1994). (See Table 6.2.) Other conditions associated with antiphospholipid antibodies include chorea (chorea gravidarum in pregnancy), migraine headaches, epilepsy, Guillain-Barré syndrome, pseudo-multiple sclerosis, transverse myelitis, livedo reticularis, skin ulcers, autoimmune hemolytic anemia, and valvular heart disease (Ordi-Ros et al., 1994; Silver & Branch, 1994). (See Table 6.3) A substantial proportion of thrombotic events related to these antibodies occur during pregnancy or with oral contraceptive use. Furthermore, pregnancy-induced hypertension (PIH), intrauterine growth restriction (IUGR), and preterm birth are common obstetrical complications in women with APS (ACOG, 1998; Silver & Branch, 1994).

Patients with APS appear to have an unusually high rate of PIH, which contributes to the high rate of preterm deliveries. Women who have early onset (less than 34 weeks) severe PIH should be tested for APS. Furthermore, uteroplacental insufficiency approaches 30 percent in pregnant women with APS, but routine antenatal testing for IUGR is not warranted, unless clinical signs are also present. Preterm deliveries occur in approximately one third of patients with APS, usually due to PIH or uteroplacental insufficiency (ACOG, 1998).

Antiphospholipid antibodies are found in 1 to 5 percent of the normal obstetrical population, most commonly at low levels (Newman, 1995). Low-level titers are of questionable significance, especially in the absence of disease, and have not been associated with pregnancy loss (Dizon-Townson & Branch, 1997; Newman, 1995; Silver & Branch 1994). Moderate or high-level aCL antibody titers or a positive LA test persisting for months or years are considered diagnostic criteria for APS (Harris, 1990; Newman, 1995). In women with recurrent pregnancy loss, lupus anticoagulant is found in 5 to 10 percent of cases and anticardiolipin antibodies in 5 to 10 percent. Approximately 70 percent of patients with lupus anticoagulant also have anticardiolipin antibodies (Newman, 1995; Silver & Branch, 1994), but the opposite is not necessarily true because fewer patients with anticardiolipin antibodies have lupus anticoagulant. The higher the anticardiolipin titers, the more likely the presence of lupus anticoagulant (Silver & Branch, 1994). Furthermore, anticardiolipin antibodies of the IgG type appear to be more specific for pregnancy loss than the IgM type (Harris, 1990). Anticardiolipin antibodies are also present in up to 50 percent of patients with the antibody that causes the false-positive test for syphilis (FP-STS), but the FP-STS is the least predictive of APS (Branch, 1991; Silver & Branch, 1994).

APS is most prevalent in patients with underlying autoimmune disease. Antiphospholipid antibodies are found in 10 to 30 percent of women with systemic lupus erythematosus (SLE) or with a history of arterial or venous thrombosis; the antibodies have also been noted in patients with other connective tissue diseases (Branch, 1991; Newman, 1995; Silver & Branch, 1994). The lupus anticoagulant was first described in 1952 in patients with SLE (ACOG, 1998). In 1957, LA was described in patients who had SLE and associated recurrent pregnancy loss, as well as in patients with unexplained clotting disorders (Patton, 1993). APS is considered *secondary* in women who have other underlying connective tissue disease (particularly SLE) and *primary* in women who do not have identifiable underlying disease. Primary APS is the most common presentation in obstetrical patients (ACOG, 1998; Branch, 1991; Newman, 1995; Ordi-Ros et al., 1994; Silver & Branch, 1994). In the vast majority of cases, patients with primary APS do not develop SLE (Branch, 1991; Ordi-Ros et al., 1994), but the clinical course may resemble SLE because complications occur at unpredictable times and are not usually related to changes in antibody levels (Ordi-Ros et al., 1994). It is also important to note that clinical signs of APS may occur before, concurrently, or after the cessation of typical SLE symptoms. Furthermore, the presence or absence of SLE does not seem to be connected with the association of antiphospholipid antibodies with fetal loss or thrombosis (Harris, 1990).

Diagnosis

Diagnosis of APS is of primary importance because treatment improves fetal outcome (Harris, 1990). Definitive diagnosis of APS requires both clinical and serologic evidence of the syndrome (Harris, 1990). Clients with at least one clinical manifestation, such as fetal loss, must also have at least one positive serologic test (See Table 6.4) (Newman, 1995; Ordi-Ros et al., 1994; Silver & Branch, 1994). Serologic tests must be positive on more than one occasion (preferably several weeks apart) for the diagnosis to be made. The diagnosis of APS is particularly difficult to make if serologic tests are borderline but clinical symptoms are present. However, APS may be the appropriate diagnosis if the symptoms have no other explanation, the test remains positive over several weeks, and there is more than one clinical feature present (Harris, 1990). If APS is suspected, both LA and aCL tests should be ordered because it is not known which one is more specific for pregnancy complications (Dizon-Townson & Branch, 1997). A false-positive serologic test for syphilis has unclear significance in the diagnosis of APS (Branch, 1991).

A phospholipid-dependent clotting assay, such as partial thromboplastin time, kaolin clotting time, or the Russell viper venom time, is used to detect the lupus anticoagulant (Bowles, 1990; Branch, 1991; Dizon-Townson & Branch, 1997; Hadi & Treadwell, 1990b). The net result is a prolonged clotting time. Factors associated with prolonged clotting time, which are not related to the presence of LA, include use of anticoagulant medications, clotting-factor deficiencies, and the presence of other, rare antibodies (Branch, 1991; Hadi & Treadwell, 1990b). At present, there is no consensus about which assay(s) should be used to diagnose LA (Dizon-Townson & Branch, 1997).

Anticardiolipin is identified by using a standardized immunoassay, usually an ELISA (enzyme-linked immunosorbent assay). Results are reported as negative, low-positive, medium-positive, or high-positive (ACOG, 1998; Branch, 1991; Dizon-Townson & Branch, 1997). Significant variation may exist between laboratories (Branch, 1991; Dizon-Townson & Branch, 1997; Newman, 1995).

Medium or high levels of IgG aCL are seen in most patients with APS, along with LA. In the absence of LA, low-positive aCL and isolated IgM aCL are of questionable significance (ACOG, 1998; Branch, 1991; Dizon-Townson & Branch, 1997).

Pathophysiology

Vasculopathy, an abnormal condition of the blood vessels, may be the result of many autoimmune conditions, including APS. The immune system produces antibody immune complexes that damage the blood vessel endothelium, causing hypoperfusion and subsequent end-organ (e.g. placenta, kidney) injury due to thrombosis and impaired circulation (Patton, 1993). Release of prostaglandins from the affected endothelium is thought to enhance this process. Prostacyclin (PGI), the "good" prosta-glandin, promotes vasodilation and inhibits platelet aggregation whereas thromboxane, the "bad" prostaglandin, causes vessel spasm and platelet aggregation, resulting in blood clots and infarction (see Figure 6.1) (Hadi & Treadwell, 1990a; Harris, 1990; Newman, 1995; Patton, 1993).

Although the pathophysiology of fetal loss in women with APS is still unclear (Hadi & Treadwell, 1990a; Harris, 1990; Silver & Branch, 1994), it is generally assumed that fetal loss in women with APS is due to placental infarction secondary to thrombosis in the uteroplacental circulation (Harris, 1990; Silver & Branch, 1994). (See Figure 6.2) In vitro, LA acts as an anticoagulant through its interaction with phospholipid, interfering with the activation of prothrombin activator complex. Conversely, it has the paradoxical effect of thrombus formation in vivo (Hadi & Treadwell, 1990a; Newman, 1995; Patton, 1993). It has been postulated that APS antibodies cause a decrease in the prostacyclin-to-thromboxane ratio, resulting in placental vascular thrombosis (Patton, 1993; Silver & Branch, 1994). Abnormal development of the uteroplacental circulation has also been cited as a possible reason for fetal loss and thrombosis. This is usually seen in women with preeclampsia and involves intimal thickening, acute atherosis, fibrinoid necrosis, and thrombosis of the spiral arteries of the placenta. These changes may occur at any time during the first or second trimesters (Harris, 1990). Other proposed mechanisms include decreased activation of protein C, platelet activation due to alteration of the lipid component of platelet membranes, and increased endothelial cell procoagulant activity (Hadi & Treadwell, 1990a; Harris, 1990; Newman, 1995; Silver & Branch, 1994). Mild thrombocytopenia usually accompanies most thromboses associated with LA, but this is rarely associated with bleeding (Hadi & Treadwell, 1990a; Patton, 1993). Anticardiolipin antibodies cause endothelial damage resulting in fibrin deposition, vascular thrombosis, and decidual and placental infarction (Newman, 1995). Other possible causes of fetal loss not related to thrombosis include decidual vasculopathy, immune complex deposition, and lymphocytotoxic antibodies against trophoblast (Silver & Branch, 1994).

Database

Subjective

- Previous history of venous or arterial thrombosis
- More than three spontaneous abortions or history of fetal death
- Systemic lupus erythematosus (see Tables 6.2 and 6.3 for associated conditions)

Objective

- Serologic evidence of LA at moderate or high titer or a positive LA test that persists for months or years

- Serologic evidence of aCL (particularly IgG) at medium-positive or high-positive level (see Table 6.4)

- Presence of FP-STS (not generally used in clinical practice; +RPR is followed up with MHATP and if negative, testing is discontinued)

- Thrombocytopenia

  NOTE: Both clinical and serologic evidence should be present for diagnosis (see introductory text)

Assessment

- Antiphospholipid syndrome

  ▶ R/O systemic lupus erythematosus

  ▶ R/O syphilis

  ▶ R/O pregnancy-induced hypertension

  ▶ R/O fetal demise

  ▶ R/O other causes of pregnancy loss:

    – Hypertensive disorders

    – Diabetes

    – Intrauterine infection

    – Cord or placental abnormalities

    – Congenital defects

    – Erythroblastosis fetalis

Plan

Diagnostic Tests

- For detection of LA

  ▶ Partial thromboplastin time (PTT)

  ▶ Kaolin clotting time

  ▶ Russell viper venom time

  ▶ Plasma clotting time

- Anticardiolipin antibody (degree of elevation is significant)

- VDRL or RPR

- Refer to introductory section for further information

Treatment/Management

- Nonpregnant

  ▶ Preconception counseling is highly recommended (ACOG, 1998).

  ▶ Baseline labs to assess the presence of anemia, thrombocytopenia, and underlying renal disease are recommended (Dizon-Townson & Branch, 1997).

  ▶ No treatment is recommended if client asymptomatic but preconception treatment may be indicated in high-risk clients.

- Pregnant

  ▶ Treatment is recommended only for patients who meet the criteria for APS, as detailed in the introductory section and Table 6.4. However, despite treatment of APS, fetal loss may still occur; preeclampsia, fetal distress, IUGR, and preterm delivery are common.

    – There is no general agreement as to optimum treatment, but, in most cases, treatment has improved pregnancy outcome.

    – Treatment is focused on suppression of the anticoagulant effect and reversal of the clotting disorder (Ordi-Ros et al., 1994).

- A single agent or any combination of the four mentioned below may be used to treat APS; regimens are to be dictated by a physician.

  ▶ Low-dose aspirin (60 to 85 mg/day p.o.)

    – Favorably increases the prostacyclin to thromboxane ratio by suppressing thromboxane production (inhibits platelet aggregation)

    – Dose is critical because thromboxane production is inhibited by low doses of ASA, whereas larger doses inhibit prostacyclin synthesis (Patton, 1993)

    – Combination therapy most effective (prednisone and ASA or heparin and ASA)

    – Usually discontinued once labor begins (Hewell & Hammer, 1997)

  ▶ Heparin

    – Prevents placental thrombosis and infarction through anticoagulant effect

    – Most widely used agent in the treatment of APS during pregnancy in combination with low-dose aspirin; has become the most widely accepted treatment of APS to prevent fetal loss in the United States (Dizon-Townson & Branch, 1997).

    – Does not cross the placenta and has not been implicated as a teratogen (Atterbury et al., 1997)

    – Initiation of use recommended after confirmation of a live embryo

    – Also useful during pregnancy and postpartum secondary to the increased risk of maternal thrombosis

- Is safe to use while breastfeeding because heparin is not secreted into breast milk (Atterbury et al., 1997; Hewell & Hammer, 1997)

- Given as subcutaneous injections two or three times daily in doses of 15,000 to 20,000 units of unfractionated sodium heparin to achieve thrombin time of 100 seconds or more and baseline PT of not more than 1.5 seconds above the control time (at least 5,000 units each as prophylaxis) (Silver & Branch, 1994)

  NOTE: Average doses of 17,000 to 25,000 units per day have been used, but the optimal dose to ensure good fetal outcome without excessive risk of osteoporosis is unknown (Dizon-Townson & Branch, 1997).

- Adverse effects

  * Bleeding

  * Osteoporosis

  * Heparin-induced thrombocytopenia (low-molecular-weight heparin is much less likely to cause heparin-induced thrombocytopenia and will likely replace unfractionated sodium heparin in the treatment of APS [ACOG, 1998]).

  NOTE: Heparin should not be used in combination with prednisone because it increases the risk of osteoporosis; the combination of heparin and prednisone has never been proven to be more effective than either agent alone (Silver & Branch, 1994).

▶ Prednisone (20 to 80 mg/day p.o.) (Newman, 1995)

- Given to suppress the immune system

- Goal is to normalize the PTT (requires 4 to 8 weeks of treatment) (Patton, 1993).

  NOTE: Most studies using prednisone and low-dose aspirin suggest benefit, with the exception of one study done in 1989 by Lockshin and coworkers (Lockshin, Druzin, & Qamar, 1989).

- Usually discontinued once labor begins (Hewell & Hammer, 1997)

- Serious side effects

  * Osteoporosis (can lead to fractures)

  * Osteonecrosis

  * Adrenal insufficiency

  * Bacterial infections

  * Glucose intolerance

  * Possible premature rupture of membranes

  * Acne and cushingoid syndrome also common

- Side effects may be minimized by use of lower doses (20 mg) or by adjusting the dose to the lowest level that will suppress the LA effect; titers need to be monitored periodically (Newman, 1995; Silver & Branch, 1994).

- Because of the potential for complications as compared to other treatment regimens, prednisone may not be considered a first-line therapy for APS (Atterbury et al., 1997).

  NOTE: Prednisone is contraindicated in women with diabetes, moderate to severe hypertension, severe preeclampsia in previous pregnancies, positive PPD (or other predisposition to infection), or symptoms of osteoporosis (Harris, 1990).

▶ Intravenous immune globulin (IVIG)

- Blocks Fc antibody receptor as well as modulates other immune effects

- Increasing number of anecdotal reports of successful pregnancy outcomes

- Maternal/fetal side effects rare but expense is greater than other regimens

- Not recommended for primary treatment without further study (Dizon-Townson & Branch, 1997)

Additional Management

- Measure maternal serum alpha fetoprotein (MSAFP); unexplained mid-trimester elevations have been associated with an increased rate of fetal loss in women with APS (Silver & Branch, 1994).

- Confirm viability with ultrasound at the initial visit before starting treatment.

  ▶ Repeat every 4 to 6 weeks starting at 18 to 20 weeks of gestation (secondary to the increased risk of uteroplacental insufficiency) (ACOG, 1998).

  ▶ Consult with physician regarding recommended frequency of ultrasound (Newman, 1995; Silver & Branch, 1994).

- Schedule office visits every 2 weeks the first and second trimesters; every 1 to 2 weeks in the third trimester (Dizon-Townson & Branch, 1997; Newman, 1995; Silver & Branch, 1994).

- Start kick counts at 28 weeks' gestation.

- Start fetal surveillance at 26 to 28 weeks' gestation, then weekly until delivery (ACOG, 1998).

  ▶ Biophysical profile may also be indicated, including amniotic fluid index (Atterbury et al., 1997; Newman, 1995; Silver & Branch, 1994)

  NOTE: An increased rate of abnormal fetal heart rate tracings have been found in women with APS.

- Surveillance for preeclampsia is indicated (Atterbury et al., 1997; Silver & Branch, 1994). See Chapter 6.13, *Hypertensive Disorders of Pregnancy*.

- Monitor platelet counts and coagulation profiles in women being treated with heparin or prednisone (Newman, 1995; Silver & Branch, 1994). Consult with a physician regarding the frequency of testing.

- Supplemental calcium (4 g daily) and vitamin D (600 to 800 units daily) is recommended during treatment with heparin to reduce the risk of osteopenia (Atterbury et al., 1997; Dizon-Townson & Branch, 1997).

- In women with SLE who have had a fetal loss, rule out severe renal impairment, congenital heart block, and severe systemic disease activity (Harris, 1990). In addition, rule out other causes of pregnancy loss, including hypertensive disorders, diabetes, intrauterine infection, cord and placental abnormalities, congenital defects, and erythroblastosis fetalis.

Consultation

- Refer client to a perinatologist once APS is suspected or confirmed.

Patient Education

- Discuss the etiology of APS in terms the client will understand.

- Explain risks associated with APS and associated treatment regimens thoroughly.

- Emphasize that fetal loss may occur even with treatment.

- This discussion is generally undertaken by the physician in charge of the client's care.

Follow-up Treatment

- See Treatment/Management section.

- If the client is on heparin, have her continue the medication during the immediate postpartum period due to increased risk of thrombosis during this time (Bolan & Alving, 1991).

- Cessation of prednisone use must be tapered postpartum.

- The Fetal Loss Registry in Utah was set up to prospectively record treatments and outcomes of women with APS (Branch, 1991). Any interested individuals or centers are eligible to participate. Direct inquiries to

  The KAPS Fetal Loss Registry
  Room 2B200 Medical Center
  50 N. Medical Drive
  Salt Lake City, UT, 84132

- Document diagnosis of APS and its management in progress notes and problem list.

Table 6.2

Syndrome Criteria

Clinical

    Thrombosis

        Arterial

        Venous

        Cerebrovascular accident

    Pregnancy Loss

        Recurrent spontaneous abortion

        Fetal death

    Thrombocytopenia

Serologic

    Lupus anticoagulant

    Anticardiolipin

        IgG $\geq$ 20 GPL units*

        IgM $\geq$ 20 MPL units*

*Numerical values assigned to standard sera.

Source: Should You Treat Women Who Have Antiphospholipid Syndrome? by Robert M. Silver and D. Ware Branch, 1994, *Contemporary OB/GYN, 40,* p. 64. Copyright 1994 by Medical Economics Publishing Company Inc. Reprinted by permission.

Table 6.3

Antiphospholipid Antibodies in Nonlupus Conditions

Rheumatic diseases
   Rheumatoid arthritis
   Systemic sclerosis
   Primary Sjogren's syndrome
   Dermato and polymyositis
   Psoriatic arthropathy
   Ankylosing spondylitis

Vasculitic diseases
   Giant cell arteritis
   Behçet syndrome
   Takayasu arteritis

Infectious diseases
   Viral infections
   Syphilis
   Lyme disease
   Leprosy
   Tuberculosis
   Q fever

Malignancies
   Solid tumors
   Leukemias and other hematologic diseases
   Lymphoproliferative diseases
   Paraproteinemias

Drug Treatments
   Phenothiazines
   Procainamide
   Ethosuximide
   Clorothiazide
   Oral contraceptives

Diabetes mellitus

Patients on dialysis

Pernicious anemia

Source: Ordi-Ros, J., Perez-Peman, P., & Monasterio, J. (1994) Clinical and therapeutic aspects associated to phospholipid binding antibodies (lupus anticoagulant and anticardiolipin antibodies). *Haemostasis, 24,* 166. Copyright 1994 by S. Karger, A.G. Reprinted by permission.

Table 6.4

Clinical and Laboratory Manifestations of Antiphospholipid Antibodies

Vascular
Venous thrombosis
Arterial thrombosis
Thrombotic endocarditis
Valvular heart disease

Obstetric
Recurrent spontaneous abortion
Intrauterine fetal demise
Fetal growth retardation
Preeclampsia
Chorea gravidarum
Postpartum serositis
Neonatal thrombosis

Neurologic
Transient ischemic attacks
Stroke
Chorea
Peripheral neuropathy
Migraine

Dermatologic
Livedo reticularis
Cutaneous necrosis
Subungual splinter hemorrhage
Superficial skin necrosis

Hematologic
Thrombocytopenia
Prothrombin deficiency

Source: Ordi-Ros, J., Perez-Peman, P., & Monasterio, J. (1994). Clinical and therapeutic aspects associated to phospholipid binding antibodies (lupus anticoagulant and anticardiolipin antibodies). *Haemostasis, 24,* 167. Copyright 1994 by S. Karger A. G. Reprinted by permission.

Figure 6.1 Anticoagulant Thombotic Effect Pathways

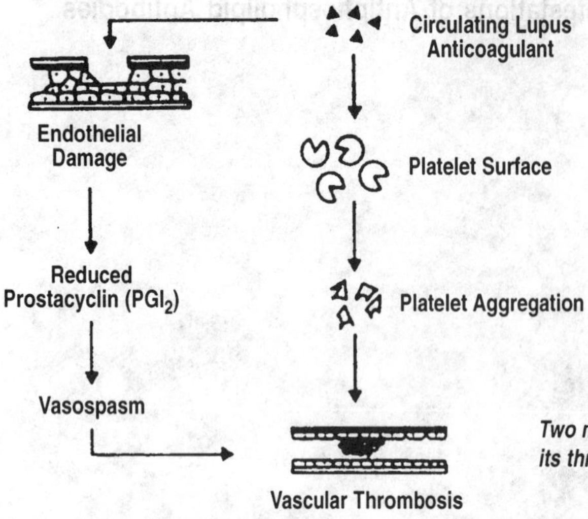

Circulating Lupus Anticoagulant

Endothelial Damage

Platelet Surface

Reduced Prostacyclin (PGI₂)

Platelet Aggregation

Vasospasm

Vascular Thrombosis

Two major pathways whereby lupus anticoagulant produces its thrombotic effect in vivo modified from Gant (19).

Source: Hadi,H.A. & Treadwell, E.L. (1990). Lupus anticoagulant and anticardiolipin antibodies in pregnancy: A review. I. Immunochemistry and clinical implications. *Obstetrical and Gynecological Survey, 45,* 781. Copyright 1990 by Williams and Wilkins. Reprinted with permission.

Figure 6.2 Fetal Loss Mechanisms

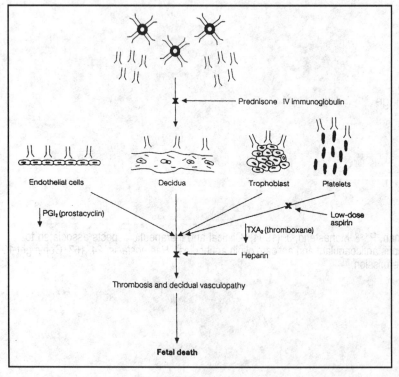

Prednisone   IV immunoglobulin

Endothelial cells

Decidua

Trophoblast

Platelets

PGI₂ (prostacyclin)

TXA₂ (thromboxane)

Low-dose aspirin

Heparin

Thrombosis and decidual vasculopathy

Fetal death

Treatment of antiphospholipid syndrome is based on countering proposed mechanisms of fetal loss, such as preventing placental thrombosis with heparin.

Source: Silver, R.M., & Branch, D.W. (1994). Should you treat women who have antiphospholipid syndrome? *Contemporary OB/GYN, 40,* 68. Copyright 1994 by Medical Economics. Reprinted with permission.

References

American College of Obstetricians and Gynecologists (ACOG). (1998). Antiphospholipid syndrome. *Educational Bulletin No. 244*. Washington, DC: Author.

Atterbury, J.L., Munn, M.B., Groome, L.J., & Yarnell, J.A. (1997). The antiphospholipid antibody syndrome: An overview. *Journal of Obstetric, Gynecologic, and Neonatal Nursing, 26*(5), 522–530.

Bolan, C.D., & Alving, B.M. (1991). Recurrent venous thrombosis and hypercoagulable states. *AFP, 44*(5), 1741–1751.

Bowles, C.A. (1990). Vasculopathy associated with the antiphospholipid antibody syndrome. *Rheumatic Disease Clinics of North America, 16*(2), 471–490.

Branch, D.W. (1991). Antiphospholipid syndrome: Laboratory concerns, fetal loss, and pregnancy management. *Seminars in Perinatology, 15*(3), 230–237.

Dizon-Townson, D., & Branch, D.W. (1997). The antiphospholipid antibody syndrome. *Primary Care Update for Ob/Gyns, 4*(3), 92–96.

Hadi, H.A., & Treadwell, E.L. (1990a). Lupus anticoagulant and anticardiolipin antibodies in pregnancy: A review. I. Immunochemistry and clinical implications. *Obstetrical and Gynecologic Survey, 45*(11), 780–785.

Hadi, H.A., & Treadwell, E.L. (1990b). Lupus anticoagulant and anticardiolipin antibodies in pregnancy: A review. II. Diagnosis and management. *Obstetrical and Gynecologic Survey, 45*(11), 786–791.

Harris, E.N. (1990). Maternal autoantibodies and pregnancy-1: The antiphospholipid antibody syndrome. *Baillière's Clinical Rheumatology, 4*(1), 53–68.

Hewell, S.W., & Hammer, R.H. (1997). Antiphospholipid antibodies: A threat throughout pregnancy. *Journal of Obstetric, Gynecologic, and Neonatal Nursing, 26*(2) 162–168.

Lockshin, M.D., Druzin, M.L., & Qamar, T. (1989). Prednisone does not prevent recurrent fetal death in women with antiphospholipid antibody. *American Journal of Obstetrics and Gynecology, 160,* 439–443.

Newman, R.B. (1995, October-November). Controversies in the management of antiphospholipid antibody syndrome (APS). *Perinatal Medicine and Nursing Conference* . Lecture presented in San Juan, Puerto Rico.

Olson, N.A. (1993). The lupus anticoagulant and pregnancy. *Journal of the American Osetopathic Association, 93*(3), 373–376.

Ordi-Ros, J., Perez-Peman, P., & Monasterio, J. (1994). Clinical and therapeutic aspects associated to phospholipid binding antibodies (lupus anticoagulant and anticardiolipin antibodies). *Haemostasis, 24,* 165–174.

Patton, D.E. (1993, March). Antiphospholipid syndrome: Lupus anticoagulant, anticardiolipin, (and certainly more to come). Lecture presented at Grand Rounds, Kaiser Permanente, San Francisco, CA.

Silver, R.M., & Branch, D.W. (1994). Should you treat women who have antiphospholipid syndrome? *Contemporary OB/GYN, 40*(6), 63–83.

Chapter 3

PERINATAL DOMESTIC VIOLENCE

Maureen T.Shannon

Lucy Newmark Sammons

Domestic violence is a syndrome involving the physical, sexual, or psychological abuse of an individual by an intimate partner or family member. A battered woman is a woman who has received physical abuse from an intimate partner at least one time during the relationship. A pattern of deliberate, severe physical abuse from the partner occurring three or more times is labeled "battered wife syndrome." Battering includes five types of interpersonal violence: physical, sexual, property, psychological, and social (Helton, 1987). Wife beating and spousal abuse are other terms referring to violence between partners in an ongoing relationship.

The type of abuse may incorporate verbal and mental abuse, with variations in severity from verbal threats to life-threatening or fatal injury. The violence tends to be cyclic in nature with successive periods of tension, emotional/psychological/physical abuse, and calm (i.e., "honeymoon period"). Signs of increasing danger include physical assault during pregnancy and threats of suicide or homicide (Helton, 1986). Because of an interrelationship between suicidal and homicidal intent, suicidal threats by either the batterer or the victim may precede an actual homicide (Walker, 1984).

Since familial violence tends to be underreported, accurate incidence statistics are difficult to obtain. Victims are found in all socioeconomic and racial groups. In the United States, domestic violence is estimated to affect 1.8 million women a year (Strauss, Gelles, & Steinmertz, 1989). The additional stresses on family dynamics during pregnancy, and later the care and demands of the newborn, may well precipitate violent episodes. Studies investigating physical abuse during pregnancy report an overall incidence between 8 and 17 percent (Centers for Disease Control and Prevention [CDC], 1994; McFarlane, Parker, & Soeken, 1996; Straus & Gelles, 1990). The nature of the episodes during pregnancy often includes sexual assault; blows to the abdomen, breasts, genitals, face and neck; choking; and broken bones. In addition to the physical trauma experienced by the woman, potential risks to the fetus include spontaneous abortion, low birthweight, preterm birth, chorioamnionitis, direct injury from abdominal blows, and fetal demise (Berenson, Wiemann, Wilkinson, Jones, & Anderson, 1994; McFarlane, Parker, Soeken, & Bullock, 1992; Parker, McFarlane, & Soeken, 1994; Ribe, Teggatz, & Harvey, 1993). Domestic violence during pregnancy is also associated with an increased incidence of maternal smoking and substance abuse, compounding the potential harm to the fetus (Amaro, Fried, Cabral, & Zuckerman, 1990; McFarlane et al., 1996).

Domestic violence is often a pattern of family dysfunction and abuse. Abusers frequently come from families where they themselves were victims of abuse. Furthermore, 53 percent of the men and 28 percent of the women in battering relationships report abusing their children (McKay, 1994; Walker, 1984). Therefore, screening for domestic violence should be incorporated into the psychosocial assessment of women, especially during pregnancy. Various methods for obtaining such information have been evaluated. One tool, the Abuse Assessment Screen (see Table 6.5), is a simple, valid, and reliable tool that can be used in various clinical settings to evaluate for domestic violence during pregnancy (McFarlane et al., 1992; McFarlane et al., 1996; Norton, Peipert, Zierler, Lima, & Hume, 1995).

Database

Subjective

- Woman reports individual or repeated incidents of physical, mental, and/or verbal abuse by her partner.

- Woman may deny or initially refuse to disclose abuse; report of how injuries occurred (e.g., "fell down") will not be consistent with nature of injuries.

- Woman may report a history of the following (American College of Obstetricians and Gynecologists [ACOG], 1989; CDC, 1994; Council on Scientific Affairs, 1993; Gazamararian et al., 1995):

  ▶ Abuse as a child or seeing her own mother abused

  ▶ Childhood in single-parent home

  ▶ Marriage before age 20

  ▶ Age 19 years or younger

  ▶ Unintended pregnancy

  ▶ Pregnancy before marriage

  ▶ Crowded living conditions

  ▶ Drug or alcohol abuse/overdose

  ▶ Suicide attempt

  ▶ Depression

- Medical/health history may reveal the following:

  ▶ Use of multiple caregivers/sites to maintain anonymity

  ▶ Frequent appointments for vague somatic complaints

  ▶ Sexual or physical assault

  ▶ Noncompliance with medical recommendations

  ▶ Failure to keep appointed office visits

  ▶ Delay in seeking medical care for injuries

  ▶ Late entry into prenatal care or lack of prenatal care

- Somatic complaints may include the following:

  ▶ Headaches

  ▶ Insomnia, violent nightmares, severe anxiety

  ▶ Choking sensation

  ▶ Hyperventilation

  ▶ Gastrointestinal symptoms

  ▶ Chest, back, or pelvic pain

- Woman may report an affirmative response to one or more of the questions listed in Table 6.5, Abuse Assessment Screen.

Objective

- The physical examination may reveal
  - ▶ Weight gain less than normal (as a result of the psychological and/or physical effects of domestic violence, or coexistent substance abuse)
  - ▶ Behavioral manifestations by the woman suggesting an abusive situation:
    - Shyness
    - Fright
    - Embarrassment or evasiveness
    - Jumpiness
    - Passivity, depression, crying or sighing
    - Anger or defensiveness
  - ▶ Signs of recent or past injury, particularly (ACOG, 1989)
    - Serious bleeding injuries
    - Broken bones, especially arms, legs, jaw, pelvis, skull or vertebrae
    - Burn injuries, as from cigarettes
    - Abdominal injury/bruising
  - ▶ Multiple injuries from different time periods may be present
- Abdominal examination may reveal a fundal height less than expected for gestational weeks if coexistent intrauterine growth restriction (IUGR).
- Partner may be resistant to leaving the client's presence throughout the health visit.

Assessment

- Domestic violence/battering
  - ▶ R/O concomitant child abuse/other family violence
  - ▶ R/O suicidal/homicidal intent (woman or her partner)
  - ▶ R/O depression
  - ▶ R/O sexual assault
  - ▶ R/O substance abuse
  - ▶ R/O IUGR
  - ▶ R/O fetal distress
  - ▶ R/O labor/preterm labor

Plan

Diagnostic Tests (Richards, 1995)

- There are no specific diagnostic tests; the problem is reliant on disclosure by woman or other family member/reliable informant.

- If injury is evident, the diagnostic tests will be determined by the nature of the injury (e.g., complete blood count [CBC], radiography, etc.).

- If fundal measurement is less than expected for gestational week, an obstetrical ultrasound should be obtained to clarify the number of gestational weeks and rule out IUGR.

Treatment/Management

- Directly ask all pregnant women if they are or have been injured/abused recently or in the past. Repeat the question(s) if circumstances warrant. Interview the woman privately if partner or children usually accompany her.

  NOTE: If the woman's partner is present, attempt to separate them so a more reliable history and physical assessment can be done. If the partner's behavior is threatening, enlisting the aid of a security officer may be necessary.

- Conduct a priority assessment of the pregnant woman who has experienced trauma, including assessment of fetal well-being (i.e., fetal heart rate [FHR], nonstress test [NST], amniotic fluid index [AFI], biophysical profile [BPP], obstetrical ultrasound, etc.), uterine contractions, vaginal bleeding, leakage of amniotic fluid, or other signs of progressing labor/imminent delivery (Bojanowski, Hill, & Martin, 1988).

- Where physical evidence will be collected for legal/forensic purposes, informed consent and specimen collection procedures should conform with local requirements. Contact local law enforcement agencies (i.e., police or sheriff's department) and/or the social service department to obtain current information about legal and forensic requirements and procedures.

- Provide care in a nonjudgmental manner, acknowledging the difficulty of disclosure, seeking assistance, leaving the abuser, or bringing legal action in a family violence situation.

- Assess the severity of the domestic situation, the woman's perception of the situation, and provide a realistic assessment of the woman's (and children's) risk of harm or death.

- Assist the woman in establishing contact with support services for women/families experiencing domestic violence (e.g., shelters; financial, social, and legal support).

- Guide the woman in the development of a "safe exit" plan if she remains where violence may recur (Helton, 1986):

  ▶ Pack essential clothing (for herself and any dependent children), toiletry articles, cash, and financial and legal papers (e.g., copy of birth certificate[s]) in a suitcase to be stored with a trusted friend.

  ▶ Keep driver's license and necessary identification papers readily available for a rapid departure.

► Predetermine a destination: friend, relative, or shelter if she is not injured; emergency room with assistance as needed by ambulance, police, or friend if she is injured.

● If the woman is currently smoking, discuss the need to stop smoking, or reduce the number of cigarettes to less than a half pack per day.

● If the woman is abusing drugs, refer her to a chemical dependency treatment program. If she is not chemically dependent, but her partner is abusing drugs, refer her partner for treatment and refer the woman to co-dependency support groups (e.g., CODA).

Consultation

● Medical consultation is required for all confirmed and highly suspicious cases of perinatal domestic violence.

● Consult with social services for provision of, or referral to, specialized resources for domestic violence; provide an emergency referral to protective services (legal, shelter, etc.) if the woman is in imminent danger.

● Obtain an emergency mental health services consultation for a woman (or the partner) who reports suicidal/homicidal intent.

● Police or social service agency notification is required if child abuse is suspected or reported by the woman.

● In some states, clinicians are required to notify police if there is suspected or documented evidence of domestic violence. Clinicians should review the domestic violence reporting laws in their states.

Patient Education

● Educate woman about cycle of violence.

► Successive periods of increased tension, battering, and calm

► Signs of increasing physical danger (Helton, 1987)

  - Battering during pregnancy

  - Involvement of weapons

  - Extension of threats or assaults to other family members

  - Observation of woman at her workplace

  - Increased jealousy

  - Forced sexual encounters

  - Decreased remorse during the calm phase

● Convey that violence is not acceptable in family living.

► It is not appropriate for problem-solving or tension release

► Family violence is **not** a woman's fault because she "deserves it" for some action she did or did not take.

- Provide written local domestic violence resource contact numbers; the National Coalition Against Domestic Violence 24-hour hotline number is 1(800) 333-SAFE (800/333-7233).

- A woman involved in a domestic violence situation may particularly benefit from educational resources that increase knowledge of her legal rights and protections, provide job skills and facilitate entry into the market place, decrease social isolation, and increase self-esteem.

- Special educational needs, if woman has opted to separate from her partner and is not settled in a permanent shelter/residence, include the following:

  - ▶ Nutritional counseling emphasizing economic and convenient foods, possible application for food supplement programs

  - ▶ Counseling about the need to maintain health care visits during pregnancy, despite potential chaotic and transient lifestyle

    - – Possible need to apply for medical financial assistance to continue prenatal care

    - – Need to maintain point of contact with provider and to follow-up on any abnormal laboratory results between office visits

- If woman stays with her partner, prenatal education of the couple should include realistic expectations of the pregnant woman's needs and anticipatory guidance regarding neonatal care and family readjustments.

- Family planning counseling is important, since unplanned or unwanted pregnancy may precipitate spousal abuse.

- Advise against the use of alcohol or drugs as stress-reducing mechanisms, especially during pregnancy because of potential fetal effects.

Follow-up

- Follow the woman as a high-risk patient, with more frequent visits, interim telephone contact, and public health nurse (PHN) visits as needed.

- Contact her pediatric care provider for appropriate follow-up of older children and neonate; contact intrapartum staff regarding domestic violence situation, so they may provide additional support to the family and be alert to any limitations/legal considerations regarding father of baby.

- Long-term care of woman and children often requires a therapy program; a combination of group and individual approaches are helpful. The batterer may be involved in therapy on his own initiative or through legal requirement.

- Continue assessment of family dynamics into the postpartum period; the additional stresses of a new infant in the home and a fatigued mother unable to respond to the needs of all family members may precipitate violence.

- Encourage clinic and office administrative staff and other providers to tolerate nonappointed visits, as scheduling permits, during disorganized periods in battered woman's life.

- Document in progress notes, in accordance with legal evidenciary standards, and problem list.

Table 6.5

Abuse Assessment Screen

Abuse Assessment Screen (Circle YES or NO for each question)

1. Have you ever been emotionally or physically abused by your partner or someone important to you?
. . . . .YES NO

2. **WITHIN THE LAST YEAR**, have you been hit, slapped, kicked, or otherwise physically hurt by someone?
. . . . .YES NO

   If YES, by whom (circle all that apply)

   Husband   Ex-husband   Boyfriend   Stranger   Other   Multiple

   Total number of times _____

3. **SINCE YOU'VE BEEN PREGNANT**, have you been hit, slapped, kicked, or otherwise physically hurt by someone? . . . . . . YES NO

   If YES, by whom (circle all that apply)

   Husband   Ex-husband   Boyfriend   Stranger   Other   Multiple

   Total number of times _____

   MARK THE AREA OF INJURY ON THE BODY MAP

   SCORE EACH INCIDENT according to the following scale:

   1 = Threats of abuse, including use of a weapon
   2 = Slapping, pushing; no injuries and/or lasting pain
   3 = Punching, kicking, bruises, cuts, and/or continuing pain
   4 = Beaten up, severe contusions, burns, broken bones
   5 = Head, internal, and/or permanent injury
   6 = Use of weapon, wound from weapon

   (If any of the descriptions for the higher number apply, use the higher number)

4. **WITHIN THE LAST YEAR**, has anyone forced you to have sexual activities?
YES   NO

   If YES, by whom (circle all that apply)

   Husband   Ex-husband   Boyfriend   Stranger   Other   Multiple

   Total number of times _____

5. Are you afraid of your partner or anyone you listed above? . . . . .YES   NO

   Name of Person Completing Form

Source: McFarlane, J., Parker, B., & Soeken, K. (1996.) Physical abuse, smoking, and substance use during pregnancy: Prevalence, interrelationships, and effects on birth weight. *Journal of Obstetrics, Gynecologic and Neonatal Nursing 25*(4), p. 314d.

Reprinted with permission.

References

American College of Obstetricians and Gynecologists (ACOG). (1989). The battered woman. (Technical bulletin no. 124.) Washington, DC: Author.

Amaro, H., Fried, L.E., Cabral, H., & Zuckerman, B. (1990). Violence during pregnancy and substance use. *American Journal of Public Health, 80* (5), 575–579.

Berenson, A.B., Wiemann, C.M., Wilkinson, G.S., Jones, W.A., & Anderson, G.D. (1994). Perinatal morbidity associated with violence experienced by pregnant women. *American Journal of Obstetrics and Gynecology, 170*(6), 1760–1769.

Bojanowski, C., Hill, K., & Martin, D. (1988). Assessment of the pregnant trauma patient. *Dimensions of Critical Care Nursing, 7*(6), 356–363.

Centers for Disease Control. (1994). Physical violence during the 12 months preceding childbirth—Alaska, Maine, Oklahoma, and West Virginia, 1990–1991. *Morbidity & Mortality Weekly Report, 43*(8), 132–1137.

Council on Scientific Affairs, American Medical Association. (1993). Adolescents as victims of family violence. *The Jounal of the American Medical Association, 270*(15), 1850–1856.

Gazmararian, J.A., Adams, M.M., Saltzman, L.E., Johnson, C.H., Bruce, F.C., Marks, J.S., Zahniser, S.C., & the PRAMS Working Group. (1995). The relationship between pregnancy intendedness and physical violence in mothers of newborns. *Obstetrics & Gynecology, 85*(6), 1031–1038.

Helton, A.S. (1986). Battering during pregnancy. *American Journal of Nursing, 86*(8), 910–913.

Helton, A.S. (1987). *Protocol of care for the battered woman.* White Plains, NY: March of Dimes Birth Defects Foundation.

McFarlane, J., Parker, B., Soeken, K., & Bullock, L. (1992). Assessing for abuse during pregnancy. *The Journal of the American Medical Association, 267*(23), 3176–3178.

McFarlane, J., Parker, B., & Soeken, K. (1996). Physical abuse, smoking, and substance use during pregnancy: Prevalence, interrelationships, and effects on birth weight. *Journal of Obstetric, Gynecologic, and Neonatal Nursing 25*(4), 313–320.

McKay, M.M. (1994). The link between domestic violence and child abuse: Assessment and treatment considerations. *Child Welfare League of America, 63*(1), 29–39.

Norton, L.B., Peipert, J.G., Zierler, S., Lima, B., & Hume, L. (1995). Battering in pregnancy: An assessment of two screening methods. *Obstetrics & Gynecology, 85*(3), 321–325.

Parker, B., McFarlane, J., & Soeken, K. (1994). Abuse during pregnancy: Effects on maternal complications and birth weight in adult and teenage women. *Obstetrics & Gynecology, 84*(3), 323–328.

Ribe, J.K., Teggatz, J.R., & Harvey, C.M. (1993). Blows to the maternal abdomen causing fetal demise: Report of three cases and a review of the literature. *Journal of Forensic Sciences, 38*(5), 1092–1096.

Richards, J. (1995). Battering/domestic violence. In W.L. Star, L.L. Lommel, & M. T. Shannon (Eds.), *Women's primary health care: Protocols for practice* (pp. 14–23). Washington, DC: American Nurses Publishing.

Straus, M.A., & Gelles, R. J. (1990). How violent are American families? In M.A. Straus & R.J. Gelles (Eds.), *Physical violence in American families: Risk factors and adaptations to violence in 8,145 familes.* New Brunswick, NJ: Transaction Publishers.

Straus, M.A., Gelles, R.J., & Steinmetz S.K. (1989). The marriage license as a hitting license. In M.A. Straus, R.J. Gelles, & S.K. Steinmetz (Eds.), *Behind closed doors. Violence in the American family* (pp. 31–50). New York: Anchor.

Walker, L.E. (1984). *The battered woman syndrome.* New York: Springer.

Chapter 4

FIRST TRIMESTER BLEEDING

Maureen T. Shannon

Vaginal bleeding during the first trimester occurs in up to 25 percent of pregnancies; approximately half of these episodes result in a spontaneous abortion (SAB). The amount of bleeding can be scant to extensive, brown to bright red in color, and may or may not be accompanied by pain. The causes of bleeding during the first trimester range in severity from minor conditions to severe, life threatening problems and include the following (Cunningham, MacDonald, Gant, Leveno, & Gilstrap III, 1993; Ghidini & Romero, 1996; McKennett & Fullerton, 1995):

- Implantation bleeding: This usually occurs approximately 1 to 2 weeks after conception and is caused by blood escaping from blood vessels in the uterine epithelium that have been eroded by the implanting fertilized ovum. The bleeding is usually scant light pink, unaccom-panied by pain, and lasts only for 1 to 2 days.

- Threatened abortion: Vaginal bleeding with or without pelvic cramping and backache during the first trimester should signal the possibility of a threatened SAB. There are no cervical changes observed in a woman with this problem (i.e., speculum examination will reveal a closed cervical os). Approximately 50 percent of threatened SABs do progress to complete SABs.

- Inevitable spontaneous abortion: When gross rupture of membranes (ROM) and cervical dilatation occurs during the first half of pregnancy, the term "inevitable spontaneous abortion" is used. Initially, this may or may not be accompanied by vaginal bleeding, pelvic cramping, or the presence of products of conception (POC) or placenta at the cervical os. However, these symptoms and clinical manifestations usually develop rapidly after the initial episode of ROM.

- Incomplete spontaneous abortion: In the majority of SABs that occur before the 10th gestational week, the fetus and placenta are expelled at the same time. However, in some instances, some placental tissue may remain within the uterine cavity causing persistent vaginal bleeding, which can be profuse. The woman usually reports the passage of tissue and clots with a history of vaginal bleeding and cramping. The bleeding and cramping will persist until all of the products of conception have been evacuated from the uterus.

- Complete spontaneous abortion: A complete SAB occurs when the uterus spontaneously evacuates itself of all of the POCs before the 20th week of gestation. The majority of complete SABs (more than 80 percent) occur within the first 12 weeks of gestation; at least 50 percent of these are due to chromosomal abnormalities of the embryo/fetus. Other etiologies include maternal disease (e.g., uncontrolled diabetes mellitus, autoimmune disorders), maternal exposure to environmental toxins (e.g., radiation exposure of more than 5 rads on the day of conception), alloimmune mechanisms, or developmental uterine defects.

- Missed spontaneous abortion: A missed SAB occurs when the products of conception are retained in the uterus for several weeks after the embryo or fetus has died. After an embryo or fetal death, the woman may report a history of signs and symptoms suggestive of a threatened SAB that appear to have resolved. However, the symptoms of pregnancy eventually disappear and the uterine size becomes smaller. Most missed SABs result in spontaneous expulsion of the POCs; however, prolonged retention of dead POCs can occur. Retention of dead POCs has been associated with an increased risk of serious coagulation problems, especially when fetal death occurs during the second trimester.

- Ectopic pregnancy: See Chapter 6.8, *Ectopic Pregnancy,* for the definition.

- Gestational trophoblastic disease (GTD) or molar pregnancy: See Chapter 6.12, *Gestational Trophoblastic Disease,* for definitions.

- Cervicitis: See Chapter 14.1, *Chlamydia,* and Chapter 14.4, *Gonorrhea,* for definitions.

- Cervical polyps: Painless bleeding, especially after coitus, that occurs early in gestation may be caused by cervical polyps, which usually increase in size during pregnancy. Cervical polyps usually appear as bright red pedunculated growths protruding from the cervical os.

- Cervical carcinoma: Painless vaginal bleeding, often after coitus, can be reported by women who have cervical carcinoma. However, a woman with this disease will have abnormal Pap smear results.

- Normal hyperemia of the cervix: Spontaneous light vaginal spotting or bleeding, which may or may not be related to coitus, can be caused by the increased vascularization of the cervix that normally occurs during pregnancy.

- Bleeding disorders (rare): Conditions such as von Willebrand's disease, idiopathic thrombocytopenia, and leukemia may be the cause of vaginal bleeding.

- Sexual assault: Forced coital activity may result in a laceration of the posterior fourchette. If instrumentation has occurred during the assault, other skin and mucous membrane trauma may result in bleeding (Richards, 1995).

The long-term consequences associated with first trimester vaginal bleeding episodes that do not result in embryo or fetal death or SABs reportedly include an increased risk of low birth weight infants, preterm deliveries, placental abnormalities (e.g., placenta previa, placental abruption), and neonatal mortality (Ghidini & Romero, 1996; Sipila, Hartidainen-Sorri, & Wendt, 1992; Williams, Mittendorf, Lieberman, & Monson, 1991).

Database

Subjective

The woman may report one or more of the following symptoms depending upon the etiology of the vaginal bleeding:

- Symptoms of pregnancy

- Vaginal bleeding that is scant to profuse; brown, pink, or bright red in color

- Abdominal pain ranging from mild cramping to severe, sharp unilateral pain

- Passage of tissue, blood clots, or grape-like vesicles (if GTD—see GTD chapter for other symptoms)

- Bleeding that occurs at specific times (e.g., postcoitally) or bleeding that is unrelated to activity

- Exposure to and symptoms of a sexually transmitted disease (see specific sexually transmitted disease chapters for symptoms)

- A history of pelvic inflammatory disease, previous ectopic pregnancy, IUD use, infertility, assisted reproduction, or adnexal surgery

- Disappearance of subjective signs and symptoms of pregnancy (in missed SABs)

- A personal or family history of a bleeding disorder

- A history of an abnormal Pap smear result, or treatment for cervical dysplasia/cancer

- Lightheadedness, dizziness, or syncope (if significant blood loss has occurred)

- Forced sexual activity

  NOTE: This information may not be elicited readily from a woman who has been sexually assaulted. Therefore, the clinician should be alert to this possibility, particularly if other evidence of emotional or physical assault is noted.

Objective

The following findings may be observed depending upon the etiology and severity of the vaginal bleeding:

- Vital signs may be within normal limits (WNL) or may demonstrate an increase in pulse and a decrease in blood pressure if significant blood loss has occurred. In such instances, do an evaluation of blood pressure and pulse for postural changes.

  NOTE: Orthostatic changes demonstrating a drop in systolic blood pressure of equal to or greater than 10 mm Hg or an increase in heart rate of equal to or greater than 10 beats per minute may be indicative of intraabdominal hemorrhage (Ghidini & Romero, 1996).

- Abdominal examination may reveal the following:

  ▶ Absence of fetal heart tones (FHTs) when auscultating with Doppler at appropriate gestational age (in missed SABs and GTD)

  ▶ Tenderness to palpation (if significant bleeding, associated with an ectopic pregnancy)

- Speculum examination may reveal the following:

  ▶ Cervical dilitation and effacement in inevitable SABs

  ▶ Presence of POCs at cervical os or in vaginal vault in incomplete SABs

  ▶ Presence of amniotic fluid in the posterior fornix or coming from the cervical os

  ▶ A bright red, pedunculated growth protruding from the cervical os, if cervical polyp is causing the bleeding

  ▶ Cervical inflammation, erythema, friability and leukorrhea, if cervicitis or if cervical neoplasia present

  ▶ Evidence of forced sexual activity including ecchymosis, edema, and/or laceration(s) at the posterior fourchette (the location of greatest stress due to stretching during forced penile penetration) (Richards, 1995)

- Bimanual examination may reveal the following:

  ▶ Cervix may be hard, with enlarged mass(es) in late stages of cervical cancer

▶ Uterine size may be:

   – Normal for dates in threatened SABs

   – Less than dates in incomplete and missed SABs, and ectopic pregnancies (after 8 weeks)

   – Well contracted in complete SABs

   – Greater than dates in GTD (50 percent of GTD cases)

▶ Unilateral sausage-like enlargement of adnexa, usually accompanied by tenderness, is sometimes palpable in ectopic pregnancies.

Assessment

• IUP ____ weeks with vaginal bleeding

  ▶ R/O implantation bleeding

  ▶ R/O postcoital bleeding associated with normal hyperemia of cervix

  ▶ R/O threatened SAB

  ▶ R/O inevitable SAB

  ▶ R/O incomplete SAB

  ▶ R/O complete SAB

  ▶ R/O missed SAB

  ▶ R/O ectopic pregnancy

  ▶ R/O GTD

  ▶ R/O cervicitis/sexually transmitted disease (STD)

  ▶ R/O cervical polyp

  ▶ R/O cervical dysplasia/cancer

  ▶ R/O intraabdominal hemorrhage

  ▶ R/O anemia due to excessive blood loss

  ▶ R/O bleeding disorder

  ▶ R/O sexual assault

Plan

Diagnostic Tests

• The following diagnostic tests may be ordered depending upon the clinical status of the woman and the possible etiology of her bleeding.

▶ Nitrazine test

- A sample of fluid is obtained from the posterior vaginal vault and is tested with nitrazine paper.

- The result may be positive (alkaline result) indicating the presence of amniotic fluid in some cases of inevitable or incomplete SABs.

  NOTE: It is important to obtain the specimen from the posterior vaginal vault and not the cervix, since contamination with cervical mucous may cause a false-positive result. False-positive results can also occur in the presence of blood, urine, vaginal discharge, or antiseptic solution (see Chapter 6.24, *Premature Rupture of Membranes*).

▶ Fern test

- A sample of fluid is obtained from the vaginal vault, is placed on a glass slide and allowed to dry. Once the sample has dried it is visualized under a microscope.

- The result may be positive (i.e., "ferning pattern") indicating the presence of amniotic fluid in some cases of inevitable or incomplete SABs.

  NOTE: A false positive result may occur if the specimen is contaminated with cervical mucous or there are fingerprints on the slide (see Chapter 6.24, *Premature Rupture of Membranes*).

▶ Wet prep of vaginal/cervical secretions may reveal evidence of vaginitis or cervicitis (see Section 14, *Vaginitis and Sexually Transmitted Diseases,* for diagnostic criteria).

▶ Order cervical cultures or rapid assay for gonorrhea and chlamydia, and serology for syphilis, as indicated.

▶ Transvaginal ultrasonography may demonstrate the presence or absence of a fetal sac, fetal heart pulsations, an extrauterine pregnancy, or evidence of GTD (Goldstein, 1994). The transvaginal sonogram should demonstrate a gestational sac when the serum ß-hCG level is equal to or greater than 2000 IU per mL. This technique is also more sensitive than abdominal sonography in demonstrating an adnexal mass or free fluid in the cul-de-sac (Goldstein, 1994; McKennett & Fullerton, 1995) (see Chapter 6.8, *Ectopic Pregnancy*).

▶ Complete blood count (CBC) or hemoglobin and hematocrit (Hgb, Hct) may reveal decreased red blood cell count or Hgb/Hct levels in women experiencing significant blood loss.

▶ Type and Rh should be obtained in a woman who has not already had these tests performed.

▶ Serum ß-hCG levels may be less than normal for weeks of gestation or may not increase (doubling of the level every 2 to 3 days is observed in a normal pregnancy).

- The serum *ß*-hCG level may be repeated every 48 hours to monitor the trend in the level.

  NOTE: Abnormally low results or a rise of less than 66 percent over 48 hours may indicate an SAB or ectopic pregnancy (Ghidini & Romero, 1996; McKennett & Fullerton, 1995) (see Chapter 6.8, *Ectopic Pregnancy*).

▶ Serum progesterone level may show less than 5 ng per mL in women experiencing a nonviable pregnancy (Carson & Buster, 1993).

▶ After consultation with a physician, coagulation studies may be ordered in a woman suspected of having a missed SAB, since disseminated intravascular coagulation (DIC) may develop—especially if it has been 5 weeks or more since death of the embryo or fetus or 5 months since her last menstrual period. The following results may be observed indicating developing DIC:

  – Platelet count less than 100,000/mm^3

  – Fibrinogen concentration less than 100 mg/dL

  – Fibrin-degradation product level equal to or greater than 20 μg/mL

  – Prothrombin time (PT) greater than upper limits of normal (ULN) (depends upon normal limits of individual laboratory)

  – Partial thromboplastin time (PTT) greater than ULN

▶ When a sexual assault is suspected or reported, laboratory tests specifically required for evidence should be obtained per forensic protocols. In most instances, women reporting sexual assault are referred to designated centers (e.g., emergency department, sexual assault center) for a complete evaluation by trained clinicians so that evidence can be properly obtained.

Treatment/Management

● In threatened SAB advise pelvic rest for at least 2 weeks after the bleeding has stopped.

● If a woman with a threatened SAB continues to have bleeding or if bleeding is accompanied by increasing pain or passage of clots or tissue, then refer her to a physician for further evaluation/intervention.

● In women with inevitable, incomplete, complete, or missed SABs, co-management with a physician is possible and guided by institution specific policies and procedures. The therapeutic options for the management of a woman experiencing an SAB should be presented to her by the clinician responsible for her care.

  ▶ Expectant management

    – Successful expectant management of women with sonographic evidence of an inevitable or incomplete SAB with retained products of conception of less than 15 mm diameter has been documented.

    – This therapeutic option was associated with a longer period of bleeding (i.e., 1 to 3 days), but there was less incidence of infection in the women randomized to the expectant management group compared to the group of women randomized to the dilatation and curettage group (Nielsen & Hahlin, 1995).

  ▶ Surgical interventions

    – This option may be indicated in some women and includes suction curettage or dilatation and curettage.

    – The physician managing the woman's care determines the most appropriate surgical intervention.

● If an ectopic pregnancy is suspected, refer immediately to a physician.

- If a woman with a threatened SAB has resolution of her symptoms, continue routine prenatal care at 2-week intervals until normal uterine growth and fetal heart tones are confirmed. Obtain an obstetrical ultrasound to confirm fetal viability.

- If anemia is present, recommend iron supplementation and high iron diet (see Chapter 9.3, *Anemia—Iron, Folate, Vitamin B_{12} Deficiency*).

- If a woman is Rh negative and she is experiencing a threatened SAB, an incomplete or complete SAB, or an ectopic pregnancy, she should be given an injection of RhoGam® within 72 hours after the completion of the SAB or termination of the ectopic pregnancy at the following doses.

  ▶ If the pregnancy is 12 or more gestational weeks, administer 300 μg IM.

  ▶ If the pregnancy is between 8 and 12 gestational weeks administer 50 μg IM.

- If the woman has vaginitis or cervicitis, she should be treated with the appropriate medication. If she has an STD, refer her partner(s) for evaluation and treatment.

- If the woman is diagnosed as having GTD, then refer her to a physician.

Consultation

- Physician consultation is warranted in women with vaginal bleeding during the first trimester when a threatened, inevitable, incomplete, missed SAB; GTD; ectopic pregnancy; or sexual assault are suspected. Co-management of women is possible depending upon the etiology of the vaginal bleeding, the stability of the woman, and the plan of care and is guided by site-specific policies and procedures.

- Transfer women with vaginal bleeding during the first trimester to physician care when GTD, ectopic pregnancy, cervical dysplasia/cancer, or significant blood loss (e.g., intraabdominal hemorrhage) are suspected/diagnosed.

- Refer for an evidentiary examination any woman who reports a sexual assault. This should be done after the woman agrees to such an evaluation.

Patient Education

- Educate the woman about the probable cause of the vaginal bleeding, the expected outcome, the plan of care, and the need for consultation/referral (if indicated).

- Provide information about any diagnostic tests that are being ordered, and interpret the results for her.

- If an SAB or ectopic pregnancy has occurred, it is important to help the woman and her partner work through any feelings of guilt and/or grief regarding their loss.

- Educate the woman regarding the importance of reporting to a clinician signs and symptoms that may indicate the development of a complication (e.g., the development of a fever, foul-smelling discharge, profuse or prolonged bleeding, passage of tissue or clots, or the development of abdominal or low-back pain).

- Educate the woman about the normal course for recovery from an SAB and the need to have follow-up evaluation of her physical (and psychological) recovery.

- If the woman is Rh negative and has had an SAB or ectopic pregnancy, educate her about the need for RhoGam® administration.

- If a woman is diagnosed with an STD, educate her about the infection, the indicated treatment and follow-up, and the need for evaluation and treatment of her partner(s). Review safer sex methods and offer counseling and voluntary human immunodeficiency virus (HIV) antibody testing whenever an STD is diagnosed.

- If a woman has experienced a sexual assault, educate her about resources available to her and refer her to appropriate psychological and legal services.

  ▶ Educate her about her legal rights and the need for a forensic examination.

  ▶ Make arrangements to facilitate such an evaluation after informed consent is obtained from the woman.

Follow-up

- If threatened SAB resolves, then the woman should return every 2 weeks for uterine growth assessment until normal growth and fetal heart tones are confirmed. Follow-up laboratory evaluations and/or obstetrical ultrasounds are per recommendation of the consulting physician.

- Follow-up evaluations of women who have experienced an inevitable, incomplete, complete, or missed SAB; GTD; ectopic pregnancies; or sexual assault are per the recommendation of the consulting physician.

- Sexually transmitted diseases are reportable conditions, and notification of the local public health department is indicated

- Suspected or documented sexual assault should be reported to the appropriate local law enforcement agency. In many communities, special sexual assault police or sheriff's divisions have been developed to help obtain the necessary forensic evidence and legal documentation in a sensitive manner. In addition, local rape crisis centers will provide an advocate for the woman to help her through this process.

- Document vaginal bleeding, its etiology, and the management thereof in the problem list and progress notes.

References

Carson, S.A., & Buster, J.E. (1993). Ectopic pregnancy. *New England Journal of Medicine, 329*(16), 1174–1181.

Cunningham, F.G., MacDonald, P.C., Gant, N.F., Leveno, K.J., & Gilstrap III, L.C. (1993). *Williams obstetrics* (19th ed., pp. 661– 690, 819–852). Norwalk, CT: Appleton & Lange.

Ghidini, A., & Romero, R. (1996). First-trimester vaginal bleeding. *Contemporary OB/GYN, 41*(11), 15–21.

Goldstein, S.R. (1994). Sonography in early pregnancy failure. *Clinical Obstetrics and Gynecology, 37*(3), 681–692.

McKennett, M., & Fullerton, J.T. (1995). Vaginal bleeding in pregnancy. *American Family Physician, 51*(3), 659–646.

Nielson, E.C., Varner, M. W., & Scott, J.R. (1991). The outcome of pregnancies complicated by bleeding during the second trimester. *Surgery, Gynecology, and Obstetrics, 173,* 371–374.

Nielsen, S., & Hahlin, M. (1995). Expectant management of first-trimester spontaneous abortion. *The Lancet, 345*(8492), 84–86.

Richards, J. (1995). Sexual assault. In W.L. Star, L.L. Lommel, & M.T. Shannon (Eds.), *Women's primary health care: Protocols for practice* (pp. 14–45, 14–54). Washington, DC: American Nurses Publishing.

Sipila, M.D.P., Hartikainen-Sorri, A.L., Oja, H., & Wendt, L. (1992). Perinatal outcome of pregnancies complicated by vaginal bleeding. *British Journal of Obstetrics and Gynaecology, 99,* 959–963.

Williams, M.A., Mittendorf, R., Lieberman, E., & Monson, R.R. (1991). Adverse infant outcomes associated with first-trimester vaginal bleeding. *Obstetrics and Gynecology, 78*(1), 14–18.

Chapter 5

SECOND AND THIRD TRIMESTER BLEEDING

Maureen T. Shannon

Vaginal bleeding during the latter half of pregnancy is reported in 4 percent of women (Mabie, 1992). It can be slight to severe; may or may not be accompanied by pain; and may be due to a number of factors including: placenta previa, abruptio placentae, preterm labor, gestational trophoblastic disease (GTD), cervicitis/vaginitis, cervical intraepithelial neoplasia/cancer, cervical polyps, trauma, or postcoital bleeding due to increased vascularization of the cervix. Of these conditions, the major causes of vaginal bleeding during the latter half of pregnancy are placenta previa (20 percent of bleeding), abruptio placentae (30 percent of bleeding), and preterm labor (Mabie, 1992; McKennett & Fullerton, 1995). This protocol will specifically address placenta previa and abruptio placentae, since information about the remainder of the factors associated with bleeding during pregnancy is presented in other chapters in this book (i.e., Chapter 6.4, *First Trimester Bleeding*, Chapter 6.25, *Preterm Labor,* and specific chapters in Section 14, *Vaginitis and Sexually Transmitted Disease.*).

Placenta Previa

Placenta previa occurs when the placenta implants very near to or completely covers the internal cervical os. The incidence of this problem is approximately 1/150 to 1/200 births. There are four classifications of this abnormality (Crane, Chun, & Acker, 1993; Lockwood, 1996):

- Total placenta previa occurs when the placenta completely covers the internal cervical os.

- Partial placenta previa occurs when the internal cervical os is partially covered by the placenta.

- Marginal placenta previa occurs when the placenta is within 2 centimeters but not covering the internal cervical os.

- Low-lying placenta occurs when the edge of the placenta is located in the lower uterine segment in close proximity to (i.e., 2 to 5 centimeters), but not reaching, the internal cervical os.

The overall incidence of placenta previa is 0.2 percent in nulliparous women and up to 5 percent in grand multiparous women (Mabie, 1992). There is variation in the incidence of this condition depending upon weeks of gestation. Approximately 45 percent of all placentas are classified as low-lying during the second trimester of pregnancy. However, at term there is a reduction in incidence noted, with only 1/150-1/200 pregnancies exhibiting some form of placenta previa. This decrease in number of reported placenta previas is due to the normal development and elongation of the lower uterine segment as pregnancy progresses with what appears to be a migration of the placental site away from the cervix to a more fundal position (Crane et al., 1993; Mabie, 1992; McKennett & Fullerton, 1995).

Risk factors that predispose a woman to the development of placenta previa include: multiparity; maternal age equal to or greater than 35 years; history of a previous cesarean section, a previous placenta previa, or a spontaneous or induced abortion; smoking; and use of cocaine (Iyasu et al., 1993; Lockwood, 1996; Taylor, Kramer, Vaughn, & Peacock, 1993; Thom, Nelson, & Vaughn, 1992). Reported complications associated with placenta previa include abruptio placentae, placenta accreta, fetal malpresentation, postpartum hemorrhage, and disseminated intravascular coagulation (DIC) (Iyasu et al., 1993; Lockwood, 1996). Although the observed maternal mortality rate is reportedly low (0.3 percent), the associated perinatal mortality rate is 8.1 percent (Iyasu et al., 1993).

Database

Subjective

- Predisposing factors (may have one or more)
  - ▶ Multiparity
  - ▶ Age 35 years or older
  - ▶ Previous cesarean section
  - ▶ Previous placenta previa
  - ▶ History of spontaneous or induced abortion
  - ▶ Smoking during pregnancy
  - ▶ Cocaine use during pregnancy
- Symptoms (may have one or more)
  - ▶ Painless, bright red vaginal bleeding which begins in the late second or the third trimester
    - – The amount of bleeding can vary from a slight amount to severe hemorrhage.
    - – Usually the first bleeding episode is mild.
  - ▶ Fatigue, lightheadedness or fainting if significant blood loss has occurred
  - ▶ Diminished or absent fetal movement with fetal compromise

Objective

Whenever a woman presents complaining of bleeding during the second or third trimester, *do not* perform a speculum or bimanual examination unless an ultrasound has been done and has documented the absence of a placenta previa.

- Woman may appear anxious, irritated, and/or apprehensive if significant blood loss has occurred.
- Vital signs may be within normal limits (WNL) or demonstrate evidence of hypovolemic shock, including a decreased blood pressure, increased pulse, and orthostatic changes.
- Skin may be pale, cold and clammy if significant blood loss has occurred
- Abdominal examination may reveal the following:
  - ▶ A soft, nontender uterus.
  - ▶ Fetal presenting part is usually not engaged, and the fetus may be in an abnormal lie (e.g., transverse, oblique, or breech).
  - ▶ Auscultation of fetal heart tones (FHTs) are usually WNL unless the woman is in shock, in

which case the FHTs may be bradycardic or tachycardic (fetal distress) or absent (fetal demise).

- Examination of the external genitalia may reveal bright red vaginal bleeding. Sanitary pad (if worn) may reveal bright red blood in varying amounts.

Abruptio Placentae

Abruptio placentae (placental abruption) occurs when a normally attached placenta separates from either a portion (partial) or all (complete) of the uterine wall prior to the birth of the fetus. This complication occurs after the 20th week of pregnancy with a reported incidence of between 1/85 to 1/200 births (Cunningham, MacDonald, Gant, Leveno, & Gilstrap III, 1993). The wide variation in the incidence figures is due to the difficulty in diagnosing the milder degrees of this complication. There are two types of abruptio placentae:

- External hemorrhage occurs when the blood escapes from between the placenta and uterine wall and flows through the cervix.

- Concealed hemorrhage (occult abruption) occurs when the bleeding is located in the central portion of the placenta and extends retroplacentally with extravasation of blood into the myometrium (Couvelaire uterus). External bleeding may or may not be present. If vaginal bleeding is observed, it is usually less than would be expected from the severity of the signs and symptoms the woman may be exhibiting. Concealed hemorrhage poses significant risk of maternal morbidity and mortality because the extent of hemorrhage can be underestimated. This can result in significant blood loss and the development of disseminated intravascular coagulation (DIC).

Risk factors associated with an increased incidence of abruptio placentae include maternal hypertension, history of a previous abruption, circumvallate placenta, sudden uterine decompression, abdominal trauma, uterine cavity abnormalities, short umbilical cord, smoking and cocaine use (Chasnoff, Burns, Schnoll, & Burns, 1985; Crane et al., 1993; Lockwood, 1996; McKennett & Fullerton, 1995; Raymond & Mills, 1993; Saftlas, Olson, Atrash, Rochat, & Rowley, 1991). Perinatal complications observed in association with this condition are intrauterine growth retardation (IUGR); fetal malformations, especially cardiac and central nervous system defects; and maternal anemia, hemorrhage, DIC, and postpartum endometritis (Mechem, Knopp, & Feldman, 1992; Raymond & Mills, 1993). Reported perinatal mortality rates range from 10 to 36 percent (Crane et al., 1993; Nielson, Varner, & Scott, 1991; Raymond & Mills, 1993).

Database

Subjective

- Predisposing factors (may have one or more)
  ▶ History of hypertension
  ▶ Cocaine use during pregnancy
  ▶ Smoking during pregnancy
  ▶ Abdominal trauma

▶ History of previous abruptio placentae

▶ History of uterine cavity abnormalities

● Symptoms (may have one or more)

▶ Vaginal bleeding occurring after the twentieth week of pregnancy

▶ Abdominal pain (mild to severe)

▶ Backache (mild to severe)

▶ Decreased or absent fetal movements

▶ Fatigue, dizziness, or lightheadedness

▶ See specific chapters for subjective data for other possible factors associated with bleeding during the second trimester (e.g., GTD, vaginitis, cervicitis, etc.).

Objective

Whenever a woman presents complaining of bleeding during the second or third trimester, *do not* perform a speculum or bimanual examination unless an ultrasound has been done and has documented the absence of a placenta previa.

● A woman may appear anxious, apprehensive, and in acute distress depending on the severity of the pain and amount of blood loss.

● Vital signs may be WNL or may demonstrate evidence of hypovolemic shock, including decreased blood pressure, increased pulse, and orthostatic changes.

● Skin may be pale, cold, and clammy if significant blood loss has occurred.

● Abdominal examination may reveal the following:

▶ Uterine irritability ranging from minimal to extreme

▶ Uterus minimally to extremely tender to palpation

▶ Increased uterine size in severe concealed abruption

▶ Uterine resting tone normal in mild abruption, increasing in severity until the uterus is hard, boardlike, and unrelaxed in severe abruptio

▶ FHTs varying between a normal rate in mild abruption, absent (fetal demise), or faint, bradycardic/tachycardic (fetal distress)

● Examination of the external genitalia may reveal dark red vaginal bleeding varying in amount from slight to severe hemorrhage; sanitary pad (if worn) may reveal bright red to dark blood in varying amounts.

● See specific protocols for the objective data for other conditions associated with bleeding during the second and third trimester (e.g., chapters about STD, GTD, abnormal cervical cytology, first trimester bleeding).

Assessment

Diagnosis, treatment and management, patient education, and follow-up follow the same course for both placenta previa and abruptio placentae.

- IUP ____ weeks or vaginal bleeding
  - ▶ R/O placenta previa
  - ▶ R/O abruptio placenta
  - ▶ R/O preterm labor
  - ▶ R/O hypovolemic shock
  - ▶ R/O fetal distress
  - ▶ R/O anemia
  - ▶ R/O cervicitis/vaginitis
  - ▶ R/O pregnancy induced hypertension/preeclampsia
  - ▶ R/O GTD
  - ▶ R/O CIN/cervical cancer
  - ▶ R/O cervical polyps
  - ▶ R/O abdominal trauma
  - ▶ R/O substance abuse

Plan

Diagnostic Tests

The following tests may be ordered after consultation with a physician.

- A complete blood count (CBC) with differential may reveal decreased red blood cell count and hemoglobin (Hgb) and hematocrit (Hct) consistent with anemia depending on the amount of blood loss.

- Coagulation studies may reveal evidence of DIC (Mechem, Knopp & Feldman, 1992):
  - ▶ Platelet count less than 100,000/mm^3
  - ▶ Fibrinogen concentration less than 100 mg/dL
  - ▶ Fibrin-degradation product level greater than 20 μg/mL
  - ▶ Prothrombin time (PT) greater than upper limits of normal (ULN) for laboratory
  - ▶ Partial thromboplastin time (PTT) greater than ULN

- Urinalysis (UA) may reveal evidence of underlying pathology (e.g., significant proteinuria in preeclampsia, blood or bilirubin in DIC).

- Transabdominal or transvaginal ultrasound should be obtained and will reveal the absence or presence of placenta previa or abruptio placentae. If abruptio placentae is documented, the sonogram may indicate the extent of the separation. When a placenta is located in the posterior portion of the uterus, the degree of abruption often cannot be determined (Crane et al., 1993; Mabie, 1992).

  NOTE: Transvaginal sonograms are more accurate than transabdominal sonograms in obtaining data about placenta previas. To have the best resolution of the image, the transducer must be placed some distance from the cervix, which also prevents aggravation of bleeding during the procedure. In addition to documenting evidence of placenta previa, transvaginal sonograms can also document the presence of placenta accreta (a condition associated with placenta previas) (Mabie, 1992; Timor-Tritsch & Monteagudo, 1993).

- Obtain blood type and Rh.

- Obtain a Betke-Kleihauer test in Rh-negative unsensitized women to determine the presence and level of fetal cells in the maternal circulation. This will determine the appropriate dose of Rh immune globulin (RhoGam®) the woman should receive.

- Transcutaneous oxygen saturation may indicate maternal hypoxia.

- External fetal monitoring should be initiated to assess fetal status and evaluate uterine activity.

Treatment/Management

- All women with second and third trimester bleeding require consultation with a physician.

- If placenta previa or abruptio placentae is diagnosed, then consult with a physician immediately.

  ▶ The plan of care for a woman with either of these conditions is determined by the consulting physician and is based on maternal and fetal status, weeks of gestation, amount of bleeding, and immediacy of delivery (i.e., active labor).

  ▶ In some clinical settings, co-management of women with placenta previa is determined by the extent of the previa, and is guided by institution specific policies and procedures.

- If the woman is in shock or the fetus is in distress *immediate* admission to the hospital is indicated (i.e., transport to labor and delivery STAT). Cardiovascular support and insertion of an intravenous line to begin fluid replacement may be necessary in some situations.

- In Rh negative women who experience second or third trimester bleeding, administration of RhoGam® is indicated. The dose can be calculated based on the results of the Kleihauer-Betke test with 10 µg of Rh immune globulin given per estimated milliliter of fetal blood (Mabie, 1992). In some settings, full-dose RhoGam® (300 µg) IM is given.

- See specific chapters for the treatment/management of other causes of vaginal bleeding during pregnancy (e.g., chapters about STD, GTN, abnormal cervical cytology, first trimester bleeding).

Consultation

- Consult with a physician whenever a woman is being evaluated for second or third trimester vaginal bleeding.

- Transfer to physician care in any woman documented to have abruptio placentae.

- Co-management of women with placenta previa is possible in some clinical settings, as determined by institution specific policies and procedures.

Patient Education

- In mild cases of placenta previa or abruptio placenta, present a complete explanation of the problems, the diagnostic tests, and need for consultation with a physician to the woman and her partner.

- In moderate to severe cases, give the woman and her partner as complete an explanation as is possible (under the circumstances) regarding her immediate treatment and prognosis. (Whenever possible this should be done by the consulting physician.)

- Emotional and psychological support of the woman and her partner during the diagnosis and treatment of these problems should be available through referrals to a social worker, psychologist, or psychiatric consultants (as indicated).

- If a fetal demise occurs, or if the infant is premature or neurologically disabled, the woman and her family will need help working through the grieving process. Initiate the appropriate referrals and interventions as soon as possible.

- Refer the families with a neurologically disabled infant to the social worker for effective utilization of the community resources available to them.

Follow-up

- Follow-up of a woman with placenta previa or abruptio placentae is determined by the consulting physician.

- Document the diagnosis of placenta previa or abruptio placentae and the management thereof in progress notes and problem list.

References

Chasnoff, I.J., Burns, W.J., Schnoll, S.H., & Burns, K.A. (1985). Cocaine use in pregnancy. *New England Journal of Medicine, 313*(11), 666–669.

Crane, S., Chun, B., & Acker, D. (1993). Treatment of obstetrical hemorrhagic emergencies. *Current Opinion in Obstetrics and Gynecology, 5*, 675–682.

Cunningham, F.G., MacDonald, P.C., Gant, N.F., Leveno, K.J., & Gilstrap III, L.C. (1993). *Williams obstetrics* (19th ed., pp. 661–690, 819–852). Norwalk, CT: Appleton & Lange.

Iyasu, S., Saftlas, A.K., Rowley, D.L., Koonin, L.M., Lawson, H.W., & Atrash, H.K. (1993). The epidemiology of placenta previa in the United States, 1979 through 1987. *American Journal of Obstetrics and Gynecology, 168*(5), 1424–1429.

Lockwood, C.J. (1996). Third trimester bleeding. In J.T. Queenan & J.C. Hobbins (Eds.) *Protocols for high-risk pregnancies* (3rd ed., pp. 567–573). Cambridge, MA: Blackwell Science.

Mabie, W.C. (1992). Placenta previa. *Clinics in Perinatology, 19*(2), 425–435.

McKennett, M., & Fullerton, J.T. (1995). Vaginal bleeding in pregnancy. *American Family Physician, 51*(3), 659–646.

Mechem, C.C., Knopp, R.R., & Feldman, D. (1992). Painless abruptio placentae associated with disseminated intravasuclar coagulation and syncope. *Annals of Emergency Medicine, 21*(7), 883–885.

Nielson, E.C., Varner, M.W., & Scott, J.R. (1991). The outcome of pregnancies complicated by bleeding during the second trimester. *Surgery, Gynecology, and Obstetrics, 173*, 371–374.

Raymond, E.G., & Mills, J.L. (1993). Placental abruption. Maternal risk factors and associated fetal conditions. *Acta Obstetricia et Gynecologica Scandinavica, 72*(8), 633–639.

Saftlas, A.F., Olson, D.R., Atrash, H.K., Rochat, R., & Rowley, D. (1991). National trends in the incidence of abruptio placentae, 1979–1987. *Obstetrics and Gynecology, 78*, 1081–1086.

Taylor, V.M., Kramer, M.D., Vaughn, T.L., & Peacock, S. (1993). Placenta previa in relation to induced and spontaneous abortion: A population-based study. *Obstetrics and Gynecology, 82*(1), 88–91.

Thom, D.H., Nelson, L.M., & Vaughn, T.L. (1992). Spontaneous abortion and subsequent birth outcomes. *American Journal of Obstetrics and Gynecology, 166*(Part 1), 111–116.

Timor-Tritsch, I.E., & Monteagudo, A. (1993). Diagnosis of placenta previa by transvaginal sonography. *Annals of Medicine, 25*(3), 279–283.

Chapter 6

BREAST MASS

Winifred L. Star

Ann-Marie McNamara

The structure and composition of a woman's breasts vary during her lifetime because of endogenous hormonal fluctuations. Hypertrophy of glandular elements of breast tissue during pregnancy and lactation may impart increased nodularity and density to the breasts. During the first trimester, lobules enlarge and fully develop; during the second trimester, secretory changes occur; and during the third trimester, fat droplets accumulate in the lobules leading to hyperplasia (Powell, 1994). These changes occur in response to changes in estrogen, progesterone, insulin, growth hormone, prolactin, and glucocorticoids. In particular, an increase in estrogen causes an increased breast size with the weight of the breast doubling during pregnancy (Powell, 1994; Scott-Connor & Schorr, 1995).

The breast changes that occur during pregnancy may make it difficult for the clinician to accurately evaluate the breasts. For example, during pregnancy fibroadenomas tend to increase in size and physiologic bloody nipple discharge is more apt to occur, both of which may be confused with breast cancer (Scott-Connor & Schorr, 1995). Eighty percent of breast lesions detected during pregnancy are benign. Of benign lesions discovered during pregnancy, 70 percent are benign lesion types found in all women (e.g., fibroadenomas) and 30 percent are lesions specific to pregnancy (e.g., lobular hyperplasia or localized breast infarcts) (Scott-Connor & Schorr, 1995).

Breast cancer during pregnancy occurs in 1 of 3,000 to 1 of 10,000 women (DiFronzo & O'Connell, 1996; Fiorica, 1994). When matched for age and stage of disease, the prognosis of women with breast cancer detected during pregnancy is no worse than for nonpregnant women (DiFronzo & O'Connell, 1996; Isaacs, 1995; Marchant, 1994; Scott-Connor & Schorr, 1995). In the past, treatment for pregnant women with breast cancer was delayed, which worsened their chances for survival (Marchant, 1994; Scott-Connor & Schorr, 1995). Currently, there is general agreement that modified radical mastectomy is the treatment of choice for women presenting with breast cancer during pregnancy. Therapeutic abortion is generally not recommended. However, it may be considered if a woman has opted for breast conservation and radiation therapy or if she has Stage III or IV cancer to allow for unrestricted treatment with radiation and chemotherapy (DiFronzo & O'Connell, 1996). When breast cancer is found later in pregnancy (i.e., third trimester), a lumpectomy or observation may be planned with further therapy carried out promptly after delivery (American College of Obstetrics [ACOG], 1991a; DiFronzo & O'Connell, 1996).

Database

Subjective

- May complain of breast lump, mass, pain, tenderness, nipple discharge, burning, itching, swelling, skin changes

- Diet may be high in methylxanthines (e.g., coffee, tea, sodas, chocolate)

- May be taking methylxanthine-containing medication (e.g., theophylline, phenothiazine)

- May have a history of trauma to the breast(s)
- May have positive family history of benign breast disease or breast cancer

Objective

- Inspection and palpation of breasts, supraclavicular areas and axillae (supine and sitting) may reveal
    - ▶ Breast fullness, nodularity, thickening, mass
    - ▶ Nipple retraction, ulceration, crusting, discharge
    - ▶ Skin dimpling (peau d'orange), erythema, edema, induration
    - ▶ Axillary or supraclavicular adenopathy
    - ▶ Accessory breast tissue (in axilla) or supernumerary nipples
- Carefully document findings using descriptive terms.
    - ▶ Terms that may be applied to description of breast tissue include thick, full, pronounced, prominent, soft, buoyant, fatty, ropey, granular, nodular, coarse, bumpy.
    - ▶ Dominant masses should be described assuming a clock position, locating the mass in distance from the base of the nipple, the dimensions measured with a centimeter tape or ruler.
        - – The consistency, presence of tenderness, shape, and mobility of the mass should also be described.
    - ▶ Skin changes of the breast and adenopathy of axillary or supraclavicular areas should be noted.

Assessment

- Breast mass (with or without associated nipple or skin changes, discharge, lymphadenopathy)
    - ▶ Hypertrophy of normal breast tissue
    - ▶ R/O benign breast disease
    - ▶ R/O fibrocystic change
    - ▶ R/O breast cancer
    - ▶ R/O cervical/dorsal radiculitis
    - ▶ R/O Tietze's syndrome (costochronditis)
    - ▶ R/O mastitis (postpartum)
    - ▶ R/O galactocele (postpartum)

Plan

Diagnostic Tests

- Technologies for evaluating the breast include
  - ▶ Mammography
    - Can be used for screening and diagnostic purposes
    - Able to identify breast cancer 85 to 90 percent of the time (Smith, 1996)
    - Can also detect calcifications, fibroadenomas, enlarged lymph nodes, galactocele, fat necrosis, nipple changes, fibrous streaks, and alterations in the density of tissue (ACOG, 1991b).

    NOTE: There is controversy over the use of mammogram during pregnancy because the increased density of the breasts that occurs during this time decreases mammographic sensitivity (Barnavon & Wallack, 1990). In general, mammograms are not useful when there is a palpable mass (DiFronzo & O'Connell, 1996).

  - ▶ Ultrasonography (B-mode scanning)
    - Used as an adjunct to mammography to help distinguish solid from cystic masses but cannot reliably detect microcalcifications (ACOG, 1991)
    - A primary noninvasive tool in evaluating clients with a breast mass and nipple discharge (Chung, Lee, Park, Lee, & Bae, 1995); can be safely used to evaluate breast masses in pregnancy (Scott-Connor & Schorr, 1995)
  - ▶ Ductography or galactography
    - Used to evaluate nipple discharge in a nonlactating breast
    - Involves cannulating the involved duct and injecting a radiopaque dye, followed by x-ray evaluation
    - Not likely to be used in pregnancy
  - ▶ Computed Tomography (CT) scan
    - Still under investigation; more sensitive than mammography in detecting axillary node metastases (Tohnosu et al., 1993)
    - May be used to guide fine needle aspiration biopsy and for preoperative wire localization of lesions (Baker, 1994; Van Gelderen, 1995)
    - Safety in pregnancy not determined
  - ▶ Magnetic Resonance Imaging (MRI)
    - Still under investigation
    - Contrast-enhanced MRI found useful in determining malignant breast masses, searching for breast tumors in dense breasts, and finding multiple foci of cancer (Davis & McCarty Jr, 1997; Kerslake et al., 1995; Schapira & Levine, 1996)
    - Poor specificity in identifying microcalcifications (Gilles et al., 1996)

- – Not recommended for use during first trimester until more information is available (ACOG, 1995)

  ▶ Diaphanography or transillumination

  - – Still under investigation as a screening procedure (Säbel & Aichinger, 1996)

- Diagnostic techniques

  ▶ Fine needle aspiration (FNA) is used as an initial technique for establishing a cytologic diagnosis of palpable breast masses

  - – Nondiagnostic/equivocal/benign FNA of dominant masses requires excisional biopsy.

  - – Most useful for masses with signs suggestive of malignancy on exam (Marchant, 1992)

  - – Absence of malignant cells on FNA does not rule out the possibility of cancer (McGrath, 1994).

  ▶ Cyst aspiration is used to withdraw fluid from suspected cystic masses.

  - – Technique is both diagnostic and therapeutic if fluid is obtained and the mass disappears.

  - – Cyst fluid may be discarded unless bloody, turbid, or opaque, in which case it should be sent for cytologic evaluation.

  - – Persistent/recurrent masses after aspiration require definitive therapy.

  ▶ Core-needle biopsy, using a cutting needle, can be performed to obtain a core of tissue for histologic diagnosis of a breast mass (although in many centers it has been replaced by FNA).

  - – Useful in cases in which FNA suggestive of carcinoma and frozen section confirmation is needed (McGrath, 1994)

  ▶ Incisional biopsy involves removal of a portion of the breast mass for histologic evaluation.

  - – Main purpose is for establishing diagnosis and providing tissue for hormone receptor assays

  - – Performed when tumor too large for complete excision (McGrath, 1994)

  ▶ Excisional biopsy is used to completely remove a discrete breast mass.

  - – Used when FNA is nondiagnostic/equivocal (or benign) and to evaluate persistent, dominant masses (Bradley & Sharp, 1995; McGrath, 1994)

NOTE: Histologic evaluation of a biopsy specimen is the only definitive procedure that leads to the diagnosis of a breast mass and is indicated in the following instances (ACOG, 1991; McGrath, 1994):

- Solid dominant mass not diagnosed as fibroadenoma
- Bloody cyst fluid on aspiration
- Failure of mass to disappear completely upon fluid aspiration
- Recurrence of cyst after one or two aspirations
- Nondiagnostic/equivocal (or benign) FNA
- Bloody nipple discharge
- Nipple ulceration or persistent crusting
- Skin edema and erythema suspicious of inflammatory breast carcinoma

Treatment/Management

- See Diagnostic Tests section.

- Ask a second examiner to corroborate breast findings, as indicated.

- Refer client to physician if a dominant breast mass is present. The specialist will determine necessary diagnostic and treatment modalities.

- Suggest elimination of methylxanthines, which has been shown to reduce symptoms in as many as 65 percent of women experiencing breast discomfort (ACOG, 1991b).

- Vitamin E and A therapy has been reported to positively influence symptoms of breast pain and swelling (ACOG, 1991b). However, there are no studies on the use of vitamin E and A during pregnancy in women with breast complaints.

  NOTE: Due to a small number of case reports suggesting that excessive doses of vitamin A ingested during pregnancy (possibly as little as 10,000 IU daily) are associated with birth defects, routine supplementation of vitamin A during pregnancy is not recommended (ACOG, 1998). See Section 1, *Preconception Health Care—An Overview,* for further information.

- Application of heat/cold may be beneficial in relieving breast pain.

- Use of a well-fitting, supportive brassiere may increase breast comfort during pregnancy.

Consultation

- Refer client to a physician for management of a palpable, dominant breast mass.

- Immediate referral to a physician-surgeon is warranted for a client with a suspicious mass. If cancer is diagnosed, obstetric care should proceed with an obstetrician. Co-management may be appropriate in certain settings.

Patient Education

- Teach or review breast self-examination (BSE).

- Discuss changes of normal breast tissue during pregnancy.

- Support and allay client's concern for positive breast findings. Discuss usual modalities for evaluation and diagnosis of breast masses during pregnancy.

- Advise against excessive doses of vitamin A (see note above).

Follow-up

- Encourage monthly BSE, starting at age 20.

- Set up a return appointment for reevaluation, as indicated, if woman has not been referred to a breast specialist.

- Follow the current American Cancer Society guidelines for routine breast screening in asymptomatic nonpregnant women (American Cancer Society, 1997):

  ▶ BSE monthly starting at age 20 years

▶ Clinical Breast Examination (CBE) every 3 years for ages 20 to 39 years, yearly after age 40 years

▶ Mammography every year starting at age 40

NOTE: Women with a personal or family history of breast cancer may need a more individualized approach to screening mammograms; seek physician consultation. For additional information on breast cancer, contact the American Cancer Society at 1(800) 227-2345.

NOTE: Controversy exists regarding screening mammography and CBE in certain age groups. The U.S. Preventive Services Task Force (1996) states that "there is insufficient evidence to recommend for or against routine mammography or CBE for women aged 40–49 or aged 70 and older" (p.73). A 1997 National Institutes of Health (NIH) consensus statement concludes "that the data currently available do not warrant a universal recommendation for mammography for all women in their forties" (NIH, 1997, p.16). (It should be mentioned, however, that two members of the panel felt routine screening for women in their forties should be actively encouraged.) The National Cancer Institute (NCI) recommends that women aged 40 and older be screened every 1 to 2 years with mammography (Taubes, 1997).

▶ For the postpartum client, mammography may not be useful due to continued breast density, which generally persists until 3 to 6 months after discontinuing breast feeding (Smith, 1996).

● Document presence of breast mass and management thereof in problem list and progress notes.

References

American Cancer Society (1997). *Cancer facts and figures.* Atlanta, GA: Author.

American College of Obstetricians and Gynecologists (ACOG) (1991a). *Carcinoma of the breast.* (Technical Bulletin No. 158). Washington, DC: Author.

American College of Obstetricians and Gynecologists (ACOG) (1991b). *Nonmalignant conditions of the breast.* (Technical Bulletin No. 156). Washington, DC: Author.

American College of Obstetricians and Gynecologists (ACOG) (1995). *Guidelines for diagnostic imaging during pregnancy.* (Committee Opinion No. 158). Washington, DC: Author.

American College of Obstetricians and Gynecologists (ACOG) (1998). *Vitamin A supplementation during pregnancy.* (Committee Opinion No. 196).Washington, DC: Author.

Baker, K.S. (1994) Ancillary breast imaging modalities. In D.E. Powell & C.S. Sterling (Eds.), *The diagnosis and detection of breast disease* (pp. 4670). St. Louis, MO: Mosby.

Barnavon, Y. & Wallack, M. (1990). Management of the pregnant patient with carcinoma of the breast. *Surgery, Gynecology & Obstetrics, 171,* 347-352.

Bradley, A.L., & Sharp, K.W. (1995). Breast disease. *Medical Clinics of North America, 79*(6), 1443–1455.

Chung, S.Y., Lee, K.W., Park, K.S., Lee, Y., & Bae, S.H. (1995). Breast tumors associated with nipple discharge. Correlation of findings on galactography and sonography. *Clinical Imaging, 19*(3), 165-171.

Davis, P.L., McCarty, K.S. Jr. (1997). Sensitivity of enhanced MRI for the detection of breast cancer: New, multicentric, residual, and recurrent. *European Radiology, 7*(Suppl. 5), 289–298.

DiFronzo, L.A., & O'Connell, T.X. (1996). Breast cancer in pregnancy and lactation. *Surgical Clinics of North America, 76*(2), 267–278.

Fiorica, J.V. (1994). Special problems. Breast cancer and pregnancy. *Obstetrics and Gynecology Clinics of North America, 21*(4), 721-732.

Gilles, R., Meunier, M., Lucidarme, O., Zafrani, B., Guinebretiere, J.M., Tardivon, A.A., Le Gal, M., Vanel, D., Neuenschwander, S., & Arriagada, R. (1996). Clustered breast microcalcifications: Evaluation by dynamic contrast-enhanced subtraction MRI. *Journal of Computer Assisted Tomography, 20*(1), 9-14.

Isaacs, J.H. (1995). Cancer of the breast in pregnancy. *Surgical Clinics of North America, 75*(1), 47-51.

Kerslake, R.W., Carleton, P.J., Fox, J.N., Imrie, M.J., Cook, A.M., Read, J.R., Bowsley, S.J., Buckley, D.L., & Horsman, A. (1995). Dynamic gradient-echo and fat-suppressed spin-echo contrast-enhanced MRI of the breast. *Clinical Radiology, 50*(7), 440-454.

Marchant, D.J. (1992). Breast disease and the gynecologist. *Current Problems in Obstetrics, Gynecology, and Fertility, 15*(1), 1–37.

Marchant, D.J. (1994). Breast cancer in pregnancy. *Clinical Obstetrics and Gynecology, 37*(4), 993-997.

McGrath, P.C. (1994). The role of the surgeon in breast disease diagnosis. In D.E. Powell & C.S. Sterling (Eds.), *The diagnosis and detection of breast disease* (pp. 76–85). St. Louis, MO: Mosby.

National Institutes of Health (NIH). (1997). Breast cancer screening for women ages 40–49. *NIH Consensus Statement, January 21–23. 15*(1), 1–35.

Powell, D.E. (1994). The normal breast: Structure, function, and epidemiology. In D.E. Powell & C.B. Stelling (Eds.), *The diagnosis and detection of breast disease* (pp. 3–20). St. Louis, MO: Mosby.

Powell, D.E., & Stelling, C.B. (1994). *The diagnosis and detection of breast disease.* St. Louis, MO: Mosby.

Säbel, M. & Aichinger, H. (1996). Recent developments in breast imaging. *Physics in Medicine and Biology, 41,* 315–368..

Schapira, D.V. & Levine, R.B. (1996). Breast cancer screening and compliance and evaluation of lesions. *Medical Clinics of North America. 80*(1), 15–26.

Scott-Connor, C.E.H. & Schorr, S.J. (1995). The diagnosis and management of breast problems during pregnancy and lactation. *The American Journal of Surgery, 170,* 401-405.

Smith, B.L. (1996). The breast. *Current Problems in Obstetrics, Gynecology and Fertility, XIX*(1), 15.

Taubes, G. (1997). NCI reverses one expert panel, sides with another. *Science, 276,* 27–28.

Tohnosu, N., Okuyama, K., Koide, Y., Kikuchi, T., Awano, T., Matsubara, H., et al. (1993). A comparison between ultrasonography and mammography, computed tomography, and digital subtraction angiography for the detection of breast cancers. *Surgery Today, 23*(8), 704-710.

U.S. Preventive Services Task Force. (1996). *Guide to clinical preventive services* (2nd ed., pp. 73–87). Baltimore, MD: Williams & Wilkins.

Van Gelderen, W.F. (1995). Computed tomography of the breast: A valuable adjunct mammography in selected cases. *Australasian Radiology, 39*(2), 176-178.

Chapter 7

CARPAL TUNNEL SYNDROME

Ellen M. Scarr

Carpal tunnel syndrome (CTS) is a common disorder caused by compression of the median nerve at the wrist. Inflammation of the wrist tendon and surrounding soft tissue, fluid shifts (e.g., edema), or anatomic changes (e.g., fractures, arthritic changes) put pressure on the median nerve within its narrow channel, resulting in paresthesias and pain in the distribution of the nerve. The dominant hand is usually involved, and, in many cases, involvement is bilateral (Ditmars, 1993; Katz, 1995).

CTS occurs more frequently in women than men, most likely because women have an anatomically smaller carpal tunnel (Putney, 1995). It is associated with diabetes, rheumatoid and gouty arthritis, hypothyroidism, collagen vascular disease, history of Colles' fracture, and activities involving repetitive wrist motion (Hunt & Osterman, 1994; Stevens, Beard, O'Fallon & Kurland, 1992).

CTS is also associated with pregnancy, where generalized edema as well as traction on the median nerve from postural changes (associated with increasing lordosis) result in median nerve compression (Ditmars, 1993; Maldonado & Barger, 1995). Hormonally induced tendinitis at the carpal tunnel may also play a role in the development of CTS during pregnancy (Kohn, 1991). The incidence in pregnancy is reported to be as high as 25 percent. CTS most often develops or worsens in the third trimester, although onset may occur earlier or later (e.g., postpartum). Preexisting CTS worsens with pregnancy (Gant & Cunningham, 1993; Mercier, 1995; Stevens et al, 1992). The prognosis for pregnancy-related CTS is good, with the majority of cases resolving by 3 months postpartum.

Database

Subjective

- Client may report history of
  - ▶ Diabetes, arthritis, thyroid disease
  - ▶ Wrist fracture, de Quervain's tendinitis, ganglion cyst, trigger finger
  - ▶ Blunt trauma, repetitive wrist movement, extensive use of hands
  - ▶ Vitamin B_6 use (excessive amounts [more than 200 to 300 mg/day] can cause toxic neuropathy) (Ditmars, 1993; Hunt & Osterman, 1994)
- Client may complain of
  - ▶ Pain, burning, tingling, and/or persistent numbness of the palmar aspect of the thumb, index finger, middle finger and/or medial half of the ring finger (median nerve distribution); rarely involves all digits; often only index and middle finger (Mercier, 1995)
  - ▶ Decreased sensitivity, stiffness, weakness or lack of coordination of involved fingers or hand (dropping items, difficulty grasping objects)
  - ▶ Pain radiating proximally to volar forearm
  - ▶ Pain coexisting in elbow, shoulder or neck

- Symptoms occur with daytime activities, or awaken client at night.

Objective

- Positive Tinel's sign (tingling along median nerve distribution with light tapping over the carpal tunnel)
- Positive Phalen's sign (numbness/tingling along median nerve distribution after active wrist flexion for 30 to 60 seconds)
- Decreased sensation to light touch along median nerve distribution
- Decreased strength of hand grip and pinch
- Clinical signs usually mildly positive in pregnancy; negative exam does not rule out CTS (e.g., diagnosis suggested by history)
- Signs of marked or prolonged median nerve compression unusual with onset of CTS in pregnancy:
  - ► Thenar atrophy (hollowing of proximal thenar muscle)
  - ► Weakness of fingers (poor thumb opposition)
- No signs of vascular insufficiency upon examination
  - ► Involved hand warm and dry
  - ► Nailbeds pink with intact capillary refill
  - ► Allen's test is negative (compression of the ulnar or radial artery after milking blood from hand does not reduce blood flow to the hand, indicating patency of contralateral artery)

Assessment

- Carpal tunnel syndrome
  - ► R/O vascular insufficiency
  - ► R/O other orthopedic causes of hand pain (e.g. de Quervain's tendinitis, ganglion cyst, wrist fracture)
  - ► R/O toxic neuropathy

Plan

Diagnostic Tests

- Electromyography (EMG) can be used to confirm diagnosis if unclear, but is rarely necessary in pregnancy.

Treatment/Management

- For mild symptoms, advise gentle range of motion of the affected hand q.i.d.
- For moderate symptoms, advise the use of a removable, soft wrist splint in the neutral position, avoiding pressure on median nerve in the mid-palm area.
- See Patient Education.

Consultation

- Consult with a physician if there are severe symptoms and/or markedly positive clinical signs.
- Steroid injection, diuretics, or evaluation for surgical repair may be indicated for severe symptoms (with physician consultation).

Patient Education

- Explain pathophysiology of CTS in pregnancy.
- Reassure client that symptoms usually resolve after delivery.
- Explain the proper use of splint(s):
  - ▶ Periodic removal during the day to prevent stiffness
  - ▶ Use of splints at night to prevent dorsiflexion of wrist and decrease nocturnal wakening from pain and paresthesias
- Assist client to identify precipitating or contributing factors that can be modified:
  - ▶ Avoid repetitive wrist motion (frequent computer use, work as cashier, typist, seamstress, musician; hobbies such as knitting, tennis, woodworking).
  - ▶ Avoid wrist flexion or extension.
  - ▶ Encourage frequent breaks from activities.
  - ▶ Encourage alternating work activities.

Follow-up

- Follow-up on symptoms at subsequent visits; if symptoms persist after 6 weeks postpartum, consider referral to orthopedist.
- Document diagnosis of CTS in progress notes and problem list.

References

Ditmars, D. (1993). Patterns of carpal tunnel syndrome. *Hand Clinics, 9*(2), 241–252.

Gant, N. & Cunningham, F. (1993). *Basic gynecology and obstetrics* (pp. 444–456). Norwalk, CT: Appleton & Lange.

Hunt, T. & Osterman, A. (1994). Complications of the treatment of carpal tunnel syndrome. *Hand Clinics, 10*(1), 63–71.

Katz, J. (1995). Regional musculoskeletal disorders. In K. Carlson, & S. Eisenstat, (Eds). *Primary care of women* (pp. 172–179). St. Louis, MO: Mosby.

Kohn, N. (1991). Neurologic diseases. In N. Gleicher (Ed.), *Principles and practice of medical therapy in pregnancy,* (2nd ed., pp. 1224–1234). Norwalk, CT: Appleton & Lange.

Maldonado, A., & Barger, M. (1995). Primary care for women: Comprehensive assessment of common musculoskeletal disorders. *Journal of Nurse-Midwifery, 40*(2), 202–215.

Mercier, L. (1995). *Practical orthopedics* (4th ed.). St. Louis, MO: Mosby.

Putney, D. (1995). Wrist, hand and finger pain. In W. Star, L. Lommel, & M. Shannon (Eds.), *Women's primary health care: Protocols for practice* (pp. 8-19–8-26). Washington, DC: American Nurses Publishing.

Stevens, J., Beard, C., O'Fallon, W., & Kurland, L. (1992). Conditions associated with carpal tunnel syndromes. *Mayo Clinic Proceedings, 67*(6), 541–548.

Chapter 8

ECTOPIC PREGNANCY

Maureen T. Shannon

The term "ectopic pregnancy" refers to the implantation of a fertilized ovum outside the normal sites within the uterine cavity. The incidence of ectopic pregnancy has been calculated to be 1/66 reported pregnancies, and is the second leading cause of maternal mortality in the United States (American College of Obstetricians & Gynecologists [ACOG], 1990a; Beckmann et al., 1995). Reported rates of ectopic pregnancy are highest in women between the ages of 15 to 19, and women over 35. Black and other racial minority women are at greater risk of ectopic pregnancies than whites (Beckmann et al., 1995; Goldner, Lawson, Xia, & Atrash, 1993; Maymon et al., 1992). Advances in the early diagnosis and conservative treatment of ectopic pregnancy, as well as a higher index of suspicion on the part of clinicians, have reduced the associated mortality rate by 90 percent during the past two decades (Goldner et al., 1993; Wyte, 1994). Despite this reduction in deaths, the occurrence of this problem has continued to escalate, resulting in significant long-term maternal sequelae, including decreased fertility and a 10 to 20 percent recurrence rate in affected women (Beckmann et al., 1995; Pernoll & Garmel, 1994).

Approximately 95 percent of ectopic pregnancies occur in the fallopian tubes. The majority of implantations are located in the ampulla (55 percent), followed by the isthmic (25 percent), fimbrial (17 percent), and interstitial areas of the tube. Extratubal implantation sites include the cornua of the uterus (rudimentary horn), ovaries, cervix, broad ligaments, or abdominal cavity. In rare instances (1 in 17,000 to 30,000 pregnancies), an ectopic pregnancy can coexist with an intrauterine pregnancy (i.e., heterotopic pregnancy) (Pernoll & Garmel, 1994).

Although the exact etiology of ectopic pregnancy is not known, several pathophysiological mechanisms have been postulated. Tubal ectopic pregnancies may be a result of an alteration in transport of a fertilized ovum caused by damage to the mucosal lining of the fallopian tube and/or fimbria (e.g., infections, inflammation, surgical procedures) (Doyle, DeCherney, & Diamond, 1991; Pernoll & Garmel, 1994). Other possible mechanisms include ovum defects (e.g., delayed or premature ovulation), zygote abnormalities, assisted reproduction technologies, mechanical interference with implantation (e.g., intrauterine devices [IUDs]), hormonal dysfunction (e.g., hyperestrogenism), and sterilization failure (Doyle et al., 1991; Pernoll & Garmel, 1994).

Therapeutic interventions currently available for the management of ectopic pregnancies include surgery, chemotherapy, and nonoperative expectant management. The treatment chosen is determined by several factors, such as the number of weeks' gestation; site of the ectopic implantation; size of ectopic, ruptured or unruptured fallopian tube; and the clinical condition of the woman (e.g., stable versus hypovolemic shock). The type of treatment chosen has been observed to have an impact on recurrence rates. Conservative interventions (e.g., expectant management, medical management, conservative surgical procedures) are associated with a lower incidence of recurrences compared to more extensive surgical procedures (Sanfilippo & Woodworth, 1992).

The most emergent complication associated with ectopic pregnancy is excessive blood loss. This occurs as a result of tubal rupture or the development of a pelvic hematocele. Consequences of excessive maternal blood loss include severe anemia, need for transfusions, development of disseminated intraavascular coagulation (DIC), or death. Persistent ectopic pregnancy is another complication that can occur when retained trophoblastic tissue continues to proliferate at the site of the implantation. It has been reported in women undergoing conservative therapeutic interventions, with an incidence as high as 20 percent after conservative surgical procedures are performed (Sanfilippo & Woodworth, 1992). Hemorrhage, continued tubal destruction, and, in rare instances, choriocarcinoma are possible sequelae of this complication (Seifer, Diamond, & DeCherney, 1991). Consequently, clinicians should suspect this problem in any woman with persistent elevation of serum human chorionic gonadotropin (hCG) levels after treatment for an ectopic pregnancy (Sanfilippo & Woodworth, 1992).

Database

Subjective

- Risk factors (woman may report a history of one or more) (Emerson & McCord, 1996):
  - ▶ Previous ectopic pregnancy
  - ▶ Tubal surgery
  - ▶ Episode of pelvic inflammatory disease (PID)
  - ▶ Infertility
  - ▶ Past or current use of an IUD
  - ▶ Use of low-dose progestins or postcoital estrogens for contraception
  - ▶ Assisted reproduction (e.g., in vitro fertilization)
  - ▶ Factors associated with uterine or tubal anatomic abnormalities (e.g., DES exposure, salpingitis)
  - ▶ Prior therapeutic abortion with complications (e.g., endometritis)
  - ▶ Induced superovulation

  NOTE: Up to 50 percent of women with ectopic pregnancies do not have an identifiable risk factor (Emerson & McCord, 1996; Pernoll & Garmel, 1994).

- Symptoms (may include one or more)
  - ▶ 90 percent of women describe some type of abdominal or pelvic pain.
    - The characteristics of the pain vary from a vague ache to a sharp, colicky pain that may be diffuse or unilateral.
    - With tubal rupture accompanied by acute blood loss, there may be acute lower quadrant pain that is intermittent and associated with backache, dizziness, and syncope.
  - ▶ Amenorrhea (40 to 95 percent of patients report a lapsed menses)
  - ▶ Abnormal vaginal bleeding (usually described as light and intermittent, but can be profuse)
  - ▶ Vertigo (if significant blood loss)
  - ▶ Syncope (if significant blood loss)
  - ▶ Shoulder pain—when hemorrhaging results in accumulation of blood under the diaphragm.
  - ▶ Breast tenderness (10 to 25 percent of patients report this symptom)

▶ Passage of decidual tissue (rare)

NOTE: Women experiencing an abdominal pregnancy may report malaise, persistent nausea and vomiting, fetal movements high in the abdomen, painful fetal movements, and decreased fetal movements (Martin & McCaul, 1990; Osguthorpe & Keating, 1988; Sanfilippo & Woodworth, 1992).

Objective

● The woman may appear to be anxious, apprehensive, or in no acute distress.

● Blood pressure may be within normal limits (WNL), decreased, and/or demonstrate postural changes.

● Pulse may be WNL, thready and/or tachycardic.

● Temperature (T) is usually WNL but 5 to 10 percent of women will have a T more than 37°C (98.6°F) (Beckman et al., 1995)

● Skin pallor may be evident

● Abdominal assessment may reveal

▶ Decreased bowel sounds if mild paralytic ileus has occurred (in women with chronic abdominal blood loss)

▶ Abdominal tenderness (present in 80 to 90 percent of women) that may be associated with rebound and guarding (Beckman et al., 1995)

▶ Cullen's sign (a periumbilical bluish discoloration), if a hemoperitoneum has occurred

▶ The uterine size will be less than expected for gestational age (with abdominal pregnancy)

▶ A distinct mass evident outside of the uterus; fetal parts may be palpated and fetal activity observed high in the abdomen (with abdominal pregnancy)

● Pelvic examination may reveal the following:

▶ Minimal to profuse amounts of blood at the introitus, in the vagina, or coming from the cervical os upon speculum examination.

▶ Bimanual examination

– Normal uterine size in approximately 70 percent of women; uterine enlargement in approximately 30 percent of women; but fetal size less than expected for weeks of gestation (Beckman et al., 1995)

– Cervical motion tenderness in 50 to 75 percent of women (Beckman et al., 1995).

– Adnexal mass in approximately 50 percent of women; there is a contralateral adnexal mass palpated in 20 percent of women (Beckman et al., 1995).

– Adnexal tenderness in 75 to 90 percent of women (may be unilateral or bilateral) (Beckman et al., 1995).

– Doughy sensation palpation of the posterior vaginal wall (pouch of Douglas) due to blood accumulation in this region.

Assessment

- Ectopic pregnancy (tubal, cervical, ovarian, abdominal, heterotopic)
  - ▶ R/O intrauterine pregnancy with inaccurate dates
  - ▶ R/O incomplete or missed spontaneous abortion
  - ▶ R/O pelvic inflammatory disease
  - ▶ R/O appendicitis
  - ▶ R/O pelvic mass
  - ▶ R/O intrauterine pregnancy with corpus luteum cyst
  - ▶ R/O ruptured corpus luteum cyst
  - ▶ R/O endometriosis
  - ▶ R/O gestational trophoblastic disease
  - ▶ R/O ureteral calculi
  - ▶ R/O depression

Plan

Diagnostic Tests

The diagnosis of an ectopic pregnancy usually involves a number of tests and procedures that are ordered based on the clinical status of the women (i.e., in shock or stable) and the point in gestation when she presents with symptoms. The significant morbidity and mortality due to hemorrhage associated with this condition requires that physician consultation be obtained when woman is suspected of having an ectopic pregnancy. The following diagnostic tests may be ordered after consultation with a physician.

- Complete blood count (CBC) with differential (may reveal leukocytosis; a decreased red blood cell [RBC] count, hematocrit, and/or hemoglobin depending upon the amount of blood lost)
- Type and Rh should be obtained
- Pregnancy tests
  - ▶ Quantitative serum beta human chorionic gonadotropin (β-hCG) radioimmunoassay. The β-hCG test is considered to be the "gold standard" pregnancy test for the evaluation of a suspected ectopic pregnancy. Results of this test are usually available 24 hours after obtaining the specimen.

    NOTE: Usually, β-hCG results are reported in international units/liter (IU/L) reflecting a standard international reference preparation to determine the hormone level. The First International Standard (1st IS) is a purified homogenous preparation that does not cross react with the alpha subunit of hCG, thus making it a more accurate test than the initial test used for this purpose (the Second International Standard [2nd IS]). Conversion of a 2nd IS level to a 1st IS level is possible by multiplying the 2nd IS value by 1.7 (Sanfilippo & Woodworth, 1992). When evaluating a woman's β-hCG level it is important to know which reference preparation has been used (especially if the test is obtained at a different clinical laboratory). For consistency and accuracy of results, the woman should have serial testing obtained at the same clinical laboratory.

–   In normal intrauterine pregnancies, the level of this hormone is expected to double every 2 days, with measurable levels possible beginning 7 to 10 days after conception; highly sensitive (99 percent).

–   Serial testing can be done to ascertain whether a normal or abnormal pregnancy is occurring.

–   Absence of abnormal results does not confirm the presence of an ectopic pregnancy; however, such results may assist the clinician in formulating a plan of care when an ectopic pregnancy is suspected.

–   ß-hCG levels that fail to demonstrate a 66 percent increase over 48 hours are reportedly associated with an ectopic pregnancy or a spontaneous abortion of an intrauterine pregnancy in 85 percent of women.

–   An abdominal pregnancy can demonstrate ß-hCG levels that are abnormally elevated for the weeks of gestation.

–   ß-hCG levels can be used in conjunction with ultrasonography to diagnose an early ectopic pregnancy. This is especially helpful in ectopic pregnancies that are at a gestational stage when tubal rupture is less likely (i.e., a pregnancy less than 10 weeks gestation). Discriminatory zones of ß-hCG levels are values at which an intrauterine gestational sac should be visualized by ultrasound (Emerson & McCord, 1996).

–   Transabdominal ultrasound demonstrates an intrauterine gestational sac in at least 90 percent of pregnant women when the ß-hCG level is between 6000 and 6500 IU/L (International Reference Preparation). Transvaginal ultrasound can demonstrate an intrauterine gestational sac at lower ß-hCG levels, specifically between 1200 and 2000 IU/L (International Reference Preparation) (Emerson & McCord, 1996; Ory, 1992).

–   When an intrauterine pregnancy is not visualized at these discriminatory zones, the pregnancy may not be viable or may be implanted at an ectopic site.

–   Visualization of an intrauterine gestational sac does not completely eliminate the possibility of an ectopic pregnancy, since heterotopic pregnancies can occur (Emerson & McCord, 1996; Sanfilippo and Woodworth, 1992).

NOTE: Discriminatory zones should be established within individual institutions depending upon the quality of ultrasonography available, the ß-hCG radioimmunoassay techniques employed, and the reference preparation used to quantify the ß-hCG values. Clinicians should ascertain the discriminatory zones utilized in their institutions as a means of accurately evaluating their obstetrical populations (Emerson & McCord, 1996).

▶ Urine human chorionic gonadotropin (ß-hCG) tests

–   Several monoclonal antibody urine tests that are ultrasensitive are available to evaluate ß-hCG levels (Tandem Icon II®, First Response®).

–   The reported false negative rate associated with these tests is 1 percent. They can reliably detect pregnancy 7 to 10 days after conception, and have the advantage of rapid screening of women when ectopic pregnancy is suspected. However, additional testing with a serum β-hCG test and ultrasonography is indicated to rule out an ectopic pregnancy.

- Serum progesterone levels

  ▶ Abnormal pregnancies, including ectopic pregnancies and spontaneous abortions, have been associated with low serum progesterone levels.

  NOTE: A single value does not confirm the diagnosis of an ectopic pregnancy; however, a low level (i.e., less than 5 ng/mL) should alert the clinician to the possibility of an abnormal pregnancy warranting further evaluation. Additionally, the result of this test is usually available the same day the specimen is obtained.

- Ultrasonography

  ▶ Abdominal ultrasound (de Crespigny, 1987; Emerson & McCord, 1996; Ory, 1992; Sanfilippo & Woodworth, 1992)

    − Suspect an ectopic pregnancy in a woman with a β-hCG level between 6000 and 6500 IU/L and an absence of an intrauterine gestational sac 6 weeks from the woman's last menstrual period (LMP) or absence of a fetal pole 7 weeks from the LMP.

    − Confirmation of a diagnosis can be made if there is evidence of a gestational sac or fetus outside of the uterine cavity.

      * An intrauterine gestational sac-like structure (i.e., a pseudogestational sac) observed in ectopic pregnancies can be misinterpreted as an intrauterine gestational sac. This finding is a result of the accumulation of blood in the uterine cavity, the development of the decidual lining without a trophoblastic rim, or the development of a thick proliferative endometrium (de Crespigny, 1987; Emerson & McCord, 1996).

  ▶ Transvaginal ultrasound (more accurate than abdominal ultrasound in locating early gestation ectopic pregnancies) (de Crespigny, 1987; Emerson & McCord, 1996; Stovall, 1994)

    − Extrauterine fetal cardiac pulsations indicates an ectopic pregnancy.

    − A sac-like ring visualized during ultrasonography is indicative of an ectopic pregnancy.

    − Echogenic fluid may indicate an ectopic pregnancy, and correlates with a hemoperitoneum in many women.

    − Fluid in the cul-de-sac may be associated with an ectopic pregnancy.

- Culdecentesis (done by the consulting physician)

  ▶ Aspiration of nonclotted blood is indicative of an ectopic pregnancy and an intraperitoneal hemorrhage.

  ▶ The possibility of an ectopic pregnancy cannot be eliminated in the absence of fluid from the cul-de-sac.

- Laporoscopy (may be necessary to confirm the site of an ectopic implantation, evaluate bleeding, and, if indicated, remove the ectopic conceptus.)

- Cervical tests for *C. trachomatis* and *N. gonorrhoeae,* as indicated.

- Clean catch midstream urine for urinalysis and culture, as indicated.

• When a woman has had a recent therapeutic abortion, the pathology report should be obtained. If there is evidence of products of conception (POCs) then the likelihood of an ectopic pregnancy is remote.

Treatment/Management

• If the woman is in shock, immediate physician management is indicated. If the woman presents in shock in an outpatient setting that is geographically remote from a hospital, then initiate procedures necessary to stabilize the woman (e.g., insertion of an IV, oxygen therapy, etc.).

• Refer all women in stable condition suspected of having an ectopic pregnancy to a physician for consultation.

▶ The therapeutic interventions for woman with an ectopic pregnancy are determined by the consulting physician and are based on the woman's physiologic status, symptoms, stage of gestation, site of implantation, and the woman's desire to maintain her fertility.

▶ The complex decision making involved in the therapeutic interventions for an ectopic pregnancy are beyond the scope of this chapter; however, a brief presentation of these options is provided in this section.

– Expectant management: Spontaneous resolution of extrauterine pregnancies has been documented (Doyle et al., 1991; Hahlin, Thorburn, & Bryman, 1995; Shaler, Peleg, Tsabari, Ramono, & Bustan, 1995; Trio, Strobelt, Picciolo, Lapinski, & Ghidini, 1995). This evidence has resulted in the offering of this option to a select group of women with ectopic pregnancies who meet strict criteria for this intervention. These criteria include:

* An initial serum β-hCG level of <2000 IU/L

* Continued decline in hCG level

* No symptoms reported by the woman

* No diagnostic evidence of tubal rupture or bleeding by ultrasound and/or laparoscopy

* Compliance with the necessary required serial testing

* Follow-up visits

NOTE: The possible complications that have been reported in association with this option include tubal rupture, hemorrhage, and persistent ectopic pregnancy.

– Medical management: Pharmacologic agents have been studied for use in the treatment of ectopic pregnancy. The success rate for this option depends upon the type of pharmacologic agent used, the method of administration (i.e., local versus systemic administration), tolerance of the agent by the woman, gestational age of the pregnancy, and size of the gestational sac.

NOTE: There has been a higher incidence of tubal patency and reproductive performance in women receiving medical treatment of ectopic pregnancy compared to women undergoing surgical therapy (Fernandez, Lelaidier, Baton, Bourget, & Frydman, 1991; Fernandez, Pauthier, Doumerc, Lelaidier, Olivennes, Ville, & Frydman, 1995; Stovall, Ling, & Buster, 1990). Complications reportedly associated with medical interventions include possible adverse effects of the selected pharmacologic agent(s), tubal rupture, hemorrhage, and persistent ectopic pregnancy. The agents studied thus far include:

* Systemic or local administration of methotrexate. This agent has demonstrated the highest efficacy rates.

* Systemic RU486 (mifepristone) and local injections of actinomycin D, potassium chloride, and prostaglandins have been evaluated and demonstrate varying efficacy rates (Brand, Gibbs, & Davidson, 1993; Deckardt, Saks, & Graff, 1993; Jusslein, 1993; Oelsner et al., 1993).

– Surgical interventions: Various surgical interventions may be considered for the treatment of an ectopic pregnancy. The decision to choose a specific procedure is based upon the status of the woman, possibility or evidence of rupture, hemorrhage, size of the gestational sac, accessibility of the ectopic implantation site, desire of the woman to maintain fertility, experience of the surgeon, and availability of various operative instruments (i.e., laparoscopic equipment). The more conservative surgical interventions are associated with less morbidity and mortality; and have a higher likelihood of maintaining tubal patency than the more extensive surgical procedures.

NOTE: Complications reported in association with the surgical procedures utilized for the treatment of an ectopic pregnancy include hemorrhage, infection, anesthesia complications, decreased tubal patency, decreased reproductive performance, persistent ectopic pregnancy, and death. The surgical procedures that may be performed for a woman experiencing an ectopic pregnancy include

* Laparoscopy with removal of the POCs and/or oviduct

* Linear salpingostomy

* Segmental resection of the fallopian tube

* Salpingectomy

* Laparotomy

* Hysteroscopy

● Women who are Rh negative and antibody screen (D^u) negative should be given $Rh(D^u)$ immune globulin at the following doses (ACOG, 1990b):

▶ $Rh(D^u)IG$ (Micro RhoGam®) 50 μg IM administered to a woman with a gestation of less than 13 weeks.

▶ $Rh(D^u)IG$ (RhoGam®) 300 μg IM administered to a woman with a gestation of more than 13 weeks.

Consultation

● Refer all women suspected of having an ectopic pregnancy to a physician for consultation. The consulting physician will determine the therapeutic interventions for the woman. Co-management with a physician is possible for women undergoing expectant or medical management.

- Consult with a psychologist or psychiatrist, if women and their partners exhibit symptoms of severe depression as a result of the pregnancy loss. This may be especially important in women/couples who had an assisted reproduction procedure to conceive, or in situations when the threat of loss of the woman's life was evident.

Patient Education

- Educate the woman with a suspected or documented ectopic pregnancy about the possible problem(s), the diagnostic tests that may be ordered, treatment options, possible complications, and follow-up.

- If the woman is exhibiting signs and symptoms of shock, then give as complete an explanation as is reasonably possible regarding her plan of care.

- Women receiving outpatient therapy (e.g., expectant or medical management) must be educated about the possibility of a sudden rupture of an ectopic pregnancy and the rapid blood loss associated with this complication.

  ▶ Give a thorough presentation of the signs and symptoms of a tubal rupture and hemorrhage.

  ▶ Advise her not to operate motor vehicles or be involved in similar activities requiring this type of concentration and responsibility because of the possibility of syncopal episodes as a result of significant blood loss if tubal rupture occurs.

  ▶ In addition, help her devise a plan for immediate access to emergency services if any signs or symptoms of a tubal rupture or hemorrhage develop and include a means of transportation to the hospital, other than driving herself, if tubal rupture or hemorrhage is suspected.

- The woman, her partner, and family should receive emotional and psychological support to help her/them work through the loss of a desired pregnancy and the implications this may have on future pregnancies.

- Educate the woman regarding her increased risk of having another ectopic pregnancy. Advise her that any time she may suspect that she is pregnant she should obtain medical evaluation due to her increased risk of a recurrence of this problem.

- Educate the woman about the signs and symptoms of possible complications following surgery for an ectopic pregnancy (e.g., infection, excessive bleeding, etc.). Ideally, this should be done by the physician performing the surgical procedure.

- Educate the Rh-negative, antibody-negative woman about the need for RhoGam® administration after an ectopic pregnancy has been terminated.

- If a woman undergoing treatment for an ectopic pregnancy does not have evidence of rubella immunity, she should be considered for rubella immunization. If the rubella immunization is to be administered, the woman should be counseled to prevent conception for at least 3 months (see below).

- Once therapy for an ectopic pregnancy has been completed, the woman should be counseled about the need to prevent conception for 3 months to allow the implantation site of the ectopic to completely recover (Ory 1992). Contraception should be provided once a thorough discussion about available options has taken place.

Follow-up

- Follow-up evaluations of and changes in the plan of care for a woman with an ectopic pregnancy are per consulting physician recommendations.

- After treatment for an ectopic pregnancy a woman should have serum ß-hCG levels monitored to assess resolution of the condition.

  - ▶ The gestation of the pregnancy and the type of therapeutic intervention determine the frequency of testing.

  - ▶ A consistent decline in serum ß-hCG level should be demonstrated (Ory, 1992).

  - ▶ If the level plateaus or begins to increase, further evaluation and possibly a change in therapy may be necessary.

- Document diagnosis of ectopic pregnancy and treatment/management thereof in problem list and progress notes.

References

American College of Obstetricians & Gynecologists (ACOG). (1990a). *Prevention of D isoimmunization.* ACOG Technical Bulletin no. 147. Washington, DC: Author.

American College of Obstetricians & Gynecologists (ACOG). (1990b). *Ectopic pregnancy.* (ACOG Technical Bulletin no. 150).Washington, DC: Author.

Beckmann, C. R. B., Ling, F. W., Barzansky, B. M., Bates, G. W., Herbert, W. N. P., Laube, D. W., & Smith, R. P. (1995). *Obstetrics and gynecology* (2nd ed., pp. 321–331). Baltimore, MD: Williams & Wilkins.

Brand, E., Gibbs, R. S., Davidson, S. A. (1993). Advanced cervical pregnancy treated with actinomycin-D. *British Journal of Obstetrics and Gynaecology, 100*(5), 491–492.

De Crespigny, L. (1987). The value of ultrasound in ectopic pregnancy. *Clinical Obstetrics and Gynecology, 30*(1), 136–147.

Deckardt, R., Saks, M. & Graff, H. (1993). Laparoscopic therapy for tubal pregnancy using prostaglandins. *Journal of Reproductive Medicine, 38*(8), 587–591.

Doyle, M. B., DeCherney, A. H., & Diamond, M. P. (1991). Epidemiology and etiology of ectopic pregnancy. *Obstetrics and Gynecology Clinics of North America, 18*(1), 1–17.

Emerson, D. S., & McCord, M. L. (1996). Clinician's approach to ectopic pregnancy. *Clinical Obstetrics and Gynecology, 39*(1), 199–222.

Fernandez, H., Lelaidier, C., Baton, C., Bourget, P., & Frydman, R. (1991). Return of reproductive performance after expectant management and local treatment for ectopic pregnancy. *Human Reproduction, 6*(10), 1474–1477.

Fernandez, H., Pauthier, S., Doumerc, S., Lelaidier, C., Olivennes, F., Ville, Y., & Frydman, R. (1995). Ultrasound-guided injection of methotrexate versus laparoscopic salpingotomy in ectopic pregnancy. *Fertility and Sterility, 63*(1), 25–29.

Goldner, T. E., Lawson, H. W., Xia, Z., & Atrash, H. K. (1993). Surveillance for ectopic pregnancy— United States, 1978–1989. *Morbidity & Mortality Weekly Report, 42*(6), 73–85.

Hahlin, M., Thorburn, J., & Bryman, I. (1995). The expectant management of early pregnancies of uncertain site. *Human Reproduction, 10*(5), 1223–1227.

Jusslein, P. (1993). Conservative treatment for ectopic pregnancy by local application of prostaglandins. *European Journal of Obstetric, Gynaecologic, & Reproductive Biology, 49,* 72–75.

Martin, J. N., & McCaul, J. F. (1990). Emergent management of abdominal pregnancy. *Clinical Obstetrics and Gynecology, 33*(3), 438–447.

Maymon, R., Shulman, A., Maymon, B. B., Bar-Levy, F., Lotan, M., & Bahary, C. (1992). *International Journal of Fertility, 37*(3), 146–164.

Oelsner, G., Admon, D., Shalev, E., Shalev, Y., Kukia, E., & Mashiach, S. (1993). A new approach for the treatment of interstitial pregnancy. *Fertility and Sterility, 59*(4), 924–925.

Ory, S. J. (1992). New options for diagnosis and treatment of ectopic pregnancy. *Journal of the American Medical Association, 267*(4), 534–537.

Osguthorpe, N. C., & Keating, C. E. (1988). Ectopic pregnancy. Surgical intervention and perioperative nursing care. *AORN Journal.,48*(2). 254–267.

Pernoll, M. L., & Garmel, S. H. (1994). Early pregnancy risks. In A. H. DeCherney & M.L. Pernoll (Eds.), *Current obstetric & gynecologic diagnosis & treatment* (8th ed., pp. 306–331). Norwalk, CT: Appleton & Lange.

Sanfilippo, J. S., & Woodworth, S. H. (1992). Ectopic pregnancy. *TeLinde's Operative Gynecology Updates, 1*(4), 1–14.

Seifer, D. B., Diamond, M. P., & DeCherney, A. H. (1991). Persistent ectopic pregnancy. *Obstetrics and Gynecology Clinics of North America, 18*(1), 153–159.

Shalev, E., Peleg, D., Tsabari, A., Romano, S., & Bustan, M. (1995). Spontaneous resolution of ectopic tubal pregnancy: Natural history. *Fertility and Sterility, 63*(1), 15–19.

Slaughter, J. L., & Grimes, D. A. (1995). Methotrexate therapy. Nonsurgical management of ectopic pregnancy. *Western Journal of Medicine, 162*(3), 225–228.

Stovall, T. G. (1994). Medical management of ectopic pregnancy. *Current Opinion in Obstetrics and Gynecology, 6*, 510–515.

Stovall, T. G., Ling, F. W., & Buster, J. E. (1990). Reproductive performance after methotrexate treatmeant of ectopic pregnancy. *American Journal of Obstetrics and Gynecology, 162*(6), 1620–1624.

Trio, D., Strobelt, N., Picciolo, C., Lapinski, R. H., & Ghidini, A. (1995). Prognostic factors for successful expectant management of ectopic pregnancy. *Fertility and Sterility, 63*(3), 469–472.

Wyte, C. D. (1994). Diagnostic modalities in the pregnant patient. *Emergency Medicine Clinics of North America, 12*(1), 9–43.

Chapter 9

ENDOMETRITIS

Ellen M. Scarr

Lucy Newmark Sammons

Postpartum endometritis (PPE), an infectious inflammation of the inner lining of the uterus, is the most common infection in the postpartum patient (Druelinger, 1994). Alternatively, it may be referred to as endomyometritis or endoparametritis, because either the myometrium, parametrium or decidua may be involved. Early PPE develops within 48 hours after delivery, generally following cesarean section, while late PPE may occur 3 days to 6 weeks postpartum, usually after vaginal delivery. Late PPE tends to be milder clinically. The incidence of PPE varies from 1 to 3 percent in uncomplicated vaginal delivery, 5 to 10 percent after elective cesarean section (before the onset of labor), to 85 to 95 percent in nonelective cesarean delivery in the high-risk patient (Calhoun & Brost, 1995; Druelinger, 1994).

The etiology of PPE is polymicrobial, usually involving vaginal organisms (Pedler & Orr, 1995). Common causative organisms include gram positive aerobes (Group A, B, D streptococcus, enterococcus), gram-negative aerobes (*Escherichia coli*, *Klebsiella*, *enterobacterium* sp., *Gardnerella vaginalis*) and anaerobes (*Bacteroides* sp., *Peptostreptococcus* sp.). *Chlamydia trachomatis* and genital mycoplasmas (*Mycoplasma hominis, Ureaplasma urealyticum*) are often responsible for late PPE. Additionally, 20 percent of patients with PPE have an associated bacteremia (Craigo & Kapernick, 1994; Druelinger, 1994). Recently, herpes simplex virus has been reported as the causative agent in several cases of postpartum endometritis (Hollier, Scott, Murphree, & Wendel, 1997).

The risks for PPE include cesarean section, chorioamnionitis, prolonged rupture of membranes, prolonged labor, and frequent vaginal exams. Whether internal fetal monitoring is a risk for PPE is controversial. Lower socioeconomic status, anemia and extremes of maternal age have also been correlated with PPE (Calhoun & Brost, 1995; Gant & Cunningham, 1993; Garite, 1990; Pedler & Orr, 1995). Extension of infection into the pelvic peritoneum can result in abscess formation, pelvic thrombophlebitis, generalized peritonitis, disseminated intravascular coagulation (DIC), septic shock and infertility.

Database

Subjective

- History may include
  - ▶ Chorioamnionitis
  - ▶ Cesarean delivery (especially surgery longer than 60 minutes, blood loss greater than 800 mL)
  - ▶ Premature/prolonged rupture of membranes (longer than 24 hours)
  - ▶ Long labor (more than 12 hours)
  - ▶ Instrumentation/other operative interference during current delivery

    ▶ Incomplete placental removal

    ▶ Perinatal hemorrhage/hematoma

- Client complains of lower abdominal pain and lower back pain.

- Postpartum temperature elevation may be preceded by constitutional changes (malaise, anorexia, myalgia, diaphoresis, or chills).

- Client may report

    ▶ Purulent or foul smelling lochia

    ▶ Constipation

- Client denies dysuria, frequency, urgency, flank pain.

Objective

- Temperature of 38° C (100.4° F) or more on any 2 of the first 10 days postpartum, excluding the first 24 hours (Musci, 1993)

- Pulse rate elevated or normal

- Observable diaphoresis/chills if virulent infection

- Abdominal tenderness, possibly rigidity

- Abnormal (increased amount, dark red/brown, malodorous) discharge may be seen at external genitalia, vaginal vault, and cervix

NOTE: Only scant, odorless lochia may be present (associated with beta-hemolytic streptococcal infection).

- Tenderness/swelling in uterus/adnexa or uterus may be soft and/or subinvoluted upon bimanual examination

- Macular rash and hypotension (suggest postpartum toxic shock syndrome [TSS])

- Paralytic ileus may be concomitant problem (signs include abdominal distention, hypoactive bowel sounds, and constipation)

- Physical examination otherwise negative for signs of localized infection or systemic disease

- Complete blood count (CBC) may reveal leukocytosis

NOTE: Leukocytosis may be present (white blood cell count up to 20,000 m^3) in the absence of infection during the normal postpartum period (Faro, 1990).

- Urine dipstick negative for leukocyte esterase, nitrites; requires catheterized specimen due to presence of lochia

Assessment

- Postpartum endometritis, early or late

    ▶ R/O cystitis

▶ R/O pyelonephritis

▶ R/O mastitis

▶ R/O severe breast engorgement

▶ R/O appendicitis

▶ R/O cesarean wound infection

▶ R/O septic pelvic thrombophlebitis

▶ R/O pelvic abscess

▶ R/O TSS

▶ R/O paralytic ileus

▶ R/O respiratory complications, pulmonary atelectasis

▶ R/O thrombophlebitis of lower extremities

Plan

Diagnostic Tests

Determined by severity of symptoms:

● Testing for *Chlamydia trachomatis*

● Blood cultures

● Cesarean wound culture

● Transcervical endometrial culture

● Urine culture

● CBC, sedimentation rate

● Ultrasound to assess for pelvic/abdominal abscess

● Computed tomography (CT) scan to assess for pelvic vein thrombosis

Treatment/Management

● Severe cases require inpatient intravenous antibiotic and fluid administration. Parenteral regimens include single agent second- and third-generation cephalosporins and newer semi-synthetic penicillins. Details of inpatient therapy are beyond the scope of this protocol.

● Outpatient use of antibiotics varies by institution and early or late-onset pathophysiology. Outpatient regimens for milder cases may include (but are not limited to) (Druelinger, 1994; Pedler & Orr, 1995):

▶ Cephalexin 500 mg p.o. q.i.d. for 7 to 10 days

▶ Ampicillin 500 mg p.o. q.i.d. for 7 to 10 days

▶ Doxycycline 100 mg p.o. b.i.d. for 7 to 10 days

NOTE: Use of doxycycline in lactating women is controversial, but gaining more acceptance.

▶ Erythromycin 500 mg p.o. q.i.d. for 7 to 10 days

▶ Clindamycin 450 mg p.o. q.i.d. for 7 to 10 days

- Increased oral fluids, if tolerated

- Analgesics for pain relief—consider lactation status (e.g., acetaminophen, acetaminophen with codeine, ibuprofen)

- If subinvolution is present, treat per subinvolution protocol

- Prevention may be enhanced by adequate diet and prevention/correction of anemia

- See also Patient Education.

Consultation

- Physician consultation required in all cases.

Patient Education

- Explain the causes and treatment approaches employed for endometritis.

- Advise bedrest in semi-Fowler's position; advise maintenance of pelvic rest until infection is resolved.

- Provide concrete suggestions for realistic management of the newborn, self-care, household, and other family members.

- Counsel regarding restorative diet and maintenance of good hydration.

Follow-up

- If symptoms worsen or fail to respond, reassess immediately.

- If adequate symptom response and good patient compliance, reassess in 48 to 72 hours.

- Public health nurse/social services referral for woman with multiple children, demanding home situation, etc.

- Document diagnosis of endometritis and treatment thereof in progress notes and problem list.

References

Calhoun, B., & Brost, B. (1995). Emergency management of sudden puerperal fever. *Obstetrics and Gynecology Clinics of North America, 22*(2), 357–367.

Craigo, S., & Kapernick P. (1994). Postpartum hemorrhage and the abnormal puerperium. In A. DeCherney & M. Pernoll (Eds.), *Current obstetric and gynecologic diagnosis and treatment* (8th ed., pp. 574–593). Norwalk, CT: Appleton & Lange.

Druelinger, L. (1994). Postpartum emergencies. *Emergency Medicine Clinics of North America, 12*(1), 219–237.

Faro, S. (1990). Postpartum endometritis. In L. Gilstrap & S. Faro (Eds.), *Infections in pregnancy* (pp. 45–54). New York: Wiley-Liss.

Gant, N., & Cunningham, F. (Eds.). (1993). *Basic gynecology and obstetrics* (pp. 381–386). Norwalk, CT: Appleton & Lange.

Garite, T. (1990). Amnionitis. In E. Quilligan & F. Zuspan, (Eds.), *Current therapy in obstetrics and gynecology* (3rd ed., pp. 190–192). Philadelphia, PA: W.B. Saunders.

Hollier, L., Scott, L., Murphree, S., & Wendel, G. (1997). Postpartum endometritis caused by herpes simplex virus. *Obstetrics & Gynecology, 89*(5, pt 2), 836–838.

Musci, T. (1993). Postpartum care. In J.Brown & W. Crombleholme, (Eds.), *Handbook of gynecology and obstetrics* (pp. 530–546). Norwalk, CT: Appleton & Lange.

Pedler, S., & Orr, K. (1995). Bacterial, fungal and parasitic infections. In W. Barron & M. Lindheimer (Eds.), *Medical disorders during pregnancy* (2nd ed., pp. 356–388). St. Louis, MO: Mosby.

Chapter 10

FETAL ARRHYTHMIAS

Maureen T. Shannon

Variations in fetal heart rate (FHR) are commonly observed as normal pregnancy progresses. Fetal cardiac activity begins approximately 22 days after conception at a rate of 90 to 100 beats per minute (bpm). The FHR then increases to approximately 170 to 180 bpm at 8 to 9 weeks' gestation and subsequently declines to approximately 140 to 150 bpm between 15 to 20 weeks' gestation. During the latter part of pregnancy, the FHR decreases until it reaches an average resting rate of 130 bpm at term, beat-to-beat variability develops, and intermittent accelerations in response to fetal movements are observed (Cullen, 1992; Ito, Magee, & Smallhorn, 1994).

By definition, a fetal arrhythmia is any irregularity of fetal cardiac rhythm not associated with a uterine contraction or a sustained rhythm outside of the parameters of 100 to 160 bpm (Cullen, 1992; Pinsky, Rayburn, & Evans, 1991). Fetal arrhythmias may occur as a primary condition or as a result of another condition (e.g., fetal distress, infection, uterine contractions, cardiac structural abnormalities) (Ito et al., 1994). Irregular FHRs are noted in 1 to 3 percent of pregnancies with 10 percent of these associated with serious fetal morbidity (Cullen, 1992; Meijboom et al., 1994). Benign FHR irregularities are usually intermittent, transient, and brief in duration (i.e., for only a few seconds). Conversely, pathological arrhythmias are usually observed for several minutes (Cullen, 1992).

Generally, fetal arrhythmias can be classified on the basis of their rate and regularity. Identification and classification of fetal arrhythmias provides a means of determining the morbidity associated with a particular fetal cardiac irregularity, and a mechanism for developing an appropriate plan of care.

Categories of Arrhythmias

Irregular rhythm

Usually these arrhythmias are intermittent, and resolve before delivery or within a few days after birth (Fyfe, Meyer, & Case, 1993). They are most often the result of an atrial ectopic beat (i.e., atrial premature beat). Occasionally an irregular rhythm may originate in the atrioventricular (AV) node, or represent a premature ventricular contraction (PVC) or a tachyarrhythmia with AV block (Cullen, 1992; Fyfe et al., 1993; Pinsky et al., 1991). Auscultation of one extra systole for every ten beats is not uncommon. In 1 to 2 percent of affected fetuses, these arrhythmias are associated with a cardiac structural abnormality; in another 1 to 2 percent of affected fetuses, a persistent arrhythmia (i.e., sustained tachycardia) may develop resulting in a subsequent problem (e.g., in utero congestive heart failure) (Cullen, 1992).

Tachycardias

Fetal tachycardia is characterized by a sustained or intermittent, regular or irregular FHR of greater than 160 bpm; and includes sinus tachycardia and supraventricular tachycardia (e.g., atrial fibrillation, atrial flutter) (Cullen, 1992; Ito et al., 1994). This arrhythmia occurs in 0.4 to 0.6 percent of all pregnancies, and is responsible for 10 percent of documented fetal arrhythmias. The majority of fetal tachycardic arrhythmias are not associated with congenital heart disease; however, in 5 to 10 percent of affected fetuses, a structural cardiac abnormality is observed (Simpson and Marx, 1994).

Possible etiologies include a reentry phenomenon involving the atria and the ventricles or a reentry pathway within the AV node (the majority of supraventricular tachycardias), maternal hyperthyroidism, maternal fever, maternal drug ingestion, and fetal distress (Cullen, 1992; Meijboom et al., 1994). Fetal tachycardias resulting from a supraventricular or ventricular focus are rare. Sustained, uncontrolled fetal tachycardias may lead to inutero cardiac failure, fetal hydrops, and fetal death and therefore require therapeutic interventions specifically targeted to interrupt the arrhythmia (Ito et al., 1994; Meijboom et al., 1994).

Bradycardias

Fetal bradycardia is characterized by a sustained or intermittent, regular or irregular FHR less than or equal to 100 bpm (Ito et al., 1994; Meijboom et al., 1994). Bradycardias account for less than 5 percent of all fetal arrhythmias (Cullen, 1992). Arrhythmias included in this category are sinus bradycardia (usually a result of fetal distress), blocked atrial ectopic beats, and complete heart block (CHB). CHB can be further classified as isolated CHB (i.e., without evidence of a structural cardiac defect) or CHB associated with a structural heart defect (Cullen, 1992; Fyfe et al., 1993; Meijboom et al., 1994). When complete heart block is present in combination with a cardiac malformation, there is a perinatal mortality rate of 80 percent (Fyfe et al., 1993). Isolated CHB may be idiopathic or a result of maternal connective tissue disease (i.e., systemic lupus erythematosis [SLE]) (Cullen, 1992; Meijboom et al., 1994).

Database

Subjective

Usually the woman will be asymptomatic, but may report a history of or symptoms indicative of a condition associated with the development of a particular fetal arrhythmia.

- Tachycardias
  - ▶ The woman may report one or more of the following:
    - Fever
    - Ingestion of a prescription or illicit drug that may cause fetal tachycardia (e.g., cocaine, methamphetamine)
    - Symptoms associated with hyperthyroidism (see Chapter 12.2, *Hyperthyroidism*)
- Bradycardias
  - ▶ The woman may report one or more of the following:
    - History of connective tissue disease (i.e., SLE)
    - Ingestion of a prescription or illicit drug (e.g., opiates, barbiturates)
    - Symptoms associated with perinatal complications that may result in fetal bradycardia (e.g., placental abruption, fetal movement, etc.)

Objective

The physical examination of the woman is usually within normal limits but may reveal clinical manifestations of an underlying condition associated with the development of a particular fetal arrhythmia. Auscultation of fetal heart rate will demonstrate an abnormal rate depending upon the existing arrhythmia.

- Fetal tachycardia

  ▶ FHR auscultation will reveal a rate of more than 160 bpm which may be regular or irregular, vary in duration, and be independent of fetal movement.

  ▶ In addition, one of the following may be documented:

    – Temperature elevation (in women with a systemic illness)

    – Clinical manifestations of hyperthyroidism (see Chapter 12.2, *Hyperthyroidism*).

- Fetal bradycardia

  ▶ FHR auscultation will reveal a rate of 100 bpm or less, which may be regular or irregular, sustained or intermittent, and may or may not be associated with uterine activity.

  ▶ In addition, one of the following may be documented:

    – Clinical manifestations of maternal SLE (e.g., joint inflammation, "butterfly" rash, splinter hemorrhages of nailbeds, etc.)

    – Evidence of possible opiate, barbiturate or other substance use associated with fetal bradycardias (e.g., somnomulence, dilated pupils, slurred speech, etc.)

    – Clinical manifestations of placental abruption (see Chapter 6.5, *Second and Third Trimester Bleeding*)

Plan

Diagnostic Tests

The following tests may be ordered after consultation with a physician.

- Ultrasound (may reveal the presence of a structural cardiac defect, fetal hydrops in situations with substantial fetal compromise)

- M-mode echocardiography (will reveal the type of arrhythmia present)

- Maternal autoantibody testing (should be ordered in any woman with documented isolated CHB) may include

  ▶ Antinuclear antibody test (will be positive in women with lupus)

  ▶ Anti-Ro antibodies (may be positive in women with connective tissue disorders)

- Thyroid function tests (will be abnormal in women with hyperthyroidism) (see Chapter 12.2, *Hyperthyroidism*)

- Antenatal fetal assessment, such as nonstress tests, amniotic fluid index, contraction stress tests (may be ordered and will range from within normal limits [WNL] to abnormal if fetal well-being is compromised)

Consultation

- Consult with a physician if any woman is suspected of or documented to have a pathological fetal arrhythmia.

- Transfer the care of women with pathological fetal arrhythmias to a physician.

Treatment/Management

The therapeutic interventions indicated in the care of a women with documented evidence of a pathologic fetal arrhythmia are the responsibility of the physician managing her care. A detailed presentation of all of the treatment options is beyond the scope of this chapter. However, a brief description of the therapeutic interventions for various fetal arrhythmias is presented in Table 6.6, Characteristics, Evaluation, and Treatment of Fetal Arrhythmias.

Patient Education

- If the woman has a documented pathologic fetal arrhythmia, discuss the reason(s) for transfer of care to a physician.

- Educate the woman with a documented pathologic fetal arrhythmia about its possible etiology, diagnostic tests indicated, therapeutic interventions available, and the prognosis. Follow-up is the responsibility of the physician managing the woman's care.

- Reassure a woman with normal diagnostic testing that the presence of a benign arrhythmia will not adversely effect her infant.

Follow-up

- Follow-up evaluations of the woman with a suspected or documented fetal arrhythmia are per recommendation of the consulting physician.

- A woman with a FHR irregularity without evidence of specific pathology should have weekly FHR auscultation, and begin weekly nonstress tests at 34 weeks' gestation (Cullen, 1992).

- Document diagnosis of fetal arrhythmia and management thereof in progress notes and problem list.

Table 6.6

Characteristics, Evaluation, and Treatment of Fetal Arrhythmias

Arrhythmia	Incidence during pregnancy	Beats per minute	Rhythm	Possible etiology	Evaluation	Treatment
Irregular Beat	1 - 3 %	120 - 160	Irregular	Atrial premature beats, ventricular premature beats, normal variant	Two dimensional/ M-mode echocardiography	Frequent auscultation, fetal movement counts, nonstress testing
Tachycardia	0.4 - 0.6 %	>160	Regular	Hyperthyroidism, fever, drugs, fetal distress	Two dimensional/ M-mode echocardiography; consider Doppler flow, thyroid testing, maternal screen for illicit and licit drugs, amniocentesis	Referral to perinatologist. Treatment: expectant management, delivery, maternal therapy for underlying condition (e.g., infection) or to control fetal arrhythmia (e.g., digoxin), and direct fetal therapy.
			Irregular	Cardiac tumor, cardiac anomaly		
Bradycardia	0.1 - 0.3 %	≤ 100	Regular	Reflex, fetal distress, atrioventricular block, complete heart block	Two dimensional/ M-mode echocardiography, Doppler flow, amniocentesis; maternal connective tissue evaluation if heart block	Referral to perinatologist. Treatment: expectant management, delivery. If maternal SLE, consider corticosteriods or immunoglobulin therapy before fetal cardiac damage occurs.
			Irregular	Complete heart block, ectopy/abnormal conduction		

Sources: Adapted from Cullen, T. (1992). Evaluation of Fetal Arrhythmias. *American Family Physician, 46*(6), 1746. Copyright 1993 by the Publications Division of the American Academy of Family Physicians. Adapted with permission.

References

Cullen, T. (1992). Evaluation of fetal arrhythmias. *American Family Physician, 46*(6), 1745–1749.

Fyfe, D.A., Meyer, K.B., & Case, C.L. (1993). Sonographic assessment of fetal cardiac arrhythmias. *Seminars in Ultrasound, CT, and MRI, 14*(4), 286–297.

Ito, S., Magee, L., & Smallhorn, J. (1994). Drug therapy for fetal arrhythmias. *Clinics in Perinatology, 21*(3), 543–572.

Meijboom, E.J., van Engelen, A.D., van de Beek, E. W., Weijtens, O., Lautenschutz, J.M., & Benatar, A.A. (1994). Fetal arrhythmias. *Current Opinion in Cardiology, 9*, 97–102.

Pinsky, W.W., Rayburn, W. F., & Evans, M. I. (1991). Pharmacologic therapy for fetal arrhythmias. *Clinical Obstetrics and Gynecology, 34*(2), 304–309.

Simpson, L.L., & Marx, G.R. (1994). Diagnosis and treatment of structural fetal cardiac abnormality and dysrhythmia. *Seminars in Perinatology, 18*(3), 215–227.

Chapter 11

GESTATIONAL DIABETES MELLITUS

Winifred L. Star

Joan R. Murphy

Definition

Gestational diabetes mellitus (GDM) is defined as glucose intolerance of variable severity with onset or initial recognition during the current pregnancy. This definition applies regardless of whether insulin is used for treatment or the condition persists after pregnancy; it does not exclude the possibility that unrecognized glucose intolerance may have antedated the pregnancy or begun concomitantly with the pregnancy (American College of Obstetrics and Gynecology [ACOG], 1994; American Diabetes Association [ADA], 1997; Avery & Rossi, 1994). In the majority of cases, glucose regulation returns to normal after delivery. At 6 weeks or more postpartum, the gestational diabetic should be reclassified as having either normoglycemia, impaired fasting glucose (IFG), impaired glucose tolerance (IGT), or diabetes (ADA, 1997).

Pathophysiology

The metabolic stress of pregnancy associated with fetal and placental growth results in various degrees of impairment of maternal carbohydrate tolerance. Both genetic and hormonal factors influence the development of GDM in susceptible individuals. In early normal pregnancy (0 to 20 weeks), estrogen/progesterone-induced metabolic alterations are reflected in hypertrophy of insulin secreting cells of the pancreas and increased insulin action at the level of muscle and adipose tissue. In the latter half of pregnancy (20 to 40 weeks), the increased level of human placental lactogen (HPL) and other placental hormones act as peripheral antagonists to the action of insulin. The sum of these hormonal changes results in a modest state of insulin resistance, increases in hepatic glucose production and mobilization of glycogen stores, and a decrease in glucose tolerance which results in higher postprandial blood glucose levels (Avery & Rossi, 1994; Hollingsworth, 1985; Nelson, 1984).

Despite the decline in glucose tolerance, most women are able to maintain normal blood glucose levels; women who are not able to do so meet the criteria for GDM (see Screening and Diagnostic Tests section). GDM develops either from an inability to meet the increased insulin needs of pregnancy or to an exaggerated resistance to insulin, or a combination of the two. Thin women with GDM tend to have a relative insulin deficiency whereas obese women tend to be more insulin resistant (Avery & Rossi, 1994). Approximately 10 percent of pregnant women may have glycosuria without aberrations in blood glucose values. The increased glomerular filtration rate (GFR) that occurs during pregnancy overcomes the renal threshold for resorbing glucose and results in renal glycosuria. This condition is more frequent in primiparas.

Diagnosis, Prevalence, and Perinatal Implications

How best to conduct screening and diagnosis for GDM will vary among clinical sites. Although the majority of obstetric practices in the United States perform universal screening, worldwide agreement about the appropriateness of this approach is lacking (Coustan, 1996). In addition, due to the absence of a clinically meaningful threshold relationship between maternal glucose values and peri-natal outcomes, diagnostic criteria will probably be determined by consensus (Sacks et al., 1995).

Depending upon the diagnostic criteria, GDM occurs in approximately 1 to 5 percent of all U.S. pregnancies or 0.15 to 12.3 percent of pregnancies worldwide (Avery & Rossi, 1994; Coustan & Carpenter, 1985). Prevalence varies markedly throughout the world and among racial and ethnic groups in the same country (ADA, 1995). There appears to be an increased risk of GDM among black, Hispanic, Native American, and Asian women, as well as those from the Indian subcontinent. (ACOG, 1994; Avery & Rossi, 1994; Moore, 1994; U.S. Preventive Services Task Force, 1996). The majority of women with GDM (75 percent) can maintain normal glucose levels through diet alone. A subgroup of gestational diabetics (10 to 15 percent) require insulin therapy to control fasting or postprandial hyperglycemia (Berry & Gabbe, 1986).

Maternal hyperglycemia increases the risk of stillbirth, macrosomia, birth trauma, and neonatal hypo-glycemia in the perinatal period (Northern California Kaiser Permanente Regional Perinatal Council, 1994). It should be noted, however, that the level of glycemia that reduces fetal and/or neonatal complications has not been established (ACOG, 1994). The relationship between glucose levels and risks of short- and long-term maternal/fetal complications likely exists on a continuum (Sacks et al., 1995). Perinatal mortality of the gestational diabetic who is euglycemic may not be increased over the general population, provided optimal obstetric care is maintained (Coustan & Carpenter, 1985; *Diabetes*, 1985; Gabbe & Landon, 1987).

The maternal/fetal risks associated with undetected GDM are significant and preventable. Perinatal mortality is a result of ketoacidosis, hypoxia, congenital anomalies, and respiratory distress syn-drome. The most common neonatal complications include macrosomia, birth trauma, hyperbili-rubinemia, hypoglycemia, hypocalcemia, and polycythemia. The incidence of macrosomia may be double that of the general population. Because of maternal hyperglycemia, fetal blood glucose levels increase and fetal hyperinsulinemia occurs. This results in increased fetal body fat and larger organ size. These infants are at greater risk for obesity and diabetes (primarily Type 2) later in life (Avery & Rossi, 1994). Maternal complications include spontaneous abortion, pyelonephritis, preterm labor and/or delivery, polyhydramnios, preeclampsia, and increased rates of cesarean section (Kitzmiller et al., 1988; Moore, 1994; Reed, 1988). Preconceptional management to achieve tight blood glucose control as well as advances in obstetrical care have led to improvement in perinatal survival and decreased perinatal morbidity.

As mentioned, the majority (90 percent) of cases of new onset diabetes diagnosed during pregnancy resolve postpartum. However, approximately 40 to 60 percent of women with GDM will develop overt diabetes mellitus at some point in their lives, often within 20 years of the initial diagnosis (ACOG, 1994; ADA, 1995; Avery & Rossi, 1994). Future risk of developing overt diabetes is greatly influenced by body weight, with the highest incidence among obese women (Reece, Homko, & Hagay, 1995). With adequate weight loss and exercise after delivery, the incidence of subsequent development of diabetes can be reduced to 25 percent (ADA, 1995).

Details of management of the *pregestational diabetic* and the *insulin-dependent* gestational diabetic are beyond the scope of this chapter, and in many settings, care of these women is primarily the re-sponsibility of the physician and a multidisciplinary team. A program entitled "Sweet Success" has established guidelines for care of women who have overt diabetes prior to pregnancy as well as for those who develop GDM. The program is administered by the State of California Health Department, Maternal and Child Health Branch. The Sweet Success guidelines for care publication can be obtained through the California Diabetes and Pregnancy Program, University of California, San Diego, 4542 Ruffner Street, Suite 130, San Diego, CA 92111 (phone: [619] 467-4990, fax: [619] 467-4993). This chapter utilizes many of the guidelines of the Sweet Success program.

Database

Subjective

- Risk factors for GDM include (Freeman, 1997; Moore, 1994; Sweet Success, 1997)

  ▶ Previous obstetric history of gestational diabetes, macrosomic infant (> 4000 gm), unexplained stillbirth, congenital anomalies

  ▶ Obesity (> 120 percent of desirable body weight)

  ▶ Family history of overt diabetes in first degree relative (i.e., parent, sibling, child)

  ▶ Age 25 years or older

  ▶ Member of certain ethnic group (see the introductory section)

  NOTE: Approximately 50 percent of women with GDM lack specific risk factors (ACOG, 1994).

- Patient is usually asymptomatic but may complain of polyuria, polydipsia, and/or polyphagia (more common in uncontrolled overt diabetes predating pregnancy)

Objective

- Physical assessment of a well-controlled gestational diabetic should be within normal limits (WNL). Variations may include

  ▶ Client that is obese and/or hypertensive

  ▶ Urine dipstick revealing glucosuria greater than 1+ on two or more occasions, or presence of ketones when GDM uncontrolled

  ▶ Evidence of bacteria on urinalysis or culture

  ▶ Uterine fundal height more than 2 cm above that expected for dates in the second or third trimester (suspect macrosomia or polyhydramnios)

- Macrosomia, polyhydramnios and/or presence of "thick placenta" may be evidenced by ultrasound in an uncontrolled gestational diabetic.

- Fetal movement should be in the normal range (ten movements within 2 hours) at 28 weeks and thereafter in an uncompromised pregnancy.

- If utilized, nonstress test (NST) should be reactive and contraction stress test (CST) negative in the absence of fetal distress. Biophysical profile (BPP) should be 8 to 10 in an uncompromised pregnancy. (See discussion of antenatal fetal surveillance in Treatment/Management section.)

- In well-controlled gestational diabetes, fasting blood glucose (FBG) should be less than or equal to 90 mg/dL and 1-hour postprandial blood glucose less than or equal to 130 mg/dL (Sweet Success, 1997).

Assessment

- Gestational diabetes mellitus (classified as either diet-controlled or requiring insulin)
  - ▶ R/O renal glucosuria
  - ▶ R/O asymptomatic bacteriuria
  - ▶ R/O urinary tract infection
  - ▶ R/O pregnancy induced hypertension/Preeclampsia
  - ▶ R/O macrosomia
  - ▶ R/O polyhydramnios
  - ▶ R/O fetal anomaly

Plan

Universal screening of all women for GDM versus *selective screening* of only those women with traditional risk factors should be decided upon by the obstetric practice. In addition, the clinical practice site must choose which criteria they wish to apply for normal threshold values.

Screening and Diagnostic Tests (See also Figure 6.3, Screening and Diagnosis of Gestational Diabetes Mellitus)

- Perform screen between 24 and 28 weeks with an oral 50-gram glucose load followed 1 hour later by a venous plasma glucose measurement. Normal value is less than 140 mg/dL (ACOG, 1994; ADA, 1997; O'Sullivan, Mahan, & Charles, 1973).

  NOTE: This test may be performed at any time of day without reference to the preceding meal; however, the sensitivity (the proportion of clients correctly identified as having GDM) is improved if the test is done while fasting (ACOG,1994). Coustan et al. (1986) recommends that if the 1-hour screen is administered to nonfasting women a value of 130 mg/dL be used as the cut-off of normal. The use of values below 140 mg/dL may improve sensitivity but decrease specificity (i.e., the proportion of clients correctly identified as *not* having GDM) (ACOG, 1994). Capillary blood measurements using glucose oxidase-impregnated test strips are not sufficiently accurate for *diagnostic* purposes and thus are not recommended for this purpose.

  - ▶ A 1-hour glucose screen can be performed earlier in pregnancy for the following categories (Northern California Kaiser Permanente Regional Perinatal Council, 1994; Sweet Success, 1997):
    - – Prior history of GDM, unexplained stillbirth, congenital anomalies or polyhydramnios
    - – Prior delivery of macrosomic infant

- Obesity (> 120 percent of desirable body weight)
- First-degree relative with diabetes
- Age 25 years or older

NOTE: If initial early screen is normal, a repeat test should be performed at 24 to 28 weeks (ACOG, 1994).

- Order a 3-hour, 100 gm oral glucose tolerance test (GTT) if the 1-hour glucose screen is 140 to 190 mg/dL (Sweet Success, 1997). This test is performed after an overnight fast of at least 8 hours and not more than 14 hours and after 3 days of unrestricted diet preparation (150 gm or more of carbohydrate/day) and physical activity. See Table 6.7, Diet Preparation for Three-Hour Glucose Tolerance Test.

  ▶ Normal values (Carpenter and Coustan, 1982):

    - Fasting = < 95 mg/dL
    - 1-hour = < 180 mg/dL
    - 2-hour = < 155 mg/dL
    - 3-hour = < 140 mg/dL

      * If *two or more* of the four values are met or exceeded, a diagnosis of GDM can be made.

  ▶ Alternatively, the following criteria may be applied (ACOG, 1994; ADA, 1997; O'Sullivan & Mahan, 1964; National Diabetes Data Group [NDDG], 1979):

    - Fasting = < 105 mg/dL
    - 1-hour = < 190 mg/dL
    - 2-hour = < 165 mg/dL
    - 3-hour = < 145 mg/dL

      * If *two or more* of the four values are met or exceeded, a diagnosis of GDM can be made.

NOTE: Both criteria are widely used in North America; however, other diagnostic criteria may be applied in other parts of the world. (Refer to the report of the Fourth International Workshop Conference on Gestational Diabetes Mellitus due to be published in 1998).

- If the 1-hour glucose screen is 191 mg/dL or more, order an FBG. If the FBG is 95 mg/dL or more, a 3-hour GTT is not required; patient is to be managed as a gestational diabetic (Sweet Success, 1997).

- If the 3-hour GTT is within normal limits between 24 and 28 weeks, consider repeating the test within 1 month if only one value of the GTT was abnormal or if the woman is at risk for the development of GDM (Avery, 1994; Coustan, 1993).

- Routine prenatal laboratory tests should be ordered at the indicated times. See Chapter 4.1, *Initial Prenatal Visit*, and Chapter 4.2, *Return Prenatal Visit*.

- Obtain urine culture and sensitivities each trimester to rule out asymptomatic bacteriuria.

- Additional laboratory tests may include (but are not limited to) lipid panel, thyroid, and renal function studies, as indicated.

Treatment/Management

- See also Patient Education and Self-monitoring section. Ideally, patient management should be coordinated closely with a multidisciplinary team, including a nurse practitioner or nurse-midwife, physician, nutritionist, clinical nurse specialist, and social worker. In some settings, care of the gestational diabetic falls exclusively to the physician.

  NOTE: Management of women with GDM differs from those with preexisting diabetes because 1) women with GDM do not have the increased risk of diabetic vasculopathy, and 2) the increased rate of congenital anomalies in offspring of women with GDM is not as prevalent as with overt diabetes. The management goal of the gestational diabetic is to normalize the level of glycemic control to the level of a nondiabetic woman, so that healthy pregnancy outcomes can be optimized (Langer, 1993). Oral hypoglycemic agents are contraindicated in pregnancy because they cross the placenta and may stimulate fetal islet cell production with subsequent release of insulin, which may increase fetal hyperinsulinemia (ACOG, 1994; ADA, 1995).

- Establish accurate dating by careful review of last menstrual period (LMP) and use of ultrasound, as indicated.

- Order routine obstetrical ultrasound between 18 and 20 weeks' gestation to screen for fetal anomalies. Repeat ultrasound to assess interval growth, the placenta, and to rule out polyhydramnios/macrosomia, as indicated.

- The following visit schedule is suggested:

  ▶ Every 2 weeks from diagnosis to 36 weeks' gestation

  ▶ Every week from 36 weeks' gestation until delivery

  ▶ More often, if indicated

- Perform routine obstetrical evaluation at each prenatal visit with careful attention to serial McDonald's measurements; BP; weight; and urine for glucose, ketones, protein, leukocyte esterase, and nitrites.

- Refer client to nutritionist for counseling regarding dietary controls. See Section 18, *Nutrition*. The goal of diet therapy is to achieve and maintain normal blood glucose levels throughout pregnancy (i.e., FBG less than or equal to 90 mg/dL, 1-hour postprandial blood glucose less than or equal to 130 mg/dL) and to achieve a steady gradual pattern of weight gain (Sweet Success, 1997).

  NOTE: Patients with only one abnormal value on the 3-hour GTT should also be referred to a nutritionist for dietary counseling. Some studies have demonstrated an association between macrosomia and one abnormal GTT value (Coustan, 1993; Lindsay, Graves, & Klein, 1989; Reese et al., 1995).

- Review client's daily food records at each prenatal visit to assess adequacy of the dietary intake and its effect on blood glucose. Adjust diet as indicated. (Depending on clinical setting, this may be done by nutritionist).

- A psychosocial evaluation should be done on all clients, preferably by a trained social worker. The assessment should include review of diabetes history, social support systems, adjustment to pregnancy, and general emotional status. The goal of psychosocial services is to assist the client in understanding and coping with the physical, emotional, and psychosocial stresses that may be encountered with GDM (Sweet Success, 1997).

- Client to perform fasting and postprandial blood capillary glucose measurements if able to master finger stick procedure. Initially, tests are performed four times a day until blood glucose control is achieved. The frequency of testing once euglycemia is maintained should be individualized according to the clinical picture. Consult with a physician.

  ▶ Patient records should be maintained on flow sheets provided for this purpose. See Table 6.8, Instructions and Flowsheet for Self-Blood Glucose and Urine Ketone Testing for Gestational Diabetics.

    – Results from the client's meter should be compared with the meter in use at the obstetrical practice. If results are significantly different, order laboratory evaluation of client's plasma glucose.

    NOTE: Laboratory results are based on plasma while glucose meter results are based on whole blood. The expected difference should be less than or equal to 15 percent (Sweet Success, 1997).

- Evaluate client's glucose records carefully. If fasting or postprandial values are consistently elevated, treatment with human insulin is required. Client to be referred to a physician.

- Fetal movement counts to be monitored by client starting at 28 weeks' gestation. See Chapter 3.5, *Antepartum Fetal Surveillance*.

- There is no current consensus regarding criteria for and timing of antenatal fetal surveillance (includes NST, BPP, amniotic fluid index) for women with well-controlled GDM, although it is generally recommended to start testing no later than 40 weeks' gestation (ACOG, 1994; ADA, 1995). Some facilities routinely order weekly surveillance beginning at 34 weeks' gestation to follow uncomplicated GDM. Earlier, more frequent testing has been recommended for women with poor glucose control or who require insulin, those with hypertension or suspected fetal growth restriction, and those with history of previous stillbirth (ACOG, 1994; Sweet Success, 1997). Consult with physician regarding antenatal fetal surveillance modalities and their frequency of use.

- Ultrasonography at term may be used to estimate fetal weight to aid in decision making regarding timing/route of delivery. It should be noted, however, that inaccuracies of 10 percent or more may occur (ACOG, 1994; ADA, 1995)

  ▶ There is no consensus as to the estimated fetal weight at which a cesarean section is recommended to avoid birth trauma (suspected birthweight in excess of 4500 grams is a reasonable threshold) (ACOG, 1994; ADA, 1995).

- Fetal lung maturity should be documented with amniocentesis if elective induction is planned prior to 39 weeks' gestation (ACOG, 1994).

- If woman is in good metabolic control, no complications exist, and fetal surveillance is WNL, spontaneous onset of labor at term may be awaited.

- If delivery has not occurred by 40 weeks, routine postdate fetal surveillance should begin twice weekly. See Chapter 6.26, *Postdate Pregnancy*, for further information.

- Induction of labor at 41 weeks' gestation is recommended for women with diet-controlled GDM (Sweet Success, 1997).

Consultation

- Client may be referred to or co-managed with a physician, depending upon the practice setting. Ideal management utilizes a multidisciplinary approach.

- Ongoing consultation with a physician is strongly suggested if a nonphysician provider assumes primary care of the gestational diabetic.

- Consult with physician regarding exercise program and contraindications.

- If fasting or postprandial blood glucose is abnormal at any time, consult with or refer to physician.

Patient Education and Self-monitoring

- Engage in basic discussion of GDM, its obstetrical and neonatal complications, and the long-term implications for the woman and her offspring. Nutrition education to be done by nutritionist. See Section 18, *Nutrition*.

- Request that client maintain daily food and beverage records (including portion sizes).

- Discuss importance of careful and close follow-up, compliance with diet recommendations and self-monitoring of blood glucose (SMBG).

- Explain the rationale and procedures for self-monitoring:

  ▶ Ketone testing of the first voided morning urine can be useful in the first few weeks of diet therapy to establish adequacy of caloric and carbohydrate intake.

    – Ketone levels should be none to trace (Sweet Success, 1997).

  ▶ Fasting and postprandial capillary blood glucose should be performed by client; frequency of testing is determined by the physician (e.g., four times a day initially—fasting, and 1 hour after breakfast, lunch, and dinner; reduction in number of daily or weekly tests based on SMBG results).

    – Assist patient in learning the proper technique for self finger-sticks and determining blood glucose readings with glucose test strips and the use of a reflectance meter.

    – Goals for blood glucose are FBG $\leq$ 90 mg/dL and 1-hour postprandial $\leq$ 130 mg/dL.

  ▶ Patient to keep accurate records on a flow sheet designed for gestational diabetes. See Table 6.8, Instructions and Flowsheet for Self-Blood Glucose Testing and Urine Ketone Testing for Gestational Diabetics.

▶ Instruct client in proper disposal of sharp equipment.

● Instruct patient on use of fetal kick count card beginning at 28 weeks' gestation. See Chapter 3.5, *Antepartum Fetal Surveillance*, for guidelines.

● Determine exercise recommendations individually and supervise the program appropriately.

▶ Optimal aerobic exercises include swimming, arm exercises, and walking. High impact or jarring exercises and contact sports should be avoided (ADA, 1995; Sweet Success, 1997).

▶ Recommended frequency of exercise is three to four times per week for 20 to 30 minutes on alternating days (6 days per week is recommended if exercising for blood glucose control) (Sweet Success, 1997).

▶ Exercise intensity should be light to moderate. Heart rate should not exceed 140 beats per minute. Also see Chapter 4.4, *Exercise During Pregnancy*.

▶ Educate the patient regarding signs/symptoms of hypoglycemia: diaphoresis, tachycardia, tremors, headache, irritability, and loss of concentration. It should be noted that hypoglycemia is generally not a problem for the diet-controlled gestational diabetic.

NOTE: The presence of uterine contractions is a contraindication to exercise. Some experts recommend monitoring fetal movements before and after exercise sessions.

● Encourage postpartum follow-up of blood glucose as discussed in Follow-up section.

● Discuss long-term health maintenance measures, such as proper diet and exercise, to reduce the occurrence of future diabetes mellitus.

● Address issues of parenting and sibling preparation, breast feeding, contraception, and other perinatal issues, as indicated by the individual client.

Follow-up

● Neonatal care provider will plan for management of the infant of the gestational diabetic, details of which are beyond the scope of this book.

● Conduct 6-week postpartum follow-up screen with an FBG or a 2-hour, 75 gm oral glucose tolerance test. Criteria for diagnoses are as follows:

▶ FBG less than 110 mg/dL—normal fasting glucose

▶ FBG between 110 and 126 mg/dL—impaired fasting glucose

▶ FBG greater than or equal to 126 mg/dL—provisional diagnosis of diabetes (must be confirmed on subsequent testing)

▶ 2-hour postload glucose less than 140 mg/dL—normal glucose tolerance

▶ 2-hour postload glucose between 140 and 199 mg/dL—impaired glucose tolerance

▶ 2-hour postload glucose greater than or equal to 200 mg/dL—provisional diagnosis of diabetes (must be confirmed on subsequent testing) (ADA, 1997).

NOTE: Use of the FBG is strongly recommended over the 2-hour test because it is easier, faster, and more convenient.

- Postpartum women diagnosed with overt diabetes should be referred to a diabetologist (Moore, 1994).

  ▶ Women with hyperglycemia near the threshold should be advised regarding individual lifestyle modifications (i.e., diet and exercise) (ADA, 1997).

  ▶ Women with a history of GDM should be screened annually for the presence of diabetes (Sweet Success, 1997).

- Encourage breast feeding. Support long-term health maintenance (especially maintenance of normal weight) in order to prevent sequelae of diabetes. Advise regarding a sensible exercise program.

- Assure that the client has identified/established a safe and effective method of contraception. Unless otherwise contraindicated, hormonal contraception (i.e., low-dose birth control pills or long-acting progestins) may be utilized in women with a history of GDM. Periodic weight, BP, glucose and lipid monitoring should be employed (Association of Reproductive Health Professionals, 1994; Kjos, 1996; The Contraception Report, 1996).

- Continue to support client with psychosocial evaluation and referrals to appropriate systems or agencies.

- Also see Chapter 4.3, *Postpartum Visit* .

- Document diagnosis of GDM in problem list and progress notes.

Table 6.7

Diet Preparation for Three-Hour Glucose Tolerance Test

Your one-hour glucose screening test was abnormal. You will need to schedule a 3-hour glucose tolerance test with the clinical laboratory. A glucose tolerance test checks how well your body responds to sugar. This test must be scheduled at a time that allows you to follow the special 3-day diet. Please call the laboratory to schedule your appointment.

In order to decrease the chance of a falsely abnormal result follow the instructions below:

1. Continue to eat regular meals and all the foods you normally enjoy.

2. For three days before the test you must include extra carbohydrate (at least 150 grams or more) in your daily food intake. To make sure you are eating enough carbohydrate you must choose extra foods.

3. Choose one item from LIST 1 and also one item from LIST 2. Eat these foods *in addition* to the usual foods you eat for three days before the test.

LIST 1	LIST 2
2 slices of bread	8 tablespoons (4 oz) raisins
2/3 cup of cooked rice	2 large apples
1 cup of cooked noodles	2 small bananas
2 corn tortillas	16 oz orange or apple juice

4. <u>EXAMPLE</u>:

Day 1   2 slices of bread
16 oz of apple juice

Day 2   1 cup of noodles
16 oz orange juice

Day 3   2 corn tortillas
2 small bananas

- On the third day of your diet, eat nothing (not even toast), and drink nothing but sips of water <u>after</u> 10:00 <u>P.M.</u>, and until the test is over.

- Please arrive at the laboratory no later than 8:30 A.M.

- First a fasting blood sample will be drawn, then you will be given a sugary liquid to drink.

- Each hour after the drink, blood will be drawn. This will be done three times. It is <u>important</u> that the blood is drawn at <u>exactly</u> one-hour intervals, so please be available at the indicated times.

- Please bring something to read or do while quietly sitting, until the test is over.

- Do not eat, smoke, or drink anything except water during the test. Sips of water should be taken only if you are very thirsty.

- After the last blood sample has been drawn, you may leave the laboratory and have your lunch.

- If you are unable to eat your usual diet, please inform your health care provider.

- Maintain your usual activity level on the days preceding the test.

Source: Adapted with permission from the University of California, San Francisco, OB Clinic.

Table 6.8

Instructions and Flowsheet for Self-blood Glucose and Urine Ketone Testing

Blood Glucose Testing

Follow instructions provided with your blood glucose meter.

Check and record your blood sugar:

_____ times a week before breakfast (fasting)

_____ times a week 1 hour after breakfast

_____ times a week 1 hour after lunch

_____ times a week 1 hour after dinner

Call _____ to report blood glucose values greater than 90 before breakfast or 130 after meals that persist for 3 days.

If you have any questions about your blood glucose meter, call the (800) number on the back of your meter for technical assistance.

Urine Ketone Testing

Follow instructions on Ketostix® container.

Check urine ketones the days you check your blood glucose.

Record the value on the chart.

Call _____ if ketones appear in your urine for 3 days.

Example

Date							
Before Breakfast Glucose (70–90)*							
Before Breakfast Urine Ketones (Negative to trace)*							
1 hr. after Breakfast Glucose (100–130)*							
1 hr. after Lunch Glucose (100–130)*							
1 hr. after Supper Glucose (100–130)*							

* Indicates Normal Values

Source: Adapted with permission from Department of Obstetrics and Gynecology, Kaiser Permanente Medical Center, San Francisco.

Figure 6.3

Screening and Diagnosis of Gestational Diabetes Mellitus (GDM)

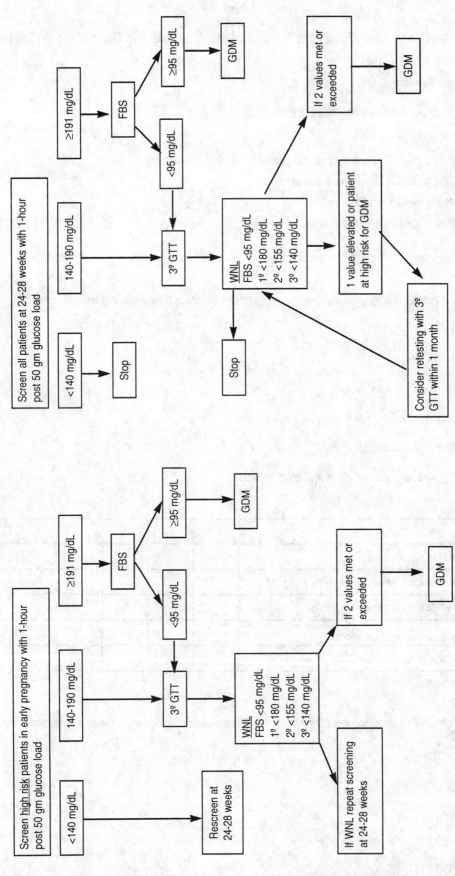

Sources: Sweet Success. (1997). *Guidelines for care.* Sacramento: State of California Health Department, Maternal and Child Health Branch. California Diabetes and Pregnancy Program.

Coustan, D.R. (1993). Methods of screening for and diagnosing of gestational diabetes. *Clinics in Perinatology, 20*(3),

Avery, M.D. & Rossi, M.A. (1994). Gestational diabetes. *Journal of Nurse-Midwifery, 39*(Suppl. 2), 9S–19S.

References

American College of Obstetricians and Gynecologists (ACOG). (1986). *Management of diabetes mellitus in pregnancy* (Technical Bulletin No. 92). Washington, DC: Author.

American College of Obstetricians and Gynecologists (ACOG). (1994). *Diabetes and pregnancy* (Technical Bulletin No. 200). Washington, DC: Author.

American Diabetes Association (ADA). (1995). *Medical management of pregnancy complicated by diabetes* (2nd ed.). Alexandria, VA: Author.

American Diabetes Association (ADA). (1997). Report of the expert committee on the diagnosis and classification of diabetes mellitus. *Diabetes Care, 20*(7), 1183–1197.

Association of Reproductive Health Professionals. (1994, January). Clinical challenges in contraception: A program on women with special medical conditions. *Clinical Proceedings.* Washington, DC: Author.

Avery, M.D., & Rossi, M.A. (1994). Gestational diabetes. *Journal of Nurse-Midwifery, 39*(Suppl. 2), 9S–19S.

Berry, J.L., & Gabbe, S.G. (1986). Diabetes mellitus in pregnancy. In R.A. Knuppel & J.E. Drukker (Eds.), *High risk pregnancy: A team approach.* Philadelphia, PA: W.B. Saunders.

Carpenter, M.V., & Coustan, D.R. (1982). Criteria for screening tests for gestational diabetes. *American Journal of Obstetrics and Gynecology, 144*, 768–773.

The contraception report. (1996). *Metabolic effects of oral contraceptives, 6(6)*, 3–14. Warren, NJ: Emron

Coustan, D.R. (1993). Methods of screening for and diagnosing of gestational diabetes. *Clinics in Perinatology, 20*(3), 593–602.

Coustan, D.R. (1996). Screening and testing for gestational diabetes mellitus. *Obstetrics and Gynecology Clinics of North America, 23*(1), 125–135.

Coustan, D.R., & Carpenter, M.W. (1985). Detection and treatment of gestational diabetes. *Clinical Obstetrics and Gynecology, 28*(3), 507–515.

Coustan, D.R., Carpenter, M.W., O'Sullivan, P.S., & Carr, S.R. (1993). Gestational diabetes: Predictors of subsequent disordered glucose metabolism. *American Journal of Obstetrics and Gynecology, 168*, 1139–1145.

Coustan, D.R., Widness, J.A., Carpenter, M. W., Rotondo, J., Pratt, D.C., & Oh, W. (1986). Should the fifty-gram, one-hour plasma glucose screening test for gestational diabetes be administered in the fasting or fed state? *American Journal of Obstetrics and Gynecology, 154*(5), 1031–1035.

Diabetes (1985). Summary and recommendations of the Second International Workshop Conference on gestational diabetes mellitus. *Diabetes, 34*(2), 123–126.

Freeman, R.B. (1997, July). *GDM: Disease or dogma?* Paper presented at the Kaiser Permanente National Obstetrics and Gynecology Conference, Maui, HI.

Gabbe, S.G., & Landon, M.B. (1987). Diabetes mellitus. In C.J. Pauerstein (Ed.), *Clinical obstetrics.* New York: John Wiley & Sons.

Harris, I., Hadden, W.C., Knowler, W.C., & Bennett, P.H. (1985). International criteria for the diagnosis of diabetes and impaired glucose tolerance. *Diabetes Care, 8*, 562–567.

Hollingsworth, D.R. (1985). Maternal metabolism in normal pregnancy and pregnancy complicated by diabetes. *Clinical Obstetrics and Gynecology, 28*(3), 457–472.

Kitzmiller, J.L., Gavin, L.A., Gin, G.D., Iverson, M., Gunderson, E., Farley, P., Cohen, H., & Sheerer, L.J. (1988 July/August). Managing diabetes and pregnancy. *Current Problems in Obstetrics, Gynecology, and Fertility, 11*(4), 107–167.

Kjos, S.L. (1996). Contraception in diabetic women. *Obstetrics and Gynecology Clinics of North America, 23*(1), 243–258.

Langer, O. (1993). Management of gestational diabetes. *Clinics in Perinatology, 20*(3), 603–617.

Lindsay, M.K., Graves, W., & Klein, L. (1989). The relationship of one abnormal glucose tolerance test value and pregnancy complications. *Obstetrics and Gynecology, 73*(1), 103–106.

Moore, T.R. (1994). Diabetes in pregnancy. In R.K. Creasy and R. Resnik (Eds.), *Maternal-fetal medicine: Principles and practice* (3rd ed., pp. 934–978). Philadelphia, PA: W.B. Saunders.

National Diabetes Data Group (NDDG). (1979). Classification and diagnosis of diabetes mellitus and other categories of glucose intolerance. *Diabetes, 28*, 1039–1057.

Nelson, D.M. (1984). Diabetes and pregnancy. In F. Arias (Ed.), *High risk pregnancy and delivery* (pp. 121–147). St. Louis, MO: C.V. Mosby.

Northern California Kaiser Permanente Regional Perinatal Council. (1994). *Diabetes and pregnancy program description and guidelines for care.* Oakland, CA: Author.

O'Sullivan, J.B., & Mahan, C.M. (1964). Criteria for the oral glucose tolerance test in pregnancy. *Diabetes, 13*, 278.

O'Sullivan, J.B., Mahan, C.M., & Charles, D. (1973). Screening criteria for high risk gestational diabetic patients. *Obstetrics and Gynecology, 116*, 895.

Reese, E.A., Homko, C.J., & Hagay, Z. (1995). When the pregnancy is complicated by diabetes. *Contemporary OB/GYN, 40*(7), 43–61.

Reed, B.D. (1988). Gestational diabetes mellitus. *Primary Care, 15*(2), 371–387.

Sacks, D.A., Greenspoon, J.S., Aby-Fadil, S., Henry, H.M., Ivolde-Tsadik, G., & Yao, J.F.F. (1995). Toward universal criteria for gestational diabetes: The 75-gram glucose tolerance test in pregnancy. *American Journal of Obstetrics and Gynecology, 172*(2), Pt. 1, 607–614.

Sweet Success. (1992). *Guidelines for care.* Sacramento, CA: State of California Health Department, Maternal and Child Health Branch, California Diabetes and Pregnancy Program.

Sweet Success. (1997). *Guidelines for care.* Sacramento, CA: State of California Health Department, Maternal and Child Health Branch, California Diabetes and Pregnancy Program.

U.S. Preventive Services Task Force. (1996). *Guide to clinical preventive services* (2nd ed., pp. 193–208). Baltimore: Williams & Williams.

Chapter 12

GESTATIONAL TROPHOBLASTIC DISEASE

Maureen T. Shannon

Gestational trophoblastic disease (GTD) is a spectrum of diseases involving the abnormal proliferation of fetal tissue resulting in the development of a benign or malignant tumor. GTD is uncommon in the United States with an incidence of 1/1500 pregnancies. However, higher rates of GTD are reported in other countries (i.e., 1/125 pregnancies in Taiwan and Mexico) (Goldstein & Berkowitz, 1994; O'Quinn & Barnard, 1994). The difference in observed rates of GTD has been attributed to socioeconomic, nutritional, and genetic factors (Goldstein & Berkowitz, 1994; Robinson, 1994; O'Quinn & Barnard, 1994).

Histologically and cytogenetically GTD can be separated into distinct disease manifestations, including hydatidiform mole, invasive mole (chorioadenoma destruens), choriocarcinoma, and placental site trophoblastic tumors (American College of Obstetricians & Gynecologists [ACOG], 1993; O'Quinn & Barnard, 1994). The clinical classification of GTD is based on the location of the tumor, and the presence and extent of metastasis (see Table 6.9, Classification of Gestational Trophoblastic Disease).

There are two different forms of hydatidiform mole, partial and complete. Each of these types has a distinct cytogenetic process resulting in characteristic histopathological findings and clinical manifestations. Partial hydatidiform moles usually have a triploid karyotype of 69 chromosomes (69,XXX or 69,XXY) derived from two paternal and one maternal haploid sets of chromosomes. Histologically, partial moles demonstrate variable and focal edematous villae and trophoblastic proliferation, with fetal tissue often present. The clinical presentation is usually a missed spontaneous abortion, with the uterine size less than expected for weeks of gestation. Medical complications (e.g., preeclampsia, hyperthyroidism, pulmonary edema) with this type of hydatidiform mole are rare, and the incidence of postmolar GTD (i.e., invasive mole) is less than 10 percent (ACOG, 1993; O'Quinn & Barnard, 1994).

Complete hydatidiform moles are usually totally derived from a paternal genome. They result from the reduplication of a paternal haploid genome of the sperm without the chromosomal complement of the ovum. Histologic examination demonstrates an absence of fetal tissue and diffuse edematous villae. Unlike partial moles, complete molar gestations are associated with the more classic clinical manifestations attributed to hydatidiform moles: uterine size larger than weeks of gestation, passage of grapelike villae, coexistent theca lutein cysts, medical complications (e.g., preeclampsia, hyperthyroidism), and an increased possibility of developing postmolar GTD (ACOG, 1993: Goldstein & Berkowitz, 1994; O'Quinn & Barnard, 1994).

Invasive moles are diagnosed when there is an elevation or a plateauing of ß-hCG levels after evacuation of a hydatidiform molar gestation. It is characterized by a persistence of edematous villi with trophoblastic proliferation, and invasion into the myometrium. Chemotherapy successfully treats this GTD condition, with metastasis rarely occurring.

Gestational choriocarcinoma comprises cytotrophoblastic and syncytiotrophoblastic elements without chorionic villi. Diagnosis is usually made histologically after a woman has undergone curettage for the evaluation and treatment of abnormal bleeding in association with molar gestations or during the postpartum period. Systemic metastasis can occur early in this condition, therefore diagnostic evaluations for the presence of metastatic lesions and the prompt initiation of chemotherapy are indicated.

Placental site trophoblastic tumors (PSTTs) are rare tumors characterized by the proliferation of cytotrophoblast cells without evidence of chorionic villi. This tumor is usually confined to the uterus, with metastasis rarely observed. PSTTs are not responsive to chemotherapy. Consequently, hysterectomy is the recommended treatment. This difference in response to chemotherapy between PSTTs and choriocarcinoma makes the histologic diagnosis extremely important, especially for women desiring future pregnancy.

The cure rate for persistent GTN of all severities is approximately 90 percent, with a cure rate of almost 100 percent being cited for low-risk cases. Early diagnosis of this disease is essential if successful treatment is to be attained.

Database

Subjective

Predisposing factors

- Maternal age less than 20 or more than 40 years

- History of previous mole

- Geographic location—the highest incidences of GTN are in areas of Asia (1/125), the South Pacific (1/173 to 1/530) and in Mexico (1/500)

Symptomatology

- Persistent dark-red or brownish vaginal bleeding, which may be minimal or profuse (over 90 percent of women with hydatidiform moles will report vaginal bleeding) during pregnancy

- Abnormal vaginal bleeding during the postpartum period resistant to usual therapeutic interventions

- Severe nausea and vomiting persisting after the 12th week of pregnancy

- Absence of fetal movement in pregnancies that continue through to the second trimester

- Passage of grapelike vesicles from vagina (up to 80 percent of women with hydatidiform moles will report this, usually by the fourth month of pregnancy)

- May be extremely fatigued due to increased loss of blood.

- May report pelvic pain or discomfort (if theca lutein cysts present)

- May report a cough or hemoptysis (if pulmonary trophoblastic embolism)

- Weight loss (in association with hyperthyroidism)

Objective

- General. Woman may appear pale, anxious, and/or apprehensive.
- Vital signs

  ▶ Blood pressure may be within normal limits (WNL), decreased (if significant blood loss), or increased (if signs of preeclampsia present).

  ▶ Pulse may be increased (due to blood loss or secondary to hyperthyroid state due to increased thyrotropin excretion by molar tissue).

  ▶ Respiratory rate may be increased (if hyperthyroid state or if pulmonary trophoblastic embolization has occurred).

  NOTE: Rarely is the volume of trophoblast transported to the lungs large enough to produce signs of pulmonary edema. Usually symptoms of pulmonary complications present postoperatively after evacuation of the molar tissue.

  ▶ Temperature is usually WNL but may be elevated if woman is experiencing thyroid storm.

- Skin may be pale (if significant blood loss) or flushed and dry (if coexistent hyperthyroid symptoms).
- Abdominal palpation may reveal uterine size not equal to dates. Fifty percent of women with GTN will have uterine size greater than dates; 25 percent will have uterine size equal to dates; and 25 percent will have uterine size less than dates.
- Auscultation for fetal heart tones (FHTs) with Doppler (beginning at appropriate weeks of gestation) will reveal an absence of FHTs.
- Signs of preeclampsia before the 24th week of pregnancy (10 to 12 percent of women) are as follows:

  ▶ Proteinuria

  ▶ Hypertension

  ▶ Edema

  ▶ Hyperreflexia

- There may be an ovarian mass due to theca lutein cysts (15 to 30 percent of women with hydatidiform moles).

Assessment

- IUP _____ weeks
- Gestational trophoblastic disease

  ▶ R/O anemia

  ▶ R/O hyperemesis gravidarum

  ▶ R/O threatened or missed spontaneous abortion

  ▶ R/O hyperthyroidism

▶ R/O IUP with inaccurate dating

▶ R/O multiple gestation

▶ R/O pneumonia

Plan

Diagnostic Tests

The following diagnostic tests should be ordered after consultation with a physician:

- Beta hCG level. The level is persistently and abnormally elevated for weeks of gestation.

  NOTE: ß-hCG levels $\geq$100,000 mIU/mL are commonly observed in the presence of hydatidiform moles.

- Obstetric ultrasound usually reveals the absence of a gestational sac and fetus, the presence of echogenic areas of villi and clots, and an enlarged ovary or ovarian cyst.

  NOTE: A partial mole may demonstrate a gestational sac and fetal pole, but an abnormal placenta (e.g., multiple cystic spaces evident).

- Chest radiograph may reveal unexplained findings (e.g., viral or fungal pneumonias) or evidence of pulmonary embolism.

- Complete blood count (CBC) may reveal decreased hemoglobin/hematocrit and red blood cell count (if there has been significant blood loss)

- Platelet count may be decreased if coagulopathy

- Liver function tests. Transaminase levels may be elevated if there is coexistent preeclampsia or coagulopathy

- Renal function tests. Blood urea nitrogen (BUN) and creatinine levels may be elevated if there is diminished renal function secondary to significant blood loss, coagulopathy, or coexistent preeclampsia.

- Thyroid studies. Elevation of T3 and T4 levels may be observed.

- Urinalysis may demonstrate proteinuria.

Treatment/Management

- Consult with a physician immediately when a woman is suspected of having GTD. The treatment of a woman with suspected or documented GTD should be managed by the consulting physician.

- The plan of care for the woman depends on the suspected or documented type of GTD and usually includes the following:

  ▶ Hydatidiform mole

  – Hospitalization for evacuation of molar tissue by suction curettage. In women who do not want future pregnancies, hysterectomy may be considered.

  – Chemotherapy is not indicated in the treatment of women with partial or complete hydatidiform mole. However, for women in whom poor follow-up is anticipated, some clinicians recommend prophylactic chemotherapy to reduce the occurrence of malignant disease (O'Quinn & Barnard, 1994).

  – Obtain serial quantitative ß-hCG levels utilizing a radioimmunoassay after evacuation of a hydatidiform mole.

    * The levels should be determined 48 hours after evacuation, every 1 to 2 weeks until the levels are normal, and then every 1 to 2 months for 6 to 12 months.

    * After successful therapy, serial quantitative ß-hCG levels usually demonstrate a 50 percent drop every week until the level reaches the normal value for nonpregnant women.

    NOTE: The definition of "normal" varies among laboratories; however, most laboratories use the value of less than 5.0 IU/L or 5.0 mIU/mL as a normal value for nonpregnant women (Fischbach, 1996).

    NOTE: A ß-hCG level that rises 50 percent over the previous value or plateaus for more than 2 weeks requires immediate evaluation for malignant postmolar GTD and the initiation of chemotherapy (ACOG, 1993; Berman & DiSaia, 1994).

  – Women experiencing hyperthyroid symptoms may require antithyroid medication for a short period until the symptoms resolve.

  – Contraception should be initiated and continued until 6 to 12 months after successful evacuation of molar tissue with serial quantitative ß-hCG determinations demonstrating sustained normal levels. *Intrauterine devices are contraindicated* because of the possibility of uterine infection and perforation. However, oral contraceptives or barrier methods can be prescribed (ACOG, 1993; O'Quinn & Barnard, 1994).

    NOTE: Oral contraceptive use does not affect the regression pattern of ß-hCG levels after treatment for hydatidiform mole; and does not increase the incidence of postmolar GTD (ACOG, 1993).

  – The woman and her partner may need assistance in coping with the psychological stress and grief they experience as a result of this diagnosis. Consider referral to a psychologist and/or support groups prior to discharge from the hospital.

▶ Invasive mole (nonmetastatic GTD)

  – In women no longer desiring future pregnancies, hysterectomy should be performed, since this procedure has been associated with a shorter duration of chemotherapy to produce a remission (ACOG, 1993).

    NOTE: The hysterectomy should be performed on the third day of chemotherapy (O'Quinn & Barnard, 1994).

  – Single-agent chemotherapy with methotrexate, dactinomycin, or etoposide should be initiated and continued until ß-hCG values reach normal levels. An additional course of chemotherapy is administered after the first normal ß-hCG value is documented (ACOG, 1993).

  – Serial quantitative ß-hCG determinations should be obtained at 2-week intervals for the first 3 months, and then monthly for the first year after completion of therapy.

  – Contraception should be continued for 12 months after therapy (see the above hydatidiform mole section).

  – Psychological assessment and therapy may be necessary for a woman undergoing treatment for this condition, and for her partner (see the above hydatidiform mole section).

▶ Metastatic GTD—low risk

  – Women meeting the low-risk criteria for metastatic GTD (see Table 6.9, Classification of Gestational Trophoblastic Disease) can be treated with single-agent chemotherapy.

  – Women who are not planning future pregnancies should consider hysterectomy in addition to chemotherapy, since this has demonstrated a decrease in the duration of chemotherapy needed to treat metastatic GTD.

  – Serial ß-hCG levels should be obtained at 2-week intervals for the first 3 months of remission and then at 1-month intervals for the first year of remission. Even though the recurrence rate after 1 year of remission is less than 1 percent, continue surveillance of ß-hCG levels every 6 months for an additional year because there is a possibility of a late recurrence.

  – Contraception should be initiated and continued for the first 12 months of remission (see the above hydatidiform mole section).

  – Psychological assessments and interventions may be necessary in women undergoing treatment for this condition, as well as their partners.

▶ Metastatic GTD—high risk

  – Women with risk factors associated with a poor prognosis should begin multiagent chemotherapy (usually with methotrexate, dactinomycin, and either chlorambucil or cyclophosphamide [MAC] or methotrexate, dactinomycin, and etoposide alternating with vincristine and cyclophosphamide [EMA/CO]).

    NOTE: Chemotherapy is continued until three consecutive normal ß-hCG levels are documented, and is then followed by three additional courses of chemotherapy to eradicate any viable tumor. The recurrence rate for women with high-risk disease, even after this regimen, is 13 percent (ACOG, 1993).

- Radiation therapy and/or surgery may be indicated in the management of cerebral or hepatic metastases.

- Primary hysterectomy has not improved the outcome for women with high-risk metastatic disease, but may be necessary in women with resistance to the usual therapeutic interventions (ACOG, 1993; O'Quinn & Barnard, 1994).

- Initiate psychological assessments and interventions for women diagnosed with this condition, as well as their partners.

- Obtain serial quantitative ß-hCG levels at the same intervals as for low-risk metastatic GTD.

- Contraception should be initiated and maintained for the first year of remission. After that time, pregnancy may be considered.

Consultation

- Consultation is required in all cases of suspected GTD.

- Transfer to physician care all women with a diagnosis of GTD.

Patient Education

- Explain the tests that are to be ordered and interpret the results.

- If a GTD diagnosis is made, then the education of the woman about the treatment options is the responsibility of the physician managing her care.

  NOTE: It is important for the woman to be educated about the good prognosis associated with this disease. The cure rate is almost 100 percent in the majority of cases that are detected early and that do not have metastasis; and future childbearing is a possibility with little risk of recurrence of GTD (1 to 2 percent).

- Some women require ongoing help to move through the grieving process (grieving the loss of a normal pregnancy and working through the threat of a major disease) and should be referred to psychologists/psychiatrists for appropriate evaluations and therapy. Referral to support groups for the woman and her partner may also be beneficial.

Follow-up

- Follow-up of a woman treated for GTD is the responsibility of the physician managing her care and includes the following:

  ▶ Serial quantitative ß-hCG levels at recommended intervals based upon the type of GTD diagnosed (see Treatment/Management section).

  ▶ Effective contraception for 6 to 12 months after the quantitative ß-hCG titers are normal (see Treatment/Management section).

▶ Immediate evaluation and treatment for malignant GTD if the serial ß-hCG levels plateau for more than 2 weeks or if a ß-hCG level rises above the previous result (ACOG, 1993).

▶ An early obstetric ultrasound if a subsequent pregnancy occurs to rule out a recurrence of GTD (ACOG, 1993).

● Document diagnosis of GTD and management thereof in progress notes and problem list.

Table 6.9

Classification of Gestational Trophoblastic Disease

I. Benign GTD
    A. Complete hydatidiform mole
    B. Partial hydatidiform mole

II. Malignant GTD
    A. Nonmetastatic GTD: No evidence of extrauterine involvement
    B. Metastatic GTD
        1. Good prognosis, low risk
            a. Duration <4 months
            b. Pretherapy levels of serum ß-hCG < 40,000 mIU/mL
            c. No evidence of brain or liver metastases
            d. GTD not associated with term gestation
            e. No prior chemotherapy
        2. Poor prognosis, high risk—presence of any of the following risk factors
            a. Duration > 4 months
            b. Pretherapy levels of serum ß-hCG >40,000 mIU/mL
            c. Evidence of brain or liver metastases
            d. GTD after term gestation
            e. Prior failed chemotherapy

Source: Adapted with permission from: American College of Obstetricians & Gynecologists (ACOG). *Management of gestational trophoblastic disease.* ACOG Technical Bulletin No. 178(March), 1993, p.5.

References

American College of Obstetricians and Gynecologists (ACOG). (1993). *Management of gestational trophoblastic disease.* ACOG Technical Bulletin No. 178. Washington, DC: Author.

Fischbach, F.T. (1996). *A manual of laboratory & diagnostic tests* (5th ed.). Philadelphia, PA: Lippincott.

Goldstein, D.P., & Berkowitz, R.S. (1994). Current management of complete and partial molar pregnancy. *Journal of Reproductive Medicine, 39*(3), 139–146.

Kohorn, E.I. (1993). Evaluation of the criteria used to make the diagnosis of nonmetastatic gestational trophoblastic neoplasia. *Gynecologic Oncology, 48*, 139-147.

O'Quinn, A.G., & Barnard, D.E. (1994). Gestational trophoblastic diseases. In A.H. DeCherney & M.L. Pernoll (Eds.), *Current obstetric & gynecologic diagnosis & treatment* (8th ed., pp. 967–976). Norwalk, CT: Appleton & Lange.

Robinson, B.J.H. (1994). Intraoperative molar pregnancy crisis. *AORN Journal, 60*(2), 193–201.

Rodriguez, G.C., Hughes, C.L., Soper, J.T., Berchuck, A., Clarke-Pearson, D.L., & Hammond, C.B. (1994). Serum progesterone for the exclusion of early pregnancy in women at risk for recurrent gestational trophoblastic neoplasia. *Obstetrics and Gynecology, 84*(5), 794–797.

Chapter 13

HYPERTENSIVE DISORDERS OF PREGNANCY

Maureen T. Shannon

Hypertensive disorders of pregnancy encompass a spectrum of conditions. There have been several attempts to classify hypertensive disorders related to or induced by pregnancy. However, these attempts have led to confusion regarding the "proper" terminology to use to describe these conditions. For the purposes of this protocol, the terminology developed by the American College of Obstetricians and Gynecologists (ACOG, 1996) will be used. According to ACOG (1996), hypertension observed during pregnancy can be caused by two distinct conditions: chronic hypertension and pregnancy-induced hypertension. Chronic hypertension is defined as hypertension that precedes pregnancy, or is evident before the twentieth week of gestation. PIH is defined as hypertension that begins after the twentieth week of gestation, unless the woman has gestational trophoblastic disease (GTD), in which case clinical manifestations of PIH may be evident during the first and early second trimesters. Clinical subsets of PIH are based upon the end-organ effects of the condition (see Definitions below). Athough chronic hypertension and PIH are considered to be separate conditions, they may coexist during pregnancy. In fact, the development of PIH is significantly increased if a pregnant woman has a history of chronic hypertension (ACOG, 1996).

The exact etiology of PIH remains unknown. Nevertheless, the pathophysiology is believed to involve the following elements: 1) generalized vasospasm resulting in an increased peripheral vascular resistance with decreased perfusion to tissues and vital organs (e.g., brain, liver, kidneys, placenta); 2) the development of vascular endothelial lesions in multiple organ systems (e.g., placenta, liver, kidneys); 3) failure of trophoblastic invasion of myometrial segments between 16–22 weeks gestation resulting in trophoblastic ischemia; and 4) endothelial injury causing alterations in the production and accumulation of prostacyclin (a potent vasodilator) and thromboxane A_2 (a vasoconstrictor) that results in abnormal vascular responses and intravascular coagulation (Byrd & Sakornbut, 1996; Cunningham, MacDonald, Gant, Leveno, & Gilstrap III, 1993; Friedman, Taylor, & Roberts, 1991; Roberts, 1994; Sibai, 1991; Sibai & Moretti, 1988). These pathophysiological events begin several months prior to the development of clinical manifestations associated with PIH, thus providing an opportunity for the development of significant maternal and fetal morbidity.

PIH is the most common hypertensive complication of pregnancy, affecting up to 10 percent of all pregnancies and 30 percent of pregnancies with multiple gestations (ACOG, 1996; Beckmann et al., 1995). It is a leading cause of both perinatal and maternal morbidity and mortality. Perinatal morbidity and mortality is the result of placental insufficiency, prematurity, and abruptio placentae (Roberts, 1994). Recognition of predisposing factors and subtle clinical signs and symptoms that a woman may exhibit during the early stages of PIH is essential in order to significantly reduce the severity of the adverse maternal and fetal outcomes associated with this disorder.

Definitions (ACOG, 1996; Frangieh & Sibai, 1996)

Pregnancy-induced hypertension

Pregnancy-induced hypertension (PIH) is a condition characterized by the development of an elevation of a woman's blood pressure during the latter half of pregnancy. PIH is categorized below.

PIH without Proteinuria and Gross Edema:

PIH without proteinuria and gross edema is defined as a sustained blood pressure (BP) of at least 140 mm Hg systolic or 90 mm Hg diastolic without proteinuria or edema.

NOTE: Blood pressure readings may vary greatly depending upon position and the type of sphygmomanometer cuff used. Ideally, a woman's BP should be obtained while sitting with her arm positioned and supported at heart level. Use a large cuff to obtain a BP in obese women.

PIH with Proteinuria and Edema (Preeclampsia)

Mild preeclampsia is defined as an increase in a woman's blood pressure to at least 140 mm Hg systolic or 90 mm Hg diastolic measured on at least two separate occasions 6 hours apart with proteinuria and/or edema measured as follows:

- Proteinuria equal to or greater than 1 gram/liter in at least two clean-catch midstream urine specimens collected 6 hours apart or greater than 300 mg total protein in a 24-hour urine collection (Frangieh & Sibai, 1996).

- Nondependent edema (equal to or greater than one-plus pitting edema after 12 hours of bed rest, or a weight gain of equal to or greater than 5 pounds in 1 week).

A severe preeclampsia diagnosis is made if one or more of the following findings occur in addition to those listed under mild preeclampsia:

- BP greater than 160–180 mm Hg systolic or greater than 110 mm Hg diastolic
- Proteinuria greater than 5 grams in a 24-hour urine collection
- Elevated serum creatinine
- Oliguria (<400 mL / 24 hours)
- Pulmonary edema
- Microangiopathic hemolysis
- Thrombocytopenia
- Impaired liver function
- Intrauterine growth retardation (IUGR)
- Oligohydramnios
- Grand mal seizures (eclampsia)
- Symptoms suggesting significant end-organ involvement (e.g., epigastric or right upper quadrant pain, headache, or visual disturbances).

HELLP Syndrome

The acronym HELLP reflects the clinical hallmarks of a syndrome which includes hypertension and hemolysis (H), elevated liver enzymes (EL), and low platelets (LP) (Sibai, 1988). It occurs in 2–12 percent of women with severe preeclampsia and has an associated perinatal mortality rate of up to 24 percent (Reubinoff & Schenker, 1991; Poole, 1993). The significant morbidity and mortality associated with this syndrome is due to prematurity, abruptio placentae, maternal disseminated intravascular coagulation (DIC), and intrauterine fetal asphyxia (Reubinoff & Schenker, 1991). There is an increased incidence of HELLP syndrome observed in women with a delayed diagnosis of pre-eclampsia (Sibai, 1986; Sibai, 1991), with up to 30 percent of affected women not manifesting symptoms until after delivery (Reubinoff & Schenker, 1991; Sibai, 1991). Early recognition of the signs and symptoms of this disorder is essential, since prompt, aggressive management is necessary to reduce the likelihood of significant maternal and perinatal morbidity and mortality.

Eclampsia

Eclampsia occurs when a preeclamptic woman develops tonic-clonic convulsions that cannot be attributed to any other cause (e.g., a pre-existing neurologic condition such as epilepsy). Approximately 25 percent of eclamptic women exhibit clinical manifestations of mild preeclampsia prior to the onset of seizures.

Chronic Hypertension Preceding Pregnancy

The diagnosis of chronic hypertension preceding pregnancy can be made when persistent hypertension due to any etiology is present before the 20th week of pregnancy and is not a result of GTD, or when hypertension continues beyond 6 weeks postpartum.

Chronic Hypertension with Superimposed PIH

Chronic hypertension of any etioloy with superimposed PIH includes superimposed preeclampsia and eclampsia. This diagnosis is made when a woman with chronic hypertension develops the signs and symptoms of preeclampsia or eclampsia.

Database

Subjective

Predisposing Factors

The woman may report one or more of the following (ACOG, 1996; Roberts, 1994; Sibai, 1991):

- Nulliparity
- Maternal age (PIH is reportedly more common in women older than 40 years of age.)

  NOTE: Although young maternal age (i.e., adolescence) has traditionally been reported as a risk factor, the independent contribution of this factor to the development of PIH is questionable (ACOG, 1996).

- African-American descent
- Family history of PIH (i.e., mother or sister of the woman)
- Antiphospholipid syndrome
- Preexisting vascular diseases—essential hypertension (20 percent of women with hypertension will develop superimposed PIH), renal disease, diabetes mellitus (up to 50 percent of women with diabetes mellitus will develop PIH)

- GTD
- Multiple gestation
- Fetal hydrops
- History of PIH
- Lower socioeconomic status (Although this has traditionally been reported as a risk factor, its independent contribution to the development of PIH is questionable [ACOG, 1996].)

Symptomatology

- PIH without proteinuria and gross edema—usually no physical complaints
- PIH with proteinuria and edema
    - ▶ Mild preeclampsia—the woman may be asymptomatic or report:
        - Edema of her fingers (e.g., tightness of rings) and/or her face (e.g., "puffy looking")
        - Excessive weight gain (e.g., 5 pounds or more in 1 week)
    - ▶ Severe preeclampsia—The woman may report one or more of the following:
        - Edema of fingers and/or face
        - Excessive weight gain (5 or more pounds in a week)
        - Severe headaches (often in the frontal or occipital areas)
        - Visual disturbances including blurred vision, "flashes of light," "spots before eyes," or blindness (due to retinal detachment)
        - Nausea, vomiting
        - Epigastric or right upper quadrant pain (pain may penetrate to the back)
        - Paresthesia of hands or feet (if significant edema)
        - Fatigue, malaise
        - Mental confusion
        - Shortness or breath or dyspnea (if coexistent pulmonary edema)
        - Hematuria
        - Ecchymosis without history of trauma
        - Abdominal pain and/or vaginal bleeding (if coexistent abruptio placentae)
        - Decreased fetal movement
    - ▶ HELLP Syndrome (see also Subjective section for severe preeclampsia and eclampsia)
        - Fatigue, malaise for a few days (up to 90 percent of women) (Reubinoff & Schenker, 1991)
        - Nausea and/or vomiting (45–85 percent of women) (Reubinoff & Schenker, 1991; Sibai, 1991)

- Epigastric or right upper quadrant pain (90 percent of women) (Reubinoff & Schenker, 1991)

- Chest pain

- Edema

- Jaundice (if significant hemolysis present)

- Prolonged bleeding (e.g., bleeding gums) (Jones, Abramowitz, Anissi, Mirwald, & Sherer, 1993)

● Eclampsia

▶ Reports loss of consciousness with drowsiness or coma following a tonic-clonic seizure (a relative or friend may describe the woman having had a seizure or "fit")

▶ May report having experienced severe dyspnea and/or shortness of breath (due to pulmonary edema)

● Chronic Hypertension

▶ May report history of hypertension prior to pregnancy

● Chronic Hypertension with Superimposed PIH

▶ See Subjective section for preeclampsia and eclampsia.

▶ May report history of hypertension prior to pregnancy.

Objective

The woman will exhibit one or more of the following clinical manifestations depending upon the severity of the disease.

● PIH without Proteinuria and Edema (ACOG, 1996; Sibai, 1991)

▶ Vital signs

- Blood pressure equal to or greater than 140 mm Hg systolic or 90 mm Hg after the 20th week gestation measured on 2 separate occasions 6 hours apart.

- Weight: normal weight gain pattern (i.e., absence of rapid excessive weight gain pattern)

- Pulse within normal limits (WNL)

- Respiratory rate WNL

▶ Neurological examination: deep tendon reflexes (DTRs) WNL

▶ Abdominal examination: fundal height WNL (i.e., usually no evidence of IUGR)

● PIH with Proteinuria and Edema (ACOG, 1996; Cunningham et al., 1993; Frangieh & Sibai, 1996; Rubeinoff & Schenker, 1991; Roberts, 1994; Sibai, 1991)

● Mild Preeclampsia

- Vital signs:

* Blood pressure (see PIH without Proteinuria and Edema section)

* Rapid, excessive weight gain equal to or greater than 5 pounds in a week

* Pulse WNL

* Respiratory rate WNL

- Skin

    * Nondependent edema (e.g., orbital, fingers, sacral) and/or pretibial edema equal to or greater than 1+

    * Absence of ecchymosis, cyanosis, jaundice

- Abdominal examination

    * Fundal height WNL for expected weeks of gestation (i.e., IUGR should not be evident with mild preeclampsia since this finding is associated with a diagnosis of severe preeclampsia)

- Neurological examination

    * Normal mentation

    * DTRs are usually WNL.

▶ Severe Preeclampsia (ACOG, 1996; Frangieh & Sibai, 1996; Reubinoff & Schenker, 1991; Sibai, 1991)

- Vital signs:

    * BP greater than 160–180 mm/Hg systolic or greater than 110 diastolic

    * Respiratory rate: May be increased and labored if coexistent pulmonary edema; or increased if significant anxiety

    * Pulse: May be increased if coexistent pulmonary edema, or if significant anxiety or epigastric discomfort.

- General: Woman may appear anxious if she is experiencing shortness of breath, dyspnea, epigastric distress, or other significant symptoms associated with severe preeclampsia.

- Skin

    * Generalized non-dependent edema, pretibial edema equal to or greater than 3+ to 4+

    * Cyanosis if coexistent pulmonary edema

    * Petechiae, ecchymosis if coexistent thrombocytopenia

    * Jaundice if significant hemolysis

- Eyes: Funduscopic examination of the eyes may reveal vascular narrowing, a decreased A:V diameter (from 3:5 to 1:2 or 1:3), or retinal detachment (rare).

- Auscultation of lungs: May reveal fine inspiratory crackles (if coexistent pulmonary edema)

- Abdominal examination

* Tenderness to palpation and/or percussion in the right upper quadrant or epigastrium

    * Fundal height less than expected for gestational weeks if coexistent IUGR

- Neurological examination

    * Woman may be confused or disoriented

    * DTRs: Hyperreflexia (3+ to 4+) with or without clonus may be present

- Urinary output is equal to or less than 400 mL /24 hours (oliguria)

▶ HELLP Syndrome (see also Objective Section for severe preeclampsia)

- Vital signs:

    * A diastolic blood pressure greater than 110 is reported in 68 percent of affected women (Reubinoff & Schenker, 1991). However, up to 20 percent of women with HELLP syndrome may not present with hypertension or significant proteinuria (ACOG, 1996; Reubinoff & Schenker, 1991).

    * Respiratory rate may be significantly increased if coexistent pulmonary edema and/or adult respiratory syndrome (ARDS).

- Skin

    * Jaundice—approximately 40 percent of patients will develop jaundice.

    * Cyanosis may be evident if coexistent pulmonary edema or ARDS

- Abdominal examination

    * Tenderness to palpation or percussion in epigastric or right upper quadrant area

    * Enlarged, firm liver

    * Ascites may be evident

● Eclampsia (see also Objective section for severe preeclampsia and HELLP syndrome)

▶ Neurological examination

- Tonic-clonic seizure(s) with coma following for varying lengths of time

- Hyperreflexia (3+ to 4+) with clonus

▶ Skin

- Jaundice

- Cyanosis may be present if coexistent pulmonary edema

- Prolonged and/or excessive bleeding if coexistent disseminated intravascular coagulation (DIC)

▶ Abdominal examination:

- Absence of fetal movement and/or fetal heart tones if fetal demise

- Chronic Hypertension (Roberts, 1994)
  - ▶ Vital signs
    - Blood pressure equal to or greater than 140 mm Hg systolic or 90 mm Hg diastolic before the 20th week of gestation (without evidence of GTN) on two separate occasions. Hypertension will persist after 6 weeks postpartum if not treated.
    - Normal weight gain pattern for pregnancy
  - ▶ Skin: Absence of gross, generalized edema
  - ▶ Neurological examination:
    - Mentation WNL
    - DTRs WNL
- Chronic Hypertension with Superimposed PIH
  - ▶ See Objective section for preeclampsia and eclampsia.
  - ▶ Hypertension persists after 6 weeks postpartum if not treated.

Assessment

- PIH (without proteinuria and edema)
- Preeclampsia—mild or severe
- Preeclampsia or eclampsia with HELLP syndrome
- Eclampsia
- R/O the following:
  - ▶ Convulsive disorder
  - ▶ Chronic hypertension
  - ▶ Chronic hypertension with superimposed PIH
  - ▶ GTD (if clinical features of preeclampsia occur before 12th week of pregnancy)
  - ▶ IUGR
  - ▶ Oligohydramnios
  - ▶ Gestational proteinuria
  - ▶ Endocrine disorders (e.g., pheochromocytoma)
  - ▶ Autoimmune disorders (e.g., antiphospholipid syndrome)
  - ▶ Liver disease (e.g., hepatitis)
  - ▶ Cholelithiasis
  - ▶ Pyelonephritis
  - ▶ Idiopathic thrombocytopenic purpura (ITP)

Plan

Diagnostic Tests

PIH without Proteinuria and Edema

- Clean catch midstream urine for dipstick testing: This test is routinely performed during prenatal visits and will be negative or trace in a woman without preeclampsia.

  NOTE: Interpret results from urinary protein dipstick testing with caution. In women with hypertension, a trace or negative result has a negative predictive value of only 34 percent. In hypertensive women with a baseline value of 3+ or 4+, the positive predictive value is only 36 percent (Meyer, Bercer, Friedman, & Sibai, 1994). False-positive results may occur in the presence of blood, vaginal secretions, low specific gravity, alkaline urine, and contamination with chlorhexidine (Byrd & Sakornbut, 1996).

- The following tests may be ordered as indicated based on clinical findings and after consultation with a physician:

  ▶ Complete blood count (CBC): Usually within normal limits (WNL) unless coexistent anemia

  ▶ Peripheral blood smear: Usually WNL

  ▶ Coagulation studies: Platelet count, fibrinogen, prothrombin time (PT), partial thromboplastin time (PTT) usually WNL

  ▶ Liver function tests: Serum aspartate aminotransferase (AST, SGOT) and serum alanine aminotransferase (ALT, SGPT) are usually WNL.

  ▶ Renal function:

  – Serum blood urea nitrogen (BUN) and creatinine usually WNL

  – 24-hour urine collection for protein and creatinine clearance WNL

  ▶ Obstetrical ultrasound: May be ordered serially (e.g., every 2 to 3 weeks) to evaluate fetal growth, and may demonstrate evidence of IUGR if significant uteroplacental insufficiency due to hypertension.

  ▶ Antenatal fetal surveillance: Weekly nonstress tests (NSTs) with amniotic fluid index (AFI), biophysical profile (BPP) or contraction stress tests (CSTs) of the fetus may be ordered beginning at 32 to 34 weeks gestation if IUGR or other problems are suspected. These tests will be abnormal if significant uteroplacental insufficiency and/or fetal compromise (see Chapter 4.3, *Antepartum Fetal Surveillance*).

Preeclampsia

Consult with a physician for a woman suspected of having preeclampsia of any severity. The consulting physician will determine the plan of care, including the indicated diagnostic tests and the appropriate intervals for testing, based upon the severity of maternal disease as well as gestational age of the fetus. The following tests are usually ordered when evaluating a woman for preeclampsia.

- Mild Preeclampsia

  ▶ Clean catch midstream urine sample for dipstick may demonstrate proteinuria equal to or greater than 1+ obtained on two separate occasions at least 6 hours apart

  ▶ 24-hour urine collection may demonstrate greater than 300 mg protein

  ▶ CBC may be WNL or may demonstrate evidence of hemoconcentration

  ▶ Peripheral blood smear may be WNL or demonstrate burr cells, spherocytes, schistocytes, and/or echinocytes (abnormal red blood cell morphological findings associated with hemolysis)

  ▶ In coagulation studies, platelet count, fibrinogen, PT, and PTT usually WNL. May demonstrate values indicative of a developing coagulopathy (e.g., platelet count values may demonstrate a gradual decline to < 100,000/mm³)

  ▶ In liver function studies, AST (SGOT), ALT (SGPT) may be WNL or elevated (21 percent of women with preeclampsia have elevated liver transaminases) (Dildy III & Cotton, 1991)

  ▶ Renal function

    – Serum creatinine may be elevated.

      NOTE: The normal value for serum creatinine during pregnancy is 0.46 ± 0.13 mg/100mL (Willett, 1994).

    – BUN may be elevated.

      NOTE: The normal value for BUN during pregnancy is 8.17 ± 1.5 mg/100mL (Willett, 1994).

    – Uric acid will increase as preeclampsia becomes more severe.

      NOTE: The normal value for uric acid ranges from 2.2 to 5.7 mg/dL (or 0.13–0.34 mmol/L). During the first and second trimesters the level is decreased, but returns to nonpregnant level during the third trimester (Willett, 1994).

  ▶ Obstetrical ultrasound: May demonstrate the presence of IUGR. If IUGR is documented, serial sonograms should be obtained every 2 to 3 weeks to assess fetal growth.

  ▶ Serial NSTs with AFIs, BPPs, and/or CSTs of the fetus to assess fetal well being and placental functioning will be abnormal in compromised fetuses or if decreased placental function.

- Severe Preeclampsia

  In addition to the diagnostic test results listed under the mild preeclampsia section the following laboratory values may be observed in a woman with severe preeclampsia.

  ▶ For clean catch midstream urine specimen: dipstick of specimen will demonstrate persistent proteinuria equal to or greater than 3+.

  ▶ A 24-hour urine will demonstrate proteinuria greater than 5 gm/24-hour; creatinine clearance will decrease over normal values observed during pregnancy.

> **NOTE:** The reference range for creatine clearance rates is 75–115 mL/min/1.73m². During normal pregnancy, creatinine clearance can increase by 40 percent (Willett, 1994).

- Coagulation studies may demonstrate decreased platelets (<100,000/mm³), increased fibrin split products if DIC or HELLP syndrome is developing.

- In liver function studies: ALT (SGPT), AST (SGOT), LDH may be elevated.

- **HELLP Syndrome**

  In addition to the diagnostic tests listed under the severe preeclampsia section the following laboratory values will be observed:

  ▶ CBC: Initially, hemoconcentration is usually observed; however, the majority of women will demonstrate a rapid, significant decrease in their hematocrits.

  ▶ Peripheral blood smear will demonstrate schistocytes, spherocytes, burr cells, and/or echinocytes.

  ▶ Platelets are usually significantly decreased (often less than 50,000/mm³).

  ▶ PT and PTT are WNL unless the woman is developing DIC.

  ▶ Fibrinogen is WNL unless the woman is developing DIC.

  ▶ Serum glucose may be significantly decreased in some women (Poole, 1993)

  ▶ In liver function studies, AST (SGOT) and ALT (SGPT) are elevated.

  ▶ In renal function studies, serum BUN and creatinine are elevated.

  ▶ Uric acid will be elevated.

Eclampsia

See laboratory values listed under Severe Preeclampsia and HELLP Syndrome.

Chronic Hypertension

- In a clean catch midstream urine specimen, dipstick for protein will be negative or trace.

- Renal function studies (e.g., serum BUN, creatinine) may be altered depending upon the severity of hypertension and any associated renal damage.

- Hematologic, coagulation, and hepatic studies (if ordered) will usually be WNL.

- Obstetrical ultrasound should be obtained if IUGR is suspected. If IUGR is documented, serial ultrasounds should be obtained every 2 to 3 weeks to assess fetal growth.

- Obtain serial NSTs with AFIs, BPPs, or CSTs beginning at 32 to 34 weeks or earlier, as indicated (e.g., suspected or documented IUGR).

Chronic Hypertension with Superimposed PIH

See diagnostic tests for mild and severe preeclampsia.

Treatment/Management

In some institutions, a reliable woman with stable, mild PIH without proteinuria and gross edema, or mild preeclampsia may be managed on an outpatient basis (Mabie & Sibai, 1996; Roberts, 1994). However, this treatment option requires co-management with a physician, since rapid progression of disease can occur.

- The following requirements must be met if a woman is to be considered a candidate for home management (ACOG, 1996; Frangieh & Sibai, 1996):

  ▶ Woman is able to comply with the clinician's management plan (see under Mild PIH/Mild Preeclampsia section).

  ▶ Diastolic pressure 100 mm Hg or less

  ▶ Systolic pressure 150 mm Hg or less

  ▶ Proteinuria less than 1gm/24 hour or less than 3+ on dipstick

  ▶ Platelet count more than 120,000/mm^3

  ▶ Normal fetal growth and antenatal fetal surveillance testing

  ▶ Absence of symptoms associated with severe preeclampsia (persistent headaches, visual disturbances, nausea, vomiting, epigastric or right upper quadrant pain, abdominal pain)

Outpatient Strategies for Stable, Mild Disease (Frangieh & Sibai, 1996)

Mild PIH/Mild Preeclampsia

- Daily blood pressure reading by the woman or a member of her family

- Daily urine dipstick to check for protein

- A platelet count, liver enzymes (AST [SGOT], ALT [SGPT]), and 24-hour urine for protein and creatinine clearance obtained weekly

- Fetal movement counts should be recorded daily beginning at 28 weeks' of gestation

- Women without evidence of worsening disease should be seen by their clinician weekly or twice weekly for evaluation of their BP, urine protein, weight, evidence of edema, deep tendon reflexes, fundal height measurement, auscultation of fetal heart tones, and symptom assessment. The symptom assessment should specifically address the following areas: development of a severe frontal or occipital headache, visual disturbances, nausea and/or vomiting, epigastric pain, abdominal pain, increased edema, decreased fetal movements.

- Weekly antenatal fetal surveillance instituted between 32 and 34 weeks' gestation (earlier, as indicated). Attempt to schedule these tests on the same day as the woman's office visit.

- A public health nurse (PHN) or home health nurse visit may be indicated if there is a question regarding the woman's ability to comply with the home management treatment plan (i.e., suspicion that BP or urine results are inaccurately measured).

- A woman exhibiting anxiety or depression should have an evaluation by a qualified clinician with appropriate therapeutic interventions initiated.

- The use of pharmacologic agents (e.g., antihypertensives) for women with mild PIH preeclampsia is not indicated. If such therapeutic regimens are being considered, consultation with a physician is warranted.

- A woman unable to comply with the above treatment plan should be hospitalized to ensure optimal care.

- A woman unresponsive to outpatient treatment (i.e., evidence of worsening maternal disease or fetal compromise) requires immediate hospitalization and transfer of care to the consulting physician. The following are indications for delivery of a woman with mild PIH/mild preeclampsia (Frangieh & Sibai, 1996):

  ▶ Gestational age more than 40 weeks

  ▶ Gestational age 37 weeks or more with: a Bishop score less than 5, fetal weight less than10th percentile, and nonreactive NST

  ▶ Gestational age 34 weeks or more with labor, rupture of membranes, vaginal bleeding, persistent headaches or visual symptoms, epigastric pain, nausea and/or vomiting, abnormal BPP

Severe Preeclampsia/HELLP Syndrome/Eclampsia

The woman with severe preeclampsia, HELLP syndrome, or eclampsia requires immediate hospitalization and physician managed care.

Chronic Hypertension

- A woman with hypertension requires co-management with a physician.

- Current opinion does not support the use of antihypertensive agents in women with diastolic pressures below 100 mm Hg, since they have not demonstrated an improvement in maternal or fetal outcome (ACOG, 1996; Sibai, Mabie, Shamsa, Villar, & Anderson, 1990).

- If antihypertensive therapy is indicated, it should be prescribed after consultation with the physician.

  ▶ In general, the first-line agent considered for use during pregnancy is alpha-methyldopa because of extensive experience and its documented fetal safety.

  ▶ Atenolol and labetalol are other acceptable medications for use during pregnancy.

  ▶ Beta-blocking agents have been associated with an increased risk of IUGR; therefore, a pregnant woman receiving a beta-blocker requires careful fetal surveillance.

  ▶ Other commonly used antihypertensive agents have not been extensively studied during pregnancy.

  ▶ A possible association with oligohydramnios and fetal/neonatal death has been reported with the use of angiotensin-converting inhibitors. Therefore, the use of these agents should be avoided.

  NOTE: Diuretics should be avoided during pregnancy because of the associated reduction in plasma volume that theoretically may result in adverse fetal effects (ACOG, 1996).

Chronic Hypertension with Superimposed PIH

Chronic hypertension with superimposed PIH requires co-management with a physician.

Consultation

- Consultation is required for any woman with evidence of hypertensive disease.

- Physician co-management of a woman with mild PIH without proteinuria or edema, mild preeclampsia, chronic hypertension, or chronic hypertension with superimposed PIH is warranted.

- Transfer to physician care all women with evidence of worsening maternal disease, fetal compromise, severe preeclampsia, HELLP syndrome, or if a woman is unreliable or noncompliant regarding her care.

Patient Education

- Educate the woman about PIH, its possible impact on maternal and fetal health, and the plan of care.

- Explain the importance of recognizing and reporting signs and symptoms of progressing preeclampsia and of other possible complications (e.g., obstetrical bleeding, preterm labor, premature rupture of membranes, etc.).

- Educate the woman about any diagnostic tests that are ordered and interpret results for her.

- Teach the woman how to count fetal movements and when to contact a clinician or the hospital about them.

- Assist with arrangements for childbirth preparation for the woman; provide anticipatory guidance regarding labor and birth.

- Review labor and birth procedures relevant to her plan of care (e.g., continuous fetal monitoring, type of analgesia/anesthesia).

- For the woman being managed as an outpatient, provide instruction in the proper techniques for blood pressure reading and urinary protein dipstick evaluations. Arrange for her to receive the necessary equipment for these evaluations.

- Reinforce the importance of complying with clinic/office, laboratory assessments, and antenatal testing appointments.

Follow-up

- If signs and symptoms of PIH are resolved after birth of the infant, schedule woman for 2- and 6-week postpartum office visits.

- If PIH persists after delivery (e.g., 24–48 hrs), schedule an office visit 1 week after birth (if no follow-up evaluation by the consulting physician is scheduled). Consult with a for any woman with evidence of persistent hypertension during her outpatient postpartum visits.

- If the infant is small for gestational age, schedule a public health nurse home visit during the first week after discharge from the hospital.

- Make sure the woman has arranged appointments for her infant's evaluations at 2 and 6 weeks after birth.

- Document hypertensive disorder and management thereof in progress notes and problem list.

References

American College of Obstetricians and Gynecologists (ACOG). (1996). *Hypertension in pregnancy.* Technical bulletin no. 219. Washington, DC: Author.

Beckmann, C. R. B., Ling, F. W., Barzansky, B. M., Bates, G. W., Herbert, W. N. P., Laube, D. W., & Smith, R. P. (1995). *Obstetrics and gynecology* (2nd ed., pp. 137-144). Baltimore, MD: Williams & Wilkins.

Byrd, J., & Sakornbut, E. (1996). Complications of pregnancy. In S. D. Ratcliffe, J. E. Byrd, & E. L. Sakornbut (Eds.), *Handbook of pregnancy and perinatal care in family practice. Science and practice* (pp. 99–133). Philadelphia, PA: Hanley & Belfus.

Cunningham, F. G., MacDonald, P.C., Gant, N. F., Leveno, K. J., & Gilstrap III, L. C. (1993). *Williams obstetrics* (19th ed., pp. 763–817). Norwalk, CT: Appleton & Lange.

Dildy III, G. A., & Cotton, D. B. (1991). Management of severe preeclampsia and eclampsia. *Critical Care Clinics, 7*(4), 829–850.

Frangieh, A. Y., & Sibai, B. M. (1996). Outpatient management of mild gestational hypertension and preeclampsia. *Contemporary OB/GYN, 41*(8), 67–78.

Friedman, S. A., Taylor, R. N., & Roberts, J. M. (1991). Pathophysiology of preeclampsia. *Clinics in Perinatology, 18*(4), 661–682.

Jones, K. A., Abramowitz, J. S., Anissi, D., Mirwald, M. A., & Sherer, D. M. (1993). Severe HELLP syndrome presenting with acute gum bleeding following toothbrushing at 38 weeks gestation. *American Journal of Critical Care, 2*(5), 395–396.

Mabie, W. C., & Sibai, B. M. (1996). Hypertensive states of pregnancy. In A. H. DeCherney & M. L. Pernoll (Eds.), *Current obstetric & gynecologic diagnosis & treatment* (8th ed., pp. 380–397). Norwalk, CT: Appleton & Lange.

Meyer, N. L., Mercer, B. M., Friedman, S. A., & Sibai, B. M. (1994). Urinary dipstick protein: A poor predictor of absent or severe proteinuria. *American Journal of Obstetrics & Gynecology, 170*(1), 137–141.

Poole, J. (1993). HELLP syndrome and coagulopathies of pregnancy. *Critical Care Nursing Clinics of North America, 5*(3), 475–487.

Reubinoff, B. E., & Schenker, J. G. (1991). HELLP syndrome–a syndrome of hemolysis, elevated liver enzymes and low platelet count complicating preeclampsia–eclampsia. *International Journal of Gynecology and Obstetrics, 36*, 95–102.

Roberts, J. M. (1994). Pregnancy-related hypertension. In R. K. Creasy & R. Resnik (Eds.), *Maternal-fetal medicine. Principles and practice* (3rd ed., pp. 804–844). Philadelphia: W. B. Saunders.

Sibai, B. M. (1988). Preeclampsia-eclampsia maternal and perinatal outcomes. *Contemporary Ob/Gyn, 32*(6), 109-118.

Sibai, B. M. (1991). Management of preeclampsia. *Clinics in Perinatology, 18*(4), 793–808.

Sibai, B. M., Mabie, W. C., Shamsa, F., Villar, M. A., & Anderson, G. D. (1990). A comparison of no medication versus methyldopa or labetalol in chronic hypertension during pregnancy. *American Journal of Obstetrics and Gynecology, 162*(4), 960–966.

Sibai, B. M., & Moretti, M. M. (1988). PIH: Still common and still dangerous. *Contemporary Ob/Gyn, 31*(2), 57-70.

Sibai, B. M., Taslimi, M. M., El-Nazar, A., Amon, E., Mabie, B. C., & Ryan, G. M. (1986). Maternal-perinatal outcome associated with the syndrome of hemolysis, elevated liver enzymes, and low platelets in severe pre-eclampsia-eclampsia. *American Journal of Obstetrics & Gynecology, 155*(3), 501-509.

Willett, G. D. (1994). *Laboratory testing in ob/gyn.* Boston: Blackwell Scientific Publications.

Chapter 14

IONIZING RADIATION

Lisa L. Lommel

Ionizing radiation (x-rays) are highly penetrating, short-wavelength electromagnetic waves with the capacity of producing ionization within tissues and subsequent electrochemical reactions (Cunningham, MacDonald, Gant, Leveno & Gilstrap, 1993). Ionizing radiation can be direct or indirect causing 1) cell death, which affects embryogenesis, 2) carcinogenesis, and 3) genetic effects of future generations from germ cell mutation (Cunningham et al., 1993). Effects of radiation on a variety of factors, including the amount of the exposure and susceptibility of the recipient.

There are several standard terms used for measuring ionizing radiation.

- Exposure: The number of ions produced by x-rays per kg of air (unit: Reontgen [R])

- Dose: The amount of energy deposited per kilogram of tissue. The traditional measurement unit is the rad; the more modern unit is the Gray [Gy] where 1 Gy = 100 rad.

- Relative effective dose: The amount of energy deposited per kilogram of tissue normalized for biological effectiveness. The traditional unit is the rem; the more modern unit is Sievert [Sv] where 1 Sv = 100 rem (Cunningham et al., 1993). When referring to diagnostic x-rays, the dose (rad) and relative effective dose (rem) are the same and can be used interchangeably. The term "mrad" is also used when referring to small doses or radiation. One mrad equals one thousandth of a rad.

Exposure of the fetus or embryo to radiation is not uncommon and is often unavoidable. Radiation exposure from the atmosphere, building materials, the ground, and naturally occurring radioisotopes account for approximately 0.075 to 0.1 of rem during gestation (National Council on Radiation Protection and Measurements [NRCP], 1977a). A routine chest x-ray accounts for less than .05 rads of exposure to the fetus (Drugan & Evans, 1988). The majority of diagnostic examinations expose the fetus to less than 5 rads (see Table 6.10, Exposure to Fetus from x-ray Studies). It has been determined that exposure of 5 rads or less presents no increased risks of pregnancy loss, congenital anomalies, mental defectiveness, or growth restriction. At levels of 5 rads or less, the risk to a fetus is not increased substantially above general risks of pregnancy loss (30 percent) and malformations (2.75 percent). At these levels, termination of the pregnancy is not recommended (American College of Obstetricians and Gynecologists, 1995; Conover, 1994; Bentur, Horlatsch, & Koren, 1991; Cunningham et al., 1993). Although not well substantiated, it has been reported that diagnostic levels (up to 5 rads) of in utero exposure increase the risk of childhood leukemia (Cunningham et al., 1993). The relative risk of childhood leukemia from fetal exposure to 1 to 2 rad has been estimated from several studies to be 1.5 to 2.0 (Cunningham et al., 1993).

Fetal exposure to ionizing radiation between 5 to 10 rads presents an unknown risk. A review of the literature describes a paucity of studies and information regarding this exposure range. It is known that for exposure levels above 10 rads, there is a substantial increase risk for intrauterine growth restriction, microcephaly, and neurologic abnormalities. Exposure to radiation above 50 rads during the first 10 to 14 days of human development is unlikely to produce congenital malformations, but there is a substantial risk of pregnancy loss. Exposure to these levels during the period of organogenesis (2 to 9 weeks) places the embryo at risk for major anatomical malformation, including mental restriction, microcephaly, and ocular abnormalities (Jankowski, 1986). During the second and third trimester, central nervous system anomalies and ophthalmic defects may occur at high doses.

The physical and biological characteristics of microwave and ultrasound energy are different from that of ionizing radiation (x-rays). The embryo is not at risk of mutagenic or carcinogenic effects from microwave radiation. Properly constructed microwave ovens do not represent a hazard during pregnancy (Burgel, 1992).

Ultrasonography uses sound waves to study anatomical features of the fetus. This procedure has greatly reduced the need for fetal exposure to x-rays. There have been no identifiable adverse effects to the fetus from diagnostic ultrasound. It is currently considered to be safe during pregnancy (Cunningham et al., 1993).

The ionizing radiation generated by a video display terminal (VDT) is emitted by the cathode ray tube and is entirely absorbed by the glass screen. Several studies could not detect measurable ionizing radiation from video display terminals (0.01 to 0.05 mrad/hr). At this level, a woman sitting at a VDT console for 30 hours a week would accumulate a maximum dose of 0.006 rads during the first trimester. Due to the minimal amount of fetal exposure, VDTs are not considered harmful (Bentur & Koren, 1991; Burgel, 1992).

Database

Subjective

- No symptoms related to exposure
- Women who may be pregnant and need diagnostic evaluation with x-rays
- Women with unknown pregnancy who were exposed to ionizing radiation
- Women at occupational risk.
  - ▶ Health care personnel who work with patients receiving x-rays
  - ▶ Those who handle radioactive material
  - ▶ Workers exposed to nuclear material on the job

Objective

- There may be no signs of exposure.
- Number or rems accumulated as determined by use of film or thermoluminescent dosimeter (TLD) badge (if in an occupation that confers risk).
- Record the type, date, and number of radiation exposures.
- Document use of protective clothing (lead equivalent) equipment.
- Determine the stage of pregnancy when radiation exposure occurred.
- Calculate the embryonic exposure.

Assessment

- Patient exposure to ionizing radiation

Plan

Diagnostic Tests

- Continue to obtain diagnostic x-rays that are essential for optimal medical care of the mother and evaluation of medical problems.

- Elective tests need not be performed on a pregnant woman, even though the risk to the embryo is small.

- Perform ultrasound to determine possible fetal anomalies if the mother has been exposed to large doses of ionizing radiation.

- Perform ultrasound between 28 and 34 weeks' gestation to rule out intrauterine growth restriction (IUGR) if exposed to large doses of ionizing radiation.

Treatment/Management

- Provide patient support and education.

- Pregnancy termination is not recommended for ionizing radiation exposure of less than 5 rads.

- For radiation exposures of more than 5 rads, consult with a physician to evaluate level of exposure and for genetic risk counseling.

Consultation

- Consult with a physician to evaluate level of embryonic exposure and need for genetic risk counseling.

Patient Education

- Advise nonpregnant women working with or in the presence of radiation (occupational exposure) that it is required they be monitored for radiation exposure by film or thermoluminescent dosimeter (TLD) badge. Maximum exposure should be no greater than 1.25 rads in 3 months or 5 rads in a year (Burgel, 1992).

- Advise pregnant women who are occupationally exposed to radiation that the exposure to the embryo/fetus should not exceed a maximum dose of 0.5 rads *for the entire pregnancy*. This is equivalent to 1.5 rads to the pregnant women because absorption of radiation by the abdominal wall usually reduces the fetal dose to 0.5 rads or less (Burgel, 1992).

  ▶ Women working in areas of radiation exposure whose fetus could receive 0.5 rads or more before birth should seek ways to reduce their exposure within their present job.

    – Request reassignment to an area of less exposure.

- Delay childbearing until a job change.

- Continue working in the present position with the awareness that there is a small risk to the unborn child.

- Advise women who are pregnant and who assist with diagnostic x-rays (radiologists, x-ray technicians, nurses) to limit radiation dose to 0.5 rads by using a 0.5 mm lead-equivalent wrap-around apron and avoiding of the radiation beam.

- Educate the patient that no special shielding precautions need to be taken during x-ray of a part away from the maternal pelvis (e.g., dental films). Shielding of the pregnant woman's abdomen is routinely done, however, in most cases.

- Reassure the patient that if she has been unshielded, radiation dose to the fetus is minuscule.

- Agencies employing workers exposed to radiation are responsible for providing employees with specific instructions on how to avoid the risks of radiation and in-utero radiation which include (Burgel, 1992)

  ▶ Shielding for x-rays

  ▶ Wearing protective clothing when working with radioactive chemicals

  ▶ Wearing long-sleeved protective uniforms

  ▶ Using protective lead-lined aprons and gloves, and protective eye wear

  ▶ Wearing personal radiation monitoring devices, which monitor individual cumulative radiation exposure, at all times during work hours

  ▶ Avoiding all unnecessary exposure to radiation sources

Follow-up

- Perform routine postpartum follow-up.
- Document exposure in progress notes and problem list.

Table 6.10

Exposure to Fetus from x-ray Studies

Head

Routine: < 50 mrad
Computerized axial tomography: < 100 mrad

Chest

Routine: < 50 mrad
Computerized axial tomography: < 1 rad
Mammography: < 50 mrad

Spine

Cervical: < 50 mrad
Thoracic: < 100 mrad
Lumbar/lumbosacral: 27–3,970 mrad

Abdominal

Upper GI series: 5–1,230 mrad
Cholecystography/cholangiography: 14–1,600 mrad
Barium enema: 28–12,600 mrad
Intravenous pyelography: 70–5,480 mrad
Pelvimetry: 220–5,480 mrad
Hysterosalpingography: 270–9,180 mrad

Extremities

Shoulder: 0.5–3.0 mrad
Other (excluding upper femur): < 50 mrad
Hips and femurs (proximal): 73–1,370 mrad

Note: mrad = one thousandth of a rad

Source: Drugan, A., & Evans, M. (1988). Exposure of the pregnant patient to ionizing radiation. *Contemporary Ob/Gyn*, *32* (4), 16–21. Reprinted with permission.

References

American College of Obstetricians and Gynecologists (ACOG) (1995). Guidelines for diagnostic imaging during pregnancy. Committee Opinion No. 158.

Bentur, Y., Horlatsch, N., & Koren, G. (1991). Exposure to ionizing radiation during pregnancy: Perception of teratogenic risk and outcome. *Teratology, 43*, 109–112.

Bentur, Y., & Koren, G. (1991). The three most common occupational exposures reported by pregnant women: An update. *American Journal of Obstetrics and Gynecology, 165*(2), 429–437.

Burgel, B.J. (1992). Pregnancy and work restrictions: Implications for occupational health nursing practice. *American Association of Occupational Health Nursing (AAOHN) Journal Update Series,* 1–8.

Conover, E. (1994). Hazardous exposures during pregnancy. *Journal of Obstetrics, Gynecologic and Neonatal Nursing, 23*(6), 524–532.

Cunningham, F.G., MacDonald, D.C., Gant, N.F., Leveno, K.J., & Gilstrap, L.C. (1993). *Williams Obstetrics* (19th Ed.) pp. 981–988. Norwalk, CT: Appleton & Lange.

Drugan, A., & Evans, M. (1988). Exposure of the pregnant patient to ionizing radiation. *Contemporary Ob/Gyn, 32*(4), 16–21.

Jankowski, C. (1986). Radiation and pregnancy: Putting the risks in proportion. *American Journal of Nursing,* 260–265.

National Council on Radiation Protection and Measurements (1977a). *Medical radiation exposure of pregnant and potential pregnant women* (NCRP Report No. 54). Washington, DC: U.S. Government Printing Office.

National Council on Radiation Protection and Measurement (1977b). *Review on NCRP radiation dose limit for embryo and fetus in occupationally exposed women* (NCRP Report No. 53). Washington, DC: U.S. Government Printing Office.

Chapter 15

INTRAUTERINE GROWTH RESTRICTION

Lisa L. Lommel

Intrauterine growth restriction (IUGR) affects 3 percent to 10 percent of all pregnancies, although up to 65 percent of all cases of IUGR are not identified until after the birth of the infant (McFarlin, 1994). The impact of fetal growth impairment is evident by the significantly higher perinatal morbidity and mortality rates compared to infants who grow normally. Neonatal morbidity associated with IUGR includes birth asphyxia, meconium aspiration, pulmonary hemorrhage, polycythemia syndrome and hypoglycemia (Pollack & Divon, 1992). The perinatal mortality is four to ten times higher in growth restricted neonates than those with normal growth patterns (McFarlin, 1994). Although the majority of full-term infants with IUGR demonstrate normal intelligence, the risk for long-term neurologic and developmental disorders is substantially increased.

Newborns weighing less than 2,500 grams at birth are classified as low birthweight according to the World Health Organization. A newborn is classified as growth restricted, or small for gestational age (SGA), when birthweight falls below the tenth percentile for gestational age. Birthweight below the fifth and third percentile, birthweight more than two standard deviations below the mean for gestational age, and a ponderal index (birthweight divided by the cube of the height) below the tenth percentile for gestational age have also been used to define intrauterine growth restriction (Craigo, 1994). However, not all fetuses below the tenth percentile will be growth restricted. Approximately 10 percent of all fetuses will be below tenth percentile and be normal but genetically or constitutionally small. It is for this reason that the diagnosis of IUGR should be defined as an increase in fetal abdominal circumference of less than 10 mm in a 2-week period. It is fetal growth, not size, that should be assessed when diagnosing IUGR. It is common clinical practice, however, to use the less-than-tenth percentile measurement as the indicator for IUGR.

Sonographic evaluation of IUGR includes the measurement of several fetal parameters. Measurements include biparietal diameter (BPD), femur length (FL), abdominal circumference (AC), head circumference (HC), estimated fetal weight (EFW) (calculated from BPD or FL and AC), total intrauterine volume (TIUV), and amniotic fluid volume (AFV). The ratios most commonly used to identify growth disturbances are the head circumference to abdominal circumference and femur length to abdominal circumference. Abdominal circumference is critical in the diagnosis of IUGR as it encompasses the liver which is the part of the fetus that most sensitively shows a change in fetal weight and growth (McFarlin, 1994).

Two types of abnormal growth patterns can be recognized using sonography in the IUGR fetus. These types of IUGR reflect differences in parameters of body length and size (see Table 6.11). Many fetuses exhibit substantial overlap between symmetric and asymmetric patterns. Therefore management decisions should not be made based on growth patterns alone (Pollack & Divon, 1992).

- Symmetrical IUGR: This type of IUGR occurs when the fetus has experienced an early and prolonged deprivation resulting from chronic maternal malnutrition, intrauterine infection, congenital malformation, fetal chromosomal anomaly, substance abuse, placental insufficiency, or multiple gestation. Fetal cell size is normal but is generally deficient throughout the body. The neonate's body and head are proportional but small (proportional growth restriction). Head circumference falls below the tenth percentile, brain size is diminished, and permanent sequelae including childhood inattention, anxiety, and behavior problems associated with poor academic performance may result.

- Asymmetrical IUGR: This type of IUGR accounts for approximately 70 percent of all cases of IUGR. It results from nutritional deficits and placental deficiency in late second and third trimesters of pregnancy caused by a variety of maternal disorders including hypoxic, vascular, renal hematologic, and environmental disorders. Diminished cell size results from atrophy of preexisting cells without a reduction in the number of cells. Head size of the neonate appears disproportionately large in relation to the body because the head growth is not restricted (disproportional growth restriction). The body contains little subcutaneous fat and appears long and emaciated. Generalized muscle wasting, poor skin turgor, sparse hair, wrinkled abdomen, and widely separated sutures are all indicative of asymmetrical IUGR. Postnatal growth and development of the infant is rapid, and the potential for normal intellectual growth is excellent.

There are a variety of socioeconomic, nutritional, and clinical factors that have been found to predict IUGR (see Data Base section). When IUGR is suspected in a pregnancy, however, a cause is identified in only a minority of cases. Even after birth, a cause for growth restriction in the SGA infant can be found in fewer than one-half of the cases.

Database

Subjective

- Socioeconomic or environmental status
  - ▶ Living at high altitudes
  - ▶ Low socioeconomic status
  - ▶ Lack of access to medical care
  - ▶ Exposure to occupational hazards
  - ▶ Substance abuse (tobacco, alcohol, drugs: methadone, cocaine, heroin, antimetabolites, anticoagulants, anticonvulsants)
- Nutrition
  - ▶ Low prepregnancy weight (strong correlation with IUGR)
  - ▶ Inadequate weight gain during pregnancy
  - ▶ Inadequate access to food
  - ▶ Personal food restrictions or food fetishes
- Medical conditions
  - ▶ Chronic hypertension (strong correlation with IUGR)
  - ▶ Diabetes mellitus
  - ▶ Renal disease
  - ▶ Autoimmune disease
  - ▶ Hemoglobinopathies

- ▶ Severe anemia
- ▶ Congenital heart condition
- ▶ Asthma
- ▶ Cystic fibrosis
- ▶ Pancreatitis
- ▶ Ileojejunal bypass
- ▶ Inflammatory bowel disease
- Maternal infections
  - ▶ Viral, such as rubella, cytomegalovirus, herpes simplex, varicella zoster
  - ▶ Bacterial, such as listeriosis, tuberculosis, poliomyelitis
  - ▶ Spirochetal (syphilis)
  - ▶ Protozoal, such as toxoplasmosis, malaria, trypanosomiasis
- Obstetrical factors
  - ▶ Previous SGA infant (recurrence risk 25 percent)
  - ▶ Previous stillborn
  - ▶ Unsure dates/late entry for prenatal care
  - ▶ Maternal age (extremes of youth or increased age)
  - ▶ Elevated maternal serum alpha-fetoprotein
- Pregnancy complications
  - ▶ Pregnancy-induced hypertension (strong correlation with IUGR)
  - ▶ Third trimester bleeding
  - ▶ Prolonged pregnancy
  - ▶ Extrauterine pregnancy
  - ▶ Placental/cord abnormalities
  - ▶ Multiple gestation
  - ▶ Poor uterine fundal growth
- Fetal chromosomal abnormalities
  - ▶ Trisomies 13, 18, 21
  - ▶ Turner's syndrome
- Fetal malformations
  - ▶ Neural tube defects
  - ▶ Congenital heart defects

- ▶ Gastrointestinal/genitourinary defects
- ▶ Skeletal dysplasias
- Review history to obtain most accurate assessment of gestational age. Include all that are appropriate. (See Table 6.12, Estimation of Gestational Age with Clinical Parameters, for a summary of accuracy of methods used to assess gestational age).
  - ▶ Recorded basal body temperature
  - ▶ Recorded last menstrual period
  - ▶ Biochemical pregnancy testing
  - ▶ Quickening
  - ▶ First trimester bimanual exam
  - ▶ Ultrasound, first or second trimester
  - ▶ Timing of in-vitro fertilization
  - ▶ Timing of ovulation induction

Objective

- Maternal weight gain less than expected
- Fundal height measurement less than expected for gestational age
  - ▶ Empty maternal bladder
  - ▶ Maternal position should be the same for each measurement
  - ▶ Preferably the same examiner at each visit or minimum number of examiners
  - ▶ All examiners should use same protocol for measuring fundal height
- Nutrition recall deficient in expected caloric intake for weight, maternal age, and gestational age
- Urine dipstick may be positive for ketones
- Sonographic evidence of an estimated fetal weight less than the tenth percentile for gestational age
  - ▶ Establishing early, accurate gestational age is critical in accurate diagnosis of IUGR.
  - ▶ Diagnosis of IUGR in third trimester with unknown gestational age is difficult due to variability of all fetal biometry measurements.
  - ▶ With unknown gestational age, fetal long bones, orbital diameter and transverse cerebellar diameter is most helpful in evaluating gestational age.
  - ▶ Abdominal circumference combined with biparietal diameter (BPD) or femur length is most helpful in evaluating for IUGR (McFarlin, 1994).
    - – Abdominal circumference less than 10th percentile for gestational age is highly for suspicious for IUGR
    - – Abdominal circumference less than 3rd percentile for gestational age is evidence for IUGR
  - ▶ Presence of oligohydramnios is suspicious for IUGR.

- Presence of clinical indicators for conditions that have been associated with IUGR (e.g., increased blood pressure in chronic hypertension, specific maternal or fetal antibodies for infectious disease, congenital malformation detected by ultrasound)

Assessment

- Intrauterine growth restriction
  - ▶ R/O inaccurate dating of pregnancy
  - ▶ R/O inaccurate fundal height measurement/estimation of fetal weight
  - ▶ R/O isolated oligohydramnios
  - ▶ R/O transverse lie
  - ▶ R/O small but normal fetus
  - ▶ Presence of condition(s) known to be associated with IUGR

Plan

Diagnostic Tests

- Perform accurate dating of gestational age as early as possible in the pregnancy, including historical information (see Subjective section), pelvic examination, earliest confirmed doptone and fetoscope auscultation of fetal heart tones, and quickening.
- Perform a sonogram before 20 weeks' gestation to confirm dates in patients at risk for IUGR or with unsure dates to determine gestational age.
- Measure uterine fundus using centimeter tape at every prenatal visit, preferably by the same examiner.
- Obtain maternal weight, blood pressure, and urine dipstick at every visit.
- As soon as IUGR is suspected, obtain a detailed ultrasound to assess for fetal anomalies and verify dating (if not already done).
- Then obtain serial sonograms approximately 3 weeks apart to estimate interval fetal growth and percentile rank of fetal weight for gestational age. Sonogram should include
  - ▶ Assessment of amniotic fluid. If decreased amniotic fluid or oligohydramnios is present once to twice weekly amniotic fluid volume evaluations should be obtained.
  - ▶ Evaluation of the placenta for maturation.
- Perform Doppler ultrasound every 2 to 4 weeks to evaluate the blood flow of the fetoplacental unit and uterine arteries.

NOTE: It has been found that growth-restricted fetuses with abnormal flow patterns are at higher risk for adverse perinatal outcome (Reed, 1995). This technique is not considered a standard of practice as yet and debate exists on how to use it with management of IUGR.

Treatment/Management

- Encourage cessation of maternal smoking, drug, or alcohol use.

- Nutritional counseling and referral to supplemental food program as indicated—see Section 18, *Nutrition*.

- Maintain adequate hydration.

- Reduce stress; perhaps change from full-time to part-time work or get assistance with children at home.

- Obtain financial assistance when appropriate.

- Initiate fetal movement counts at 28 weeks—see Chapter 3.5, *Antepartum Fetal Surveillance*.

- Schedule weekly (or more often, as indicated) nonstress tests and biophysical profiles—see Chapter 3.5, *Antepartum Fetal Surveillance,* for when to initiate testing.

- Manage and treat the conditions known to be associated with IUGR.

- Schedule amniocentesis to determine fetal lung maturity or rule out chromosomal abnormality as appropriate.

- Delivery may be necessary when maternal illness is aggravated by the pregnancy (i.e., pre-eclampsia/eclampsia), when fetal growth is poor or absent, oligohydramnios develops, or there is evidence of fetal distress with nonreassuring fetal function test.

- Continue fetal monitoring during labor and delivery.

Consultation

- Consultation with a physician is required for suspected IUGR.

- Refer patient to a physician when IUGR is diagnosed. Consider co-management with a physician if appropriate.

Patient Education

- See Treatment/Management section.

- Avoid using the term "intrauterine growth retardation" when talking with patients. Use the terms slow fetal growth, growth restriction, or small for gestational age.

  ▶ Explain that a small fetus does not always mean there is a problem.

  ▶ Explain the causes of IUGR.

- Discuss the plan of care with the patient, including an explanation of tests and interpretation of results.

- Encourage compliance with nutrition, hydration, stress reduction, and substance cessation to enhance fetal intrauterine environment.

- Encourage patients to attend all provider and antenatal testing appointments.

- Explain how to obtain fetal movement counts.

- Encourage a well-balanced, high-caloric, high-protein diet.
- Advise the patient to rest as much as possible in the lateral recumbent position.

Follow-up

- Patient requires more frequent evaluations, depending upon gestation and severity of disease.
- Refer to nutritionist for diet counseling.
- Refer to social worker for assistance with socioeconomic problems.
- Refer to public health nurse. as appropriate.
- Document IUGR in progress notes and problem list.

Table 6.11

Clinical Classification of IUGR

	Type I: Symmetrical	Type II: Asymmetrical
Incidence	25%	75%
Causes	"Intrinsic," genetic anomalies, "Extrinsic," TORCH teratogens, severe malnutrition (?), drugs, smoking, alcohol	"Extrinsic" utero placental insufficiency (i.e., maternal disorders)
Timing of insult	< 28 weeks' gestation	> 28 weeks' gestation
Cell number	Decreased (hypoplastic)	Normal
Cell size (hypotrophic)	Normal	Decreased
Head size	Microcephalic	Usually normal
Brain size	Decreasd	Usually normal
Liver, thymus size	Decreasd	Decreased
Brain/liver weight ratio (Normal 3:1)	Normal	Increased > 6:1
Placental growth	Frequently normal, though cell number decreasd	Decreased
Congenital anomalies	Frequent	Rare
Ponderal index	Normal	Decreased
Ultrasound evaluation		
BPD	Small	Early-Normal/Late-Small
A C	Small	Small
HC:AC ratio	Normal	Early-Increased Late-Normal
Doppler		
Umbilical and aortic resistance index	Increased	Increased
Carotid resistance index	Increased "No brain spairing"	Decreased "Brain spairing"
Postnatal catch-up growth	Poor	Good

Source: Brar, H.S., & Rutherford, S.E. (1988). Classification of intrauterine growth retardation. *Seminars in Perinatology*, *12* (1), 2–10. Reprinted with permission.

Table 6.12

Estimation of Gestational Age with Clinical Parameters

Estimating Gestational Age	Accuracy	
In-vitro fertilization	<1	day
Ovulation induction	3–4	days
Recorded basal body temperature chart	4–5	days
Ultrasound, crown-rump length, 6–14 weeks	± 5–7	days
First trimester bimanual examination	± 1	week
Ultrasound biparietal diameter before 20 weeks	± 5–7	days
Ultrasound gestational sac diameter, 5–6.5 weeks	± 1.5	weeks
Ultrasound biparietal diameter 20–26 weeks	± 1.6	weeks
Recorded last menstrual period	± 2.5	weeks
Ultrasound biparietal diameter 26–30 weeks	3–4	weeks
Last menstrual period, from memory	4–5	weeks
Ultrasound biparietal diameter >30 weeks	3–4	weeks

Source: McFarlin, B.L. (1994) Intrauterine growth retardation: Etiology, diagnosis and management. *Journal of Nurse Midwives, 39*(2), 525–655. Reprinted with permission.

References

Brar, H.S., & Rutherford, S.E. (1988). Classification of intrauterine growth retardation. *Seminars in Perinatology, 12*(1), 2–10.

Craigo, S.D. (1994). The role of ultrasound in the diagnosis and management of intrauterine growth retardation. *Seminars in Perinatology, 18*(4), 292–304.

Hadlock, F.P. (1994). Ultrasound determination of menstrual age. In P. W. Callen (Eds) *Ultrasonography in Obstetrics and Gynecology.* Philadelphia, PA; W. B. Saunders.

McFarlin, B.L. (1994). Intrauterine growth retardation: Etiology, diagnosis and management. *Journal of Nurse-Midwifery, 39*(2), 52S–65S.

Pollack, R.N. & Divon, M.Y. (1992). Intrauterine growth retardation: Definition, classification, and etiology. *Clinical Obstetrics and Gynecology, 35*(1), 99–107.

Reed, K.L. (1995). Using doppler ultrasound to detect fetal problems. *Contemporary OB/GYN, 40*(12), 15–28.

Witler, F.R. (1993). Perinatal mortality and intrauterine growth retardation. *Current Opinion in Obstetrics and Gynecology, 5*, 56–59.

Chapter 16

KETONURIA

Lisa L. Lommel

Ketonuria is the presence of ketones excreted in the urine as metabolic end-products of fatty acid metabolism. Fats are used when glucose is unavailable to the body's cells. The three ketone bodies in the urine are acetone, acetoacetic acid, and beta-hydroxybutyric acid. Clinically available strips and tablets are available to test for the presence of acetoacetic acid. The unavailability of glucose as an energy source is usually due to inability to transport glucose to the cells, as in diabetes, or because insufficient amounts of glucose exist in the body. Since insulin is necessary for transport of glucose to the cells, ketonuria in the pregnant, diabetic patient indicates an insulin/glucose imbalance. Testing the urine for the presence of ketones is often used to monitor diabetes in pregnancy. Ketonuria due to insufficient amounts of glucose in the body may be the result of fasting, heavy exercise, or the inability of the pregnant woman to maintain food intake because of nausea and vomiting.

Database

Subjective

- History of diabetes
- Dieting, fasting, pica
- Nausea and vomiting
- Hyperemesis gravidarum
- Excessive exercise
- May feel weak and anxious with dry lips, mouth and throat

Objective

- Ketonuria (range of trace to large, as identified by dipstick)
- Weight loss
- Vomiting
- Failure to gain weight
- Signs of dehydration
    - ▶ Decreased skin turgor
    - ▶ Dry mucous membranes
    - ▶ Ketones on breath
    - ▶ Increased pulse rate and temperature
- Document type, amount, and frequency of exercise

Assessment

- Ketonuria trace to large
  - ▶ R/O diabetes
  - ▶ R/O hyperemesis gravidarum
  - ▶ R/O dieting/Pica
  - ▶ R/O excessive exercise
  - ▶ R/O hyperthyroidism

Plan

Diagnostic tests

- Perform a urine dipstick for ketones and glucose.
  - ▶ Trace = 5 mg/dL
  - ▶ Small = 15 mg/dL
  - ▶ Moderate = 40 mg/dL
  - ▶ Large = 50-160 mg/dL

  NOTE: Trace false-positive results may occur with high specific gravity/low pH urines or highly pigmented urines (Detmer, McPhee, Nicoll & Chou, 1992).

- Obtain patient weight.
- Obtain a 24-hour diet recall.
- Serum acetone may be ordered if significant ketonuria is present.
- Screen all patients for diabetes routinely at 24 to 28 weeks.
- Earlier screening may be indicated for patients who present with ketones on urine dipstick.

Treatment/Management

- Prescribe an adequate diet.
- Provide an antiemetic for severe nausea and vomiting. See Chapter 5.12, *Nausea/Vomiting*.
- Decrease the amount of exercise, when excessive.
- Refer to labor and delivery unit for IV hydration if severe hyperemesis.
- Refer to Chapter 5.12, *Nausea/Vomiting*, Chapter 5.13, *Pica*, and Chapter 6.11, *Gestational Diabetes*.
- Refer those patients practicing pica to a nutritionist.

Consultation

- Consult with a physician in cases of excessive, prolonged nausea and vomiting or persistent significant ketonuria.

Patient Education

- Explain the physiology of ketonuria and ensure that the patient knows that ketonuria is of concern during pregnancy.

- Discuss the value of adequate exercise; but emphasize the problems that may be associated with excessive and/or prolonged exercise.

- Explain the importance of adequate nutritional intake and the problems of dieting or fasting during pregnancy.

- Patients practicing pica require an understanding of its meaning during pregnancy.

Follow-up

- Document the presence of ketonuria in problem list and progress notes.

References

Detmer, W. M., McPhee, S. J., Nicoll, D. & Chou, T. M. (1992). *Pocket guide to diagnostic tests*. Connecticut: Appleton and Lange.

Wallach, J. (1992). *Interpretation of diagnostic tests* (5th ed.). Boston, MA: Little Brown and Company.

Chapter 17

MALPRESENTATION

Maureen T. Shannon

Malpresentation is defined as the fetal presention other than cephalic. There are different types of abnormal fetal presentations including breech presentations, transverse lie, deflection abnormalities, and compound presentations. Many factors have been noted to contribute to fetal malpresentation including placenta previa, contracted pelvis, uterine abnormalities, multiple gestations, fetal congenital malformations, and oligohydramnios. Some fetal malpresentations, such as a deflection abnormality or a compound presentation, do not become apparent until labor has started. However, other abnormal fetal presentations are clinically evident during the antepartum period and should be diagnosed antenatally so that obstetrical interventions such as external version or an elective cesarean section can be discussed.

Types of Presentation

The following is a description of the various fetal malpresentations, a brief description of their incidences, and risks associated with each type.

Breech Presentation

The fetus is in a longitudinal lie with the fetal buttocks, knees or feet as the presenting part, and the fetal sacrum is the denominator (Collea, 1994). The incidence of singleton breech presentations declines as gestational age advances, with a reported incidence of 35 percent in pregnancies at 28 weeks gestation compared to 2 to 4 percent in pregnancies at or beyond 36 weeks' gestation (Bowes Jr., 1994; Collea, 1994). In multiple gestations, breech presentations are more common because multiple fetuses may prevent position changes that would accommodate a cephalic presentation. In twin gestations, the incidence of breech presentations is 25 percent for twin A and 50 percent for twin B. These percentages increase with additional fetuses (Collea, 1994). Intrapartum risks to the fetus associated with breech presentations include prolapse of the umbilical cord, entrapment of the after-coming head, and birth trauma (Bowes Jr., 1994; Collea, 1994).

There are four types of breech presentations:

1. Complete breech presentation occurs when the fetal thighs and knees are flexed. The fetus appears to be in a tailorsitting position. The incidence of complete breech presentation in singleton pregnancies in which the fetus weighs more than 2,500 grams is 10 percent (Collea, 1994).

2. Frank breech presentation occurs when the fetal thighs are flexed and the knees are extended. The incidence is 65 percent of singleton breech presentations in which the fetus weighs more than 2,500 grams (Collea, 1994).

3. Footling breech presentation can be single or double and occurs when the fetal thigh(s) and knee(s) extends and one or both of the feet present(s). The incidence of a footling breech presentation in a pregnancy in which a fetus weighs more than 2,500 grams is 25 percent (Collea, 1994).

4. Kneeling breech presentation occurs when the fetal thighs are extended, the knees are flexed, and the knees are the presenting part. A kneeling breech can be single or double.

Transverse Lie

This fetal position occurs when the long axis of the fetus is perpendicular to the mother's body. Often the fetal shoulder is over the pelvic inlet and the term shoulder presentation (or acromion presentation) is used. The incidence of transverse lie is approximately 1 in 300 births (Bowes Jr., 1994). Prematurity, increased parity, placenta previa, and premature rupture of membranes (PROM) are factors that have been associated with transverse lie. The reported perinatal mortality rate ranges from 3.9 to 24 percent, and is attributed to the high incidence of low birth weight infants with shoulder presentations and umbilical cord prolapse in term infants (Bowes Jr., 1994).

Oblique Lie

An oblique lie occurs when the fetal head or breech is in the maternal iliac fossa. This is usually a transitory presentation that evolves into either a transverse or longitudinal lie (e.g., a cephalic or breech presentation) when labor begins.

Deflection Abnormalities

Brow and face presentations are classified as deflection abnormalities and are different degrees of deflection of cephalic presentations. Each of these abnormalities has an incidence of 1 in 500 births; the diagnosis is usually made during labor (Bowes Jr., 1994). Often deflection abnormalities diagnosed early in labor will correct themselves as labor progresses. Etiologic factors reportedly associated with deflection abnormalities include anencephaly, prematurity, premature rupture of membranes, cephalopelvic disproportion, and increased parity (Bowes Jr., 1994). There is an increased perinatal mortality rate observed in pregnancies with deflection abnormalities compared to cephalic presentations. This is attributed to the higher rates of prematurity, fetal anomalies, and birth trauma secondary to manipulation during vaginal delivery associated with this complication (Bowes Jr., 1994; Collea, 1994).

Compound Presentation

A compound presentation occurs when one or more fetal limbs prolapse into the lower uterine segment alongside the presenting part. The incidence of compound presentations is low, reportedly 1 in approximately 1,200 pregnancies (Bowes Jr., 1994; Collea, 1994). The most common compound presentation is a fetal hand prolapsing alongside the cephalic presenting part. In breech presentations prolapse of an upper extremity is the most common compound presentation reported (Collea, 1994). Spontaneous retraction of the prolapsed extremity often occurs during labor. Prematurity, grand multiparity, hydramnios, multiple gestations, and cephalopelvic disproportion are prediposing factors associated with this abnormal presentation. A perinatal mortality rate of 25 percent has been reported in pregnancies complicated by compound presentations, with umbilical cord prolapse, prematurity, and traumatic vaginal birth significantly contributing to this perinatal loss rate (Bowes Jr., 1994; Collea, 1994).

Database

Subjective

- In breech presentations, the woman may report one or more of the following:
  ▶ Feeling fetal movements in the lower abdomen
  ▶ Painful "kicking" in her cervical or rectal area(s)
  ▶ If a primigravida, not feeling the fetus "drop" before the onset of labor
  ▶ Increased pressure in upper abdominal quadrants or under ribs (from fetal head)
- In a transverse or oblique lie the woman may report one or more of the following:
  ▶ Feeling fetal movements in right or left side
  ▶ If a primigravida, not feeling the fetus "drop" before the onset of labor (unless the oblique lie converts to a cephalic or breech presentation)
- Deflection abnormalities
  ▶ If a primigravida, may not feel the fetus "drop" before the onset of labor
- Compound presentation
  ▶ If a primigravida, may not feel the fetus "drop" before the onset of labor

Objective

- Breech presentation
  ▶ Leopold's maneuvers will reveal the fetal head (harder and more globular than the buttocks, ballotable) in the fundus and a soft, irregular, nonballotable mass lying over the pelvis. The presenting part often is not engaged.
  ▶ Fetal heart tones (FHTs) are usually heard most distinctly above the umbilicus.
  ▶ Vaginal examination will usually reveal that the presenting part is not engaged and is soft without suture lines or fontanelles. If cervical dilitation has occurred, the anal orifice or a foot of the fetus may be felt.
  ▶ Obstetrical ultrasound will confirm the presence of a suspected breech presentation.
- Transverse or oblique lie
  ▶ Leopold's maneuvers will reveal that neither the fetal head nor the buttocks are palpable in the uterine fundus or over the pelvis. The fetal head will be felt in one of the mother's sides with the fetal buttocks palpated in the opposite side.
  ▶ The appearance of the abdomen is asymmetrical and wider than usual.
  ▶ Measurement of the uterine fundus will usually reveal that it is lower than expected for the weeks of gestation.
  ▶ The FHTs are usually heard below the umbilicus.
  ▶ Upon vaginal examination (done only if no history of second or third trimester bleeding or if previous sonographic evaluation has ruled out the possibility of a placenta previa), neither the

fetal head nor buttocks can be felt by the examiner, and the presenting part is not engaged. Occasionally, an examiner may feel a fetal shoulder, back, hand, or rib cage.

► Obstetrical ultrasound will confirm the presence of a suspected transverse or oblique lie.

• Deflection abnormalities (usually diagnosed during labor)

► Leopold's maneuvers may reveal the fetal head to be extended or hyperextended. The presenting part may not be engaged.

► If the lamboidal sutures and the posterior fontanelle are not identified by a vaginal examination during labor, a deflection abnormality should be suspected. Face presentations can be identified when the anterior fontanelle or an orbit are palpated during the bimanual examination (Bowes Jr., 1994).

► Obstetrical ultrasound may confirm the presence of a deflection abnormality.

• Compound presentations (usually diagnosed during labor)

► Leopold's maneuvers may reveal a breech presentation or a transverse lie. The presenting part may not be engaged.

► Vaginal examination may reveal the presence of a fetal extremity adjacent to the presenting part.

► The FHT's are usually heard the loudest above the umbilicus if the fetus is in a breech presentation.

► Obstetrical ultrasound will confirm the presence of a compound presentation.

Assessment

• IUP ___ weeks
  ► R/O breech presentation
  ► R/O transverse lie
  ► R/O oblique lie
  ► R/O deflection abnormality
  ► R/O compound presentation
  ► R/O cephalopelvic disproportion
  ► R/O umbilical cord prolapse

Plan

Diagnostic Tests

• Order an ultrasound whenever an abnormal fetal presentation is suspected during the last 5 weeks of pregnancy.

• If a spontaneous conversion of an abnormal fetal presentation to a cephalic or vertex presentation is suspected 5 weeks before term, then order ultrasound to confirm this.

Treatment/Management

- The incidence of breech presentations decreases weekly from approximately 35 percent at 28 weeks gestation to between 2 to 4 percent at term. If a breech presentation, transverse lie or oblique lie is present at 35 to 36 weeks gestation, then order an ultrasound to confirm this presentation. Prior to this time, an ultrasound may not be warranted due to the high probability that a spontaneous conversion of breech presentations and transverse lies will occur prior to 36 weeks gestation.

- In recent years, several studies have reported the successful conversion of breech presentations to cephalic presentations by external version under tocolysis after 36 to 37 weeks gestation (Bowes Jr., 1994; Collea, 1994; Flamm, Fried, Lonky, & Giles, 1991; Gemer & Segal, 1994; Zhang, Bowes Jr., & Portney, 1993). Therefore, refer a woman with a breech presentation or transverse lie to a physician who is qualified and experienced in this technique as soon as this presentation is confirmed by sonogram after 35 weeks.

- RhoGAM® (Rh immune globulin) 300 µg IM should be administered to Rh negative women prior to external version.

Consultation

- Consult with a physician (required) in all abnormal presentations that occur from 35 to 36 weeks gestation and are confirmed by obstetrical ultrasound.

- Physician evaluation and education of a woman with an abnormal presentation is essential so that she can explore all of the options available to her (e.g., external version, if not contraindicated; the possibility of a vaginal breech delivery or cesarean section).

Patient Education

- Reassure the woman with a breech presentation or a transverse or oblique lie early in the third trimester that most of these presentations spontaneously convert to a cephalic presentation as the pregnancy progresses.

- Educate the woman about the need for a obstetrical ultrasound if a malpresentation is suspected at 35 to 36 weeks' gestation.

- Educate the woman regarding the need for a referral for external version if a malpresentation is confirmed by obstetrical ultrasound after 35 weeks gestation.

- Educate the woman regarding her options (e.g., external version, cesarean section, vaginal breech birth) if an abnormal presentation is confirmed after 35 weeks gestation.

- If external version is planned, educate the woman about the procedure (e.g., need for hospitalization and external fetal monitoring, tocolytics). Informed consent should be obtained by the physician prior to the procedure, after risks versus benefits have been discussed.

Follow-up

- Continue routine prenatal follow-up of a woman with an abnormal fetal presentation that has spontaneously converted to a cephalic presentation or of a woman who has undergone successful external version.

- Co-management with a physician is indicated for those women whose abnormal fetal presentation cannot be corrected by external version or women who do not want this procedure attempted.

- Document fetal malpresentation and attempts at external version in progress notes and problem list.

References

Bowes Jr., W.A. (1994). Clinical aspects of normal and abnormal labor. In R.K. Creasy & R. Resnik (Eds.), *Maternal-fetal medicine. Principles and practice* (3rd ed., pp. 527–557). Philadelphia, PA: W.B. Saunders.

Collea, J.V. (1994). Malpresentation and cord prolapse. In A.H. DeCherney & M.L. Pernoll (Eds.), *Current obstetrics & gynecologic diagnosis and treatment* (8th ed., pp. 410–427). Norwalk, CT: Appleton & Lange.

Flamm, B.L., Fried, M. W., Lonky, N.M., & Giles, W.S. (1991). External cephalic version after previous cesarean section. *American Journal of Obstetrics and Gynecology, 165*(2), 370–372.

Gemer, O., & Segal, S. (1994). Incidence and contribution of predisposing factors to transverse lie presentation. *International Journal of Gynecology and Obstetrics, 44,* 219–221.

Zhang, J., Bowes, Jr., W.A., & Portney, J.A. (1993). Efficacy of external cephalic version: A review. *Obstetrics and Gynecology, 82*(2), 306–312.

Chapter 18

MASTITIS—PUERPERAL

Lisa L. Lommel

Lucy Newmark Sammons

Puerperal infectious mastitis is an infection of the lactating breast. The term "congestive mastitis" may be used to refer to noninfectious mastitis or breast engorgement. Simple, early breast engorgement is treated by suppressing of lactation with binding and mild analgesia if lactation is not desired, or by thorough breast emptying if lactation is being established. This discussion of mastitis, however, focuses on sporadic puerperal mastitis, which is a nonepidemic breast infection during the puerperium.

The most common sporadic (nonepidemic) organism causing puerperal mastitis is *Staphylococcus aureus*. Other common skin inhabitants, including *Micrococcus dyogenes, Streptococcus*, and *Hemophilus species,* or occasionally *Escherichia coli*, may also be responsible. The offending bacteria usually are from the infant's nose and throat, but may be from nursery or hospital personnel, the mother's hands, or circulating blood. In several cases, bilateral mastitis has been reported to be caused by group B *Streptococcus* and is associated with disease in the infant (Melnikow & Bedinghaus, 1994).

The incidence of puerperal mastitis is about 2.5 percent of lactating women, with reported ranges of 2.1 to 33 percent (Dahlen, 1993). Of these women, 5 to 11 percent will go on to develop a breast abscess (Dahlen, 1993). The responsible pathogen may enter the breast at the site of a nipple injury, such as cracking or abrasion. Milk stasis or a clogged milk duct predisposes to a noninfectious inflammation that can develop into infectious mastitis. Hence, infection is commonly seen at the time of weaning or with incomplete breast emptying.

Mastitis is generally differentiated from a clogged duct by suddenness of onset, fever, systemic symptoms, and local findings (Olsen & Gordon, 1990). Characteristic flu-like symptoms have led to the traditional warning that influenza in the nursing mother is mastitis until proven otherwise. Recurrence of mild mastitis suggests the presence of a predisposing factor, such as inadequate drainage of the breast due to poorly emptying lobules or ducts, poor letdown, breast constriction from clothing or feeding technique, poor infant positioning, ineffectual infant sucking, missed feedings, mother-baby separation, or maternal fatigue or stress (Ogle & Davis, 1988). Recurrent severe mastitis suggests ductal abnormalities or a persistent lobular problem, chronic nipple fissures or cracks, or inadequate antibiotic therapy (Lawrence, 1994).

Database

Subjective

- Patient complains of diffuse myalgias, fatigue, chills, and fever.
- Breast is tender. There is usually a unilateral painful area or lump, often in the outer quadrant of breast.
  - ▶ Tenderness persists through and between feeding periods.
  - ▶ Breast may be hard, warm, and reddened.

▶ Pain may be aggravated when infant nurses.

● Occurs more commonly in

▶ Primiparous women

▶ First two months postpartum, peaking in incidence between second and fourth weeks; rarely occurs before fifth postpartum day

▶ Women with a history of

    − Weaning

    − Interruption of regular nursing

    − Failure to empty breasts adequately

    − Cracked nipples

    − Improper nursing technique

Objective

● Fever, often high (greater than 38.5°C)

● Tachycardia (common)

● Breast examination

▶ Affected area(s) usually have increased warmth, redness, tenderness, swelling; erythematous lobule often in outer quadrant (often a wedge-shaped area)

▶ Crack or abrasion of nipple common

▶ Breast may be distended with milk, indurated

▶ Absence of pitting edema and fluctuation (wavy impulse felt on palpation produced by vibration of underlying fluid, which would indicate abscess formation)

● Blood count, if done, shows leukocytosis.

● Remainder of physical exam within normal limits

Assessment

● Mastitis, infectious puerperal

▶ R/O clogged duct, milk stasis, non-infectious mastitis

▶ R/O breast abscess

▶ R/O other breast disease, inflammatory carcinoma

▶ R/O viral syndrome

▶ R/O other types of infection (e.g., endometritis, cystitis)

▶ R/O toxic shock syndrome

Plan

Diagnostic Tests

- Microscopic and microbiologic laboratory analysis of secreted milk for bacterial count and leukocyte count is possible, and may contribute to differential diagnosis, but is rarely employed. Infectious mastitis milk will show evidence of greater than 10^3 bacterial colonies/mL and greater than 10^6 WBCs (Dahlen, 1993).

- Perform other tests as needed to rule out alternate pathology.

Treatment/Management

- Advise the woman to continue emptying the breasts, either by nursing or with pump.

- Advise application of moist heat.

- Encourage rest periods.

- Encourage increased fluids by mouth.

- Institute antibiotic therapy in all suspected cases of mastitis to decrease risk of abscess formation. Choice of antomicrobial therapy should consider streptococcus and staphlococci as causative organism. In cases of bilateral mastitis, streptococcus has been shown to be the most common organisms (Melnikow & Bedinghaus, 1994). Begin therapy with (Nieybl, 1996; Lawrence, 1994):

  - ▶ Penicillin 250 mg p.o. q.i.d. for 10 to 14 days

  - ▶ In penicillin-sensitive patients, substitute with erythromycin 250 mg p.o. q.i.d. for 10 to 14 days

  - ▶ If penicillin-resistant producing staphylococci is suspected, substitute with dicloxacillin 250 to 500 mg p.o. q.i.d. for 10 to 14 days.

- Suggest using an over-the-counter analgesic/antipyretic. Acetaminophen is preferred over aspirin/acetyl-salicylic acid if the woman is still breastfeeding, because breakdown products from aspirin compete for bilirubin binding sites, putting the infant at risk for kernicterus. Neonates tolerate acetaminophen well (Lawrence, 1994).

- See also Patient Education section.

Consultation

- Medical consultation for suspected abscess or other breast pathology

- Refer to a lactation consultant/specialist, if indicated, for expanded education

Patient Education

- Explain cause of mastitis and rationale for therapeutics employed.

- Advise continuation of nursing during antibiotic treatment. Suggest emptying the breast(s) by nursing or use of breast pump to prevent milk stasis. Initially, frequent nursing (every 1 to 2 hours) will promote good drainage; defer weaning, if planned, to reduce risk of abscess formation.

- Measures to reduce discomfort while nursing from sore breast include immersion of breast in warm water before nursing. Nursing on unaffected side first until let down occurs may be less painful. Apply warm compresses to breast.

- Advise woman to continue taking full course of antibiotics although symptom relief may occur within a few days.

- Woman should be alert to signs of infection in the infant (e.g., umbilical cord and mouth in cases of thrush).

- Preventive measures include

  ▶ Good breast hygiene

  ▶ Prevention, early detection, and care of nipple fissures, milk stasis, or clogged ducts

  ▶ Use of variety of positions to enhance emptying

  ▶ Avoidance of constrictive clothing (especially bras)

  ▶ Avoidance of prolonged intervals between nursing and unrelieved gorgement

  ▶ Regular handwashing practices

  ▶ Gradual weaning

- After antibiotic treatment, problems with sore nipples or breast pain may indicate *Candida albicans* infection, which would require reevaluation by a provider.

- Explore rest-promoting and stress-reduction strategies, particularly around infant-feeding periods.

- Encourage liberal fluid intake, especially water.

Follow-up

- Client is to contact provider if she does not experience symptom relief in 24 to 36 hours. Failure to achieve relief may indicate the infectious organism is not sensitive to the prescribed antibiotic, or abscess formation may have occurred.

- Document problem in progress notes and problem list.

References

Dahlen, H. (1993). Lactation mastitis. *Nursing Times, 89*(36), 38–40.

Lawrence, R.A. (1994). *Breastfeeding: A guide for the medical professional* (3rd ed.). St. Louis, MO: C.V. Mosby.

Melinikow, J. & Bedinghaus, J.M. (1994). Management of common breastfeeding problems. *The Journal of Family Practice, 39*(1), 56–64.

Niebyl, J.R. (1996). Treating breast infections. *Contemporary OB/GYN, 41*(2), 11–12.

Ogle, K.S., & Davis, M. (1988). Mastitis in lactating women. *The Journal of Family Practice, 26*(2), 139–144.

Olsen, C. & Gordon, R.E. (1990). Breast disorder in nursing mothers. *American Family Physician, 41*(5), 1509–1516.

Chapter 19

MITRAL VALVE PROLAPSE

Maureen T. Shannon

Mitral valve prolapse (MVP) is the protrusion of one or both mitral leaflets into the left atrium during ventricular contraction. It is the most common congenital cardiac lesion affecting between 5 and 10 percent of the general population with a female to male ratio of 2:1 (Savage et al., 1983). In one prospective study, 17 percent of women between 20 and 29 years of age had evidence of MVP, with the incidence declining to 7.5 percent in women ages 50 to 59 (Savage et al., 1983).

One proposed etiology of MVP is that enlargement of one or both of the mitral valve leaflets results in a superior, posterior displacement of the leaflets during systole (Cowles & Gonik, 1990). Another is that it is caused by an autosomal dominant connective tissue abnormality with myxomatous degeneration of the mitral leaflets and redundant chordae tendinae (Biswas & Perloff, 1994; Cowles & Gonik, 1990; Shabeti, 1994). MVP may occur as an isolated clinical condition or in association with other hereditary conditions, including Marfan's syndrome, Ehlers-Danlos syndrome, osteogenesis imperfecta, and Hurler's syndrome (Cowles & Gonik, 1990).

The hallmark clinical finding of MVP is the presence of a midsystolic click during auscultation of the heart. However, this finding can be intermittent and can vary depending upon the woman's position. A mid- or late systolic murmur may also be evident, indicating the presence of mitral regurgitation. In pregnant women, the normal cardiovascular changes associated with advanced pregnancy can diminish or eliminate auscultory or echocardiographic evidence of MVP (American College of Obstetricians and Gynecologists [ACOG], 1992; Cowles & Gonik, 1990; Haas, 1976; Rayburn, LeMire, Bird, & Buda, 1987; Shabeti, 1994).

In the vast majority of cases, MVP is asymptomatic and benign (Savage et al., 1983); however, it has been associated with complications such as mitral insufficiency, infective endocarditis, ruptured chordae tendineae, transient ischemic attacks, cerebrovascular accidents, arrhythmias, and, rarely, sudden death (Braverman, Bromley, & Rutherford, 1991; Cowles & Gonik, 1990; Shabeti, 1994; Wong, Giuliani, & Haley, Jr., 1990). Asymptomatic, benign MVP is not associated with an increase in maternal or perinatal morbidity or mortality (ACOG, 1992; Cowles & Gonik, 1990; Shabeti, 1994). The use of prophylactic antibiotics for normal vaginal births in women with MVP is controversial. In general, women with asymptomatic MVP without evidence of mitral regurgitation do not need prophylactic antibiotic therapy for normal labors and vaginal births; however, prophylactic antibiotic therapy is recommended for women with MVP and evidence of valvular regurgitation (Biswas & Perloff, 1994; Shabeti, 1994).

Database

Subjective

- Usually asymptomatic
- May report a personal or family history of MVP
- May report symptoms of fatigue, palpitations, dyspnea, anxiety, lightheadedness, syncope

- May report experiencing retrosternal chest pain of varying severity that is unrelated to exercise and unresponsive to rest

Objective

- Blood pressure is usually within normal limits (WNL); however, a decrease may be observed.
- Heart-rate is usually WNL but may be tachycardic with occasional ectopic beats.
- Auscultation of heart may reveal a midsystolic click (a high-pitched, crisp sound between S_1 and S_2) that increases in intensity when patient is sitting, standing or in a left lateral decubitus position. A mid- or late-systolic murmur may also be evident.

Assessment

- Probable mitral valve prolapse
  - ▶ R/O mitral regurgitation
  - ▶ R/O arrhythmias
  - ▶ R/O hemic murmur of pregnancy
  - ▶ R/O other hereditary disorders (e.g., Marfan's syndrome)

Plan

Diagnostic Tests

The following tests may be ordered after consultation with a physician:

- EKG may reveal low or inverted T waves in the inferior or lateral precordial leads with or without S-T depression (Cowles & Gonik, 1990).
- Echocardiography may reveal evidence of displacement of the mitral leaflets into the left atrium during ventricular contraction, chordal rupture, and/or annular dilitation (Cowles & Gonik, 1990).
- Holter monitoring is recommended in individuals with recurrent or sustained tachyarrhythmias and/or syncopal episodes and may reveal atrial or ventricular arrhythmias (Gottlieb, 1987).
- Women with pronounced symptoms should have thyroid function tests obtained prior to the initiation of antiarrhythmic agents to rule out hyperthyroidism as a possible cause of their symptoms (Shabeti, 1994).

Treatment/Management

- Consult with a physician (required) in all women being evaluated for MVP. Transfer to physician care all women with MVP who are symptomatic or who have echocardiogram results demonstrating significant valvular regurgitation.

- The use of an anti-arrhythmic medication (e.g., beta blockers such as propranalol) is indicated in women with symptomatic MVP and should be prescribed and managed by the physician consultant.

- Prophylactic antibiotics during labor and delivery for women with MVP and mitral regurgitation should be prescribed by the physician consultant.

Consultation

- Consult with a physician (required) in all women suspected of having MVP.

Patient Education

- Education of the woman diagnosed with MVP should include information about MVP, the diagnostic tests ordered and their results, and the fact that there are no adverse maternal or fetal effects known to occur in patients with asymptomatic MVP.

- In women with symptomatic MVP or significant valvular regurgitation, explain the plan of care and the reasons for transferring their care to a physician.

- Reassure women with asymptomatic MVP about their prognoses, emphasizing that between 5 and 10 percent of the population have this condition and the majority of these people do not develop any significant problems.

- Educate the woman about signs and symptoms that should be reported to a clinician for further evaluation (e.g., palpitations, ectopic or "skipped" beats, excessive fatigue, lightheadedness, syncope, chest pain).

- Hormonal contraceptives or intrauterine devices may be considered for contraception in women with asymptomatic MVP without evidence of valvular regurgitation or a history of thrombotic complications (Sullivan & Lobo, 1993).

- Discuss the familial tendency of MVP and recommend screening of other family members for this condition.

Follow-up

- Follow-up evaluations of women with MVP who are symptomatic is determined by the physician managing their care.

- Follow-up care of women with asymptomatic MVP involves only routine prenatal visits unless symptoms develop that require more immediate evaluation.

- Document MVP and indicate treatment thereof in problem list and progress notes.

References

American College of Obstetricians and Gynecologists (ACOG). (1992). Cardiac disease in pregnancy. *ACOG Technical Bulletin No. 168*. Washington, DC: Author.

Biswas, M.K., & Perloff, D. (1994). Cardiac, hematologic, pulmonary, renal & urinary tract disorders in pregnancy. In A. DeCherney & M. Pernoll (Eds.), *Current obstetric & gynecologic diagnosis & treatment* (8th ed., pp.428–468). Norwalk, CT: Appleton & Lange.

Braverman, A.C., Bromley, B.S., & Rutherford, J.D. (1991). New onset ventricular tachycardia during pregnancy. *International Journal of Cardiology, 33* , 409–412.

Cowles, T., & Gonik, B. (1990). Mitral valve prolapse in pregnancy. *Seminars in Perinatalogy, 14*(1), 34–41.

Gottlieb, S.H. (1987). Mitral valve prolapse: From syndrome to disease. *American Journal of Cardiology, 60*, 53J–58J.

Haas, J.M. (1976). The effect of pregnancy on the midsystolic click and murmur of the prolapsing posterior leaflet of the mitral valve. *American Heart Journal, 92*(2), 407–408.

Rayburn, W F., LeMire, M.S., Bird, J.L., & Buda, A.J. (1987). Mitral valve prolapse. Echocardiographic changes during pregnancy. *Journal of Reproductive Medicine, 32*(3), 185–187.

Savage, D.D., Garrison, R.J., Devereux, R.B., Castelli, W.P., Anderson, S.J., Levy, D., McNamara, P. M., Stokes, J., Kannel, W.B., & Feinleib, M. (1983). Mitral valve prolapse in the general population. 1. Epidemiologic features: the Framingham Study. *American Heart Journal, 186*(3), 571–576.

Shabeti, R. (1994). Cardiac diseases. In R.K. Creasy & R. Resnik (Eds.), *Maternal-fetal medicine. Principles and practice* (3rd ed., pp. 768–791). Philadelphia, PA: W.B. Saunders.

Sullivan, J.M., & Lobo, R.A. (1993). Considerations for contraception in women with cardiovascular disorders. *American Journal of Obstetrics & Gynecology, 168*(6), 2006–2011.

Wong, M.C.W., Giuliani, M.J., & Haley, Jr., E.C. (1990). Cerebrovascular disease and stroke in women. *Cardiology, 77* (Suppl. 2), 80–90.

Chapter 20

MULTIPLE GESTATION

Ellen M. Scarr

Lucy Newmark Sammons

Twins are the most commonly occurring multiple gestations, with an overall incidence of about 1 in 80 pregnancies in the United States. Twins developing from two separately released and fertilized ova are labeled dizygotic, double-ovum, or fraternal twins. Rates of dizygotic twinning are higher in certain groups (Keith, Lopez-Zeno, & Luke, 1993; Lynch, 1992):

- Women with a personal or familial (maternal) history of multiple ovulation/dizygotic twinning
- Blacks
- Larger and taller women
- Those who have recently ceased using oral contraceptives
- Those using fertility-enhancing drugs
- Those of increasing age and parity

Dizygotic twinning is less common in Asians and during periods of malnourishment. Twins developing from a single fertilized ovum are known as monozygotic, single-ovum, or identical twins. Monozygotic twins are of the same sex, account for a third of all United States-born twins, and have a worldwide incidence of about 1/250 pregnancies, unaffected by known risk factors (Gant & Cunningham, 1993; Marinoff, 1993; Pernoll & Benson, 1994).

In twin pregnancies, variations in the placenta and membranes occur, determined by the timing of embryonic division. All dizygotic twins and 30 percent of monozygotic twins have two separate (or a single fused) placentas, with two chorions and two amnions (dichorionic-diamniotic). Seventy percent of monozygotic twins have a single placenta, with one chorion and two amnions (monochorionic-diamniotic). Rarely, monozygotic twins have a single placenta, one chorion, and one amnion (monochorionic-monoamniotic) (Marinoff, 1993; Pernoll & Benson, 1994).

Combinations of dizygotic and monozygotic processes may be involved in higher order multifetal pregnancies. Triplets, for example, may develop from one, two, or three ova (Pernoll & Benson, 1994). The incidence of naturally occurring triplets is 1/7,925 live births, but with the widespread use of ovulation-inducing drugs and assisted reproduction technology, triplets occur in 1/1,411 live births in the United States. Grand multifetal pregnancies, those with four or more embryos, have also increased with advances in reproductive technology. There are more than 50 intact quintuplet sets alive in the United States (Keith et al., 1993).

Certain maternal and fetal risks increase with multiple gestation. Most (75 percent) monochorionic placentas have vascular anastomoses between the fetal circulations; there is a risk of twin-twin transfusion syndrome via these arteriovenous shunts. Monochorionic-monoamniotic twins have a less than 50 percent chance of survival because cord entanglement diminishes placental-fetal blood flow (Pernoll & Benson, 1994). Monochorionic-monoamniotic twins in which very late division of the zygote occurs will be conjoined (Siamese twins). Other fetal risks in multiple gestation pregnancies that are increased include the following:

- Spontaneous abortions, often with reabsorption of one fetus and continued viability of the other(s)

- Increased incidence of congenital anomalies

- Placenta previa and abruptio

- Cord accidents

- Increased morbidity and mortality (three times that of singleton pregnancies) secondary to prematurity, intrauterine growth restriction, birth trauma, and maternal anemia

Multiple gestation increases maternal risks for anemia (iron deficiency, folate deficiency, acute blood loss), pregnancy-induced hypertension (PIH), urinary tract infections (UTIs), hydramnios, premature rupture of the membranes, abnormal fetal presentation (locked twins, breech presentation), operative delivery, and antepartum and postpartum hemorrhage (Elliott, 1992; Keith et al., 1993; Makowski, 1990; Neilson, 1992).

The greatest cause of the increased morbidity in multigestational offspring is related to prematurity and its associated complications. Thirty to fifty percent of twins, and eighty-seven percent of triplets are born before 37 weeks (Baldwin, 1994; Garcia & Gall, 1990). The emphasis in care of multifetal pregnancies is early detection so that these potential complications can be either prevented or minimized, if possible.

Database

Subjective

- Client may have the following predisposing risk factors:

  ▶ Use of drugs causing ovarian hyperstimulation or infertility technology involving transfer of multiple fertilized ova

    - Clomiphene citrate

    - Human gonadotropins (hMG, hCG)

    - In-vitro fertilization (IVF)

    - Gamete intrafallopian transfer (GIFT)

  ▶ Personal or familial (maternal) history of dizygotic twins

  ▶ Race (black)

  ▶ Increased age or parity

  ▶ Recent cessation of oral contraceptives

  ▶ Large or tall frame

- Client may report the following:

  ▶ Exaggerated or prolonged nausea and vomiting

▶ Sensations of excessive fetal movement

▶ Sensation of feeling larger than expectation for gestational age

Objective

- Fundal height measurements greater than expected for gestational date; particularly, a discrepancy of 4 cm or more in second and third trimester

- Palpation of multiple fetal parts or more than two fetal poles

- Simultaneous auscultation of more than one distinct fetal heart sound

- Client may demonstrate the following:

  ▶ Rapid weight gain pattern

  ▶ Anemia (due to additional fetal demands)

  ▶ Elevated blood pressure, which is especially suspicious for multiple gestation if onset is before 20 weeks' gestation

- Maternal serum alpha-fetoprotein (MSAFP) results higher than expected for singleton pregnancy

  NOTE: Human placental lactogen (HPL), β-hCG, estriol, and pregnanediol levels may all be elevated, but these are less indicative of multiple gestation.

- Multiple gestation confirmed by ultrasound performed for routine screening or other indication

Assessment

- Multiple gestation

  ▶ R/O size-date discrepancy due to inaccurate dating, hydramnios, uterine myomas, or adnexal mass

  ▶ R/O discordant twin syndrome

  ▶ R/O intrauterine growth restriction

  ▶ R/O hydatidiform mole (may co-exist with normal fetus)

  ▶ R/O maternal complications: Anemia, hypertension, polyhydramnios

  ▶ R/O preterm labor

Plan

Diagnostic Tests

- Ultrasound examination to determine multiple gestation and assess fetal status

  ▶ Number of placentas, location of placenta (increased risk of placenta previa)

  ▶ Number of membranes (dichorionic-diamniotic, monochorionic-diamniotic)

  ▶ Fetal sex (same sex increases likelihood of monozygosity)

- Complete blood count (CBC) to assess for maternal anemia

Treatment/Management

- Initiate preterm birth prevention program, serial cervical examinations; consider using an ambulatory monitor. See Chapter 6.25, *Preterm Labor.*
- Initiate fetal assessment program, which may include the following:
  - ▶ Weekly nonstress testing (NST) in third trimester (by 32 weeks)
  - ▶ Biophysical profiles for discordant or nonreactive NSTs
  - ▶ Continuous wave Doppler ultrasound to assess intrauterine growth restriction
  - ▶ Serial ultrasound examinations (every 3 to 4 weeks starting between 24 and 26 weeks), which are necessary to monitor fetal growth and detect potential malpresentation prior to birth, as well as part of biophysical profile
  - ▶ Daily fetal movement counts (important from 28 weeks on, but may be difficult to attribute to an individual fetus; see Chapter 3.5, *Antepartum Fetal Surveillance*).
- Suggest activity reduction or bed rest, as indicated; clinic-specific routines vary by site regarding this controversial aspect of management.
- Establish nutritional support.
  - ▶ An addition of at least 300 kcal/day above singleton pregnancy recommendations
  - ▶ Prenatal vitamin and mineral supplementation daily, including 1 mg folic acid
  - ▶ Iron supplement of 60 to 100 mg/day (modify depending on individual hematologic status, nutritional stores, and dietary patterns)
  - ▶ Weight gain goal of 40–60 pounds; optimal level not known. See Section 18, *Nutrition.*
- Fetal pulmonary lung maturation may be difficult to assess.
  - ▶ Lecithin-sphingomyelin ratios may normally exceed 2 by 32 weeks (vs. 36 weeks in singleton pregnancies). Values may vary among fetuses.
  - ▶ Corticosteroids may be used to stimulate fetal lung maturity if preterm delivery is imminent.
- Routine prophylactic tocolytic agents and elective cerclage do not appear to be justified for twin pregnancy (Jones, Sbarra & Cetrulo, 1990; Marinoff, 1993).
- When systemic tocolytics are required to prevent premature delivery in multiple gestations, monitor client more carefully, since risk of complications (e.g., pulmonary edema) appears higher than in singleton pregnancy
  - ▶ Magnesium sulfate or calcium-channel blockers (e.g., nifedipine) may be preferred over β-adrenergics (Coyne, 1993; McCombs, 1995; Nageotte, 1990).
- Because of high fetal mortality in monoamniotic twins, hospitalization with intensive monitoring may be initiated as early as 25 weeks (Marinoff, 1993).
- See also Patient Education.

Consultation

- Physician consultation is required for management of multiple gestation pregnancy.

  ▶ Care may be undertaken in high-risk obstetrical setting utilizing multidisciplinary approach (e.g., nutritionist, social services, obstetric clinical nurse specialist).

  ▶ Co-management with physician may be possible at some sites.

- Pediatric provider to be alerted when labor imminent for optimal neonatal care.

Patient Education

- Explain the work-up and diagnostic procedures for multiple gestation pregnancy.

  ▶ When diagnosis is confirmed, assure that woman understands the implications for herself and her babies in terms of potential complications and their early detection/management.

- Reinforce preterm birth prevention strategies.

- Advise that continuation of sexual intercourse to term may be permissible (Neilson & Mutambira, 1989).

- Reinforce activity restrictions, which may be imposed from 25 to 34 weeks, and clarify the extent of restriction (bed rest, modified bed rest, minimum 10 hours rest at night and 2 hours during the day, or frequent resting with avoidance of exertional activity, etc.).

- Assist in planning for household maintenance.

  ▶ Nutritious meal preparation

  ▶ Disability income

  ▶ Child care

  ▶ Childbirth and homecoming preparation

- Emphasize cessation of tobacco use, as indicated.

- Postpartal care of the infants, especially feeding and scheduling, and household maintenance, especially cleaning and cooking, may well be problematic during the first 3 months (Neifert & Thorpe, 1990). Make plans for assistance well before delivery.

- Explore family reactions to multiple additions to family life.

  ▶ Work with family to develop their own resources.

  ▶ Contact additional financial, social, and community resources needed prenatally and postpartally.

  ▶ In addition to institutional and local services, assistance may be obtained by contacting the following organizations:

    - Twin Line, P.O. Box 10066, Berkeley, CA 94709; (510) 524-0863

    - National Organization of Mothers of Twins Clubs, Inc., P.O. Box 23188, Albuquerque, NM 87192

    - The Triplet Connection, P.O. Box 99571, Stockton, CA 95209; (209) 474-0885

- Provide symptom-specific education for discomforts of pregnancy, e.g., nausea and vomiting, increased esophageal reflux, fatigue and insomnia, shortness of breath, varicosities (see specific chapters).

- Support breastfeeding if selected.

  ▶ Discuss scheduling patterns (simultaneous, individual, complete demand, modified demand, alternating or same-side breast), desirability of piston electric breast pump after feedings to establish adequate milk supply, positioning, and maternal nutritional needs (Neifert & Thorpe, 1990; Sollid, Evans, McClowry, & Garrett, 1989).

  ▶ Referral to lactation support group or lactation specialist may be valuable.

Follow-up

- Follow client every 2 weeks to 28 weeks, then weekly, or as needed.

- Refer client to social services, public health nursing, specialty support groups, and other services prenatally and postpartally, as needed.

- Document multiple gestation in progress notes and problem list.

References

Baldwin, V. (1994). *Pathology of multiple pregnancies.* New York: Springer-Verlag.

Coyne, B. (1993). Obstetric and surgical complications of pregnancy. In J. Brown & W. Crombleholm (Eds.), *Handbook of gynecology and obstetrics* (pp. 363–379). Norwalk, CT: Appleton & Lange.

Elliott, J. (1992). Amniocentesis for twin-twin transfusion syndrome. *Contemporary OB-GYN, 37*(8), 30–47.

Gant, N. & Cunningham, F. (Eds.). (1993). *Basic gynecology and obstetrics* (pp. 421–425). Norwalk, CT: Appleton & Lange.

Garcia, P., & Gall, S. (1990). Multiple pregnancy. In J. Scott, P. SiSaia, C. Hammond, & W. Spellacy (Eds.), *Danforth's obstetrics and gynecology* (6th ed., pp. 381–401). Philadelphia, PA: J.B. Lippincott.

Jones, J.M., Sbarra, A.J., & Cetrulo, C.L. (1990). Antepartum management of twin gestation. *Clinical Obstetrics and Gynecology, 33*(1), 32–41.

Keith, L., Lopez-Zeno, J., & Luke, B. (1993). Triplet and higher order pregnancies. *Contemporary OB/GYN, 38*(6), 36–50.

Lynch, L. (1992). Twins in older women: Amniocentesis detects Down syndrome. *Contemporary OB/GYN, 37*(10), 33–44.

Makowski, E. (1990). Twin pregnancy. In E. Quilligan & F. Zuspan (Eds.), *Current therapy in obstetrics and gynecology* (3rd ed., pp. 290–292). Philadelphia, PA: W.B. Saunders.

Marinoff, D. (1993). Multiple gestation. In J. Brown & W. Crombleholm (Eds.), *Handbook of gynecology and obstetrics* (pp. 447–461). Norwalk, CT: Appleton & Lange.

McCombs, J. (1995). Update on tocolytic therapy. *Annals of Pharmacotherapy, 29*(5), 515–522.

Nageotte, M.P. (1990). Prevention and treatment of preterm labor in twin gestation. *Clinical Obstetrics and Gynecology, 33*(1), 61–68.

Neifert, M., & Thorpe, J. (1990). Twins: Family adjustment, parenting, and infant feeding in the fourth trimester. *Obstetrics and Gynecology, 33*(1), 102–115.

Neilson, J. (1992). Abnormalities of fetal growth. In A. Calder & W. Dunlop (Eds.), *High risk pregnancy* (pp. 362–386). Oxford, England: Butterworth-Heineman.

Neilson, J.P., & Mutambira, M. (1989). Coitus, twin pregnancy, and preterm labor. *American Journal of Obstetrics and Gynecology, 160*(2), 416–418.

Pernoll, M., & Benson, R. (1994). Multiple pregnancy. In A. DeCherney & M. Pernoll (Eds.), *Current obstetric and gynecologic diagnosis and treatment* (8th ed., pp. 357–367). Norwalk, CT: Appleton & Lange.

Sollid, D.T., Evans, B.T., McClowry, S.G., & Garrett, A. (1989). Breastfeeding multiples. *The Journal of Perinatal and Neonatal Nursing, 3*, 46–63.

Chapter 21

OLIGOHYDRAMNIOS

Lisa L. Lommel

Oligohydramnios is defined as a deficiency in the amount of amniotic fluid for gestational age. The amount of amniotic fluid is estimated to increase progressively throughout pregnancy to a peak of about 1,000 mL by 33 to 35 weeks' gestation. At that time, the volume begins to decline until it reaches an average of about 800 mL by 38 weeks. After 38 weeks, the volume normally drops by 150 mL weekly (Devoe & Ware, 1994; Skovgaard & Silnonek, 1993).

Oligohydramnios is confirmed by ultrasound in one of two ways. The first method measures the diameter of the largest single pocket of fluid of the maximum vertical pocket (MVP). Using this method, oligohydramnios is defined variably as a pocket no larger than 0.5, 1, 2 or 3 cm. (Skovgaard & Silvonek, 1993). The more commonly used method, the amniotic fluid index (AFI), which correlates slightly better with actual oligohydramnios than MVP. It is the sum, in centimeters, of the largest pocket of fluid in each of the four quadrants of the maternal abdomen that is free of cord. Normal values for gestational age are reported in centimeters plus or minus a standard deviation. Using this method, severe oligohydramnios is defined as an AFI of less than 5 cm. Moderate oligohydramnios is defined as an AFI between 5.1 and 8.0 cm. Normal fluid values are 8.1 to 24.0 cm. (Moore, 1996).

The estimated incidence of oligohydramnios is between 0.5 to 5.5 percent of all pregnancies, depending on the population tested and the criteria for diagnosis (Peipert & Donnenfeld, 1991).

A variety of fetal and maternal conditions are associated with oligohydramnios. Fetal conditions include chromosomal abnormalities, congenital anomalies (particularly the renal system), intrauterine growth restriction, intrauterine fetal demise, postdates pregnancy, and premature and prolonged rupture of membranes. Maternal conditions associated with oligohydramnios include uteroplacental insufficiency, drug use (prostaglandin synthetase inhibitors and angiotensin converting enzyme inhibitors), placental abruption and twin-to-twin transfusion syndrome. Idiopathic oligohydramnios, also contributes to an unknown number of cases (Peipert & Donnenfeld, 1991).

When oligohydramnios occurs in early pregnancy, adhesions between the amnion and part of the fetus may occur (amniotic bands), causing serious deformities, including musculoskeletal malformation or amputation. Pulmonary hypoplasia due to compression of the fetal thorax by the uterus, which prevents chest wall excursion and lung expansion, is also a consequence of oligohydramnios in early pregnancy (Moore, 1996). In late pregnancy, the incidence of cord compression and fetal distress is increased in the presence of small fluid volume. In most cases of oligohydramnios the skin of the newborn appears dry, leathery, and wrinkled.

Perinatal morbidity and mortality is significantly increased in pregnancies complicated by oligohy-dramnios. In addition to the elevated risks which the conditions associated with oligohydramnios present, risk of perinatal morbidity and mortality are further increased in cases presenting in early pregnancy and with very low levels of amniotic fluid. The finding of oligohydramnios always warrants a search for a cause. Close antenatal surveillance is indicated.

Database

Subjective

- Small uterine size
- Previous growth-restricted pregnancy or risk factor for intrauterine growth restricted (IUGR)
- Postdate pregnancy
- Continuous, slow fluid leakage from vagina
- Uterine contractions

Objective

- Obstetrical data review to rule out inaccurate dating
- Uterine size small for gestational age
- Fetal outline easily felt through the abdominal wall
- Incidental finding on ultrasound
- Vaginal fluid ph 7 to 7.5 (positive nitrazine test) and positive fern test-indicated if rupture of the membranes suspected
- Position, dilatation, effacement, and consistency of the cervix, if membranes not ruptured

Assessment

- Oligohydramnios
  - ▶ R/O IUGR
  - ▶ R/O inaccurate dating
  - ▶ R/O fetal anomaly
  - ▶ R/O preterm labor
  - ▶ R/O rupture of membranes

Plan

Diagnostic Tests

- Obtain ultrasound to
  - ▶ Assess amniotic fluid volume
  - ▶ Assess fetal growth
  - ▶ Rule out presence of fetal malformation, particularly fetal renal and uretal anomalies
- Nitrazine and fern test to rule out rupture of membranes as indicated

Treatment/Management

- Monitor weight gain

- Compare changes in fundal height

- Conduct antenatal surveillance (e.g., NST or CST with AFIs, biophysical profile) weekly or twice weekly beginning at 34 to 36 weeks or as soon as oligohydramnios is diagnosed. See Chapter 3.5, *Antenatal Fetal Surveillance.*

- Prescribe rest in lateral recumbent position.

- For preterm labor. see Chapter 6.25, *Preterm Labor.*

- Initiate fetal movement counts at 28 weeks. See Chapter 3.5, *Antepartum Fetal Surveillance.*

- Maintain maternal hydration and nutrition.

- Encourage relaxation, visualization, and other stress management techniques, as indicated.

- For intrauterine growth restriction, see Chapter 6.15, *Intrauterine Growth Restriction or Small for Gestational Age.*

- For postdates, see Chapter 6.26, *Postdate Pregnancy.*

Consultation

- Refer client to a physician in all cases of oligohydramnios.

- Co-management with a physician may be appropriate.

Patient Education

- Discuss the need for close prenatal surveillance and tests that will be used.

- Provide information regarding etiology of the condition.

- Provide anticipatory guidance and counseling when a fetal anomaly has been identified by sonography.

- Educate the client regarding the signs and symptoms of preterm labor and rupture of membranes, with an emphasis on prompt reporting by the client.

- Explain how to record fetal movement counts.

Follow-up

- Document the presence of oligohydramnios and other obstetrical/fetal complications in problem list and progress notes.

References

Devoe, L.D., & Ware, D.J. (1994). Oligohydramnios: Definition and diagnosis. *Contemporary OB/GYN*, Sept., 31–40.

Moore, T.R. (1996). Oligohydramnios. *Contemporary OB/GYN, 41*(9), 15–24.

Peipert, J.F., & Donnenfeld, A.E. (1991). Oligohydramnios: A review. *Obstetrical and Gynecological Survey, 46*(6), 325–339.

Skovgaard, R.L., & Silvonek, A.L. (1993). Oligohydramnios, literature review and case study. *Journal of Nurse-Midwifery, 38*(4), 208–215.

Chapter 22

POLYHYDRAMNIOS

Lisa L. Lommel

Polyhydramnios is defined as the excessive quantity of amniotic fluid in the amniotic sac. Antepartum ultrasound is utilized to make the diagnosis. Via ultrasound, the amniotic fluid index (AFI) is obtained by measuring the vertical diameter of the largest amniotic fluid pocket in each of the four quadrants of the uterus. The AFI equals the sum of these four values. The two most common definitions of polyhydramnios utilize the amniotic fluid index. The first definition assigns gestational age-adjusted norms for the AFI with polyhydramnios defined as an AFI greater than the 97.5 percentile for the corresponding gestational age (see Table 6.13) (Moore & Cayle, 1990). It is this definition that is more widely accepted. The second definition defines polyhydramnios as a sum of these four values that is greater or equal to 24 cm (normal is 8 to 23 cm.) (Moise, 1993).

Acute polyhydramnios is the very sudden increase of amniotic fluid over the course of a few days that occurs before the 24th week of gestation. Chronic polyhydramnios is the gradual increase of amniotic fluid and is more commonly diagnosed than acute polyhydramnios. The incidence of polyhydramnios (chronic) is estimated to be between 0.13 to 3.2 percent of all pregnancies (Moise, 1993). The incidence varies depending on the criteria used for diagnosis.

The causes of polyhydramnios vary involving many maternal and fetal conditions. A review of several studies indicates that up to 60 percent of the cases of polyhydramnios may be idiopathic; 20 percent may be related to fetal malformations, 8 percent to multiple gestation, 5 percent to maternal diabetes; and 9 percent are due to miscellaneous causes (Kramer, Van den Veyver & Kirshon, 1994). Fetal malformations associated with polyhydramnios include gastrointestinal obstructions (esophageal or duodenal atresia) when there is decreased swallowing or gastrointestinal absorption of the amniotic fluid, central nervous system abnormalities (anencephaly, spina bifida, and hydrocephaly), skeletal dysplasias, cardiac anomalies, and urinary and reproductive tract anomalies. Fetal chromosomal abnormalities are also associated with polyhydramnios. Other factors include isoimmunization and maternal syphilis.

Perinatal mortality is higher in the more severe cases of polyhydramnios, especially if accompanied by a fetal malformation. Premature rupture of membranes, premature labor and delivery, and mal-presentation and prolapse of the cord further increase perinatal mortality. The most frequent maternal complications are discomfort from the distended uterus, placental abruption, uterine dysfunction, and postpartum hemorrhage.

Database

Subjective

- Multiple pregnancy
- Maternal diabetes mellitus
- Dyspnea
- Generalized edema, especially of lower extremities

- Rapid enlargement of the abdomen

- Maternal discomfort from distended uterus and/or decreased mobility

- Regular/irregular uterine contractions

- With chronic polyhydramnios, symptoms are commonly well-tolerated.

- With acute polyhydramnios (before 24 weeks) symptoms may be severe: able to breathe only when upright, oliguria from uterine obstruction, severe edema.

Objective

- Obstetrical data review to rule out inaccurate dating

- Uterine size large for dates, rapid enlargement of the abdomen

- Generalized edema, especially of the lower extremities

- Palpation of excessive fluid in the uterus

- Difficulty in palpating fetal parts and position; difficulty in palpating any part of the fetus in severe polyhydramnios

- Difficulty in hearing fetal heart tones

- Uterine contractions felt with abdominal palpation

- Ultrasound shows increased volume of amniotic fluid

- Position, dilation, consistency, and effacement of the cervix

Assessment

- Size greater than dates
    - R/O Polyhydramnios
    - R/O inaccurate dating
    - R/O diabetes mellitus
    - R/O multiple pregnancy
    - R/O macrosomia
    - R/O fetal anomaly
    - R/O irregular antibody
    - R/O preterm labor

Plan

Diagnostic Tests

- Ballot for fetal parts.

- Screen for irregular antibodies by indirect Coombs test.
- Screen for syphilis.
- Obtain 1-hour glucose screen to rule out diabetes mellitus.
- Obtain ultrasound to
  - ▶ Demonstrate increased amniotic fluid status (see Table 6.13, Amniotic Fluid Index Values for Normal Pregnancies)
  - ▶ Assess fetal growth
  - ▶ Rule out presence of malformation, multiple fetuses, macrosomia, fetal hydrops or malpresentation
- Consider fetal echocardiogram to rule out congestive heart failure with physician consultation.

Treatment/Management

- Monitor weight gain.
- Compare changes in fundal height.
- Manage mild to moderate idiopathic polyhydramnios with physician consultation and/or referral.
  - ▶ Maintain the pregnancy until 37 weeks or the L/S ratio indicates fetal lung maturity.
  - ▶ Maintain partial bed rest.
- Manage moderate to severe polyhydramnios in a woman with respiratory distress or marked uterine irritability by referring her to a physician.
- Treatment may include therapeutic amniocentesis to withdraw excessive amniotic fluid.

  NOTE: As much as 1,500 to 2,000 mL fluid may be withdrawn at the rate of 50 mL per hour. Serial amniocenteses increases risk of abruption, infection, premature rupture of the membranes and premature labor. Fluid reaccumulates in 1 to 2 weeks (Moise, 1995).

- Indomethacin (prostaglandin synthase inhibitor) is currently being used in cases of symptomatic polyhydramnios in singleton pregnancies.
  - ▶ Indomethacin's significant therapeutic effect is a decrease in fetal urine production.
  - ▶ Major fetal risks include constriction of the fetal ductus arteriosus.
  - ▶ Major maternal risks include its antipyretic activity (masking infection), depressive effect on platelet function (increasing bleeding risk), and exacerbation of hypertension (Moise, 1995).
- Observe the client for signs of congestive heart failure.
- Initiate fetal movement counts at 28 weeks. See Chapter 3.5, *Antepartum Fetal Surveillance* for fetal movement count protocol.
- Perform a sterile pelvic exam if membranes rupture to rule out cord prolapse.
- For preterm labor see Chapter 6.25, *Preterm Labor*.

Consultation

- Refer client to a physician for management in all cases of polyhydramnios.

Patient Education

- Provide information regarding etiology of the condition.

- Discuss the need for close prenatal surveillance and the tests that will be used.

- Provide sensitive emotional support to the mother and her partner when an antenatal diagnosis of fetal anomaly has been made.

- Educate the client regarding signs and symptoms of preterm labor and rupture of membranes with emphasis on prompt reporting by the client.

- Explain how to record fetal movement counts. See Chapter 3.5, *Antepartum Fetal Surveillance*.

Follow-up

- Document the presence of polyhydramnios and other obstetrical/fetal complications in problem list and progress notes.

Table 6.13

Amniotic Fluid Index Values for Normal Pregnancies

Amniotic Fluid Index Percentile Values

Week	2.5th	5th	50th	95th	97.5th	Number
16	73	79	121	185	201	32
17	77	83	127	194	211	26
18	80	87	133	202	220	17
19	83	90	137	207	225	14
20	86	93	141	212	230	25
21	88	95	143	214	223	14
22	89	97	144	216	235	14
23	90	98	146	218	237	14
24	90	98	147	219	238	23
25	89	97	147	221	240	12
26	89	97	147	223	242	11
27	85	95	146	226	245	17
28	86	94	146	228	249	25
29	84	92	145	231	254	12
30	82	90	145	234	258	17
31	79	88	145	238	263	26
32	77	86	144	242	269	25
33	74	83	143	245	274	30
34	72	81	142	248	278	31
35	70	79	140	249	279	27
36	68	77	138	249	279	39
37	66	75	135	244	275	36
38	65	73	132	239	269	27
39	64	72	127	226	255	12
40	63	71	123	214	240	64
41	63	70	116	194	216	162
42	63	69	110	175	192	30

Source: Moore, T.R., & Cayle, J.E. (1990). The amniotic fluid index in normal human pregnancy. *American Journal of Obstetrics and Gynecology, 162,* 1168–1173. Reprinted with permission.

References

Cunningham, F.G., MacDonald, P.C., Gant, N.F., Leveno, K.J., & Gilstrap, L.C. (1993). *Williams Obstetrics* (19th ed.) pp. 734–740. Connecticut: Appleton & Lange.

Kramer, W.B., Van den Veyver, I.B., & Kirshon, B. (1994). Treatment of polyhydramnios with indomethacin. *Clinics in Perinatology, 21*(3), 615–630.

Moise, K.J. (1993). Polyhydramnios: Problems and treatment. *Seminars in Perinatology, 17*(3), 197–209.

Moise, K.J. (1995). Indomethacin as treatment for symptomatic polyhydramnios. *Contemporary OB/GYN,* 40(5), 53–60.

Moore, T.R., & Cayle, J.E. (1990). The amniotic fluid index in normal human pregnancy. *American Journal of Obstetrics and Gynecology, 162,* 1168–1173.

Chapter 23

POSTPARTUM DEPRESSION

Ellen M. Scarr

Lucy Newmark Sammons

Mood disturbances occurring postpartum are commonly categorized into three classifications of increasing severity: "blues," depression, and psychosis. Postpartum blues, with a prevalence of 50 to 80 percent, is a mild affective syndrome that usually begins 2 to 3 days postpartum, peaks 5 to 7 days postpartum, and begins to resolve by the second week. Occasionally symptoms persist into the fourth or fifth week (Sichel, 1995). Symptoms of the blues include sadness, tearfulness, crying spells, irritability, anxiety, mood swings, confusion, fatigue, and sleep and appetite disturbances. Causative factors include postpartum fatigue, increased burdens and responsibilities, and changing or absolute hormonal levels (estrogens, progesterone, prolactin, cortisol, norepinephrine, serotonin and tryptophan.) A self-limited disorder, consequences are generally benign, except when symptoms persist or worsen (Diket & Nolan, 1997; Novy, 1994). Postpartum blues has been correlated with the subsequent development of postpartum depression (Cooper & Murray, 1997; Pariser, Nasrallah, & Gardner, 1997).

Postpartum depression (PPD) occurs in 10 to 15 percent of women (O'Hara, 1995). It is characterized by depressed mood, some functional impairment, lack of affectionate bonding between mother and infant, and symptoms associated with depression, such as changes in sleeping and eating, excessive fatigue, psychomotor agitation or retardation, feelings of worthlessness, suicidal ideation, and loss of interest in pleasurable activities. Negative life events (e.g., loss of a loved one, poor marital support, divorce, financial difficulties) occurring during pregnancy or early in the postpartum period show the most promising link to date with PPD. A personal history of a mood disorder and/or a family history of depression may increase a woman's risk of PPD. Recent research suggests thyroid dysfunction may also contribute to PPD (Pariser et al., 1997). Despite numerous studies, there is inconclusive evidence linking demographic variables (age, marital status, social status, education), obstetric variables (parity, difficult pregnancy, delivery complications), or biochemical variables (hormonal levels, beta-endorphins, electrolytes, tryptophan) with PPD (O'Hara, 1995). Symptoms of PPD may appear 1 week to 1 year after delivery; the duration varies from weeks to months (Diket & Nolan, 1997). Consequences appear to include increased likelihood of additional depression for the woman, particularly in subsequent pregnancies, and risk for emotional, cognitive, or social problems for her children (Cooper & Murray, 1997).

Postpartum psychosis is characterized by severely impaired functional ability, often accompanied by agitation, hallucinations, delusions, paranoia, or severe mood depression. Suicidal or homicidal ideation may also be present. The incidence of postpartum psychosis is approximately 1–2/1000 births; most episodes occur 1 to 4 weeks after birth, but may appear up to 90 days postpartum (O'Hara, 1995; Sichel, 1995). Puerperal psychosis appears to be associated with first-time pregnancy, unmarried status, personal history of manic-depressive illness, and family history of psycho-pathology. Treatment may include psychotropic and electroconvulsive therapy, and hospitalization (Pariser et al., 1997).

Database

Subjective

- Client or her family report symptoms of depression.
  - ▶ Sad, depressed, or lowered mood
  - ▶ Mood swings
  - ▶ Crying episodes
  - ▶ Sleeping disturbances, such as insomnia or excessive fatigue/hypersomnia
  - ▶ Eating changes, such as loss of appetite
  - ▶ Confusion or inability to concentrate
  - ▶ Inability to perform usual roles as mother, wife, or employee
  - ▶ Loss of interest in usual sources of pleasure (anhedonia)
  - ▶ Feelings of worthlessness or inappropriate guilt
  - ▶ Anger or hostility towards infant, other children, or partner
- May complain of weight gain or loss, intolerance to cold or heat, changes in bowel function
- Possible predisposing factors include the following:
  - ▶ Stressful life event during pregnancy and/or puerperium
    - – Loss of loved one (fetus, newborn, spouse, parent, other child)
    - – Illness in spouse, parent, or child
    - – Financial difficulties
    - – Job loss
    - – Move of household
  - ▶ Problematic interpersonal relationships, particularly partner relationship, divorce, abandonment
  - ▶ Inadequate social support from partner, family, and friends
  - ▶ History of sexual abuse and/or domestic violence
  - ▶ Personal history includes poor psychological adjustment before and during pregnancy, high levels of anxiety, neurotic behavior, and depression or emotional distress
  - ▶ Personal and/or family history of psychopathology, particularly depression

Objective

- May appear unkempt, personal grooming not maintained
- Verbal/nonverbal responses may be inappropriate (e.g., flat or agitated affect, no eye contact)
- May demonstrate inappropriate weight loss or weight gain
- Thyroid exam within normal limits (no enlargement outside the range of normal for pregnancy, no nodules or tenderness)

Assessment

- Postpartum blues (benign) or postpartum depression
  - ▶ R/O postpartum psychosis or other psychopathology
  - ▶ R/O organic etiology (e.g., thyroid dysfunction)
  - ▶ R/O bereavement response
  - ▶ R/O substance abuse

Plan

Diagnostic Tests

- There are no specific diagnostic tests.
- Consider thyroid testing (2 to 4 percent of postpartum women are hypothyroid, which may present with symptoms similar to depression [Sichel, 1995]).

Treatment/Management

- For postpartum blues, no definitive treatment is required since it is a self-limited syndrome.
  - ▶ Provide client education and support (see Patient Education).
  - ▶ Monitor woman for successful resolution.
- For postpartum depression, refer client to physician supervision.
  - ▶ Treatment may include conventional chemotherapy (e.g., antidepressants, possibly anxiolytics) or psychotherapy, with emphasis on inclusion of spouse/partner (Robinson & Stewart, 1993; Sichel, 1995).
- See also Patient Education.

Consultation

- Postpartum depression, psychosis, or suspicion of other psychopathology requires medical/psychiatric consultation.
- Presence of thoughts, dreams, or actions suggesting injury to self or others, particularly infant, requires immediate psychiatric consultation and/or referral to crisis unit or suicide prevention.

Patient Education

- Explain the causes and treatment approaches employed for the relevant level of postpartum depressed mood.

- Advise client that additional psychological support may be indicated should she develop thoughts suggesting injury to herself or others.

- Assure woman of availability of continued routine or emergency services if they are needed.

- Involve family members and key support people; this is an integral aspect of prevention, identification, and management of postpartum mood disorders (Martell, 1990).

- For postpartum blues

  ▶ Reassure the woman that this mood alteration is self-limited, benign, and considered to be without future consequences for her or her family.

  ▶ Assist the woman and her family to identify and mobilize resources to meet demands of infant and child care, family relationships, work, household maintenance, and social and leisure activities.

- Foster strategies to promote postpartum well-being.

  ▶ Avoid overload with non-essential tasks.

  ▶ Obtain plenty of rest and sleep.

  ▶ Maintain communication and share feelings with partner, family and friends.

  ▶ Reduce responsibilities without eliminating social and recreational interests.

  ▶ Avoid major life changes in pregnancy or early postpartum period.

Follow-up

- Assure that patient/family have access to health care providers on a 24-hour basis for crisis management should need arise.

- Contact client and family to reassess mood and functional status within 1 week of first report. If symptoms are persisting or increasing in severity, evaluate further.

- Refer the client to social services, financial services, mental health care professionals, public health nursing, community support groups, etc., as needed, for assistance in coping and adjustment to demands of the puerperium

- Communicate with pediatric providers for appropriate follow-up of children in cases of severe depression or other psychopathology.

- No additional care is required for resolved postpartum blues.

- For postpartum depression and severe psychopathology, document in progress notes and problem list.

References

Cooper, P., & Murray, L. (1997). Prediction, detection, and treatment of postnatal depression. *Archives of disease in childhood, 77*(2), 97–99.

Diket, A., & Nolan, T. (1997). Anxiety and depression: Diagnosis and treatment during pregnancy. *Obstetrics and Gynecology Clinics of North America, 24*(3), 535–558.

Martell, L. (1990). Postpartum depression as a family problem. *MCN-The American Journal of Maternal-Child Nursing, 15,* 90–93.

Novy, M. (1994). The normal puerperium. In A. DeCherney & M. Pernoll (Eds.), *Current obstetric and gynecologic diagnosis and treatment* (8th ed., pp. 240–274). Norwalk, CT: Appleton & Lange.

O'Hara, M. (1995). Childbearing. In M. O'Hara, R. Reiter, S. Johnson, A. Milburn & J. Engeldinger (Eds.), *Psychological aspects of women's reproductive health.* New York: Springer Publishing Co.

Pariser, S., Nasrallah, H., & Gardner, D. (1997). Postpartum mood disorders: Clinical perspectives. *Journal of Women's Health, 6*(4), 421–343.

Robinson, G., & Stewart, D. (1993). Postpartum disorders. In D. Stewart & N. Stotland (Eds.), *Psychological aspects of women's health care* (pp. 115–138). Washington, DC: American Psychiatric Press.

Sichel, D. (1995). Postpartum psychiatric disorders. In K. Carlson & S. Eisenstat (Eds.), *Primary care of women,* (pp. 394–399). St. Louis, MO: Mosby.

Chapter 24

PREMATURE RUPTURE OF MEMBRANES

Winifred L. Star

Premature rupture of membranes (PROM) is defined as rupture of the membranes prior to the onset of labor. Preterm PROM (PPROM) indicates membrane rupture prior to 37 completed weeks' gestation (259 days from the onset of the last menstrual period). Prolonged rupture of membranes refers to rupture of membranes for more than 24 hours. The latent period is the interval between the rupture of membranes and the time labor ensues. An inverse relationship exists between gestational age at the time of membrane rupture and the duration of the latency period (i.e., latency periods tend to be longer in preterm pregnancies with PROM) (American College of Obstetricians and Gynecologists [ACOG], 1988; Allen, 1991; Harlass, 1991; King, 1994).

Incidence of PROM varies between 3 percent and 18.5 percent. PPROM complicates approximately 1 to 2 percent of all pregnancies and is responsible for about 30 to 40 percent of all premature deliveries. Spontaneous onset of labor following PROM occurs within 24 hours in over 90 percent of term pregnancies. With PROM at 28 to 34 weeks, 50 percent of clients are in labor within 24 hours and 80 to 90 percent within one week; prior to 26 weeks, about half the clients begin labor within a week (ACOG, 1988; Arsat & Garite, 1991; Garite, 1994; King, 1994).

The etiology of PROM is multifactorial and has been evaluated from the standpoint of infection, nutritional status, lifestyle risks, local membrane insult, and predisposing physiologic and anatomic abnormalities (French & McGregor, 1996; Shubert, Diss, & Iams, 1992) (see the Subjective section). It is postulated that infection is a major etiologic agent in the pathogenesis of PPROM (Shubert et al., 1992). Bacteria can weaken fetal membranes and lead to prostaglandin synthesis (Allen, 1991). Group B streptococcus (GBS), *Neisseria gonorrhoeae*, *Chlamydia trachomatis*, *Trichomonas vaginalis*, *Mycoplasma hominis, Ureaplasma urealyticum, Prevotella* species, *Gardnerella vaginalis*, and common vaginal bacteria (as in bacterial vaginosis [BV]) have all been implicated in the pathogenesis of membrane rupture (Allen, 1991; French & McGregor, 1996; Garite, 1994; McGregor, French, & Seo, 1993; Pauerstein, 1987). The consequences and complications associated with PROM are (Garite, 1994)

- Maternal infection (chorioamnionitis, endometritis, pelvic cellulitis)

- Fetal/neonatal infection (septicemia, pneumonia, urinary tract infection, local infection)

- Premature labor and delivery

- Hypoxia and asphyxia from umbilical cord compression

- Increased cesarean section rates

- Fetal deformation

Preterm infants are more likely to succumb to infectious complications. At term, the incidence of infection following PROM increases as the latency period increases (Garite, 1994). In the preterm pregnancy the greater concern is neonatal respiratory distress syndrome (RDS), with an incidence of about 50 percent in gestations under 33 weeks (Maxwell, 1993). Neonates born at less than 28 weeks' gestation are at increased risk for pulmonary hypoplasia; oligohydramnios that accompanies PPROM potentiates this problem and contributes to fetal deformation (Richards, 1991). Most cases of perinatal mortality consequent to PPROM are secondary to RDS, intraventricular hemorrhage (IVH), and/or necrotizing enterocolitis (NEC) (Garite, 1994).

The management of PROM is still controversial with respect to aggressive versus expectant management and the use of modalities, such as tocolytics and corticosteroids. In 1994, the National Institutes of Health (NIH) released a consensus statement on the effect of antenatal steroids for fetal maturation on perinatal outcomes. The issue of corticosteroid therapy in the presence of PPROM was addressed:

> "The use of antenatal corticosteroids to reduce infant morbidity in the presence of PPROM remains controversial . . . Strong evidence from observational studies suggests that, even in the presence of PPROM, the incidence of neonatal mortality and IVH is reduced when corticosteroids are used. Although the risk of neonatal infection associated with antenatal corticosteroid use in the face of PPROM may be increased, the magnitude of the increase is small. Because of the effectiveness of antenatal corticosteroids in reducing mortality and IVH in fetuses less than 30 to 32 weeks' gestation, antenatal corticosteroid use is appropriate in the absence of chorioamnionitis." (NIH, 1994, p. 7)

Despite these NIH conclusions, experts demand further clinical trials to evaluate potential risks and benefits of corticosteroids in the subset of clients with PPROM (ACOG, 1994; Imseis & Iams, 1996) In 1996, the Centers for Disease Control and Prevention (CDC) issued recommendations for preventing perinatal group B streptococcal infection, which includes guidelines regarding the use of intrapartal prophylactic antibiotics in the setting of prolonged rupture of membranes (CDC, 1996).

Database

Subjective

Risk factors for PROM or PPROM

- Previous PPROM or preterm delivery
- Cervical incompetence
- Cervical cerclage; previous cervical operations/procedures (e.g., conization, mechanical dilatation); cervical injury or lacerations
- Cervical shortening, funneling, or dilation
- Diethylstilbestrol (DES) exposure
- Cervical/vaginal infection
- Elevated vaginal pH
- Bleeding during pregnancy
- History of midtrimester pregnancy loss
- Multiple gestation
- Polyhydramnios
- Placental pathology (abruptio placentae, placenta previa, marginal cord insertion)

- Prenatal diagnostic procedures (amniocentesis, chorionic villus sampling (CVS)
- Smoking
- Cocaine use
- Hypertension, diabetes
- Poor nutritional status (low ascorbic acid, zinc, copper levels)
- Abnormalities in collagen content of membranes/cervix
- Ehlers-Danlos syndrome (group of heritable connective tissue diseases)
- Lower socioeconomic status

Symptomatology

- Sudden gush or leakage of clear fluid from the vagina, a "popping" sensation, or a constant wetness
- Vaginal discharge, bloody show, watery discharge (common presenting symptom in premature cervical dilation of women with incompetent cervix), pelvic pressure or "heaviness," menstrual-like cramping, painless uterine contractions
- Fever, chills, increased pulse rate, abdominal/pelvic pain, malodorous vaginal discharge (symptoms of chorioamnionitis, more common with increased duration of PROM)

History

- Establish the time of the rupture or onset of leaking.
- Targeted history questions attempt to separate out other sources of fluid loss, such as semen, urine, cervical mucus, leukorrhea, etc.
  - ▶ Ascertain if there is an odor of urine on the undergarments or bedclothes.
  - ▶ Ask about timing of last coital event, history of vaginal infection and/or use of intravaginal medication (or douche), and history of incontinence.
- Query client regarding signs/symptoms of chorioamnionitis.
- Obtain complete past and present obstetric, gynecologic, and medical history:
  - ▶ History of prenatal diagnostic procedures (e.g., CVS, amniocentesis)
  - ▶ History of surgical procedures (e.g., cervical cerclage, cervical dilation, conization)
  - ▶ Sexual history, including number of partners
  - ▶ History of vaginal infections and sexually transmitted diseases (STDs)
  - ▶ History of medical illness
  - ▶ Assessment of nutritional status
  - ▶ Lifestyle and habits

Objective

- Initial evaluation may occur in the ambulatory setting or the hospital. Invasive procedures should be performed in the hospital. Client should be managed by a physician.

- Establish gestational age by review of last menstrual period (LMP), early pregnancy test, early uterine sizing, prenatal records, ultrasound findings, prenatal examinations.

- Depending on weeks of gestation, perform Leopold's maneuvers and McDonald's measurements to assess fetal lie and gestational age of the fetus; establish fetal heart tones and rate.

- Assess maternal BP, temperature, heart rate and respirations for signs of infection; palpate uterus for contractions/tenderness to assess for labor/signs of infection.

  NOTE: Objective signs of infection include maternal/fetal tachycardia; maternal fever (≥100.4° F [> 38° C]) (best diagnostic marker); uterine tenderness; purulent/malodorous vaginal discharge; and leukocytosis (with left shift).

- Observe client's perineum: it may appear moist; dribbling of clear fluid may be seen coming from the vagina.

- Perform a *sterile speculum* examination.

  ▶ Vagina may appear moist or wet.

  ▶ Observe for prolapse of umbilical cord in vagina and for membrane prolapse at cervical os.

  ▶ Observe for visible cervical structural abnormalities (e.g., cervical collar, hood).

  ▶ Observe for presence of amniotic fluid (AF) in the posterior fornix; note its color and odor. If no fluid is readily seen, ask the client to bear down (Valsalva's maneuver) or cough and observe for a gush or leaking of fluid from the cervical os (gentle fundal pressure may also be used). Observation of a pool of fluid ("pooling") in the posterior vaginal fornix or visualization of fluid coming from the cervical os strongly suggests ROM.

  NOTE: If pooling of fluid is noted, draw-up the fluid in a syringe; it may be sent for phosphatidylglycerol [PG] analysis later.

  ▶ Touch a sterile cotton swab to the posterior vaginal pool then rub onto nitrazine paper. A blue color change (pH 7.0 to 7.5) is considered a positive nitrazine test, which can be indicative of the presence of amniotic fluid.

  NOTE: False-positive readings may result from alkaline urine, blood, vaginal discharge/infection, cervical mucus, semen, soap, glove powder, lubricant jelly, tap water, or antiseptic solution. False-negative results (10 percent of cases) may occur due to decreased efflux of AF with prolonged rupture (over two hours) or if there is an intermittent high leak (King, 1994).

  ▶ Place a sample of fluid from the posterior fornix onto a glass slide and allow to air dry for 5 to 7 minutes. Under low-power microscopy observe for presence of a delicate, discrete ferning pattern.

  NOTE: False positives may result from a cervical mucus sample or from fingerprints on the glass slide. False negatives may occur with the presence of blood, meconium, cervical/ vaginal infections or if there is an intermittent, high leak or prolonged rupture (over 2 hours) (King, 1994).

▶ If initial sterile speculum examination is negative, place client in semi-Fowler's position and repeat the examination in 30 minutes to 1 (or more) hour(s) using Valsalva's maneuver and gentle fundal pressure.

● **Do not** perform a digital cervical examination if PROM has been confirmed. Sterile speculum examination alone can provide an accurate assessment of cervical dilation and effacement (Lewis & Dunnihoo, 1995).

● Utilize ultrasound to assess the following:

▶ Cervical length, dilatation, and funneling

▶ Gestational age

▶ Amniotic fluid level

▶ Placental location and grade

▶ Pelvic abnormalities

▶ Fetal position

▶ Fetal anomalies.

NOTE: If oligohydramnios is identified by ultrasound, keep in mind that other causes besides ROM may be involved; in addition, a normal level of AF does not exclude ROM (Davidson, 1991).

● See Diagnostic Tests section for further information.

Assessment

● PROM or PPROM

▶ R/O other causes of fluid leakage (e.g., vaginal discharge, urine, semen)

▶ R/O umbilical cord prolapse

▶ R/O STD

▶ R/O bacterial vaginosis

▶ R/O group B streptococcal colonization

▶ R/O chorioamnionitis

▶ R/O oligohydramnios

▶ R/O preterm labor/labor

▶ R/O cervical incompetence

▶ R/O fetal anomalies/fetal demise

Plan

Diagnostic Tests

- Perform sterile speculum examination. See Objective section.

- Fetal lung maturity may be assessed via lecithin/sphingomyelin (L/S) ratio, PG measurements, foam stability index, and fetal lung maturity (FLM) assay.

    ▶ Fluid from the vaginal pool or cervical os may be aspirated for the presence of PG. If significant bacterial contamination is not present, vaginal sample may also be used to assess L/S ratio (Beazley & Lewis, 1996).

    ▶ Amniocentesis (performed by physician) for determination of L/S ratio, PG, and FLM may be attempted.

- Lower vaginal (or vaginal and anorectal) culture for group B streptococcus should be obtained. See Chapter 10.3, *Group B Streptococcus,* for information on obtaining culture. Cervical samples for *C. trachomatis* and *N. gonorrhoeae* testing may also be obtained, as indicated.

- Wet mount may be performed.

- Other diagnostic tests may include but not be limited to the following:

    ▶ Intra-amniotic dye injection (e.g., indigo carmine, Evans blue, fluorescein) into amniotic cavity when diagnosis unclear but highly suspicious for ROM

    ▶ White blood cell (WBC) count and C-reactive protein (CRP) to assess maternal infection

    ▶ Gram stain and culture of AF; AF glucose determination (via amniocentesis) to assess intra-amniotic infection

    ▶ External tocodynamometry for monitoring contractions

    ▶ Continuous fetal heart rate monitoring, nonstress test (NST), biophysical profile (BPP) to assess for fetal distress and impending infection

- Additional diagnostic modalities utilized to assess upper genital tract abnormalities may include hysterosalpingography and hysteroscopy.

    NOTE: In women with a history of in utero exposure to DES, the following defects may be identified: T-shaped uterus or other uterine-cavity shape abnormalities, intrauterine synechiae/diverticula, or fallopian tube structural abnormalities.

- See Objective section for additional information.

Treatment/Management

General/preventive management principles

- Carefully review OB/GYN history for risk factors that predispose to PROM. Women with a history of cervical incompetence, PPROM, or midtrimester pregnancy loss in a previous pregnancy should be evaluated by a physician in the current pregnancy.

- Screen for and treat STDs and BV in women at risk for PROM. Refer partners of women with STDs for appropriate treatment. Carefully evaluate women with symptoms of vaginitis. (See Section 14, *Vaginitis and Sexually Transmitted Disease.*)

- Screen all clients for asymptomatic bacteriuria and treat accordingly. See Chapter 13.1, *Asymptomatic Bacteriuria.*

- Serial clinical cervical examination (by same examiner) and serial ultrasonographic assessment of the cervix for length and dilatation may be performed in women at risk for or with a history suggestive of cervical incompetence (Parisi, 1994). Note the position, consistency, length (in centimeters), and status of the external/internal os (i.e., closed, or degree of dilatation in centimeters) on clinical examination.

    NOTE: It should be kept in mind that both primigravidas and multigravidas can have cervical dilation of 1 to 2 cm in the mid to late second trimester.

Management of acute PROM

Women with confirmed PROM should be referred to a physician. Medical management should be individualized. Interventions will be summarized below. Details of inpatient evaluation and treatment/ management are beyond the scope of this chapter.

PROM at Term (36 Weeks and Beyond) (ACOG, 1988; Garite, 1994; Greenwald, 1993)

The goal of management is delivery.

- Labor ensues spontaneously within 24 hours in 90 percent of cases.

- Women in active labor should be allowed to progress and managed routinely. Cesarean section is performed for the usual indications.

- Women not in labor should be evaluated for infection and fetal distress. In the absence of infection or fetal distress, client may be managed expectantly or undergo induction of labor.

- Patients with signs of chorioamnionitis should be treated for infection and delivered. Cesarean section is performed for the usual indications.

- Patients with signs of fetal distress should be delivered either vaginally or by cesarean section based on the specific case presentation.

- See Chapter 10.3, *Group B Streptococcus,* for information on the use of intrapartal prophylactic antibiotics.

Preterm PROM (25 to 35 Weeks) (ACOG, 1988; Arsat & Garite, 1991; Garite, 1994; Greenwald, 1993; Mercer, 1997; Mercer & Arheart, 1996)

Management goals are to prolong gestation if client is not in labor, is not infected, and has no evidence of fetal distress. Use of tocolytic agents and corticosteroids remains controversial. See Chapter 10.3, *Group B Streptococcus*, for information on intrapartal prophylactic antibiotics. Refer also to the National Institutes of Health (1994) reference.

- Between 25 and 30 weeks' gestation

  ▶ Expectant management in hospital with assessment/observation for infection, signs of labor, and fetal distress. After initial hospital stay, home management may be possible if client meets certain criteria.

  ▶ Delivery is indicated for chorioamnionitis, irreversible fetal distress, or spontaneous labor.

  ▶ Antibiotics are given for clinical infection and may also be used as an adjunctive treatment to expectant management.

  ▶ Cesarean section is performed for the usual indications.

- Between 31 and 35 weeks' gestation

  ▶ Patients in labor are allowed to progress.

  ▶ Nonlaboring clients are evaluated for fetal lung maturity and infection.

  ▶ If assessment reveals mature lung profile or incipient infection, delivery is undertaken.

  ▶ Antibiotics are given for clinical infection and may also be utilized as an adjunctive treatment to expectant management.

  ▶ Cesarean section is performed for the usual indications.

Previable/Preterm PROM Less than 25 Weeks)(ACOG, 1988; Arsat & Garite, 1991; Garite, 1994; Greenwald, 1993; Lewis & Mercer, 1996; Schucker & Mercer, 1996)

- If labor or infection is present client should be delivered.

- Termination of pregnancy is an option; leave the decision to the client/couple after discussion with the physician regarding the maternal/fetal issues.

- Expectant management at home is also an option provided there is no infection. (Further studies are needed to evaluate the benefits and risks of outpatient expectant management.)

  ▶ Maternal risks must be understood (e.g., infection, sepsis, abruption) as well as outcomes for the fetus (e.g., neurologic morbidity, fetal deformation syndrome, pulmonary hypoplasia).

  ▶ After initial hospital evaluation, client may be discharged home with the following instructions:

    – Remain on bed rest.

    – Avoid intercourse.

    – Check temperature regularly (adjunctive antibiotic therapy may be utilized).

    – Monitor self for contractions.

  ▶ At 25 to 26 weeks (possibly 23 to 24 weeks depending upon case-particulars) client may be admitted to hospital for daily fetal evaluation and interventions, as indicated.

ROM Following Invasive Prenatal Diagnostic Procedures (Kaiser Permanente Medical Center, San Francisco, 1994)

- Perform sterile speculum evaluation. See Objective section.

- Refrain from digital cervical examination.

- Send vaginal cultures for group B streptococcus (STD cultures may also be considered, as indicated).

- Utilize ultrasonography to document residual amniotic volume; repeat in 1 week to reassess volume.

  NOTE: The majority of clients will stop leaking by third day and reestablish normal amniotic fluid volume within 1 week of rupture. Oligohydramnios persisting more than 1 week after ROM is a poor prognostic sign: Counsel client about risks (amnionitis, pulmonary hypoplasia, amniotic band syndrome). Pregnancy termination may be a consideration.

- Hospitalize the woman to rule out chorioamnionitis if she is febrile or has uterine tenderness.

- Home management is appropriate if the client is afebrile, nontender, and considered reliable to assess self for signs of infection.

  ▶ Temperature should be taken twice a day; if more than 100.6° F (>38.1° C), call provider.

  ▶ If malaise, myalgia, foul-smelling vaginal discharge, bleeding, or increasing pelvic pain/cramps develop, call provider.

  ▶ Maintain bed rest and pelvic rest. If leakage has stopped and normal amniotic fluid is reestablished, client may return to normal activities 1 week after membrane rupture.

  ▶ Reassure client that prognosis is generally excellent if ROM occurs after amniocentesis: In over 80 percent of clients, membranes appear to "seal over" and pregnancy outcomes are normal.

Consultation

- Physician consultation is required in all cases of suspected or confirmed ROM and in clients at risk for or with a history suggestive of cervical incompetence.

- Management of PROM/PPROM is directed by the physician.

Patient Education

- Discuss risk factors and etiology of PROM/PPROM and implications for mother and baby.

- Discuss diagnostic tests to be utilized if ROM is suspected.

- Educate the client regarding signs of infection (e.g., fever, chills, foul smelling discharge) and signs/symptoms of preterm labor (see Chapter 6.25) when PROM/PPROM is diagnosed. Emphasize the importance of bed rest/pelvic rest in a client who is being considered for expectant management at home and ensure that she understands the components of self-care and assessment. Medical management plans, ideally, should be discussed with the client by the physician in charge of her care.

- Counsel client regarding the role of infection, smoking, substance use/abuse, and diet if there is a prior history of PROM/PPROM.

- Review nutritional status and advise regarding the adequacy of the diet; recommend multivitamin, iron, and calcium supplements, if necessary.

- Discuss safer sex practices as indicated.

- Advise avoidance of strenuous exercise and heavy exertion for the current pregnancy in women with a prior history of PPROM (Regenstein & Main, 1992).

Follow-up

- The follow-up schedule is determined by the physician or high-risk team according to clinical presentation.

- Refer to social services, as indicated.

  ▶ Client may need assistance with financial and child care arrangements if hospitalized or on bed rest.

  ▶ Ongoing psychosocial support is important for women with PPROM or those who may be anticipating a preterm delivery.

- If the client is to be managed at home, make referral to public health nurse or home care team.

- The genetic counselor should be notified in the event the client has had rupture of membranes after a prenatal diagnostic procedure.

- The neonatal care team will assume responsibility for care of the newborn.

- Primary obstetrical care provider may resume care of client in the postpartum period, as indicated by her condition and preference.

- The diagnosis of incompetent cervix as a cause of PPROM needs to be considered in planning for future pregnancy: Refer client to physician for preconceptional anticipatory guidance.

- Document PROM/PPROM and its management on the problem list and in progress notes. In addition, document GBS carrier status and/or the presence of BV or an STD as indicated.

REFERENCES

Allen, S R. (1991). Epidemiology of premature rupture of the fetal membranes. *Clinical Obstetrics and Gynecology, 34*(4), 685–693.

American College of Obstetricians and Gynecologists (ACOG). (1988). *Premature rupture of membranes.* (Technical Bulletin No. 115). Washington, DC: Author.

American College of Obstetricians and Gynecologists (ACOG). (1994). *Antenatal corticosteroid therapy for fetal maturation.* (Committee Opinion No. 147). Washington, DC: Author.

Arsat, T., & Garite, T.J. (1991). Management of preterm premature rupture of membranes. *Clinical Obstetrics and Gynecology, 34(4)*, 730–741.

Beazley, D., & Lewis, R. (1996). The evaluation of infection and pulmonary maturity in women with premature rupture of the membranes. *Seminars in Perinatology, 20*(5), 409–417.

Centers for Disease Control and Prevention (CDC). (1996). Prevention of perinatal group B streptococcal disease: A public health perspective. *Morbidity and Mortality Weekly Report, 45*(RR–7), 1–24.

Davidson, K.M. (1991). Detection of premature rupture of the membranes. *Clinical Obstetrics and Gynecology, 34*(4), 715–722.

French, J.L., & McGregor, J.A. (1996). The pathobiology of premature rupture of membranes. *Seminars in Perinatology, 20*(5),344–368.

Garite, T.J. (1994). Premature rupture of the membranes. In R. K. Creasy & R. Resnik (Eds.), *Maternal-fetal medicine: Principles and practice* (3rd ed., pp. 625–638). Philadelphia, PA: W.B. Saunders.

Greenwald, J.L. (1993). Premature rupture of the membranes: Diagnostic and management strategies. *American Family Physician, 48*(2), 293–306.

Harlass, F.E. (1991). The use of tocolytics in clients with preterm premature rupture of the membranes. *Clinical Obstetrics and Gynecology, 34*(4), 751–758.

Kaiser Permanente Medical Center, San Francisco. (1994). *Management after invasive PND procedures.* Internal memorandum.

King, T. (1994). Clinical management of premature rupture of membranes. *Journal of Nurse-Midwifery, 39*(2, Suppl.), 81S–90S.

Lewis, D.F., & Dunnihoo, D.R. (1995). Digital vaginal examinations after PROM: What consequences? *Contemporary OB/GYN, 40*(1), 33–40.

Lewis, R., & Mercer, B.M. (1996). Selected issues in premature rupture of the membranes: Herpes, cerclage, twins, tocolysis, and hospitalization. *Seminars in Perinatology, 20*(5), 451–461.

Maxwell, G.L. (1993). Preterm premature rupture of membranes. *Obstetrical and Gynecological Survey, 48*(10), 576–583.

McGregor, J.A., French, J.I., & Seo, K. (1993). Premature rupture of membranes and bacterial vaginosis. *American Journal of Obstetrics and Gynecology, 169*(2, Pt. 2), 463–466.

Mercer, B.M. (1997). Antibiotic therapy for preterm rupture of membranes. *Contemporary OB/Gyn, 42*(3), 57–68.

Mercer, B.M., & Arheart, K.L. (1996). Antibiotic therapy for preterm premature rupture of the membranes. *Seminars in Perinatology, 20*(5), 426–438.

National Institutes of Health (NIH). (1994). The effect of antenatal steroids for fetal maturation on perinatal outcomes—Interim draft statement. *NIH Consensus Statement, Feb 28–Mar 2, 12*(2), 1–24.

Parisi, V.M. (1994). Cervical incompetence. In R.K. Creasy & R. Resnik (Eds.), *Maternal-fetal medicine. Principles and practice* (3rd ed., pp. 453–466). Philadelphia, PA: W.B. Saunders.

Pauerstein, C.J. (1987). *Clinical obstetrics* (pp. 367–381). New York: John Wiley and Sons.

Regenstein, A.C., & Main, D.M. (1992). Antenatal care of the client with previous preterm premature rupture of membranes. *Obstetrics and Gynecology Clinics of North America, 19*(2), 387–395.

Richards, D.S. (1991). Complications of prolonged PROM and oligohydramnios. *Clinical Obstetrics and Gynecology, 34*(4), 759–768.

Schucker, J.L., & Mercer, B.M. (1996). Midtrimester premature rupture of the membranes. *Seminars in Perinatology, 20*(5), 389–400.

Shubert, P.J., Diss, E., & Iams, J.D. (1992). Etiology of preterm premature rupture of membranes. *Obstetrics and Gynecology Clinics of North America, 19*(2), 251–263.

Chapter 25

PRETERM LABOR

Winifred L. Star

Joan R. Murphy

Preterm labor leading to preterm birth is the single most important problem facing obstetrics today and remains the leading cause of perinatal morbidity and mortality (Creasy, 1989; Iams & Creasy, 1988; Garite & Lockwood, 1996). Low birth weight accounts for more than 60 percent of the mortality not attributable to anatomic or chromosomal congenital defects; 6.7 percent of infants are low birth weight and 1 percent are very low birth weight (less than 1500 gm). Over the last several decades, the incidence of low birth-weight infants has not decreased consistently nor has the rate of premature deliveries changed since the 1950s (Garite & Lockwood, 1996). The United States ranks nineteenth in the world in infant mortality, a rate comparable to many developing countries (Gibbs, Romero, Hillier, Eschenbach, & Sweet, 1992).

Preterm labor is defined as the onset of regular contractions resulting in cervical change between 20 and 37 completed weeks of pregnancy (114 to 259 days gestation). A preterm birth is any delivery that occurs prior to 37 completed weeks of pregnancy (less than 259 days from the last menstrual period [LMP]) (Wheeler, 1994). The true incidence of preterm delivery is not well documented and depends upon the population studied; estimates range between 5 and 10 percent of births in developed countries (American College of Obstetricians and Gynecologists [ACOG], 1995; Creasy, 1989).

Preterm births are responsible for the majority of neonatal deaths in newborns without anomalies. Developmental delay, vision and hearing impairment, chronic lung disease, and cerebral palsy are also disproportionately increased with preterm birth (ACOG, 1995). Respiratory distress syndrome and intracranial bleeding are the primary neonatal complications (Arias, 1984; Creasy, 1994).

Multiple factors contribute to preterm labor and delivery, many of which are poorly understood. In the majority of cases, the etiology of preterm labor is unknown (ACOG, 1995). It appears that equal numbers of preterm births are caused by preterm labor (PTL), preterm premature rupture of membranes (PPROM), or maternal/fetal complications (Gomez, Romero, Edwin, & David, 1997; Main, 1988). Increasing evidence indicates that infection and inflammation in the upper reproductive tract arising from lower tract infection, abnormal colonization, or bacterial vaginosis may cause from 20 to 40 percent of preterm births (Gibbs & Eschenbach, 1997; Gibbs et al., 1992; McGregor, French, & Witkin, 1996). Associated organisms may include *Chlamydia trachomatis*, *Gardnerella vaginalis*, Group B streptococcus, *Trichomonas vaginalis, Ureaplasma urealyticum, Mycoplasma hominis, Fusobacterium* species, and various anaerobes (Creasy, 1994; Gomez et al., 1997). In addition, certain infectious organisms (e.g., *Listeria monocytogenes, Treponema pallidum*, mycobacteria) may reach the intrauterine environment by transplacental passage from the maternal circulation and induce preterm labor (Creasy, 1994). Evolving understanding of the pathogenesis of preterm labor has led to the development of various approaches for identifying women at risk.

Preterm Birth Prevention

The various components of preterm birth prevention programs include (a) identification and close observation of clients at risk for preterm labor and delivery, (b) client education regarding the signs and symptoms of preterm labor and self-detection of uterine contractions, (c) home uterine activity monitoring, (d) staff education regarding the problem of preterm labor and the signs and symptoms, and (e) prompt treatment with tocolysis once the diagnosis is made. Selected facets of preterm birth prevention will be further discussed below.

Several risk-scoring systems for preterm labor are in use today. Risk scoring helps identify clients at risk for preterm labor/delivery; however, the systems currently available are not discriminating enough to identify the approximately 50 percent of clients who have spontaneous preterm deliveries. The positive predictive value has been less than 20 percent. Because risk factors vary from population to population, the systems cannot be reliably transferred from one population to another without prospective testing. The significance of prior pregnancy complications as predictors of preterm labor/delivery make these scoring systems more accurate for multigravidas. Additional means of identifying high-risk patients (e.g., biochemical/biophysical tests) need to be developed (ACOG, 1995; Creasy, 1989; Iams & Creasy, 1988; Wheeler, 1994).

Measurement of fetal fibronectin (fFN) in cervical and vaginal secretions has shown promise in the prediction of preterm birth. Fetal fibronectin is a protein present in fetal tissue throughout pregnancy; it is released into the cervix and vagina if disruption of the amniotic membranes occurs. Fetal fibronectin appears in cervicovaginal secretions in normal pregnancies with intact membranes at term. Detection of fFN prior to membrane rupture may be a marker for preterm labor. Further investigational studies are needed to determine the clinical utility of this test in prevention of preterm birth (Ascarelli & Morrison, 1997; Garite & Lockwood, 1996; Wheeler, 1994).

Home uterine activity monitoring (HUAM) is a system of care that involves daily use of a tocodynamometer to detect uterine contractions in conjunction with telephone contact by trained nursing staff. Its purpose is to allow earlier detection of preterm labor and, therefore, earlier treatment to prevent preterm birth (Goepfert & Goldenberg, 1996). However, it has not been clearly proven that HUAM can actually affect the rate of preterm delivery and substantial controversy exists regarding the benefit of its use with high-risk groups (ACOG, 1995). Certain studies indicate that the daily nurse contact may be the major factor in improving outcome rather than use of the monitor (ACOG, 1995; Cotton, Kayne, Zhang, & Heeren, 1995; Lantz & Porter, 1995). Use of HUAM and subsequent treatment for preterm labor has the potential for substantially increasing costs; thus, further studies are needed to address these issues (ACOG, 1995). The American College of Obstetricians and Gynecologists concludes that "data are insufficient to support a benefit from HUAM in preventing preterm birth" (ACOG, 1996a, p. 6). As understanding of the pathogenesis of spontaneous preterm birth improves, so does the possibility of more direct approaches and interventions to prevent this pregnancy complication (Goepfert & Goldenberg, 1996).

Database

Subjective

- Risk factors (ACOG, 1995; Creasy, 1994):
  - ▶ Demographic factors
    - – Age less than 20 or more than 35 years
    - – Race (black)

- Single status
- Low socioeconomic/educational status

▶ Behavioral factors

- Smoking
- Substance use/abuse (particularly cocaine)
- Poor nutrition
- Underweight status
- Inadequate weight gain in pregnancy
- Lack of/inadequate prenatal care
- Strenuous, physically demanding employment
- Psychological stress

▶ Medical/obstetrical factors

- Prior preterm birth (recurrence risk 17 to 47 percent; risk increases with the number of previous preterm deliveries and decreases with the number of term deliveries)
- One or more spontaneous second trimester abortions
- Uterine anomaly
- Cervical incompetence (congenital, iatrogenic)
- Cervical length ≤ 25 mm (by transvaginal ultrasound) (Iams et al., 1996)
- Diethylstilbestrol (DES) exposure (especially if associated cervical/uterine anomaly)
- Cone biopsy
- Multiple first-trimester induced abortions
- Second trimester induced abortion
- Multiple gestation (10 percent of all preterm births)
- Leiomyomata (multiple, large)
- First trimester bleeding
- Vaginal/cervical/intrauterine infection
- Uterine irritability
- Cervical effacement or dilatation
- Preterm premature rupture of membranes (direct antecedent of 30 to 40 percent of preterm births)
- Antepartum hemorrhage due to placenta previa, abruptio placentae, or abnormally implanted placenta
- Polyhydramnios/oligohydramnios
- Abdominal surgery in second or third trimester

- Renal disease
- Asymptomatic bacteriuria with underlying renal disease
- Pyelonephritis
- Pregnancy induced hypertension/Preeclampsia
- Systemic infection
- Diabetes complicated by polyhydramnios
- Assisted reproductive technologies (ART)
- Unexplained elevation of maternal serum alpha-fetoprotein (MSAFP)
- Hypovolemia
- Pituitary adenoma

▶ Additional possible risk factors
- Asthma
- Hyperthyroidism
- Heart disease
- Obstetric cholestasis
- Hepatitis
- Anemia (< 9 gm/100 mL)

▶ Fetal factors
- Anencephaly associated with polyhydramnios
- Renal agenesis associated with oligohydramnios
- Multiple congenital anomalies
- Central nervous system anomalies
- Antepartum fetal compromise/death

Subjective

- Signs and symptoms
  ▶ Menstrual–like cramps
  ▶ Low, dull backache (intermittent or constant)
  ▶ Rhythmic or persistent pelvic pressure
  ▶ Abdominal cramping
  ▶ Diarrhea
  ▶ Uterine contractions or "balling-up" of uterus (i.e., uterus rises up and hardens, then softens; often painless)

▶ Increase or change in vaginal discharge (watery, bloody, or mucosal)

▶ Fluid leaking from vagina

▶ Vaginal bleeding or spotting

▶ Overall sense of not feeling well

▶ Fever (if patient has systemic illness)

NOTE: Routinely question client regarding signs and symptoms of preterm labor and document in prenatal chart. This should be done at every prenatal visit, especially after 20 weeks.

Objective

● Identify maternal risk factors through comprehensive history taking and use of a preterm labor risk assessment tool (see Table 6.15, Risk Assessment for Preterm Labor). Complete the screen at the initial prenatal visit and, as indicated, if risk factors develop in the pregnancy. Refer high-risk clients to a formal preterm birth prevention program, if available, in the obstetrical practice.

● Document baseline cervical status at initial obstetric examination. Record position, consistency, length in centimeters, and status of the external and internal os (i.e., closed, or degree of dilation in centimeters).

● Assess routine OB clinical parameters at each visit.

● Identify presence or absence of uterine contractions by palpation of the uterus and/or with use of the tocodynamometer as indicated.

● Identify presence or absence of cervical change by gentle digital cervical examination as indicated.

▶ Comment on position, consistency, length, and status of the external/internal os.

▶ Assess status of lower uterine segment and station of presenting part.

▶ If the patient has a history of preterm birth, begin cervical examinations when preterm labor started in previous pregnancies or at 28 weeks, whichever comes first. In primiparous patients, begin at the onset of symptoms.

▶ Serial cervical examinations should be done by the same examiner whenever possible.

NOTE: Digital examination should be avoided in the presence of ruptured membranes. If rupture of membranes is suspected, perform a sterile speculum examination to assess for amniotic fluid leakage and do a visual inspection of the cervix to evaluate effacement/ dilation. If vaginal bleeding occurs during the second or third trimester, digital examination should be deferred until absence of placenta previa is documented (see Chapter 6.24, *Premature Rupture of Membranes*).

● Perform additional physical examination components as indicated by client complaints and concerns.

Assessment

- Preterm labor
  - ▶ R/O normal fetal activity
  - ▶ R/O gastrointestinal activity
  - ▶ R/O irritable uterus
  - ▶ R/O dehydration
  - ▶ R/O PROM/PPROM
  - ▶ R/O asymptomatic bacteriuria
  - ▶ R/O cystitis
  - ▶ R/O pyelonephritis
  - ▶ R/O chorioamnionitis
  - ▶ R/O vaginitis/cervicitis
  - ▶ R/O sexually transmitted disease (STD)
  - ▶ R/O uterine/cervical anomaly
  - ▶ R/O fetal pathologic condition

Plan

Diagnostic Tests

- Screen for asymptomatic bacteriuria with urine culture.

- Screen for *Neisseria gonorrhoeae, Chlamydia trachomatis,* and group B streptococcus.

- Perform a wet mount to assess for *Trichomonas vaginalis* and bacterial vaginosis.

- Perform sterile speculum examination with testing for rupture of membranes, as indicated (see Chapter 6.24, *Premature Rupture of Membranes*).

  - ▶ If rupture of membranes is ruled out, gentle digital cervical examination may be undertaken to assess position, consistency, length, and status of the external/internal os.

  - ▶ With intact membranes and documented contractions, preterm labor is diagnosed if cervical change is documented or the cervix is 2 or more centimeters dilated or 80 percent or more effaced (Creasy, 1994).

- Use ultrasound to confirm/establish gestational age and to assess presence of abnormalities of the uterus, cervix, fetus, placenta.

  - ▶ Transvaginal ultrasound may be used to determine cervical length and assess for funneling of the cervix (Iams, 1994; Parisi, 1994).

- Employ tocodynamometry to assess presence or absence of uterine contractions. Use electronic fetal monitoring (EFM), as indicated, to assess fetal heart rate, variability, accelerations, and decelerations.

- Refer client for amniocentesis to diagnose fetal maturity (assessment of lecithin/sphingomyelin [L/S] ratio and phosphatidylglycerol [PG]), as indicated.

  ▶ Bacteriologic studies of the amniotic fluid may be done to rule out chorioamnionitis, as indicated.

- Order lupus anticoagulant (associated with recurrent pregnancy loss, preterm delivery, and abruption), as indicated (Lubbe & Wiggins, 1985).

- May order serum collagenase or C-reactive protein levels (not routinely used).

  ▶ Prolongation of pregnancy for 7 days or longer has been associated with maternal C-reactive protein values of up to 0.8 ng/dL; greater values predict delivery within 7 days (Iams, 1994).

- Test for fetal fibronectin in cervicovaginal secretions as available per site-specific practice.

  ▶ Concentrations greater than or equal to 50 ng/mL (at 20 to 37 weeks' gestation) place woman at high risk for preterm labor (Ascarelli & Morrison, 1997).

  NOTE: The fetal fibronectin enzyme immunoassay kit was recently approved by the Food and Drug Administration. If used, membranes should be intact, cervical dilation should be less than 3 cm, and sampling should be performed no earlier than 24 weeks, 0 days and no later than 34 weeks, 6 days of gestation (ACOG, 1997).

- Order other laboratory tests as indicated by history or physical findings (e.g., CBC, clotting studies, etc.).

Treatment/Management

- Preterm labor prevention ideally begins before conception by attempting to correct for maternal risk factors.

- Perform routine prenatal care with special attention to

  ▶ Regular prenatal visits

  ▶ Avoidance of overexertion

  ▶ Stress reduction

  ▶ Avoidance of smoking/substance use

  ▶ Good nutrition

  ▶ Identification and treatment of bacteriuria, vaginal/cervical infections

  ▶ Prompt evaluation of febrile illness

  ▶ Careful evaluation/treatment of all medical complications

  ▶ Patient education regarding preterm labor

- Use the preterm labor risk assessment tool at initial OB visit and, as indicated, if risk factors develop. If any risk factor is identified, begin preterm labor surveillance and education.

  ▶ See client every 2 weeks (or more often, as indicated) until 36 weeks and then weekly until delivery.

▶ A careful history should be undertaken at each visit and a gentle digital cervical examination performed, as indicated.

● In identified at-risk patients (i.e., history of preterm labor, preterm delivery, multiple gestation), recommend reduction of physical and sexual activity in the late second and early third trimesters.

▶ Ideally, client should be on modified bed rest if experiencing frequent contractions (bathroom privileges, up for meals and shower).

▶ Bed rest may need to be maintained until 36 weeks or until signs/symptoms of PTL abate completely (there are no studies regarding the efficacy of bed rest in preventing preterm labor in high-risk singleton pregnancies (ACOG, 1995; Wheeler, 1994).

▶ Alternatives to intercourse/orgasm may be suggested.

▶ Avoidance of breast stimulation is warranted.

▶ HUAM is not recommended by ACOG (ACOG, 1996a).

● In patients with irritable uteri, suggest decreased activity and increased hydration, as well as the possibility of a modified work schedule, as indicated.

NOTE: Pregnant women whose occupation entails prolonged periods of standing and long work hours may be at increased risk for preterm birth and the delivery of a low-birth-weight infant (Gabbe & Turner, 1997).

● Serial ultrasound examination of cervical length and dilatation may be performed in the early second trimester in women with prior second trimester pregnancy loss or with a history suggestive of cervical incompetence (Parisi, 1994).

▶ Cervical cerclage should be reserved for clients with cervical incompetence (identified by a history of rapid, painless cervical effacement and dilatation resulting in second trimester pregnancy loss) or for women who have sufficient cervical change without uterine activity in the current pregnancy (ACOG, 1996b; Iams & Creasy, 1988; Parisi, 1994).

● Hospital admission is indicated for rupture of membranes, vaginal bleeding related to placenta previa or abruptio placentae, diagnosis of preterm labor with cervical change, or strong suspicion of preterm labor. Inpatient management details are beyond the scope of this chapter.

● Tocolytic therapy in the hospital may be initiated provided the following criteria are met (Pernoll, 1994):

▶ Gestational age between 20 and 34 weeks (may be used up to 36 to 37 weeks' gestation if intensive neonatal care is not available)

▶ Membranes intact

▶ Cervical dilatation less than 4 cm, effacement less than 80 percent

▶ Fetus apparently healthy

Although tocolysis is commonly used, there are no data to suggest that these agents improve any index of long-term perinatal morbidity or mortality. (ACOG, 1995). Full discussion regarding inpatient management of the woman on tocolytic therapy is beyond the scope of this chapter. Dosage regimens will be dictated by the physician in charge of the patient's care. Contraindications to tocolytic therapy are listed in Table 6.14 and in the drug section below.

▶ Commonly used tocolytic agents

   – Magnesium sulfate is an intracellular calcium antagonist. Its combined use with beta-mimetics may increase both efficacy and adverse effects.

      * Side effects include nausea/vomiting, headache, flushing, sense of warmth, dry mouth, urinary retention, visual changes, weakness, lethargy, vasodilation, respiratory depression, cardiac arrest, and death.

      * Fetal/neonatal effects include respiratory depression, hypotonia, drowsiness, bony abnormalities, congenital rickets (Iams, 1994; Wheeler, 1994).

      * Dosage is 4 to 6 gm IV bolus, then 1 to 3 gm/hour (R. Field, M.D., personal communication, May 13, 1996).

      * Contraindications include hypocalcemia, myasthenia gravis, and renal failure (ACOG, 1995).

   – Terbutaline is a beta-mimetic. Its action results in myometrial relaxation; it is most effective in prolonging pregnancy for 24 to 48 hours; there appears to be no decrease in neonatal morbidity or mortality (ACOG, 1995; Wheeler, 1994).

      * Side effects include tachycardia, pulmonary edema, hyperglycemia, hypokalemia, fluid retention, anxiety and jitteriness, increased systolic BP, decreased diastolic BP, mild palpitations, flushing, chest pain, cardiac arrhythmias, and myocardial ischemia (Creasy, 1994).

      * Fetal/neonatal effects include tachycardia, hypoglycemia, hyperinsulinemia, hypocalcemia, hypotension, and hydrops.

      * Dosage is 0.010 to 0.080 mg/minute IV, 2.5-5.0 mg p.o. every 2 to 4 hours, or 0.250 to 0.500 mg IM or SC every 3 to 4 hours (Creasy, 1994; R. Field, M.D., personal communication, May 13, 1996; Mercer & Lewis, 1997).

      * Contraindications to beta-mimetics include maternal cardiac rhythm disturbance or other cardiac disease, poorly controlled diabetes, thyrotoxicosis, or hypertension (ACOG, 1995).

   NOTE: A terbutaline pump can administer pulsatile, low-dose, subcutaneous infusion of terbutaline and release intermittent high-dose boluses when increased uterine activity is present. The total daily dose is less than oral dose; no current evidence to support its use (ACOG, 1995; Niebyl, 1993).

   – Ritodrine is a beta-mimetic similar to terbutaline. It is not commonly used because of an increased risk of maternal side effects (e.g., tachycardia, hypotension, apprehension, chest tightness/pain, pulmonary edema).

      * Dosage is 0.050 to 0.350 mg/minute IV, 20 mg p.o. every 2 to 4 hours, or 5 to 10 mg IM every 2 to 4 hours (Creasy, 1994; R Field, M.D., personal communication, May 13, 1996).

   NOTE: In the United States, only parenteral ritodrine is now available since the manufacturer discontinued distribution of tablets in 1995 (Cunningham et al., 1997).

Ritodrine and terbutaline are the only Federal Drug Administration–approved tocolytic agents (Mercer & Lewis, 1997). See contraindications to beta-mimetics above.

- Nifedipine is a calcium channel blocker. While usually well-tolerated by mother, it may cause maternal hypotension. It is considered a second-line drug when primary therapy has failed (AGOG, 1995).

  * Side effects include facial flushing, nausea, headache, hypotension, tachycardia, hepatotoxicity, vasodilation, decreased peripheral resistance, and decreased uteroplacental perfusion (Wheeler, 1994).

  * There are no known adverse fetal or neonatal effects.

  * Dosage is 10-20 mg p.o. every 4-6 hr (Iams, 1994; R. Field, M.D., personal communication, May 13, 1996).

  * Contraindications include maternal liver disease (AGOG, 1995).

- Indomethacin is a prostaglandin synthesis inhibitor. While usually well-tolerated by mother, potential risks to fetus are main concern (Niebyl, 1993). It is considered a second-line drug when primary therapy has failed (AGOG, 1995).

  * Side effects include nausea/vomiting, diarrhea, headache, thrombocytopenia, dizziness, depression, psychosis, serious allergic reaction (Creasy, 1994; Wheeler, 1994).

  * Fetal/neonatal effects include premature closure of ductus arteriosus (not recommended for use after 32 weeks), primary pulmonary hypertension (increased incidence with use longer than 5 days) and decreased urine output (Niebyl, 1993).

  * Dosage is 25 to 50 mg p.o. every 6 hours; an initial dose of 50 to 100 mg may be in the form of a rectal suppository (Iams, 1994; R. Field, M.D., personal communication, May 13, 1996).

  * Contraindications include peptic ulcer disease or gastrointestinal bleeding, asthma, coronary artery disease, coagulation disorders, hepatic or renal insufficiency, oligohydramnios, and suspected fetal cardiac/renal anomaly (ACOG, 1995; Creasy, 1994).

- Antibiotic therapy for women in preterm labor is not routinely employed to prolong pregnancy.

  ▶ Specific therapy for vaginitis and STDs should be undertaken, as indicated (refer to appropriate chapters).

  ▶ Standard practices should be applied regarding group B Streptococci prophylaxis (see Chapter 10.3, *Group B Streptococcus*) (Gibbs & Eschenbach, 1997).

  ▶ Also see Chapter 6.24, *Premature Rupture of Membranes.*

- Corticosteroid therapy may be utilized for women at risk of preterm delivery to enhance fetal organ system maturation, as indicated (ACOG, 1994; ACOG, 1995;Creasy, 1994). Regimens include

▶ Betamethasone 12 mg IM, 2 doses given 24 hours apart

OR

▶ Dexamethasone 6 mg IM, 4 doses given 12 hours apart (National Institutes of Health, [NIH], 1994).

● Women admitted for suspected preterm labor who do not demonstrate cervical change and whose contractions cease may be discharged from the hospital to be further evaluated with regular frequent OB visits.

● Also see Chapter 6.24, *Premature Rupture of Membranes*, Chapter 10.3, *Group B Streptococcus*, and Section 14, *Vaginitis and Sexually Transmitted Diseases*.

Consultation

● Consultation is mandatory if preterm labor is suspected or confirmed, or if PROM is evidenced.

▶ May refer client to a high-risk OB team if available, or to a physician for primary management.

▶ Co-management with physician is also feasible.

Patient Education

● Encourage good self-care during pregnancy.

▶ Pay attention to adequate nutrition and fluid intake.

▶ Avoid extreme physical activity and fatigue.

▶ Minimize psychological stress.

▶ Keep regular prenatal appointments.

▶ Promptly report problems.

● Educate pregnant women regarding the risk factors for premature delivery, and encourage them to make necessary lifestyle changes in an attempt to prevent this outcome.

▶ Prolonged standing and walking should be avoided if woman is at risk for preterm birth (Gabbe & Turner, 1997).

● Intensive education/counseling is mandatory for clients at risk for or with suspected preterm labor. At many facilities, client education materials are available on the subject of preterm birth prevention.

● Educate the client regarding the signs and symptoms of preterm labor as described in the Subjective section. Be sure she understands these.

● Teach self-detection and timing of uterine contractions.

- Establish criteria for notification of the health care provider:
  - ► Regular uterine contractions 15 minutes apart or closer or more than four contractions in 1 hour
  - ► Vaginal bleeding or leaking of fluid
  - ► Other signs/symptoms of preterm labor

- Stress importance of compliance with bed rest and the reporting of signs and symptoms of preterm labor.

- Offer suggestions for meal planning if on bed rest. See Section 18, *Nutrition*.

- Review danger signs of pregnancy relative to spontaneous abortion, preeclampsia, and placenta previa/abruptio placentae.

- Provide Labor & Delivery suite, emergency, and health care provider phone numbers.

Follow-up

- Assess presence or absence of signs/symptoms of preterm labor at each visit.
  - ► Assess compliance with and side effects of tocolytic medication as indicated.
  - ► Alter dosage regimen, depending on side effects (consult with physician).

- Tocolytic medications should be discontinued if the client experiences severe side effects or is unable to tolerate the medication and when the patient completes 36 weeks of pregnancy. Alteration in dosage regimen also may be indicated, depending on side effects.
  - ► Long-term terbutaline therapy may adversely affect glucose tolerance; consult with physician regarding need for repeating the oral glucose screening test.

- Perform gentle serial cervical examinations at each prenatal visit and as indicated in clients at risk for or with signs/symptoms of preterm labor.

- Review the following with client at each visit and have her verbalize her understanding.
  - ► Signs and symptoms of preterm labor
  - ► Self-detection and timing of uterine contractions
  - ► Criteria for notification of health care provider

- Assess activity level and compliance with bed rest regimen, as indicated.

- Advance activity slowly, as indicated by history and cervical examination.

- Support need for sexual expression exclusive of breast stimulation (and possibly intercourse and orgasm) when preterm labor is a risk.

- Assess social situation and support systems.
  - ► Refer to social services or public health nurse, as indicated.
  - ► Assist with child care arrangements, as necessary, if client is on bed rest.

- Client to be referred to Labor & Delivery if preterm labor is suspected or confirmed or in cases of PROM.

- Preterm delivery may precipitate an emotional crisis for the client and family. Provide support for the normal responses of grief, guilt, and anxiety.

- Make client aware that one preterm delivery places her at risk for another; therefore, in future pregnancies, early and comprehensive prenatal care should be sought.

- Refer partners of pregnant women with sexually transmitted diseases for appropriate treatment.

- Document diagnosis of preterm labor and management thereof in progress notes and problem list. Document high-risk status for preterm labor with the aid of a risk assessment tool, as available, and include form in client's prenatal record.

Table 6.14

Contraindications to Tocolytic Inhibition of Preterm Labor

Absolute contraindications	Severe pregnancy-induced hypertension Severe abruptio placentae Severe bleeding from any cause Chorioamnionitis Fetal death Fetal anomaly incompatible with life Severe fetal growth retardation
Relative contraindications	Mild chronic hypertension Mild abruptio placentae Stable placenta previa Maternal cardiac disease Hyperthyroidism Uncontrolled diabetes mellitus Fetal distress Fetal anomaly Mild fetal growth retardation Cervix more than 5 cm dilated

Source: Creasy, R.K. (1994). Preterm labor and delivery. In R.K. Creasy and R. Resnik (Eds.), *Maternal-Fetal Medicine: Principles and Practice* (3rd ed., pp. 494–520). Philadelphia, PA: W.B. Saunders. Reprinted by permission.

Table 6.15

Risk Assessment for Preterm Labor

Name: _____

Gravidy _____ (# of pregnancies) Parity _____ (# of deliveries > 20 weeks)

FACTORS   1st Visit   Rescreen

1. Preterm delivery <34 weeks last delivery (PTL, PROM)   ☐   ☐
2. Preterm labor at <34 weeks with term delivery last delivery   ☐   ☐
   (requiring parenteral tocolytics)
3. Uterine anomaly - nullipara (didelphys, bicornuate, or septum)   ☐   ☐
4. DES exposure - nullipara   ☐   ☐
5. Cone biopsy - no subsequent term delivery   ☐   ☐
6. ≥ 2nd trimester abortions, 2 or more (spontaneous or therapeutic)   ☐   ☐
7. Drug use continuing during current pregnancy (cocaine or amphetamines)   ☐   ☐
8. Multiple gestation   ☐   ☐
9. Incompetent cervix (cerclage in place)   ☐   ☐
10. Abdominal surgery this pregnancy (after 18 weeks)   ☐   ☐
11. Polyhydramnios at < 34 weeks (pocket > 10 cm or AFVI > 30 cm)   ☐   ☐
12. Cervical dilation > 1 cm before 32 weeks   ☐   ☐
13. Cervical length ≤ 25 mm by vaginal ultrasound (24–32 weeks)   ☐   ☐
14. Uterine irritability (admission to R/O PTL)   ☐   ☐
15. Preterm labor this pregnancy (cervix ≥ 1 cm dilated)   ☐   ☐
16. NO RISK FACTOR PRESENT   ☐   ☐

(1) Initial Screen (Complete at First Visit)   (2) Rescreen (As indicated if risk factors develop)

Date ☐☐-☐☐-☐☐   Date ☐☐-☐☐-☐☐

☐ High Risk*   ☐ High Risk*
Preterm birth prevention referral   Preterm birth prevention referral

                        ☐ Yes ☐ No   ☐ Yes ☐ No
_____ MD/RNP   _____ MD/RNP

*High risk if any factor present

Source: Danbe, K. & Dyson, D. (1993). Kaiser Permanente Northern California Regional Perinatal Nursing Service Center. Adapted with permission.

References

American College of Obstetricians and Gynecologists (ACOG). (1994). *Antenatal corticosteroid therapy for fetal maturation.* (Committee Opinion No. 147). Washington, DC: Author

American College of Obstetricians and Gynecologists (ACOG). (1995). *Preterm labor* (Technical Bulletin No. 206). Washington, DC: Author.

American College of Obstetricians and Gynecologists (ACOG). (1996a). *Home uterine activity monitoring* (ACOG Committee Opinion No. 172). Washington, DC: Author.

American College of Obstetricians and Gynecologists (ACOG). (1996b). *Procedure: Cervical cerclage* (Criteria Set Number 17). Washington, DC: Author.

American College of Obstetricians and Gynecologists (ACOG). (1997). *Fetal fibronectin preterm labor risk test.* (ACOG Committee Opinion No. 187). Washington, DC: Author.

Arias, F. (1984). Preterm labor. In F. Arias (Ed.), *High risk pregnancy and delivery* (pp. 37–62). St. Louis, MO: C. V. Mosby.

Ascarelli, M.H., & Morrison, J.C. (1997). Use of fetal fibronectin in clinical practice. *Obstetrical and Gynecological Survey, 52*(4), S1–S12.

Colton, T., Kayne, H.L., Zhang, Y., & Heeren, T. (1995). A meta-analysis of home uterine activity monitoring. *American Journal of Obstetrics & Gynecology, 173,* 1499–1505.

Creasy, R.K. (1989). Preterm labor and delivery. In R.K. Creasy & R. Resnik (Eds.), *Maternal-fetal medicine: Principles and Practice* (2nd ed., pp. 477–504). Philadelphia, PA: W.B. Saunders.

Creasy, R.K. (1994). Preterm labor and delivery. In R.K. Creasy & R. Resnik (Eds.), *Maternal-fetal medicine: Principles and Practice* (3rd ed., pp. 494–520). Philadelphia, PA: W. B. Saunders.

Cunningham, F.G., McDonald, P.C., Gant, N.F., Levano, K.J., Gilstrap III, L.C., Hankins, G.D.V., & Clark, S.L. (1997). *Williams Obstetrics* (20th ed., pp. 797–826). Stamford, CT: Appleton & Lange.

Danbe, K., & Dyson, D. (1993). *Preterm Labor Screen.* Kaiser Permanente Northern California Regional Perinatal Nursing Service Center.

Gabbe, S.G., & Turner, L.P. (1997). Reproductive hazards of the American lifestyle: Work during pregnancy. *American Journal of Obstetrics and Gynecology, 176*(4), 826–832.

Garite, T.J., & Lockwood, C.J. (1996). A new test for diagnosis and prediction of preterm delivery. *Contemporary OB/GYN, 41*(1), 77–93.

Gibbs, R.S., & Eschenbach, D.A. (1997). Use of antibiotics to prevent preterm birth. *American Journal of Obstetrics and Gynecology, 177*(2), 275–380.

Gibbs, R.S., Romero, R., Hillier, S.H., Eschenbach, D.A., & Sweet, R.L. (1992) A review of premature birth and subclinical infection. *American Journal of Obstetrics and Gynecology, 166* 1515–1528.

Goepfert, A.R., & Goldenberg, R.L. (1996). Prediction of prematurity. *Current Opinion in Obstetrics and Gynecology, 8,* 417–427.

Gomez, R., Romero, R., Edwin, S.S., & David, C. (1997). Pathogenesis of preterm labor and preterm premature rupture of membranes associated with intra-amniotic infection. *Infectious Disease Clinics of North America, 11*(1), 135–176.

Grimes, D.A., & Schultz, K.F. (1992). Randomized controlled trials of home uterine activity monitoring: A review and critique. *Obstetrics & Gynecology, 79*(1), 137–142.

Hamilton, M.P.R., Abdalla, H.I., & Whitfield, C.R. (1985). Significance of raised maternal serum alpha-fetoprotein in singleton pregnancies with normally formed fetuses. *Obstetrics and Gynecology, 65*(4), 465–470.

Iams, J.D. (1994). Delaying labor with tocolysis. *Contemporary OB/GYN, 39*(11), 69–75.

Iams, J.D., & Creasy, R.K. (1988). Prevention of preterm birth. *Clinical Obstetrics and Gynecology, 31*(3), 599–615.

Iams, J.D., Goldenberg, R.L., Meis, P.J., Mercer, B.M., Moawar, A., Das, A., Thom, E., McNellis, D., Cooper, R.L., Johnson, F., Roberts, J.M. (1996). The length of the cervix and the risk of spontaneous preterm delivery. *New England Journal of Medicine, 334*, 567–572.

Iams, J.D., Johnson, F.F., & O'Shaughnessy, R.W. (1988). A prospective random trial of home uterine activity monitoring in pregnancies at increased risk of preterm labor. *American Journal of Obstetrics and Gynecology, 159*(3), 595–603.

Katz, M., Gill, P.J., & Newman, R.B. (1986). Detection of preterm labor by ambulatory monitoring of uterine activity: A preliminary report. *Obstetrics and Gynecology, 68*(6), 773–778.

Katz, M., & Scheerer, L.J. (1988). Ambulatory monitoring of uterine contractions. *Clinical Obstetrics and Gynecology, 31*(3), 616–634.

Lantz, M.E., & Porter, K.B. (1995). Home uterine activity monitoring: Update on the literature. *The Female Patient, 20,* 80–88.

Laros, R. (1988). *Preterm labor screen.* San Francisco: University of California.

Lipshitz, J., & Brown, R.L. (1986). Preterm labor. In R.A. Knuppel & J.E. Drukker (Eds.), *High risk pregnancy: A team approach* (pp. 303–324). Philadelphia, PA: W.B. Saunders.

Lubbe, W.F., & Wiggins, G.C. (1985). Lupus anticoagulant and pregnancy. *American Journal of Obstetrics and Gynecology, 153*(3), 322–327.

Main, D.M. (1988). The epidemiology of preterm birth. *Clinical Obstetrics and Gynecology, 31*(3), 521–532.

McGregor, J.A. (1987). Preventing preterm birth caused by infection. *Contemporary Ob/Gyn, 29*(4), 33–42.

McGregor, J.A., French, J.I., & Witkin, S. (1996). Infection and prematurity: Evidence-based approaches. *Current Opinion in Obstetrics and Gynecology, 8,* 428–432.

Mercer, B.M., & Lewis, R. (1997). Preterm labor and preterm premature rupture of membranes. *Infectious Disease Clinics of North America, 11*(1), 177–201.

National Institutes of Health (NIH). (1994). The effect of antenatal steroids for fetal maturation on prenatal outcomes: Interim draft statement. *NIH Consensus Statement Online 1994 Feb. 28–Mar. 2; 12*(2) 1–24.

Niebyl, J.R. (1993). Preventing preterm labor with tocolytics. *Contemporary OB/GYN, 38*(3), 21–33.

Parisi, V.M. (1988). Cervical incompetence and preterm labor. *Clinical Obstetrics and Gynecology, 31*(3), 585–598.

Parisi, V.M. (1994). Cervical incompetence. In R.K. Creasy & R. Resnik (Eds.), *Maternal fetal medicine: Principles and Practice* (3rd ed., pp. 453–466). Philadelphia, PA: W.B. Saunders.

Pernoll, M.L. (1994). Late pregnancy complications. In A.H. De Cherney & M.L. Pernoll (Eds.), *Current obstetric and gynecologic diagnosis and treatment* (pp. 331–343). Norwalk, CT: Appleton & Lange.

Romero, R., & Mazor, M. (1988). Infection and preterm labor. *Clinical Obstetrics and Gynecology, 312*(3), 553–584.

Wheeler, D.G. (1994). Preterm birth prevention. *Journal of Nurse-Midwifery, 39*(Suppl. 2), 66s–80s.

Chapter 26

POSTDATE PREGNANCY

Lisa L. Lommel

There are various terms to describe pregnancy that continues past the estimated date of delivery. *Postdate* and *post-term* pregnancy are used to describe pregnancy that exceeds 42 weeks (294 days) from the onset of the last normal menstrual period. This term includes patients with uncertain dates. *Prolonged pregnancy* is used to describe pregnancy that is well documented by ovulation or conception to have exceeded 294 days (Woods, 1994). The term *postmature* is used to describe the maturity of the neonate, which cannot be assessed until after birth (Woods, 1994).

The incidence of postdate pregnancy, based on menstrual data, is reported to be 3 to 12 percent of all pregnancies (American College of Obstetricians and Gynecologists [ACOG], 1989). Early confirmatory ultrasound dating decreases the incidence to 1 to 2 percent (Woods, 1994). Inaccurate dating of pregnancies and irregularity of ovulation accounts for the variation in incidence of postdate pregnancy. Seventy percent of postdate pregnancies are misdiagnosed term pregnancies. Early and accurate evaluation of the patient is important to determine the estimated date of delivery. The known date of the last menstrual period (LMP) is considered to be the best clinical predictor of date of delivery. If the last menstrual period is unknown, additional clinical and physical parameters should be collected to aid in the date determination.

The risk of morbidity and mortality is increased in the postdate pregnancy. The leading causes of neonatal morbidity occur in relation to placental insufficiency (dysmaturity/postmaturity, fetal distress, birth asphyxia, meconium aspiration, and low Apgar scores) and macrosomia (fractures, neurologic injuries of the shoulder). Neonatal mortality is slightly increased in pregnancies lasting more than 42 weeks. This mortality is most demonstrable when the postdate pregnancy coexists with certain high-risk conditions, such as hypertension and diabetes (Sulik & Greenwald, 1994). It is also known that pregnancies complicated by fetal malformation have an increased incidence of postdatism, which subsequently elevates fetal mortality rates.

Maternal morbidity in the postdate pregnancy is increased primarily due to an increased incidence of cesarean section. The sequelae of cesarean section may increase the risk of postpartum hemorrhage, vaginal and rectal lacerations, and endometritis (Sulik & Greenwald, 1994).

Management of postdate pregnancy focuses on assessment of fetal well-being with induction for signs of fetal distress. Perinatal morbidity is twice as high in postdate pregnancies that are associated with other high-risk factors (i.e. hypertension, diabetes). Thus, these pregnancies should not be allowed to progress to beyond 42 weeks (Kilpatrick, 1994).

Database

Subjective

- Maternal factors associated with postdate pregnancy
  - ▶ LMP induced by oral contraceptives

- ▶ Uncertain dating of pregnancy

- ▶ History of postdate pregnancy

- ▶ Primigravida

- ▶ Symptoms may include decreased fetal movement

- Fetal factors associated with postdate pregnancy (Cunningham, MacDonald, Gant, Leveno, & Gilstrap, 1993)

  - ▶ Anencephaly

  - ▶ Fetal adrenal hypoplasia

  - ▶ Absence of the fetal pituitary

  - ▶ Placental sulfatase deficiency

  - ▶ Extrauterine pregnancy

Objective

- Maternal weight loss

- Decreasing fundal height secondary to oligohydramnios and fetal wastage

- Decreasing abdominal girth secondary to reduced amounts of amniotic fluid

- Data review

  - ▶ Accuracy of LMP, including history of regular/irregular menses

  - ▶ Predicted ovulation by temperature, coital records, and/or ovulation predictor kit

  - ▶ Oral contraceptive use

  - ▶ Positive pregnancy test 5 to 6 weeks after LMP

  - ▶ Ultrasound before 20 weeks gestation that agrees with LMP (accurate to ± one week when performed between 6 and 12 weeks' gestation)

  - ▶ Findings on pelvic examination before 12 weeks' gestation

  - ▶ Date of fetal heart tones first heard with the electronic Doppler (at 10 to 12 weeks)

  - ▶ Date of fetal heart tones first heard with the fetoscope

  - ▶ Date of first fetal movement (usually 16 to 19 weeks' gestation in primigravidas)

  - ▶ Fundal heights measured between 16 and 34 weeks' gestation

- Result of ultrasound, nonstress test (NST), contraction stress test (CST) or biophysical profile (BPP)

- Position, dilatation, effacement, and consistency of the cervix after 40 weeks

- Station of the presenting part after 40 weeks

Assessment

- Intrauterine pregnancy greater than 42 weeks
  - ▶ Size equals date, is greater than date, is less than date
  - ▶ R/O oligohydramnios
  - ▶ R/O fetal anomaly

Plan

Diagnostic Tests

- See Chapter 3.4, *Ultrasound*. Ultrasound may be obtained to
  - ▶ Confirm gestational age particularly if seen for the first time in late pregnancy or labor.

    Note: Ultrasound after the second trimester is associated with an error of ±2 weeks.
  - ▶ Determine placental function.
  - ▶ Assess amniotic fluid volume. Oligohydramnios correlates highly with perinatal morbidity and mortality. See the information about amniotic fluid index in Chapter 6.21, *Oligohydramnios*.
  - ▶ Rule out congenital anomaly.
  - ▶ Estimate fetal weight/size.
- Obtain a nonstress test (NST) to evaluate fetal well-being. See nonstress test information in Chapter 3.5, *Antepartum Fetal Surveillance*.
- Obtain a contraction stress test (CST) if the NST is nonreactive. The nipple stimulation contraction stress test (NSCST) is more commonly used than the oxytocin challenge test (OCT). See contraction stress test information in Chapter 3.5, *Antepartum Fetal Surveillance*.
- Obtain a biophysical profile (BPP) to evaluate fetal heart reactivity, fetal breathing movements, fetal muscular tone, fetal body movements, and amniotic fluid volume. See BPP protocol.
- Initiate fetal movement counts on all postdate pregnancies. See fetal movement count information in Chapter 3.5, *Antepartum Fetal Surveillance*.
- Amniocentesis may be conducted by a physician to assess amniotic fluid color and the lecithin/sphingomyelin (L/S) ratio.

Treatment/Management

- Begin twice-weekly NST, amniotic fluid index (AFI) assessment, and cervical exam at 41.5 weeks' gestation (Kilpatrick, 1994)
  - ▶ Refer client to a physician for management if NST or AFI is abnormal (an AFI of less than 5.0 cm, NST with any decelerations or no accelerations)
- ▶ Refer to a physician for induction if cervix is favorable. A Bishop's score greater than 5 is indicative of favorability. See Table 6.16, Bishop Scoring System.

- If macrosomia is suspected (estimated fetal weight less than 4,500 grams) refer to physician. May obtain ultrasound to confirm, as appropriate.

- Patients not in labor by 43 weeks should be managed by a physician for induction.

- Assess fetal movement counts at every visit.

- Patients with other high-risk factors (i.e., hypertension, diabetes) should not be allowed to progress beyond 42 weeks' gestation. Refer to a physician at term.

Consultation

- Consult with and refer to a physician after 41.5 weeks' gestation.

- Refer to a physician at term any patient who has additional high-risk factors.

Patient Education

- Discuss postdate pregnancy and its implications.

- Explain how to obtain fetal movement counts and their importance on postdate pregnancies.

- Counsel regarding the tests that will be performed and their use in fetal surveillance.

- Explain labor induction, if appropriate.

Follow-up

- Closely evaluate the newborn resulting from a postdate pregnancy. Assess for signs of hypoglycemia (especially in infants more than 4,000 grams), hypothermia in the dysmature infant, and consequences of meconium aspiration.

- Perform routine postpartum follow-up for mother and infant at appropriate intervals.

- Document postdatism in progress notes and problem list.

Table 6.16

Bishop Scoring System

Score	Cervical dilatation (%)	Cervical effacement (%)	Station	Cervical consistency	Position
0	Closed	0–30	-3	Firm	Posterior
1	1–2	40–50	-2	Medium	Midposition
2	3–4	60–70	-1, 0	Soft	Anterior
3	≥ 5	≥ 80	+1, +2		

References

American College of Obstetricians and Gynecologists (ACOG) (1989). *Diagnosis and management of post-term pregnancy* (Technical Bulletin No. 130). Washington, DC: Author.

Cunningham, F.G., MacDonald, D.C., Gant, N.F., Leveno, K.J., & Gilstrap, L.C. (1993). *Williams Obstetrics* (19th ed.) pp. 871–875. Norwalk, CT: Appleton & Lange.

Kilpatrick, S.J. (1994). Management of the post-term pregnancy: Still a major dilemma? In Department of OB, GYN, and Reproductive Sciences at UCSF (Chair), *Antepartum & Intrapartum Management.* Symposium conducted in San Francisco.

Sulk, S.M., & Greenwald, J.L. (1994). Evaluation and management of postdate pregnancy. *American Family Physician, 49*(5), 1177–1188.

Wood, C.L. (1994). Postdate pregnancy update. *Journal of Nurse-Midwifery, 39*(2), 110S–122S.

Chapter 27

PROTEINURIA

Lisa L. Lommel

Protein is excreted in the urine (proteinuria) when the renal system is stressed by disease or infection. However, small amounts (trace to 1+) may be found in a "clean catch" specimen contaminated by vaginal secretions or blood. Large amounts of protein (2 to 4+) is a common characteristic of renal dysfunction. In the pregnant client, proteinuria may indicate a kidney or bladder infection, a sign of preeclampsia, or chronic/acute renal disease.

Albumin is the primary protein of clinical significance excreted in all of these conditions. The dipstick method is used most often to monitor for proteinuria in the pregnant client. Prenatal clients should have their urine evaluated for protein at every prenatal visit.

Database

Subjective

- Usually asymptomatic

- Pain or burning on urination, urgency, frequency, fever and/or chills if urinary tract (UTI) infection present

- Flank or suprapubic pain with a urinary tract infection (UTI)

- Headache, visual disturbances, epigastric pain, decreased urinary output, generalized edema may be present with preeclampsia

- Vaginal discharge, accompanying signs and symptoms of vaginitis may be present

- Patient may have a history of chronic renal disease

Objective

- Amount of protein recorded on dipstick, trace to 4+

- Elevated temperature, rapid pulse with UTI

- CVA or suprapubic tenderness with UTI

- Positive leukocyte esterase, nitrites and/or hemoglobin on dipstick with UTI

- Positive urine culture with UTI

- Elevated blood pressure with preeclampsia

- Sudden weight gain with preeclampsia

- Edema of hands, feet, and/or face with preeclampsia

- Hyperreflexia with preeclampsia
- Positive wet mount/culture for vaginitis

Assessment

- Proteinuria, 1 to 4+
  - ▶ R/O UTI or pyelonephritis
  - ▶ R/O preeclampsia
  - ▶ R/O vaginal contamination with normal flora
  - ▶ R/O vaginitis
  - ▶ R/O renal disease

Plan

Diagnostic Tests

- Obtain clean-catch urine specimen and dipstick for protein. False-negative readings can be caused by highly buffered alkaline urine (Detmer, McPhee, Nicoll & Chou, 1992).
  - ▶ 1+ = 30 mg/dL
  - ▶ 2+ = 100 mg/dL
  - ▶ 3+ = 300 mg/dL
  - ▶ 4+ ≥ 2,000 mg/dL
- If initial dipstick is positive for protein (≥ 1+), obtain clean-catch urine specimen and repeat dipstick.
- If unable to obtain clean-catch urine in presence of subjective and/or objective signs and symptoms, obtain catheterized urine specimen and dipstick.
- If repeat dipstick is positive for protein (≥ 1+), obtain complete urinalysis and urine culture with sensitivities.
- Assess for preeclampsia (see Chapter 6.13, *Hypertensive Disorders of Pregnancy*).
- Obtain vaginal wet mounts and cultures as indicated.
- For persistent proteinuria of 1 to 4+ order:
  - ▶ Serum creatinine and uric acid
  - ▶ 24-hour urine for total protein, creatinine, and creatinine clearance

Treatment/Management

- If repeat dipstick contains trace to 1+ protein, initiate routine follow-up, as indicated.
- If repeat urine dipstick contains ≥ 2+ protein, refer to the following protocols for management.
  - ▶ See chapters in Section 13, Asymptomatic Bacteriuria, Cystitis, and Pyelonephritis.

▶ See Chapter 6.13, Hypertensive Disorders of Pregnancy.

▶ See Chapter 14.7, Vaginitis.

Consultation

- Consult with physician when there is persistent proteinuria (≥ 1+), recurrent UTI, or possible preeclampsia.

Patient Education

- Explain the need for a clean-catch urine specimen and the method of collection.

- Stress the importance of perineal hygiene to prevent UTI.

- See the Patient Education sections of Chapter 13.1, *Asymptomatic Bacteriuria;* Chapter 13.2, *Cystitis;* Chapter 13.3, *Pyelonephritis;* and Chapter 14.7, *Vaginitis.*

Follow-up

- Evaluate the patient's urine for proteinuria at each visit.

- Document in progress notes and problem list if a significant, on-going problem.

References

Detmer, W.M., McPhee, S.J., Nicoll, D., & Chou, T.M. (1992). *Pocket guide to diagnostic tests.* Connecticut: Appleton and Lange.

Wallach, J. (1992). *Interpretation of diagnostic tests.* (5th ed.). Boston, MA: Little Brown and Company.

Chapter 28

SEIZURES

Ellen M. Scarr

A seizure is a paroxysmal episode of disturbed central nervous system (CNS) function, caused by abnormal cerebral neuronal activity and resulting in an alteration in consciousness (Cascino, 1994). The etiology of seizures is usually unknown, but may be caused by infections (meningitis, encephalitis), metabolic alterations (hypocalcemia, hypoglycemia), toxic substances (mercury, lead, CO_2, drugs), head trauma, cerebral vascular abnormalities (arteriovenous malformation [AVM], cerebrovascular accident [CVA]) or neoplasms. Recurrent seizures are known as epilepsy, a disorder which affects 0.5 to 1 percent of the population and is genetically linked; more than 40 percent of patients with epilepsy have a family history of seizures (Buehler & Stempel, 1992; Dreifuss, 1995; Gilstrap & Little, 1992; Yerby, 1993).

Seizures are classified by clinical and electrophysiologic localization of seizure activity; patients may have partial or generalized seizures, or a combination of both. Grand mal (tonic-clonic) seizures are characterized by a total loss of consciousness, a tonic phase (rigid extremities, apnea), then a clonic phase (relaxation and contraction of the skeletal muscles). Postictal confusion and drowsiness are common. More than 70 percent of epileptics have grand mal seizures. Petit mal (absence) seizures involve only brief alterations in consciousness, often lasting less than 10 seconds. There is no motor activity and individuals are often unaware of the seizure. Ten percent of epileptics have petit mal seizures; these rarely persist beyond adolescence. Focal seizures are usually motor seizures that start with localized, peripheral twitching, commonly of the face, foot or hand. They may remain localized or progress and become more generalized. Psychomotor seizures are characterized by subjective mood disturbances or visual disturbances. They are often associated with autonomic activity (salivation, pupillary dilation, flushing) and automatisms (involuntary lip smacking, chewing). The term "status epilepticus" refers to recurrent seizure activity without full recovery of consciousness between events or continuous seizure activity for more than 30 minutes. A "convulsion" refers to a seizure with primarily motor involvement (Buehler & Stempel, 1992; Treiman, 1993).

Up to half of pregnant women with a history of epilepsy suffer an increase in seizure frequency during pregnancy, 5 to 10 percent experience reduced seizure activity, and the remainder experience no change (Buehler & Stempel, 1992; Cartlidge, 1995). Women whose seizures are poorly controlled prior to pregnancy are most likely to sustain more seizures while pregnant. Factors that contribute to an increase in seizure activity during pregnancy include decreased absorption of anti-epileptic drugs (AEDs) from the gastrointestinal tract (due to vomiting), increased liver and renal clearance of AEDs, metabolic changes, increased blood volume, increased fatigue and sleep disturbances, anxiety and emotional stress, and noncompliance with medications, often because of nausea or worry about drug effects on the fetus (Cartlidge, 1995; Paulson & Paulson, 1990; Shuster, 1994; Yerby, 1993).

Seizures threaten the well-being of both the mother and fetus, particularly generalized tonic-clonic seizures and status epilepticus. Maternal physical injury, accidental drowning and aspiration are potential hazards during seizure activity. Generalized seizures may cause fetal bradycardia, hypoxia, intrauterine growth restriction, premature rupture of membranes (PROM), abruption and premature delivery. The rate of stillbirth and neonatal mortality is twice normal.

Congenital malformations in fetuses of mothers with seizure disorders occur more frequently, not only as a result of an increased inherited risk but also from the effects of AEDs, all of which are potentially fetotoxic. (See Table 6.16, Potential Toxic Effects of Commonly Used Anticonvulsants.) There is a 6 to 8 percent chance of birth defects (particularly orofacial clefts, cardiac anomalies, and neural tube defects) in fetuses exposed in utero to AEDs, which represents a two- to threefold increase over that of the general population (Abbott, 1994; American College of Obstetricians and Gynecologists [ACOG], 1996; Cartlidge, 1995; Paulson & Paulson, 1990; Treiman, 1993). Fetuses of women who are taking more than one AED are probably at greatest risk for defects (Delgado-Escueta & Janz, 1992). Children born to women with seizures have higher rates of learning disabilities and delayed language development (Yerby, 1993). See Section 2, *Genetic Counseling,* for further discussion of anti-epileptic drugs.

Database

Subjective

- Obtain prepregnant seizure history
  - ► Type(s) of seizure
  - ► Age at onset
  - ► Etiology, if known (trauma, infection, exposure to toxic substances)
  - ► Frequency of seizure activity
  - ► Known precipitants (fatigue, illness/fever, menses, stress, alcohol, visual or auditory stimuli [Aminoff, 1995])
  - ► Prodromal symptoms, if any (headache, mood changes, malaise, twitching)
  - ► Results of neurologic testing
  - ► Medication history
    - – Current medication
    - – Recent medication(s) used (particularly at time of conception)
    - – Serum drug levels
    - – Efficacy of medication on seizure frequency
- Denies symptoms of preeclampsia (headache, generalized or nondependent edema)

Objective

- Vital signs are within normal limits (afebrile, blood pressure without elevation)
- Interval weight gain is appropriate
- Neurological examination nonfocal
- No facial, hand or generalized edema
- Urine dipstick is negative for proteinuria

Assessment

- Seizure disorder
  - ▶ R/O preeclampsia/eclampsia
  - ▶ R/O metabolic abnormalities
  - ▶ R/O cerebral vascular abnormalities
  - ▶ R/O cerebral neoplasm
  - ▶ R/O drug withdrawal
  - ▶ R/O infection

Plan

Diagnostic Tests

- Offer maternal serum alpha-fetoprotein (MSAFP) screen or triple marker screen at 15 to 20 weeks' gestation
- Give patients on valproic acid or carbamazepine a choice of screening tests to assess for neural tube defects:
  - ▶ Amniocentesis (for amniotic fluid AFP and acetylcholinesterase [ACHE])
    - OR
  - ▶ MSAFP/triple marker screen

In addition, offer these patients an early ultrasound at 12 to 13 weeks' gestation to rule out anencephaly.

- Offer ultrasound at 16 to 20 weeks' gestation to all patients to rule out spina bifida.
  - ▶ Repeat ultrasound at 22 to 24 weeks' gestation to rule out cardiac and oral cleft anomalies (Delgado-Escueta & Janz, 1992; Eller, Patterson, & Webb, 1997; Liporace, 1997).
- Obtain monthly free-plasma drug levels (the free level is chemically active).

Treatment/Management

- After physician consultation, consider discontinuation of AED if woman has been seizure free for 2 years or more.
- If an AED is required, the goal is monotherapy. Avoid high levels of medication if possible, particularly in the first trimester. See Table 6.17, Commonly Used Anticonvulsants During Pregnancy.

NOTE: While all AEDs are fetotoxic, it is best to avoid valproic acid and carbamazepine if possible. The risk of a neural tube defect is estimated to be 1 to 2 percent with these drugs (Buehler & Stempel, 1992; Eller, Patterson, & Webb, 1997; Liporace, 1997).

- Supplement diet with folic acid 0.4 to 1.0 mg per day p.o. (400 to 1000 micrograms per day) throughout pregnancy.

  NOTE: Ideally, folic acid intake should begin before conception. AEDs (especially phenytoin) decrease folic acid, which may be associated with the development of neural tube defects. Check serum folate levels prior to conception, if possible, or in the first trimester: A low serum folate level will increase the risk of spontaneous abortion and/or fetal anomalies. If the folate level is low, higher folic acid doses are recommended (e.g., 4.0 mg per day p.o.) (Liporace, 1997; Public Health Service, 1992; Rayburn, 1992).

- Prescribe vitamin K supplementation (20 mg per day p.o.) in last 2 weeks of pregnancy to prevent hemorrhage (AEDs interfere with vitamin K transfer) (Kohn, 1991; Liporace, 1997).

- Maintain therapeutic AED levels in last month of pregnancy to prevent seizures in labor and delivery.

Consultation

- Refer client to genetic counseling early in pregnancy to discuss risks of congenital malformation, AED syndromes, and learning disabilities.

- Consult with a physician if there is increased frequency of seizure activity or new onset of seizures in pregnancy.

- Involve a neurologist in management of AEDs; notify neurologist of impending delivery because client is at risk for increased seizure activity during labor.

- Notify pediatrician of impending delivery because the fetus is at risk for hemorrhage, drug withdrawal, and congenital malformations.

Patient Education

- Ideally, counseling of the woman with seizures begins before conception, with modification of drug therapy, as necessary, and full education about known risks.

- Reassure client that more than 90 percent of fetuses are not affected by maternal seizure disorders.

- Encourage client to avoid known triggers of seizure activity.

- Encourage client to obtain adequate sleep, maintain adequate nutrition.

- Encourage compliance with AED therapy; avoid the use of other medications.

- Include family/friends in management of seizure activity.

  ▶ Protect the woman.

  ▶ Lay her on her side to prevent aspiration.

  ▶ Maintain her airway.

- Reinforce driving restrictions for clients with seizure activity within the last year.

Follow-up

- Client must notify provider of increased frequency of seizure activity or problems with AED compliance.

- Continue ongoing assessment of seizure control at follow-up visits.

- Document history of seizure disorder in progress notes and problem list. Make note of all current seizure medications.

Table 6.16

Potential Toxic Effects of Commonly Used Anticonvulsants

Medication	Maternal Effects	Characteristic Potential Fetal/Neonatal Effects
Carbamazepine	Drowsiness, leukopenia, ataxia, mild hepatotoxicity	Facial dysmorphisms, neural tube defects, hypoplasia of distal phalanges
Phenobarbital	Drowsiness, ataxia	Neonatal withdrawal, neonatal coagulopathy
Phenytoin	Nystagmus, ataxia, hirsutism, gingival hyperplasia, megaloblastic anemia	Facial clefting, hypoplasia of distal phalanges, hypertelorism, neonatal coagulopathy
Primidone	Drowsiness, ataxia, nausea	Neonatal withdrawal, neonatal coagulopathy
Valproic acid	Ataxia, drowsiness, alopecia, hepatotoxicity, thrombocytopenia	Facial dysmorphisms, neural tube defects

Source: American College of Obstetricians and Gynecologists (ACOG). (1996). *Seizure disorders in pregnancy.* (Technical Bulletin No. 231). Washington, DC: Author. Reprinted with permission.

Table 6.17

Commonly Used Anticonvulsants During Pregnancy

Medication	Therapeutic Level (mg/L)	Nonpregnant Dosage*	Usual Half-Life
Carbamazepine	4–10	600–1,200 mg/d in 3 or 4 divided doses	36 h (initially) 16 h (with chronic therapy)
Phenobarbital	15–40	90–180 mg/d in 2 or 3 divided doses	100 h
Phenytoin	10–20 (total) 1–2 (free)	300–500 mg/d in single or divided doses†	Average 24 h
Primidone	5–15	750–1,500 mg/d in 3 divided doses	8 h
Valproic acid	50–100	550–2,000 mg/d in 3 or 4 divided doses	Average 13 h

* Due to changes in volume of distribution and metabolism, dosages in pregnancy are often higher. The dosages must be individualized and may be dramatically higher than those listed.

† If a total dose greater than 300 mg is needed, dividing the dose will result in a more stable serum concentration.

Source: American College of Obstetricians and Gynecologists (ACOG). (1996). *Seizure disorders in pregnancy.* (Technical Bulletin No. 231). Washington, DC: Author. Reprinted with permission.

References

Abbott, J. (1994). Medical disorders during pregnancy. *Emergency Medicine Clinics of North America*, *12*(1), 115–28.

American College of Obstetricians and Gynecologists (ACOG). (1996, December). *Seizure disorders in pregnancy* (Technical Bulletin No. 231). Washington, DC: Author.

Aminoff, M. (1995). Nervous system. In L. Tierney, S. McPhee, & M. Papadakis (Eds.) *Current medical diagnosis and treatment* (34th ed., pp. 827–883). Norwalk, CT: Appleton & Lange.

Buehler, B., & Stempel, L. (1992). Anticonvulsant therapy during pregnancy. In W. Rayburn & F. Zuspan (Eds.), *Drug therapy in obstetrics and gynecology* (3rd ed., pp. 147–163). St. Louis, MO: Mosby.

Cartlidge, N. (1995). Neurologic disorders. In W. Barron & M. Lindheimer (Eds.), *Medical disorders during pregnancy* (2nd ed., pp. 430–450). St. Louis, MO: Mosby.

Cascino, G. (1994). Epilepsy: Contemporary perspectives on evaluation and treatment. *Mayo Clinic Proceedings, 69*, 1199–1211.

Delgado-Escueta, A., & Janz, D. (1992). Consensus guidelines: Preconception counseling, management, and care of the pregnant woman with epilepsy. *Neurology, 42*(Suppl. 5), 149–160.

Dreifuss, F. (1995). Prevention as it pertains to epilepsy. *Archives of Neurology, 52*(4), 363–366.

Eller, D., Patterson, C., & Webb, G. (1997). Maternal and fetal implications of anticonvulsant therapy during pregnancy. *Obstetrics and Gynecology Clinics of North America, 24*(3), 523–534.

Gilstrap, L., & Little, B. (Eds.). (1992). *Drugs and pregnancy.* New York: Elsevier Science.

Kohn, N. (1991). Neurologic diseases. In N. Gleicher (Ed.), *Principles and practice of medical therapy in pregnancy* (2nd ed., pp. 1224–1234). Norwalk, CT: Appleton & Lange.

Liporace, J. (1997). Women's issues in epilepsy: Menses, childbearing, and more. *Postgraduate Medicine, 102*(1), 123–138.

Paulson, G., & Paulson, R. (1990). Seizure disorders in pregnancy. In E. Quilligan & F. Zuspan (Eds.), *Current therapy in obstetrics and gynecology* (3rd ed., pp. 273–277). Philadelphia, PA: W.B. Saunders.

Public Health Service. (1992). Recommendations for the use of folic acid to reduce the number of cases of spina bifida and other neural tube defects. *Morbidity and Mortality Weekly Report, 41*(RR-14), 1–7.

Rayburn, W. (1992). Drugs for fetal therapy. In W. Rayburn & F. Zuspan (Eds.), *Drug therapy in obstetrics and gynecology* (3rd ed., pp. 32–44). St. Louis, MO: Mosby.

Shuster, E. (1994). Seizures in pregnancy. *Emergency Medicine Clinics of North America, 12*(4), 1013–1025.

Treiman, D. (1993). Current treatment strategies in selected situations in epilepsy. *Epilepsia, 34*(Suppl. 5), S17–S23.

Yerby, M. (1993). Epilepsy and pregnancy: New issues for an old disorder. *Neurologic Clinics, 11*(4), 777–786.

Chapter 29

SIZE/DATES DISCREPANCY

Maureen T. Shannon

A size/dates (S/D) discrepancy exists when the uterine size (by clinical parameters) is either smaller or larger than is expected based on a woman's *known* last normal menstrual period (see Table 6.12, Estimation of Gestational Age with Clinical Parameters in Chapter 6.15, *Intrauterine Growth Restriction or Small for Gestational Age*). There are two categories for size/dates discrepancies: 1) the uterine size is smaller than dates by the last menstrual period (LMP) or 2) the uterine size is larger than dates by LMP (Nichols, 1987).

Assessment of uterine size as it relates to gestational age is an essential component of prenatal care, since significant discrepancies between these may indicate perinatal complications (e.g., intrauterine growth restriction, hydramnios, oligohydramnios, abnormal fetal presentation, etc.). Prior to 20 weeks gestation, anatomic landmarks are used to assess uterine growth. At 8 weeks the uterine fundus is just at the symphysis pubis; at 12 weeks the uterus is palpable above the symphysis pubis and is now an abdominal organ; at 16 weeks the uterine fundus is midpoint between the symphysis pubis and the umbilicus; and at 20 weeks the fundus is palpable at the umbilicus (Pernoll & Taylor, 1994). Beginning at 20 weeks through 36 weeks, the fundal height in centimeters (cm) should approximate the gestational age in weeks (Beckmann et al., 1995).

Database

Subjective

- If the LMP is unknown or uncertain, the subjective signs and symptoms of pregnancy may not correlate with the estimated gestational age.
- The woman may state that she feels more or less pregnant than her estimated gestational age.
- The woman may note a rapid abdominal growth rate (in acute hydramnios or in ovarian cysts).
- The woman may report an increased or decreased nutritional intake.
- The woman may report a history of uterine fibroids or Rh disease.
- The woman may have a family history of diabetes, multiple gestations, hypertension, or pre-eclampsia.
- In multiple gestation pregnancies, the woman often reports a great deal of fetal movement.
- See subjective data contained in specific chapters for intrauterine growth restriction (IUGR), gestational trophoblastic disease (GTD), gestational diabetes mellitus (GDM), and polyhydramnios.

Objective

- In true S/D discrepancy, serum or urine pregnancy tests are positive at the appropriate times.
- In true S/D discrepancy, the bimanual examination of the uterus done during the first trimester will usually correlate with the woman's known LMP.

- McDonald's measurements are 3 cm less than or 3 cm greater than what is expected for dates (Nichols, 1987).

- Estimates of fetal weight are less than or greater than expected for gestational age.

- Two or more distinct fetal heart tones (FHTs) are noted by simultaneous auscultation done for 1 minute by two examiners (in multiple gestations).

- Absence of FHTs after the 12th week by dates (in molar pregnancy, missed spontaneous abortions, or inaccurate dating)

- Obstetrical ultrasound may reveal IUGR, fetal macrosomia, fetal anomalies, excessive amniotic fluid, multiple gestations, etc.

- Maternal weight gain may be significantly increased or decreased for that point in the pregnancy.

- Fetus may be palpated in a transverse or oblique lie.

- Distended bladder of woman may be palpated.

- See objective data contained in specific chapters for IUGR, GTD, polyhydramnios, Rh isoimmunization, etc.

Assessment

- IUP with size less than dates or size greater than dates
  - ▶ R/O inaccurate dating
  - ▶ R/O transverse or oblique lie
  - ▶ R/O IUGR
  - ▶ R/O excessive/inadequate weight gain
  - ▶ R/O polyhydramnios
  - ▶ R/O multiple gestation
  - ▶ R/O gestational trophoblastic disease
  - ▶ R/O gestational diabetes mellitus
  - ▶ R/O fetal macrosomia
  - ▶ R/O fetal anomalies
  - ▶ R/O maternal fibroids, ovarian cysts, or tumors

Plan

Diagnostic Tests

- Obstetrical ultrasound may be indicated to
  - ▶ Help calculate gestational age
  - ▶ Determine fetal size and growth patterns

   ▶ Assess the presence of some fetal anomalies

   ▶ Determine the presence of multiple fetuses

   ▶ Assess the amount of amniotic fluid

   ▶ Eliminate the presence of GTD

   ▶ Evidence of a missed abortion

   ▶ Confirm a fetal malpresentation

- Radioimmunoassay HCG level should be obtained in suspected GTD or missed abortion

- A glucose screen should be obtained on every pregnant woman between 24 to 28 weeks gestation, and a 3-hour glucose tolerance test done in women with abnormal screens (see Chapter 6.11, *Gestational Diabetes Mellitus*).

- Order nonstress tests (NST), amniotic fluid volume index (AFI), contraction stress tests (CST), and/or biophysical profile (BPP) of the fetus for women with high-risk pregnancies (e.g., IUGR, postterm pregnancies, multiple gestations, polyhydramnios, etc.)

Treatment/Management

- Review the woman's pregnancy landmarks (e.g., date of LMP and possible conception, when subjective symptoms began, date of quickening, etc.) and the clinical parameters in the chart to confirm gestational age.

- Establish an accurate gestational age as soon as possible—ideally by the end of the first trimester.

- Ideally, measurement of the fundal height should be done by the same clinician at each prenatal visit. The manual technique employed to assess fundal height should be as follows: Measurements should be made with a centimeter tape with the measurement starting at the upper border of the symphysis pubis along the curvilinear surface of the abdomen to the top of the uterine fundus (Euans, Connor, Hahn, Rodney, & Arheart, 1995; Pernoll & Taylor, 1994).

NOTE: A study investigating the accuracy of manual compared to ultrasound fundal height measurements determined that manual measurements were as reliable as ultrasound measurements in both normal weight and obese women (Euans et al., 1995).

- If a S/D discrepancy of greater than or less than 3 cm is documented, have the woman return in one week for another measurement.

- Order an ultrasound exam initially on all pregnant patients with unknown or uncertain LMPs, women taking medications that are associated with irregular menses and/or anovulation (e.g., psychotropic medications, hormonal contraceptives, etc.) just before or during the possible time of conception, or if a S/D discrepancy of greater than or less than 3 cm is documented.

- See specific chapters for the treatment/management of IUGR, multiple gestation, polyhydramnios, Rh isoimmunization, etc.

Consultation

- Consultation is required if S/D discrepancy is due to a suspected or documented abnormality (e.g., IUGR, multiple gestation, fetal anomalies, etc.).

- Refer woman to physician care if S/D discrepancy is based on an abnormality. In some high risk situations (e.g., IUGR) a woman will be co-managed with a physician.

Patient Education

- Education and counseling of a woman should be based upon the underlying cause of the S/D discrepancy.

  ▶ If an abnormality is found, then the counseling of the woman is based upon the underlying problem (e.g., IUGR).

  ▶ If no abnormality is found and fetal growth is within normal limits, then reassurance of the women is all that is indicated.

- Educate the woman about the various tests that are being ordered, and interpret the test results for her.

- Obtain nutrition counseling if the maternal weight gain is either less than or greater than expected.

Follow-up

- If S/D discrepancy evaluation reveals no problems and fetal growth is WNL, then prenatal care should proceed routinely.

- If S/D discrepancy evaluation reveals an abnormality, then follow-up is per protocol for the specific problem (e.g., IUGR).

- Document S/D discrepancy and evaluation thereof in progress notes and problem list.

References

Beckmann, C. R. B., Ling, F. W., Barzansky, B. M., Bates, G. W., Herbert, W. N. P., Laube, D. W., & Smith, R. P. (1995). *Obstetrics and gynecology* (2nd ed.). Baltimore, MD: Williams & Wilkins.

Euans, D. W., Connor, P. D., Hahn, R. G., Rodney, W. M., & Arheart, K. L. (1995). A comparison of manual and ultrasound measurements of fundal height. *The Journal of Family Practice, 40*(3), 233-236.

Nichols, C. (1987). Clinical management for size/dates discrepancy. *Journal of Nurse-Midwifery, 30*(1), 15-24.

Pernoll, M. L., & Taylor, C. M. (1994). Normal pregnancy & prenatal care. In A. H. DeCherney & M. L. Pernoll (Eds.), *Current obstetric & gynecologic diagnosis & treatment* (8th ed., pp. 183-201). Norwalk, CT: Appleton & Lange.

Chapter 30

SUBINVOLUTION

Lisa L. Lommel

Lucy Newmark Sammons

Subinvolution is the delayed or incomplete return of the uterus to normal dimensions following childbirth. To evaluate the extent of involution, perform palpation of the uterus. Normally, uterine fundal height moves from midway between the umbilicus and symphysis after third-stage labor to the level of the bony pelvis by 2 weeks postpartum to nonpregnant uterine size at 4 to 6 weeks postpartum. Endometrial regeneration is complete by the third week, except at the placental site, where regeneration is complete about 6 weeks after delivery (Novy, 1994).

Common causative or contributing factors of subinvolution are endometritis, retained placental fragments, uterine overdistention from multiple gestation or polyhydramnios, fibroids, absence of lactation, or inadequate uterine drainage (Druelinger, 1994). Recent use of immunohistochemical techniques suggest that subinvolution of the uterus is caused by a delay in return to normal of the uteroplacental arteries, possibly due to an abnormal interaction between maternal uterine cells and the fetal trophoblast (Andrew, Bulmer, Morrison, Wells, & Buckley, 1993).

Database

Subjective

- Client describes greater quantity and longer duration of bloody vaginal discharge than normal.

- Symptoms occur 1 week to several months postpartum, with maximal occurrence in the second week (Khong & Khong, 1993).

- Contributing/risk factors may include the following:

  ▶ History of heavy blood loss in early postpartum period

  ▶ Difficulty with placental delivery

  ▶ Increased maternal age

  ▶ Multiparity

  ▶ Current endometritis

  ▶ History of polyhydramnios, fibroids, or multiple gestation in current pregnancy

  ▶ History of subinvolution in previous pregnancy

  ▶ Absence of lactation

- Hemorrhage, that may be abrupt in onset

- Client may have symptoms of anemia; see Chapter 9.3, *Anemia—Iron, Folate, and Vitamin B$_{12}$ Deficiency.*

Objective

- Uterus enlarged, soft, boggy, possibly retrodisplaced
- Uterus generally freely movable
- Cervical os is patulous.
- Continuation of lochia rubra beyond the second to third week postpartum
- May have signs of concomitant infection (see Chapter 6.9, *Endometritis*).
- May have signs of anemia (see Chapter 9.3).

Assessment

- Subinvolution
  - ▶ R/O postpartum hemorrhage
  - ▶ R/O retained placental fragments
  - ▶ R/O fibroids
  - ▶ R/O inadequate uterine drainage
  - ▶ R/O endometritis
  - ▶ R/O chronically inverted uterus
  - ▶ R/O gestational trophoblastic neoplasia (GTN)
  - ▶ R/O anemia

Plan

Diagnostic Tests

- There are no definitive diagnostic tests. Considered a diagnosis of exclusion.
- Obtain hemoglobin/hematocrit to assess anemia due to blood loss.
- Obtain other tests, as indicated for suspicion of concomitant pathology, e.g., complete blood count (CBC), sedimentation rate, beta-hCG, gonorrhea culture, endometrial biopsy

Treatment/Management

- Initial treatment includes assessment and stabilization of the patient's hemodynamic status.
- For patients with heavy bleeding, refer to a physician immediately.
- Refer for medical treatment for causative factor, as indicated.
  - ▶ Retained placental fragments
  - ▶ Fibroids

▶ Endometritis (see Chapter 6.9, *Endometritis*)

▶ Gestational trophoblastic neoplasia (GTN) (see Chapter 6.12, *Gestational Trophoblastic Disease*)

- For patients without excessive bleeding, retained placental fragments, endometritis or GTN consider outpatient management with ergot preparation.

▶ Methylergonovine maleate 0.2 mg 1 tab p.o. every 6 hours for 6 doses (Druelinger, 1994; Craigo & Kapernick, 1994)

- Nonsteroidal anti-inflammatory drugs may decrease discomfort and decrease bleeding.

Consultation

- Consult and/or refer to rule out underlying pathology.

Patient Education

- Explain causes and therapeutic approaches for subinvolution.

- Discuss preventive measures, including enhancing normal uterine drainage by ambulation and upright positioning.

- Advise patient that ergot medications may produce uterine cramping.

- Alert patient to signs of further complications.

▶ Bleeding unresponsive to medication

▶ Increased bleeding, fever or chills

▶ See also Chapter 6.9, *Endometritis*

- Advise patient to maintain pelvic rest and nonstrenuous ambulation.

Follow-up

- Patient must contact provider if further complications occur or with failure to respond to therapy.

- In absence of other morbidity, reevaluate involution in 1 to 2 weeks.

- Document subinvolution in progress notes and problem list.

References

Andrew, A.C., Bulmer, J.N., Morrison, L., Wells, M., & Buckley, C.H. (1993). Subinvolution of the uteroplacental arteries: An immunohistochemical study. *International Journal of Gynecologic Pathology, 12*(1), 28–33.

Craigo, S.D., & Kapernick, P.S. (1994). Postpartum hemorrhage & the abnormal puerperium. In A.H. DeCherney & M.L. Pernoll (Eds.) Current obstetric & gynecologic diagnosis & treatment (8th ed.), (pp. 574–593). Norwalk, CT: Appleton & Lange.

Druelinger, L. (1994). Postpartum emergencies. *Emergency Medicine Clinics of North America, 12*(1), 219–237.

Khong, T.Y., & Khong, T.K. (1993). Delayed postpartum hemorrhage: A morphologic study of causes and their relation to other pregnancy disorders. *Obstetrics & Gynecology, 82*(1), 17–22.

Novy, M.J. (1994). The normal puerperium. In A.H. DeCherney & M.L. Pernoll (Eds.), *Current obstetric and gynecologic diagnosis and treatment* (8th ed.) (pp. 216–245). Norwalk, CT: Appleton & Lange.

CHAPTER 31

SUBSTANCE ABUSE

Susan L. Adams

Lucy Newmark Sammons

Substance abuse in pregnancy has the potential to cause serious health problems for women and their fetuses. Substances under consideration include

- Alcohol and tobacco (legal substances)

- Legally available, prescribed drugs, such as barbiturates (downers) or narcotic analgesics

- Legally available nonprescription substances (such as nicotine, caffeine, and over-the-counter drugs)

- Illegal drugs or chemicals, particularly

  > Cocaine and its derivatives (crack, rock, hubba, freebase or base, coke, snow)

  > Heroin (smack, H, horse, china white)

  > PCP (angel dust)

  > Amphetamines (uppers)/methamphetamines (crank, speed, ice, meth, crystal)

  > Marijuana (pot, weed, grass, joint)

The United States Department of Health and Human Services (US-DHHS) estimated that a significant number of women of childbearing age were active substance users. The 1995 National Household Survey Estimates on Drug Abuse estimated that 82.3 percent of the American population over the age of 12 years had used alcohol at some time in their lives and 32.4 percent (72.4 million) of the American population over the age of 12 years had used illicit substances at some time in their lives (US-DHHS, 1995).

Based on the 1995 estimates, approximately 73 percent of women between the ages of 18 and 34 used alcohol within the previous year, more than 35 percent of women between age 18 and 34 used tobacco within the previous year, and 22.7 percent of women ages between 18 and 25 and 10.6 percent of women between ages 26 and 34 reported that they used illicit drugs within the previous year. Overall, 9.3 percent of white women, 5.9 percent of Hispanic women, and 7.7 percent of black women used illicit substances in the previous year. This data was based on a U.S. population of 82.7 million white women, 13 million black women, 9.9 million Hispanic women, and 4.4 million "other" women. Substance abuse may vary with geographic location. For example, women who lived in the western region were more likely to use illicit substances than in other regions, although all regions were affected. Overall, there was an approximately 2 percent decrease in use compared to 1994 statistics (US-DHHS, 1994; US-DHHS, 1995).

Legal substances such as alcohol and tobacco are socially accepted and more frequently used than illicit substances such as crack cocaine. However, the abuse of legal, as well as illegal, substances is associated with adverse health consequences.

Alcohol abuse during pregnancy is associated with fetal alcohol syndrome (FAS) and fetal alcohol effects syndrome (FAE). One ounce of hard liquor, or the equivalent, each day may be enough to cause fetal damage. Tobacco has been associated with an increased risk for miscarriage and fetal demise, low birth-weight babies, and a fivefold risk for sudden infant death syndrome (SIDS). Unfortunately, many women who use illicit substances are also using alcohol and tobacco, thus possibly compounding the effects on their fetuses.

While incidence figures for maternal perinatal substance abuse vary depending on geographic location, rigor of assessment protocols, the reliability and validity of toxicologic screening, and legal reporting practices, estimates for perinatal substance use are in the range of 10 to 17 percent (Chasnoff, Landress, & Barrett, 1990; Frank, Zuckerman, & Amaro, 1988; Jessup & Roth, 1988; US-DHHS, 1994;Vega, Kolody, Hwang, & Noble, 1993). Chasnoff, et al. (1990) demonstrated the inequities in reporting practices. They found equivalent rates of perinatal substance exposure in both public and private clinical settings, yet public clinic clients were more likely to be reported for their substance use than private practice clients and African-American women were ten times more likely to be reported than white women. Chasnoff's group postulated that variations in reporting were possibly explained by several factors. These included the type of obstetrical care that women received (public vs. private), physical manifestations of drug use in women and their newborns, physician knowledge base, physicians who consider some substances more harmful than others (cocaine vs. marijuana), fear of adverse patient reactions to reporting, fear of the loss of future referrals, and finally, the preconception that substance abuse, especially during pregnancy, is a problem that affects minority groups, urban populations, and lower socioeconomic groups.

Prenatal drug and alcohol abuse have multiple deleterious effects on the mother, and on her baby before and after birth (see Table 6.18). Major potential maternal sequelae are cardiac, liver, and gastrointestinal (GI) damage, hypertension (HTN), preterm labor and birth (PTL and PTB), spontaneous abortion (SAB), placental abruption, cerebrovascular accident (CVA), and cardiac arrest. In addition, polydrug use and the addictive lifestyle subject the woman to increased risk of acquiring sexually transmitted diseases (STDs), gynecologic disorders, hepatitis, nutritional disorders, and infection with the human immunodeficiency virus (HIV) (Chasnoff, 1991; Dombrowski & Sokol, 1990; Lindsay, Peterson, & Boring, et al., 1992; Puentes, 1990; Robins & Mills, 1993).

Major potential fetal/neonatal adverse outcomes include FAE, FAS, addiction and acute withdrawal, stillbirth, intrauterine growth restriction (IUGR), low birth weight (LBW) and other consequences of prematurity, congenital anomalies, seizure disorders, meconium aspiration, multiple behavioral and feeding problems, developmental and learning disabilities, and increased rate for SIDS (Robins & Mills, 1993). Long-term effects for many substances, with the exception of alcohol, are unknown. There is evidence that the social environment of exposed children may be a stronger predictor of long-term sequelae than the actual fetal exposure (Black, Schuler, & Nair, 1993).

Database

Subjective

- Client may admit to current and/or past substance abuse; alternately, a substance abuser may deny chemical dependency or addictive behaviors.

▶ The way the interview is conducted will determine the thoroughness of the history. It is not sufficient to simply ask, "Are you using drugs, alcohol or tobacco?" Many deny use. It is quite possible that during that particular moment or day they were not using.

▶ Further questioning is required if there is an initial negative response such as, "Have you *ever* in your life used alcohol? (Allow the opportunity for response after naming each substance.) Tobacco? Marijuana? Cocaine?" etc.

▶ If there is a yes response inquire about the age of first use, the amount used per day, week, or month, periods of abstinence, route of administration (oral, nasal, inhaled, injectable). Quantify as best as possible with type and amount (e.g., "number of drinks" can be conceptualized as shot glass size servings or quarts of hard liquor). Maternal and fetal outcomes are more worrisome for women who drink a quart of vodka per day when compared with women who drink two ounces of wine per day.

● Medical history may include

▶ Unexplained obstetrical/neonatal complications possibly associated with substance abuse (e.g., PTL, abruptio placentae, fetal death, congenital anomalies, FAS, IUGR, LBW infant, SIDS)

▶ Use of mood-altering prescriptive drugs

▶ Undocumented "seizure disorder," blackouts

▶ Symptoms of withdrawal may include fatigue, headache, flu-like symptoms, nausea, pelvic cramps that are similar to early pregnancy symptoms (Ronkin, Fitzsimmons, Wapner, & Finnegan, 1988)

▶ Victim of physical or sexual abuse (e.g., adult survivor of child physical and/or sexual abuse, past domestic violence or other assaults, rape)

▶ Menstrual irregularities, history of infertility

▶ Recent multiple STDs

● Current obstetric care behavior may present as

▶ Late unexplained registration for prenatal care or admission to labor and delivery—without any prenatal care

▶ Noncompliance with keeping prenatal appointments or obtaining ordered laboratory tests, especially if coupled with frequent labor and delivery or emergency room drop-in visits

● Personal/family/partner psychosocial history may indicate

▶ Family or partner substance abuse

▶ Family-of-origin risk factors

 – Alcoholism

 – Substance abuse

 – Psychiatric illness

 – Incest

 – Others

▶ Psychiatric care history

    – Inpatient or outpatient treatment

    – Suicide attempt

▶ Incarceration or arrest; drunk driving violations

▶ Social instability or chaotic lifestyle

    – Multiple, changing addresses and contact telephone numbers

    – Homelessness

    – Physical and/or abusive conflict in interpersonal relationships

▶ Previous child(ren) cared for by foster parent or someone other than woman herself, or previous involvement with Child Protective Services (CPS)

▶ Vagueness or evasiveness in revealing history

Objective

● Client may demonstrate signs of current intoxication or drug use:

▶ Substance odor on breath or clothing (e.g., alcohol, tobacco, marijuana, crack)

▶ Chronic cough, may be productive and include black sputum

▶ Eye signs, as evaluated by general observation (Tennant, 1988)

    – Pupil size measurement

    – Pupil light reactivity

    – Testing for nystagmus

    – Testing for convergence

NOTE: These will vary from normal to abnormal depending on substance of abuse.

▶ Unable to maintain eye contact

▶ "Nodding" in and out of sleep during the interview

▶ Behavior inappropriate, bizarre, or agitated

▶ Behavior combative, disruptive, abusive, threatening violence

▶ Demonstrated mood swings, emotional lability

▶ Speech slurred

▶ Unkempt appearance and poor hygiene

● Medical indicators suggestive of current or history of substance abuse—physical examination or laboratory studies indicating (Chasnoff, 1987; Jessup & Roth, 1988)

▶ General appearance of physical exhaustion, poor orientation

▶ Cirrhosis, hepatitis

▶ Pancreatitis

▶ Hypertension

▶ Gastrointestinal tract (GI) inflammation

▶ Hematological disorders

▶ Indicators of inadequate nutritional stores or current deficiency (e.g., malnutrition)

▶ Cardiac arrhythmias, endocarditis, or other related cardiac disease

▶ Cellulitis

▶ Phlebitis

▶ STDs, including HIV infection

▶ Septicemia

▶ Pneumonia

▶ Positive tuberculosis screen

▶ Withdrawal symptoms

▶ Signs of drug use on skin

   – Observable track marks (can be along any vein including areas of the breasts, feet, and hands, but usually noted in the antecubital area)

   – "Popping" marks (circular skin scars)

   – Abscesses

   – Edema, particularly in extremities

▶ Inflamed or indurated nasal mucosa

▶ Toxicology screen, if obtained, is positive

● Current problematic pregnancy indicators may include

▶ Signs of preterm labor

▶ Abruptio placentae

▶ Inactive or hyperactive fetus

▶ Inadequate weight gain

▶ Vaginal bleeding or spotting

▶ Ultrasonic evidence of IUGR, oligohydramnios, or placental or congenital abnormalities

Assessment

● Substance abuse of specific drug/chemical or polydrug combination prior to or during current pregnancy

▶ R/O IUGR

▶ R/O drug withdrawal

▶ R/O congenital abnormalities

▶ R/O anemia

▶ R/O STDs (including HIV infection)

▶ R/O vaginitis

▶ R/O other infections (e.g., cellulitis, bronchitis, pneumonia, endocarditis)

▶ R/O liver disease (including hepatitis B and C)

▶ R/O malnutrition

▶ R/O tuberculosis

▶ R/O other general medical and obstetric complications associated with substance abuse

Plan

Diagnostic Tests

● Toxicology screen for identification/quantification of drugs of abuse after informed consent by the woman.

NOTE: Laboratories will vary as to which screening tests are available. Follow local specifications regarding sampling from urine, blood, or gastric sampling, and the volume of specimen required.

▶ Always advise women that their urine is being tested for drugs or alcohol and the reason for testing (for example, "You have had a problem with drug abuse in the past and I would like to randomly test your urine to document the progress of your recovery efforts" or "Our policy at this institution is to test all women for drug and alcohol use at random times throughout the pregnancy." She should provide her verbal consent. Information about what will happen if the test is positive should be provided. This policy of informed testing is better suited to gaining trust and building a therapeutic alliance with the woman than covert testing to "catch her in the act," which could force her to "go underground" and not receive prenatal care (Poland, Dombrowski, Ager & Sokol, 1993).

▶ Archie (1992) and the U.S. Department of Health and Human Services (1993) list the approximate duration that drugs can be detected in urine. See Table 6.19.

● Other test modalities may include radioimmunoassays (RIA) of maternal hair and neonatal meconium for cocaine and illicit drug use.

● Where heavy alcohol intake is known or suspected obtain liver function tests.

● Obtain a complete blood count (CBC) with indices.

● Record urine dipstick ketone bodies.

● Order obstetrical ultrasound at approximately 18 to 20 weeks of pregnancy for dating and to determine fetal status.

● STD evaluation (gonorrhea, syphilis, chlamydia, human papilloma virus, herpes, trichomonas).

● Conduct HIV antibody screening (after patient consents).

- Conduct tuberculosis screening (See Chapter 10.10).
- Conduct hepatitis B and hepatitis C screening.

Treatment/Management

- Assess *all* pregnant women for alcohol and substance abuse.
- Where risk factors are present, obtain screening test for drugs of abuse at intake or as soon as risk is apparent.
  - ▶ Obtain woman's consent; document if woman refuses to consent.
  - ▶ Repeat toxicology screens each trimester or as indicated by previous results and interval history.
- Medically supervised detoxification may be required for some substances, such as alcohol, benzodiazepines, and opiates, and will depend on the amount of consumption, the duration of use, and the use of other substances (Jessup & Green, 1987; Schuckit, 1995).

  NOTE: Rapid elimination of large doses of alcohol, benzodiazepines, or opiates could lead to GI symptoms, hallucinations, and seizures (Jessup & Green, 1987; Schuckit, 1995).
- Opiate-addicted women may be treated with methadone maintenance regimens, which will vary depending on the intensity of withdrawal symptoms. Methadone-maintained women should not be abruptly terminated from their maintenance dose while pregnant because this is associated with a higher risk of fetal demise. If detox is attempted, it should ideally occur slowly during the second trimester and under strict medical management. Dosages may need to be increased for some women as their pregnancies advance and if withdrawal symptoms develop because of altered renal clearance. However, split dosing methadone can be tried before increasing to a higher dose.
- Encourage HIV antibody screening at intake with repeat testing, as indicated. Explain risk factors and prevention methods.
- Screen for STDs at subsequent visits pending interval history of high risk exposures.
- Order additional obstetrical ultrasound, as indicated.
- Teach kick counts after 28 weeks. (The baby should move four times within an hour or ten times within 2 hours after eating to indicate fetal well-being).
- Order other fetal surveillance modalities such as nonstress tests (NSTs), biophysical profiles (BPPs) and/or serial ultrasounds, as indications arise (see Chapter 3.5, *Antepartum Fetal Surveillance*).
- Refer to appropriate treatment program(s) (see Follow-up section).
- Provide prenatal vitamins with additional supplemental calcium (as indicated by dairy intake) and additional supplemental iron (as indicated by CBC).
- Attempt to establish a trusting relationship with the woman through
  - ▶ Continuity of care by a consistent provider
  - ▶ An honest, caring, and nonjudgmental approach
  - ▶ Provision of information based on facts as they are known

> ▶ Acknowledgment of any progress in the recovery process

> ▶ Assurance of confidentiality as allowed by law

- Provide contraceptive counseling and services consistent with woman's preferences and lifestyle. Emphasize the importance of safer sex practices.

- See also Patient Education section.

Consultation

- Medical consultation and management by a multidisciplinary team is ideally required for confirmed cases of perinatal substance abuse.

- Refer to social services, as indicated.

- Obtain a nutritional consult, if indicated by serious nutritional deficits or eating disorders.

Patient Education

- Educate all women about the effects of alcohol and substance abuse on themselves and their babies, during and after pregnancy, in a factual and nonjudgmental manner.

- Educate the client regarding beneficial effects for herself and her baby of immediate cessation of substance abuse.

- Educate women with identified substance abuse about the specific maternal and infant complications for which they are at risk. Early warning signs should be periodically reviewed.

- Inform woman of possible urine screening for drugs during the antepartum and delivery periods and the potential involvement of CPS if drug or alcohol abuse is detected at birth (if notification procedures are employed at site).

  NOTE: Legal requirements and interpretations vary by institution and by state.

- Provide and reinforce preterm labor detection and preterm birth prevention information (see Chapter 6.25, *Preterm Labor*).

- Inform the woman of the potential effects of drug and alcohol transmission through breast milk if nursing is being considered; breastfeeding is contraindicated for most substances if the mother continues to abuse them (Chasnoff, 1987; Novy, 1987).

Follow-up

- One of the most important components in the plan is the continued surveillance for substance use during pregnancy. This should be done in a caring and nonjudgmental way that builds trust, encourages recovery, and provides information leading to healthy outcomes for the woman, her baby, and the family.

- Refer to available outpatient and inpatient treatment programs, with particular reference to antenatal/postpartum services; self-help groups such as alcoholics/cocaine/narcotics anonymous for the woman and her family members.

- Refer to social services for evaluation.

- Refer for nutritional consultation, as indicated.

- Refer to pediatric care provider prenatally, with identification of high-risk status.

- Refer to public health nursing services prenatally and postnatally, as needed.

- Refer women to prenatal education programs and parenting classes. Women who are active substance abusers during pregnancy should be referred to infant CPR courses in view of increased SIDS risk (especially for tobacco and cocaine users).

- Follow woman at 2 to 3 week intervals, or more often if needed, to 36 weeks, then weekly.

- Placement of infant with mother or with CPS will depend upon

  ▶ Nature and extent of substance abuse

  ▶ Other covariants (e.g., homelessness, previous history of involvement with CPS, and lack of stable supports in the environment)

  ▶ Compliance with treatment programs, local, legal and hospital policies

  ▶ Availability of alternate supportive services

- Document the dates and nature of known substance exposures on problem list and whether or not the woman agrees to random urine toxicology screening.

- Document the education, counseling, and referrals in the progress notes.

Table 6.18

Maternal, Fetal, and Neonatal Associated Risks with Substance Exposure

Substance[1,2,3]	Maternal Associated Risks	Fetal/Neonatal Associated Risks
Alcohol	GI damage, liver damage (cirrhosis), CNS depression, heart disease, diabetes, breast cancer, anovulation, amenorrhea, infertility, SAB, stillbirths, preterm labor (PTL), withdrawal (DT seizures)	Intrauterine growth retardation (IUGR), low birth weight (LBW), prematurity, FAE, FAS, CNS depression, neurobehavioral sequelae, malignant neoplasms (acute myeloid leukemia before age 2), withdrawal (jitters, tremors, difficult to soothe)
Tobacco	Heart and lung disease (esp. lung CA, emphysema, bronchitis, asthma), CNS stimulation, impaired fertility, PTL, abnormal placenta, abruptio placentae, ruptured membranes, withdrawal	IUGR, LBW, prematurity, SAB/stillborn, congenital malformations (heart, cleft, palate, hernia, CNS abnormalities), 5x higher risk SID's, asthma, bronchitis, pneumonia, and slightly lower intelligence
Marijuana	CNS depression, respiratory depression, impaired fertility	Possible IUGR and LBW, possible similar risks as with tobacco
Amphetamines	CNS and cardiovascular stimulation, anorexia and malnutrition, insomnia	IUGR, LBW, prematurity, abnormal sleep, withdrawal (jitters, tremors, difficult to soothe)
Cocaine	CNS and cardiovascular stimulation, HTN, stroke, MI, anorexia, malnutrition, insomnia, abruptio placentae, SAB, stillborn, premature rupture of membranes, and PTL	IUGR, LBW, prematurity, stroke, birth defects (GU, GI, heart, extremities), abnormal sleep/breathing, increased risk for SID's, withdrawal (jitters, tremors, difficult to soothe)
Opiates (heroin, morphine, codeine, Percodan, etc.)	CNS depression, anemia, hepatitis, infections (e.g., endocarditis, cellulitis), amenorrhea, infertility, HTN, SAB, PTL, withdrawal (flu-like symptoms)	Stillborn, IUGR, LBW, prematurity, strabismus, disturbed sleep, poor feeding, neurobehavioral sequelae, withdrawal
PCP	Hallucination, memory & speech problems, potential for self-inflicted harm, paranoia, psychotic episodes, seizures	Microcephaly, neurobehavioral sequelae, withdrawal
Prescription Drugs A) Tranquilizers (benzodiazepines) B) Barbiturates	Withdrawal	A) Cleft lip/palate (4x increased risk), third trimester exposure related to neonatal apnea, hypotonia, and hypothermia A) & B) CNS depression, poor muscle tone, poor suck, delayed gross motor development, withdrawal

[1] Substance abuse in general is associated with an increased risk of sexually transmitted infections, including HIV. The risk for HIV increases with injection use and sharing needles.

[2] Substances can be passed through the breast milk thus continuing infant exposure.

[3] Multiple substance exposure compounds and complicates the associated maternal, fetal, and neonatal risks.

Sources: Chasnoff, I.J. (1991). *Drugs, alcohol, pregnancy, and parenting.* Boston: Kluwer Academic Publishers; Jessup, M. (1992). *Drug dependency in pregnancy: Managing withdrawal.* North Highlands, CA: State of California, Department of General Services Publication Section; Puentes, A.J. (1990). *Maternal/Fetal/Neonatal Effects of Substances Commonly Abused by Pregnant Women.* San Jose, CA: Santa Clara County Substance Abuse Services; Roth, P. (1991). *Alcohol and drugs are women's issues. Vol. I. A review of the issues.* NJ: Women's Action Alliance & The Scarecrow Press ; TERIS. (1995). *The Teratogen Information System - Database, Vol. 88.* Washington, D.C.: University of Washington, Micromedex. United States Department of Health and Human Services (US-DHHS). (1994). *Alcohol, tobacco, and other drugs may harm the unborn.* Rockville, MD: Office for Substance Abuse Prevention.

Table 6.19

Duration of Drug Detection in Urine

Substance	Time
Alcohol	12 hours
Amphetamines	24–72 hours
Barbiturates	10–30 days
Cannabinoids (Marijuana)	3–30 days
Cocaine	24–72 hours
Heroin (detected as Morphine)	24 hours
Methadone (dose dependent)	3 days
Opiates (in general)	2–4 days
Methaqualone (Quaaludes)	4–24 days
Phencyclidine (PCP)	3–10 days
Benzadiazapine (Diazepam)	4 days–several weeks

NOTE: Urinary retention times vary by drug, patient's physical condition and hydration, and route and frequency of drug use (Dombrowski & Sokol, 1990; Ronkin et al., 1988).

Sources: Archie, C.L. (1992). Obstetric management of the addicted pregnant woman. In M. Jessup (Ed.), *Drug dependency in pregnancy: Managing withdrawal* (pp. 37–58). North Highlands, CA: State of California, Department of General Services Publications Section.; US-DHHS (1993); *United States Department of Health and Human Services (US-DHHS). (1993)* Pregnant, Substance-using women: Treatment improvement protocol (TIP) Series 2. Pub # (SMA) 93–1993, p. 30–52. Rockville, MD: Substance Abuse and Maternal Health Services Administration, Center for Substance Abuse Treatment (CSAT).; Ruggerio, R. (personal communication, May 1996).

References

Archie, C.L. (1992). Obstetric management of the addicted pregnant woman. In M. Jessup (Ed.), *Drug dependency in pregnancy: Managing withdrawal* (pp. 37–58). North Highlands, CA: State of California, Department of General Services Publications Section.

Black, M., Schuler, M., & Nair, P. (1993). Prenatal drug exposure: Neurodevelopmental outcome and parenting environment. *Journal of Pediatric Psychology, 18*(5), 605–620.

Chasnoff, I.J. (1987). Perinatal effects of cocaine. *Contemporary Ob/Gyn, 29*(5), 163–179.

Chasnoff, I.J. (1991). *Drugs, alcohol, pregnancy, and parenting.* Boston: Kluwer Academic Publishers.

Chasnoff, I.J., Landress, H.D., & Barrett, M.E. (1990). The prevalence of illicit drug or alcohol use during pregnancy and discrepancies in mandatory reporting in Pinellas County, Florida. *The New England Journal of Medicine, 322*(17), 1202–1206.

Dombrowski, M.P., & Sokol, R.J. (1990). Cocaine and abruption. *Contemporary Ob/Gyn, 35*(4), 13–19.

Frank, D.A., Zuckerman, B.S., Amaro, H., Aboagye, K., Bauchner, H., & Cabral, H. (1988). Cocaine use during pregnancy: Prevalence and correlates. *Pediatrics, 82*(6), 888–895.

Jessup, M. (1992). *Drug dependency in pregnancy: Managing withdrawal.* North Highlands, CA: State of California, Department of General Services Publication Section.

Jessup, M., & Green, J. (1987). Treatment of the pregnant alcohol-dependent woman. *Journal of Psychoactive Drugs, 19*(2), 193–203.

Jessup, M., & Roth, R. (1988). Clinical and legal perspectives on prenatal drug and alcohol use: Guidelines for individual and community response. *Medicine and Law, 7,* 377–389.

Lindsay, M.K., Peterson, H.B., Boring, J., Gramling, J., Willis, S., & Klein, L. (1992). Crack cocaine: A risk factor for human immunodeficiency virus infection Type I among inner-city populations. *Obstetrics & Gynecology, 80*(6), 981–984.

Novy, M.J. (1987). The normal puerperium. In M.L. Pernoll & R.C. Benson (Eds.), *Current obstetric and gynecologic diagnosis and treatment 1987* (pp. 216–245). Norwalk, CT: Appleton & Lange.

Poland, M.L., Dombrowski, M.P., Ager, J.W., & Sokol, R.J. (1993). Punishing pregnant drug users: Enhancing the flight from care. *Drug & Alcohol Dependence, 31,* 199–203.

Puentes, A.J. (1990). *Maternal/Fetal/Neonatal Effects of Substances Commonly Abused by Pregnant Women.* San Jose, CA: Santa Clara County Substance Abuse Services.

Robins, L.N. & Mills, J.L. (1993). Effects of in utero exposure to street drugs. *American Journal of Public Health, 83*(Supplement), 1–32.

Ronkin, S., Fitzsimmons, J., Wapner, R., & Finnegan, L. (1988). Protecting mother and fetus from narcotic abuse. *Contemporary Ob/Gyn, 31*(3), 178–187.

Roth, P. (1991). *Alcohol and drugs are women's issues. Vol. I. A review of the issues.* NJ: Women's Action Alliance & The Scarecrow Press.

Schuckit, M.A. (1995). *Drug and alcohol abuse. A clinical guide to diagnosis and treatment.* New York: Plenum Medical Book Company.

Tennant, F. (1988). The rapid eye test to detect drug abuse. *Postgraduate Medicine, 84*(1), 108–114.

TERIS. (1995). *The Teratogen Information System Database, Vol. 88.* Washington, DC: University of Washington, Micromedex.

United States Department of Health and Human Services (US-DHHS). (1993) Pregnant, Substance-using women: Treatment improvement protocol (TIP) Series 2. Pub # (SMA) 93–1993, p. 30–52. Rockville, MD: Substance Abuse and Maternal Health Services Administration, Center for Substance Abuse Treatment (CSAT).

United States Department of Public Health and Human Services (US-DHHS). (1994, July). *National Household Survey on Drug Abuse: Population Estimates.* Advance report number 7. Rockville, MD: U.S. Department of Health and Human Services.

United States Department of Health and Human Services (US-DHHS). (1994). *Alcohol, tobacco, and other drugs may harm the unborn.* Rockville, MD: Office for Substance Abuse Prevention.

United States Department of Health and Human Services (US-DHHS). (1995). *National Household Survey on Drug Abuse: Population Estimates.* Rockville, MD: Author.

Vega, W.A., Kolody, B., Hwang, J., & Noble, A. (1993). Prevalence and magnitude of perinatal substance exposures in California. *The New England Journal of Medicine, 329*(12), 850–854.

Chapter 32

TRIAL OF LABOR: VAGINAL BIRTH AFTER CESAREAN SECTION (VBAC)

Lisa L. Lommel

Until recently, women who had had a previous cesarean section were advised to have a repeat cesarean. This practice was encouraged for fear of uterine rupture during subsequent labor. This belief prevented health care providers from offering a trial of labor and vaginal birth after cesarean section (VBAC). It is currently believed that risk of VBAC had been overestimated and the trend toward trial of labor is now increasing.

In the United States, the rate of cesarean section was 22.8 percent in 1993 compared with 24.7 percent in 1988. Fortunately, the rate of cesarean sections appears to be slowly decreasing compared to the dramatic increases during the 1970s and early 1980s (Clarke & Taffel, 1995). The primary cesarean rate remained stable from 1988 to 1993 at 16.3 cesareans per 100 women with no history of a previous cesarean (Clarke & Taffel, 1995). Another promising trend is that 25.4 percent of women who had a previous cesarean gave birth vaginally in 1993 compared to 12.6 percent in 1988 (Clarke & Taffel, 1995). In the United States, the overall success rate for women attempting vaginal birth after cesarean section is 74 percent (Clemenson, 1993).

To accomplish the Department of Health and Human Service's national goal for the year 2000 of an overall cesarean rate of 15 percent, the VBAC rates must continue to increase and the primary cesarean rate must be reduced by 50 percent (Clarke & Taffel, 1995; Public Health Service, 1991).

In 1991, the American College of Obstetrician and Gynecologist (ACOG) Committee on Obstetrics, Maternal and Fetal Medicine, formulated guidelines for vaginal delivery after a previous cesarean birth. The report recommends that women with one previous cesarean delivery and a low-transverse scar should be counseled to attempt VBAC. In addition, women with two or more previous cesareans (with low-transverse scar) may also attempt VBAC. The two only absolute contraindications to VBAC include a known or strongly suspected classic uterine incision and patient refusal of the procedure following full discussion and disclosure. ACOG also recommends individual assessment, which is necessary in cases with missing risk data: previous low vertical uterine incision, unknown type of uterine incision, multiple gestation, breech presentation, or estimated fetal weight over 4,000 grams (ACOG, 1988, reaffirmed 1991).

The advantages of VBAC over repeat cesarean include shorter hospital stay, more rapid maternal recovery, lower medical costs, opportunity to experience natural childbirth, a decreased risk associated with surgery, and lower risk of infection. The disadvantages of a trial of labor for VBAC include the possibility that a cesarean section may still be required, preventing advanced scheduling, and the increased risk of uterine rupture. Published estimates of complete uterine rupture range from 0.18 to 0.6 percent with no serious maternal or neonatal complications (Clemenson, 1993). In properly selected patients, careful management of vaginal birth after cesarean entails less maternal and fetal risk than the risks associated with an elective repeat cesarean delivery.

Database

Subjective

- History of previous cesarean section(s) with low-transverse uterine incision
- Pregnant women desires VBAC

Objective

- Review obstetrical data to rule out inaccurate dating.
- Assess fetal size, position, and presentation.
- Document pelvic size and adequacy.
- Document previous low-transverse scar from medical records (obtain operative report, if possible).
- No absolute contraindications for VBAC with low-transverse incision.

  NOTE: Patients with previous low vertical incision, unknown type of incision, multiple gestation, breech presentation or estimated fetal weight greater than 4,000 grams require physician referral to confirm eligibility.

Assessment

- Previous low-transverse cesarean section desires VBAC
  - ▶ Uterine size equal to dates and/or sonogram
  - ▶ No absolute contraindications for vaginal delivery

Plan

Diagnostic Tests

- Obtain ultrasound as early as possible in the pregnancy to confirm dates.
- Perform electronic fetal and uterine monitoring during labor.

Treatment/Management

- Discuss option for trial of labor in patients who meet criteria for VBAC.
- Initiate fetal movement counts at 28 weeks. See fetal movement count protocol in Chapter 3.5, *Antepartum Fetal Surveillance.*
- Continue routine prenatal care.
- Perform electronic fetal and uterine monitoring in labor.
- See that emergency cesarean delivery is available within 30 minutes from the time the decision is made until the surgical procedure is begun (ACOG, 1988, reaffirmed 1991).

Consultation

- Physician consultation may be required to confirm eligibility for trial of labor with no absolute contraindications.

- Refer to a physician in cases in which risk data is lacking: whether previous incision is a low-vertical uterine incision, unknown type of uterine incision, multiple gestation, breech presentation, or estimated fetal weight greater than 4,000 grams (ACOG, 1988, reaffirmed 1991).

Patient Education

- Explain the risks and benefits of VBAC to the client and her partner.

- Encourage the client and her partner to attend VBAC classes, if available, and become informed about VBAC.

- Explain what may be expected during labor, including electronic fetal monitoring

- Discuss situations that may necessitate a repeat cesarean delivery.

- Discuss pain medication options and alternative pain-relieving measures, especially with patients who have a fear of labor pain.

Follow-up

- Schedule a routine 6-week postpartum visit.

- Document that the patient is to undergo a trial of labor for VBAC with no absolute contraindications and document outcome in progress notes and problem list.

References

American College of Obstetricians and Gynecologists (ACOG) (1988, reaffirmed 1991). *Guidelines for vaginal delivery after a previous cesarean birth* (Committee Opinion No. 64). Washington, DC: Author.

Clarke, S.C., & Taffel, S. (1995). Changes in cesarean delivery in the United States, 1988 and 1993. *Birth, 22*(2), 63–67.

Clemenson, N. (1993). Promoting vaginal birth after cesarean section. *American Family Physician, 47*(1), 139–144.

Public Health Service (1991). *Healthy People 2000: National Health Promotion and Disease Prevention Objective.* DHHS Publication No. (PHS) 91–50212. Washington, DC: US Department of Health and Human Services.

Chapter 33

VENOUS THROMBOEMBOLIC DISEASE

Ellen M. Scarr

Venous thromboembolic disease, characterized by blood clot formation in a vein, complicates 0.2 to 2.0 percent of pregnancies and remains a leading cause of maternal mortality (Bates & Ginsberg, 1997; Biswas & Perloff, 1994). Normal hematologic changes, which serve to protect against postpartum hemorrhage, subsequently place the pregnant woman at twice the normal risk for venous thrombosis. Blood hypercoagulability, caused by an increase in factors VII, VIII, IX, X, XII, and fibrinogen, is compounded by a decrease in naturally occurring anticoagulants (e.g., protein S and tissue plasminogen activator) and inhibition of the fibrionolytic system (Toglia & Weg, 1996). Platelet activation is thought to increase during pregnancy (Toglia & Nolan, 1997). Additional factors that contribute to the risk of venous thrombosis formation are listed in the Subjective section.

Thromboembolism occurs with equal frequency in the antepartum and postpartum periods (ACOG, 1997). Venous thrombosis most often develops in the superficial or deep veins of the legs, or deep veins of the pelvis. A thrombus may begin in a small calf vein, then extend proximally to the iliac or femoral veins. Thrombus formation in hypertrophied uterine veins can extend to iliac and pelvic veins. Thrombophlebitis refers to the symptomatic form of venous thrombosis. Superficial thrombophlebitis occurring in the saphenous veins of the legs is the most common thrombophlebitis in the antepartum and postpartum period and is unlikely to embolize to the lungs, although it may signal an underlying hypercoagulability (O'Shaughnessy, 1990). Deep vein thrombosis (DVT) occurs in the deep veins of the legs or pelvis, and may be the result of a superficial thrombophlebitis. Recent data suggests most DVTs (75 percent) occur antenatally, half of those by 15 weeks gestation (Toglia & Nolan, 1997).

Septic thrombophlebitis usually occurs in the early postpartum period and refers to a pelvic thrombus that has sustained bacterial invasion and frequently showers bacteria-laden emboli. Originating most commonly from ovarian veins (40 percent), uterine or iliac veins, the incidence of septic thrombophlebitis is 1/2,000 deliveries (Biswas & Perloff, 1994). Pulmonary embolism, the leading cause of maternal mortality, has an incidence of 1/2,000 and usually results from a thromboembolus in deep pelvic or leg veins, although it can be caused by an amniotic fluid embolism or air embolism (Goldhaber, 1995). Two-thirds of pulmonary emboli occur postpartum, commonly after Cesarean section (Toglia & Nolan, 1997). Pulmonary embolism is frequently the sequelae of asymptomatic thromboembolic disease; 50 percent of women who die after pulmonary embolus have no symptoms of thromboembolism. Cerebral venous thrombosis, which usually involves the largest of the cerebral venous sinuses (the superior sagittal sinus), occurs infrequently in the postpartum period (1/2,500 to 1/10,000 deliveries) (Cartlidge, 1995; Terhaar & Kaut, 1993).

Database

Subjective

- Predisposing factors

    ▶ Obstetric factors (ACOG, 1997; Brown & Hiett, 1996; Schmidt & Hall, 1995; Toglio & Nolan, 1997)

- Hormone-induced relaxation of smooth muscle (which increases venous capacitance, and thereby, stasis)

- An overall increase in circulating blood volume

- Compression of the inferior vena cava and iliac veins by the gravid uterus (which promotes venous pooling)

- Multiparity

- Local damage to pelvic veins during placental separation (vaginal or operative delivery)

- Instrument-assisted delivery

- Operative delivery (increases risk 9 fold)

- Infection/sepsis

▶ Genetic factors (ACOG, 1997; Bates & Ginsberg, 1997; de Boer, Buller, ten Cate & Levi, 1992; Rosendaal, 1996; Toglia & Nolan, 1997)

- Mutation of factor V gene (which leads to activated protein C resistance [ACPR], increasing risk of thrombus 7 to 8 fold)

- Underlying congenital deficiencies of normal coagulation inhibitors (antithrombin III, protein C and protein S)

- Increased levels of factor VIII

- A family history of thromboembolism

▶ Personal history/Risk behaviors (Goldhaber, 1995; Letsky, 1992; O'Shaughnessy, 1990)

- Personal history of thromboembolism (women with a history of DVT have a 10 to 20 percent chance of recurrence during pregnancy)

- Obesity

- Maternal age greater than 35

- Anemia

- Hypertension

- Trauma

- Cigarette smoking

- Prolonged bed rest

● Symptomatology

▶ Superficial thrombophlebitis

- The patient may complain of pain, tenderness, swelling, heat, and/or redness of the affected area.

▶ Deep vein thrombosis

- Most patients asymptomatic

    – May complain of pain, tenderness, swelling, heat, redness of affected area (swelling associated with DVT is usually unilateral, with rapid onset)

    – May complain of pain above hip

    – May have a fever

▶ Septic thrombophlebitis

    – Occurs postpartum

    – Fever, often with "picket fence" curve, with range from 98.6° F to 105.8° F (37.0° C to 41.0° C) and no response to antibiotics (Biswas & Perloff, 1994)

    – May complain of lower abdominal pain

▶ Pulmonary Embolus

    – Chest pain, pleuritic pain, shortness of breath, dyspnea on exertion, cough

    – May note occasional hemoptysis

    – May complain of abdominal pain (from diaphragmatic irritation)

    – May complain of feeling apprehensive

▶ Cerebral venous thrombosis

    – Headache

    – May have fever

    – Others may notice decreased level of consciousness or unusual seizure activity

NOTE: The common presence of physiologic leg edema, leg cramps, and dyspnea make clinical diagnosis of thromboembolic phenomena difficult.

Objective

● Superficial thrombophlebitis

    ▶ Vital signs within normal limits (WNL)

    ▶ Leg edema, erythema, discoloration of affected area

    ▶ Palpable, cord-like superficial vein; may be tender

    ▶ May note venous distention of subcutaneous vessels

● Deep vein thrombosis

    ▶ Vital signs WNL

    ▶ Leg edema, erythema, discoloration, and tenderness of affected area

    ▶ May have palpable cord

    ▶ May have positive Homan's sign (pain with dorsiflexion of the foot) but usually considered to have little diagnostic value

- Septic thrombophlebitis
  - ▶ Elevated temperature, without localizing signs
  - ▶ Increased pulse and respiratory rate
  - ▶ Diffuse lower abdominal tenderness or pain on palpation
  - ▶ Pelvic examination WNL or tender, firm, thrombosed vessels in vaginal fornices may be palpable
- Pulmonary embolism
  - ▶ Vital signs—tachycardia, tachypnea, hypotension
  - ▶ Hypoxemia—decreased oxygen saturation with oximetry
  - ▶ Cardiac examination reveals S_3, prominent P_2, left parasternal heave, friction rub, increased jugular venous distension (JVD), cyanosis
  - ▶ Lung examination may reveal splinting, crackles, or rales
  - ▶ Examination of extremities may reveal evidence of DVT
  - ▶ Patient appears anxious
- Cerebral venous thrombosis
  - ▶ May have signs of increased intercranial pressure (elevated BP, decreased pulse, pupillary changes)
  - ▶ Decreased level of consciousness; may be comatose
  - ▶ May have mild fever

Assessment

- Venous thromboembolic disease
  - ▶ Superficial thrombophlebitis
  - ▶ Deep vein thrombosis
  - ▶ Septic thrombophlebitis
  - ▶ Pulmonary embolism
  - ▶ Cerebral venous thrombosis
  - ▶ R/O varicosities
  - ▶ R/O musculoskeletal injury
  - ▶ R/O physiologic leg edema
  - ▶ R/O postpartum endometritis

▶ R/O pyelonephritis

▶ R/O adnexal mass, torsion

▶ R/O pneumonia, pleural effusion, asthma exacerbation

▶ R/O myocardial infarction

▶ R/O pericarditis/endocarditis

▶ R/O malaria, gram negative sepsis

Plan

Diagnostic Tests

● Superficial or deep vein thrombosis

    ▶ Noninvasive testing is preferred, although it is less reliable in the second half of pregnancy.

        – High resolution compression ultrasound (useful with symptomatic proximal DVT—not calf)

        – Doppler ultrasound (study of choice [ACOG, 1997])

            * Scans large leg veins for blood flow patterns

            * Most sensitive/specific for proximal DVT (less so for calf)

            * Less accurate late in pregnancy due to decreased venous flow

        – Impedance plethysmography (IPG)

            * Detects volume changes in leg veins

            * Sensitive for proximal DVT, not isolated calf DVT

            * Less accurate late in pregnancy due to decreased venous flow

            * May pick up isolated iliac vein thrombus not found on ultrasound

        – Venogram

            * Invasive, expensive

            * Most accurate for diagnosing DVT, but used cautiously in pregnancy because of fetal exposure to minimal radiation (ACOG, 1997)

            * Small risk of post-venogram DVT

            * Use if other tests are equivocal (ACOG, 1997)

        – I-fibrinogen scan

            * Contraindicated in pregnancy, exposes fetus to radiation

            * Sensitive for calf vein thrombus, use in postpartum only

- Septic thrombophlebitis
  - ▶ Blood cultures
  - ▶ Ultrasound to rule out pelvic abscess
  - ▶ Computed tomography (CT) scan (may identify large pelvic vein thrombosis)
- Pulmonary embolism
  - ▶ Chest x-ray usually normal or nonspecific (effusion, atelectasis)
  - ▶ Ventilation/Perfusion (V/Q) Scan (initial test, minimal fetal exposure to radiation)
  - ▶ Pulmonary arteriogram ("gold standard," used if V/Q scan nondiagnostic; some fetal exposure to radiation)
  - ▶ Arterial blood gas (ABG) (may show pO_2 less than 70, with normal or decreased CO_2, but normal ABG does not rule out pulmonary embolism)
  - ▶ Electrocardiogram (ECG) (reveals tachycardia, may show right heart strain [right axis deviation] and/or nonspecific T-wave inversions)
- Cerebral venous thrombosis
  - ▶ Magnetic resonance imaging scan (MRI)

Treatment/Management

- Superficial thrombophlebitis
  - ▶ Bed rest, local moist heat, elevate affected leg
  - ▶ Support stockings (see Chapter 5.15, *Varicosities*)

    NOTE: Details of treatment/management of DVT, septic thrombophlebitis, pulmonary embolism, and cerebral venous thrombosis are beyond the scope of this chapter. See Consultation section.

Consultation

- ▶ Consult with a physician for women with history of thromboembolic disease, who may require prophylactic anticoagulation during pregnancy.
- ▶ Consultation for suspected DVT, septic thrombophlebitis, pulmonary embolism or cerebral venous thrombosis is mandatory.
- ▶ Refer to a physician for confirmed DVT, septic thrombophlebitis, pulmonary embolism, or cerebral venous thrombosis for anticoagulation; surgical intervention may be indicated.

Patient Education

▶ Educate the client about pathophysiology of thromboembolism with clear explanation of warning signals indicating worsening of condition.

▶ Advise avoidance of use of nonsteroidal antiinflammatory drugs (NSAIDs) during pregnancy.

▶ Encourage compliance with management plan.

Follow-up

▶ Assess superficial thrombophlebitis at each subsequent visit.

▶ Assess for signs/symptoms of DVT at subsequent visits.

▶ Notify Labor & Delivery staff of antepartum thrombophlebitis.

▶ Document venous thromboembolic conditions in progress notes and problem list.

References

American College of Obstetricians and Gynecologists. (1997). *Thromboembolism in pregnancy* (Technical Bulletin No. 234). Washington, DC: Author.

Bates, S., & Ginsberg, J. (1997). Thrombosis in pregnancy. *Current Opinion in Hematology, 4*(5), 335–343.

Biswas, M., & Perloff, D. (1994). Cardiac, Hematologic, pulmonary, renal and urinary tract disorders in pregnancy. In A. DeCherney, & M. Pernoll (Eds.), *Current obstetric and gynecologic diagnosis and treatment* (8th ed., pp. 428–467). Norwalk, CT: Appleton & Lange.

Brown, H., & Hiett, A. (1996). Deep vein thrombosis and pulmonary embolism. *Clinical Obstetrics and Gynecology, 39*(1), 87–100.

Cartlidge, N. (1995). Neurologic disorders. In W. Barron & M. Lindheimer (Eds.), *Medical disorders during pregnancy* (2nd ed., pp. 430–450). St. Louis, MO: Mosby.

de Boer, K., Buller, H., ten Cate, J., & Levi, M. (1992). Deep vein thrombosis in obstetric patients: Diagnosis and risk factors. *Thrombosis and Haemostasis, 67*(1), 4–7.

Goldhaber, S. (1995). Thromboembolic disease in pregnancy. In K. Carlson & S. Eisenstat (Eds.), *Primary care of women* (pp. 375–379). St. Louis, MO: Mosby.

Letsky, E. (1992). Thromboembolism. In A. Calder & W. Dunlop (Eds.), *High risk pregnancy*, (pp. 94–138). Oxford, England: Butterworth-Heineman.

O'Shaughnessy, R. (1990). Venous thromboembolic disease in pregnancy. In E. Quilligan & F. Zuspan (Eds.), *Current therapy in obstetrics and gynecology* (3rd ed., pp. 293–295). Philadelphia, PA: W.B. Saunders.

Rosendaal, F. (1996). Thrombosis in the young: Epidemiology and risk factors. *Thrombosis and Haemostasis, 78*(1), 1–6.

Schmidt, G., & Hall, J. (1995). Pulmonary disease. In W. Barron & M. Lindheimer (Eds.), *Medical disorders during pregnancy* (2nd ed., pp. 168–195). St. Louis. MO: Mosby.

Terhaar, M., & Kaut, K. (1993). Perinatal superior sagittal sinus venous thrombosis. *Journal of Perinatal and Neonatal Nursing, 7*(1), 35–48.

Toglia, M., & Nolan, T. (1997). Venous thromboembolism during pregnancy: A current review of diagnosis and management. *Obstetrical and Gynecologic Survey, 52*(1), 60–72.

Toglia, M., & Weg, J. (1996). Venous thromboembolism during pregnancy. *The New England Journal of Medicine, 335*(2), 108–114.

SECTION 7
DERMATOLOGICAL CONDITIONS

Chapter 1

HERPES GESTATIONIS

Maureen T. Shannon

Herpes gestationis is a rare autoimmune condition of pregnancy and of trophoblastic disease (Black, 1994; Shornick & Black, 1992). Despite its name, there is no causal relationship between this condition and the herpes virus. The clinical manifestations of this disorder are immunologically induced and mediated by an IgG antibasement membrane antibody (a C3 complement component).

Herpes gestationis is characterized by intense pruritis (itching) that is followed several days to weeks later by the eruption of extremely pruritic blisterlike lesions in the second or third trimester (Hayashi, 1990). The lesions usually begin as erythematous, urticarial papules or plaques that develop vesicles or bullae peripherally/circumferentially (Black, 1994; Hayashi, 1990; Rapini & Jordan, 1994; Shornick & Black, 1992).

Initially, the pruritis and lesions are distributed over the client's abdomen and trunk, but can progress to involve the entire cutaneous surface of her body sparing the face and mucosa (Shornick & Black, 1992). The lesions may coalesce to form circular patterns. Eventually the vesicles and bullae crust and heal without scarring. The lesions will persist until delivery with regression occurring within a few weeks postpartum.

Opinions vary regarding the possible increased perinatal mortality associated with this disease. Reports of increased maternal and perinatal mortality may have been secondary to sepsis or infection. However, there have been reports of placental insufficiency associated with an increased incidence of prematurity and small-for-gestational-age infants (Black, 1994; Shornick & Black, 1992). In most instances, herpes gestationis resolves without adverse effects to the mother or infant (Rapini & Jordon, 1994). Herpes gestationis lesions can develop in approximately 5 percent of infants born to women with this condition, but the lesions usually regress spontaneously without complications (Rapini & Jordon, 1994).

Postpartum recurrence of the skin eruptions has been reported in 50 to 70 percent of affected women. The exacerbations usually begin within 48 hours after delivery and can persist for several weeks. Breast-feeding women have a reportedly shorter duration of symptoms compared to non–breast-feeding women (Hayashi, 1990; Rapini & Jordon, 1994). The condition has also been noted to recur in subsequent pregnancies, during oral contraceptive use, and during menstrual cycles.

Database

Subjective

- May report a history of herpes gestationis in a previous pregnancy
- Complains of severe itching of trunk and abdomen in the second or third trimester (can occur during the first trimester if a recurrent episode)
- May report development of erythematous papules, plaques, or blisters

Objective

- Observation of erythematous urticarialike papules, vesicles, or bullae on abdomen and/or trunk, initially, and on other cutaneous surfaces after the initial eruption

- May have signs of secondary infection of lesions (rare)

Assessment

- Herpes gestationis

  ▶ R/O erythema multiform

  ▶ R/O papular dermatitis of pregnancy

  ▶ R/O pemphigus vulgaris

  ▶ R/O impetigo herpetiformis

  ▶ R/O herpes zoster

  ▶ R/O disseminated herpes simplex

  ▶ R/O bullous drug eruption

Plan

Diagnostic Tests

The following laboratory evaluations may be obtained after consultation with a physician.

- Histologic examination of skin biopsy

  ▶ May reveal eosinophilic spongiosis and subepidermal separation

  ▶ Basal keratinocytes may demonstrate focal necrosis (Black, 1994; Rapini & Jordon, 1994)

- Serum IgG1 level (may be increased)

- Direct immunofluorescence (IF) of serum during acute disease reveals linear band of C3 complement basal membrane deposition (Black, 1994)

- Indirect complement-added immunofluorescence may demonstrate "IgG that fixes to the basement membrane zone [BMZ]" (Shornick & Black, 1992, p. 63)

Treatment/Management

- Consult with a physician in all cases of suspected herpes gestationis.

  ▶ Transfer of care is indicated for women diagnosed with severe forms of this condition.

  ▶ Co-manage women with a physician in less severe forms of this condition.

- In mild to moderate cases, symptomatic treatment may include cool compresses or oatmeal baths to help reduce pruritis

- Systemic antihistamines may be prescribed to help relieve pruritic symptoms. Agents may include

  ► Diphenhydramine 25–50 mg p.o. every 6 hours p.r.n.

  ► Hydroxyzine HCL 10–50 mg p.o. every 6 hours p.r.n.

  NOTE: Antihistamines should be avoided during the first trimester because limited and conflicting data suggest that teratogenic effects may result from first-trimester use. In addition, the use of antihistamines during the last 2 weeks of pregnancy has been associated with retrolentel fibroplasia in premature infants (Briggs, Freeman, & Yaffe, 1994). Advise the woman about the antihistamine-associated symptom of drowsiness and the need to avoid activities requiring alertness and concentration (i.e., driving motor vehicles).

- A topical steroid preparation may be prescribed to help reduce inflammation (Goldstein & Goldstein, 1992).

  ► Hydrocortisone 1 percent cream/lotion applied to the affected areas b.i.d. or t.i.d. (a low potency topical preparation)

  ► Triamcinolone acetonide 0.1 percent cream applied to affected areas b.i.d. or t.i.d. (a moderately potent topical preparation)

- In severe cases, pharmacologic management by the physician may include systemic cortico-steroid therapy after the risks versus the benefits of such therapy have been considered and discussed with the woman.

  ► Use of systemic corticosteroids reduces symptoms and helps decrease the formation of new vesicles.

  ► The usual regimen is prednisone 40 mg p.o. daily in divided doses during active disease.

    – Taper the dose to a lower level for maintenance once suppression of vesicle formation has occurred.

    – Taper prednisone by reducing the dose by 5 mg every 2 to 3 days until the lowest dose necessary to maintain control and prevent pruritic symptoms is attained (Rapini & Jordon, 1994).

  NOTE: Women requiring chronic systemic steroids during pregnancy need parenteral steroid administration during labor. In addition, infants born to women on corticosteroid therapy should be evaluated for adrenal insufficiency (Rapini & Jordon, 1994).

Consultation

- Consult with an obstetrician/perinatalogist for all women suspected of having herpes gestationis.

- Consultation with a dermatologist may be necessary, depending upon the severity of the condition and indicated treatment(s).

Patient Education

- Educate the woman about the cause of this dermatologic condition, how it progresses during the pregnancy, the likelihood of complete regression without complications or scarring a few weeks after delivery, and the possibility of recurrence in subsequent pregnancies, during menstrual cycles, or if oral contraceptives are used.

- Discuss the very remote possibility that the infant may have similar lesions after birth that usually regress without scarring or complications.

- Discuss proper skin hygiene and the signs and symptoms of secondary infection of lesions.

- When systemic corticosteroid therapy is indicated, have this treatment option presented by the consulting physician.

Follow-up

- Follow-up evaluations of women with herpes gestationis is per physician recommendation and depends upon the severity of the condition and the pharmacologic agent(s) prescribed.

- Document diagnosis of herpes gestationis and management thereof in problem list and progress notes.

References

Black, M.M. (1994). New observations on pemphigoid 'Herpes' gestationis. *Dermatology, 189*(Suppl), 50–51.

Black, M.M., & Stephens, C.J.M. (1991). The specific dermatoses of pregnancy: The British perspective. *Advances in Dermatology, 7*, 105–127.

Borradori, L., & Saurat, J.H. (1994). Specific dermatoses of pregnancy. Toward a comprehensive view. *Archives of Dermatology, 130*, 778–780.

Briggs, G.G., Freeman, R.K., & Yaffe, S.J. (1994). *Drugs in pregnancy and lactation* (4th ed.). Baltimore, MD: Williams & Wilkins.

Errickson, C.V., & Matus, N.R. (1994). Skin disorders of pregnancy. *American Family Physician, 49*(3), 605–610.

Goldstein, B.G., & Goldstein, A.O. (1992). *Practical dermatology*. St. Louis: Mosby Year Book.

Hayashi, R.H. (1990). Bullous dermatoses and prurigo of pregnancy. *Clinical Obstetrics and Gynecology, 33*(4), 746–753.

Rapini, R.P., & Jordon, R.E. (1994). The skin and pregnancy. In R.K. Creasy R. Resnik (Eds.), *Maternal-fetal medicine: Principles and practice* (3rd ed., pp. 1101–1111). Philadelphia: W.B. Saunders Company.

Reece, A., Hobbins, J.C., Mahoney, J.J., & Petrie, R.H. (1995). *Handbook of medicine of the fetus & mother* (pp. 433–435). Philadelphia, PA: J.B. Lippincott.

Shornick, J.K., & Black, M.M. (1992). Fetal risks in herpes gestationis. *Journal of the American Academy of Dermatology, 26*(1), 63–68.

Chapter 2

IMPETIGO HERPETIFORMIS

Maureen T. Shannon

Impetigo herpetiformis is a very rare dermatologic condition similar to, if not a form of, generalized pustular psoriasis (Holm & Goldsmith, 1991; Rapini & Jordon, 1994). The actual etiology of this condition is unknown; however, eruption has been associated with hypocalcemia during pregnancy and with hypoparathyroidism after surgical procedures (Moynihan & Ruppe, 1985; Stewart, Battaglini-Sabetta & Millstine, 1984; Holm & Goldsmith, 1991). It can occur at any time during pregnancy, but most frequently begins during the third trimester (Holm & Goldsmith, 1991; Rapini & Jordon, 1994).

Impetigo herpetiformis is characterized by the abrupt eruption of painful erythematous plaques and patches that are rapidly covered with sterile, crusting pustules (Holm & Goldsmith, 1991; Rapini & Jordon, 1994). The distribution of the eruptions can involve any part of the body; however, 90 percent of women usually develop initial lesions in the periumbilical area with progression to the lower abdomen, inner thighs, inguinal areas, axilla, and between the breasts (Black & Stephens, 1991). Painful lesions of the oral mucosa can also develop. Systemic manifestations usually accompany each eruption and include fever, diarrhea, malaise, vomiting, arthralgias, lethargy, leukocytosis, hypocalcemia, and splenomegaly (Holm & Goldsmith, 1991). In rare instances, women may experience delirium, tetany, and convulsions in association with hypocalcemia (Rapini & Jordon, 1994). This condition usually spontaneously regresses after delivery, but can recur in subsequent pregnancies, usually at an earlier point in gestation. Current treatment regimens have demonstrated good prognosis for the mother. However, an increased incidence of stillbirths has been reported in association with this condition (Rapini & Jordon, 1994).

Database

Subjective

- May report one or more of the following:
    - ▶ History of a similar condition occurring during a previous pregnancy
    - ▶ Personal or family history of psoriasis
    - ▶ History of a painful red rash with pustules (may be anywhere on the body)
    - ▶ Lethargy
    - ▶ Tender joints at onset of eruption
    - ▶ Painful oral lesions
    - ▶ Fever
    - ▶ Vomiting
    - ▶ Malaise
    - ▶ Diarrhea

Objective

- Observation of erythematous papules or plaques with superficial pustules on the axilla, lower abdomen, groin, inner thighs, or in mouth (however, lesions may be observed anywhere on the body)

- Temperature (will be elevated during acute eruption)

- Joints may be tender to palpation during acute eruption

- Splenomegaly on palpation of abdomen

Assessment

- Impetigo Herpetiformis
  - ▶ R/O herpes gestationis
  - ▶ R/O pemphigus vulgaris

Plan

Diagnostic Tests

- The following tests may be ordered, as indicated, after consultation with a physician:
  - ▶ White blood cell count (WBC) (will be elevated with an increased neutrophil count)
  - ▶ Erythrocyte sedimentation rate (ESR) (will increase during acute eruptions)
  - ▶ Serum calcium (will be decreased)
  - ▶ Serum chemistry panel (may reveal an electrolyte imbalance if associated with severe dehydration)
  - ▶ Culture of pustules (no growth of bacteria or viruses unless there is secondary infection of the lesions)

- Histologic examination
  - ▶ Biopsies obtained early during lesion formation usually demonstrate "epidermal and upper dermal edema with perivascular lymphohistiocytic infiltrate" (Black & Stephens, 1991, p. 107).
  - ▶ Biopsies of the lesions during later phases of the condition reveal the presence of spongiform pustules (Errickson & Matus, 1994).

Treatment/Management

- Consultation with a physician is mandatory because women diagnosed with this condition may require hospitalization for fluid and electrolyte replacement, administration of systemic corticosteroids, and close maternal/fetal surveillance.

- Transfer care to a physician if hospitalization is required.

- Symptomatic treatment may include
  - ▶ Application of wet compresses to the lesions
  - ▶ Topical fluorinated steroid applications
    - – Fluocinonide 0.05 percent cream applied to lesions b.i.d.
    - – Halcinonide 0.1 percent cream applied to lesions b.i.d.
- Systemic corticosteroid administration is the treatment of choice.
  - ▶ Prednisone 20 to 40 mg daily to suppress new lesion formation.
  - ▶ Once this has been achieved, the prednisone dose should be tapered down to a maintenance dose of 10 mg p.o. daily (Black & Stephens, 1991).

    NOTE: Women requiring chronic systemic corticosteroid therapy during pregnancy will need parenteral corticosteroids during labor. In addition, infants born to women on corticosteroid therapy should be evaluated for adrenal insufficiency (Rapini & Jordon, 1994).
- Medication for pain relief may be necessary and should be prescribed in consultation with a physician.
- Initiate fetal movement counts at 28 weeks' gestation.
- Initiate antenatal fetal surveillance (e.g., nonstress tests, amniotic fluid index, contraction stress tests) between 32 to 34 weeks' gestation.

Consultation

- Consult with an obstetrician/perinatalogist for all women with suspected impetigo herpetiformis.
- Consult with a dermatologist, depending upon the severity of the condition and response to treatment.

Patient Education

- Discuss the probable course of impetigo herpetiformis, its treatment, and its possible recurrence in future pregnancies.
- Discuss proper skin hygiene and the signs and symptoms of secondary infection of the lesions.

Follow-up

- Follow-up evaluations of patients diagnosed with this condition are per physician recommendation.
- Document diagnosis of impetigo herpetiformis and management thereof in problem list and progress notes.

References

Abrams, R.S. (1989). *Handbook of medical problems during pregnancy* (pp. 91–111). Norwalk, CT: Appleton & Lange.

Black, M.M., & Stephens, C.J.M. (1991). The specific dermatoses of pregnancy: The British perspective. *Advances in Dermatology, 7,* 105–127.

Errickson, C.V., & Matus, N.R. (1994). Skin disorders of pregnancy. *American Family Physician, 49*(3), 605–610.

Holm, A.L., & Goldsmith, L.A. (1991). Impetigo herpetiformis associated with hypocalcemia of congenital rickets. *Archives of Dermatology, 127,* 91–95.

Moynihan, G.D., & Ruppe, J.P. (1985). Impetigo herpetiformis and hypoparathyroidism. *Archives of Dermatology, 121,* 1330–1331.

Rapini, R.P., & Jordon, R.E. (1994). The skin and pregnancy. In R.K. Creasy R. Resnik (Eds.), *Maternal-fetal medicine: Principles and practice* (3rd ed., pp. 1101–1111). Philadelphia, PA: W. B. Saunders Company.

Stewart, A.F., Battaglini-Sabetta, J., & Millstine, L. (1984). Hypocalcemia-induced pustular psoriasis of von Zumbusch. *Annals of Internal Medicine, 100,* 677–680.

Chapter 3

INTRAHEPATIC CHOLESTASIS OF PREGNANCY

Maureen T. Shannon

Intrahepatic cholestasis of pregnancy (ICP), also known as pruritis gravidarum, is a pregnancy-associated liver disease with a reported incidence of 0.02 to 2.0 percent, although in Chile and Scandinavia the reported incidence is as high as 10 percent (Errickson & Matus, 1994; Rapini & Jordon, 1994; Reyes & Simon, 1993). The etiology and pathophysiology of this condition is not known. The most probable explanation is the presence of an inherited abnormality in sex steroid metabolism (i.e., estrogen) or hepatic response to increased estrogen levels, or a combination of both of these factors in affected individuals (Reyes, 1992; Reyes & Simon, 1993; Riely, 1994). The interaction of these factors results in intrahepatic cholestasis with the accumulation of bile salts in the serum and skin (Errickson & Matus, 1994; Khandelwal & Malet, 1994). Additional influences from environmental or metabolic factors may contribute to and modulate clinical symptoms.

Although symptoms may be reported during the first trimester, the majority of women with this condition experience the onset of symptoms during the third trimester. It is characterized by generalized pruritis without evidence of skin lesions, other than excoriations. Approximately 2 to 3 weeks after the pruritis begins, mild jaundice may be observed in a small percentage of patients. Regression of pruritis gravidarum occurs shortly after delivery but can recur in 50 percent of subsequent pregnancies (Rapini & Jordon, 1994). Exacerbation of symptoms, especially in women with a history of icterus, can occur with the use of oral contraceptives (Rapini & Jordan, 1994). There have been reports of increased incidence of cholelithiasis in women who have experienced ICP (Reyes, 1992). Although maternal outcome is generally good, there have been reports of an increased incidence of perinatal morbidity including amniotic fluid meconium, prematurity, fetal distress, and lower birth weights in infants born to women with this condition (Reyes, 1992; Rioseco et al., 1994).

Database

Subjective

- History of intrahepatic cholestasis in previous pregnancies
- Mild to severe itching, often increasing at night
- May report yellow skin, sclera
- May report nausea, vomiting, anorexia, and lassitude
- May report dark urine

Objective

- Direct observation of the skin reveals no lesions where pruritis is reported
- May observe excoriation of skin in areas where pruritis is reported
- May observe jaundice of skin, sclera

- ❯ Liver edge may be palpated and be slightly tender (Reyes, 1992)
- Fundal height may be less than expected for gestational week of pregnancy.

Assessment

- Intrahepatic cholestasis of pregnancy
  - ▶ R/O hepatitis
  - ▶ R/O biliary obstruction
  - ▶ R/O scabies
  - ▶ R/O allergic reaction

Plan

Diagnostic Tests

The following laboratory tests may be ordered after consultation with a physician:

- Serum choleglycine (bile acids).
  - ▶ This test should be done in a fasting state.
  - ▶ If elevated, it is diagnostic of ICP (Reece, Hobbins, Mahoney, & Petrie, 1995).
- Alkaline phosphatase
  - ▶ Values may be 2 to 4 times the normal nonpregnant values.
- Total bilirubin
  - ▶ Value may be increased but is usually less than 5 mg/dL.
- 5'-nucleotidase
  - ▶ Elevation above upper limits of normal is indicative of ICP (Reece et al., 1995).
- Hepatitis screen
  - ▶ Is within normal limits (WNL) unless coexistent hepatitis exposure/infection.
- Serum transaminases
  - ▶ Values may be elevated two to ten times above the upper limits of normal (Reyes, 1992).

Treatment/Management

- Symptomatic treatment to reduce pruritis
  - ▶ Lukewarm oatmeal baths p.r.n.
  - ▶ Avoidance of warmth (i.e., tight-fitting clothing, hot showers/baths)

- ▶ Antihistamines (in moderate to severe itching)

    - Diphenhydramine 25 to 50 mg p.o. every 6 hours p.r.n.

    - Hydroxyzine HCL 10 to 50 mg p.o. every 6 hours p.r.n.

    NOTE: Antihistamines should be avoided during the first trimester because the limited and conflicting data suggest that teratogenic effects may result from first-trimester use. In addition, the use of antihistamines during the last 2 weeks of pregnancy has been associated with retrolental fibroplasia in premature infants (Briggs, Freeman, & Yaffe, 1994). Advise the woman about the antihistamine-associated symptom of drowsiness and the need to avoid activities requiring alertness and concentration (i.e., driving motor vehicles).

- Systemic therapy to reduce the level of bile salts may be prescribed after consultation with a physician.

    - ▶ In the United States, the pharmacologic agent used is cholestyramine.

    NOTE: A reduction in pruritis will not be noted until approximately 2 weeks of therapy with this medication.

    - ▶ If there is little or no response to the minimum daily dose, the frequency of administration may be increased.

        - The usual dose is cholestyramine 9 gm packet mixed in 4 to 6 ounces of liquid p.o. daily (up to t.i.d.)

    NOTE: Commonly reported side effects include anorexia, nausea, constipation, bloating, and an unpleasant taste in the mouth. Other medications must be taken 1 hour before or 4 hours after the administration of cholestyramine. In some women, cholestyramine may increase the malabsorption of fat-soluble vitamins and result in hypoprothrom-binemia due to inadequate vitamin K levels (Reyes, 1992). Fetal intracranial hemorrhage, presumably due to the use of cholestyramine during pregnancy to treat intrahepatic cholestasis, has been reported (Sadler, Lane, & North, 1995).

- Laboratory tests to evaluate the possibility of hypoprothrombinemia prior to and every 2 to 4 weeks after the initiation of cholestyramine

    - ▶ The tests usually ordered for this purpose include a platelet count and prothrombin and partial prothrombin levels.

- Antenatal fetal surveillance

    - ▶ Daily fetal movement counts beginning at 28 weeks' gestation

    - ▶ Weekly nonstress test with amniotic fluid index should be initiated at 32 weeks gestation

    NOTE: Early delivery of infants by 38 weeks, or by 36 weeks in women with jaundice, has reportedly reduced adverse perinatal outcomes (Rioseco et al., 1994; Reyes, 1992). This decision is the responsibility of the consulting physician.

Consultation

- Consult with a physician in all suspected cases of intrahepatic cholestasis.
- Co-manage with the consulting physician if there is no evidence of biliary obstruction.

Patient Education

- Include in the education session the etiology of this condition, diagnostic tests that have been ordered and their results, probable course of this condition, anticipated remission after delivery, and possibility of recurrence in subsequent pregnancies or with use of oral contraceptives.

- The signs and symptoms of preterm labor should be presented. See Chapter 6.25, *Preterm Labor*.

- Discuss nonpharmacologic therapy to reduce the itching (e.g., oatmeal baths and the avoidance of tight-fitting clothing).

- Discuss medication options (including the risks versus benefits of the medications and possible side effects).

  ▶ Inform those women who are initiating cholestyramine therapy that 2 weeks of administration is necessary before a reduction in pruritis will be noted.

  ▶ Also, inform the women about the need for laboratory evaluations to monitor for any change in their blood clotting ability.

- Educate the woman about the potential adverse effects of this condition on her fetus and the need for close fetal surveillance during the third trimester.

Follow-up

- Follow-up patient evaluation is per physician recommendation and is determined by whether or not cholestatic jaundice is evident.

- Document ICP and management in problem list and progress notes.

References

Abrams, R.S. (1989). *Handbook of medical problems during pregnancy* (pp. 91–111). Norwalk, CT: Appleton & Lange.

Briggs, G.G., Freeman, R.K., & Yaffe, S.J. (1994). *Drugs in pregnancy and lactation* (4th ed.). Baltimore, MD: Williams & Wilkins.

Errickson, C.V., & Matus, N.R. (1994). Skin disorders of pregnancy. *American Family Physician, 49*(3), 605–610.

Khandelwal, M., & Malet, P.F. (1994). Pruritis associated with cholestasis. A review of pathogenesis and management. *Digestive Diseases and Sciences, 39*(1), 1–8.

Rapini, R.P., & Jordon, R.E. (1994). The skin and pregnancy. In R.K. Creasy R. Resnik (Eds.), *Maternal-fetal medicine. Principles and practice* (3rd ed., pp. 1101–1111). Philadelphia: W. B. Saunders Company.

Reece, A., Hobbins, J.C., Mahoney, J.J., & Petrie, R.H. (1995). *Handbook of medicine of the fetus & mother* (pp. 433–435). Philadelphia: J.B. Lippincott.

Reyes, H. (1992). The spectrum of liver and gastrointestinal disease seen in cholestasis of pregnancy. *Gastroenterology Clinics of North America, 21*(4), 905–921.

Reyes, H., & Simon, F.R. (1993). Intrahepatic cholestasis of pregnancy: An estrogen-related disease. *Seminars in Liver Disease, 13*(3), 289–301.

Riely, C.A. (1994). Hepatic disease in pregnancy. *The American Journal of Medicine, 96*(Suppl. 1A), 18S–22S.

Rioseco, A.J., Ivankovic, M.B., Manzur, A., Hamed, F., Kato, S.R., Parer, J.T., & Germain, A.M. (1994). Intrahepatic cholestasis of pregnancy: A retrospective case-control study of perinatal outcome. *Obstetrics & Gynecology, 170*(3), 890–895.

Sadler, L.C., Lane, M., & North, R. (1995). Severe fetal intracranial haemorrhage during treatment with cholestyramine for intrahepatic cholestasis of pregnancy. *British Journal of Obstetrics and Gynaecology, 102*(Feb), 169–170.

Chapter 4

PAPULAR DERMATITIS OF PREGNANCY

Maureen T. Shannon

Papular dermatitis of pregnancy, a rare pruritic condition of unknown etiology, can occur anytime during pregnancy. The characteristic eruption of this condition consists of discrete, single erythematous papules with hemorrhagic crusts that are approximately 3 to 5 mm in diameter. The papules are usually distributed over the woman's trunk and extremities, appear excoriated (secondary to the pruritis), and heal within 10 days after eruption, leaving areas of postinflammatory hyperpigmentation. This condition is also characterized by elevated urinary chorionic gonadotropin levels, decreased plasma cortisol levels, and decreased urinary estriol levels during the last trimester (Spangler & Emerson, 1971). These findings have led to its categorization as a distinct clinical entity. However, some investigators believe that this condition is probably a more severe form of prurigo gestationis (prurigo of pregnancy) (Borradori & Saurat, 1994; Errickson & Matus, 1994). Papular dermatitis of pregnancy abates with delivery or during the early postpartum period; however, it may recur in subsequent pregnancies. Initial reports regarding whether an increased fetal loss is associated with this dermatologic condition are controversial.

Database

Subjective

- History of papular dermatitis of pregnancy occurring in a previous pregnancy
- Severe itching
- Eruption of papules on body
- Hyperpigmentation at sites where papules have healed

Objective

- Discrete, individual erythematous papules with excoriation throughout body
- Hyperpigmented areas where papules have healed

Assessment

- Papular dermatitis of pregnancy
  - ▶ R/O allergic reaction
  - ▶ R/O pruritic urticarial papules and plaques of pregnancy (PUPPP) syndrome
  - ▶ R/O scabies
  - ▶ R/O xerosis

Plan

Diagnostic Tests

- The following laboratory test results may confirm the diagnosis:

  ▶ Urinary chorionic gonadotropin level (increased during the third trimester)

  ▶ Plasma cortisol level (decreased during the third trimester)

  ▶ Urinary estriol level (decreased during the third trimester)

  ▶ Histologic examination of skin lesion biopsies (nonspecific)

Treatment/Management

- Consult with a physician. Because initial reports about this condition indicated a possible increased fetal loss associated with it, co-manage the case with a physician.

- Pharmacologic therapy should be determined by the physician and usually includes high doses of systemic corticosteroids. Medications for the relief of pruritis may be prescribed:

  ▶ Diphenhydramine 25 to 50 mg p.o. every 6 hours p.r.n.

  ▶ Hydroxyzine HCL 10 to 50 mg p.o. every 6 hours p.r.n.

    NOTE: Antihistamines should be avoided during the first trimester because the limited and conflicting data suggest that teratogenic effects may result from first-trimester use. In addition, the use of antihistamines during the last 2 weeks of pregnancy has been associated with retrolental fibroplasia in premature infants (Briggs, Freeman, & Yaffe, 1994). Advise the woman about the antihistamine-associated symptom of drowsiness and the need to avoid activities requiring alertness and concentration (i.e., driving motor vehicles).

- Nonpharmacologic therapy can include the following:

  ▶ Oatmeal baths (Aveeno baths) to decrease the pruritis

  ▶ Wearing of loose-fitting clothing to reduce skin irritation

Consultation

- Consult with a physician in *all* suspected cases of papular dermatitis of pregnancy.

Patient Education

- Discuss the course of the condition, treatment options, and the possible recurrence in subsequent pregnancies.

- The clinician providing the woman's care should present the information regarding the questionable association of this condition with an increased incidence of fetal loss.

- Review proper skin hygiene techniques and the signs and symptoms of secondary infection of lesions.

Follow-up

- Follow-up evaluation of papular dermatitis of pregnancy is per physician recommendation.
- Document diagnosis of papular dermatitis and management thereof in problem list and progress notes.

References

Abrams, R.S. (1989). *Handbook of medical problems during pregnancy* (pp. 91–111). Norwalk, CT: Appleton & Lange.

Borradori, L., & Saurat, J.H. (1994). Specific dermatoses of pregnancy: Toward a comprehensive view? *Archives of Dermatology, 130*, 778–780.

Briggs, G.G., Freeman, R.K., & Yaffe, S.J. (1994). *Drugs in pregnancy and lactation* (4th ed.). Baltimore, MD: Williams & Wilkins.

Errickson, C.V., & Matus, N.R. (1994). Skin disorders of pregnancy. *American Family Physician, 49*(3), 605–610.

Spangler, A.S., & Emerson, K. (1971). Estrogen levels and estrogen therapy in papular dermatitis of pregnancy. *American Journal of Obstetrics & Gynecology, 110*, 534–537.

Chapter 5

PRURIGO GESTATIONIS

Maureen T. Shannon

Prurigo gestationis, a dermatologic condition of unknown etiology, occurs in up to 2 percent of pregnancies. In many women with this condition, a genetic predisposition to atopic dermatitis has been reported (Rapini & Jordon, 1994). The condition is characterized by the eruption of small, discrete, excoriated pruritic papules or nodules on the extensor surface of the patient's extremities, and occasionally on her abdomen, back, trunk, and shoulders (Errickson & Matus, 1994; Rapini & Jordon, 1994). The eruptions usually begin during the latter half of the second trimester through the beginning of the third trimester. This condition spontaneously regresses after delivery, although this process may take up to 3 months, and it may recur in subsequent pregnancies. There are no known associated maternal or fetal complications (Errickson & Matus, 1994; Rapini & Jordon, 1994).

Database

Subjective

- History of this condition in a previous pregnancy
- History of atopic dermatitis
- Itching
- Development of a papulelike rash or nodules on the extensor surfaces of the extremities and, possibly, the abdomen, back, trunk, and shoulders
- Reports that the symptoms began after the 20th week of pregnancy

Objective

- Observation of erythematous, excoriated papular lesions or nodules on the extensor surfaces of the extremities
    - ▶ May also observe the eruption on the abdomen, back, trunk, and shoulders

Assessment

- Prurigo gestationis
    - ▶ R/O papular dermatitis of pregnancy
    - ▶ R/O allergic reaction
    - ▶ R/O scabies
    - ▶ R/O pruritic urticarial papules and plaques of pregnancy (PUPPP) syndrome

Plan

Diagnostic Tests

- No specific diagnostic tests will confirm diagnosis.

  ▶ However, tests may be ordered to rule out other dermatologic conditions, as indicated.

Treatment/Management

- Symptomatic treatment for the relief of pruritis and discomfort may include

  ▶ Calamine lotion applied to affected areas

  ▶ Oatmeal baths to reduce discomfort

  ▶ Wearing loose-fitting clothing to decrease skin irritation

- Generally, topical corticosteroids of mild to moderate potency can be used when other symptomatic treatment fails. Such therapy may include (Rapini & Jordon, 1994)

  ▶ Hydrocortisone 1 percent cream/lotion applied b.i.d. to the affected areas (low-potency topical preparation)

  ▶ Triamcinolone acetonide 0.1 percent cream applied b.i.d. to affected areas (moderate potency topical preparation)

- Systemic corticosteroid therapy is rarely necessary and should be initiated only after consultation with a physician.

  ▶ The dose should be determined by the physician consultant.

  NOTE: Infants born to women who have used systemic corticosteroids during pregnancy should be monitored for adrenal insufficiency (Rapini & Jordon, 1994).

- Systemic antihistamines may help reduce pruritic symptoms that persist after topical steroid treatment has been attempted. Such therapy may include

  ▶ Diphenhydramine 25 to 50 mg p.o. every 6 hours p.r.n.

  ▶ Hydroxyzine HCL 10 to 50 mg p.o. every 6 hours p.r.n.

  NOTE: Antihistamines should be avoided during the first trimester because the limited and conflicting data suggest that teratogenic effects may result from first-trimester use. In addition, the use of antihistamines during the last 2 weeks of pregnancy has been associated with retrolental fibroplasia in premature infants (Briggs, Freeman, & Yaffe, 1994). Advise the woman about the antihistamine-associated symptom of drowsiness and the need to avoid activities requiring alertness and concentration (i.e., driving motor vehicles).

Consultation

- Consult with a physician, if necessary, to rule out other dermatologic conditions.

- Consultation with a physician is warranted in any woman being considered for systemic corticosteroid therapy.

Patient Education

- Include information regarding the expected course of this condition and its regression after delivery, the possibility of recurrence in subsequent pregnancies, and the fact that it is not associated with any adverse maternal or fetal complications.

- If pharmacologic treatment is being considered, educate the woman about options available to her, including the risks versus benefits of specific medications and side effects associated with the medication(s).

- Review proper skin hygiene to decrease the likelihood of secondary infection of lesions.

Follow-up

- Continue routine prenatal follow-up visits.

- Document diagnosis of prurigo gestationis and management thereof in problem list and progress notes.

References

Abrams, R.S. (1989). *Handbook of medical problems during pregnancy* (pp. 91–111). Norwalk, CT: Appleton & Lange.

Briggs, G.G., Freeman, R.K., & Yaffe, S.J. (1994). *Drugs in pregnancy and lactation* (4th ed.). Baltimore, MD: Williams & Wilkins.

Errickson, C.V., & Matus, N.R. (1994). Skin disorders of pregnancy. *American Family Physician, 49*(3), 605–610.

Rapini, R.P., & Jordon, R.E. (1994). The skin and pregnancy. In R.K. Creasy R. Resnik (Eds.), *Maternal-fetal medicine. Principles and practice* (3rd ed., pp. 1101–1111). Philadelphia, PA: W.B. Saunders Company.

Chapter 6

PRURITIC URTICARIAL PAPULES AND PLAQUES OF PREGNANCY

Maureen T. Shannon

Pruritic urticarial papules and plaques of pregnancy (PUPPP) syndrome is a dermatologic condition of unknown etiology that begins in the third trimester and slowly regresses during the first few weeks postpartum. Reports of an increased incidence in twin gestations have led to etiologic theories involving abdominal distention with a resulting lymphohistiocytic inflammatory reaction (Becket & Goldberg, 1991; Carli, Tarocchi, Mello, & Fabbri, 1994). Another theory postulates a maternal response to circulating paternal factors, with desensitization developing in subsequent pregnancies (Weiss, Derm, & Hull, 1992).

PUPPP syndrome, the most common dermatosis specific to pregnancy, is characterized by the development of discrete erythematous papules, plaques, and urticarial patches over the abdomen, thighs, and occasionally the buttocks, legs, and arms. These pruritic eruptions are rarely seen above the midthorax, and are never present on the face. PUPPP syndrome is observed primarily in primigravida and recurrence in subsequent pregnancies is rare. There are no adverse maternal, fetal, or neonatal outcomes associated with this condition.

Database

Subjective

- Itching of abdomen, thighs, buttocks, legs, and/or arms beginning in the third trimester.

- Development of hivelike or vesicular lesions over the abdomen, thighs, buttocks, arms, and/or legs

Objective

- Discrete erythematous papules, plaques, and hivelike patches on the abdomen, thighs, buttocks, arms, and/or legs

- A thin pale halo surrounding the papules (Goldstein & Goldstein, 1992)

- Absence of a similar eruption on the mucous membranes, face, neck, and upper trunk

Assessment

- PUPPP syndrome
  - ▶ R/O allergic reaction
  - ▶ R/O papular dermatitis of pregnancy
  - ▶ R/O herpes gestationis
  - ▶ R/O allergic reaction
  - ▶ R/O scabies
  - ▶ R/O intrahepatic cholestasis of pregnancy

Plan

Diagnostic Tests

- No specific laboratory evaluations can further confirm the diagnosis.

- Tests can be ordered to rule out other possible diagnoses.

Treatment/Management

- Consult with a physician to confirm the diagnosis and rule out other possible dermatologic conditions (e.g., herpes gestationis).

- Symptomatic treatment for the alleviation of pruritic symptoms may include

  ▶ Lukewarm oatmeal baths for 20 to 30 minutes b.i.d.

  ▶ Avoidance of warmth (i.e., tight-fitting clothing, warm or hot showers or baths) to decrease skin irritation.

- Application of a topical antipruritic agents (e.g., calamine lotion) may relieve itching if mild to moderate pruritis is being experienced by the woman.

- If symptomatic therapy is unsuccessful in reducing pruritis, topical corticosteroid therapy may be initiated:

  ▶ Hydrocortisone 1 percent cream/lotion applied to affected areas b.i.d. to t.i.d. (a low-potency topical preparation)

  ▶ Triamcinolone acetonide 0.1 percent cream applied to affected areas b.i.d. to t.i.d. (a moderate potency topical preparation)

- Systemic antihistamines can be prescribed to help reduce symptoms. The most commonly prescribed antihistamines include

  ▶ Diphenhydramine 25 to 50 mg p.o. every 6 hours p.r.n.

  ▶ Hydroxyzine HCL 10 to 50 mg p.o. every 6 hours p.r.n.

NOTE: Antihistamines should be avoided during the first trimester because the limited and conflicting data suggest that teratogenic effects may result from first-trimester use. In addition, the use of antihistamines during the last 2 weeks of pregnancy has been associated with retrolental fibroplasia in premature infants (Briggs, Freeman, & Yaffe, 1994). Advise the woman about the antihistamine-associated symptom of drowsiness and the need to avoid activities requiring alertness and concentration (i.e., driving motor vehicles).

- The treatment of PUPPP syndrome rarely requires the use of systemic corticosteroids, which should be prescribed only *after* consultation with a physician.

  ▶ The usual regimen prescribed is prednisone 40 mg p.o. daily for 2 days with tapering of the dose by 5 mg every 1 to 2 days. If several weeks of systemic corticosteroid therapy is needed, prescribing a dose every other day is an option (Rapini & Jordon, 1994).

  NOTE: Infants born to women who have received systemic steroids during pregnancy should be monitored for adrenal insufficiency (Rapini & Jordon, 1994).

Consultation

- Consultation with a physician may be indicated to confirm diagnosis, rule out other dermatologic conditions, and determine if topical and/or systemic corticosteroids or antihistamines are indicated.

Patient Education

- Educate the woman about the course of PUPPP syndrome, treatment options, and the fact that it probably will not recur in subsequent pregnancies.
- Reassure the woman that the condition will not adversely affect her or her fetus.
- Review proper skin hygiene to decrease the possibility of secondary infection of the lesions.

Follow-up

- Continue routine prenatal follow-up visits.
- Document diagnosis of PUPPP syndrome and management thereof in problem list and progress notes.

References

Abrams, R.S. (1989). *Handbook of medical problems during pregnancy* (pp. 91–111). Norwalk, CT: Appleton & Lange.

Beckett, M.A., & Goldberg, N.S. (1991). Pruritic urticarial plaques and papules of pregnancy and skin distention. *Archives of Dermatology, 127*, 125–130.

Black, M.M., & Stephens, C.J.M. (1991). The specific dermatoses of pregnancy: The British perspective. *Advances in Dermatology, 7*, 105–127.

Briggs, G.G., Freeman, R.K., & Yaffe, S.J. (1994). *Drugs in pregnancy and lactation* (4th ed.). Baltimore, MD: Williams & Wilkins.

Carli, P., Tarocchi, S., Mello, G., & Fabbri, P. (1994) Skin immune system activation in pruritic urticarial papules and plaques of pregnancy. *International Journal of Dermatology, 33*(12), 884–885.

Goldstein, B.G., & Goldstein, A.O. (1992). *Practical dermatology*. St. Louis, MO: Mosby Year Book.

Rapini, R.P., & Jordon, R.E. (1994). The skin and pregnancy. In R.K. Creasy R. Resnik (Eds.), *Maternal-fetal medicine. Principles and practice* (3rd ed., pp. 1101–1111). Philadelphia, PA: W.B. Saunders Company.

Weiss, R., Derm, S.A., & Hull, P. (1992). Familial occurrence of pruritic urticarial papules and plaques of pregnancy. *Journal of the American Academy of Dermatology, 26*(5), 715–717.

SECTION 8

GASTROINTESTINAL CONDITIONS

Chapter 1

ABDOMINAL PAIN—ACUTE

Lisa L. Lommel

Appendicitis

Appendicitis is the most frequently nonobstetric emergency during pregnancy. The incidence of appendicitis is not increased in pregnancy; however, the course of appendicitis is changed because of the delay in diagnosis, leading to a rate of perforation two to three times that of nonpregnant women (Smoleniec & James, 1993). The delay in diagnosis is usually due to the difficulty in differentiating the signs and symptoms of appendicitis from pregnancy related complaints (Witlin & Sibai, 1996).

Obstruction of the appendiceal lumen by a fecalith, inflammation, foreign body, or neoplasm is thought to initiate appendicitis. Although mucosal ulceration has been identified as an antecedent to obstruction in many cases, it is not known whether the cause of ulceration obstruction of the lumen is by infection or swelling. Once the obstruction occurs, there is inflammation and secretion of mucus, which, in turn, distends the appendix, causing pain, necrosis, and, if not removed, perforation.

Perforation is a serious complication because it can contaminate the peritoneal cavity, causing intra-abdominal sepsis. The maternal and fetal mortality rates are significant, 17 percent and 43 percent respectively, when perforation occurs (Smoleniec & James, 1993).

Database

Subjective

- Negative history of appendectomy

- Right lower to middle quadrant vague abdominal pain although atypical pain is common

- Anorexia, malaise, constipation, or, sometimes, diarrhea, nausea, and vomiting develop

- Patient can usually point to specific area of maximal tenderness

- Depending on location of appendix, other symptoms may occur:

  ▶ Appendix adjacent to the bladder—urinary frequency and dysuria

  ▶ Retrocecal or pelvic appendix—minimal or absent abdominal tenderness and positive tenderness in flank or on rectal examination

Objective

- Temperature normal or slightly elevated (37.2° to 38° C; 99° to 100° F). (25 percent are afebrile)

- Temperature above 38.3° C (101° F) may indicate perforation

- Tachycardia present with elevation of temperature

- Elevated WBC count, 10,000/μL and 20,000/μL with an increase in neutrophils

  NOTE: Physiologic leukocytosis with a variation in the range of neutrophilia is common during pregnancy, making it an unreliable prediction for appendicitis (Smoleniec & James, 1993)

- Microscopic hematuria and pyuria may be present

- Light palpation or percussion can identify a point of maximal tenderness in right lower quadrant of abdomen to right upper quadrant or flank, depending on stage of pregnancy

- Rebound tenderness and muscle rigidity in right lower quadrant to right upper quadrant of abdomen or flank depending on stage of pregnancy (although both are much less demonstrable as pregnancy progresses)

- Rectal and vaginal tenderness usually present, particularly in early pregnancy

- Diminished or absent bowel sounds

- Rigidity and tenderness of abdomen increased as disease progresses

- Signs of perforation

  ▶ Increasing pain, tenderness, and spasm followed by evidence of generalized peritonitis or a localized abscess

  ▶ Increasing temperature, malaise, tachycardia, and WBC

  ▶ Diagnosis of appendicitis using ultrasound made by demonstrating lack of peristalsis and lack of compressibility of the appendix (Witlin & Sibai, 1996). If the appendix cannot be seen, appendicitis cannot be excluded.

Assessment

- Acute appendicitis

  ▶ R/O gastroenteritis

  ▶ R/O ruptured graafian follicle or corpus luteum cyst

  ▶ R/O round ligament pain

  ▶ R/O pyelonephritis

  ▶ R/O abruptio placentae

  ▶ R/O chorioamnionitis

  ▶ R/O acute cholecystitis

  ▶ R/O endometritis

  ▶ R/O labor (term or preterm)

  ▶ R/O adenexal torsion

  ▶ R/O ectopic pregnancy

  ▶ R/O salpingitis

  ▶ R/O other renal disease

Plan

Diagnostic Tests

- Symptoms, clinical findings, and progression of disease over time are hallmark in diagnosing appendicitis, although the diagnosis can often be obscured by pregnancy-related complaints.

  ▶ Urinalysis is helpful in ruling out genitourinary symptoms that can mimic appendicitis.

  ▶ High-resolution, real-time ultrasound has an overall accuracy of 96 percent for the diagnosis of acute appendicitis.

- During close observation, abdominal and rectal exams, WBC count, and differential should be repeated periodically for signs of disease progression

Treatment Management

- In pregnancy, once appendicitis is suspected, a diagnostic laparotomy is recommended (Witlin & Sibai, 1996).

- During close observation, patient should be resting and given nothing by mouth. No laxatives or narcotics should be prescribed; these will interfere with assessment for disease progression.

- Refer the client to a surgeon immediately once a strong suspicion or diagnosis of appendicitis is made.

- Conduct antepartum fetal surveillance pre- and postsurgery (nonstress test), as indicated.

Consultation

- Consult with a physician for diagnosis.
- Refer the woman to a surgeon in cases of suspected appendicitis.

Patient Education

- Explain disease process, progression, and treatment plan.
- Advise patient about the probability of surgery if diagnosis is made.
- Teach patient regarding signs and symptoms of preterm labor and kick counts.

Follow-up

- Follow up, as indicated, by surgical team.
- Perform fetal surveillance testing and uterine activity monitoring, as indicated for suspicion of diagnosis and postsurgery when there is a suspicion of appendicitis.
- Document problems in progress notes and problem list.

Cholecystitis

Cholecystitis is an inflammation of the gallbladder that occurs most often when a stone becomes lodged in the ampulla or in the cystic duct. Inflammation and pressure develop behind the obstruction as a result of continued secretion. Chronic cholecystitis is secondary to continued inflammation of the gallbladder. An acute cholecystitis attack is usually preceded by a history of previous symptomatic episodes.

Pregnancy may increase the incidence of cholelithiasis by altering gallbladder contractility and by changing bile lithogenicity. During pregnancy, the fasting, residual, and average gallbladder volumes are increased and the emptying rate of the gallbladder is diminished. These changes are thought to increase gallstone formation. Studies have shown that the risk of gallstones increases with the number of pregnancies (Connon, 1994; Scott, 1992). The incidence of acute cholecystitis is not increased in pregnancy.

Database

Subjective

- Chronic cholecystitis
  - ▶ Recurrent episodes of sudden onset, intermittent, or constant, right hypochondriac, or epigastric "colicky" pain, building to a maximum within 1 hour, lasting 1 to 4 hours, radiating to left or right scapula
  - ▶ Dark urine or light, clay-colored stools may occur
- Acute cholecystitis
  - ▶ Sudden onset of severe, usually constant, right hypochondriac or epigastric pain, subsiding in 12 to 18 hours
  - ▶ May have nausea and vomiting
  - ▶ Dark urine, light, clay-colored stools may occur

NOTE: Though ingestion of fatty foods or large amounts of food, with subsequent flatulence, epigastric heaviness, belching, heartburn, and upper abdominal pain were thought to be precipitatory factors in cholecystitis symptoms, studies show that these associations are probably incidental.

Objective

- Chronic cholecystitis
  - ▶ Mild or absent right upper-quadrant abdominal tenderness
  - ▶ Jaundice may be present
- Acute cholecystitis
  - ▶ Right upper-quadrant abdominal tenderness with guarding and rebound tenderness
  - ▶ Jaundice (occurs in 25 percent of cases)

▶ Moderately elevated WBC count

▶ Alkaline phosphatase

▶ Positive Murphy's sign

▶ Elevated temperature

▶ HIDA (99m dimethylimino-diacetic acid imaging agent) scan may show obstructed cystic duct. Substantially less than 1cGy radiation dose to the fetus (Moore, 1994) (see Chapter 6.14, *Ionizing Radiation Exposure*)

▶ Ultrasound may show gallstones or a thickened gallbladder (97 percent sensitive in demonstrating stone in the gallbladder)

Assessment

● Cholecystitis—acute or chronic.

▶ R/O peptic ulcer disease

▶ R/O pancreatitis

▶ R/O hepatitis

▶ R/O appendicitis

▶ R/O diverticulitis

▶ R/O right lower-lobe pneumonia

▶ R/O irritable bowel syndrome

▶ R/O HELLP syndrome

▶ R/O severe preeclampsia

▶ R/O acute viral hepatitis

▶ R/O pyelonephritis

▶ R/O kidney stones

Plan

Diagnostic Tests

▶ WBC count (will be moderately elevated)

▶ Total serum bilirubin, serum transaminase, serum amylase, alkaline phosphatase, and liver function studies

▶ Ultrasound of the gallbladder

▶ Antepartum fetal assessment, as indicated

Treatment/Management

- Referral to a physician is warranted for decision regarding surgical or nonsurgical treatment.

- In the first trimester, medical management is indicated (and preferable).

  ▶ Treatment of uncomplicated acute cholecystitis should be managed conservatively, particularly in the first trimester. This may include

    - Fat-restricted diet
    - Bed rest
    - Broad spectrum IV antibiotics
    - NPO
    - NG tube
    - IV hydration
    - Analgesic relief of pain
    - TPN may be needed

    NOTE: There is no experience with oral bile salts or lithotripsy in pregnancy, and they are currently not recommended.

  ▶ Operative surgery in the first trimester is associated with a fetal loss rate of up to 5 percent.

    NOTE: It is recommended that a cholecystectomy be considered before pregnancy in client with symptomatic gallstones.

- In the second trimester: medical vs surgical management

  ▶ There is no known increase in total mortality with operative surgery in the second trimester (Scott, 1992).

- In the third trimester the best treatment is medical management with postpartum surgery.

  ▶ Operative surgery is associated with an increased risk of preterm delivery in the third trimester (Smoleniec & James, 1993).

Consultation

- Refer the client to a physician to decide whether surgical or nonsurgical treatment is indicated.

Patient Education

- See the Treatment/Management section.
- Explain disease process progression and management plan.
- Advise the client about what to expect if surgery is necessary.

Follow-up

- Follow up, as indicated, by case presentation.
- Document problems in progress notes and problem list.

Diarrhea

Diarrhea is defined as an increase in frequency, fluidity (70 to 90 percent water), and volume (greater than 200 grams/day) of bowel movements. The average daily stool weight is 100 to 150 grams per day with a water content of 60 to 70 percent (Knauer 1993).

The pathophysiologic mechanisms of diarrhea include (Knauer 1993)

- Osmotic diarrhea: excess water-soluble molecules in the bowel lumen causing increased nonabsorbable intraluminal water (as seen in lactose deficiency, magnesium-containing cathartics)

- Secretory diarrhea: increased secretion and decreased absorption of electrolytes (as caused, for example, by cholera and bile salt enteropathy)

- Exudative diarrhea: impairment in colonic absorption with intestinal loss of serum proteins, blood, mucus, or pus (as associated with ulcerative colitis, and shigellosis)

- Anatomic rearrangement: decreased absorption surface (can be caused by subtotal colectomy or gastrocolic fistula)

- Motility disturbances: decreased contact time (as in hyperthyroidism, irritable bowel syndrome)

Diarrhea is *not* exacerbated by pregnancy, but there may be an increased incidence of episodes of diarrhea due to the effects of relaxin, a substance released by the placenta to relax smooth muscle contractions. Relaxin's effect on the gastrointestinal smooth muscle (causing diarrhea) can be seen in preterm or term labor when its release is increased to quiet the contractions (West, Warren, & Cutts, 1992). However, most causes of diarrhea are the same as in the nonpregnant patient, (i.e., drugs, alterations in diet, malabsorption, food poisoning and infections) (Baron, Ramirez, & Richter, 1993).

The evaluation of diarrhea in a pregnant woman must include assessment of fetal well-being. Fetal tachycardia and an abnormal nonstress test is often the first sign of significant maternal-fetal hypovolemia. Significant volume depletion in a pregnant patient may be missed because of the increased intravascular volume. Consequently, diarrhea should always be evaluated in a pregnant client followed by appropriate management and follow-up (Torbey & Richter, 1995).

Database

Subjective

- Symptoms may include
  - ▶ Loose liquid stools
  - ▶ Blood, mucus, pus, or grease in stools

- ▶ Urgency to defecate
- ▶ Increase in frequency of stools
- ▶ Abdominal pain
- ▶ Cramping before, during, and/or after defecation
- ▶ Increase in flatulence
- ▶ Abdominal bloating
- ▶ Fever
- ▶ Nausea, vomiting
- ▶ Weight loss
- ● Historical evidence and symptoms of common causes of diarrhea include (Knauer 1993)
  - ▶ Recent travel or exposure to others with diarrhea
  - ▶ Psychogenic factors, such as nervousness or anxiety
  - ▶ Drugs
    - – Ingestion of magnesium-containing antacids, laxatives, or antibiotics

    NOTE: Pseudomembranous colitis develops when normal bowel flora is suppressed by broad-spectrum antibiotic use, allowing *Clostridium difficile* to proliferate, producing mild to severe, profuse watery stools.

  - ▶ Infection
    - – Usually abrupt onset
    - – Associated symptoms: headache, anorexia, fever, nausea, vomiting, malaise, myalgia

    NOTE: Diarrhea of viral etiology has incubation period of 48 to 72 hours and lasts 1 to 3 days (primarily enterovirus or Norwalk virus)

  - ▶ Dietary factors
    - – Excessive intake of fruits, caffeine-containing foods, alcohol, or herbal teas
    - – Lactase deficiency with intolerance to milk (produces bloating and cramping)
    - – Malnutrition
    - – Food allergy (diarrhea after ingestion of certain foods)
  - ▶ Other intestinal factors
    - – Fecal impaction (suggested by period of absent stools)
    - – Symptoms of diarrhea may actually indicate incontinence
    - – Malabsorption syndrome—malabsorption of carbohydrates or fats (steatorrhea)
  - ▶ Gastrointestinal surgery
    - – Dumping syndrome causes sweating, lightheadedness, tachycardia, and diarrhea following food ingestion

- See Chapter 8.2, *Chronic Abdominal Pain;* Section 12, *Thyroid Conditions;* Chapter 10.2, *Hepatitis A, B, C, D, and E;* and Chapter 6.11, *Gestational Diabetes Mellitus.*

Objective

- Postural vital sign changes, elevation in temperature, and weight loss (depending on the extent of dehydration secondary to diarrhea).

- Fetal tachycardia

- Abnormal NST

- Abdominal exam may reveal

  ▶ Abdominal tenderness, guarding, rebound

  ▶ Increased bowel sounds (or decreased, as in cases of fecal impaction)

- Rectal examination as indicated

Assessment

- Diarrhea

  ▶ R/O dehydration

  ▶ R/O preterm labor

  ▶ R/O laxative overuse

  ▶ R/O irritable bowel disease

  ▶ R/O malabsorption

  ▶ R/O thyroid disease

Plan

Diagnostic Tests

- Usually no diagnostic testing is recommended if history and physical examination suggest viral illness.

- For history and clinical findings suggestive of bacterial or parasitic infection, obtain

  ▶ Stool culture

  ▶ Stool for ova and parasites

  ▶ Stool examination for leukocytes

  ▶ Stool for occult blood

- Sigmoidoscopy is recommended when blood or pus is present, if unable to attribute diarrhea to acute bacterial infection

- Clients with recent history of antibiotic ingestion should have stools examined for *C. difficile* toxin

- Stool alkalization test is indicated for suspected laxative abuse (The paper will turn pink in presence of phenolphthalein, a common ingredient in laxatives).

- Sudan stain tests fat in stool if fat malabsorption is present.

  ▶ If fat is present, obtain a 72-hour quantitative stool-fat determination.

- CBC and serum electrolytes may be indicated for evaluation of moderate to severe dehydration.

Treatment/Management

- Acute diarrhea of short duration is managed by restriction of food (not fluid) intake for 24 hours.

  ▶ Oral hydration should be encouraged with solutions rich in electrolytes and sugar, such as 8 oz. of fruit juice, with pinch of table salt and teaspoon of honey or sugar taken every hour.

  ▶ Nondiet cola drinks that have lost their carbonation may be ingested.

  ▶ Fluid replacement via intravenous line may be indicated with moderate to severe dehydration or with associated nausea and vomiting.

  ▶ Food can slowly be added as tolerated, starting with broth-based soups, gelatin, tea, toast, or crackers, moving to bananas, baked potato, rice, and applesauce. Slowly increase protein intake and, lastly, fats. Limit milk-product intake until complete recovery.

- Monitor fetal well-being with nonstress testing with amniotic fluid index (AFI) or biophysical profile as appropriate for gestation.

- Monitor the client for signs and symptoms of preterm labor.

- In cases of chronic diarrhea, the best management strategy is to treat underlying condition.

  ▶ Reevaluate need for drugs causing diarrhea.

  ▶ Eliminate foods causing diarrhea (e.g., caffeine, milk products).

  ▶ Initiate vitamin therapy for patients with malnutrition and steatorrhea.

  ▶ Dumping syndrome may respond to small, frequent feedings.

  ▶ Pseudomembranous colitis responds to antibiotic therapy.

  ▶ Advise discontinuation of chronic laxative use.

  ▶ See Chapter 6.11, *Gestational Diabetes Mellitus*; Chapter 8.2, *Chronic Abdominal Pain*; Chapter 10.2, *Hepatitis A, B, C, D, and E*; and Section 12, *Thyroid Conditions*.

- Diarrhea of psychogenic origin may be managed with psychotherapy.

- Antidiarrheal agents, if appropriate.

  ▶ Kaolin and pectin: over-the-counter drug, prescribe as directed on package.

  ▶ Narcotic analogs

  – Loperamide: human data is limited; not found to be teratogenic in animals. (Torbey & Richter, 1995).

    NOTE: This agent should be avoided if client has infectious diarrhea because it may worsen or prolong the course or conditions that increase the risk of toxic megacolon.

- Antibiotic therapy is appropriate for certain types of bacterial and parasitic infections. Physician consultation is recommended.
- Viral gastroenteritis infections causing diarrhea are usually self-limiting and can be treated with rehydration and kaolin and pectin.

Consultation

- When the client has acute severe diarrhea and is unable to maintain oral hydration, refer her to a physician.
- Consult with a physician in cases of chronic diarrhea when unable to establish diagnosis.
- Consult with a physician when considering antibiotic therapy for bacterial or parasitic infection.

Patient Education

- Educate the client regarding pathophysiology and management of diarrhea.
- Advise the client to continue with hydration throughout recovery period.
- Advise clients with possible contagious diarrhea to maintain good

  hygiene (i.e., wash hands with soap and water after using the bathroom).
- To relieve perineal discomfort teach the client to
  - ▶ Take two to three sitz baths/day.
  - ▶ Gently dry perineal area with absorbent cotton.
  - ▶ Avoid use of soap in perineal area
  - ▶ Clean perineal area with witch hazel pads.
- Advise patient that a short course of 0.5 percent to 1 percent hydrocortisone cream to perianal inflammation may be helpful.
- Advise the client to avoid narcotic therapy in the treatment of diarrhea.
- Teach patient the signs and symptoms of preterm labor. See Chapter 6.25, *Preterm Labor*.
- See Chapter 6.11, *Gestational Diabetes Mellitus*; Chapter 8.2, *Chronic Abdominal Pain*; Chapter 10.2, *Hepatitis A, B, C, D, and E*; and Section 12, *Thyroid Conditions*.

Follow-up

- Follow up as indicated by case presentation.
- Document any significant or ongoing problems in progress notes and problem list.

References

Baron, T.H., Ramirez, B., & Richter, J. E. (1993). Gastrointestinal motility disorders during pregnancy. *Annals of Internal Medicine, 118,* 366–375.

Connon, J. (1994). Gastrointestinal complications. In G.N. Burrow & T.F. Ferris (Eds.), *Medical complications during pregnancy.* (4th ed.) (pp. 285–291). Philadelphia, PA: W.B. Saunders.

Knauer, C.M. (1993). Alimentary tract. In L.M. Tierney, S.J. McPhee, M.A. Papadakis, and S. A. Schroeder (Eds.), *Current medical diagnosis and treatment.* (35th ed.) (pp. 451–502). Norwalk, CT: Appleton & Lange.

Moore, P.J. (1994). Maternal physiology of pregnancy. In A.H. DeCherney & M.L. Pernoll (Eds.), *Current obstetric and gynecologic diagnosis and treatment.* (8th ed.) (pp. 146–152). Norwalk, CT: Appleton & Lange.

Scott, L.D. (1992). Gallstone disease and pancreatitis in pregnancy. *Gastroenterology Clinics of North America, 21*(4), 803–815.

Smoleniec, J.S., & James, D.K. (1993). Gastro-intestinal crisis during pregnancy. *Digestive Disease, 11,* 313–324.

Torbey, C.F., & Richter, J.E. (1995). Gastrointestinal motility disorders in pregnancy. *Seminars in Gastrointestinal Disease, 6*(4), 203–216.

West, L., Warren, J., & Cutts, T. (1992). Diagnosis and management of irritable bowel syndrome, constipation, and diarrhea in pregnancy. *Gastroenterology Clinics of North America, 21*(4), 793–801.

Witlin, A.G., & Sibai, B.M. (1996). When a pregnant patient develops appendicitis. *Contemporary OB/GYN, 41*(2), 15–30.

Chapter 2

CHRONIC ABDOMINAL PAIN

Lisa L. Lommel

Gastroesophageal Reflux and Heartburn

Gastroesophageal reflux disease (GERD) results from regurgitation of gastric contents into the esophagus. The mechanisms involved in reflux are due to a permanently or intermittently incompetent lower esophageal sphincter, and inability of the esophagus to generate peristaltic wave action that would prevent acid and pepsin from coming in contact with the mucosa (Knauer, 1993).

Hormonal, neural, anatomic, and dietary factors are involved in the function of the lower esophageal sphincter. Many individuals experience gastrointestinal symptoms at some time but the frequency and duration will distinguish physiologic reflux from gastroesophageal reflux disease.

Heartburn is the most common symptom of gastroesophageal reflux, as well as other disorders (see the Peptic Ulcer Disease section). It presents as a retrosternal burning sensation and is due to irritation from reflux of stomach acid into the esophagus.

Reflux esophagitis refers to inflammation of the esophagus secondary to injury of the mucosa by refluxed acid, pepsin, or bile. Complications can include pain, bleeding, ulcers, and strictures.

Gastroesophageal reflux with resulting heartburn affects 30 to 50 percent of all pregnancies. Symptoms may present in pregnancy as an exacerbation of preexisting disease, but most often initial onset of symptoms begin during pregnancy. The majority of clients are most affected with symptoms in the third trimester and are relieved of their symptoms postpartum (Torbey & Richter, 1995).

The pathophysiology of GERD alters in pregnancy, although its exact cause is not known. A decrease in lower esophageal sphincter (LES) pressure is thought to be the primary cause of symptoms. The increase in progesterone and estrogen during pregnancy initiates smooth muscle relaxation of the LES causing further exacerbation of symptoms. Progesterone also slows gastrointestinal transit time, which may increase GERD symptoms. Last, the enlarging gravid uterus contributes to symptoms by increasing gastric pressure and delaying gastric emptying (Torbey & Richter, 1995; Niewiarowski & Fisher, 1993).

Maternal morbidity and mortality is increased in the women with GERD who require anesthesia during delivery because there is an increased risk of aspiration. Several studies are under way to look at drug therapy to reduce reflux during obstetric anesthesia. Fetal morbidity and mortality is not significantly increased with maternal GERD (Torbey & Richter, 1995).

Database

Subjective

- The client reports heartburn characterized by retrosternal, intermittent aching, burning 30 to 60 minutes after eating.

► Symptoms are more evident after a large meal.

► Symptoms radiate upward toward the throat into the back.

► Symptoms are increased when lying down, bending over, or exercising.

► Symptoms awaken the client at night.

► Can mimic cardiac ischemia with chest heaviness or pressure.

► Symptoms are relieved by drinking water, milk, or taking antacids.

- The client reports gastroesophageal reflux characterized by regurgitation of food or fluid, especially at night

  ► She may awaken with coughing or strangling sensation.

  ► She may soil the pillow by regurgitation or water brash (i.e., regurgitation and increased saliva).

- Tobacco, alcohol, chocolate, peppermint, citrus fruits, coffee, tea, colas, and foods with high fat or carbohydrate content induce symptoms (decrease lower esophageal sphincter tone)

- The client reports pain or difficulty swallowing (usually indicates long-term reflux with inflammation and/or stricture).

- Hiatal hernia, recurring or persistent vomiting, obesity, ascites, tight binders, or girdles may increase symptoms.

- History of scleroderma or diabetes mellitus may predispose client to reflux.

- The client reports hoarseness or morning laryngitis (can be caused by severe reflux).

- There may be hematemesis and melena.

- Symptoms commonly present in third trimester and/or worsen as pregnancy progresses.

- Clients whose symptoms initially present in pregnancy are often symptom-free after delivery.

- Hyperemesis gravidarum may aggravate symptoms.

Objective

- Physical examination is unremarkable.

- Decreased hematocrit and hemoglobin may be present with bleeding.

Assessment

- Gastroesophageal reflux

- Heartburn

  ► R/O peptic ulcer disease

  ► R/O ischemic heart disease

  ► R/O esophageal spasm

▶ R/O esophageal infection in immunocompromised host

▶ R/O cholelithiasis

▶ R/O diabetes mellitus

▶ R/O anemia

Plan

Diagnostic Tests

- Diagnosis of reflux usually made if symptoms are typical with absence of clinical findings for other diseases.

- Test stool for occult blood, as indicated.

- Order a CBC, as indicated (may reveal decreased hemoglobin/hematocrit if there is associated bleeding).

- Barium swallow or upper GI should be avoided because of radiation risk to the fetus. Endoscopy is safe in pregnancy (Torbey & Richter, 1995).

- Consider endoscopy with biopsy to assess extent of damage due to esophageal disease if symptoms are not improved with therapeutic trial or there is suspicion of

  ▶ Other causative disorders (e.g., peptic ulcer, dyspepsia)

  ▶ Dysphagia

  ▶ Significant weight loss

  ▶ Occult blood loss

- Determine esophageal reflux and acid clearing time with 24-hour pH probe recordings (considered safe in pregnancy and used for evaluation of atypical symptom presentation).

  ▶ Most sensitive and specific test but expensive and not universally available

  ▶ Helpful in assessing

    — Noncardiac chest pain to determine if reflux episodes are associated with typical pain

    — Clients presenting with pulmonary or ear, nose, and throat symptoms

    NOTE: Esophageal reflux pain can mimic cardiac symptoms; there is a possibility of concomitant cardiac disease. Diagnostic tests for cardiac disease should be obtained if suspected (e.g., sequential EKGs, enzyme determinations).

Treatment/Management

- In the absence of suspicion of other disorders, therapeutic trial is appropriate in clients with suspected reflux.

- Begin treatment with conservative measures including the following (Richter, 1995):

  ▶ Avoid foods high in fats or carbohydrates.

▶ Avoid large meals in evening or late-night snacks.

▶ Avoid lying down after meals.

▶ Elevate head of bed up to 6 inches.

▶ Avoid cigarettes, alcohol, coffee, colas, peppermint, citrus, and spicy foods.

▶ Avoid tight belts, girdles, bending over, heavy lifting.

● Clients with symptoms unrelieved by the preceding measures or those with mild to moderate symptoms may consider antacid trial.

NOTE: Antacids relieve pain discomfort by neutralizing acid, inactivating pepsin, binding bile salts, and stimulating gastric bicarbonate secretion. There is no evidence that antacids are teratogenic, although first-trimester use of any drug should always be carefully weighed.

▶ Aluminum hydroxide/magnesium hydroxide mixtures, 15 to 30 mL p.o. 2 hours after meals and at bedtime

– Side effects of aluminum may be constipation, phosphate deficiency, and osteoporosis.

– Side effects of magnesium may be diarrhea and should not be used in clients with renal insufficiency.

NOTE: Use combination preparations or alternate preparations to manage gastrointestinal symptoms.

▶ A mixture of aluminum hydroxide, magnesium hydroxide, and calcium carbonate, 15 to 30 mL p.o. 1 and 3 hours after meals and at bedtime (liquid form of antacid is more effective than tablet form)

NOTE: Calcium carbonate alone is not recommended for treatment because of calcium-induced gastric hypersecretion.

▶ Sodium bicarbonate is not recommended because of its high sodium content.

● In clients with symptoms unrelieved by the preceding measures, or for those with mild to moderate symptoms consider sucralfate. The goal is to control the client's symptoms with the least amount of medication.

▶ Sucralfate (a mucosal protective agent), 400 mg p.o. after dinner (Torbey & Richter, 1995).

NOTE: Antacids can be used concomitantly but not within 1 hour of sucralfate. Sucralfate may have side effects such as constipation and inhibition of the absorption of digoxin, tetracycline, phenytoin, and cimetidine.

● Clients with symptoms unrelieved by the preceding measures or for those with moderate to severe symptoms H_2 blockers may be considered. Physician consultation is warranted. The goal is to control the client's symptoms with the least amount of medication.

▶ Cimetidine, 800 mg p.o. daily after dinner

– Side effects may be galactorrhea, skin rashes, leukopenia, agranulocytosis, hepatitis, elevated serum creatinine and interaction with many drugs (Knauer, 1993). See *The Physician's Desk Reference (PDR)*.

NOTE: Cimetidine inhibits gastric secretion stimulated by food, gastrin, histamine, and caffeine. Avoid taking at same time as antacids, separate them by at least 1 to 2 hours. In pregnancy, the recommendation is to maintain single daily dosing.

▶ Ranitidine, 150 mg p.o. every 12 hours *or* 300 mg p.o. after dinner

    – Side effects may be diarrhea, dyspepsia, loss of libido, dizziness, or mental confusion (Knauer, 1993).

- If therapeutic trial does not improve symptoms, or with moderate to severe symptoms, consider endoscopy to rule out malignancy, stricture and to determine extent of esophagitis. Physician consultation/referral is warranted.

Consultation

- Consult when the client's symptoms are not relieved by conservative measures.
- Consult with a physician for atypical symptoms and if therapeutic trial does not improve symptoms.
- Consult with or refer to a physician for evaluation of relapse of symptoms.
- Refer to a physician when there is a suspicion of organic disorders.
- Refer to a physician for endoscopy.

Patient Education

- See the Treatment/Management section.
- Explain the pathophysiology of reflux, the chronic and recurrent nature of the disease, the aggravating factors, and the necessity of following conservative measures even throughout therapeutic trial.
- Advise client to continue with medication and conservative measures as prescribed, even after symptoms have subsided.
- Advise client regarding a nutritious diet. (See Section 18, *Nutrition.*)
- Advise client to avoid straining when defecating.
- Assist client in cessation of alcohol intake and smoking. Refer to appropriate support services, as indicated (Alcoholics Anonymous, Nicotine Anonymous, American Cancer Society, etc.).
- Instruct client in methods of stress reduction.

Follow-Up

- Reevaluate the client in 4 to 6 weeks after initiation of treatment and 4 to 6 weeks postpartum.
- At every visit, reinforce adherence to conservative measures.

- Withdraw one pharmacologic agent at a time to assist in determination of minimum maintenance treatment.

  NOTE: Up to 45 percent of clients relapse after discontinuation of medication. Some clients may require a maintenance dose of a particular drug.

- Review the American Cancer Society's recommendations for early detection of cancer in asymptomatic people (American Cancer Society [ACS], 1993).

  ▶ Sigmoidoscopy: every 3 years beginning at age 50 years

  ▶ Stool guaiac: yearly beginning at age 50 years

  ▶ Digital rectal examination: yearly beginning at age 40 years

  NOTE: The ACS suggests a digital rectal examination of all women during their annual gynecological visit.

- Document problems in progress notes and problem list.

Inflammatory Bowel Disease

Inflammatory bowel disease (IBD) refers to any intestinal inflammatory condition that is chronic in nature. The two most common inflammatory conditions are ulcerative colitis and Crohn's disease. Similarities of these two conditions include

- Clinical presentation
- Average age at onset between 15 and 40 years
- Higher incidence in Caucasians (particularly Jewish Caucasians) in developed western countries
- Slightly higher incidence in females
- Family clustering

The cause of IBD is unknown. Pathogenesis is thought to involve many factors, including autoimmune factors, collagen disorders, genetic factors, infections, psychogenic factors, environmental factors, drugs, and weakened gastrointestinal defenses.

Ulcerative colitis affects the mucosal and submucosal layers of the distal colon and rectum. It is characterized by ulcer lesions lining the entire colon tissue. The most common extracolonic manifestations of ulcerative colitis include arthritis, skin and eye lesions, and liver disease. Complications include hemorrhage, pericolitis, toxic dilatation, perforation, and colon cancer.

The course of IBD during pregnancy is related to disease activity before conception; pregnancy does not significantly alter the periods of quiescence or exacerbations. In pregnant clients who are in remission at the time of conception, approximately 30 percent will experience an exacerbation of their disease, which usually occurs in the first trimester. If the disease is active at the onset of pregnancy, it will most likely continue to be active or even worsen during pregnancy. It is therefore recommended that active IBD be treated and allowed to go into remission prior to a planned pregnancy (Korelitz, 1992). Overall, long-term prognosis does not seem to be altered by pregnancy (Connon, 1994; Weeks & Freeman, 1993).

The rate of maternal and fetal morbidity and mortality associated with IBD increases depending upon disease severity. Maternal risks correlate with disease complications as outlined above. Fetal risks include a 2 to 30 percent risk of preterm birth or growth restriction and the consequences of pharmacologic therapy and surgery, if indicated (Calhoun, 1992; Weeks & Freeman, 1993).

Ulcerative Colitis

Database

Subjective

In *mild* cases, ulcerative colitis symptoms include

- ▶ One to four semiformed stools per day
- ▶ Minimal blood in stools
- ▶ No systemic symptoms
- In *moderate to severe* cases, symptoms include
  - ▶ Frequent liquid stools
  - ▶ Blood and/or pus in stools
  - ▶ Abdominal cramping
  - ▶ Nocturnal diarrhea
  - ▶ Mild fever during exacerbations
  - ▶ Weight loss
  - ▶ Symptoms of dehydration to varying degrees
- Client has history of intolerance to dairy products.
- Constipation, tenesmus and anal incontinence may be present when only rectum is involved.
- Symptoms characterized by exacerbations and remissions. Remissions may last from months to years.
- Symptoms of associated manifestations may be arthritis, skin and eye lesions, and liver disease.
- Symptoms of complications may be present for hemorrhage, pericolitis, toxic dilatation, perforation, and carcinoma.

Objective

- Clinical findings depend on severity of illness.
- In *mild* cases, findings may include
  - ▶ Slight abdominal tenderness or normal abdominal examination
  - ▶ Loss of normal vascular pattern and mild to moderate diffuse inflammation (revealed by colonoscopy)
- ▶ Normal laboratory value

- In *moderate to severe* cases, findings may include
  - ▶ Abdominal tenderness especially along the course of the colon
  - ▶ Irritation, hemorrhoids, fissures and spasm (revealed by rectal examination)
  - ▶ Signs of dehydration and undernutrition of varying degrees
  - ▶ Fever
  - ▶ Continuous, granulomatous, superficial ulcerations (revealed by colonoscopy)
- Laboratory findings reflect severity of disease
  - ▶ Decreased hemoglobin (Hgb) and hematocrit (Hct) reflecting amount of blood loss
  - ▶ White blood count (WBC) and erythrocyte sedimentation rate (ESR) elevated (in severe cases and those with complications)
  - ▶ Decrease potassium, magnesium, and sodium (amount of decrease reflects severity)
  - ▶ Decreased albumin, calcium, and total protein (in severe cases)
  - ▶ Abnormal liver function studies (in severe cases)
  - ▶ Positive blood in stool
  - ▶ Stool negative for bacteria and parasites
- Client may present with enlarged lymph nodes.
- Clinical findings of associated manifestations may present as arthritis, skin and eye lesions, and liver disease.
- Clinical findings of complications may present as hemorrhage, pericolitis, toxic dilatation, perforation, and carcinoma.

Assessment

- Ulcerative colitis
  - ▶ R/O Crohn's disease
  - ▶ R/O infectious colitis (bacterial, viral, fungal, parasitic)
  - ▶ R/O drug-induced colitis
  - ▶ R/O diverticular disease
  - ▶ R/O irritable bowel syndrome
  - ▶ R/O carcinoma

Plan

Diagnostic Tests

- Ulcerative colitis diagnosis is usually made by clinical presentation and sigmoidoscopy and confirmed by biopsy.

  ▶ Colonoscopy may determine extent of disease.

  ▶ Risks to the pregnancy with these diagnostic tests are minimal.

- Ultrasonography or computed tomographic (CT) scan of abdomen may detect abdominal mass, abscess, or obstruction.

- CBC should be obtained as baseline.

- ESR should be obtained as baseline.

- Depending on severity of disease obtain

  ▶ Electrolytes

  ▶ Total protein, albumin

  ▶ Liver function studies

- Obtain stool culture, ova and parasites, and occult blood testing

- Additional testing may be warranted to rule out extraintestinal manifestations of the disease.

- Additional testing may be warranted to rule out complications of the disease.

Treatment/Management

- Hospitalization is warranted for moderate to severe disease or major complications.

- Majority of clients with mild disease can be managed on outpatient basis.

- Diet should be altered during exacerbations and may be of benefit as a general measure

  ▶ Try elimination of lactose containing foods (milk products).

  ▶ Try a low-residue diet eliminating raw fruits and vegetables, fruit juices.

  ▶ Clients with steatorrhea should have low-fat diet (less than 80 gm/day).

  ▶ Undernourished clients should have a balanced high-calorie (2,500 to 3,000 kcal/day) and high-protein (120 to 150 g/day) diet.

  ▶ To aid in decreased absorption of fat soluble vitamins a multivitamin with iron, calcium, and magnesium should be taken.

    NOTE: Megavitamin therapy is not advised.

  ▶ Folic acid supplementation (1 mg/day) is warranted when intake of green leafy vegetables and fresh fruits is poor or when sulfasalazine therapy is being taken.

  ▶ Prescribe parenteral vitamin B_{12} therapy, as indicated.

► Prescribe parenteral iron therapy, as indicated.

  NOTE: Oral therapy is usually not well tolerated.

► With severe exacerbations, prescribe elemental supplements (Ensure ®, Vivonex ®), or total parenteral alimentation may be warranted to rest the bowel.

  NOTE: Home parenteral nutrition is widely available as an alternative to hospitalization.

- Pharmacologic therapy for mild to moderate ulcerative colitis.

  ► Sulfa antibiotic and 5-aminosalicylic acid (sulfasalazine) (reduces frequency and severity of recurrent ulcerative colitis)

    − Can be used safely in pregnancy, although first trimester use of any drug should be carefully considered (Korelitz, 1992; Weeks & Freeman, 1993; Calhoun, 1992; Connon, 1994).

      NOTE: Twenty-five percent of clients experience intolerable side effects. The alternate preparations (mesalamine and olsalazine) are associated with increased efficacy and fewer side effects.

    − Recommend 1 mg/day folate supplementation when using this drug (Linn & Peppercorn, 1992).

    − Initiate therapy with 2 gm/day in divided doses (q.i.d.) with meals and increase dosage as tolerated over several days to 4 gm/day; then decrease to smallest dosage that maintains symptom control (usually 2 g/day) and continue for at least 1 year to maintain remission (Ruymann & Richter, 1995).

    − Side effects can be

      * Headache

      * Dyspepsia

      * Anorexia

      * Fever

      * Rash

      * Hemolytic anemia

      * Leukopenia

      * Folate deficiency

      * Exacerbation of colitis

      * Reversible male infertility due to effects on spermatogenesis

      NOTE: Gastric side effects can be reduced by using enteric coated tablets and taking with food. Mild allergic reactions can be managed through desensitization, (i.e. give low daily dose of 10 to 250 mg, increasing slowly every 3 to 7 days to therapeutic level) (Cooke, 1991)– See the *Physician's Desk Reference* (*PDR*).

- Contraindications include history of severe allergy to sulfa drugs. May be advisable to temporarily discontinue therapy 2 to 3 days before expected delivery and resume after delivery to reduce fetal bilirubinemia (Connon, 1994).

▶ If sulfasalazine fails to achieve control in mild to moderate cases or in acute cases, add prednisone.

▶ For round-the-clock symptoms, give prednisone, 40 mg/day p.o. in divided doses, then change to AM dosage for 7 to 10 days until symptom control is achieved; then decrease by 5 to 10 mg every 2 weeks and taper off, if possible, depending on disease activity

- Can be used safely in pregnancy, although first trimester use of any drug should be carefully considered (Korelitz, 1992; Weeks & Freeman, 1993; Calhoun, 1992; Connon, 1994).

NOTE: Prednisone is not effective in maintaining remission (Linn & Peppercorn, 1992).

- Side effects are dose related and include

  * Adrenal suppression

  * Bone thinning

  * Mood alterations

  * Weakened resistance to infection

  * Impaired glucose tolerance

  * Cushingoid appearance

- See *PDR*.

- Pharmacologic therapy for moderate to severe disease: Refer to a physician for management.

- Pharmacologic therapy for mild ulcerative proctitis (disease confined to rectosigmoid)

▶ 5-aminosalicylic acid enema (Mesalamine®), 3 gm/100 cc enema per rectum at bedtime for 2 to 6 weeks. (Foam preparation is easier to retain but more expensive).

- Administer in left lateral position and retain overnight, if possible.

NOTE: Relapse is almost 100 percent after complete discontinuation. Recommend taper to every other or every third night.

- Found to be more effective than prednisone enemas (Linn & Peppercorn, 1992).

- Side effects: Similar to oral preparation but to varying degrees; also anal irritation and mucosal sensitivity to varying degrees. See *PDR*.

▶ Prednisone enema, 60 cc (100 mg hydrocortisone) enema per rectum at bedtime for 14 nights (Foam preparation available).

- Administer in left lateral position and retain overnight, if possible. Taper to every other or every third night (Cooke, 1991).

- Side effects (systemic absorption and associated side effects with prolonged use)

  * Adrenal suppression

* Bone thinning

* Mood alteration

* Weakened defense against infection

* Impaired glucose tolerance

* Cushingoid appearance

–See *PDR*

- If mild diarrhea persists during ulcerative colitis remission consider trial of psyllium hydrophilic colloid 1 teaspoon in 8 oz. water p.o. every day or b.i.d. (Ruymann & Richter, 1995).

- Even during pregnancy, surgery may be indicated with ulcerative colitis in cases unresponsive to medical therapy or involving intractable bleeding, unresponsive toxic megacolon, disabling strictures, or carcinoma (Cooke, 1991).

Consultation

- Consult for management of mild to moderate disease.

- Refer to a gastrointestinal specialist for diagnosis and to evaluate extent of disease.

- Refer if unresponsive to medical therapy or for moderate to severe disease.

- Refer for colonoscopy and x-ray procedures.

- Refer to a psychotherapist, as indicated, for anxiety or depression.

- Refer or consult with a nutritionist for education.

- Refer to appropriate specialist for evaluation of extraintestinal manifestations.

Patient Education

- See the Treatment/Management section.

- Explain pathogenesis, treatment plan, chronicity, and course of the disease. Include the client's partner and family in education.

- Discuss the client's concerns regarding conception, pregnancy, and childbearing.

- Counsel women with ulcerative colitis to postpone pregnancy until remission of about 1 year.

- Advise women considering pregnancy that there is an increased risk of preterm delivery and low birth weight. Approximately 30 percent of women have exacerbations during pregnancy and postpartum.

- Discuss concerns regarding incontinence, cancer, and social isolation.

- Provide supportive relationship and observe for signs of depression associated with chronic illness.

- Advise client regarding nutritious diet. See special indications under in the Treatment/Management section.

- Suggest a regular exercise program.

- Encourage small, regular, frequent meals.

- Advise elimination of caffeine-containing foods.

- Advise discontinuing smoking and alcohol intake. Refer to appropriate services if indicated (American Cancer Society for smoking cessation, Alcoholics Anonymous, etc.).

- Teach medication adjustment within a prearranged set of guidelines and limits to allow a more active role in care.

- Refer clients to The Crohn's and Colitis Foundation of America (CCFA) to provide additional education and support services to clients and families. (Toll-free number [800] 932-2423).

Follow-up

- The client should be followed closely during exacerbations.

- During remission, evaluations are warranted every 3 to 6 months to document

    - Number of exacerbations (if any)

    - Weight

    - Results of proctoscopy or sigmoidoscopy

    - Laboratory results (Hgb, ESR, and albumin)

- After 5 to 10 years post diagnosis, colonoscopy with directed biopsy should be performed every 2 years because there is an increased incidence of colorectal cancer after 7 to 10 years with ulcerative colitis involving the entire colon.

- Testing for occult blood in stool as an indicator of malignancy is inappropriate as many clients with IBD experience blood loss.

- Document ongoing problems in progress notes and problem list.

Crohn's Disease

Database

Subjective

- Symptom onset is subtle. The client may notice associated manifestations (weight loss) before GI symptoms.

- Symptoms may include

    ▶ Diarrhea

    ▶ Lesions in the mouth, soft palate, or perianal area.

    ▶ Abdominal cramping and tenderness

    ▶ Steatorrhea in cases of bile salt malabsorption

- Symptoms are not usually associated with passage of blood.
  - ▸ If small bowel is involved symptoms may include
    - – Fatigue
    - – Fever (higher than in ulcerative colitis)
    - – Right lower-quadrant cramping pain (more severe than in ulcerative colitis)
    - – Nausea and vomiting
    - – Weight loss and undernutrition
- Symptoms are characterized by exacerbations and remissions.
- Variable symptoms of arthritis, ankylosing spondylitis, skin and eye lesions, cholelithiasis, and nephrolithiasis (see appropriate chapters) may be present as associated manifestations.
- Complications may present as variable symptoms of stenosis, enteric or perianal fistulas, abdominal or perianal abscess, perforation, and perianal suppuration (see appropriate chapters).

Objective

- Clinical findings depend on severity of illness.
- The client may present with
  - ▸ Aphthoid ulcers in mouth, soft palate or perianal area
  - ▸ Anal fissures, fistulas, hemorrhoids or abscesses
  - ▸ Rectovaginal fistulas
  - ▸ Enlarged lymph nodes
  - ▸ Fever
  - ▸ If small bowel is involved
    - – Mid-abdominal and right lower quadrant tenderness
    - – Right lower quadrant fullness or mass reflecting adherent loops of bowel
  - ▸ Varying degrees of undernutrition depending on severity
  - ▸ Deep, ulcerated fissures not continuous with areas of normal mucosa (revealed by colonoscopy)
- Laboratory findings reflect severity of disease:
  - ▸ Macrocytic anemia (vitamin B_{12} malabsorption)
  - ▸ Decreased hemoglobin and hematocrit
  - ▸ Normal or elevated WBC
  - ▸ Elevated ESR
  - ▸ Decreased total protein and albumin in severe cases
  - ▸ Positive or negative blood in stool
  - ▸ Stool negative for bacteria or parasite

- Clinical findings of associated manifestation may be present for arthritis, ankylosing spondylitis, skin and eye lesions, cholelithiasis and nephrolithiasis
- Clinical findings of complications may be present for stenosis, enteric or perianal fistulas, abdominal or perianal abscess, perforation, and perianal suppuration

Assessment

- Crohn's disease
    - ▶ R/O ulcerative colitis
    - ▶ R/O infectious colitis (bacterial, viral, fungal, parasitic)
    - ▶ R/O drug-induced colitis
    - ▶ R/O diverticular disease
    - ▶ R/O irritable bowel syndrome
    - ▶ R/O carcinoma

Plan

Diagnostic Tests

- Crohn's disease diagnosis is usually made by clinical presentation and contrast x-ray of large and small bowel. Approximate fetal radiation exposure for each upper GI or barium enema study is 600 to 800 mrads which is below the 5 to 10 rad exposure level at which risk of fetal injury is increased (Weeks & Freeman, 1993). Maternal and fetal benefits from diagnosis should outweigh risk of exposure.

- See Diagnostic Tests section under ulcerative colitis.

Treatment/Management

- Hospitalization is warranted for moderate to severe disease.
- See diet recommendations in the Treatment/Management section for ulcerative colitis.
    - ▶ In addition, for Crohn's disease, try a low-fiber diet by eliminating nuts, seeds, tough meat, and cole slaw to reduce risk of obstruction.
- Pharmacologic therapy for mild to moderate disease of small bowel
    - ▶ Prednisone
        - – For round-the-clock symptoms 60 mg/day p.o. in divided dose, then change to AM dose and continue until symptoms controlled (may be as long as 4 months)
        - – An every-other-day dose may be sufficient.
            - * Taper by decreasing 5 to 10 mg every few weeks.

- Side effects are dose related and include

  * Adrenal suppression

  * Bone thinning

  * Mood alteration

  * Weakening defense against infection

  * Impaired glucose tolerance

  * Cushingoid appearance

- See *PDR.*

NOTE: Prednisone is not effective in maintaining remission (Linn & Peppercorn, 1992).

- Pharmacologic therapy for colonic Crohn's disease

  ▶ Begin sulfasalazine, 2 gm/day in divided doses (q.i.d.) with meals and increase as tolerated over several days to 4 gm/day; continue for 4 to 8 weeks.

    - See indications, side effects, and contraindications as per ulcerative colitis treatment.

    NOTE: Sulfasalazine will not prevent relapse in Crohn's disease (Ruymann & Richter, 1995).

  ▶ If no response to sulfasalazine switch to metronidazole.

    - 10 to 20 mg/kg/day p.o. (e.g., 250 mg to 500 mg t.i.d.) and continue for a 4-week trial; if satisfactory response, continue for 4 to 6 months, then stop if symptoms have ceased (Ruymann & Richter, 1995).

    - Side effects include

      * Altered taste

      * Paresthesia of hands and feet

      * Peripheral neuropathy

      * Epileptic seizures

      * Abdominal complaints

      * Ingestion of alcohol may produce Antabuse® affect

      * Considered mutagenic

    - See *PDR.*

    NOTE: Large-scale studies have shown no evidence of fetal complications with use of metronidazole (Korelitz, 1992). However, use in the first trimester is not recommended because of possible cytotoxic effects found in animals (Mabie, 1992).

  ▶ If inadequate response to metronidazole switch to prednisone. See pharmacologic therapy of Crohn's disease (with mild to moderate disease of the small bowel) (Ruymann & Richter, 1995).

- Pharmacologic therapy for perianal Crohn's disease
  - ▶ Metronidazole:
    - – 15 to 20 mg/kg/day p.o. (may be increased up to 50 mg/kg/day if necessary) (Cooke, 1991).
    - – Side effects include
      - * Altered taste
      - * Paresthesia of hands and feet
      - * Peripheral neuropathy
      - * Epileptic seizures
      - * Abdominal complaints
      - * Ingestion of alcohol may produce Antabuse affect
      - * Considered mutagenic
    - – See *PDR*.

    NOTE: Relapse occurs following discontinuation.
- Surgery may be indicated with Crohn's disease in cases of intestinal obstruction, abscess formation, bladder or vaginal fistula, or intractable bleeding or diarrhea.

  NOTE: There is a high recurrence rate (70 percent after 15 years) after surgery for Crohn's disease (Cooke, 1991).

Consultation

- Consult for management of mild to moderate disease.
- Refer to a gastrointestinal specialist for diagnosis and to evaluate extent of disease.
- Refer if unresponsive to medical therapy or for moderate to severe disease.
- Refer for colonoscopy and x-ray procedures.
- Refer to a psychotherapist, as indicated, for anxiety or depression.
- Refer or consult with a nutritionist for education.
- Refer to appropriate specialist for evaluation of extraintestinal manifestations.

Patient Education

- See the Treatment/Management section.
- Explain pathogenesis, treatment plan, chronicity, and course of the disease. Include the client's partner and family in education.
- Discuss the client's concerns regarding conception, pregnancy, and childbearing.

- Advise women considering pregnancy that there is an increased risk of preterm delivery and low birth weight. Approximately 30 percent of women have exacerbations during pregnancy and postpartum.

- Discuss concerns regarding incontinence, cancer, and social isolation.

- Provide supportive relationship and observe for signs of depression associated with chronic illness.

- Advise client regarding nutritious diet. See special indications in the Treatment/Management section.

- Suggest a regular exercise program.

- Encourage small, regular, frequent meals.

- Advise elimination of caffeine-containing foods.

- Advise discontinuing smoking and alcohol intake. Refer to appropriate services if indicated (American Cancer Society for smoking cessation, Alcoholics Anonymous, etc.).

- Teach medication adjustment within a prearranged set of guidelines and limits to allow a more active role in care.

- Refer clients to The Crohn's and Colitis Foundation of America (CCFA) to provide additional education and support services to clients and families. (Toll-free number [800] 932-2423).

Follow-up

- The client should be followed closely during exacerbations.

- During remission, evaluations are warranted every 3 to 6 months to document

    - Number of exacerbation (if any)

    - Weight

    - Results of proctoscopy or sigmoidoscopy

    - Laboratory results (Hgb, ESR, and albumin)

- Upper-gastrointestinal and small bowel x-ray with colonoscopy should be performed every two years because in Crohn's disease of the colon, cancer risk increases with increasing area of involvement and longer duration. In small bowel disease, risk increases with longer duration.

- Testing for occult blood in stool as an indicator of malignancy is inappropriate as many clients with IBD experience blood loss.

- Document ongoing problems in progress notes and problem list.

Irritable Bowel Syndrome

Irritable bowel syndrome (IBS) is a disturbance of bowel motor activity characterized by constipation and/or diarrhea, abdominal pain, hypersecretion of colonic mucus, dyspeptic symptoms and varying degrees of anxiety or depression (Knauer, 1993). Nonpropulsive colonic contractions and slow-wave myoelectric activity predisposes to constipation and discomfort. Diarrhea is due to the increased contraction of the small bowel and colon and decreased activity in the large colon causing a pressure gradient.

Psychological stress is thought to be a major component in this syndrome: Affected individuals experience more severe colonic symptoms at times of stress than nonaffected individuals. Low-residue diet is also suspected in the pathogenesis of this disorder. Intolerance to lactose or sugar may also predispose some individuals.

The incidence of irritable bowel syndrome is not significantly altered by pregnancy, although the emotional significance of pregnancy may increase symptoms. The pathogenesis of IBS in pregnancy is not clearly understood. It is thought, however, that the increased level of progesterone in pregnancy serves as a smooth-muscle relaxant responsible for intestinal hypomotility with resultant episodes of constipation. Elevated prostaglandin levels in pregnancy have also been implicated in bowel symptom changes causing intestinal hypermotility with resultant episodes of diarrhea (West, Warren, & Cutts, 1992). Maternal and fetal morbidity and mortality has not been evaluated in irritable bowel syndrome.

Database

Subjective

- A detailed history is key in diagnosis, attempting to identify the symptom complex consistent with irritable bowel syndrome.

- The client has long-term history of symptoms, which are symptoms not steadily progressive, and may include

    ▶ Varying degrees of bloating, nausea, vomiting, flatulence, anorexia, foul breath, heartburn, weakness, palpitations

    ▶ Constipation alternating with diarrhea

    ▶ Passage of mucus with or without stool

    ▶ Episodic or continuous abdominal pain of varying degrees

    ▶ Abdominal pain associated with urge to defecate or passage of flatus, pain is relieved when passage is completed

        – Pain may radiate to left chest or arm (gas in splenic flexure)

    ▶ Symptoms exacerbated by ingestion of large or fatty meals, foods that produce gas (beans, cabbage), stimulant foods (containing caffeine), medication, hormonal changes that occur at menses, and psychological stress

    ▶ Absent nocturnal symptoms

- Commonly, there is a history of headaches, joint pain, allergies, lack of mental concentration, fatigue, anxiety, depression, nervousness or emotional disturbances.

- The client may have history of cathartic and enema use.

Objective

- The client may appear anxious or depressed.

- Abdominal exam may reveal abdominal tenderness of varying degrees, especially along the course of the colon.

- Sigmoidoscopy may show increased spasm and mucus in the colonic lumen.

Assessment

- Irritable bowel syndrome
  - ▶ R/O inflammatory bowel disorder
  - ▶ R/O gastroenteritis
  - ▶ R/O lactase deficiency
  - ▶ R/O psychological disorder
  - ▶ R/O other causes of chronic diarrhea

Plan

Diagnostic Tests

- Diagnosis is commonly made by identifying symptom complex as consistent with irritable bowel syndrome and excluding other abnormalities.
  - ▶ CBC, as indicated.
  - ▶ Stool for occult blood, as indicated.
  - ▶ Stool examination for ova and parasites, as indicated.
  - ▶ Stool examination for bacteria, as indicated.
  - ▶ Consider obtaining serum electrolytes, liver and thyroid function studies.
  - ▶ Sigmoidoscopy or radiographic study of gastrointestinal system may be indicated to rule out other disorders.

Treatment/Management

- Conservative management with stool-bulking agents, a high-fiber diet, and behavioral therapy is recommended for pregnant clients.
  NOTE: Medications including anticholinergic and antispasmodic agents are contraindicated in pregnancy (West, Warren, & Cutts, 1992).

- There is no specific diet that will prove helpful to all clients.
  - ▶ Consider eliminating certain food when there is a suspicion of intolerance (i.e., lactose-containing foods, such as milk and milk products) on a trial basis for 1 to 2 weeks and evaluate for symptom improvement.

- ▶ Increase dietary fiber (grains, vegetables, fruits)
- ▶ Psyllium or methylcellulose may be of benefit (see Chapter 5.2, *Constipation*)
- ▶ Reduce fat intake, intake of gas-producing foods, and sorbitol-containing products.
- ▶ Avoid food stimulants, such as caffeine-containing products.

- Psychotherapy may benefit individuals with signs of psychiatric conditions. Many antidepressant drugs are contraindicated in pregnancy. A psychiatric referral would be indicated.

- Hypnotherapy, biofeedback or other structured relaxation techniques may be helpful.

Consultation

- Physician consultation may be needed for irritable bowel syndrome treatment plan.
- Refer to a physician for sigmoidoscopy or radiographic studies.
- Refer to a physician, if indicated, for disabling symptoms or refractory diarrhea.
- Refer to a psychotherapist for clients with serious psychopathology.
- Refer to a psychiatrist if psychoactive medication is being considered.
- Refer for hypnotherapy or biofeedback, as indicated.

Patient Education

- Explain pathophysiology, etiology, and management plan.
- Explain that the disorder is chronic and recurring and a cure cannot be expected; the management plan is to identify and modify factors that exacerbate symptoms.
- Provide support to the client. Acknowledge symptoms, address client fears, and provide reassurance.
- Discuss psychological and environmental factors that predispose or exacerbate symptoms. Assist the client in reducing these factors.
  - ▶ Suggest keeping a diary of daily factors that seem to exacerbate symptoms.
  - ▶ Assist the client in stress- and anxiety-reducing measures.
- Advise eating smaller, more frequent meals.
- Encourage a nutritious diet, high in fiber and with reduced food stimulants.
- Advise increasing water intake.
- Advise client to discontinue all nonessential medications that affect bowel function, especially laxatives or enemas.
- For clients with constipation, see Chapter 5.2, *Constipation*.

Follow-up

- Evaluate the client at regular intervals.
  - ▶ Assist client by providing a supportive relationship.
  - ▶ Assist client in recognizing periods of increased stress.
- Document problems in progress note and problem list.

Peptic Ulcer Disease

Peptic ulcer disease refers to a group of related ulcerative diseases of the upper gastrointestinal tract. These disorders are duodenal ulcer (80 percent of peptic ulcer disease), gastric ulcer, and Zollinger-Ellison syndrome. Approximately 95 percent of duodenal ulcers occur in the duodenal bulb or cap. The remaining 5 percent are between the duodenal bulb and the ampulla. Duodenal ulcers are two to three times more common than gastric ulcers. The majority of gastric ulcers are found within 6 cm of the pylorus at or near the lesser curvature on the posterior wall of the stomach.

Peptic ulcer disease is thought to be the result of an imbalance between the acid-pepsin secretion and mucosal defenses. Gastric acid and pepsin secretion, elevated in individuals with duodenal ulcers, is relatively normal in individuals with gastric ulcers. Gastric emptying is also accelerated in individuals with duodenal ulcers, causing greater acid exposure of the duodenal mucosa before neutralization of the acid can occur (Goroll, 1995).

Mucosal defense mechanisms are important in protecting the upper gastrointestinal tissue from excess secretions. Specifically, mucus secretion, bicarbonate production, mucosal blood flow, and cellular repair mechanisms are factors in mucosal defense. Prostaglandin E_2 is important in mucous production and bicarbonate secretion and repair. Prostaglandin E_2 has been found to be decreased in individuals with active ulcer disease.

Peptic ulcer results when the protective factors of the mucosal defense mechanisms are outweighed by the aggressive factors of acid/pepsin. Mucosal defense failure is thought to play a larger role in gastric ulcer development than hypersecretion (Knauer, 1993). The role of *Helicobacter pylori* is now well known as a major precipitant to peptic ulcer disease. The organism does not cause ulcers, but it makes the mucosa more susceptible to the injurious actions of acid and pepsin. *H. pylori* has been found in over 95 percent of cases of new onset duodenal ulcer and ulcer recurrence, and its prevalence increases with age. Treatment of *H. pylori* increases the healing time of ulcers and decreases recurrence rates (Goroll, 1995). Detection of *H. pylori* is not recommended in pregnancy because treatment of the organism is not considered safe in the pregnant client.

New onset of peptic ulcer disease in pregnancy is uncommon and preexisting ulcers tend to become asymptomatic or the overall signs and symptoms of peptic ulcer disease tend to decrease. The improvement in symptoms is primarily due to progesterone, which lowers the levels of basal and stimulated acid secretions from the stomach. In addition, there is an increase in mucous output, which offers a protective coating to the stomach and duodenum. The placenta is also a rich source of histamine, which antagonizes the action of histamine at the parietal cell level. The decrease in histamine action causes a drop in gastric acid production (Calhoun, 1992).

Complications of peptic ulcer disease include refractoriness to therapy, perforation, obstruction, and hemorrhage. There is a greater incidence of malignancy and mortality—as a result of hemorrhage—with gastric ulcers than there is with duodenal ulcers. In pregnancy, perforation, obstruction, or hemorrhage necessitates rapid surgical exploration to prevent maternal and fetal mortality. If activation of a previously asymptomatic ulcer does occur, it is usually in the postpartum period, at which time the ulcer can become penetrating (Hess, Morrison, & Hess, 1994).

Database

Subjective

- A general history of peptic ulcer disease may include
  - ▶ Symptoms that are chronic and/or recurrent
  - ▶ High stress level
  - ▶ Large-volume alcohol or coffee ingestion, smoking, glucocorticosteroid or nonsteroidal anti-inflammatory (NSAID) use
  - ▶ Family member with ulcer disease

    NOTE: Peptic ulcer disease rarely occurs during pregnancy (1:4000 deliveries) but appears to be more common when there is associated preeclampsia (Hess, Morrison, & Hess, 1994).

- Duodenal ulcers
  - ▶ Symptoms may include
    - – Recurrent, episodic, epigastric pain occurring 30 minutes to 3 hours after food ingestion
      - * Sharp, gnawing, burning, or aching with abdominal pressure or "hunger sensation"
      - * May radiate below costal margins to back
      - * Relieved within a few minutes by food, antacids, or vomiting (which usually consists of small quantities of highly acid gastric juices)
  - ▶ Symptoms are usually absent before breakfast, worsening over the day.
  - ▶ Client is most symptomatic between 12:00 midnight and 2:00 AM.
  - ▶ Changes in character of pain or symptoms may indicate complication.
    - – Symptoms of penetration
      - * Constant pain, not relieved by food or antacid
      - * Radiation to back or either upper quadrant of the abdomen
    - – Symptoms of obstruction
      - * Accentuated pain, not relieved by food
      - * Epigastric fullness, and vomiting of undigested food after meals

- Symptoms of perforation
  * Acute onset of epigastric pain, radiating to shoulder or right lower quadrant, sometimes with nausea and vomiting
  * Pain lessens after a few hours
- Symptoms of hemorrhage
  * Sudden onset of weakness, faintness, dizziness
  * Sudden onset of chills
  * Moist skin
  * Desire to defecate
  * Red or tarry stools
  * Hematemesis

- Gastric ulcers
  ▶ Symptoms may be atypical, vague, or absent.
    - Gnawing, burning, aching, pain described as "hunger pangs" referred to left subcostal region
      * Occurs 30 to 60 minutes after a meal or may be precipitated by a meal
      * In contrast to duodenal ulcer, antacids less consistently helpful in relieving symptoms
      * Nausea and vomiting are common
  ▶ Symptoms may come and go over time

Objective

- Epigastric tenderness and muscle guarding common with peptic ulcers
- Rigid abdomen, rebound tenderness, and initially hyperactive bowel sounds (progressing to hypoactive then absent), fever, leukocytosis, tachycardia (may be signs of perforation)
- Postural hypotension/tachycardia, mucosal pallor, and positive occult blood in stools may be signs of hemorrhage)

  NOTE: Anemia may be present, although considered a late sign

- Fetal tachycardia and abnormal fetal nonstress tests

Assessment

- Peptic ulcer disease, either duodenal or gastric ulcer
  ▶ R/O gastric ulcer or duodenal ulcer
  ▶ R/O reflux esophagitis

▶ R/O ulcer perforation

▶ R/O hemorrhage

▶ R/O gastritis

▶ R/O gastric carcinoma

▶ R/O irritable bowel syndrome

Plan

Diagnostic Tests

- Diagnosis is most often made on clinical findings.

- Routine endoscopy during pregnancy is usually unnecessary and should be postponed except in those clients who fail to respond to symptomatic management (Connon, 1994).

- Do not make the diagnosis of *H. pylori* with endoscopy during pregnancy; treatment is safest in the nonpregnant, nonnursing client (Michaletz-Onody, 1992).

- CBC to evaluate for anemia (a late sign), as indicated.

- Obtain stool occult blood tests, as indicated.

Treatment/Management

- Management can proceed from clinical findings except in individuals with suspicion of complication (bleeding, perforation, obstruction). Refer to physician.

- Nonsystemic treatment

  ▶ Antacids relieve pain discomfort by neutralizing acid, inactivating pepsin, binding bile salts and stimulation of gastric bicarbonate secretion.

  NOTE: There is no evidence that antacids are teratogenic although first trimester use of any drug should always be carefully weighed (Calhoun, 1992). Also, the liquid form of antacids is more effective than tablet form.

  – Aluminum hydroxide/magnesium hydroxide mixtures, 15 to 30 mL p.o. 2 hours after meals and at bedtime

    * Side effects

      • Aluminum can cause constipation, phosphate deficiency, and osteoporosis.

      • Magnesium can cause diarrhea and should not be used in clients with renal insufficiency.

      • Use combination preparations or alternate preparations to manage gastrointestinal symptoms.

  – Calcium carbonate, aluminum hydroxide, magnesium hydroxide mixtures, 15 to 30 mL p.o. 1 and 3 hours after meals and at bedtime

  NOTE: Calcium carbonate alone is not recommended because it induces gastric hypersecretion.

- Sodium bicarbonate is not recommended in treatment of peptic ulcer disease because of its high sodium content.

▶ Sucralfate is a mucosal protective agent that adheres to areas of duodenal and gastric ulcers. It is minimally systemically absorbed.

NOTE: Sucralfate is as effective with duodenal ulcers as antacids and H_2 antagonists.

- Dose: 1 g, 30 to 60 minutes p.o. before meals and at bedtime or 2 g, p.o. 30 to 60 minutes before breakfast and dinner.

NOTE: Antacids can be used concomitantly but not within 1 hour of sucralfate.

- Side effects

  * Constipation

  * Inhibits absorption of digoxin, tetracycline, phenytoin, cimetidine.

- Systemic treatment

  ▶ Consider a histamine H_2-receptor antagonist (cimetidine and ranitidine) in the client who is unresponsive to antacid therapy, if the benefits of use outweigh the risks.

  - Histamine H_2-receptor antagonists: potent inhibitors of basal and stimulated gastric acid secretion.

    * Cimetidine, 300 mg p.o. q.i.d., before meals and at bedtime *or* 400 mg p.o. b.i.d. *or* 800 mg p.o. daily after dinner.

      • Side effects can be the rare effects of galactorrhea, skin rashes, leukopenia, agranulocytosis, hepatitis, elevated serum creatinine, and interactions with warfarin, propranolol, benzodiazepines, phenytoin, theophylline compounds, and other drugs metabolized by hepatic microsomes (potentiates their effects) (Knauer, 1993). See the *PDR*.

    NOTE: Cimetidine inhibits gastric secretion stimulated by food, gastrin, histamine and caffeine. Avoid taking at same time as antacids; separate ingestion by at least 1 to 2 hours. In pregnancy, the recommendation is to maintain single daily dosing.

    * Ranitidine, 150 mg p.o. every 12 hours *or* 300 mg p.o. after dinner.

      • Side effects can be diarrhea, dyspepsia, loss of libido, dizziness, and mental confusion (Knauer, 1993).

    NOTE: Ranitidine is more potent than cimetidine and interferes less with other drugs.

  ▶ Pharmacologic treatment of *H. pylori* is *not* recommended in pregnancy and can usually be postponed until after delivery (Michaletz-Onody, 1992).

  ▶ Diet has not been shown to be a factor in the incidence or healing of ulcers (Knauer, 1993).

  ▶ Client should cease smoking and alcohol consumption.

  ▶ Client should discontinue or limit use of aspirin, NSAIDs, and steroids.

▶ Client should restrict caffeine intake, including coffee, tea, and cola beverages—regular or decaffeinated.

- Management by a physician is warranted in cases of obstruction, subacute bleeding and perforation.

- Hemorrhage and acute perforation constitute a medical emergency. Refer to an emergency service and physician.

Consultation

- Consult with the physician therapeutic management in clients with complicated disease unresponsive to antacids.

- Refer to a physician immediately those clients with cases of suspected obstruction, acute hemorrhage, or perforation.

Patient Education

- Explain the risk factors, chronic and recurrent nature of the disease, physiology, treatment regimes, and consequences of inadequate treatment.

- Advise clients not to take antacids with meals.

- Encourage client to get adequate rest and sleep.

- Advise client regarding a nutritious diet (see Section 18, *Nutrition*) and regular meal intake. A bland or milk diet is not necessary.

- Encourage limiting only those foods that cause discomfort (fatty foods, alcohol, chocolate, caffeine).

- Encourage small, frequent meals.

- Advise client to avoid eating immediately before bedtime, which may help eliminate nocturnal discomfort.

- Advise client to separate liquid ingestion from mealtime.

- Encourage client to restrict intake of coffee, tea, and cola beverages.

- Advise client to elevate the head of the bed at night with 6-inch blocks.

- Assist client to discontinue alcohol and smoking. Refer to appropriate support services if necessary (Alcoholic Anonymous, Nicotine Anonymous, and American Cancer Society, etc.).

- Assist client in finding stress reduction measures.

Follow-up

- Reevaluate client 4 to 6 weeks after initiation of treatment.

- Most duodenal ulcers heal in 4 to 6 weeks of treatment. Treatment of active disease for 4 to 8 weeks or until symptoms resolve. Then switch to maintenance therapy for another 4 to 8 weeks.

- After delivery, refer to a physician for endoscopy those clients

  ▶ Whose symptoms worsen during pregnancy

  ▶ With duodenal ulcers whose symptoms do not resolve after 4 to 6 weeks of therapy

  ▶ With gastric ulcers after 12 weeks of therapy to document healing and rule out gastric cancer

- Employ the American Cancer Society's recommendations for early detection of cancer in asymptomatic people (American Cancer Society (ACS), 1993):

  ▶ Sigmoidoscopy every 3 years beginning at age 50 years

  ▶ Stool guaiac yearly beginning at age 50 years

  ▶ Digital rectal examination yearly beginning at age 40 years

  NOTE: The ACS suggests a digital rectal examination of all women during their annual gynecological visit.

- Document in progress notes and problem list.

References

American Cancer Society (ACS). (1993). Summary of American Cancer Society recommendations for the early detection of cancer in asymptomatic people. Professional Education Publications. Philadelphia, PA: J.B. Lippincott.

Calhoun, B.C. (1992). Gastrointestinal disorders in pregnancy. *Obstetrics and Gynecology Clinics of North America 19*(4), 733–744.

Connon, J. (1994). Gastrointestinal Complications. In G.N. Burrow & T.F. Ferris (Eds.), *Medical complications during pregnancy* (4th ed.) (pp. 285-291). Philadelphia, PA: W.B. Saunders Company.

Cooke, D.M. (1991). Inflammatory bowel disease: Primary health care management of ulcerative colitis and Crohn's disease. *Nurse Practitioner, 16*(8), 27–39.

Goroll, A.H. (1995). Management of peptic ulcer disease. In A.H. Goroll, L.A. May, & A.G. Mulley (Eds.), *Primary care medicine* (3rd ed.) (pp. 382–392). Philadelphia, PA: J.B. Lippincott.

Hess, L.W., Morrison, J.C., & Hess, D.B. (1994). General medical disorders during pregnancy. In A. H. DeCherney & M. L. Pernoll (Eds.), *Current obstetric & gynecologic diagnosis and treatment* (8th ed.) (pp. 468–492). Norwalk, CT: Appleton & Lange.

Knauer, C.M. (1993). Alimentary tract. In L.M. Tierney, S.J. McPhee, M.A. Papadakis, & S.A. Schroeder (Eds.), *Current medical diagnosis and treatment* (8th ed.) (pp. 451–537). Norwalk, CT: Appleton & Lange.

Korelitz, B.I. (1992). Inflammatory bowel disease in pregnancy. *Gastroenterology Clinics of North America, 21*(4), 827–834.

Linn, F.V. & Peppercorn, M.A. (1992). Drug therapy for inflammatory bowel disease: Part 1. *The American Journal of Surgery, 164*, 85–89.

Mabie, W.C. (1992). Obstetric management of gastroenterologic complications of pregnancy. *Gastroenterology Clinics of North America, 21*(4) 923–935.

Medical Economics Data. (1998). *Physicians' Desk Reference* (52nd ed.). Montvale, NJ: Author.

Michaletz-Onody, P.A. (1992). Peptic ulcer disease in pregnancy. *Gastroenterology Clinics of North America, 21*(4), 817–826.

Niewiarowski, T., & Fisher, R.S. (1993). Effects of upper GI dysomotility in pregnancy. *Contemporary OB/GYN, 38*(2), 67–82.

Richter, J.M. (1995). Approach to the patient with heartburn and reflux. In A.H. Goroll, L.A. May, and A.G. Mulley (Eds.), *Primary care medicine* (3rd ed.) (pp. 344–348). Philadelphia, PA: J.B. Lippincott.

Ruymann, E.W., & Richter, J.M. (1995). Management of inflammatory bowel disease. In A. H. Goroll, L. A. May, & A. G. Mulley (Eds.), *Primary care medicine* (3rd. ed.) (pp. 416–425). Philadelphia, PA: J. B. Lippincott.

Torbey, C.F., Richter, J.E. (1995). Gastrointestinal motility disorders in pregnancy. *Seminars in Gastrointestinal Disease, 6*(4), 203–216.

Weeks, J.W., & Freeman, R.K. (1993). Inflammatory bowel disease in pregnant women. *Contemporary OB/GYN, 38*(4), 41–53.

West, L., Warren, J., & Cutts, T. (1992). Diagnosis and management of irritable bowel syndrome, constipation, and diarrhea in pregnancy. *Gastroenterology Clinics of North America, 21*(4), 793–801.

SECTION 9
HEMATOLOGIC CONDITIONS

Chapter 1

ABO INCOMPATIBILITY/IRREGULAR ANTIBODIES

Lisa L. Lommel

There are four major blood groups that belong to the ABO blood group system: A, B, AB, and O. Red blood cells have either antigen A (type A blood), antigen B (type B blood), antigen A and B (type AB blood), or no antigen (type O blood) on the surface of their cells. The antigens are all capable of inducing antibody production in an individual who does not have that antigen.

ABO Incompatibility

ABO incompatibility occurs in approximately 20 percent of all pregnancies. The majority of these cases are in blood group O mothers carrying a group A or B fetus. The group O mother has naturally occurring anti-A and anti-B antibodies in her blood that can adhere to fetal red blood cells causing hemolysis. Because anti-A and anti-B antibodies are derived from immunoglobulin M (IgM), which does not readily pass from mother to fetus, and because fetal red cells have a diminished number of A and B antigenic sites, fewer than 5 percent of ABO incompatible pregnancies actually develop hemolytic disease (Cunningham, MacDonald, Gant, Leveno & Gilstrap, 1993). ABO incompatibility provides partial protection to Rh (D) isoimmunization in the Rh (D)-negative woman. The mechanism is thought to involve the removal of fetal red blood cells from the maternal circulation at a faster rate in ABO-incompatible women, which lowers the effective dose of antigen (Duerbeck & Seeds, 1993). See Chapter 9.8, *Rh (D) Isoimmunization*.

There is no definitive diagnostic test available for prenatal diagnosis of ABO incompatibility. The direct Coombs test (neonatal antibody screen) may be positive or negative and maternal antibodies are variable. The usual criteria for diagnosis of hemolysis due to ABO incompatibility is accomplished in the post-natal period and include

1) the major blood group of the mother is O, with anti-A and anti-B in her serum, while the neonate is group A, B, or AB

2) the onset of neonatal jaundice within the first 24 hours after birth

3) anemia, reticulocytosis, and erythroblastosis of varying degrees, and

4) other causes of hemolysis have been excluded (Cunningham et al., 1993).

ABO incompatibility can manifest as a range of hemolytic disease, and there can be little laboratory evidence of red cell sensitization to severe disease. In most cases, it presents in the neonate within 24 hours after birth with jaundice and variable elevation of the indirect bilirubin. Management of ABO hemolytic disease in the newborn (HDN) includes bilirubin surveillance and phototherapy. Exchange transfusion is necessary in only 1 percent of cases and serious fetal sequelae are rare.

Irregular Antibodies

Irregular antibodies occur in 1 to 2 percent of all pregnancies and are responsible for approximately 2 percent of hemolytic disease in the newborn. Antenatal diagnosis for irregular antibodies is accomplished by an indirect Coombs test to screen for abnormal antibodies in maternal serum. The pathogenesis, management, and sequelae of HDN caused by irregular antibodies are similar to Rh erythroblastosis fetalis (see Chapter 9.8, *Rh (D) Isoimmunization*). Sources of sensitization are also similar to those of the Rh antigen (i.e., fetal blood and/or transfused blood). The major difference between irregular antibodies and Rh disease is the involvement of *both* IgG and IgM class antibodies. The IgG antibodies readily cross the placenta allowing fetal antigen to enter the maternal blood circulation resulting in varying degrees of erythroblastosis fetalis which can lead to fetal death. As mentioned above, since the IgM antibodies do not cross the placenta, they pose no threat to the fetus and require no follow-up. Also, unlike Rh disease, there is not prophylactic immune globulin to prevent isoimmunization to irregular antibodies (Moise, 1994). Table 9.1, Hemolytic Disease Due to Irregular Antibodies, outlines the known irregular antigens associated with HDN and the grade of severity of the disease caused by each antigen. Also, unlike Rh disease, there is no phophylactic immune globulin to prevent isoimmunization to irregular antibodies (Moise, 1994).

Database

Subjective

- ABO incompatibility
  - ▶ Asymptomatic
  - ▶ 40 to 50 percent of cases occur in primigravidas
  - ▶ History of ABO incompatibility in previous pregnancy with an 87 percent recurrence rate (Cunningham et al., 1993).
- Irregular antibodies
  - ▶ Asymptomatic
  - ▶ History of irregular antibody

Objective

- ABO incompatibility
  - ▶ Most often a blood type O mother
- Irregular antibodies
  - ▶ Positive antibody screen for irregular antibodies
  - ▶ If maternal screen is positive for antibody, capable of causing HDN, document presence or absence of antigen in father of the baby.

Assessment

- ABO incompatibility
  - ▶ Rh-positive or Rh-negative mother with ABO incompatibility

  NOTE: This assessment is usually made after delivery with neonatal presentation of HDN

- Irregular antibodies
  - ▶ Rh-positive or Rh-negative mother with irregular antibody with either
    - – Irregular antibody not proven to cause HDN
    - – Irregular antibody capable of causing HDN
      - * Father of baby negative or positive to the antigen

Plan

Diagnostic Tests

- Obtain blood type, Rh type, and antibody screen at first prenatal visit on all patients.
- No specific tests available to detect ABO incompatibility prenatally.
- If the initial antibody screen is negative in Rh-positive clients, a repeat antibody screen in later pregnancy is not usually recommended.
- Repeat antibody screen at 26 to 27 weeks' gestation in Rh-negative women.
- If antibody screen is positive, the antibody should be identified by the laboratory.
- Obtain blood type and screen for antigen in the father of the baby (if the woman is positive for an antibody capable of causing HDN).

Treatment/Management

- Women with antibodies not proven to cause HDN require no further management, except for type and crossmatch before delivery (compatible blood may be difficult to find).
- Women with HDN-causing antibodies and with partners who are antigen negative for that specific antibody, require no further management.
- Women with HDN-causing antibodies and fetuses whose fathers who are positive for the same specific antigens should be monitored by amniotic fluid analysis and *not* by indirect Coombs titers because Coombs titers do not always correlate with fetal status and neonatal outcome (American College of Obstetricans and Gynecologists [ACOG], 1990).

Consultation

- Refer to physician if client has irregular antibody capable of causing HDN and the father is positive for that specific antigen.

Patient Education

- If the mother is blood type O
  - ▶ Explain the etiology and risk of ABO incompatibility.

▶ Explain the process of HDN and treatment/management plans for the newborn after delivery.

● If the patient is antibody-screen positive

▶ Give her a card identifying her Rh type, blood type, and irregular antibody.

▶ Advise the patient to alert health care providers of her antibody status in the event of future pregnancies or blood transfusion.

▶ Explain the risks for the fetus and management plans for the pregnancy.

▶ Explain the importance of obtaining a screen from the father of the baby.

▶ Discuss the implications of a positive maternal and paternal antibody screen for subsequent pregnancies.

Follow-up

● Assure that the infant has adequate medical follow-up after delivery.

● Document the presence of irregular antibodies amd Rh status in progress notes and problem list.

Table 9.1

Hemolytic Disease Due to Irregular Antibodies

Blood Group System	Antigens Related to Hemolytic Disease	Severity of Hemolytic Disease	Proposed Management
Lewis		Not a proved cause of hemolytic disease of the newborn	
I		Not a proved cause of hemolytic disease of the newborn	
Kell	K	Mild to severe with hydrops fetalis	Amniotic fluid bilirubin studies
	k	Mild	Expectant
	Ko	Mild	Expectant
	Kp^a	Mild	Expectant
	Kp^b	Mild	Expectant
	Js^a	Mild	Expectant
	Js^b	Mild	Expectant
Duffy	Fy^a	Mild to severe with hydrops fetalis	Amniotic fluid bilirubin studies
	Fy^b	Not a cause of hemolytic disease of the newborn	
	Fy^3	Mild	Expectant
Kidd	Jk^a	Mild to severe	Amniotic fluid bilirubin studies
	Jk^b	Mild to severe	Amniotic fluid bilirubin studies
	Jk^3	Mild	Expectant
MNSs	M	Mild to severe	Amniotic fluid bilirubin studies
	N	Mild	Expectant
	S	Mild to severe	Amniotic fluid bilirubin studies
	s	Mild to severe	Amniotic fluid bilirubin studies
	U	Mild to severe	Amniotic fluid bilirubin studies
	Mi^a	Moderate	Amniotic fluid bilirubin studies
	Mt^a	Moderate	Amniotic fluid bilirubin studies
	Vw	Mild	Expectant
	Mur	Mild	Expectant
	Hut	Mild	Expectant
Lutheran	Lu^a	Mild	Expectant
	Lu^b	Mild	Expectant
Diego	Di^a	Mild to severe	Amniotic fluid bilirubin studies
	Di^b	Mild to severe	Amniotic fluid bilirubin studies
Xg	Xg^a	Mild	Expectant
P	$PP_1P^k(Tj^a)$	Mild to severe	Amniotic fluid bilirubin studies
Public Antigens	Yt^a	Moderate to severe	Amniotic fluid bilirubin studies
	Yt^b	Mild	Expectant
	Lan	Mild	Expectant
	En^a	Moderate	Amniotic fluid bilirubin studies
	Ge	Mild	Expectant
	Jr^a	Mild	Expectant
	Co^a	Severe	Amniotic fluid bilirubin studies
	Co^{a-b-}	Mild	Expectant

(continued)

Hemolytic Disease Due to Irregular Antibodies (continued)

Blood Group System	Antigens Related to Hemolytic Disease	Severity of Hemolytic Disease	Proposed Management
Private antigens	Batty	Mild	Expectant
	Becker	Mild	Expectant
	Berrens	Mild	Expectant
	Biles	Moderate	Amniotic fluid bilirubin studies
	Evans	Mild	Expectant
	Golzales	Mild	Expectant
	Good	Severe	Amniotic fluid bilirubin studies
	Heibel	Moderate	Amniotic fluid bilirubin studies
	Hunt	Mild	Expectant
	Jobbins	Mild	Expectant
	Radin	Moderate	Amniotic fluid bilirubin studies
	Rm	Mild	Expectant
	Ven	Mild	Expectant
	Wright[a]	Severe	Amniotic fluid bilirubin studies
	Wright[b]	Mild	Expectant
	Zd	Moderate	Amniotic fluid bilirubin studies

Source: Weinstein, L. (1982). Irregular antibodies causing hemolytic disease of the newborn: A continuing problem. *Clinical Obstetrics and Gynecology*, *25* (2), 321–329. Reprinted with permission.

References

American College of Obstetricians and Gynecologists (ACOG), Committee on Obstetrics: Maternal and Fetal Medicine (1990). *Management of isoimmunization in pregnancy* (Technical Bulletin Number 148). Washington, DC: Author.

Cunningham, F.G., MacDonald, P.C., Gant, N.F., Leveno, K.J., & Gilstrap, L.C. (1993). *Williams Obstetrics* (19th Ed.) pp. 1004–1013. Norwalk, CT: Appleton & Lange.

Duerbeck, N.B. & Seeds, J.W. (1993). Rhesus immunization in pregnancy: A review. *Obstetrical and Gynecological Survey, 48*(12), 801–810.

Moise, K.J. (1994). Changing trends in the management of red blood cell alloimmunization in pregnancy. *Archives of Pathology and Laboratory Medicine, 118,* 421–428.

Pernoll, M.L. (1994). Late pregnancy complications. In A.H. DeCherney & M.L. Pernoll (Eds.) *Current Obstetric and Gynecologic Diagnosis and Treatment* (pp. 331–343). Norwalk, CT: Appleton & Lange.

Weinstein, L. (1982). Irregular antibodies causing hemolytic disease of the newborn: A continuing problem. Clinical Obsterics and Gynecology, 25(2), 321–329.

CHAPTER 2

ALPHA THALASSEMIA

Winifred L. Star

The thalassemias are a "heterogeneous group of inherited disorders of hemoglobin synthesis characterized by absent or diminished synthesis of one or the other of the globin chains of hemoglobin A" (Nathan, 1992, p. 205). The major normal adult hemoglobin (Hb), Hb A, is made up of two alpha and two beta globin chains. Minor adult hemoglobin, Hb A_2, is composed of two alpha and two delta globin chains. A small percentage of adult hemoglobin is Hb F or fetal hemoglobin, which is composed of two alpha and two gamma globin chains. Normally, a person has four functioning alpha globin genes, two beta globin genes, two delta globin genes, and four gamma globin genes (Nathan, 1992).

Alpha thalassemia syndromes are genetic disorders affecting the production of the alpha globin chains of normal hemoglobin (most often due to deletions, although point mutations also exist) (Globin Gene Disorder Working Party, 1994). There are four possible states resulting from reduced (alpha$^+$ thalassemia) or absent (alpha^0 thalassemia) globin chain production: (1) silent carrier state (1-gene deletion, alpha thalassemia 2), (2) alpha thalassemia minor (or alpha thalassemia trait) (2-gene deletion, alpha thalassemia 1), (3) Hb H disease (3-gene deletion), or (4) alpha thalassemia major (4-gene deletion). The clinical picture of alpha thalassemia is defined by the number of genes deleted (Stein, Berg, Jones, & Detter, 1984).

The silent carrier state is undetectable without specialized DNA studies; there is no existing clinical or hematologic abnormality in this state. Individuals with alpha thalassemia trait have benign, lifelong, mild microcytic, hypochromic anemia with no clinical disease. Alpha thalassemia trait may coexist with a beta globin chain abnormality without adversely affecting (and occasionally improving) the clinical picture (e.g., alpha thalassemia trait/beta thalassemia trait).

Hemoglobin H disease results in a chronic mild to moderate hemolytic anemia with high levels of Hb H (four beta chains) and Hb Bart's (four gamma chains). Complications such as splenomegaly, gallstones, increased risk for infection, jaundice, and leg ulcers may develop if the anemia worsens. Also, pregnancy may worsen the anemia and increase complications. Transfusions may be indicated in severely anemic states (State of California Department of Health Services & Children's Hospital, Oakland, 1992).

In alpha thalassemia major, no alpha globin chains of hemoglobin are produced; thus a fetus cannot make Hb F or normal adult hemoglobin, resulting in the production of Hb Bart's (four gamma chains) and lethal hydrops fetalis (Maberry, Klein, Boehm, Warren, & Gilstrap, 1990) (although there have been rare reports of short-term survival with this condition [Beaudry et al., 1986; Bianchi et al., 1986]). Serious obstetrical complications may arise in a woman carrying an affected fetus: anemia, spontaneous abortion, premature labor, pregnancy induced hypertension, polyhydramnios, placenta previa, abruptio placentae, intrauterine fetal demise, congestive heart failure, and postpartum hemorrhage (Hsia, 1991; Maberry et al., 1990; Stein et al., 1984). Fetuses become severely anemic and have progressive edema; they are usually stillborn or die soon after birth (Stein et al., 1984).

Asians with alpha thalassemia trait have two missing genes on the same chromosome, whereas blacks most commonly have the missing genes on different chromosomes. Because of the location of the gene deletions in blacks, Hb H disease is very rare and alpha thalassemia major has yet to be documented in this population (Fischel-Ghodsian, 1990; Kazazian Jr., 1990). Asians, however, are at risk of producing offspring with serious alpha thalassemia disorders, as described above. This becomes significant for preconceptional counseling and screening during pregnancy.

Less commonly, alpha thalassemia is a result of *nondeletional defects* (mainly point mutations). An important form of nondeletional alpha thalassemia is associated with the hemoglobin variant, Hb Constant Spring, commonly found in southeast Asia (Hill, 1992). When this hemoglobin is inherited with 2-gene deletion alpha thalassemia, Hb H disease can result (Fishleder, 1992).

Countries in which alpha thalassemia is prevalent include China, the Philippines, Malaysia, Thailand, Cambodia, Laos, Vietnam, Myanmar (Burma), India, Sri Lanka, and Indonesia. African and American blacks, Middle Easterners, and Native Americans also may have certain forms of alpha thalassemia. Obstetrical care of women from these different ethnic groups should be culturally appropriate, utilizing interpreters when necessary and as available.

Database

Subjective

- Descendant of population at risk for alpha thalassemia syndromes.

- May be aware of abnormal laboratory results or anemia in the past or provide history of alpha thalassemia trait.

- Client is asymptomatic in alpha thalassemia trait or silent carrier state. An estimated 25 to 30 percent of African-Americans are silent carriers and 3 percent have alpha thalassemia trait (Kazazian Jr., 1990).

- With Hb H disease, client may have fatigue and general discomfort or complaints related to hepatosplenomegaly and/or gallstones or may have characteristic thalassemia facies resulting from bone marrow expansion. Transfusion history or history of splenectomy may be obtained in some individuals with Hb H disease. Disorder is mild in blacks and very rarely seen in this population.

- Complete family, medical, and pregnancy history is important.

Objective (See Table 9.2, Laboratory Values in Selected Anemias or Hemoglobinopathies.)

- Silent carrier state

  ▶ No clinical signs. Generally cannot be detected by routine laboratory tests; gene mapping leads to definitive diagnosis

  ▶ Mean corpuscular volume (MCV) may be 78–80 fL, or in normal range

  ▶ Mean corpuscular hemoglobin (MCH) may be borderline low; all other laboratory parameters within normal limits

- Alpha thalassemia trait

  ▶ Hb normal or decreased

  ▶ Red blood cell (RBC) count normal or increased

  ▶ MCV less than 80 fL (70–75 fL range)

- ▶ MCH less than 26 pg (mean 22 pg)
- ▶ Mean corpuscular hemoglobin concentration (MCHC) around 31 gm/dL
- ▶ Mentzer index (MVC/RBC) usually less than 13
- ▶ Hemoglobin electrophoresis
  - – Hb A, Hb A2, and Hb F normal unless there is concomitant beta globin chain abnormality or Hb H disease
    - – Hb Constant Spring may also be seen
- ▶ Red cell morphology shows microcytosis, hypochromia, anisocytosis, poikilocytosis
- ▶ Iron studies within normal limits unless coexistent iron deficiency
- Hemoglobin H Disease
  - ▶ Hb 7–10 gm/dL range
  - ▶ MCV less than 80 fL
  - ▶ MCH less than 26 pg
  - ▶ Reticulocytes 5 to 10 percent
  - ▶ Peripheral blood smear shows small misshapen red cells, microcytosis, hypochromia, and targeting
  - ▶ Hemoglobin electrophoresis (of fresh blood) shows 5 to 30 percent Hb H (or when blood incubated with brilliant cresyl blue (BCB) stain, multiple small inclusions form in the red cell); Hb A2 decreased; Hb Bart's may be present in small amounts
- Alpha thalassemia major
  - ▶ Hb Bart's, small amounts of Hb H and Hb Portland
  - ▶ Generally incompatible with life
- Other hemoglobin variants
  - ▶ Alpha thalassemia trait can be associated with any beta chain variant.
    - – Sickle cell/alpha thalassemia trait—electrophoresis shows Hb AS but percent of S less than usual; MCV decreased.
    - – Additional beta chain variants associated with alpha thalassemia include beta thalassemia trait, Hb C, Hb E, and Hb J Bangkok.

    NOTE: The clinical picture of Hb H with Hb E trait or Hb S trait is similar to Hb H disease alone (Wintrobe, 1981).

Assessment

- Alpha thalassemia trait
- Hb H disease
  - ▶ R/O coexistent iron deficiency anemia

▶ R/O concomitant hemoglobinopathy

▶ R/O hemoglobinopathy in father of baby

Plan

Diagnostic Tests

- See Figure 9.1, Evaluation for Anemia/Hemoglobinopathies.

- Maternal diagnostic tests include

  ▶ Complete blood count (CBC) with RBC indices

  ▶ Hemoglobin electrophoresis with quantitative A_2 and F, as indicated

  ▶ Serum iron, serum ferritin, transferrin saturation as indicated

  NOTE: The diagnosis of alpha thalassemia is one of exclusion of the microcytic anemias; HbA_2, HbF, and iron studies are within normal limits. Serum iron less than 30 $\mu g/dL$, serum ferritin less than 12 $\mu g/dL$, and transferrin saturation less than 15 percent are indicative of iron deficiency (American College of Obstetricians and Gynecologists [ACOG], 1993). Confirmation and precise definition of alpha thalassemia trait can only be done by DNA analysis (Fischel-Ghodsian, 1990).

- The use of a BCB dye study on freshly drawn blood may be used to confirm the diagnosis of Hb H disease.

  NOTE: Hb H is a very unstable hemoglobin and precipitates rapidly; therefore electrophoresis and dye study must be done quickly on fresh blood samples. Laboratories may require advance notice to allow for appropriate set-up. Presence of a beta chain abnormality reduces sensitivity of BCB study (Stein et al., 1984).

- If client is not black or of mixed ancestry and has alpha thalassemia trait or Hb H disease, offer laboratory screen for father of baby (CBC and hemoglobin electrophoresis with quantitative A_2 and F). Partner screening is usually accepted when couple understands potential risks to the pregnancy. Discuss possibility of nonpaternity prior to the tests being performed.

- DNA analysis is available for prenatal diagnosis; the technique used depends on which hemoglobin is being sought and laboratory capabilities (ACOG, 1993; Kazazian Jr., 1990). Fetal DNA may be obtained via chorionic villus sampling (CVS), amniocentesis, or percutaneous umbilical cord blood sampling (PUBS).

  NOTE: Alpha thalassemia major is most common among individuals of Asian descent and is quite rare outside this ethnic group. Prenatal diagnosis is generally offered to Asian couples when both members have alpha thalassemia trait since most of these couples have a 25 percent risk of a fetus with alpha thalassemia major. Most couples do not pursue prenatal diagnosis for Hb H disease because the condition is not perceived to be severe enough to justify elective abortion (Fischel-Ghodsian, 1990; Kazazian Jr., 1990). Prenatal diagnostic techniques are generally discussed with client/couple by genetic counselor.

- Cord-blood electrophoresis and newborn screening tests are also used to diagnose neonatal hemoglobinopathies. In some states, hemoglobin testing is part of routine newborn screening.

Treatment/Management

- Ideally, identification of alpha thalassemia occurs preconceptionally in the primary care setting. Thus, inappropriate therapy is avoided (i.e., administering unnecessary iron), counseling about the disorder can take place, and partner screening can be offered.

- There is no treatment for silent carrier state or alpha thalassemia trait. Prenatal care generally proceeds as with an unaffected client.

- Routine iron supplementation (physiologic doses) may be provided. No active intervention is needed to increase Hb concentration if it remains in the range expected for this type of thalassemia (White et al., 1985). If iron deficiency anemia is diagnosed, treat according to guidelines in Chapter 9.3, *Anemia—Iron, Folate, and Vitamin B$_{12}$ Deficiency*.

- With Hb H disease, anemia usually worsens in pregnancy (Hb may decrease to 4–5 gm/dL); therefore transfusion may be necessary in some cases. Consult with physician if anemia becomes severe.

- If client and partner have been diagnosed with alpha thalassemia trait and there is risk of alpha thalassemia major in the fetus, prompt referral to a genetic counselor is indicated. In nonblack couples, if mother of the baby has alpha thalassemia trait and baby's father is unavailable for or declines screening, referral is also in order.

  NOTE: In the black population, because of the chromosomal location of the absent genes in alpha thalassemia trait, there has yet to be a documented case of alpha thalassemia major in the offspring when both parents have the trait.

- Management of a pregnancy in which it has been established that the fetus has alpha thalassemia major and a decision has been made to continue the pregnancy will not be covered in this chapter. This is a high-risk situation and the patient should be referred to a perinatologist or obstetrician.

Consultation

- None required in alpha thalassemia trait with mild anemia. Consult with a physician for severe anemia. Consider physician referral or co-management in these cases.

- Consultation is advised for Hb H disease; consider referral to or co-management with obstetrician, especially if anemia worsens during pregnancy.

- Consultation with a hematologist may be indicated for severe anemia or for assessment of complicated or confusing laboratory results.

- Refer to a genetic counselor in cases where both client and partner have alpha thalassemia trait and the pregnancy is at risk. Genetic consultation is also in order if the mother has been diagnosed with the trait and the baby's father is unavailable for or has declined screening.

- In the rare case that a couple decides to continue a pregnancy complicated by a fetus with alpha thalassemia major, client should be referred to an obstetrician or perinatologist for care.

Patient Education

- Discuss the function of hemoglobin and the benign nature of alpha thalassemia *trait*. Clarify differences between alpha thalassemia trait, Hb H disease, and alpha thalassemia major. Utilize patient education materials if available.

- Educate clients that they cannot presume the father of the baby does not have a hemoglobin disorder merely because he is "healthy" or has had "blood tests that were normal." Documentation of laboratory results (i.e., CBC and hemoglobin electrophoresis with quantitative A_2 and F) on the baby's father is necessary for accurate and specific education regarding prenatal risk if the mother of baby has a hemoglobin disorder.

- Discuss prenatal implications if both members of a (nonblack) couple have alpha thalassemia trait: Most often there is a 25 percent chance that fetus will have alpha thalassemia major (generally incompatible with life), 25 percent chance for a normal fetus, and 50 percent chance for a fetus with alpha thalassemia trait.

- Discuss other possible combinations for the offspring as indicated. In general

  ▸ Silent carrier x normal → normal (50 percent) and silent carrier (50 percent) (silent carrier state not generally detectable by ordinary laboratory tests)

  ▸ Silent carrier x trait → trait (25 percent), normal (25 percent), Hb H (25 percent), silent carrier (25 percent) (silent carrier state not generally detectable by ordinary laboratory tests).

  ▸ Trait x normal → trait (50 percent), normal (50 percent) (Nathan, 1992)

  NOTE: A fetus may be at risk for Hb H disease if one parent has alpha thalassemia trait and the other has apparently normal hemoglobin because the presence of silent carrier state cannot be ruled out in the normal partner unless gene mapping studies are done. In addition, a small number of nonblacks with alpha thalassemia trait have the same deletion pattern as blacks (i.e., gene deletion on opposite chromosomes); thus the above recurrence risks may not always hold true. Risk for other hemoglobin variants in offspring may exist, depending on parent's types. Education and counseling must be individualized based on case presentation, and, in most instances, will be undertaken by the genetic counselor.

- Explore pros and cons of prenatal diagnosis fully with the couple if the pregnancy is at risk. Generally, specifics will be provided by the genetic counselor; a joint appointment with obstetrical care provider and counselor may be appropriate.

- Give reassurance that Hb H disease in an offspring will be mild enough that prenatal diagnosis is unwarranted. However, if the couple has had a child with severe Hb disease and wants to avoid birth of another child with this condition, prenatal diagnosis should not be denied (Fischel-Ghodsian, 1990).

- Obstetrical risks to the woman carrying an affected fetus should be outlined (see Introduction). Pregnancy should be managed by a physician.

- If severe anemia develops, the physician responsible for her care should discuss the possible need for blood transfusion with client.

Follow-up

- Ensure prompt appointment with a genetic counselor if both members of the couple have alpha thalassemia trait (or other significant hemoglobin variants) and the pregnancy is at risk. Also advise genetic counseling if mother of baby has a hemoglobin disorder and father of baby is unavailable for or declines screening, or when client/couple desire(s) comprehensive education about hemoglobinopathies, even if there is no significant risk to the offspring.

- If fetus has been diagnosed with alpha thalassemia major, review postdiagnosis options carefully to enable couple to make an informed decision regarding the pregnancy (i.e., termination or preparation for an affected child). Specifics usually are provided by the genetic counselor. Pregnancy termination is sought in a majority of cases where fetus has alpha thalassemia major; rarely, some couples may choose to continue the pregnancy. In this case, client should be referred to an obstetrician or perinatologist for care. Prenatal referral to a hematologist and/or pediatrician to discuss neonatal interventions may also be appropriate.

- Provide ongoing emotional support for a client/couple facing the birth of a child with a significant hemoglobinopathy. Refer to social services and community resources, if indicated.

- If prenatal testing reveals that the fetus does not have a significant hemoglobin disorder, educate the couple so they understand that this does not mean the baby will be "perfect." The risk of birth defects in the general population is about 2 to 4 percent.

- Newborn screening is indicated for at-risk pregnancies. Consult your state's protocols regarding initial screening and recommended follow-up.

- Advise the client to make note of her hemoglobin disorder and alert future health care providers of this history. Preconception counseling is indicated for women with hemoglobinopathies to provide information on risks associated with the specific disorder during pregnancy, including maternal morbidity, perinatal loss, and effects of treatment that may be indicated. In addition, preconceptional counseling for future pregnancies is indicated in the event a client has a different partner.

- Document diagnosis of hemoglobin disorder in client/partner in progress notes and problem list.

  ▶ Comment on fetal diagnosis, as indicated.

  ▶ Make note of any pregnancy complications.

  ▶ Also include in documentation whether partner was unavailable for/declined screening and the offering of genetic counseling.

Table 9.2

Laboratory Values in Selected Anemias or Hemoglobinopathies

Factor	Iron Deficiency Anemia	Folic Acid Deficiency Anemia	Alpha Thalassemia Trait	Beta Thalassemia Trait	Sickle Cell Trait (Hb As)	G6PD Deficiency
Hb	↓a	↓	↓	↓	N	↓*
Hct	↓a	↓	↓	↓	N	↓*
RBC	↓	↓	Nl or ↑	Nl or ↑	N	↓*
MCV	↓	↑	↓	↓	N	N
MCH	Nl or ↓	Nl or ↓	↓	↓	N	N
MCHC	N	Nl or ↓	↑	↓	N	N
Retic	Nl or ↓b	Nl or ↓c	↑	Nl or ↑	N	↑*
Iron/Ferritin	↓	N	Nl or ↑	Nl or ↑	N	N
Transferrin Saturation	< 15%	N	Nl or ↑	Nl or ↑	N	N
Other findings	Microcytosis, hypochromia, target cells may be present. Platelets may be ↑ or ↓. Hb A_2 may be ↓	Macrocytosis. Folate ↓. LDH ↑. Serum bilirubin ↑	Nl A, A_2 & F. Microcytosis, hypochromia, aniso/poikilocytosis. Hb Constant spring may be seen	Nl Hb A. Hb A_2 ↑. Hb F may be ↑. Microcytosis, hypochromia, aniso/poikilocytosis, target cells, basophilic stippling	Hb A & S. S = 30-40% (if HbS↓ may have alpha thalassemia or iron/folate deficiency). Hb A_2 may be ↑	Bilirubin ↑ in some variants. *during hemolysis

(CONTINUED)

a Follow onset of treatment, level should return to normal in 4-6 weeks, with increase beginning at 2 weeks.

b In severe cases reticulocytosis can be seen after 7-10 days of iron therapy.

c Reticulocytosis should be seen after 7 days of folate therapy.

Nl = normal   ↑ = increase or increased   ↓ = decrease or decreased

BCB = Brilliant cresyl blue

Table 9.2 (cont.)

Laboratory Values in Selected Anemias or Hemoglobinopathies

Factor	Hb C Trait (Hb AC)	Hb D Trait (Hb AD)	Hb E Trait (Hb AE)	Hb C Disease (Hb CC)	Hb E Disease (Hb EE)	Hb H Disease	Sickle Cell Disease (Hb SS)	Hb SC
Hb	NI	NI	NI or slight ↓	↓	Slight ↓	NI or ↓	↓	↓
Hct	NI	NI	NI or slight ↓	↓	Slight ↓	NI or ↓	↓	↓
RBC	NI	NI	Slight ↑	Shortened life span	Slight ↑	NI or ↓	Shortened life span	NI Indices
MCV	NI	NI	↓	↓	↓	↓	NI	NI
MCH	NI	NI	↓	NI or ↓	↓	↓	NI	NI
MCHC	NI	NI	NI	NI or ↓	NI or ↓	↓	NI	NI
Retic	NI	NI	NI	Slight ↑	NI	↑	↑	↑
Iron/Ferritin	NI	NI	NI	NI	NI	NI	NI	NI
Transferrin Saturation	NI	NI	NI	NI	NI	NI	NI	NI
Other findings	Hb C 30-50%, rest Hb A Hb A2 slight ↑ 10-30% target cells Negative solubility test	Hb A & D Normal smear Negative solubility test	Hb E 20-40%, rest Hb A Target cells	Hb A absent Hb C major fraction Hb F slight ↑ Occasional microcytosis, hypochromia Target cells >90% Hb crystals	Hb A absent Hb E 92-98% Hb F NI or ↑ Target cells microcytosis, leptocytosis, basophilic stippling	Hb H 5-30% Hb A2 ↓ Hb Bart's may be present Target cells Positive BCB prep	Hb S 80-90% Hb A absent, NI A2 Hb F 0-20% Poikilocytosis, anisocytosis, sickled & target cells, spherocytes, basophilic stippling, Howell-Jolly bodies, polychromasia, bilirubin ↑	Equal amounts Hb S & C Hb A absent Hb F NI or slight ↑ Target cells Rare sickled cells

NI = normal   BCB = Brilliant cresyl blue   ↑ = increase or increased   ↓ = decrease or decreased

SOURCE: Patterson, K.A. (1986). In J.D. Neeson & K.A. Mays (Eds.), *Comprehensive Maternity Nursing* (p.502). Philadelphia, PA: J. Lippincott Co. Adapted with permission.

Chapter 2

647

Figure 9.1

Evaluation for Anemia/Hemoglobinopathies

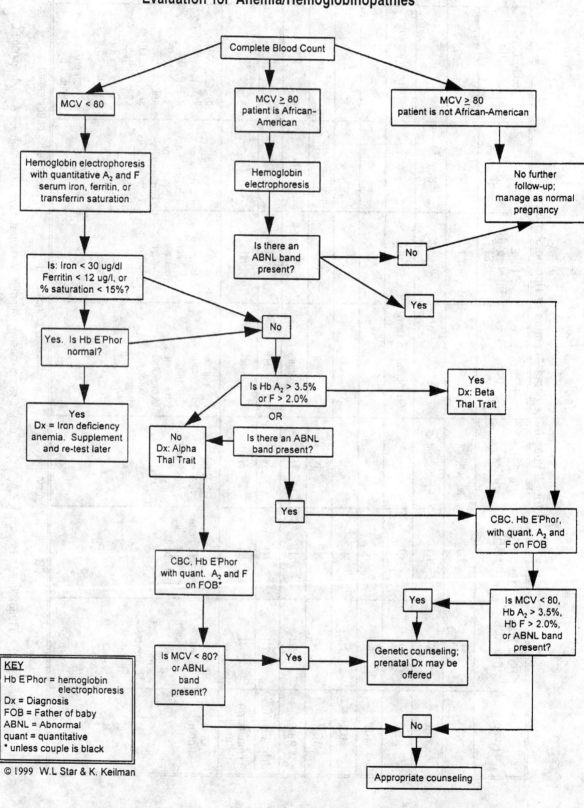

KEY
Hb E'Phor = hemoglobin electrophoresis
Dx = Diagnosis
FOB = Father of baby
ABNL = Abnormal
quant = quantitative
* unless couple is black

© 1999 W.L Star & K. Keilman

REFERENCES

American College of Obstetricians and Gynecologists (ACOG). (1993). *Hemoglobinopathies in pregnancy*. (Technical Bulletin No. 185). Washington, DC: Author.

Beaudry, M.A., Ferguson, D.J., Pearse, K., Yanofsky, R.A., Rubin, E.M., & Kan, Y.W. (1986). Survival of a hydropic infant with homozygous alpha-thalassemia-1. *The Journal of Pediatrics, 108*(5, Pt. 1), 713–716.

Bianchi, D.W., Beyer, E.C., Stark, A.R., Saffan, D., Sachs, B.P., & Wolfe, L. (1986). Normal long-term survival with alpha-thalassemia. *The Journal of Pediatrics, 108*(5, Pt. 1), 716–718.

Fischel-Ghodsian, N. (1990). Prenatal diagnosis of hemoglobinopathies. *Clinics in Perinatology, 17*(4), 811–828.

Fishleder, A.J. (1992). Prenatal hemoglobinopathy screening. *Journal of the American Medical Association, 268*(2), 266.

Globin Gene Disorder Working Party of the BCSH General Haematology Task Force. (1994). Guidelines for the fetal diagnosis of globin gene disorders. *Journal of Clinical Pathology, 47*, 199–204.

Hill, A.V.S. (1992). Molecular epidemiology of the thalassemias (including haemoglobin E). *Baillière's Clinical Haematology, 5*(1), 209–238.

Hsia, Y.E. (1991). Detection and prevention of important alpha-thalassemia variants. *Seminars in Perinatology, 15*(1, Suppl. 1), 35–42.

Kazazian, H.H. Jr. (1990). The thalassemia syndromes: Molecular basis and prenatal diagnosis in 1990. *Seminars in Hematology, 27*(3), 209–228.

Maberry, M.C., Klein, V.R., Boehm, C., Warren, T.C., & Gilstrap, L.C. (1990). Alpha thalassemia: Prenatal diagnosis and neonatal implications. *American Journal of Perinatology, 7*(4), 356–358.

Nathan, D.G. (1992). The thalassemias. In W.S. Beck (Ed.), *Hematology* (5th ed., pp. 205–222). Cambridge, MA: The MIT Press.

State of California Department of Health Services, & Children's Hospital, Oakland. (1992). *Sickle cell educator/counselor training program: Course manual*. Berkeley, CA: State of California, Department of Health Services, Genetic Disease Branch.

Stein, J., Berg, C., Jones, J. ., & Detter, J. . (1984). A screening protocol for a prenatal population at risk for inherited hemoglobin disorders: Results of its application to a group of Southeast Asians and Blacks. *American Journal of Obstetrics and Gynecology, 150*(4), 333–341.

White, J. ., Richards, R., Byrne, M., Buchanan, T., White, Y.S. ., & Jelenski, G. (1985). Thalassemia trait and pregnancy. *Journal of Clinical Pathology, 38*, 810–817.

Wintrobe, M. (1981). The thalassemias and related disorders: Quantitative disorders of hemoglobin synthesis. In M. Wintrobe (Ed.), *Clinical hematology* (8th ed., pp. 869–894). Philadelphia, PA: Lea & Febiger.

Chapter 3

ANEMIA—IRON, FOLATE, AND VITAMIN B$_{12}$ DEFICIENCY

Winifred L. Star

A brief explanation of the physiological effects of pregnancy on blood volume is helpful to the understanding of anemia. Hemodilutional effects of pregnancy account for normal lowering of hemoglobin and hematocrit values. Expansion of intravascular volume starts at 6 weeks' gestation, peaks at about 28 to 34 weeks, and plateaus until term. Red blood cell production increases at about 12 weeks and continues throughout pregnancy. Plasma volume expansion is faster and greater than red blood cell production with a resultant lowering of hemoglobin and hematocrit, a condition termed "physiological anemia." Because of individual variations in plasma volume expansion, true anemia during pregnancy is difficult to diagnose based on the hemoglobin and hematocrit values alone. (See Table 9.4, Normal Hemoglobin and Hematocrit During Pregnancy.)

Anemia exists when there is a decrease in the amount of hemoglobin necessary to maintain the normal requirements of tissues for oxygen (Harvey, 1980). It is precisely defined as a hemoglobin concentration more than two standard deviations below the mean for healthy women of the same age, sex, and stage of pregnancy (Institute of Medicine [IOM], 1990). The prevalence of anemia in pregnancy is relatively low in the United States but certain segments of the population may be at risk (e.g., adolescents, recent immigrants, those living in poverty) (Beard, 1994; IOM, 1993).

Iron deficiency anemia, the most common cause of true anemia during pregnancy, refers to anemia associated with laboratory evidence of iron depletion, based on the results of one or more tests (i.e., low serum ferritin, low transferrin saturation, or elevated erythrocyte protoporphyrin). National data suggest that less than 2 percent of nonpregnant women aged 20 to 44 years have iron deficiency anemia; the prevalence among pregnant women is unknown (U.S. Preventive Services Task Force, 1996). Causes of iron deficiency anemia include inadequate dietary intake, inadequate absorption of ingested iron due to low bioavailability or malabsorption syndromes, increased iron demands due to accelerated erythropoiesis, and acute/chronic blood loss (Engstrom & Sittler, 1994). Iron depletion generally progresses through three stages: 1) depletion of iron stores, 2) impaired hemoglobin production (iron deficiency without anemia), and 3) iron deficiency anemia (IOM, 1990). A number of pregnant women with iron deficiency anemia will have lower plasma volume expansions; thus, their hemoglobin/hematocrit values may remain in the normal range (Dimperio, 1988).

The status of pre-pregnant iron stores and the inadequacy of the average American diet contribute to an iron-deficient state in many women. Iron requirements are higher in gravidas with depleted stores at the onset of pregnancy (Hercberg & Galan, 1992). The total iron requirement during pregnancy is over 1000 mg, with the greatest need occurring during the second half (6 mg/day) due to increased red blood cell mass and the demands of the growing fetus. Blood loss during delivery and in the puerperium, in addition to iron loss through lactation, contribute to iron deficiency. Despite increased gastrointestinal absorption in the latter trimesters, an unsupplemented diet will not provide more than one to two thirds of the normal requirements for iron. The recommended dietary allowance (RDA) for iron during pregnancy is 30 mg/day* (Food and Nutrition Board, 1989). There is still debate over whether routine iron supplementation improves the outcome of pregnancy for mother or fetus (Beard, 1994). Infants of iron-

---

* Value as of this writing. The reader should check the most current RDA or Dietary Reference Intake (DRI) values.

deficient mothers appear to have lower cord-blood ferritin levels and may be at greater risk for developing iron deficiency later in infancy (Williams & Wheby, 1992).

The second leading cause of anemia and the major cause of megaloblastic anemia in pregnancy is folate deficiency, which is most likely to be revealed in late pregnancy or postpartum. Although the prevalence of folate deficiency among U.S. pregnant women has not been clearly determined, it is thought that two-thirds of anemic women are folate-deficient during pregnancy (Beck, 1992; IOM, 1990). Folate is particularly important for cell division and growth, and requirements increase during pregnancy and lactation. Low reserves of folic acid due to inadequate dietary intake prior to pregnancy and the increased daily requirements of this vitamin during pregnancy contribute to the deficiency (Bailey, 1990; Beck, 1992). In addition, any condition that creates a folate demand above normal requirements (e.g., multiple pregnancy, hemolytic anemia, infection, lactation) will add to the risk of folate deficiency anemia. Smoking, alcohol consumption, and specific types of drugs (e.g., anticonvulsants, oral contraceptives) may also impair folate status (Bailey, 1990; Beck, 1992). Folate deficiency may be associated with other vitamin deficiencies (e.g., vitamin B$_{12}$) and may also be caused by intestinal malabsorption. Overcooking contributes to the loss of folic acid from food; poor absorption of the vitamin is rare. The RDA for folate during pregnancy is 0.4 mg/day[*] (Food and Nutrition Board, 1989).

Folic acid supplementation has been shown to reduce the risk of neural tube defects. It is recommended that all women planning pregnancy take a daily multivitamin supplement containing folic acid at a dose of 0.4 to 0.8 mg, beginning at least one month prior to conception and continuing through the first trimester (Centers for Disease Control and Prevention [CDC], 1992; U.S. Preventive Services Task Force, 1996). A woman planning pregnancy who has had a previous pregnancy affected by a neural tube defect should begin folic acid supplementation at 4 mg/day (unless contraindicated) 1 to 3 months prior to conception and continuing through the first trimester; this regimen has been shown to reduce the recurrence risk of neural tube defects (CDC, 1991; U.S. Preventive Services Task Force, 1996). (See Treatment/Management section for further discussion.)

Anemia due to vitamin B$_{12}$ deficiency is usually due to abnormalities of gastrointestinal (GI) function as seen in older persons (e.g., malabsorption associated with inadequate production of intrinsic factor as in pernicious anemia, pancreatic insufficiency, and disorders of the ileum); thus, this deficiency is not an important cause of anemia during pregnancy (IOM, 1990; Nexo, Hansen, Rasmussen, Lindgren, & Grasbeck, 1994; Williams & Wheby, 1992). Dietary vitamin B$_{12}$ deficiency is very rare unless an individual has been following a strict vegetarian diet for many years. During pregnancy, there is a normal physiologic fall in serum B$_{12}$ concentration, which returns to normal by 6 weeks postpartum. Supplementation of the diet with B$_{12}$ does not prevent this fall in serum levels. Women who enter pregnancy with suboptimal animal protein intake may have significantly reduced B$_{12}$ stores, and, with increased fetal demands, B$_{12}$ deficiency could ensue (Metz, McGrath, Bennett, Hyland, & Bottiglieri, 1995). Pregnancy requirements for vitamin B$_{12}$ can be met easily by body stores or diets that contain modest amounts of animal proteins; vegetarian diets that include eggs, milk, and cheese provide adequate amounts for pregnancy. The RDA for vitamin B$_{12}$ during pregnancy is 2.2 µg[*] (Food and Nutrition Board, 1989).

Traditionally, it has been taught that maternal anemia is associated with suboptimal fetal outcome; however, data supporting this concept are scarce (Laros, 1994). Studies in industrialized countries have shown a two- to threefold increased risk of preterm delivery, low birth weight, and perinatal mortality in

---

[*] Value as of this writing. The reader should check the most current RDA or Dietary Reference Intake (DRI) values.

women with moderate to severe anemia (hemoglobin less than 9–10 g/dL) (Scholl & Hediger, 1994; U.S. Preventive Services Task Force, 1996). While profound maternal anemia can adversely affect the fetus, it appears that the "margin of safety" is large (Laros, 1994). Women with very severe anemia (i.e., hemoglobin less than 6–7 g/dL) are at risk for high output cardiac failure (Williams & Wheby, 1992). Normally expanded blood volume (i.e., third trimester hemodilution) is a good prognosticator of a low rate of adverse pregnancy outcomes (Scholl & Hediger, 1994).

Database

Subjective

- Inquire regarding ethnicity.

- Obtain complete medical, obstetrical, dietary, medication, habits, environmental, and family history.

- Ask about signs and symptoms of anemia and other medical problems that may cause anemia (see below).

  ▶ Risk factors for iron/vitamin deficiencies

    - Lower socioeconomic status

    - Underweight status

    - Adolescence

    - African-American, Hispanic, Native American, or Asian ethnicity

    - Multiparity

    - Closely spaced pregnancies (less than 2 years from birth to conception)

    - Multiple gestation

    - Cesarean section in prior pregnancy

    - Major surgery in last year

    - Chronic infectious process

    - Malabsorptive states

    - Blood loss (menstrual, GI, genitourinary [GU])

    - Parasitic infection (except pinworms)

    - Poor weight gain

    - Eating disorders

    - Bowel disorders

    - Inadequate nutritional intake, inadequate intake of supplements

    - Strict vegetarian diet

- Alcohol abuse, smoking
- Human immunodeficiency virus (HIV) infection
- Certain drugs

    * Anticonvulsants (e.g., phenytoin, primidone, phenobarbital)

    * Folic acid antagonists (e.g., trimethoprim)

    * Oral contraceptives

    * Barbiturates

    * Antacids and H$_2$ blockers

    * Nonsteroidal anti-inflammatory drugs (NSAIDs)

        NOTE: All the above medications may decrease folic acid absorption or affect metabolism.

    * Aspirin (may cause GI bleeding).

- Blood donation
- Long-distance running; intense, prolonged endurance training
- Personal or family history of anemia

▶ Obstetrical complications that may be associated with anemia

- Spontaneous abortion
- Intrauterine growth restriction
- Abruptio placentae
- Pregnancy induced hypertension, preeclampsia/eclampsia
- Neural tube defects
- Preterm delivery
- Stillbirth
- Low birth weight infants
- Neonatal death
- Delayed wound healing, decreased resistance to infection
- Postpartum hemorrhage

● Symptomatology: Client generally asymptomatic; with severe or rapid onset of anemia may complain of

▶ Fatigue, weakness, increased need for sleep

▶ Lightheadedness, vertigo, syncope

▶ Visual disturbances, headaches, tinnitus

▶ Mood changes, irritability, anxiety, confusion, forgetfulness, loss of concentration

▶ Cold intolerance

▶ Easy bruising

▶ Brittle nails; rough, dry skin

▶ Sore or beefy red, smooth tongue; dry mouth

▶ Anorexia, nausea/vomiting, heartburn, dyspepsia, dysphagia, abdominal pain, diarrhea

▶ Weight loss

▶ Pica (craving for ice, starch, clay, dirt, or type of food [i.e., brittle, crunchy])

▶ Epistaxis, hematemesis, melena, hematochezia

▶ Menorrhagia

▶ Exertional dyspnea, orthopnea, chest pain, palpitations, tachycardia

▶ Paresthesias—neurologic syndrome of vitamin B_{12} deficiency, consists of

  – Symmetric paresthesias in feet and fingers

  – Associated disturbances of vibratory sense and proprioception

  – Later, spastic ataxia (Beck, 1992; Nexo et al., 1994)

▶ Neuropsychiatric symptoms (Nexo et al., 1994)

  – Slow cerebration

  – Confusion or memory changes

  – Delirium

  – Depression

  – Acute psychotic states

  – Manic or schizophrenic states

NOTE: These symptoms are often the only sign of vitamin B_{12} deficiency (Nexo et al., 1994).

Objective

● See Table 9.2, Laboratory Values in Selected Anemias or Hemoglobinopathies, and Table 9.4, Normal Hemoglobin and Hematocrit During Pregnancy.

● Obtain height and weight. Calculate desirable body weight (DBW).

● Physical examination will usually be within normal limits (WNL), but may reveal one or more of the following if anemia is severe (Engstrom & Sittler, 1994):

  ▶ Vital signs

    – Orthostatic changes in blood pressure, pulse

    – Tachycardia

► Extremities/lymph nodes

- Mild cyanosis

- Peripheral edema

- Leg ulcers

- Lymphadenopathy

► Eyes

- Pale/jaundiced conjunctiva

- Papilledema

- Retinal hemorrhage

► Skin

- Pallor

- Slight jaundice

- Purpura

- Petechiae

- Spider angiomas

- Ulcers

► Hair

- Thin or split

- Brittle

- Graying

► Nails

- Brittle

- Ridging

- Koilonychia (spoon-shape)

► Mouth/lips

- Dry or cracked

- Cheilosis

- Glossitis

- Angular stomatitis

► Heart

- Tachycardia or gallop

- Systolic heart murmur

▶ Lungs

   – Crackles

▶ Abdomen

   – Hepatomegaly

   – Splenomegaly

   – Masses

   – Ascites

▶ Pelvis

   – Usually WNL for stage of pregnancy

   – Sources of bleeding from the genital tract should be assessed

▶ Rectum

   – Hemorrhoids

▶ Musculoskeletal

   – Tenderness over ribs, sternum, vertebrae

▶ Neurological

   – Loss of positional/vibratory sense

   – Positive Romberg

   – Gait changes

   – Peripheral neuropathy

● Normal laboratory values

NOTE: Values tend to vary from one laboratory to another. Values to follow are referenced from: Northern California Kaiser Permanente Regional Laboratory, the University of California San Francisco Laboratory; Rodak, 1995; and Tinkle, 1997).

▶ Hemoglobin (Hb):

   – For 12 to 15 years: 11.8–15.5 g/dL (118–155 g/L)

   – For 15+ years: 12.0-15.5 g/dL (120-155 g/L)

▶ Hematocrit (Hct): 36–46 percent

NOTE: Due to the physiologic hemodilution of pregnancy changes in Hb/Hct must be evaluated according to the week of gestation and trimester. Refer to Table 9.4, Normal Hemoglobin and Hematocrit During Pregnancy.

▶ Red blood cell (RBC) count: 4.0-5.2 x 10^{12}/ L

▶ Red cell indices

  – MCV

    * For 12 to 18 years, 78–98 fL

    * For 18+ years, 80–100 fL

  – MCH

    * For 12 to 18 years, 25–34 pg

    * For 18+ years, 26–34 pg

  – MCHC

    * For 12 to 18+ years, 310-360 g/L

▶ Reticulocytes: 0.5–2%; absolute count: 42–148 x 10^9/ L

▶ Ferritin: 4–161 µg/L

▶ Iron: 40–170 µg/dL (7–30 µmol/L)

▶ Iron binding capacity: 200–450 µg/dL (Massey, 1992)

▶ Transferrin: 216–399 mg/dL

▶ Transferrin saturation: 16–60 percent (ratio of serum iron to iron-binding capacity)

▶ Folate (serum): 2.7–21.0 ng/mL

▶ Folate, RBC: 238–756 µg/L (539–1717 nmol/L)

▶ Vitamin B$_{12}$: 209-961 ng/L (154–709 pmol/L); or 224–1300 pg/mL

▶ Free erythrocyte protoporphyrins (FEP): less than 35 µg/dL (less than 0.62 µmol/L whole blood)

▶ Hemoglobin electrophoresis

  – Hb A is 95 percent or more

  – Hb A$_2$ is less than 3.3 percent

  – Hb F is less than 2 percent

● Laboratory changes consistent with iron deficiency:

▶ Iron depletion

  – Normal hemoglobin/hematocrit

  – Serum iron normal or slightly decreased

  – Serum ferritin low

  – Transferrin saturation normal

▶ Iron deficiency without anemia

  – Normal (or near normal) hemoglobin/hematocrit

  – Serum iron and serum ferritin low

- – Transferrin saturation less than 16 percent
- – Free erythrocyte protoporphyrin elevated

▶ Iron-deficiency anemia

- – Hemoglobin/hematocrit low
- – Red blood cell count (RBC) decreased
- – Reticulocytes may be normal or low (in severe anemia, reticulocytosis can be seen after 7 to 10 days of iron therapy)
- – MCV less than 80 fL (usually between 70–79 fL) (microcytosis)
- – MCH less than 26 pg (hypochromia)
- – Serum iron low
- – Serum ferritin low (levels less than 12 µg/L)
- – Transferrin saturation less than 16 percent
- – Serum transferrin receptors increased
- – Iron-binding capacity increased
- – Free erythrocyte protoporphyrin elevated (also increased in lead poisoning or in infectious/inflammatory conditions of more than 1 week duration)
- – Platelets may be normal, decreased or increased
- – Peripheral red blood smear: microcytosis, hypochromia, polychromatophilia, basophilia, poikilocytosis, anisocytosis, and target cells
- – Red cell distribution width (RDW) increased
- – Serum bilirubin may be low

- Laboratory changes consistent with folate deficiency anemia:

▶ Hemoglobin/hematocrit decreased

▶ Serum folate and RBC folate decreased (less than 3 ng/mL and less than 160 ng/mL, respectively)

▶ MCV more than 96–100 fL

NOTE: Macrocytosis may be masked by iron deficiency or thalassemia; thus, the combination of microcytic and macrocytic anemias may yield a normal MCV.

▶ MCH 33–35 pg

▶ Hypersegmentation of polymorphonuclear leukocytes, ovalocytes, nucleated red cells, hypersegmentation of neutrophils

▶ Reticulocytes normal or decreased (reticulocytosis should be observed after 7 days of folate therapy)

- Laboratory changes consistent with vitamin B_{12} deficiency anemia:

▶ Hemoglobin/hematocrit decreased

▶ Serum B$_{12}$ decreased

▶ Serum folate usually elevated (unless there is coexisting folate deficiency)

▶ MCV greater than 96–100 fL

NOTE: Macrocytosis may be masked by iron deficiency or thalassemia; thus, combined microcytic and macrocytic anemia may yield normal MCV.

▶ MCH 33-35 pg

▶ Leukopenia and/or thrombocytopenia

▶ Granulocytes with multilobulated nuclei

▶ Reticulocytes decreased (abrupt reticulocytosis begins several days after the start of therapy)

▶ Serum methylmalonic acid (MMA) and hemocysteine (Hcy) levels may be elevated.

NOTE: MMA and Hcy are B$_{12}$ metabolites that increase in true, tissue B$_{12}$ deficiency. Check with local laboratory for normal values.

- Laboratory changes also secondary to megaloblastic anemia:

  ▶ Serum bilirubin—slight to moderate increases

  ▶ Serum LDH—marked elevation

  ▶ Serum potassium—occasionally decreased

  ▶ Serum uric acid—decreased

  ▶ Bone marrow examination shows megaloblastic changes

Assessment

- R/O iron deficiency anemia

- R/O folate and vitamin B$_{12}$ deficiency anemia

- R/O hemodilutional effect of pregnancy

- R/O thalassemia/concomitant hemoglobinopathy

- R/O other causes of anemia as indicated (e.g., G6PD deficiency, bone marrow failure, sideroblastic anemia, hemolytic diseases, blood loss [from GI/GU tract], acute/chronic infection, chronic disease, disorders of porphyrin/heme synthesis, malabsorptive syndromes, parasitic infection, endocrine abnormalities, drug-induced/inherited disorders of DNA synthesis, alcoholism)

- R/O hemoglobinopathy in father of baby, if indicated

Plan

Diagnostic Tests

- See Figure 9.1, Evaluation for Anemia/ Hemoglobinopathies

- Complete blood count (CBC) with RBC indices (at initial prenatal visit; repeat at 24 to 28 weeks). Hemoglobin and hematocrit may be used for screening in certain settings.

- Additional laboratory tests to evaluate iron status may include but not be limited to
  - ▶ Serum ferritin
  - ▶ Serum iron
  - ▶ Iron-binding capacity
  - ▶ Transferrin saturation
  - ▶ Erythrocyte protoporphyrin
  - ▶ Transferrin receptor concentration (a new indicator, may be available only in some laboratories)

NOTE: As of this writing, serum ferritin has the best sensitivity and specificity for diagnosing iron deficiency anemia. An overnight fast is recommended prior to drawing blood for iron or folate levels. Inflammatory processes may be responsible for increases in ferritin and erythrocyte protoporphyrin, and/or decreases in hemoglobin, serum iron, and transferrin saturation. The presence of at least two abnormal values among the various tests for iron deficiency improves the accuracy of the diagnosis (Hercberg & Galan, 1992; IOM, 1993). It is not cost-effective to order more than two to three tests to detect iron deficiency (IOM, 1993).

- Hemoglobin electrophoresis, as indicated
- If MCV greater than 80 fL, order serum folate or RBC folate (more accurate) and serum B_{12} to rule out folate or vitamin B_{12} deficiency

NOTE: Serum folate declines in normal pregnancy by about one-half that of prepregnancy values at term. Normal levels rule out folate deficiency as cause of anemia. Also, B_{12} levels normally decline during pregnancy (Williams & Wheby, 1992).

- Reticulocyte count, as indicated
- Additional tests that may be indicated to rule out hemolysis (Laros, 1994)
  - ▶ Direct Coombs' test
  - ▶ Osmotic fragility
  - ▶ Total bilirubin
  - ▶ G6PD
- Stool for occult blood should be obtained if GI bleeding is suspected as the cause for iron deficit; stool for ova and parasites may also be indicated.
- Urinalysis, as indicated.
- Bone marrow examination (via aspiration or biopsy) rarely indicated but may be helpful in evaluating severe macrocytic anemia
- Upper GI endoscopy is used for diagnosing gastric atrophy.

Treatment/Management

- See Table 9.5, Treatment/Management for Iron Deficiency Anemia in Pregnancy.
- Anemia should be diagnosed and treated as soon as possible (Scholl & Hediger, 1994). Goals of

therapy are to eliminate symptoms (if present), correct the deficiency, and replenish the stores (Lops, Hunter, & Dixon, 1995).

- Perform a thorough dietary history to screen for nutritional deficiencies. Refer client to nutritionist, as indicated. See Section 18, *Nutrition,* for information on multivitamin supplementation during pregnancy.

- Lower-income pregnant and lactating women who lack resources to purchase adequate food can be referred to the federal Supplemental Food Program for Women, Infants, and Children (WIC). Food stamp programs, and state programs may also be available to women who meet certain criteria. Refer client to social services, as indicated.

- Iron deficiency anemia

  ▶ For *prevention* of iron-deficiency anemia, 30 mg p.o. of elemental iron/day in the second and third trimesters is recommended (American College of Obstetricians and Gynecologists [ACOG], 1993; Niebyl, 1996). This dose is available separately or contained in prenatal vitamins. Iron doses are expressed in terms of elemental iron or in terms of the iron compound (IOM, 1993):

    – 30 mg elemental iron is equivalent to

      * 90 mg ferrous fumarate

      * 150 mg ferrous sulfate

      * 250 mg ferrous gluconate

    – 60 mg elemental iron is equivalent to

      * 180 mg ferrous fumarate

      * 300 mg ferrous sulfate

      * 500 mg ferrous gluconate

  NOTE: Support for the practice of routine iron supplementation is based on extrapolation from an incomplete database and evidence that it results in important clinical benefits in healthy pregnant women without anemia is limited (IOM, 1993; U.S Preventive Services Task Force, 1996).

  ▶ In the first trimester

    – If the hemoglobin is 11.0 g/dL or greater and ferritin is greater than 20 μg/L iron, supplementation is not indicated.

    – Prescribe 30 mg elemental iron/day when the hemoglobin is 9.0–10.9 g/dL and ferritin is 12–20 μg/L, or the hemoglobin is 11.0 g/dL or greater with ferritin 20 μg/L or less.

    – Prescribe 60 to 120 mg elemental iron/day when the hemoglobin is 9.0–10.9 g/dL and ferritin is less than 12 μg/L.

    – Obtain medical evaluation when hemoglobin is less than 9.0 g/dL or between 9.0–10.9 g/dL and ferritin is greater than 30 μg/L.

    – At subsequent visits evaluate hemoglobin. If there is no response to iron supplementation, refer client for additional medical evaluation. If hemoglobin is normal for that stage of pregnancy, lower the iron dose to 30 mg/day (IOM, 1993).

NOTE: The ferritin test is more precise in determining iron deficiency. In settings where it is impractical or too costly to perform, the Hb/Hct values can be used (IOM, 1993).

▶ In the second trimester

- Prescribe 30 mg elemental iron/day when the hemoglobin is 10.5 g/dL or greater with ferritin of 20 µg/L or less; if ferritin is greater than 20 µg/L, no treatment is needed.

- Prescribe 60 to 120 mg of elemental iron/day when the hemoglobin is 9.0–10.4 g/dL and ferritin is less than 12 µg/L.

- Obtain medical evaluation if hemoglobin is less than 9.0 g/dL (IOM, 1993).

NOTE: Serum ferritin concentration declines during the second trimester, but the measurement can be useful in assisting with the interpretation of the hemoglobin value (IOM, 1993).

▶ In the third trimester

- Prescribe 30 mg elemental iron/day when the hemoglobin is 11.0 g/dL or more.

- Prescribe 60 to 120 mg elemental iron/day when the hemoglobin is 9.0–10.9 g/dL.

- Obtain medical evaluation if hemoglobin is less than 9.0 g/dL (IOM, 1993).

NOTE: Iron deficiency anemia should *not* be treated with multiple doses of prenatal vitamins; rather, supplemental iron (as above) should be used (Engstrom & Sittler, 1994). Divided doses increase absorption. Also, certain minerals (e.g., calcium, magnesium) may significantly impair iron absorption; therefore, supplemental iron should not be ingested along with a prenatal vitamin/mineral tablet (Dimperio, 1988). If the source of supplemental iron is going to be a single daily vitamin/mineral tablet it is preferable to prescribe one that has no more than 250 mg of calcium and to select one with 60 mg iron (Allen, 1994; IOM, 1993).

▶ Iron supplementation may interfere with zinc absorption; thus, assessment of zinc status may be indicated. Rich food sources of zinc should be recommended: wheat germ, oysters, lobster, liver, meat, cheese, milk, nuts, peanut butter, whole wheat (Dimperio, 1988). When therapeutic iron doses (60-120 mg) are prescribed, a multivitamin/mineral supplement that contains 15 mg of zinc and 2 mg of copper is recommended (Allen, 1994; IOM, 1990).

▶ Parenteral iron therapy is rarely necessary. Indications include malabsorption, intolerance of oral intake or failure to take tablets, iron losses exceeding maximal oral replacement, inflammatory bowel/ulcer disease (Massey, 1992; Reich, 1984). Iron dextran is the available preparation. Consult with clinical pharmacist regarding dosage and administration.

● Folate deficiency anemia

▶ Folate deficiency anemia during pregnancy should be treated with oral folic acid supplementation; the recommended dosage is 1–2 mg/day (Williams & Wheby, 1992). Refer client to nutritionist for counseling.

▶ See the introduction for discussion regarding folic acid supplementation and prevention of neural tube defects. High intakes of folic acid (i.e., 4 mg/day) should be obtained from supplements containing only folic acid *not* from multiple doses of prenatal vitamins (1 mg folic acid tablets are available by prescription).

NOTE: Folate in excess of 1 mg/day may mask vitamin B_{12} deficiency and have adverse effects on individuals with untreated vitamin B_{12} deficiency (usually undiagnosed pernicious anemia). Effects include aggravation of parasthesias, numbness, ataxia and vibratory sense loss (Chanarin, 1994). Vitamin B$_{12}$ status should be assessed prior to initiating folate therapy (Bailey, 1992). Consult with a physician, if warranted.

- Vitamin B$_{12}$ deficiency anemia

  ▶ Vitamin B$_{12}$ deficiency can be prevented by a diet that contains animal protein. A strict vegetarian (especially if she has been one for more than 3 years without dietary animal sources) should probably take a vitamin supplement that contains vitamin B$_{12}$ (2.0 µg/day), and vitamin D (10 µg/day) and be supplemented with iron as above (Dimperio, 1988; IOM, 1990). Refer these individuals to a nutritionist for counseling during pregnancy.

  ▶ Clients with pernicious anemia or ileal disease should be followed by a physician. Details of management of these conditions are beyond the scope of this chapter.

Consultation

- Consult with a physician if the hemoglobin is less than 10.0 g/dL or hematocrit is less than 30%, or if client fails to respond to iron/vitamin supplementation.

- Manage women who are clearly iron and/or vitamin-deficient based on laboratory indices in consultation with a physician and nutritionist.

- Women with pernicious anemia or ileal disease should be managed by a physician.

- Consult with a hematologist when the laboratory picture is complicated or confusing.

Patient Education

- General

  ▶ Encourage good health maintenance, proper nutrition and good eating habits, and adequate weight gain during pregnancy. An individual's health beliefs need to be taken into account.

  ▶ Discuss implications of anemia and alert the client to signs and symptoms of iron/vitamin deficiency.

  ▶ Explain the goals of therapy in iron/vitamin-deficiency anemia (see Treatment/Management section). Advise that preventing or treating anemia helps reduce fatigue and increases ability to adapt to delivery (IOM, 1993).

  ▶ Provide information on nutrient-dense foods. Iron/vitamin supplements are used in conjunction with improvements in diet.

  ▶ Because some studies have indicated an increased risk of preterm delivery in anemic clients, ensure patient education regarding preterm labor signs and symptoms. See Chapter 6.25, *Preterm Labor.*

  ▶ Discuss the possibility of blood transfusion for clients with severe anemia who may require replacement during delivery or in the puerperium.

- Iron deficiency anemia

  ▶ Show how iron deficiency can be prevented by a diet that includes lean meat, poultry, fish, legumes, whole/enriched grains, cereals, nuts, dried fruit, and molasses. Food (especially acidic foods) cooked in iron pots take up iron from the pot (Gutierrez, 1994; Hercberg & Galan, 1992; IOM, 1993). See Section 18, *Nutrition,* for additional information.

▶ Discuss how best to take iron supplements (i.e., between meals or at bedtime with water or vitamin C-rich juice—not tea, coffee or milk). If not tolerated without food, iron may be taken with meat, fish, poultry, or vitamin C-rich foods.

NOTE: If 120 mg elemental iron/day is prescribed, recommend divided doses (60 mg p.o. b.i.d.) (IOM, 1993).

▶ Provide information on intake of substances that interfere with iron absorption (e.g., coffee, tea, carbonated beverages, whole grains, bran, oxalates [spinach], dairy/soy products, dried beans, egg yolk, certain minerals [zinc, calcium, magnesium, cadmium], starch/clay) (Gutierrez, 1994; Hercberg & Galan, 1992; IOM, 1993).

▶ Discuss side effects of iron supplementation, which are usually dose related: nausea, constipation, diarrhea, abdominal cramps, bloating, heartburn, black or tarry stool, skin rash, stained teeth from liquid iron (use straw, avoid swishing in mouth).

▶ For clients who are having difficulty tolerating iron supplements due to GI distress offer these suggestions:

  − Start slowly and build up to prescribed dosage.

  − Take with meals or at bedtime.

  − Crush tablet and blend with fruit drink.

  − Try enteric-coated, liquid, chewable or slow-release preparations (slow-release tablets are better absorbed with meals).

▶ Warn clients to keep iron in child-proof containers and out of reach of children!

● Folate deficiency anemia

▶ Advise that folic acid deficiency can be prevented by a diet rich in dark green vegetables, citrus fruit, liver, legumes, whole-grains, and fortified cereals. A well-balanced prenatal multivitamin supplement that contains 0.4-0.8 mg of folic acid can also be used (Food and Nutrition Board, 1989; Gutierrez, 1994; Lops et al., 1995). See Section 18, *Nutrition,* for additional information.

▶ Educate the client regarding the prevention of neural tube defects. See the Introduction.

● Vitamin B_{12} deficiency anemia

▶ Advise that vitamin B_{12} deficiency can be prevented by a diet that contains animal protein (see Section 18, *Nutrition*). Clients with pernicious anemia or ileal disease will be followed by a physician.

Follow-up

● Laboratory tests:

▶ As a general rule, order hemoglobin and hematocrit (or CBC) approximately one month after initiating therapy.

▶ Reticulocyte count may be ordered as indicated.

▶ Serum folate (or RBC folate) or serum B_{12} levels may be ordered several months after beginning therapy for folate or vitamin B$_{12}$ deficiencies, respectively. Consult with physician for additional tests that may be necessary.

▶ Offer laboratory screening (CBC and hemoglobin electrophoresis) for the father of the baby if mother has a hemoglobinopathy.

▶ Refer couple to genetics if there is evidence of a hemoglobinopathy in both members.

NOTE: Following onset of therapy for iron deficiency anemia, Hb/Hct should return to normal within 4 to 6 weeks, with the increase starting at 2 weeks. Repletion of iron stores may take 4 to 6 months (Massey, 1992; Williams & Wheby, 1992). Ideally, the end-point of iron therapy should be determined by serum ferritin, with oral iron discontinued when the value rises above 50 μg/L (Cook, 1994). Reticulocytosis will be apparent within 7 to 10 days of initiating therapy for iron, folate, and vitamin B$_{12}$ deficiencies. Four to five weeks of folic acid therapy will usually reverse folate deficiency anemia and replenish stores. Body stores of vitamin B$_{12}$ can hold up to a 3-year reserve (Goroll, May, & Mulley, 1995; Marin, 1995).

● Assess routine obstetrical parameters with an eye toward possible complications.

● Assess client's progress with recommendations for improved nutrition. Confer with nutritionist as needed.

● Carefully assess whether the woman is taking her supplements and if she is tolerating them. Provider should consider changing the form of iron (e.g., ferrous gluconate vs. ferrous sulfate; liquid or time-released form) to improve client tolerance, as indicated (Dimperio, 1988). A stool softener may be necessary for individuals with severe constipation (e.g., docusate sodium 100 to 200 mg p.o./day) (Niebyl, 1996).

● If the client is not responding to iron/vitamin therapy based on follow-up laboratory indices, *other causes of anemia must be ruled out!* Consult with a physician. Failure to respond to treatment may be due to incorrect diagnosis, failure to take supplement(s), continued loss of iron (usually due to blood loss), chronic infection or inflammatory condition, concurrent lead poisoning, undiagnosed thalassemia, malabsorption (rare) (Marin, 1995; Reich, 1984).

● Supplemental iron may be discontinued at the time of delivery unless iron deficiency anemia continued throughout the pregnancy or the woman is at high risk for iron deficiency. In these cases iron supplementation should continue for at least 4 to 6 weeks postpartum (IOM, 1993).

● Treatment for folate deficiency anemia should continue for several weeks after delivery (Williams & Wheby, 1992).

● Strict vegetarians may continue their vitamin supplement after delivery. Women with vitamin B$_{12}$ deficiency secondary to pernicious anemia or ileal disease should be followed by a physician.

● Women with risk factors for anemia (e.g., anemia continued throughout pregnancy, history of excessive blood loss during delivery, multiple births, etc.) should have laboratory tests to assess for anemia at the 6-week postpartum visit. Results are interpreted with same criteria as for nonpregnant women. See Table 9.6, Prevention & Treatment of Iron Deficiency Anemia in Nonpregnant Women.

● Continued good nutrition is important in the postpartum period. The prenatal multivitamin supplement may be continued if the diet is inadequate.

● Document anemia status and indicated therapy in progress notes and problem list.

Table 9.4

Normal Hemoglobin and Hematocrit During Pregnancy

Weeks gestation	Hemoglobin (g/dL)	Hematocrit (%)
12	11.0	33.0
16	10.6	32.0
20	10.5	32.0
24	10.5	32.0
28	10.7	32.0
32	11.0	33.0
36	11.4	34.0
40	11.9	36.0

Source: Centers for Disease Control and Prevention. (1989). CDC criteria for anemia in children and child-bearing women. *Morbidity and Mortality Weekly Report, 38*, 400–404.

Table 9.5

Treatment/Management for Iron Deficiency Anemia in Pregnancy

First Trimester

- If Hb ≥ 11.0 g/dL and ferritin >20 µg/L, no treatment needed.

- If Hb 9.0–10.9 g/dL and ferritin 12–20 µg/L *or* if Hb ≥ 11.0 g/dL and ferritin is ≤ 20 µg/L, prescribe 30 mg supplemental iron/day.

- If Hb 9.0–10.9 g/dL and ferritin is < 12 µg/L, prescribe 60–120 mg supplemental iron/day.

- Refer for medical evaluation if Hb < 9.0 g/dL *or* Hb 9.0–10.9 and ferritin is > 30 µg/L at initial visit.

- Evaluate Hb at subsequent visits. If WNL for stage of pregnancy, client may reduce iron to 30 mg/day. If no response, refer for medical evaluation.

Second Trimester

- If Hb ≥ 10.5 g/dL with ferritin ≤ 20 µg/L, prescribe 30 mg supplemental iron/day. If ferritin > 20 µg/L, no therapy needed.

- If Hb 9.0–10.4 g/dL and ferritin < 12 µg/L, prescribe 60–120 mg supplemental iron/day.

- Refer for medical evaluation if Hb < 9.0 g/dL.

Third Trimester

- If Hb ≥ 11.0 g/dL, prescribe 30 mg supplemental iron/day.

- If Hb 9.0-10.9 g/dL, prescribe 60–120 mg supplemental iron/day.

- Refer for medical evaluation if Hb < 9.0 g/dL.

Postpartum

- Supplemental iron may be discontinued at delivery (at 4–6 weeks postpartum if anemia continued throughout/after pregnancy or client at increased risk for iron deficiency).

- Screen women at high risk for iron deficiency at the 6-week postpartum visit (risk factors include anemia continued throughout pregnancy, excessive bleeding during delivery, and multiple births). Hb/Hct results are interpreted with same criteria as for nonpregnant women. See Table 9.6.

Source: Adapted with permission from *Iron deficiency anemia: Recommended guidelines for the prevention, detection, and management among U.S. children and women of childbearing age* (pp. 24–25). Copyright 1993 by the National Academy of Sciences. Courtesy of the National Academy Press, Washington, DC.

Table 9.6

Prevention & Treatment of Iron Deficiency Anemia in Nonpregnant Women

Prevention

- Most women do not require iron supplements.

- Woman who are planning a pregnancy and are at increased risk of iron deficiency can take an iron-folate combination supplement containing iron at about 30 mg and folate at 0.4 mg/day.

- In women with increased risk of nutrient deficiencies, consider a multivitamin-mineral supplement that contains about 30 mg of elemental iron.

Treatment

- If Hb is no more than 2 g/dL below the normal cutoff value (see below) treat with about 60 mg elemental iron b.i.d. (total daily dose 120 mg). Provide dietary advice.

- After 1 to 2 months recheck Hb/Hct. If no response is noted (i.e., an increase of at least 1.0 g/dL Hb or 3 percent Hct) check serum ferritin & consider other causes of anemia. (Anemia + ferritin of < 15 µg/L suggest iron deficiency.)

- If response has been noted, continue therapeutic iron dose for 2 to 4 months or until Hb is 12.0 g/dL. After that time iron dose may be reduced to about 30 mg/day for 6 months.

- A repeat serum ferritin within normal limits is recommended before terminating iron therapy to determine repletion of iron stores.

- Blacks may have slightly lower Hb levels (average of 0.8 g/dL less), thus may be incorrectly suspected of having iron deficiency anemia. In addition, normal Hb/Hct values need to be adjusted for altitude and cigarette smoking. See below.

- Severe anemia is unusual; if present, further evaluation is warranted!

Parameter	Non-smoker	10–20 cigarettes/day	21-40 cigarettes/day	Altitude > 5,000 ft
Hb (g/dL)	12.0	12.3	12.5	12.5
Hct (%)	36.0	37.0	37.5	37.5

Source: Adapted with permission from *Iron deficiency anemia: Recommended guidelines for the prevention, detection, and management among U.S. children and women of childbearing age* (pp. 22–23). Copyright 1993 by the National Academy of Sciences. Courtesy of the National Academy Press, Washington, DC.

REFERENCES

Allen, L.H. Nutritional supplementation for the pregnant woman. *Clinical Obstetrics and Gynecology, 37*(3), 587–595.

American College of Obstetricians and Gynecologists (ACOG). (1993). *Nutrition during pregnancy.* (Technical Bulletin No. 179). Washington, DC: ACOG.

Bailey, L.B. (1990). Folate status assessment. *Journal of Nutrition, 120,* 1508–1511.

Bailey, L.B. (1992). Evaluation of a new Recommended Dietary Allowance for folate. *Journal of the American Dietetic Association, 92,* 463–468.

Beard, J.L. (1994). Iron deficiency: assessment during pregnancy and its importance in pregnant adolescents. *American Journal of Clinical Nutrition, 59*(Suppl.), 502S–510S.

Beck, W.S. (1992). Megaloblastic anemias II. Folic acid deficiency. In W.S. Beck (Ed.), *Hematology* (5th ed., pp. 113–132). Cambridge, MA: The MIT Press.

Centers for Disease Control and Prevention (CDC). (1989). CDC criteria for anemia in children and child-bearing women. *Morbidity and Mortality Weekly Report, 38*(22), 400–404.

Centers for Disease Control and Prevention (CDC). (1991). Use of folic acid for prevention of spina bifida and other neural tube defects—1983-1991. *Morbidity and Mortality Weekly Report, 40*(30), 513–516.

Centers for Disease Control and Prevention. (1992). Recommendations for the use of folic acid to reduce the number of cases of spina bifida and other neural tube defects. *Morbidity and Mortality Weekly Report, 41*(RR-14), 1–7.

Chanarin, I. (1994). Adverse effects of increased dietary folate. Relation to measures to reduce the incidence of neural tube defects. *Clinical Investigation Medicine, 17*(3), 244–252.

Cook, J.D. (1994). Iron-deficiency anemia. *Baillière's Clinical Haematology, 7*(4), 787–804.

Dimperio, D. (1988). *Prenatal nutrition: Clinical guidelines for nurses.* White Plains, NY: March of Dimes Birth Defects Foundation.

Engstrom, J.L., & Sittler, C.P. (1994). Nurse-midwifery management of iron-deficiency anemia during pregnancy. *Journal of Nurse-Midwifery, 39*(2, suppl.), 20S–34S

Food and Nutrition Board, National Academy of Sciences—National Research Council. (1989). *Recommended dietary allowances* (10th ed.). Washington, DC: National Academy Press.

Goroll, A.H., May, L.A., & Mulley, A.G. (1995). *Primary care medicine* (3rd ed., pp. 447–455, 468–472). Philadelphia, PA: J.B. Lippincott.

Gutierrez, Y.M. (1994). *Nutrition in health maintenance and health promotion for primary care providers.* San Francisco: University of California, San Francisco, School of Nursing.

Harvey, A. (1980). *The principles and practice of medicine* (20th ed., pp. 476–522). New York: Appleton-Century-Crofts.

Hercberg, S., & Galan, P. (1992). Nutritional anaemias. *Baillière's Clinical Haematology, 5*(1), 143–159.

Institute of Medicine (IOM). (1990). *Nutrition during pregnancy. Weight gain. Nutrient supplements.* Washington, DC: National Academy Press.

Institute of Medicine (IOM), Food and Nutrition Board, Committee on the Prevention, Detection, and Management of Iron Deficiency Anemia U.S. Children and Women of Childbearing Age. (1993). *Iron deficiency anemia: Recommended guidelines for the prevention, detection, and management among U.S. children and women of childbearing age.* Washington, DC: National Academy Press.

Laros, R.K., Jr. (1994). Maternal hematologic disorders. In R.K. Creasy & R. Resnik (Eds.), *Maternal-Fetal Medicine. Principles and practice* (3rd ed., pp. 905–933). Philadelphia, PA: W. B. Saunders.

Lops, V.R., Hunter, L.P., & Dixon, L. . (1995). Anemia in pregnancy. *American Family Physician, 51*(5), 1189–1197.

Marin, M.M. (1995). Anemia. In W.L. Star, L.L. Lommel, & M.T. Shannon (Eds.), *Women's primary health care: Protocols for practice* (10-3–10-17). Washington, DC: American Nurses Publishing.

Massey, A.C. (1992). Microcytic anemia. *The Medical Clinics of North America, 76*(3), 549–566.

Metz, J., McGrath, K., Bennett, M., Hyland, K., & Bottiglieri, T. (1995). Biochemical indices of vitamin B_{12} nutrition in pregnant patients with subnormal serum vitamin B_{12} levels. *American Journal of Hematology, 48*, 251–255.

Nexo, E., Hansen, M., Rasmussen, K., Lindgren, A., & Grasbeck, R. (1994). *Scandinavian Journal of Clinical Laboratory Investigation, 54*(Suppl. 219), 61–76.

Niebyl, J.R. (1996). Iron therapy in pregnancy. *Contemporary OB/GYN, 41(3)*, 146–150.

Reich, P.R. (1984). *Hematology* (2nd ed.). Boston: Little, Brown & Co.

Rodak, B.F. (1995). *Diagnostic hematology.* Philadelphia, PA: W.B. Saunders.

Scholl, T.O., & Hediger, M.L. (1994). Anemia and iron-deficiency anemia: compilation of data on pregnancy outcome. *American Journal of Clinical Nutrition, 59*(Suppl.), 492S–501S.

Tinkle, M. (1997) Folic acid and food fortification: Implications for the primary care provider. *The Nurse Practitioner, 22*(3), 105–114.

U.S. Preventive Services Task Force. (1996). *Guide to clinical preventive services* (2nd ed., pp. 231-246, 467–483). Baltimore, MD: Williams & Wilkins.

Williams, M.D., & Wheby, M.S. (1992). Anemia in pregnancy. *The Medical Clinics of North America, 76*(3), 631–647.

Chapter 4

BETA THALASSEMIA

Winifred L. Star

The thalassemias are a "heterogeneous group of inherited disorders of hemoglobin synthesis characterized by absent or diminished synthesis of one or the other of the globin chains of hemoglobin A " (Nathan, 1992, p. 205). The major normal adult hemoglobin (Hb), Hb A, is made up of two alpha and two beta globin chains. Minor adult hemoglobin, Hb A$_2$, is composed of two alpha and two delta globin chains. A small percentage of adult hemoglobin is Hb F or fetal hemoglobin, which is composed of two alpha and two gamma globin chains. Normally, a person has four functioning alpha globin genes, two beta globin genes, two delta globin genes, and four gamma globin genes (Nathan, 1992).

Beta thalassemia is a hereditary condition characterized by decreased production (beta$^+$) or absence (beta^0) of the beta chains of hemoglobin. Most cases arise from point mutations of the beta globin genes, rather than deletions (as in the case of alpha thalassemia). There are about 100 different mutations responsible for beta thalassemia; thus, there is considerable phenotypic variation, depending on the nature of the mutations involved. The severity of the phenotype depends mainly on the amount of underproduction of beta globin chains (Fischel-Ghodsian, 1990).

In beta thalassemia minor or trait (heterozygous beta^0 or beta$^+$ thalassemia), individuals carry one gene for the production of the usual number of beta chains and one gene for the production of a decreased number. A 25 percent decrease in beta globin chains produces no clinical signs; a mild microcytosis and hypochromia will appear on a blood smear. A 50 percent reduction results in significant microcytosis, hypochromia, targeting, mild anemia, and occasionally, hepatosplenomegaly (Fischel-Ghodsian, 1990).

In pregnancy, women with heterozygous beta^0 thalassemia may develop significant anemia due to rapid drops in hematocrit, and transfusion may be required (American College of Obstetricians and Gynecologists [ACOG], 1996). Hematological values are the lowest in the later second and early third trimester, mainly due to hemodilution (Savona-Ventura & Bonello, 1994). Women with beta$^+$ thalassemia trait generally have uncomplicated pregnancies with mild to no anemia (ACOG, 1996). In a study by White et al. (1985) of beta thalassemia heterozygotes during pregnancy, no increased maternal or fetal morbidity and no associated abnormality of placental function was observed. In addition, premature labor is not known to be increased in patients with this form of thalassemia trait (Savona-Ventura & Bonello, 1994).

In beta thalassemia major (Cooley's anemia) (homozygous beta^0 or beta$^+$ thalassemia) individuals have two defective beta globin genes; there is greatly reduced or no beta globin chain production and the clinical picture is more severe. Hemolytic anemia begins within a few months after birth and a regular transfusion program is necessary. Iron overload (hemosiderosis) occurs due to the transfusion regimen and damages major organs. Progressive hepatosplenomegaly and bony structure abnormalities develop, and infection is common. Physical growth and development are below normal; however, intellectual development is unaffected. Sexual development is severely delayed and reproductive axis failure usually leads to infertility. With optimal treatment, including blood transfusions and iron chelation, individuals may live to young or middle adulthood (Bunn, Forget, & Ranney, 1977; Fischel-Ghodsian, 1990; Kazazian Jr., 1991). Pregnancy in persons with beta thalassemia major has been rarely reported due to their shortened life span and reduced fertility; if pregnancy does occur, however, it may pose deleterious consequences for mother and fetus (e.g., severe anemia, chronic hypoxia, myocardial hemosiderosis, cardiac arrhythmias, congestive heart failure) (Savona-Ventura & Bonello, 1994).

Thalassemia intermedia, a milder form of beta thalassemia major with a variable reduction in beta chain production, results in a disease spectrum from mild to moderate anemia to a thalassemia major syndrome. (The term is used to refer to either severe heterozygous beta thalassemia or mild homozygous beta thalassemia.) The majority of individuals with thalassemia intermedia have moderate anemia requiring occasional transfusion. Hepatosplenomegaly, bony deformities, and hemosiderosis leading to endocrinologic abnormalities may also exist (Fischel-Ghodsian, 1990). Particularly character-istic to this thalassemia is recurrent leg ulceration, folate deficiency, symptomatic extramedullary hemopoietic tumors in the chest and skull, gallstones, and susceptibility to infection (Savona-Ventura & Bonello, 1994). It is expected that improvements in treatment regimens will make it possible for more women with homozygous thalassemia to become pregnant. A review of the literature will be important for clinicians in caring for these women.

An interacting thalassemia may exist when an individual acquires a thalassemia gene for a given globin chain on one chromosome and a gene for a structural variant of the same type of globin chain on the other chromosome. The clinical severity of this condition approaches that of homozygosity for the abnormal hemoglobin (Bunn et al., 1977). Examples of this are sickle/beta thalassemia, a form of sickle cell anemia with a variable course ranging from severe sickle cell disease to a symptom-free state (more rare), and Hb E/beta thalassemia, with variable manifestations but often mimicking homozygous beta thalassemia (Bunn et al., 1977; Savona-Ventura & Bonello, 1994; Stein, Berg, Jones, & Detter, 1994). A *noninteracting* thalassemia occurs when a beta chain abnormality is inherited with a structural variant for another globin chain (e.g., alpha); the clinical severity of the condition is similar to the heterozygous state for the structural variant (Bunn et al., 1977).

The spectrum of beta thalassemia has been found in almost all populations; those at greatest risk are people of Mediterranean origin (especially Greeks and Italians), Southeast Asians, Pakistanis and Indians, and North Africans. To a lesser extent, beta thalassemia is also present in those of African, Caribbean, or Central American descent (ACOG, 1996). Beta thalassemia major is less severe in the African and African-descended population than in Mediterraneans or Asians (State of California Department of Health Services & Children's Hospital, Oakland, 1992). Obstetrical care of women from these different ethnic groups should be culturally appropriate utilizing interpreters when necessary and as available.

This chapter addresses prenatal screening for beta thalassemia and the database and treat-ment/management plan for women with beta thalassemia trait. It is beyond the scope of this chapter to discuss all the clinical presentations associated with beta thalassemia and with beta thalassemia in association with beta chain structural variants (although a brief description of laboratory findings in these conditions is presented). Refer to a current textbook for additional information.

Database

Subjective

- Descendant of population at risk for beta thalassemia syndromes.

- May be aware of abnormal lab results, or anemia in the past, or provide history of beta thalassemia trait.

- Clients with beta thalassemia *trait* are generally asymptomatic.

- Complete family, medical, and pregnancy history is important.

Objective

- See Table 9.2, Laboratory Values in Selected Anemias or Hemoglobinopathies.

- Beta thalassemia trait (minor)

  - ▶ Heterozygous state

  - ▶ Physical findings vary among races

    - – Majority of individuals have no abnormal physical signs.

    - – Liver or spleen enlargement has been seen in some cases (Weatherall & Clegg, 1981).

  - ▶ Mild anemia: hemoglobin 1 to 2 gm/dL lower than normal for age and sex (10 to 11 gm/dL is usual in most nonpregnant women; may be lower during pregnancy)

  - ▶ Red blood cell (RBC) count may be increased above the normal range

  - ▶ Mean corpuscular volume (MCV) less than 80 fL (55–75 fL range)

  - ▶ Mean corpuscular hemoglobin (MCH) less than 26 pg (16–25 pg range)

  - ▶ Peripheral blood smear typically shows

    - – Microcytosis

    - – Hypochromia

    - – Anisocytosis

    - – Poikilocytosis

    - – Targeting and basophilic stippling of the red cells (Bunn et al., 1977)

  - ▶ Hb A_2 increased: 3.5 to 7 percent

  - ▶ May have slightly elevated Hb F (50 percent of cases): 2 to 5 percent

  - ▶ Bone marrow may show mild erythroid hyperplasia

  - ▶ Iron studies normal unless coexistent iron deficiency

- Beta thalassemia major and intermedia

  - ▶ Homozygous beta^0 thalassemia

    - – Severe anemia present

- – Hb A absent

- – Variable amounts of Hb A$_2$, the remainder Hb F (about 98%)

▶ Homozygous beta$^+$ thalassemia

- – Severe anemia present

- – Variable amounts of Hb A, Hb F increased (about 70%)

- – Hb A$_2$ normal, decreased or increased

▶ Thalassemia intermedia

- – Moderate to severe anemia (Hb around 6–9 gm/dL)

- – Marked anisocytosis, hypochromia, target cells, basophilic stippling

- – Electrophoresis variable—most common feature Hb F (around 20 percent) (Savona-Ventura & Bonello, 1994; Wintrobe, 1981)

● Beta thalassemia with beta chain structural variants

▶ Sickle/beta^0 thalassemia

- – Sickled cells, red cell microcytosis, hypochromia, targeting, basophilic stippling

- – MCV mean 68 fL, MCH mean 20 pg

- – Hb S major hemoglobin, Hb F variably increased, Hb A absent, Hb A$_2$ elevated (differentiated from sickle cell anemia by low MCV, elevated Hb A$_2$ and Hb F)

▶ Sickle/beta$^+$ thalassemia

- – Hb A 25 percent, Hb S 70 percent, Hb F increased, Hb A$_2$ elevated (distinguished from Hb AS on electrophoresis by more Hb S than Hb A)

▶ Hb C-beta thalassemia

- – Morphology like beta thalassemia trait but more target cells

- – Hb C predominant, Hb F increased

- – Hb A$_2$ cannot be separated from Hb C, thus A$_2$ levels are indeterminate

▶ Hb E-beta thalassemia

- – Hematologic features of thalassemia major

  * Marked microcytosis (MCV in 50 fL range), marked hypochromia

  * Severe anemia (Hb <8 gm/dL)

  * Teardrops, target cells

  * Hb F 15 to 40 percent, rest Hb E (State of California Department of Health Services & Children's Hospital, Oakland, 1992; Wintrobe, 1981).

Assessment

- Beta thalassemia trait
  - ▶ R/O beta thalassemia variant
  - ▶ R/O concomitant hemoglobinopathy
  - ▶ R/O coexistent iron and/or folate deficiency anemia
  - ▶ R/O hemoglobinopathy in father of baby

Plan

Diagnostic Tests

- See Figure 9.1, Evaluation for Anemia/Hemoglobinopathies.
- Maternal diagnostic tests include
  - ▶ Complete blood count (CBC) with RBC indices
  - ▶ Hemoglobin electrophoresis with quantitative A_2 and F as indicated
  - ▶ Serum iron, serum ferritin, transferrin saturation, serum folate or RBC folate as indicated

  NOTE: The diagnosis of beta thalassemia is generally made by the presence of a low MCV and MCH, *plus* elevated Hb A_2 with or without elevated Hb F. Serum iron less than 30 µg/dL, serum ferritin less than 12 µg/mL, and transferrin saturation less than 15 percent indicate iron deficiency. Iron deficiency anemia can cause a decrease in Hb A_2 in a patient with beta thalassemia trait; thus, the A_2 levels in beta thalassemia with coexistent iron deficiency may fall in the normal range and confuse the laboratory picture of the thalassemia. In cases of iron deficiency anemia where microcytosis and hypochromia persist after iron replacement, suspect beta thalassemia. Hb A_2 will return to elevated levels in beta thalassemia patients after correction of a coexistent iron deficiency. Lastly, the Mentzer index (MCV/RBC) is usually less than 13 in thalassemia, but greater than 14 in iron deficiency anemia.

- If maternal beta thalassemia trait is diagnosed, offer screening for father of the baby; order a CBC and hemoglobin electrophoresis. Discuss the possibility of nonpaternity prior to the tests being performed.
- If both members have beta thalassemia trait (or other significant hemoglobin variant), client/couple may opt for prenatal diagnosis to evaluate the fetus. If both parents have an identifiable mutation, prenatal diagnosis of beta thalassemia is possible via DNA analysis (ACOG, 1996; Kazazian, Jr., 1991).

  NOTE: A diagnostic problem may exist when one parent has thalassemia trait and the other has a borderline MCV and Hb A_2 (silent carrier alleles exist in Asian Indian and Mediterranean populations). In this situation, laboratory tests on the parents of the possible carrier may need to be carried out. DNA studies may be indicated if one member of the couple is suspected to have carrier values because there may be a risk to the fetus of a significant thalassemia, in which case, the couple may opt for prenatal diagnosis (Kazazian, Jr. et al., 1990).

- Fetal DNA may be obtained via chorionic villus sampling or amniocentesis, or percutaneous umbilical cord blood sampling (PUBS). Prenatal diagnostic techniques are generally explained to the client/couple by the genetic counselor.

- Cord blood electrophoresis and newborn screening tests are also used to diagnose neonatal hemoglobinopathies. In some states, hemoglobin testing is a routine part of the newborn screening program.

Treatment/Management

- Ideally, identification of beta thalassemia occurs in the primary care setting prior to conception. By so doing, inappropriate therapy is avoided (i.e., administering of unnecessary iron), counseling about the disorder can take place, and partner screening can be offered.

- If both client and partner have been diagnosed with beta thalassemia trait (or other significant hemoglobin variant), refer them to a genetic counselor promptly. If the mother of the baby has beta thalassemia trait and the father of the baby is unavailable for or has declined screening, a referral is also in order.

- There is no specific treatment for maternal beta$^+$ thalassemia trait; prenatal care generally proceeds as with an unaffected client (Perry & Morrison, 1990).

- Clients with beta^0 thalassemia trait may require co-management with or referral to a physician, depending on the severity of anemia. Transfusion is rarely required for severe anemia not responding to therapy. If transfusion becomes necessary, the women should be counseled about the risks of this procedure by the physician responsible for her care.

- If there is coexisting iron deficiency anemia, treat according to protocol. See Chapter 9.3, *Anemia— Iron, Folate, and Vitamin B$_{12}$ Deficiency,* for regimens.

  NOTE: Iron therapy should be reserved for cases of demonstrable iron deficiency anemia so as not to risk iron overload and hepatotoxicity (ACOG, 1996).

- Supplement folic acid as for a normal pregnancy. If megaloblastic anemia due to folate deficiency exists, supplement according to protocol. See Chapter 9.3, *Anemia—Iron, Folate, and Vitamin B$_{12}$ Deficiency,* for regimens.

- Management of a pregnant woman with homozygous beta thalassemia will not be covered in this chapter; this is a high-risk pregnancy and client should be referred to a perinatologist.

Consultation

- Consultation is not required in beta thalassemia trait with mild anemia. Physician consultation is advised for clients with severe anemia; consider physician referral or co-management in these cases.

- Consult with a hematologist for an assessment of complicated or confusing laboratory results.

- An obstetrician or perinatologist should care for women with homozygous beta thalassemia, sickle/beta thalassemia, or Hb E/beta thalassemia. Referral to a hematologist may also be in order.

- Refer to a genetic counselor in cases where both the client and the father of the baby have beta thalassemia trait or in situations where one parent is an identified carrier and the other has borderline laboratory values. If the mother has beta thalassemia trait and the baby's father is unavailable for or has declined screening, a referral is also in order.

Patient Education

- Discuss the function of hemoglobin and the benign nature of beta thalassemia trait. Be sure to clarify the difference between *trait* and *disease*. Utilize patient education materials if available.

- Help clients to understand that they cannot presume the father of the baby does not have a hemoglobin disorder merely because he seems "healthy" or has had "blood tests that were normal." Documentation of the father's laboratory results (i.e., CBC and hemoglobin electrophoresis with quantitative A_2 and F) on the baby's father is necessary for accurate and specific education regarding prenatal risk when the mother of the baby has a hemoglobin disorder.

- Discuss prenatal implications if diagnosis of beta thalassemia trait is made in both parents: a 25 percent ($1/4$) chance that the fetus will have beta thalassemia major.

  NOTE: Risk for other hemoglobinopathies in offspring may exist based on the results of the parents' screens (e.g., if one parent affected with beta thalassemia trait and the other parent has sickle cell trait, there is a 25 percent ($1/4$) chance that the fetus will have sickle/beta thalassemia. Individualized education and counseling based on the case presentation, in most instances, will be performed by the genetic counselor.

- If diagnosis of beta thalassemia trait is made in both client and partner, explore the pros and cons of prenatal diagnosis with the couple. Generally, the genetic counselor will conduct the discussion based on specifics; a joint appointment with obstetrical care provider and counselor may be appropriate.

Follow-up

- Ensure a prompt appointment with a genetic counselor if both members of the couple have beta thalassemia trait (extended family studies may be needed before prenatal diagnosis can be made). Also advise genetic counseling when the mother of the baby has a hemoglobin disorder and the baby's father is unavailable for or has declined screening, or when client/couple desire(s) comprehensive education about hemoglobinopathies even if there is no significant risk to the offspring.

- If the fetus has been diagnosed with a significant hemoglobin disorder, review postdiagnosis options carefully to enable the couple to make a decision regarding the pregnancy (i.e., termination or preparation for an affected child). Specifics are usually provided by the genetic counselor.

- If the decision has been made to continue a pregnancy in which the fetus has a significant hemoglobinopathy, refer client/couple to a hematologist and/or pediatrician to discuss childhood interventions. There is much phenotypic variation of beta thalassemia disorders and disease complexity may differ from case to case. Providers should be aware of current treatment/management strategies available for a child affected with thalassemia major.

- Provide ongoing emotional support for the client/couple facing the birth of a child with a significant hemoglobinopathy. Refer to appropriate social services and community resources.

- If prenatal testing reveals no hemoglobin disorder, it is important for the couple to understand that "normal" results do not guarantee a "perfect" baby. The general population risk of birth defects is around 2 to 4 percent.

- Newborn screening is indicated for at-risk pregnancies. Consult your state's protocols regarding initial screening and recommended follow-up.

- Advise client to make note of her hemoglobin disorder and alert future health care providers of this history. Advise preconception counseling for the woman with a hemoglobinopathy to provide information on the risks associated with the disorder during pregnancy, including maternal morbidity, perinatal loss, and effects of treatment. In addition, preconception counseling for future pregnancies is indicated in the event she has a different partner.

- Document diagnosis of hemoglobin disorder in client/partner in progress notes and problem list.

  ▶ Comment on fetal diagnosis, as indicated.

  ▶ Make note of any pregnancy complications.

  ▶ Also include in documentation whether partner was unavailable for/declined screening and the offering of genetic counseling.

References

American College of Obstetricians and Gynecologists (ACOG). (1996). Hemoglobinopathies in pregnancy. (Technical Bulletin No. 220). Washington, DC: Author.

Bunn, H.F., Forget, B.G., & Ranney, H.M. (1977). *Human hemoglobinopathies*. Philadelphia: W.B. Saunders.

Esposito, N.W. (1992). Thalassemias: Simple screening for hereditary anemias. *Nurse Practitioner, 17*(2), 50–61.

Fischel-Ghodsian, N. (1990). Prenatal diagnosis of hemoglobinopathies. *Clinics in Perinatology, 17*(4), 811–828.

Kazazian, H.H., Jr. (1991). Prenatal diagnosis of beta thalassemia. *Seminars in Perinatology, 15*(3, Suppl. 2), 15–24.

Kazazian, H.H., Jr., Dowling, C.E., Boehm, C.D., Warren, T.C., Economou, E.P., Katz, J., & Antonarakis, S.E. (1990). Gene defects in beta thalassemia and their prenatal diagnosis. *Annals New York Academy of Sciences, 612*, 1–14.

Nathan, D.G. (1992). The thalassemias. In W.S. Beck (Ed.), *Hematology* (5th ed., pp. 205–222). Cambridge, MA: The MIT Press.

Perry, K.G., & Morrison, J.C. (1990). The diagnosis and management of hemoglobinopathies during pregnancy. *Seminars in Perinatology, 14*(2), 90–102.

Savona-Ventura, C., & Bonello, F. (1994). Beta thalassemia syndromes and pregnancy. *Obstetrical and Gynecological Survey, 49*(2), 129–137.

State of California Department of Health Services, & Children's Hospital, Oakland. (1992). *Sickle cell educator/counselor training program: Course manual*. Berkeley, CA: State of California. Department of Health Services, Genetic Disease Branch.

Stein, J., Berg, C., Jones, J.A., & Detter, J.C. (1984). A screening protocol for a prenatal population at risk for inherited hemoglobin disorders: Results of its application to a group of Southeast Asians and Blacks. *American Journal of Obstetrics and Gynecology, 150*(4), 333–341.

Weatherall, D.J., & Clegg, J.B. (1981). *The thalassemia syndromes* (3rd ed.). Oxford, England: Blackwell Scientific Publications.

White, J.M., Richards, R., Byrne, M., Buchanan, T., White, Y.S., & Jelenski, G. (1985). Thalassemia trait and pregnancy. *Journal of Clinical Pathology, 38*, 810–817.

Wintrobe, M. (1981). The thalassemias and related disorders: Quantitative disorders of hemoglobin synthesis. In M. Wintrobe (Ed.), *Clinical hematology* (8th ed., pp. 869–894). Philadelphia: Lea & Febiger.

Chapter 5

GLUCOSE-6-PHOSPHATE DEHYDROGENASE (G6PD) DEFICIENCY

Maureen T. Shannon

Glucose-6-phosphate dehydrogenase (G6PD) deficiency is an X-linked hereditary erythrocyte enzyme deficiency that is passed on to the male offspring of female carriers (Biswas & Perloff, 1994; Laros, 1994; Willett, 1994). Although there are more than fifty variants of this disorder, the major types include Type A (found in blacks) and the Mediterranean type (found in Greeks, Sardinians, and Sephardic Jews) (Laros, 1994). In the United States, 12 percent of black males and 3 percent of black females reportedly have this deficiency (Biswas & Perloff, 1994; Laros, 1994).

Although the female carriers are usually asymptomatic, this enzyme deficiency can result in an acute, usually mild, hemolytic anemia when the affected person ingests oxidant drugs (e.g., sulfonamides, nitrofurantoin, primaquine) or certain foods (e.g., fava beans); or is exposed to viral or bacterial infections. Up to two thirds of women affected by this deficiency will have hematocrits less than 30 percent (Biswas & Perloff, 1994). Also, there is reportedly an increased incidence of urinary tract infections in this population of women (Biswas & Perloff, 1994). Overall, 5 percent of affected male offspring have neonatal hyperbilirubinemia. However, there is a significant increase in the incidence of hyperbilirubinemia (up to 50 percent) observed in affected male infants who have an older sibling with a history of neonatal jaundice (Laros, 1994). In addition, fetal exposure to maternal ingestion of oxidant medications may cause other adverse perinatal outcomes, including fetal hemolysis, fetal hydrops, and fetal death (Biswas & Perloff, 1994). Hemolysis has also been observed in affected breastfed infants after their mothers ingested oxidant medications or fava beans (Laros, 1994).

Database

Subjective

- Usually the woman is asymptomatic.
- She may report fatigue (especially if she also has iron deficiency anemia).

Objective

- Vital signs, maternal weight gain, and fundal height are within normal limits (WNL)
- Laboratory results will reveal evidence of G6PD, see Diagnostic Tests section and Table 9.2, *Laboratory Values in Selected Anemias or Hemoglobinopathies*.

Assessment

- G6PD deficiency
  - ▶ R/O iron deficiency anemia
  - ▶ R/O hemoglobinopathy
  - ▶ R/O asymptomatic bacteriuria

Plan

Diagnostic Tests

- Complete blood count (CBC) will reveal decreased erythrocytes, hematocrit, and hemoglobin levels with a normal mean corpuscular volume (MCV) unless a coexisting anemia or hemoglobinopathy is present.

- Iron studies are WNL unless a coexisting iron deficiency anemia is present (see Chapter 9.3, *Anemia—Iron, Folate, and Vitamin B_{12} Deficiency*).

- G6PD level results will be less than normal values established by a specific laboratory.

- Hemoglobin electrophoresis with quantitative A_2 and F should be ordered when the MCV is less than 80. Results will be WNL unless a coexistent hemoglobinopathy is present.

- Total bilirubin level may be elevated if significant hemolysis.

- Ehrlich stain presence of at least five or more Heinz bodies in 40 percent of the blood cells suggests G6PD deficiency.

- Urine culture obtained on an initial specimen may reveal a coexistent asymptomatic bacteriuria.

Treatment/Management

- Routine prenatal care should continue.

- If there is coexistent iron deficiency anemia, initiate iron supplementation per protocol (see Chapter 9.3, *Anemia—Iron, Folate, and Vitamin B_{12} Deficiency*).

- If there is coexistent hemoglobinopathy, initiate plan of care appropriate to specific disorder (see appropriate hemoglobinopathy chapters in Section 9).

- Long dipstick of urine should be performed at each visit to screen for asymptomatic bacteriuria.

- If bacterial infections requiring antibiotic therapy develop, avoid the use of oxidant medications (e.g., sulfonamides, nitrofurantoin, etc.).

- Transfusions are rarely indicated in affected pregnant women but when necessary should be ordered by the consulting physician.

Consultation

- Consultation is not required unless severe anemia exists.

Patient Education

- Explain and interpret laboratory test results to the woman and discuss the importance of partner screening.

- Educate the woman about G6PD deficiency and factors that may trigger an acute hemolytic anemia (e.g., sulfonamides, nitrofurantoin, primaquine, fava beans, etc.).

- Educate the woman and her partner about the possible effects on the fetus and neonate.

Follow-up

- Obtain prenatal screening for the woman's partner to evaluate for G6PD.

- Recommend that the woman and her partner talk with a pediatrician before the birth of their infant to establish rapport and discuss possible implications (during neonatal and infancy periods) if the infant has G6PD deficiency.

- Arrange a routine 6-week post-partum follow-up for the woman (see Chapter 4.3, *The Postpartum Visit*).

- Document diagnosis of G6PD deficiency and management thereof in progress notes and problem list.

References

Biswas, M.K., & Perloff, D. (1994). Cardiac, hematologic, pulmonary, renal, and urinary tract disorders in pregnancy. In A.H. DeCherney & M.L. Pernoll (Eds.), *Current obstetric & gynecologic diagnosis & treatment* (8th ed., pp.428–468). Norwalk, CT: Appleton & Lange.

Fischbach, F. (1996). *A manual of laboratory & diagnostic tests* (5th ed.). Philadelphia, PA: Lippincott.

Laros, R.K. (1994). Maternal hematologic disorders. In R.K. Creasy & R. Resnik (Eds.), *Maternal-fetal medicine. Principles and practice* (3rd ed., pp. 905–933). Philadelphia, PA: W.B. Saunders Company.

Willett, G.D. (1994). *Laboratory testing in OB/GYN*. Boston: Blackwell Scientific Publications.

Chapter 6

HEMOGLOBINS C, D, and E

Winifred L. Star

Hemoglobins C, D, and E are *qualitative* hemoglobin (Hb) variants. This means that a *structural variation* has occurred, resulting in a change in the type of hemoglobin produced. Normal adult hemoglobin is composed of Hb A (two alpha chains and two beta chains), and small amounts of Hb A$_2$ (two alpha chains and two delta chains) and Hb F (two alpha chains and two gamma chains).

Hemoglobin C

Hemoglobin C contains a lysine substitution on the sixth position of the beta globin chain where glutamic acid normally occurs. The heterozygous state for Hb C, Hb C trait, or Hb AC is clinically silent and produces no threat to health. The structurally altered hemoglobin causes a decreased solubility within cells and a targetlike appearance due to a distorted cell membrane. The hemoglobin concentration is within the range of normal but red cell mass and red cell survival may be decreased. Hb C is found in about 2 to 3 percent of African-Americans and at a higher frequency in West and North Africans (the carrier rate may be as high as 25 percent), and may also be found in Mediterranean populations (particularly those from southern Sicily) (American College of Obstetricians and Gynecologists [ACOG], 1996; Wintrobe, 1981). In the homozygous state (Hb C disease or Hb CC), a mild to moderate anemia exists; there is increased risk for jaundice, splenomegaly and gallstones, and infection can trigger aplastic episodes (State of California Department of Health Services & Children's Hospital, Oakland, 1992; Wintrobe, 1981). Approximately one out of 5,000 to 6,000 African-Americans may be affected with Hb CC (Wintrobe, 1981; Young, 1984). During pregnancy, it has been observed that women with Hb C syndromes have little morbidity except for mild to moderate anemia (Maberry, Mason, Cunningham, & Pritchard, 1990).

The genetic significance of maternal Hb C is the possibility of interaction with a paternal hemoglobin disorder. If Hb C is present in the mother *and* the father has Hb S, the offspring is at risk for sickle cell-hemoglobin C disease (Hb SC). Hemoglobin SC is the second-most prevalent form of sickle cell disease affecting 1:833 African-Americans (ACOG, 1996; State of California Department of Health Services & Children's Hospital, Oakland, 1992). Clinical manifestations of Hb SC are similar to sickle cell anemia (Hb SS) but usually less severe, with fewer vaso-occlusive episodes. Retinal thrombosis and necrosis of the femoral head are more common in Hb SC, however (State of California Department of Health Services & Children's Hospital, Oakland, 1992; Wintrobe, 1981). The probabilities of preterm labor and intrauterine growth restriction are increased in women with sickle cell disease. Pregnant women with sickle cell disease also face morbidity from pneumonia, pyelonephritis, cholecystitis, pulmonary emboli, and skin infections (ACOG, 1996).

Hb C may also interact with beta thalassemia to produce Hb C/beta thalassemia, characterized by a mild to moderate hemolytic anemia and splenomegaly (Bunn, Forget, & Ranney, 1977).

Hemoglobin D

Hemoglobin D contains a substitution of glutamic acid by glutamine on the 121st position of the beta globin chain. Hemoglobin D trait (Hb AD) has no associated clinical, hematological, or physiological abnormalities. There are many variants of Hb D: Hb D-Punjab (also known as Hb D-Los Angeles) is the most common, occurring in 1 to 3 percent of West Indians and in small numbers in European communities with ties to the Indian subcontinent. Hemoglobin D disease (Hb DD), which can be confused with doubly heterozygous Hb D/beta^0 thalassemia, is characterized by mild hemolytic anemia and mild to moderate splenomegaly (Wintrobe, 1981).

The genetic significance of maternal Hb D is the potential interaction with Hb S in a father. An offspring with Hb SD disease suffers from hemolytic anemia with vaso-occlusive phenomena, although less severe on average than Hb SS (ACOG, 1996; State of California Department of Health Services & Children's Hospital, Oakland, 1992).

Hemoglobin E

Hemoglobin E is caused by a substitution of lysine for glutamic acid in the 26th position of the beta globin chain. The structurally abnormal beta chains are also produced in a slightly reduced amount (Stein, Berg, Jones, & Detter, 1984). Hemoglobin E is the most common structural variant in southeast Asia; an estimated 30 million people from Laos, Cambodia, Thailand, and Vietnam are affected. It is the third most common variant worldwide (Hurst, Tittle, Kleman, Embury, & Lubin, 1983; Lorey, Cunningham, Shafer, Lubin, & Vichinsky, 1994; Wintrobe, 1981). Before the influx of southeast Asians to the United States, Hb E was rarely seen (incidence of only one in 10,000 African-American newborns) (Ramahi, Lewkow, Dombrowski, & Bottoms, 1988). Although Hb E prevalence has increased in the U.S, it remains infrequent among blacks and whites (McGhee & Payne, 1995).

Hemoglobin E occurs in homozygous and heterozygous forms in combination with normal hemoglobin, beta thalassemia, hemoglobin S, and hemoglobin C (Ramahi et al., 1998). The heterozygous state, Hb E trait or Hb AE, is associated with a moderate microcytosis, mild erythrocytosis, and targeted erythrocytes; there is usually no anemia or reticulocytosis. Hemoglobin E disease (Hb EE) is characterized by a microcytic, normochromic anemia; some affected persons have mild splenomegaly, but usually no other physical abnormalities. A rare double heterozygous S/E hemoglobinopathy has also been described. This state shares several features in common with S/beta thalassemia: mild microcytosis with target cells, splenomegaly, and Hb S of 60 to 70 percent (Ramahi et al., 1988).

The genetic significance of maternal Hb E is the possibility of interaction with paternal hemoglobin traits that may result in severe disease in the offspring. An example of this is Hb E/beta thalassemia, which produces marked microcytosis, severe anemia (often transfusion-dependent), and splenomegaly (Hurst et al., 1983). Both E/beta thalassemia and S/E hemoglobinopathies may have detrimental obstetrical effects. Early neonatal deaths and fetal anomalies have been reported, and Hb E/beta thalassemia clients may have morbidity as severe as those with sickle cell disease (ACOG, 1996). Close antenatal surveillance is warranted in these conditions (Ramahi, et al., 1988).

Hemoglobin AE or Hb EE may be associated with alpha thalassemia trait. The clinical significance of these combined syndromes requires further study.

Database

Subjective

- Descendent of population at risk for hemoglobin disorders

- May have awareness of abnormal laboratory results or anemia in the past, or provide a history of having hemoglobin C, D, or E.

- Hemoglobin C

  ▶ Hb C trait (Hb AC) is clinically benign. There are no adverse effects during pregnancy (ACOG, 1996).

  ▶ Hb C disease (Hb CC) clinical features may include

    - Increased incidence of cholelithiasis

    - Mild intermittent abdominal pain, arthralgia, and headache but the association with the hemoglobinopathy is unclear (Wintrobe, 1981)

    - See Objective section for additional clinical presentations

  ▶ Pregnancy is usually uneventful in Hb C syndromes (Maberry et al., 1990).

  ▶ Hb SC disease clinical features may include

    - Episodic abdominal/skeletal pain

    - Increased incidence/severity of infectious illness

    - Complications of sickling (Wintrobe, 1981)

    - See Objective section for additional clinical presentations

- Hemoglobin D

  ▶ Hb D trait (Hb AD) is clinically benign.

  ▶ Hb SD disease is characterized by vaso-occlusive phenomena, but less severe than sickle cell anemia.

  ▶ Doubly heterozygous states for Hb D and Hb S are clinically silent with one exception: Hb D-Punjab + Hb S (Hb SD-Punjab), which produces symptoms that mimic mild sickle cell anemia (Wintrobe, 1981).

- Hemoglobin E

  ▶ Hb E trait (Hb AE) is clinically benign.

  ▶ Hb EE disease (Hb EE) is generally a benign condition.

  ▶ Hb E/beta thalassemia is a thalassemia major condition with variable severity in affected individuals with complications including

    - Splenomegaly (which may require splenectomy)

    - Increased susceptibility to infection

- – Hypoplastic crisis

- – Chronic transfusion-dependent anemia (results in chronic iron overload requiring chelation therapy) (Hurst et al, 1983)

▶ Hb S/E is relatively benign but may be associated with increased risk of fetal complications (see Introduction).

▶ Hb AE or Hb EE + alpha thalassemia: clinical significance requires further study.

Objective

- See Table 9.2, Laboratory Values in Selected Anemias or Hemoglobinopathies.

- Hemoglobin C

  ▶ Hemoglobin C trait (Hb AC)

    - – No anemia

    - – Hb electrophoresis

      * 30 to 50 percent Hb C (Note: Hb C may be reduced if there is coexistent alpha thalassemia. See also Note in Hb E trait section.)

      * 50 to 60 percent Hb A

      * Hb A_2 slightly increased

    - – 10 to 30 percent target cells on smear

    - – Negative solubility test (sickledex or sickle prep)

  ▶ Hemoglobin C disease (Hb CC)

    - – Splenomegaly (usually asymptomatic but spontaneous rupture has been reported)

    - – Aplastic episodes triggered by infection (State of California Department of Health Services & Children's Hospital, Oakland, 1992)

    - – Mild to moderate hemolytic anemia

      * Hb 10 to 12 gm/dL

      * Mean hematocrit 33 percent

    - – More than 90 percent target cells on smear, occasional spherocytes, hemoglobin "crystals" present

    - – Decreased MCV

    - – Slightly elevated reticulocytes (2 to 6 percent)

    - – Hb electrophoresis

      * Major fraction Hb C

      * Hb A absent

* Hb F slightly increased (more Hb F [to 22 percent] in coexistent alpha thalassemia)

▶ Sickle-hemoglobin C disease (Hb SC)

- Splenomegaly

- Splenic infarction and acute splenic sequestration

- Proliferative retinopathy

- Aseptic necrosis of the femoral head

- Acute chest syndrome secondary to fat emboli after bone marrow infarction (most commonly seen in the last months of pregnancy)

- Moderate hemolytic anemia

* Hb 9 to 12 gm/dL

- Red blood cell (RBC) indices, white blood cell (WBC) count and leukocyte differential within normal limits (WNL)

- Reticulocytes increased

- 50 percent target cells on smear, rare sickled cells, hemoglobin "crystals" present

- Hb electrophoresis

* Equal amounts Hb S and C

* Hb A absent

* Hb F normal or slightly increased

● Hemoglobin D

▶ Hemoglobin D trait (Hb AD)

- Normal blood smear

- Negative solubility test (sickledex or sickle prep)

▶ Hemoglobin D disease (Hb DD)

- Mild to moderate splenomegaly

- Mild hemolytic anemia

- Hb electrophoresis

* 95 percent Hb D

* Hb A absent

* Hb A_2 and Hb F WNL

▶ Hemoglobin SD disease (Hb SD)

- Hemolytic anemia

- Doubly heterozygous states for Hb S and Hb D clinically silent *except* for Hb D-Punjab + Hb S, which produces mild hemolytic anemia

- Hemoglobin E
  - ▶ Hemoglobin E trait (Hb AE)
    - Moderate microcytosis (MCV reduced 15 percent, mean 65 fL)
    - Hb is often WNL but may be slightly low
    - Slight erythrocytosis, targeted erythrocytes
    - Usually no reticulocytosis
    - Smear resembles thalassemia trait
    - Hb electrophoresis
      * 20 to 40 percent Hb E
      * Rest Hb A (Hb E may be reduced if there is coexistent alpha thalassemia or iron deficiency, confusing the diagnosis.)

      NOTE: Hb E migrates to the same position as Hb C on cellulose acetate electrophoresis. Samples showing Hb C should be repeated on citrate agar electrophoresis where Hb E will migrate with Hb A instead. Isoelectric focusing techniques permit identification of Hb E by single electrophoresis, but this may not be widely available (Hurst et al., 1983).
  - ▶ Hemoglobin E disease (Hb EE)
    - Associated with mild splenomegaly in some individuals
    - Marked microcytosis (MCV reduced 30 percent)
    - Mild anemia: Hb 10 to 12 gm/dL
    - Mild erythrocytosis
    - Blood smear with target cells, microcytosis, leptocytosis, and basophilic stippling
    - Hb electrophoresis
      * 92 to 98 percent Hb E
      * Hb A absent
      * Hb F WNL or slightly increased
  - ▶ Hemoglobin E/beta thalassemia
    - Splenomegaly
    - Marked microcytosis (MCV in 50s).
    - Anemia (may be severe)
    - Smear shows marked hypochromia, microcytosis, teardrops and target cells

- Hb electrophoresis

  * Usually Hb E and variable amounts of Hb F

  * Elevated Hb A_2 not readily identified because it migrates in same position as Hb E.

  NOTE: Hb EE and E/beta thalassemia can not be distinguished by electrophoresis.

▶ Hemoglobin S/E

  - Mild splenomegaly.

  - Mild anemia, microcytosis

  - Target cells on smear

  - Hb S 60 percent, Hb E 30 percent

▶ Hemoglobin AE/EE + alpha thalassemia trait

  - Microcytosis

  - Relative proportion of Hb E reduced by coexistent alpha thalassemia

  NOTE: Gene mapping studies are necessary to confirm existence of alpha thalassemia in this group (Hurst et al., 1983; Wintrobe, 1981).

Assessment

● Hemoglobin C, Hemoglobin D, or Hemoglobin E

  ▶ R/O concomitant hemoglobinopathy

  ▶ R/O coexistent iron deficiency anemia

  ▶ R/O anemia secondary to other causes (e.g., parasites)

  ▶ R/O hemoglobinopathy in father of baby

Plan

Diagnostic Tests

● See Figure 9.1, Evaluation for Anemia/Hemoglobinopathies

● Maternal diagnostic tests include

  ▶ Complete blood count (CBC) with RBC indices

  ▶ Hemoglobin electrophoresis with quantitative A_2, and F, as indicated

  ▶ Serum iron, serum ferritin, and transferrin saturation, as indicated

● Offer a screen for father of the baby (CBC and hemoglobin electrophoresis with quantitative A_2 and F) if mother has Hb C, D, or E.

● DNA testing can be utilized to diagnose fetal hemoglobinopathies as indicated.

  ▶ DNA from fetal cells can be obtained via amniocentesis, chorionic villus sampling or percutaneous umbilical cord blood sampling (ACOG, 1996).

▶ Prenatal diagnostic techniques are generally discussed with the client/couple by the genetic counselor.

● Cord blood electrophoresis or newborn screening tests are also used to diagnose neonatal hemoglobinopathies. In some states, hemoglobin testing is a routine part of the newborn screening program.

Treatment/Management

● Obstetrical care of women from various ethnic groups should be culturally appropriate, utilizing interpreters when necessary and as available.

● Hemoglobin C, D, and E traits are asymptomatic and require no therapy. Clients with hemoglobinopathies resulting in severe anemia, sickling, or other complications should be managed by a physician.

● Refer client to a genetic counselor if it is determined that the fetus may be at risk for a significant hemoglobinopathy based on the hemoglobin types of the client and partner. If the mother of the baby has a hemoglobin disorder and the baby's father is unavailable for or has declined screening, a referral is also in order.

Consultation

● Usually no consultation is indicated for benign hemoglobin traits.

● If a significant hemoglobinopathy is found in the mother, consult with a physician. The client may be co-managed, depending on the severity of the condition and the presence or absence of complications.

● Refer couples at risk for a fetus with a significant hemoglobinopathy for genetic counseling. Also refer the mother to genetic consultation if she has a hemoglobin disorder and the baby's father is unavailable for or has declined screening.

● Consult with a hematologist for assessment of complicated or confusing laboratory results.

Patient Education

● Discuss the benign nature of the hemoglobin trait; clarify differences between trait and disease. Utilize patient education materials if available.

● Impress upon the parents that they cannot presume the father of the baby does not have a hemoglobin disorder merely because he seems "healthy" or has had "blood tests that were normal." Documentation of the father's laboratory results (i.e., CBC and hemoglobin electrophoresis with quantitative A_2 and F) is necessary for accurate and specific education regarding prenatal risk when it has been determined that the mother of the baby has a hemoglobin disorder.

● Discuss the prenatal implications when both client and partner have been diagnosed with a hemoglobin disorder. Education and counseling must be individualized, based on the case presentation, and, in most instances, will be undertaken by the genetic counselor.

- Explore fully the pros and cons of prenatal diagnosis with the couple at risk for a significant hemoglobinopathy in their offspring. Generally, specifics will be provided by the genetic counselor; a joint appointment with obstetrical care provider and counselor may be appropriate. Following discussion, some couples may elect to defer testing until after delivery (newborn screening or cord blood electrophoresis).

Follow-up

- Ensure prompt appointment with a genetic counselor if both members of the couple have a hemoglobin disorder that may pose risk for a significant fetal hemoglobinopathy. Genetic counseling is also advisable if the mother of the baby has a hemoglobin disorder and the baby's father is unavailable for or has declined screening, or when the patient/couple desires comprehensive education about hemoglobinopathies even if there is no significant risk to the offspring.

- If a significant hemoglobin disorder has been diagnosed in the fetus, review postdiagnosis options carefully to enable the couple to make a decision regarding the pregnancy (i.e., termination or preparation for an affected child). Specifics are usually provided by the genetic counselor.

- Provide ongoing emotional support for the client/couple facing the birth of a child with a significant hemoglobinopathy.

  ▶ Refer them to social services and community resources, if indicated.

  ▶ Refer them to a hematologist and/or pediatrician before delivery to discuss childhood interventions, if appropriate.

- If prenatal testing reveals that the fetus does not have a significant hemoglobinopathy, it is important for the couple to understand that this does not mean the baby will be "perfect." The general population risk of birth defects is 2 to 4 percent.

- Newborn screening is indicated for at-risk pregnancies. Consult your state's protocols regarding initial screening and recommended follow-up.

- Advise the client to make note of her hemoglobin disorder and alert future health care providers of this history.

  ▶ Preconception counseling is indicated for the woman with a hemoglobinopathy to provide information on the risks associated with the disorder during pregnancy, including maternal morbidity, perinatal loss, and effects of treatment that may be indicated.

  ▶ In addition, preconception counseling for future pregnancies is indicated in the event she has a different partner.

- Document diagnosis of hemoglobin disorder in client/partner in progress notes and problem list.

  ▶ Comment on fetal diagnosis, as indicated.

  ▶ Make note of any pregnancy complications.

  ▶ Also include in documentation whether partner was unavailable for/declined screening and the offering of genetic counseling.

References

American College of Obstetricians and Gynecologists. (ACOG). (1996). Hemoglobinopathies in Pregnancy. (Technical Bulletin No. 185). Washington, D.C.: Author

Bunn, H.F., Forget, B.G., & Ranney, H.M. (1977). *Human hemoglobinopathies*. Philadelphia, PA: W.B. Saunders.

Hurst, D., Tittle, B., Kleman, K.M., Embury, S.H., & Lubin, B.H. (1983). Anemia and hemoglobinopathies in Southeast Asian refugee children. *The Journal of Pediatrics, 102*(5), 692–697.

Lorey, F., Cunningham, G., Shafer, F., Lubin, B., & Vichinsky, E. (1994). Universal screening for hemoglobinopathies using high-performance liquid chromatography: Clinical results of 2.2 million screens. *European Journal of Human Genetics, 2*, 262–271.

Maberry, M.C., Mason, R.A., Cunningham, G., & Pritchard, J.A. (1990). Pregnancy complicated by hemoglobin CC and B-beta-thalassemia. *Obstetrics & Gynecology, 76*(3, Pt. 1), 324–327.

McGhee, D., & Payne, M. (1995). Hemoglobinopathies and hemoglobin defects. In B.F. Rodak (Ed.), *Diagnostic hematology* (pp. 261–262). Philadelphia, PA: W. B. Saunders.

Ramahi, A.J., Lewkow, L.M., Dombrowski, M.P., & Bottoms, S.F. (1988). Sickle cell E hemoglobinopathy and pregnancy. *Obstetrics & Gynecology, 71*(3, Pt. 2), 493–495.

State of California Department of Health Services, & Children's Hospital, Oakland. (1992). *Sickle cell educator/counselor training program: Course manual.* Berkeley, CA: State of California: Department of Health Services, Genetic Disease Branch.

Stein, J.S., Berg, C., Jones, J.A., & Detter, J. (1984). A screening protocol for a prenatal population at risk for inherited hemoglobin disorders: Results of its application to a group of southwest Asians and blacks. *American Journal of Obstetrics and Gynecology, 150*(4), 333–341.

Wintrobe, M. (1981). Hemoglobinopathies S, C, D, E, and O. In M. Wintrobe (Ed.), *Clinical hematology* (8th ed.). Philadelphia, PA: Lea & Febiger.

Young, J.S. (1984). Hemoglobin S and other common hemoglobin variants: Sickle cell anemia, sickle cell trait, hemoglobin C, alpha thalassemia, beta thalassemia. (Sickle Cell Disease Branch of the National Heart, Lung, and Blood Institute Grant No. HL 209 85-07). Sickle Cell Anemia Research and Education, Inc.

Chapter 7

HEMOGLOBIN S AND SICKLE CELL TRAIT

Winifred L. Star

Hemoglobin S is formed when glutamic acid in the number six position of the beta globin chain is substituted by the amino acid valine; the alpha chain is normal. Sickle cell trait or hemoglobin (Hb) AS, occurs when a person has one gene for normal Hb A (two alpha, two beta chains) and one gene for Hb S (two alpha, two beta S chains). The amount of Hb A in a person with Hb AS is sufficient to prevent sickling under most physiological conditions. Sickle cell trait is the most common hemoglobin disorder in the United States, with 1 in 14 African Americans carrying the Hb S gene. The trait also occurs in Mediterranean (Greek and Italian), East Indian, Middle Eastern, and Latin American populations (American College of Obstetricians and Gynecologists [ACOG], 1996; State of California Department of Health Services & Children's Hospital, Oakland, 1992).

It is important to recognize that sickle cell trait is *not* a disease. The condition does not produce anemia and its presence offers some protection against malaria. Problems associated with sickle cell trait are occasional hematuria and hyposthenia (impaired renal concentrating ability). In addition, in rare instances, splenic infarction can occur at altitudes greater than 8,000 feet . Some studies have suggested that persons with sickle cell trait are at greater risk for sudden death under *extreme* conditions, such as severe dehydration, malnutrition, and physical overexertion and exhaustion (Kark, Posey, Schumacher, & Ruehle, 1987); however, this risk is relatively small (State of California Department of Health Services & Children's Hospital, Oakland, 1992). During pregnancy, unless hypoxia or infection are complicating factors, outcome is generally normal for a woman with sickle cell trait (ACOG, 1996). There is, however, a twofold increase in the rate of urinary tract infection (UTI) in women with the condition; thus, screening for asymptomatic bacteriuria and preventing pyelonephritis during pregnancy is important (ACOG, 1996; Laros, 1994). Iron deficiency anemia may also develop and supplementation should be advised after the diagnosis is made by appropriate laboratory testing (Laros Jr., 1994).

The genetic significance of maternal Hb S is the possibility of combination with a hemoglobin disorder in the father of the baby, which may cause a significant sickle cell *disease* variant in the offspring. For example, Hb S may (1) coexist with another globin variant (e.g., Hb SC, SD), (2) be present with one of the many types of thalassemia (e.g., Hb S/beta thalassemia syndromes), or (3) interact with a thalassemic hemoglobinopathy (e.g., Hb S/E) (Kinney & Ware, 1994). Various clinical manifestations of sickle cell disease can occur with these compound heterozygous states; thus, partner screening should be offered during pregnancy if a woman has Hb S.

Sickle cell anemia (Hb SS) occurs when an individual inherits two genes for Hb S, one from each parent. It is the most severe and prevalent type of sickle cell disease in the United States, affecting one in 625 African Americans (Vichinsky, Hurst, & Lubin, 1988). Clinical manifestations of this disorder include hemolytic anemia, systemic manifestations (e.g., growth impairment, susceptibility to infection, varying types of anemic crises), and chronic organ damage from repeated vaso-occlusive episodes (Weatherall & Clegg, 1981). Women with sickle cell disease may face serious complications during pregnancy, including severe anemia, vaso-occlusive crises, pneumonia, pyelonephritis, cholecystitis, pulmonary emboli, skin infections, preterm labor, intrauterine growth restriction, and stillbirth (AGOG, 1996). (See also the chapters on thalassemia and the hemoglobins C, D, and E for information on other forms of sickle cell disease.)

Guidelines for care in this chapter focus on the clinical presentation and obstetrical management of women with sickle cell trait. Sickle cell disease and the numerous clinically significant compound heterozygous conditions that involve Hb S will not be covered herein (although a brief description of laboratory findings for some of these conditions is presented). Pregnant women with sickle cell disease should be referred to an obstetrician or perinatologist for care. Obstetrical care of women from various ethnic groups should be culturally appropriate, utilizing interpreters when necessary and as available.

Database

Subjective

- Descendant of population at risk for Hb S
- May have awareness of diagnosis of sickle cell trait
- People with sickle cell trait are generally asymptomatic; history of UTIs, hematuria, pyelonephritis in pregnancy may be reported.
- Complete family, medical, and pregnancy history is important. Assess the client's knowledge regarding sickle cell trait and sickle cell disease.

Objective

- See Table 9.2, Laboratory Values in Selected Anemias or Hemoglobinopathies.
- Sickle cell trait
  - ► Complete blood count (CBC) is within normal limits (WNL).
  - ► Red blood cell (RBC) morphology WNL. If coexistent iron deficiency anemia or thalassemia, RBC indices may reveal low mean corpuscular volume (MCV) and low mean corpuscular hemoglobin (MCH).
  - ► Hemoglobin electrophoresis shows about 30 to 40 percent Hb S and 55 to 65 percent Hb A; Hb A_2 and Hb F are WNL. If there is coexistent thalassemia or iron/folate deficiency, the percentage of Hb S is less than usual (Bunn, 1992; McGhee & Payne, 1995).
  - ► Iron studies are WNL unless iron deficiency anemia coexists.
  - ► Urinalysis may show microscopic evidence of hematuria and/or bacteriuria. Urine culture may be positive for significant pathogen.
- Compound heterozygous states
  - ► Sickle cell/alpha thalassemia trait: electrophoresis shows Hb AS but percent of S less than usual; MCV decreased.
  - ► Sickle-hemoglobin C disease (Hb SC): moderate hemolytic anemia (Hb 9–12 gm/dL); RBC indices, white blood cell (WBC) count and leukocyte differential WNL; reticulocytes increased; fifty percent target cells on smear, rare sickled cells, hemoglobin "crystals." (See NOTE in hemoglobin S/E section below.)

▶ Sickle/beta^0 thalassemia: sickled cells, red cell microcytosis, hypochromia, targeting, basophilic stippling; MCV mean 68 fL, MCH mean 20 pg; Hb S major hemoglobin, Hb F variably increased, Hb A absent, Hb A$_2$ elevated (distinguishable from sickle cell anemia by low MCV, elevated A$_2$ and Hb F).

▶ Sickle/beta$^+$ thalassemia: Hb A 25 percent, Hb S 70 percent, Hb F increased, Hb A$_2$ elevated (distinguished from Hb AS on electrophoresis by more Hb S than Hb A).

▶ Hemoglobin S/E: mild anemia, microcytosis; target cells on smear; Hb S 60 percent, Hb E 30 percent.

NOTE: Hb E migrates to the same position as Hb C on cellulose acetate electrophoresis. Samples showing Hb C should be repeated on citrate agar electrophoresis where Hb E will migrate with Hb A instead. Isoelectric focusing techniques permit identification of Hb E by single electrophoresis, but this may not be widely available (Hurst, Tittle, Kleman, Embury, & Lubin, 1983).

▶ See Chapter 9.6, *Hemoglobin C, D, and E* and the thalassemia Chapters 9.2 and 9.4, for additional information.

Assessment

● Sickle cell trait

▶ R/O concomitant hemoglobinopathy

▶ R/O coexistent iron/folate deficiency anemia

▶ R/O asymptomatic bacteriuria

▶ R/O hemoglobinopathy in father of baby

Plan

Diagnostic Tests

● See Figure 9.1, Evaluation for Anemia/Hemoglobinopathies.

● Maternal diagnostic tests include

▶ CBC with RBC indices.

▶ Hemoglobin electrophoresis with quantitative A$_2$ and F to be ordered for all blacks at first prenatal visit. Other ethnic groups may be considered for screening.

NOTE: Solubility tests (i.e., sickledex, sickle prep) *cannot* distinguish between sickle cell trait and disease, *do not* detect other hemoglobin traits, and *should never be used alone to diagnose a hemoglobin variant.* These tests may be positive for presence of S hemoglobin; however, false-negative results can occur if the percentage of Hb S is very low (less than 10 percent, as with newborns) or the patient is very anemic (Hb less than 7 gm/dL). False positive results may occur if blood contains excessive white blood cells, lipids, or proteins (State of California Department of Health Services & Children's Hospital, Oakland, 1992).

▶ Serum iron, serum ferritin, transferrin saturation, serum folate or RBC folate as indicated.

- If electrophoresis shows presence of Hb S in the mother, offer screen for the father of the baby (CBC and hemoglobin electrophoresis with quantitative A_2 and F). Discuss the possibility of nonpaternity prior to the tests being performed.

- DNA testing can be utilized to diagnose fetal hemoglobinopathies as indicated. DNA from fetal cells can be obtained via amniocentesis, chorionic villus sampling (CVS), or percutaneous umbilical cord blood sampling (PUBS) (ACOG, 1996). Prenatal diagnostic techniques are generally discussed with the client/couple by the genetic counselor.

- Cord blood electrophoresis or newborn screening tests are also used to diagnose neonatal hemoglobinopathies. In some states, hemoglobin testing is a routine part of the newborn screening program.

Treatment/Management

- Ideally, identifying sickle cell trait occurs preconceptionally in the primary care setting. By so doing, counseling about the carrier state can take place and partner screening can be offered. Women with sickle cell disease require intensive preconception counseling about the implications and ramifications of their disease; refer them to a specialist in this area.

- There is no treatment for sickle cell trait. Order urinalysis and culture each trimester and as indicated by urine dipstick to rule out asymptomatic bacteriuria; treat accordingly (see Chapter 13.1, *Asymptomatic Bacteriuria.*)

- If there is coexistent iron or folate deficiency anemia, treat according to protocol (see Chapter 9.3, *Anemia—Iron, Folate, and B_{12} Deficiency.*)

- If both client and partner have been diagnosed with sickle cell trait, prompt referral to a genetic counselor is indicated. If the mother of the baby has sickle cell trait (or another significant hemoglobin variant) and the baby's father is unavailable for or has declined screening, a referral is also in order.

- Details of obstetrical management of women with sickle cell disease will not be covered in this chapter.

Consultation

- Consultation is not usually required for patients with sickle cell trait. If complications arise consult with or refer to a physician.

- If a client has severe anemia secondary to other causes, consider physician referral or co-management.

- Refer women with sickle cell disease to an obstetrician or perinatologist for prenatal care. Referral to a hematologist may also be in order. Consult with a hematologist, if indicated, for assessment of complicated or confusing laboratory results.

- Refer couples at risk for a fetus with a significant hemoglobinopathy for genetic counseling. Genetic counseling is also in order if the mother of the baby has a hemoglobin disorder and the baby's father is unavailable for or has declined screening.

Patient Education

- Discuss the function of hemoglobin and the generally benign nature of sickle cell trait.

  ▶ Explain the rare possibility of complications associated with sickle cell trait under certain conditions (see Introduction).

  ▶ Clarify differences between sickle cell trait and sickle cell disease.

  ▶ Utilize education materials if available.

- Educate the client regarding the increased risk of UTI during pregnancy. Advise her to report signs/symptoms of infection promptly. Discuss the need for routine screening (urinalysis/culture each trimester) to rule out asymptomatic bacteriuria.

- Impress upon the parents that they should not presume the father of the baby does not have a hemoglobin disorder merely because he seems "healthy" or has had "blood tests that were normal." Documentation of laboratory results (i.e., CBC and hemoglobin electrophoresis with quantitative A_2 and F) on the baby's father is necessary for accurate and specific education regarding prenatal risk when the mother of the baby has a hemoglobin disorder.

- Discuss the prenatal implications if both the woman and her partner have sickle cell trait: 25 percent ($^1/_4$) chance that the fetus will have sickle cell anemia.

  ▶ Risk for other hemoglobinopathies in offspring may exist based on the results of the parent's screen.

  ▶ Individualize education and counseling, based on the case presentation (undertaken by the genetic counselor in most instances).

- If diagnosis of sickle cell trait (or other significant hemoglobin variant) is made in both the woman and her partner, explore the pros and cons of prenatal diagnosis with the couple.

  ▶ Generally, specifics will be provided by the genetic counselor; a joint appointment with obstetrical care provider and counselor may be appropriate.

  ▶ Following discussion, some couples may elect to defer testing until after delivery (cord blood electrophoresis or newborn screening).

- If the partner is unavailable for screening, advise the woman with sickle cell trait that there is a 1/40 risk for an affected fetus if the father of the baby is black. In addition, counsel the client about the availability of prenatal diagnosis.

Follow-up

- Ensure prompt appointment with a genetic counselor if both members of the couple have sickle cell trait. Also advise genetic counseling if the mother of the baby has trait and the baby's father is unavailable for or has declined screening, or when the client/couple desire(s) comprehensive education about hemoglobinopathies even if there is no significant risk to the offspring.

- If a significant hemoglobinopathy has been diagnosed in the fetus, review postdiagnosis options carefully to enable the couple to make a decision regarding the pregnancy (i.e., termination or preparation for an affected child). The genetic counselor usually supplies the specifics.

- Provide ongoing emotional support for the client/couple facing the birth of a child with a significant hemoglobinopathy.

  ▶ Refer them to social services and community resources, if indicated.

  ▶ Refer them to a hematologist and/or pediatrician before delivery to discuss childhood interventions, if appropriate.

- If prenatal testing reveals that the fetus does not have a significant hemoglobinopathy, it is important for the couple to understand that this does not mean the baby will be "perfect." The general population risk of birth defects is 2 to 4 percent.

- Newborn screening is indicated for at-risk pregnancies. Consult your state's protocols regarding initial screening and recommended follow-up.

- Advise the client to make note of her hemoglobin disorder and alert future health care providers of this history.

  ▶ Preconception counseling is indicated for the woman with a hemoglobinopathy to provide information on the risks associated with the disorder during pregnancy, including maternal morbidity, perinatal loss, and the effects of treatment that may be indicated.

  ▶ In addition, preconception counseling for future pregnancies is indicated in the event she has a different partner.

- Document diagnosis of hemoglobin disorder in client/partner in progress notes and problem list.

  ▶ Comment on fetal diagnosis as indicated.

  ▶ Make note of any pregnancy complications.

  ▶ Also include in documentation whether partner was unavailable for/declined screening and the offering of genetic counseling.

References

American College of Obstetricians and Gynecologists. (1996). Hemoglobinopathies in pregnancy. (Technical Bulletin No. 220). Washington, DC: Author.

Bunn, H.F. (1992). Hemoglobin II. Sickle cell anemia and other hemoglobinopathies. In W.S. Beck (Ed.), *Hematology* (5th ed., pp. 187–204). Cambridge, MA: The MIT Press.

Hurst, D., Tittle, B., Kleman, K.M., Embury, S.H., & Lubin, B.H. (1983). Anemia and hemoglobinopathies in Southeast Asian refugee children. *The Journal of Pediatrics, 102*(5), 692–697.

Kark, J.A., Posey, D.M., Schumacher, H.R., & Ruehle, C.J. (1987). Sickle-cell trait as a risk factor for sudden death in physical training. *New England Journal of Medicine, 317*(13), 781–787.

Kinney, T.R., & Ware, R.E, (1994). Compound heterozygous states. In S.H. Embury, R.P. Hebbel, N. Mohandas, & M.H. Steinberg (Eds.), *Sickle cell disease: Basic principles and clinical practice* (pp. 437–451). New York: Raven Press.

Laros, R.K. Jr. (1994). Maternal hematologic disorders. In R.K. Creasy & R. Resnik (Eds.), *Maternal-fetal medicine: Principles and Practice* (3rd ed., pp. 905–933). Philadelphia, PA: W.B. Saunders.

McGhee, D., & Payne, M. (1995). Hemoglobinopathies and hemoglobin defects. In B.F. Rodak (Ed.), *Diagnostic hematology* (pp. 260). Philadelphia, PA: W. B. Saunders.

State of California Department of Health Services, & Children's Hospital, Oakland. (1992). *Sickle cell educator/counselor training program. Course manual.* Berkeley, CA: State of California. Department of Health Services, Genetic Disease Branch.

Vichinsky, E., Hurst, D., & Lubin, B. (1988, Feb.). Update on sickle cell disease. *Hospital Medicine*, 131–149.

Weatherall, D.J., & Clegg, J.B. (1981). *The thalassaemia syndromes* (3rd ed.) Oxford, England: Blackwell Scientific Publications.

Chapter 8

Rh (D) ISOIMMUNIZATION

Lisa L. Lommel

The Rh factor is an inherited antigen confined to the surface of red blood cells. There are five major antigens determining Rh status: C, DX, E, c, and e. The presence of the D antigen determines an individual's Rh-positive status. The absence of the D antigen determines an individual's Rh-negative status. The presence of a positive test for D^u indicates that the mother's red blood cells carry a varient of the D-antigen and can be considered D-positive (American College of Obstetricians and Gynecologists (ACOG, 1990). The Rh antigens C, c, E, and e are less immunogenic than D antigen. Ninety-eight percent of hemolytic disease in the newborn (HDN) is caused by RhD isoimmunization. While the c antigen causes the most severe erythroblastosis fetalis (ACOG, 1990).

The major antigen D, or Rh factor, is of concern when an Rh-negative mother is carrying an Rh-positive fetus. Rh (D) isoimmunization may occur following 1) incompatible blood transfusion or 2) fetomaternal blood cell exchange between a mother and incompatible fetus. With isoimmunization, the Rh-negative woman produces IgG antibodies in response to Rh-positive, fetal red blood cells entering the maternal circulation. These antibodies readily cross the placenta and destroy the Rh-positive fetal red blood cells causing hemolytic disease in the newborn (HDN). ABO incompatibility (see Chapter 9.1, *ABO Incompatibility/Irregular Antibodies*) confers some protection against D isoimmunization because fetal red cells entering the mother usually are rapidly destroyed before they elicit an antigenic response. With incompatibility there is a 2 percent chance of D isoimmunization by 6 months' gestation, while a D-negative woman who delivers a D positive ABO-compatible infant has a 16 percent chance of developing isoimmunization (Cunningham, MacDonald, Gant, Leveno & Gilstrap, 1993).

Hemolytic disease of the newborn (HDN) can vary from mild to severe. The severity of HDN depends on several factors:

- The maternal immune response to the fetal blood antigen

- The amount of antigen infused into maternal circulation

- The ABO group of the fetus (see ABO Incompatibility/Irregular Antibody protocol)

- The gestational age at which maternal antibody response and hemolysis become significant (Cunningham et al., 1993).

The severity of HDN in subsequent pregnancies of Rh-positive fetuses is usually equal to or greater than that of the previous pregnancy (ACOG, 1990).

A severe form of HDN, erythroblastosis fetalis, occurs when destruction of fetal red blood cells exceeds production. Erythroblastosis fetalis is usually manifested by neonatal anemia, kernicterus, and generalized edema (hydrops fetalis). Hydrops fetalis is the result of accelerated destruction of fetal red blood cells, which causes severe anemia and tissue hypoxia. The perinatal mortality rate for hydrops fetalis is high. It is diagnosed by the presence of edema, anemia, hepatomegaly, splenomegaly, and placental enlargement. Early intervention, before the onset of hydrops fetalis, greatly improves neonatal outcome.

Administering D immunoglobulin within 72 hours of exposure to antigen can prevent the formation of antibodies and has been effective in reducing the incidence of Rh isoimmunization. However, although Rh isoimmunization can be prevented, it still occurs because of failure to administer D immunoglobulin at the appropriate time or failure to administer an adequate dose (Vomund & Witter, 1994). D immunoglobulin is not useful if the mother has already developed D-antigen antibodies. It is important to screen all pregnant women for Rh status and offer antenatal and postpartum D immunoglobulin to nonsensitized Rh-negative mothers to prevent isoimmunization in subsequent pregnancies.

Pregnancies complicated by Rh isoimmunization should be managed by a physician. Management includes serial amniocenteses to evaluate the level of bilirubin in the amniotic fluid. High levels of bilirubin measured in conjunction with fetal gestational age (Liley graph) can estimate the future severity of hemolytic disease of the newborn. Fetuses that are considered severely affected may need to undergo intrauterine fetal transfusions to reduce the risk of death until sufficient pulmonary maturity exists for delivery.

Database

Subjective

- History of Rh-negative status
  - ▶ Membership in a genetic pool with a high Rh-negative probability (Basques of Spain, 34 percent; Caucasians, 15 percent; African-Americans, 8 percent; Asians and American Indians, <1 percent) (Duerbeck & Seeds, 1993)
- Rh-negative woman with history of fetal-maternal hemorrhage caused by
  - ▶ Vaginal or cesarean delivery (as little as 0.1 mL of fetal blood in the maternal circulation can produce an immune response)
  - ▶ Amniocentesis
  - ▶ Chorionic villi sampling
  - ▶ Ectopic pregnancy
  - ▶ Antepartum hemorrhage
  - ▶ Manual removal of the placenta
  - ▶ Placenta previa
  - ▶ Abruptio placentae
  - ▶ External version
  - ▶ Pregnancy induced hypertension/preeclampsia
  - ▶ Fetal demise
  - ▶ Multiple pregnancy
  - ▶ Abdominal trauma
  - ▶ Traumatic delivery
- History of previous pregnancy with rising titers and /or affected fetus or infant

- History of blood transfusion
- Father-of-baby's Rh type unknown or different from mother
- Usually asymptomatic

Objective

- Nonsensitized Rh-negative mother
- Sensitized Rh-negative mother
- Presence or absence of rising antibody titer
- Documentation of father Rh type

Assessment

- Rh-negative mother, sensitized or non-sensitized
- Rh-positive father or status unknown
- Rising antibody titer
- Document procedures performed or events causing increased risk of fetal-maternal hemorrhage in the pregnancy

Plan

Diagnostic Tests

- Blood type, Rh type, and antibody screen (indirect Coombs test) at first visit on all patients
- Non-sensitized, Rh-negative women
  - ▶ Screen father of baby for blood type and Rh type (if certain of paternity), otherwise assume Rh-positive
  - ▶ Antibody screen of Rh-negative mothers at 26 to 27 weeks' gestation
- Sensitized, Rh-negative women
  - ▶ Obtain antigen status and zygosity of father of the baby; If unobtainable, assume antigen positive

Treatment/Management

- Nonsensitized, Rh-negative
  - ▶ If the father of the baby is Rh-negative, no further testing is necessary. The fetus will be Rh-negative.

▶ If the father of the baby is Rh-positive or if his status is unknown, administer 300 µg of D immunoglobulin (RhoGam) at 28 to 29 weeks' gestation to patients whose antibody screen is negative at 26 to 28 weeks.

NOTE: Administration of 300 µg of D immunoglobulin protects against approximately 30 mL of fetal whole blood or 15 mL of fetal red blood cells in the maternal circulation.

▶ Administer 300 µg of D immunoglobulin to women who undergo a second-trimester amniocentesis. These patients should also receive the standard dose of 300 µg of D immunoglobulin at 28 to 29 weeks' gestation.

▶ Administer 300 µg of D immunoglobulin to women who undergo a third-trimester amniocentesis when delivery is not expected within 48 hours of the procedure.

   – If delivery occurs within 21 days and examination of maternal blood (Keihauer-Betke test) following delivery does not show excessive fetal red blood cells or if the indirect Coombs test is negative, additional D immunoglobulin is not needed (ACOG, 1996).

   – If delivery occurs within 48 hours, only a standard postpartum dose of 300 µg is recommended unless it is confirmed the newborn is D positive.

▶ Administer 300 µg of D immunoglobulin to patients who have a spontaneous or therapeutic abortion after 12 weeks' gestation.

NOTE: A dose of 50 µg of D immunoglobulin is adequate in pregnancies terminated before 13 weeks' gestation, ectopic pregnancies, or after chorionic villi sampling.

▶ Administer 300 µg of D immunoglobulin to women who undergo percutaneous umbilical cord blood sampling unless the fetal blood is found to be D negative.

▶ Administer 300 µg of D immunoglobulin to women who undergo extensive manipulation of the fetus (external cephalic version or percutaneous puncture) in the second or third trimester.

▶ Administer 300 µg of D immunoglobulin to patients whose D type is in question (i.e., a D-negative, D^u-positive mother in which the positive D^u status cannot be ruled out to be the result of circulating D^u-positive fetal red blood cells) (ACOG, 1996; Duerbeck & Seeds, 1993).

▶ If 300 µg of D immunoglobulin is given at 28 to 29 weeks' gestation, a repeat antibody titer at 36 weeks is not recommended. Approximately 20 percent of antibody titers performed at 36 weeks will be positive due to passively acquired antibodies from D immunoglobulin.

▶ Administer 300 µg of D immunoglobulin within 72 hours after delivery to patients whose newborns are found to be Rh-positive after cord blood sampling.

▶ If a patient experiences a high-risk pregnancy or delivery, which is known to be associated with greater amounts of fetal to maternal bleeding (i.e., abruptio placentae, placenta previa, cesarean delivery, intrauterine manipulation, manual removal of placenta), screening should be done to test for the number of fetal cells in the maternal circulation. After calculating the volume of the fetal-maternal bleed (Kleihauer-Betke test), give additional D immunoglobulin in the amount of 300 µg for every 30 mL of fetal blood or 15 mL of fetal red blood cells detected (ACOG, 1996).

• Sensitized Rh-negative

▶ Refer woman to a physician.

Consultation

- Physician management is *required* for isoimmunized patients.

Patient Education

- Discuss Rh factor and implications for the fetus.

- Explain to woman the risks and benefits of D immunoglobulin immunization.

- Provide woman with a card that identifies her as Rh-negative, including documentation of any D immunoglobulin immunizations received.

- Advise woman to alert her health care providers that she is Rh-negative in the event of future pregnancies or blood transfusions.

- Advise woman that reaction to D immunoglobulin is rare and is usually localized to the site of injection. A slight temperature elevation may be experienced.

- Discuss the risks to the fetus, need for amniocentesis, possibility of intrauterine transfusions, and management by MD in Rh-isoimmunized patients.

Follow-up

- Document Rh-negative status in progress notes and problem list to alert intrapartum staff to administer D immunoglobulin postpartum to non-sensitized patients whose infants are Rh-positive

References

American College of Obstetricians and Gynecologists, Committee on Obstetrics: Maternal and Fetal Medicine (1990). *Prevention of D isoimmunization* (Technical Bulletin No. 147). Washington, DC: Author.

American College of Obstetricians and Gynecologists, Committee on Obstetrics: Maternal and Fetal Medicine (1996). *Management of isoimmunization in pregnancy* (Educational Bulletin No. 227). Washington, DC: Author.

Cunningham, F.G., MacDonald, P.C., Gant, N.F., Leveno, K.J., & Gilstrap, L.C. (1993). *Williams Obstetrics* (19th Ed.) pp. 1004–1013. Norwalk, CT: Appleton & Lange.

Duerbeck, N. & Seeds, J.W. (1993). Rhesus immunization in pregnancy: A review. *Obstetrical and Gynecological Survey, 48*(12), 801–810.

Vomund, S.L., & Witter, S.E. (1994). Advanced techniques for the treatment of severe isoimmunization. *Maternal-Child Nursing, 19,* 18–23

SECTION 10

INFECTIOUS DISEASES

Chapter 1

CYTOMEGALOVIRUS

Winifred L. Star

Cytomegalovirus (CMV), a member of the herpesvirus family with many strains, is the most common cause of congenital viral infections in humans. Congenital CMV infection occurs in 0.5 to 2.5 percent of newborns in the United States—about 40,000 cases annually. The infection is a leading cause of deafness and a significant contributor to learning disabilities in this country (Raynor, 1993). Although the virus is widespread, serious illness is produced only in fetuses and the immunodeficient or immunosuppressed host (Gibbs & Sweet, 1994).

CMV is not highly contagious and the spread of infection requires close or intimate contact with infected secretions (Stagno & Cloud, 1994). The virus can be transmitted via body fluids (blood, semen, oropharyngeal secretions, cervical/vaginal secretions, urine, saliva, breast milk, tears), feces transplacentally, and through blood-product transfusion or bone-marrow or organ donation. Similar to herpes simplex virus, CMV may become latent after primary infection and be reactivated at a later time. Fifty to 85 percent of reproductive-age females have serologic evidence of prior CMV infection and are immune; among susceptible women the attack rate is about 2 to 6 percent per year (Ghidini & Lynch, 1994). Maternal immunity does not prevent the reactivation of CMV during pregnancy nor does it reliably prevent fetal transmission; approximately 1 to 2 percent of women with immunity develop recurrent infection during pregnancy (Alford, Stagno, & Pass, 1990; Ghidini & Lynch, 1994).

Most individuals with acute infection are asymptomatic. Occasionally, an acute mononucleosis-like syndrome presents. Other rare findings are a Guillain-Barré-like syndrome, pneumonia, aseptic meningitis, myocarditis, thrombocytopenia, and anemia (Scott, Hollier, & Dias, 1997).

Congenital infection is the result of transplacental transmission of CMV during either primary or recurrent maternal infection. Primary infection occurs in approximately 0.7 to 4.1 percent of pregnancies, with an estimated 40 percent intrauterine transmission risk. Symptomatic congenital CMV is more often associated with primary maternal infection, with infection during the first 20 weeks of gestation resulting in more severely affected infants. Spontaneous abortion and fetal loss may also occur in pregnant women with primary infection. Due to the high prevalence of maternal seropositivity, most congenitally infected infants are born to mothers with recurrent infection. The risk of transmission with recurrent maternal infection is between 0.2 and 1.8 percent. Congenital infections from recurrent maternal CMV are less likely to be clinically apparent (American College of Obstetricians and Gynecologists [AGOG], 1993; Andersson, 1990; Gibbs & Sweet, 1994; Nelson & Demmler, 1997; Scott et al., 1997; Stagno, 1995; Stagno et al., 1982; Stagno & Whitley, 1985).

Of infants infected by maternal primary infection, 85 to 90 percent exhibit no signs of clinical infection at birth, but 5 to 15 percent go on to develop neurodevelopmental sequelae, which usually appear within the first 2 years of life. Abnormalities may include sensorineural deafness (most common), microcephaly, motor defects, dental defects, chorioretinitis, and mental retardation. The remaining 10 percent of infected newborns will have cytomegalic inclusion disease (CID) at birth, which typically presents with hepatosplenomegaly, microcephaly, jaundice, and petechiae. Mortality among the most severely affected may be as high as 30 percent. Surviving CMV-infected infants have serious sequelae, which may include hepatitis, thrombocytopenia, sensorineural hearing loss, spastic plegias, chorioretinitis, microcephaly, cerebral calcifications, mental retardation, and other neuropsychologic abnormalities

(Alford et al., 1990; Britt, Pass, Stagno, & Alford, 1991; Gibbs & Sweet, 1994; Peckham, 1991; Raynor, 1993; Stagno, 1995).

If congenital infection occurs as a result of recurrent maternal infection, the majority of infected infants will be asymptomatic at birth, but about 5 to 10 percent will develop sequelae (usually hearing loss) (Fowler, Stagno, & Pass, 1993; Pass, 1991; Raynor, 1993; Urang, 1990). Preexisting maternal antibody is a strong determinant of favorable clinical outcome for the infant (Hanshaw, 1994). Congenital infection has also been associated with increased incidence of premature rupture of membranes and preterm delivery.

Infant perinatal infection with CMV may be acquired from multiple sources: during the course of delivery from exposure to infected maternal secretions, via breast-milk, or (iatrogenically) from transfused blood products (Alford et al., 1990). Approximately 10 percent of seropositive women excrete CMV during delivery and 30 to 50 percent of newborns whose mothers have genital infection at the time of birth will acquire the virus (Gibbs & Sweet, 1994). Forty to 60 percent of infants breast-fed by a CMV-positive mother for more than 1 month will become infected (Leguizamon & Reece, 1997). Incubation for perinatally acquired CMV infection is 4 to 12 weeks; the vast majority of infants are asymptomatic, although CMV pneumonitis may develop in early infancy (Alford et al., 1990; Raynor, 1993). In general, perinatal transmission as a means of infant CMV acquisition is usually without clinical consequence except in extremely low-birth-weight infants, who may develop severe disease (Gibbs & Sweet, 1994; Stagno & Cloud, 1994).

CMV infection from a public health standpoint requires consideration. Sources of infection may include day-care centers (urine and saliva of infected children are the two most important sources). Seroprevalence is higher in young children in grouped-care settings and these children may act as potential sources of infection for day-care-center workers, as well as for pregnant mothers and infant siblings. On the other hand, working in health care does not appear to significantly increase the risk of infection due, most likely, to the attention paid to universal precautions and rigorous hygiene measures in these settings (Canadian Paediatric Society, 1990; Isaacs, 1991; Pass, 1991; Stagno, 1995; Stagno & Cloud, 1994).

Database

Subjective

- Seroprevalence increases with age; infection-acquisition patterns vary widely according to ethnic, socioeconomic, occupational, and geographic factors. Patient may report history of seropositivity.

- Infection in adults is generally asymptomatic.

- Approximately 10 percent of clients with acute infection present with a mononucleosis-like syndrome.

  ▶ Abrupt onset of spiking temperature, chills

  ▶ Nausea, mild diarrhea

  ▶ Headache, malaise, myalgia, fatigue

  ▶ Mild sore throat, cough

Objective

- Possible maternal signs during symptomatic infection
  - ▶ Elevated temperature (low- or high-grade), increased pulse rate
  - ▶ Mild pharyngitis
  - ▶ Cervical or generalized lymphadenopathy
  - ▶ Papular rash of trunk
  - ▶ Splenomegaly, hepatomegaly (rarely)
  - ▶ Localized granulomas, occasionally
- Clinical findings of congenitally infected newborns with CID are discussed in the introductory section.
- See Diagnostic Tests section.

Assessment

- Maternal exposure to cytomegalovirus
  - ▶ R/O cytomegalovirus infection
  - ▶ R/O mononucleosis
  - ▶ R/O acute retroviral syndrome
  - ▶ R/O hepatitis A, B, and C
  - ▶ R/O congenital cytomegalovirus infection
  - ▶ R/O other perinatal infections: toxoplasmosis, rubella, herpes simplex virus infection, syphilis

Plan

Diagnostic Tests

- Diagnosis of maternal infection is rare due to the subclinical nature of disease in the majority of cases.
- Principal tests used for diagnosis are *serology* and *viral isolation*
  - ▶ Acute infection is evidenced by seroconversion with serial CMV-IgG determinations *or* by a significant (fourfold or greater) rise in IgG titer from acute and convalescent sera.

    NOTE: Specimens should be collected 3 to 4 weeks apart and tested in parallel; no change in antibody levels occurs with recurrent infection.

  - ▶ Presence of CMV-IgM may indicate recent infection (levels equal to at least 30 percent of the IgG value)

    NOTE: Antibody may persist for up to 18 months; thus, precise determination of onset of infection is difficult. High titer IgG and presence of nonspecific serum factors (e.g., rheumatoid factor) may interfere with IgM assays. Ten percent of women with recurrent infection have IgM antibodies; 20 percent of primary infections are not accompanied by IgM antibodies (Centers for Disease Control and Prevention [CDC], 1992; Scott et al., 1997).

▶ Viral isolation from urine, saliva, or vaginal or cervical secretions may be attempted; positive culture does not differentiate primary from recurrent infection.

● Additional laboratory tests that can aid in diagnosis of clients with symptomatic infection may include

▶ Heterophile (negative)

▶ White blood cell count, differential (will indicate lymphopenia or leukocytosis with a higher number of atypical lymphocytes on peripheral smear)

▶ Platelets (indicative of thrombocytopenia)

▶ Liver function tests (will show elevations [usually mild]) in total bilirubin, alkaline phosphatase, AST, ALT, LDH)

NOTE: Hepatic abnormalities are usually of a few weeks duration and gradually disappear.

▶ Cerebrospinal fluid (CSF) (increased levels of protein) (Alford et al., 1990; Yow, 1990)

● If there is clinical or laboratory evidence of maternal CMV infection, consultation with a physician is imperative. The following procedures may be offered for fetal assessment/diagnosis:

▶ Ultrasound. Findings may include

   – Microcephaly

   – Fetal ascites or hydrops

   – Cerebral ventriculomegaly or hydrocephalus

   – Pleural or pericardial effusion

   – Hepatosplenomegaly

   – Cystic/calcified lesions in brain/liver/placenta

   – Increased bowel echodensity

   – Oligohydramnios or polyhydramnios

   – Intrauterine growth restriction (Ghidini & Lynch, 1994; Nelson & Demmler, 1997; Raynor, 1993)

▶ Amniocentesis, cordocentesis. Various laboratory techniques can be utilized for determination of CMV infection in amniotic fluid or fetal blood (e.g., DNA studies, anti-CMV IgM, viral cultures and other laboratory analyses [complete blood count with differential and platelets, liver enzymes, and total IgM]).

NOTE: Amniotic fluid viral culture is presently the most commonly used method to diagnose fetal infection. Prenatal diagnosis of fetal CMV infections is most useful in pregnancies that have demonstrated ultrasonographic evidence of fetal disease plus clinical or laboratory findings suggestive of maternal infection (Nelson & Demmler, 1997).

● Detection of CMV-IgM antibody in cord or neonatal blood is strong presumptive evidence of congenital infection (Hanshaw, 1994). (About 80 percent of congenitally infected neonates have IgM antibody in the first few months of life.)

NOTE: False positives and negatives may occur; thus, attempts to isolate virus from the infant should be pursued (see below).

- CMV-IgG antibody titers may be followed for the first 6 to 12 months after birth to determine whether immunity was acquired passively from the mother or actively by infection of the infant. (Passive antibody from mother usually disappears by 9 months.)

- Culture of fresh urine is the most reliable means of diagnosis of congenital CMV in the neonate. (Cultures may also be obtained from the newborn's saliva, nasopharynx, conjunctiva, or spinal fluid.)

  NOTE: Diagnosis of congenital CMV must be accomplished in first 2 to 3 weeks of life because virus recovered after this time may indicate acquired infection.

- Perinatally acquired infections are diagnosed (preferably) by tissue culture 3 to 12 weeks after exposure; urine/saliva (and other body fluid) cultures from the newborn should be negative in the first 2 weeks of life (Stagno, 1995).

Treatment/Management

- Routine screening of pregnant women, family members, day-care staff, or hospital staff for CMV infection is generally *not* recommended (American Academy of Pediatrics, 1994; Canadian Paediatric Society, 1990; Isaacs, 1991).

  NOTE: If testing is performed, women found to be seronegative should be provided with information to prevent CMV-acquisition (see Patient Education section).

- Women with symptoms suggestive of CMV infection should be screened for CMV with urine and cervical cultures. Serologic studies as described in Diagnostic Tests also may be employed (Urang, 1990).

- When maternal infection has been diagnosed, the client can be referred to a physician for further management.

- As of this writing there are no established treatment guidelines for CMV infection during pregnancy. Ganciclovir has been used in adults/neonates with CMV infection, but further studies regarding its efficacy and safety are needed. Research continues on the development of a vaccine. Treatment of the "mono-like" syndrome in the mother is purely symptomatic.

- The option of pregnancy termination should be presented in cases of confirmed fetal infection and fetal abnormalities (Stray-Pederson, 1993). However, families should be counseled that in the absence of unequivocal evidence of severe fetal disease, the vast majority of fetuses of primarily infected mothers (more than 80 to 90 percent, depending on the clinical setting) will be unaffected or only mildly affected (K. P. Beckerman, M.D., personal communication, October 8, 1996).

- Breastfeeding generally should not be restricted in a CMV-infected woman.

  ▶ Mother should understand that although CMV can be excreted in breast milk, it is rarely a concern for a healthy infant (premature infants are at higher risk for morbidity).

  ▶ Storing breast milk at -20° C will reduce but not eliminate infectivity (Stagno, 1995).

- Thorough evaluation of a congenitally infected infant should be carried out by the pediatric team. Details are beyond the scope of this chapter.

Consultation

- Consult with a physician in all cases of suspected CMV infection. Depending upon site-specific practice, client may be managed by the obstetrician or perinatologist.

- In complicated cases, consultation with an infectious disease expert may be warranted.

Patient Education

- When maternal CMV is diagnosed, provide information on the means of transmission, potential risk of congenital infection, disease sequelae, the assessment tools available for diagnosis of fetal infection, and information about pregnancy termination, as indicated.

    NOTE: It is often difficult to provide meaningful information about fetal risks due to the limitations of maternal IgM antibody screening for diagnosing primary versus recurrent infection. Women should be reassured that even with primary infection, risk of fetal harm is low (Scott et al., 1997). In many cases the physician caring for the client will carry out the education and counseling.

- Education regarding prevention of CMV transmission should be undertaken, especially if a woman has a child in day-care, works in such a setting, or is a health care worker. Discussion should include the following points:

    ▶ Use good hand-washing technique, especially after changing child's diaper, after assisting child with use of toilet, and before eating.

    ▶ Dispose of diapers promptly and separate diapering area from food preparation area.

    ▶ Clean surfaces promptly (including toys) if they have been contaminated with urine or saliva.

    ▶ Avoid kissing children on the mouth or nuzzling children with saliva on their faces.

    ▶ Use good hand-washing and hygiene practices, universal precautions, and latex gloves in hospital settings (ACOG, 1993; American Academy of Pediatrics, 1994; Canadian Paediatric Society, 1990; Isaacs, 1991).

- Safer sex guidelines should be addressed, as indicated.

Follow-up

- Referrals to psychological, social, and other support services are important considerations if the infant has significant congenital CMV disease and associated sequelae thereof.

- Infants with congenital CMV infection require close long-term follow-up by the pediatric team.

- Client should understand that there is a potential risk of congenital CMV infection in subsequent pregnancies. Counseling a woman who has given birth to an infant with CMV is difficult as the incidence of recurrence is not known.

- Document CMV status in problem list and progress notes. Comment on perinatal findings, as appropriate.

References

Alford, C.A., Stagno, S., & Pass, R.F. (1990). Congenital and perinatal cytomegalovirus infections. *Reviews of Infectious Diseases, 12*(Suppl. 7), S745–S753.

American Academy of Pediatrics. (1994). *1994 Red book: Report of the Committee on Infectious Diseases* (23rd ed., pp. 173–177). Elk Grove Village, IL: Author.

American College of Obstetricians and Gynecologists (ACOG). (1993). Perinatal viral and parasitic infections. (Technical Bulletin #177). Washington, DC: Author.

Andersson, J. (1990). Cytomegalovirus infection in pregnancy. *Scandinavian Journal of Infectious Disease, 71*, 67–70.

Britt, W.J., Pass, R.F., Stagno, S., & Alford, C.A. (1991). Pediatric cytomegalovirus infection. *Transplantation Proceedings, 23*(3, Suppl. 3), 115–117.

Canadian Paediatric Society. Infectious Diseases and Immunization Committee. (1990). Cytomegalovirus infection in day-care centres: Risks to pregnant women. *Canadian Medical Association, 142*(6), 547–549.

Centers for Disease Control and Prevention (CDC). (1992). Cytomegalovirus. Fax document #362303. Atlanta: Author

Chandler, S.H., Alexander, E.R., & Holmes, K.K. (1985). Epidemiology of cytomegalovirus infection in a heterogeneous population of pregnant women. *Journal of Infectious Diseases, 152*, 249–256.

Fowler, K.B., & Pass, R.F. (1991). Sexually transmitted diseases in mothers of neonates with congenital cytomegalovirus infection. *Journal of Infectious Disease, 164*, 259–264.

Fowler, K.B., Stagno, S., & Pass, R.F. (1993). Maternal age and congenital cytomegalovirus infection: Screening of two diverse newborn populations. *Journal of Infectious Disease, 168*, 552–556.

Ghidini, A., & Lynch, L. (1994). Management strategies for congenital infections. *The Mount Sinai Journal of Medicine, 61*(5), 376–388.

Gibbs, R.S., & Sweet, R.L. (1994). Clinical disorders. In R.K. Creasy, & R. Resnik (Eds.), *Maternal-fetal medicine. Principles and practice* (3rd ed., pp. 661–664). Philadelphia, PA: W.B. Saunders.

Hanshaw, J.B. (1994). Congenital cytomegalovirus infection. *Pediatric Annals, 23*(3), 124–128.

Isaacs, D. (1991). Cytomegalovirus infection and hospital staff. *Paediatric Child Health, 27*, 317–318.

Leguizamon, G., & Reece, E.A. (1997). Is serologic screening for all pregnant women for cytomegalovirus warranted? *Contemporary OB/GYN, 42* (8), 49–62.

Nelson, C.T., & Demmler, G.J. Cytomegalovirus infection in the pregnant mother, fetus, and newborn infant. *Clinics in Perinatology, 24* (1), 151–160.

Pass, R. F. (1991). Day-care centers and the spread of cytomegalovirus and parvovirus B19. *Pediatric Annals, 20(8)*, 419–426.

Peckham, C.S. (1991). Cytomegalovirus infection: Congenital and neonatal disease. *Scandinavian Journal of Infection, 78,* 82–87.

Raynor, B.D. (1993). Cytomegalovirus infection in pregnancy. *Seminars in Perinatology, 17(6),* 394–402.

Scott, L.L., Hollier, L.M., & Dias, K. (1997). Perinatal herpes virus infections: Herpes simplex varicella, and cytomegalovirus. *Infectious Disease Clinics of North America, 11*(1), 27–53.

Stagno, S. (1995). Cytomegalovirus. In J. S. Remington, & J. O. Klein (Eds.), *Infectious diseases of the fetus and newborn infant* (4th ed., pp. 312–353). Philadelphia, PA: W.B. Saunders.

Stagno, S., & Cloud, G.A. (1994). Working parents: The impact of day care and breast-feeding on cytomegalovirus infections in offsprings. *Proceedings of the National Academy of Science, 91,* 2384–2389.

Stagno, S., Pass, R.F., Dworsky, M.E., Henderson, R.E., Moore, E.G., Walton, P.D., & Alford, C.A. (1982). Congenital cytomegalovirus infection: the relative importance of primary and recurrent maternal infection. *New England Journal of Medicine, 306,* 945–949.

Stagno, S., & Whitley, R.J. (1985(. Herpesvirus infections of pregnancy, part 1: Cytomegalovirus and Epstein-Barr virus infections. *New England Journal of Medicine, 313,* 1270–1274

Stray-Pederson, B. (1993). New aspects of perinatal infections. *Annals of Medicine, 25,* 295–300.

Urang, A. (1990). Cytomegalovirus infection in pregnancy. *Journal of Nurse-Midwifery, 35(5),* 299–306.

Yow, M.D. (1990, March). CMV infection in young women. *Hospital Practice,* 61–79.

Chapter 2

HEPATITIS A, B, C, D, AND E

Lisa L. Lommel

Viral hepatitis is a systemic infection that primarily affects the liver. The most common causes of viral hepatitis are the 1) hepatitis A virus (HAV), 2) hepatitis B virus (HBV), 3) hepatitis delta virus (HDV), and 4) two different non-A, non-B hepatitis (NANB) viruses, hepatitis C virus (HCV) and hepatitis E virus (HEV).

Hepatitis A Virus (HAV)

Also known as "infectious hepatitis," hepatitis A has an incubation period of 2 to 6 weeks and is transmitted by fecal-oral routes, commonly with contaminated food or drinking water. HAV transmission occurs rarely through contaminated blood, but perinatal transmission has not been demonstrated. However, neonates born to mothers with early, acute HAV infection may contract the disease in the neonatal period and suffer a severe case of the disease (Simms & Duff, 1993). Stool is infectious during the late incubation period and through the first week of illness when transaminase levels peak. Infectivitiy ceases before the onset of jaundice.

Hepatitis A is more common in young children, who often have mild or subclinical cases. Adults commonly present with jaundice. Hepatitis A does not cause a chronic state but 1 percent of cases may progress to fulminant hepatitis. The course of hepatitis is not altered by pregnancy nor is there an increased risk of poor pregnancy outcome, unless the mother is very ill. No adverse fetal effects have been identified (Simms & Duff, 1993).

Hepatitis B Virus (HBV)

Also known as "serum hepatitis," hepatitis B has an incubation period varying from 2 to 6 months and is transmitted through a break in the skin, contact with mucous membranes or their effluvia, or parenteral or perinatal exposure. Approximately 10 percent of adults contracting hepatitis B become chronic carriers, defined by abnormal aminotransferase levels and histopathological findings that persist longer than 6 months. Approximately 25 to 30 percent of chronic carriers will progress to liver cirrhosis with an increased risk of hepatocellular carcinoma.

There are two subclasses of chronic HBV hepatitis, chronic persistent hepatitis (CPH) and chronic active hepatitis (CAH), both of which maintain the ability to transmit the virus. The distinction between these two categories is made by liver biopsy and is characterized by the extent of liver involvement; CAH extends beyond the portal area and has a poorer prognosis.

The course of HBV does not manifest differently in the pregnant woman. There are no teratogenic syndromes associated with acute HBV infection in pregnancy, and pregnancy outcomes are no different from women without HBV in pregnancy (Pastorek, 1993).

Perinatal transmission of hepatitis B virus from mother to fetus is one of the most efficient modes of infection. Transmission most often occurs in mothers who develop acute hepatitis infection late in the third trimester or during the intrapartum and postpartum period; the fetus or infant is exposed to hepatitis B surface antigen (HBsAg) via positive vaginal secretions, blood, amniotic fluid, saliva, and breast milk (American College of Obstetricians and Gynecologists [ACOG], 1992). However, transmission of the virus through the placental membrane is thought to be rare because of the relatively large size of the virus. Neonatal infection is also rare when maternal hepatitis infection is resolved during the first and second trimesters.

Infants born to mothers who are positive for both HBsAG and hepatitis B e antigen (HBeAG), which denotes a highly infectious state, have a 90 percent chance of acquiring perinatal hepatitis B infection. It is estimated that more than 90 percent of infants so infected will become chronic carriers. Twenty-five percent of chronic carriers die from primary hepatocellular carcinoma or cirrhosis of the liver (ACOG, 1992).

Routine screening for HBsAG on all pregnant women is recommended. In addition, routine immunization of all infants is currently recommended, with the additional administration of hepatitis B immune globulin to infants born to HBsAG-positive mothers. This regime has been found to be 85 to 95 percent effective in preventing neonatal infection when given correctly. Screening and vaccination of susceptible household members and sexual partners of hepatitis B carriers is also recommended.

Hepatitis D Virus (HDV)

Hepatitis D (delta hepatitis) is caused by either a co-infection (acute hepatitis D virus [HDV] simultaneous with acute hepatitis B virus [HBV]) or a superinfection (acute HDV superimposed on a hepatitis B carrier); that is hepatitis D can occur only in the presence of HBV. HDV is most commonly transmitted through parenteral routes (intravenous drug use and multiple transfusions). Perinatal transmission has been reported, although it is rare because neonatal prophylaxis against HBV assures effective immunity against hepatitis D.

The majority of HDV coinfection is self-limiting. Approximately 5 percent of patients with delta co-infection develop chronic infection. Approximately 80 percent of patients with superinfection develop chronic hepatitis. Approximately 75 percent of patients with chronic delta hepatitis develop cirrhosis. The course of hepatitis D is not altered by pregnancy nor is there an increased risk of poor pregnancy outcome unless the mother is very ill. No adverse fetal effects have been identified (Simms & Duff, 1993).

Non-A, Non-B Hepatitis

Hepatitis C Virus (HCV)

Hepatitis C has an incubation period varying from 6 to 12 weeks. It is primarily transmitted through the parenteral route (blood transfusion and intravenous drug use) and is the primary cause of post-transfusion non-A, non-B hepatitis (95 percent). Information regarding the incidence of perinatal transmission is conflicting. There have been identified, although infrequent, cases. Some studies have suggested an increased incidence of vertical transmission with maternal HIV infection (Simms & Duff, 1993). Acute hepatitis C virus (HCV) infections are usually mild. Approximately 50 percent of patients with HCV develop chronic hepatitis, and approximately 20 percent of those develop cirrhosis. Hepatitis C is also a frequent cause of community acquired (sporadic) hepatitis. Anti-HCV antibody cannot be detected until 6 to 8 weeks after onset of clinical hepatitis, which makes testing undesirable for diagnosis of acute HCV infection. The course of hepatitis C is not altered by pregnancy nor is there an increase risk of poor pregnancy outcome unless the mother is very ill. Chronic active hepatitis is associated with an increased incidence of prematurity and intrauterine growth restriction (Simms & Duff, 1993). There is no vaccine available for prevention of this disease.

Hepatitis E Virus (HEV)

Hepatitis E has an incubation period of 6 weeks and is transmitted by the fecal-oral route. Hepatitis E virus (HEV) is one of the primary causes of viral hepatitis in developing countries. In the United States, the only cases that have been reported were acquired in endemic countries. Hepatitis E appears most often in the 15- to 39-year-old age group; it is more common in males, but the highest incidence is in pregnant females. The virus is shed in stool in the late incubation period and early acute phase. Shedding decreases before peak alanine amniotransferase (ALT). It does not cause chronic liver disease but 1 to 2 percent of cases are fatal. In pregnancy, case fatality can be as high as 20 percent. If the mother survives the acute phase of illness, fetal outcome is not adversely affected. Perinatal transmission is not know to occur.

General Hepatitis Information

Database

Subjective

- Symptoms are extremely variable from asymptomatic to fulminating disease.

- Common symptoms and discomforts of pregnancy can mimic symptoms of hepatitis.

- General symptoms in the prodromal phase may include the following:

  ▶ Abrupt or insidious onset

  ▶ Malaise, fatigue

  ▶ Myalgia, arthralgia

  ▶ Upper respiratory symptoms (nasal discharge, pharyngitis)

  ▶ Headache

  ▶ Photophobia

  ▶ Anorexia

  ▶ Nausea, vomiting

  ▶ Weight loss

  ▶ Diarrhea or constipation

  ▶ Fever rarely over 39.5° C/103.1° F

  ▶ Altered taste and smell with distaste for smoking

- General symptoms in the icteric phase may include the following:

  ▶ Jaundice (usually appears 5 to10 days after symptom onset when prodromal symptoms begin to diminish)

- ▶ Lack of jaundice
- ▶ Right upper quadrant/epigastric pain aggravated by jarring or exertion
- ▶ Dark urine, clay-colored stools present with jaundice
- ▶ Intensified prodromal symptoms (with onset of jaundice) followed by symptom improvement
- General symptoms in the convalescent phase may include the following:
  - ▶ Disappearance of jaundice
  - ▶ Return of appetite
  - ▶ Resolving abdominal pain
- Acute illness subsides after 2 to 3 weeks and is gone by 6 to 8 weeks.

Assessment

- Viral hepatitis

Plan

Diagnostic Tests

- The following tests should be performed at least twice a week until enzyme levels have reached plateaus and then weekly until they normalize (Mishra & Seeff, 1992):
  - ▶ Alanine amniotransferase (ALT; formerly SGPT) and aminotransferase (AST; formerly SGOT)
  - ▶ Complete blood count (CBC)
  - ▶ Prothrombin time (PT)
  - ▶ Bilirubin
  - ▶ Albumin/globulin
  - ▶ Urinalysis

Treatment/Management

- Pregnancies complicated by acute viral hepatitis are usually managed on an outpatient basis.
- Supportive therapy is a mainstay of treatment with acute viral hepatitis.
- Adequate nutrition should be encouraged with small, frequent meals containing high protein and low fat.
- Maintain adequate hydration.
- Bed rest has not been proven to alter disease course.
- Physical activity should be encouraged as tolerated; take care to avoid hepatic injury.
- Eliminate hepatotoxic agents (e.g., medications and alcohol).

- Hospital management is indicated when there is

  ▶ intractable nausea and vomiting

  ▶ Severe anemia

  ▶ Prolonged prothrombin time

  ▶ Low serum albumin

  ▶ Serum bilirubin greater than 15 mg/100 mL

  ▶ Associated conditions such as diabetes

  ▶ Encephalopathy or coagulopathy

- Antepartum fetal surveillance should be employed, when appropriate, for severe maternal disease compromising fetal health.

Consultation

- Physician consultation is required for acute hepatitis or abnormal liver function tests.

- Refer to a physician all patients who

  ▶ Are immunocompromised

  ▶ Have difficult-to-manage underlying chronic disorders

  ▶ Have severe symptoms unable to provide adequate caloric and fluid intake

  ▶ Have worsening symptoms

  ▶ Have clinical manifestations of fulminant disease

- Refer patients with chronic hepatitis to a physician to determine specific diagnosis.

  ▶ Patients with chronic persistent hepatitis may be followed in consultation with the physician.

  ▶ Patients with chronic active hepatitis should be managed by a physician.

Patient Education

- Teach patient and family about risk factors, pathophysiology, management plan, state of infectivity, and prophylaxis availability of hepatitis vaccines.

- Advise an infected patient regarding transmission precautions until period of infectivity has passed.

- Inform patient of perinatal and sexual transmissibility, as appropriate, for hepatitis B, D and C.

- Inform patient that hepatitis virus infection does not increase risk for fetal abnormalities.

- Patients with a carrier or chronic state should be advised to continue antitransmission precautions.

- Teach patient good personal hygiene:

  ▶ Wash hands with soap after using the bathroom.

▶ Dispose of tampons, peripads, bandages in plastic bags.

▶ Use separate drinking cups, utensils, razors, toothbrushes, manicure sets.

● Advise patient not to prepare or serve food to others.

● Advise patient that intimate contact (sharing of bodily fluids) should be avoided.

● Advise patient that male sex partners should use condoms.

● Dental dams and female condoms should also be advised as appropriate.

● Advise thorough handwashing for those who come in contact with infected utensils, bedding, or clothing.

● Educate intravenous drug users to clean their needles properly with bleach; discuss availability of new needles through needle exchange services in the area.

● Educate health care workers to properly dispose of blood, blood products, and needles (do not recap them, special waste containers should be available). Employ universal precautions at all times.

● Explain the importance of immunoprophylaxis for infant and exposed contacts with hepatitis B and D.

● Advise that breastfeeding is not contraindicated if the infant was immunized against hepatitis B.

● Advise patient regarding a nutritious diet. See Section 18, *Nutrition*.

● Advise patient regarding measures to reduce nausea (small frequent meals, carbohydrates).

● Advise patient to engage in regular physical activity, as tolerated, but to avoid becoming overtired.

● Advise patient to omit hepatotoxic agents (e.g., hepatotoxic drugs and alcohol).

● Advise patient to inform all health care providers regarding hepatitis infection status.

Follow-up

● Patient should be evaluated at 2 weeks after diagnosis and in 3 months for repeat laboratory studies.

▶ Patient may need to be evaluated more often, depending on symptomatology.

▶ Patient with persistent symptoms or laboratory abnormalities beyond 12 weeks should be monitored every 4 weeks with:

－ ALT and AST

－ Bilirubin

－ PT

－ Albumin/globulin

－ Serologic marker for virus type

● Refer a patient with persistent symptoms or abnormal lab values for longer than 6 months to a physician.

- Patients with chronic hepatitis should be followed by a physician. In particular, patients with chronic active hepatitis should be followed closely.

- A public health nurse referral may assist the family with preventive care and teaching in the home.

- Report HBsAG-positive pregnant women to the local and/or state health department to ensure that they are entered into a case-management system and that appropriate prophylaxis is provided for their infants (CDC, 1998).

- Referral to drug treatment program if patient actively using drugs.

- Document hepatitis status in progress notes and problem list.

Hepatitis A

Database

Subjective

- Risk factors include

  - Recent foreign travel

  - Exposure to individual with hepatitis

  - Child in day care center

  - Residency or employment in institutions for mentally handicapped

  - Intravenous drug use

  - Ingestion of raw shellfish

- Forty percent of individuals have no identifiable risk factor.

- Ninety percent of adults will exhibit symptoms as listed above under General Hepatitis Information.

Objective

- Aminotransferase elevations (in the hundreds) may precede or coincide with onset of prodromal symptoms.

- Bilirubin elevation is five to ten times normal

- Laboratory tests are usually normal after 9 weeks.

Assessment

- Hepatitis A

  - R/O hepatitis B

  - R/O hepatitis D

  - R/O hepatitis C

▶ R/O hepatitis E

▶ R/O infectious mononucleosis

▶ R/O cytomegalovirus infection

▶ R/O herpes simplex virus infection

▶ R/O drug-induced liver disease

▶ R/O toxoplasmosis

▶ R/O severe preeclampsia

▶ R/O acute fatty liver

▶ R/O biliary tract disease

▶ R/O Epstein-Barr virus infection

▶ R/O human immunodeficiency virus and Infection

Plan

Diagnostic Tests

● See Table 10.1, Serological markers for hepatitis A and Figure 10.1, Course of Hepatitis A Infection.

▶ IgM antibody to HAV (anti-HAV) will develop early in acute infection and persist for 6 to 12 months.

▶ IgG anti-HAV will indicate previous exposure to HAV, noninfectivity, and immunity to recurring HAV infection.

● ALT will peak at onset of clinical disease and return to normal after 3 months.

Treatment/Management

● Hepatitis A is self-limiting. Supportive measures are recommended.

● Hospitalization may be necessary if there is dehydration because of nausea and vomiting or with fulminant hepatitis A.

● Hepatitis A vaccine or immune globulin (IG) is recommended for all susceptible persons traveling to or working in developing countries.

▶ Hepatitis A vaccine (Havrix®)

– Dosage for adults over 18 years old is 1440 ELISA units (ELU), which is a volume of 1.0 mL, IM into the deltoid now and 6 to 12 months later (for a total of two doses) (CDC, 1998).

▶ Hepatitis A vaccine (VAQTA)

– Dosage for adults over 17 years old is 50 units IM into the deltoid now and 6 months later (for a total of two doses) (CDC, 1996).

- Screening for total antibodies to HAV (anti-HAV) in travelers who are likely to have had a prior HAV infection may be useful to determine susceptibility and eliminate unnecessary vaccination or IG prophylaxis of already immune persons.

- Protection is assumed by 4 weeks after receiving initial vaccine dose. The second dose 6-12 months later is necessary for long-term protection.

  NOTE: Data on the persistence of antibody after vaccine are limited. Estimates from models suggest that protective levels of anti-HAV could persist for at least 20 years (CDC, 1996).

- Since the hepatitis A vaccine is produced from inactivated HAV, the theoretical risk to a developing fetus is probably low when the vaccine is administered to a pregnant woman. There is currently no animal or human data to determine the safety of hepatitis A vaccination during pregnancy (CDC, 1996).

- Hepatitis A vaccine should not be administered to persons with a history of hypersensitive reaction to components in the vaccine (i.e., alum or the preservative 2-phenoxyethanol).

- Give immune globulin in the following circumstances:

  ▶ Travelers who are allergic to a vaccine component or elect not to receive the vaccine should receive immune globulin.

  ▶ If traveling to intermediate or high-risk areas less than 4 weeks after initial dose of vaccine, also give immune globulin (0.02 mL/kg) but at a different injection site.

  ▶ Give immune globulin 0.02 mL/kg IM within 2 weeks of arrival in an endemic area for a stay of less than 3 months (CDC, 1996).

  ▶ If staying longer than 3 months, recommended dosage is immune globulin 0.06 mL/kg IM every 5 months (CDC, 1996).

  ▶ Preexposure prophylaxis is recommended in pregnancy when traveling to endemic areas of Asia, Africa and India where hygiene standards are not strictly controlled. Pregnancy is not a contraindication to using immune globulin (CDC, 1996).

- Hepatitis A vaccine is recommended for all susceptible persons traveling to or working in developing countries.

- Postexposure prophylaxis is recommended in pregnancy when there has been a known exposure.

  ▶ Immune globulin 0.02 mL/kg IM (Knauer, 1993).

  ▶ Infants of mothers who may be infectious at or soon after delivery are also candidates for immune globulin.

NOTE: Prophylaxis is 80-95 percent effective in preventing symptomatic hepatitis if given within 2 weeks of exposure (CDC, 1998).

Consultation

- See Consultation section under General Hepatitis Information, above.

Patient Education

- See Patient Education section under General Hepatitis Information, above.

Follow-up

- See Follow-up section under General Hepatitis Information, above.
- Document hepatitis A status in progress notes and problem list.

Hepatitis B

Database

Subjective

- Risk factors include (Center for Disease Control and Prevention [CDC], 1998):
  ► Health or public safety worker exposed to blood or blood products
  ► Hemodialysis staff or patients
  ► Illegal drug users, including injection-drug users and users of illegal noninjected drugs
  ► Recipients of high-risk blood products or multiple transfusions
  ► Female partners of sexually active bisexual men
  ► Sexually active heterosexual women, including those who
    – Recently had another sexually transmitted disease (STD) diagnosed
    – Had more than one sex partner in the preceding 6 months
    – Received treatment in an STD clinic
    – Are prostitutes
  ► Inmate of a long-term correctional institution
  ► Employee or patient in institution for developmentally disabled
  ► Sexual and household contacts with HBsAG carriers
  ► Traveler to endemic areas planning extended stay or intimate contact with locals
  ► Adoptee or contact with an adoptee from countries where HBV infections are endemic
  ► Neonate has an HBsAG mother who has not received routine immunization
- Symptoms may include those listed under General Hepatitis Information.
- Thirty to 40 percent experience icteric phase.
- Five to 10 percent of cases may be complicated by urticaria, skin rashes, and joint pains.

- May present with cholestatic illness with pruritus lasting longer than 1 month.

   NOTE: Fulminant hepatitis is a complication most commonly associated with hepatitis B, with symptoms of liver failure, encephalopathy, ascites and coagulopathy.

- Symptoms of chronic persistent hepatitis vary from asymptomatic to various degrees of fatigue, malaise, and anorexia.

- Symptoms of chronic active hepatitis include jaundice (20 percent) and amenorrhea (risk for infertility).

Objective

- Five to 10 percent may present with urticaria, maculopapular rash, fever, polyarthritis and arthralgia.

- May present with cholestatic illness with marked jaundice and elevation of serum alkaline phosphatase and cholesterol.

- Fulminant hepatitis is more commonly associated with hepatitis B, presenting with signs of liver failure, encephalopathy, ascites, and coagulopathy.

- Aminotransferase is elevated in hundreds to thousands IU/L depending on disease severity.

- Laboratory tests are usually normal by 16 weeks.

- Clinical signs for chronic persistent hepatitis are usually absent. Intermittent or persistent aminotransferase elevation two to three times normal.

- Signs for chronic active hepatitis include

  ▶ Multiple spider nevi

  ▶ Acne

  ▶ Hirsutism

  ▶ Multiple system involvement (lungs, bowels, kidneys, joints)

  ▶ Coombs-positive hemolytic anemia

  ▶ Absent hepatitis B antibody markers

Assessment

- Hepatitis B

  ▶ R/O hepatitis A

  ▶ R/O hepatitis D

  ▶ R/O hepatitis C

  ▶ R/O hepatitis E

  ▶ R/O infectious mononucleosis

  ▶ R/O cytomegalovirus infection

▶ R/O herpes simplex virus infection

▶ R/O drug-induced liver disease

▶ R/O toxoplasmosis

▶ R/O severe preeclampsia

▶ R/O acute fatty liver

▶ R/O biliary tract disease

▶ R/O Epstein-Barr virus infection

▶ R/O human immunodeficiency virus and Infection

Plan

Diagnostic Tests

- Obtain HBsAG on all pregnant women during early prenatal period.

- If HBsAG is positive, obtain HBeAG, anti-HBe and anti- HBc IgM antibody, and alkaline phosphatase.

- See Table 10.2, Serologic Markers for Acute Hepatitis B, and Figure 10.2, Course of Acute Hepatitis B Infection.

  ▶ Hepatitis B surface antigen (HBsAG) indicates infection or, if present for longer than 6 months, chronic hepatitis.

  ▶ IgM antibody to HBcAG (anti-HBc) indicates acute infection (high titer).

  ▶ IgG anti-HBc indicates chronic disease if HBsAG is positive or prior exposure if HBsAG is negative.

  ▶ Antibody to hepatitis B virus surface antigen (anti-HBs) indicates that the individual has immunity.

  NOTE: There is a "window period" between time that HBsAG is cleared and anti-HBs appears. Infectivity has been demonstrated during this period. If the first HBsAg is negative in early pregnancy and the mother could possibly be in the window period of infection after exposure to hepatitis or she engages in high-risk behavior during pregnancy (e.g., parenteral drug use), a repeat HBsAG should be obtained in the third trimester.

  ▶ The presence of HBeAG indicates an acute infectious state denoting a more highly replicative chronic infection associated with increased infectivity and liver disease.

  ▶ Antibody to HBeAG (anti-HBe) indicates convalescence or ongoing infection.

- ALT will peak at the onset of clinical disease and return to normal after 4 to 5 months.

- See Figure 10.3, Course of Chronic HBV.

  ▶ HBsAG persists for longer than 6 months

- A liver biopsy is indicated for diagnosis of chronic hepatitis to distinguish between chronic persistent and chronic active hepatitis (usually reserved until postpartum in pregnant patients).

Treatment/Management

- There is no specific treatment for acute or chronic infection. Several studies are under investigation.

- Vaccine dosages (Knauer, 1993)

  ▶ Hepatitis B recombinant vaccine (Recombivax HB®) 10 µg IM in deltoid immediately and at 1 to 2 and 4 to 6 months later, for a total of three doses (CDC, 1998)

    OR

  ▶ Hepatitis B recombinant vaccine (Engerix-B®) 20 µg IM in deltoid immediately and at 1 to 2 and 4 to 6 months later, for a total of 3 doses (CDC, 1998)

- Immunoprophylaxis is recommended in pregnancy for all individuals at risk for infection. See risk factors in the Hepatitis B Subjective section.

  ▶ Vaccine recipients must have a negative HBsAG and HBcAb before immunization.

  ▶ Adolescents who have not previously received three doses of hepatitis B vaccine should have the hepatitis B vaccine series completed (CDC, 1991).

  NOTE: Up to 95 percent of properly immunized individuals will develop protective levels of antibody (Nowicki & Balisteri, 1993a).

- The Immunization Practices Advisory Committee (ACIP) of the U.S. Department of Health and Human Services recommends routine hepatitis B vaccination of all infants (Advisory Committee on Immunization Practices, American Academy of Pediatrics, 1996).

  ▶ Infants born to mothers negative for hepatitis B surface antigen (HBsAG) should receive 2.5 µg of Recombivax HB or 10 µg of Engerix-B. A second dose is recommended at age 1 to 2 months, and the third dose at 6 months.

  ▶ Infants born to HBsAG-positive mothers should receive 0.5 mL hepatitis B immune globulin (HBIG) within 12 hours of birth, and either 5 µg of Recombivax HB or 10 µg of Engerix-B at a separate site. A second dose is recommended at age 1 to 2 months and the third dose at 6 months of age.

  ▶ Infants born to mothers whose HBsAG status is unknown should receive either 5 µg of Recombivax HB or 10 µg of Engerix-B within 12 hours of birth. The second dose of vaccine is recommended at age 1 month and the third dose at 6 months of age.

- Post-exposure prophylaxis is recommended if a pregnant woman sustains a needlestick or transmucosal inoculation.

  ▶ Blood should be drawn from the "donor" and recipient and analyzed for HBV markers.

  ▶ Also consider HCV and HIV antibody status if the donor is at risk for these viruses.

  ▶ After the blood is drawn, give the recipient hepatitis B immunoglobulin (H-BIG®, Hep-B-Gammagee®, HyperHep®) 0.06 mL/kg IM within 7 days of exposure and again 30 days after the first vaccination (Knauer, 1993).

  ▶ If the donor is negative for HBsAG and recipient is negative for HBsAG and anti-HBs begin immunization with Hepatitis B recombinant vaccine (Recombivax HB)

    – 10 mg IM within 7 to 14 days of exposure and at 1 and 6 months.

- Immunocompromised and hemodialysis patients are considered to be poor responders to vaccine. It is recommended that if these individuals are again exposed to hepatitis B that they receive postexposure hepatitis B immunoglobulin.

   NOTE: Protective antibody levels persist for more than 3 years in adults. Protection against HBV appears to be evident for more than 5 years even with declining antibody levels. Efficacy of a 10-year booster is currently under investigation (Nowicki & Balisteri, 1993a).

Consultation

- See Consultation section under General Hepatitis Information, above.

Patient Education

- See Patient Education section under General Hepatitis Information, above.
- Inform patient of perinatal and sexual transmissibility, as appropriate, of hepatitis B.
- Explain importance of immunoprophylaxis for infant and exposed contacts with hepatitis B.
- Advise that breastfeeding is not contraindicated if the infant was immunized against hepatitis B.

Follow-up

- See Follow-up section under General Hepatitis Information, above.
- Document hepatitis B status in progress notes and problem list.

Hepatitis D

Database

Subjective

- Risk factors are the same as for hepatitis B.
- Prodromal symptoms may include those listed under General Hepatitis Information.
- With co-infection, a single episode of acute hepatitis may occur or a biphasic illness that is characterized by two sets of symptoms.
- Approximately 3 percent of patients with co-infection develop fulminant hepatitis (see under hepatitis B symptoms).
- Superinfection is characterized by symptoms of acute hepatitis (see Hepatitis B) in a previously asymptomatic carrier.

Objective

- With co-infection of HBV, a single episode of acute hepatitis may occur or a biphasic illness characterized by two sets of signs and aminotransferase peaks.

- Superinfection is characterized by signs of acute hepatitis and elevated aminotransferase level in a previously asymptomatic carrier (see Hepatitis B).

- Approximately 3 percent of patients will develop fulminant hepatitis (see Hepatitis B).

Assessment

- Hepatitis D
  - ▶ R/O hepatitis A
  - ▶ R/O hepatitis B
  - ▶ R/O hepatitis C
  - ▶ R/O hepatitis E
  - ▶ R/O infectious mononucleosis
  - ▶ R/O cytomegalovirus infection
  - ▶ R/O herpes simplex virus infection
  - ▶ R/O drug-induced liver disease
  - ▶ R/O toxoplasmosis
  - ▶ R/O severe preeclampsia
  - ▶ R/O acute fatty liver
  - ▶ R/O Biliary tract disease
  - ▶ R/O Epstein-Barr virus infection
  - ▶ R/O human immunodeficiency virus and Infection

Plan

Diagnostic Tests

- See Table 10.3, Serologic Markers for Hepatitis C, D and E, and Figure 10.4, Acute HDV-HBV Co-infection that Resolves.
  - ▶ Determine whether there is antibody to HDV (anti-HDV) along with the hepatitis B markers HBsAG and IgM anti-HBc.
    - – Rising titers of anti-HDV indicate acute infection.
    - – Sustained high titer of anti-HDV indicates chronic hepatitis D infection. A single or biphasic aminotransferase peak may occur.

- Hepatitis D superinfection is diagnosed by
  - ▶ HBsAG and anti-HDV in absence of IgM anti-HBc.
  - ▶ Elevated aminotransferase level in previous asymptomatic carrier

Treatment/Management

- There is no effective treatment for hepatitis D
- Immunoprophylaxis is the same as for hepatitis B.

Consultation

- See Consultation section under General Hepatitis Information, above.

Patient Education

- See Patient Education section under General Hepatitis Information, above.
- Inform patient of perinatal and sexual transmissibility, as appropriate, of hepatitis D.
- Explain importance of immunoprophylaxis for infant and exposed contacts with hepatitis D.

Follow-up

- See Follow-up section under General Hepatitis Information, above.
- Document hepatitis D status in progress notes and problem list.

Hepatitis C

Database

Subjective

- Risk factors include
  - ▶ Receiving blood or blood products
  - ▶ Intravenous drug use
  - ▶ Hemodialysis
  - ▶ Female partners of sexually active bisexual men
  - ▶ HIV-positive, high-risk mothers (the most common vertical transmission factor)

    NOTE: Perinatal transmission and transmission through sexual intercourse are uncommon.
- Patients are most often asymptomatic.

- Symptoms may include those listed previously under General Hepatitis Information, although they usually present in a milder form than HBV infections.

- Only approximately 25 percent develop jaundice.

Objective

- Physical findings may include those listed under General Hepatitis Information, although they usually present in a milder form.

- Transferase levels have a lower peak than in HBV or HAV infection.

- Alanine aminotransferase (ALT) levels show 3 patterns:

  ▶ Monophasic (single ALT elevation with complete resolution conferring a 42 percent risk of chronic disease).

  ▶ Polyphasic, the most common pattern (tends to have fluctuating levels, with 87 percent risk of chronic disease)

  ▶ Plateau (expect persistent elevation with a 95 percent risk of chronic infection) (Nowicki & Balisteri, 1993b).

Assessment

- Hepatitis C
  ▶ R/O hepatitis A
  ▶ R/O hepatitis B
  ▶ R/O hepatitis D
  ▶ R/O hepatitis E
  ▶ R/O infectious mononucleosis
  ▶ R/O cytomegalovirus infection
  ▶ R/O herpes simplex virus infection
  ▶ R/O drug-induced liver disease
  ▶ R/O toxoplasmosis
  ▶ R/O severe preeclampsia
  ▶ R/O acute fatty liver
  ▶ R/O Biliary tract disease
  ▶ R/O Epstein-Barr virus infection
  ▶ R/O human immunodeficiency virus and Infection

Plan

Diagnostic Tests

- See Table 10.3, Serologic Markers for Hepatitis C,D and E, and Figure 10.5: Hepatitis C: From Acute to Chronic.

- Universal screening is not recommended. Consider screening members of high-risk populations (intravenous drug users, prostitutes, women with HIV infection, partners of HCV-positive men and patients with a history of acute hepatitis).

- Antibody to HCV (anti-HCV) is positive in 95 percent of patients with posttransfusion hepatitis and in 50 percent of those with sporadic infection.

- Presence of anti-HCV in serum can be detected as early as 6 to 8 weeks or as late as 1 year after onset of clinical manifestations (Knauer, 1993).

- Test sequential samples over 6 to 9 months, if indicated.

- An anti-HCV test is not applicable for diagnosis of acute hepatitis C infection.

- Presence of HCV-RNA is the best means of confirming diagnosis.

- Whether an individual is in a recovery or chronic carrier state cannot be determined.

- ALT may be fluctuating, especially in chronic hepatitis, but may be monophasic or plateau like.

Treatment/Management

- There is no effective treatment for acute hepatitis C.

- Interferon alfa-2b as been approved for treatment of chronic hepatitis C.

- No immunoprophylaxis is available.

Consultation

- See Consultation section under General Hepatitis Information, above.

Patient Education

- See Patient Education section under General Hepatitis Information, above.

- Inform patient of perinatal and sexual transmissibility, as appropriate, of hepatitis C.

Follow-up

- See Follow-up section under General Hepatitis Information, above.

- Document hepatitis C status in progress notes and problem list.

Hepatitis E

Database

Subjective

- Exposure to endemic areas is a risk factor.
- Symptoms may include those listed previously under General Hepatitis Information.

  NOTE: Majority of infections are self-limited and do not cause persistent viremia.

Objective

- Physical findings may include those listed under General Hepatitis Information, although they usually present in a milder form.

Assessment

- Hepatitis E
  - ▶ R/O hepatitis A
  - ▶ R/O hepatitis B
  - ▶ R/O hepatitis D
  - ▶ R/O hepatitis C
  - ▶ R/O infectious mononucleosis
  - ▶ R/O cytomegalovirus infection
  - ▶ R/O herpes simplex virus infection
  - ▶ R/O drug-induced liver disease
  - ▶ R/O toxoplasmosis
  - ▶ R/O severe preeclampsia
  - ▶ R/O acute fatty liver
  - ▶ R/O Biliary tract disease
  - ▶ R/O Epstein-Barr virus infection
  - ▶ R/O human immunodeficiency virus and Infection

Plan

Diagnostic Tests

- See Table 10.3, Serologic Markers for Hepatitis C,D, and E.
- Diagnosis is made by epidemiologic and serologic exclusion of other agents (HAV, HBV, HCV, cytomegalovirus, Epstein-Barr virus).

- Identification of hepatitis E virus antigen (HEAg) in the liver is not suitable for routine screening.

Treatment/Management

- There is no effective treatment available.
- No immunoprophylaxis is available.

Consultation

- See Consultation section under General Hepatitis Information, above.

Patient Education

- See Patient Education section under General Hepatitis Information, above.

Follow-up

- See Follow-up section under General Hepatitis Information, above.
- Document hepatitis E status in progress notes and problem list.

Figure 10.1   Course of Hepatitis A Infection

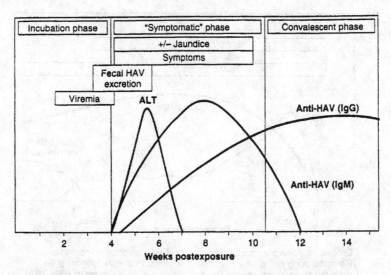

In HAV infection, IgM antibody to HAV begins to rise as symptoms develop, and detectable titers persist for about 4 months. IgG antibody appears later, and its presence confers immunity.

Source: Nowick, M.J. & Balisteri, W.F. (1993a) Hepatitis A through E: New viruses, new problems. *Contemporary OB/GYN, 38*(5), 49–72. Reprinted with permission.

Figure 10.2   Course of Acute Hepatitis B Infection

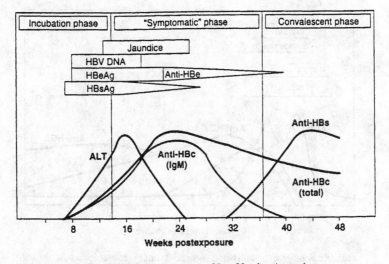

There is often a "window period" in weeks 25 to 30, after the surface antigen disappears and before anti-HBs appears. During this period, HBV infection can still be detected by the presence of antibody to the core antigen (anti-HBc).

Source: Nowick, M.J. & Balisteri, W.F. (1993a) Hepatitis A through E: New viruses, new problems. *Contemporary OB/GYN, 38*(5), 49–72. Reprinted with permission.

Figure 10.3   Course of Chronic HBV

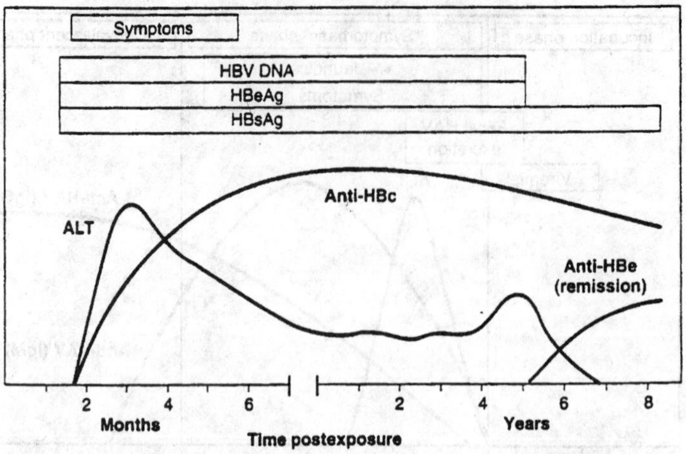

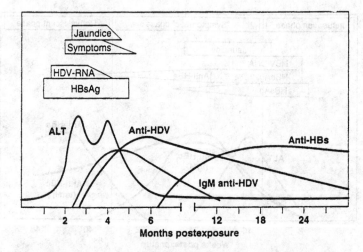

Chronic HBV infection can be diagnosed if HBsAg persists for more than 6 months along with clinical evidence of hepatitis. Viral replication must be ongoing. It can be documented by the presence of the e antigen or HBV-DNA in the serum and an absence of anti-HBs. Remission occurs with clearance of HBeAg and the appearance of anti-HBe.

Source: Nowick, M.J. & Balisteri, W.F. (1993a) Hepatitis A through E: New viruses, new problems. *Contemporary OB/GYN, 38*(5), 49–72. Reprinted with permission.

Figure 10.4   Acute HDV-HBV Coinfection that Resolves

Simultaneous infection with hepatitis B and D viruses (coinfection) is usually self-limited. Only 5% of cases progress to chronic hepatitis. The diagnosis is confirmed by rising titers of total anti-HDV along with transient IgM anti-HDV and a positive test for IgM antibody to the hepatitis B core antigen (IgM anti-HBc). The latter would follow HBsAg.

Source: Nowick, M.J. & Balisteri, W.F. (1993b) Three important new hepatitis viruses: C, D, and E. *Contemporary OB/GYN, 38*(6), 71–88. Reprinted with permission.

Figure 10.5 Hepatitis C: From Acute to Chronic

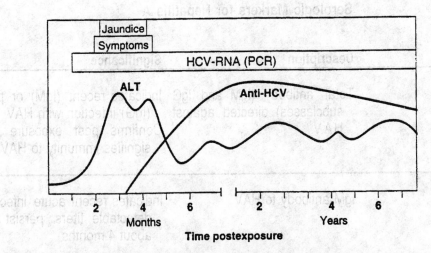

When acute HCV infection progresses to chronic disease, anti-HCV may not be detectable for up to 12 months, and its presence does not imply protection from infection. Fluctuating alanine aminotransferase (ALT) patterns are common. In some patients with chronic disease, HCV–RNA has been detected in liver tissue by polymerase chain reaction (PCR).

Source: Nowick, M.J. & Balisteri, W.F. (1993b) Three important new hepatitis viruses: C, D, and E. *Contemporary OB/GYN, 38*(6), 71–88. Reprinted with permission.

Table 10.1

Serologic Markers for Hepatitis A

Marker	Description	Significance
Anti-HAV	Total antibody (IgM and IgG subclasses) directed against HAV	Indicates recent (IgM) or past (IgG) infection with HAV Confirms past exposure and signifies immunity to HAV
Anti-HAV-IgM	IgM antibody to HAV	Indicates recent acute infection detectable titers persist for about 4 months
Anti-HAV-IgG	IgG antibody to HAV	Signifies previous HAV infection; confers immunity

Source: Nowicki, M.J. & Balisteri, W.F. (1993a). Hepatitis A through E: New viruses, new problems. *Contemporary OB/GYN, 38*(5), 49-72. Reprinted with permission.

Table 10.2

Serologic Markers for Hepatitis B

Markers	Description	Significance
HBsAG	Hepatitis B surface antigen; found on the surface of the intact virus and in serum as free particles (tubular or spherical)	Indicates infection with HBV (acute) or chronic) Precedes biochemical or clinical evidence of infection Presence for more than 6 months indicates chronic infection
HBcAg	Hepatitis B core antigen; found within the core of the intact virus	Not detectable in serum; found only in liver tissue
HBeAg	Hepatitis B e antigen; a soluble antigen produced during self-cleavage of the core antigen	Indicates active HBV infection Signifies high infectivity Persistence for 6 to 8 weeks suggests chronic carrier state and/ or chronic liver disease
HBV DNA	DNA of the hepatitis B virus	Indicates active HBV infection (acute and chronic) Indicates high levels of viral replication, infectivity, and high probability of liver dis-ease
Anti-HBs	Antibody to HBV surface antigen with (HBsAg); subclasses IgM (early) and IgG	Indicates clinical recovery from HBV infection and signifies immunity Protective
Anti-HBc	Total antibody to HBV core antigen (HBcAg)	Indicates active HBV infection (acute and chronic)
Anti-HBc-IgM	IgM antibody to core antigen	Early index of acute HBV infection; appears during on-set of symptoms Rises during acute phase then declines; persists for about 1 to 2 months Detectable in window period after surface antigen disappears
Anti-HBc-IgG	IgG antibody to core antigen	Appears later and may persist for years if viral replication continues
Anti-HBe	Antibody to HBV e antigen (HBeAG)	Indicates clearance of HBeAG

Source: Nowicki, M.J. & Balisteri, W.F. (1993a). Hepatitis A through E. New viruses, new problems. *Contemporary OB/GYN, 38*(5), 49-72. Reprinted with permission.

Table 10.3

Serologic Markers for Hepatitis C, D, and E

Marker	Description	Significance
HEPATITIS C VIRUS (HCV)		
Anti-HCV	Antibody to specific portion of the HCV genome infection	Indicates active infection with HCV. Present in acute and chronic Not protective
HCV-RNA	RNA of the hepatitis C virus	Detectable in serum and liver by polymerase chain reaction Best means of confirming infection with HCV
HEPATITIS D (DELTA) VIRUS (HDV)		
HDAg	Hepatitis D antigen	Detected in acute HDV infection by RIBA and ELISA
Anti-HDV	Total antibody to the hepatitis D virus	Indicates exposure to HDV Patient may transmit HDV infection
HDV-RNA	RNA of the hepatitis D virus	Present in serum/liver
HEPATITIS E VIRUS (HEV)		
HEAg	Hepatitis E antigen	Research tool at present; can be found in liver, bile, and stool during incubation period and symptomatic phase of infection
Anti-HEV	Antibody to the hepatitis E virus	Research tool at present; found in serum during acute illness Immunity to infection may not be complete

Source: Nowicki, M.J. & Balisteri, W.F. (1993b). Three important new hepatitis viruses: C, D, and E. *Contemporary OB/GYN, 38*(6), 71–88. Reprinted with permission.

References

American College of Obstetricians and Gynecologists (ACOG). (1992). Hepatitis in Pregnancy. (Technical Bulletin No. 174). Washington, DC: Author.

Advisory Committee on Immunization Practices, American Academy of Pediatrics. (1996). Recommended Childhood Immunization Schedule—United States, January–June 1996. *Morbidity and Mortality Weekly Report, 44*(51 & 52), 940–943.

Balisteri, W.F. (1988). Viral hepatitis. *Pediatric Clinics of North America, 39,* 637-649.

Centers for Disease Control and Prevention. (1991). Hepatitis B virus: A comprehensive strategy for eliminating transmission in the United States through universal childhood vaccination. Recommendations of the Immunization Practices Advisory Committee (ACID). *Morbidity and Mortality Weekly Report, 40* (1), 43–45.

Centers for Disease Control and Prevention. (1995). Health Information for International Travel 1995. Atlanta, GA: Author.

Centers for Disease Control and Prevention. (1998). 1998 guidelines for treatment of sexually transmitted diseases. *Morbidity and Mortality Weekly Report, 47*(1), 98–104.

Knauer, C.M. (1993) Liver, biliary tract and pancreas. In L. M. Tierney, S.J. McPhee, M.A. Papadakis, and S.A. Schroeder (Eds.), *Current medical diagnosis and treatment* (35th ed., pp. 503–537). Norwalk, CT: Appleton and Lange.

Mishra, L., & Seeff, L. (1992). Viral hepatitis, A through E, complicating pregnancy. *Gastroenterology Clinics of North America, 21*(4), 873–887.

Nowicki, M.J. & Balisteri, W.F. (1993a) Hepatitis A through E: New viruses, new problems. *Contemporary OB/GYN , 38*(5), 49–72.

Nowicki, M.J. & Balisteri, W.F. (1993b) Three important new hepatitis viruses: C, D and E. *Contemporary OB/GYN , 38*(6), 71–88.

Pastorek II, J.E. (1993). The ABCs of hepatitis in pregnancy. *Clinical Obstetrics and Gynecology, 36*(4), 843–854.

Simms, J. & Duff, D. (1993) Viral hepatitis in pregnancy. *Seminars in Perinatolgy, 17*(6) 384–393.

Chapter 3

GROUP B STREPTOCOCCUS

Winifred L. Star

Group B streptococcus (GBS), or *Streptococcus agalactiae*, is a facultative gram-positive diplococcus with several known serotypes (Ia, Ib/c, Ia/c, II, III, IV, V, VI, and VII). GBS infection is the leading cause of neonatal sepsis and meningitis; approximately 7,600 episodes of sepsis occur in newborns in the United States annually (rate of 1.8/1,000 live births) (American College of Obstetricians and Gynecologists [ACOG], 1996). The number of cases of GBS disease exceeds the number of congenital infections attributed to toxoplasma, rubella, herpes, and syphilis (Baker & Edwards, 1995).

Colonization with GBS during pregnancy occurs in 5 to 30 percent of women. Prevalence determination is dependent on geographic location, age, gravidy, duration of gestation, sites cultured, and culture methods (Gibbs & Sweet, 1994). Vaginal carriage patterns in pregnancy may be either transient, intermittent, or chronic; anorectal carriage is more constant (Gibbs & Sweet, 1994; Katz, 1993; Yancy & Duff, 1993). Rectal carriage of GBS provides a reservoir for recurrent vaginal colonization and may also contribute to GBS as a urinary tract pathogen (Baker & Edwards, 1995). Fluctuations in the presence of the organism may make antibiotic therapy difficult to evaluate; resolution of the organism may occur without therapy (Eschenbach, 1985). Cultures performed during gestation may not predict colonization status at the time of labor and antenatal antibiotic prophylaxis does not consistently reduce maternal colonization (Dinsmoor, 1990, Gardner et al., 1979). Vertical transmission to the fetus generally occurs during labor and delivery with increased rates in neonates with mothers who have dense vaginal colonization (Boyer & Gotoff, 1988).

Maternal morbidity from group B streptococcus infection may include urinary tract infection, chorioamnionitis, postpartum endomyometritis (usually associated with cesarean delivery), endometritis-associated bacteremia, and wound infection. Controversy exists over whether GBS causes premature rupture of membranes (PROM) or preterm labor (PTL). One to 5 percent of urinary tract infections in pregnancy may be caused by GBS (Gibbs & Sweet, 1994; Dinsmoor, 1990). Gravidas with GBS colonization of the urinary tract appear to be more prone to PROM and PTL. Second and third trimester fetal loss has also been associated with heavy colonization of GBS as manifest by GBS bacteriuria (Katz, 1993). Evidence from selected studies shows an increased rate of preterm rupture of membranes and preterm labor/delivery in women with GBS bacteriuria and, when bacteriuria is eradicated, a lowering of the rate (Møller, Thomsen, Borch, Dinesen, & Zdravkovic, 1984; Thomsen, Mørup, & Hansen, 1987). The association between preterm labor and GBS colonization from the genital tract is much weaker (Eriksen & Blanco, 1993).

Neonatal clinical syndromes of early- or late-onset disease may occur following GBS transmission from mother to fetus. Vertical transmission rates range from 29 to 85 percent (mean 51 percent); however, only 1 to 2 percent of neonates develop clinical disease (Baker & Edwards, 1995; Katz, 1993). Incidence of early-onset infection ranges from 0.7 to 3.7 per 1,000 live births. Early-onset infection predominantly affects the neonates of mothers with complications known to be associated with risk for neonatal sepsis, including, preterm labor, prolonged rupture of membranes (i.e., more than 18 hours) prior to delivery, chorioamnionitis, multiple births, and maternal fever (Baker & Edwards, 1995). The most common clinical manifestations of early-onset disease in neonates are pneumonia, septicemia, and meningitis, which usually occur within the first few hours or days of life (mean onset 20 hours) but may develop anytime in the first week (Baker & Edwards, 1995; Eriksen & Blanco, 1993; Gibbs & Sweet, 1994;

Dinsmoor, 1990). Overall mortality of early-onset disease is 15 percent; however, with GBS sepsis, which has a rapid, fulminating course, mortality can occur in up to 50 percent of cases (Eriksen & Blanco, 1993; Fletcher & Gordon, 1990; Noya & Baker, 1992).

Late-onset disease, with a more gradual onset, presents after the first week of life (mean onset 24 days) and may occur beyond 12 weeks of age. Incidence estimates are 0.5 to 1.8 per 1,000 live births. Meningitis is the presenting clinical manifestation in the majority of affected infants but multiple sites of localized infection may also exist. Factors playing a role in late-onset infection include nosocomial or community acquisition and vertical mother-infant transmission (less likely). The mortality rate is generally lower than that of early-onset disease (2 to 6 percent); however, 25 to 50 percent of surviving infants with meningitis will have permanent neurological sequelae (e.g., mental retardation, speech/language delays, spastic quadriplegia, cortical blindness, deafness, seizures, and hydrocephalus) (Baker & Edwards, 1995; ACOG, 1993; Gibbs & Sweet, 1994; Dinsmoor, 1990).

Several strategies for the prevention of early-onset GBS disease in newborns have been proposed over the years. In May 1996, the Centers for Disease Control and Prevention (CDC) issued recommendations for the prevention of perinatal disease based on clinical risk factors or antenatal culture results. These recommendations form the basis for the guidelines presented in this chapter. Ongoing research is needed to further define the most effective strategies. Active immunization aimed at pregnant women seems to have the best prospect of controlling early- and late-onset disease, however, a vaccine is currently not available to the medical community (Institute of Medicine, 1985; Ohlsson & Myhr, 1994).

Database

Subjective

- Predisposing/risk factors for GBS colonization or infection may include (Baker & Edwards, 1995):
  - ▶ 20 years of age or younger
  - ▶ Lower parity
  - ▶ Hispanic woman of Caribbean origin; African-American woman
  - ▶ First half of menstrual cycle
  - ▶ Sexually active woman
  - ▶ Intrauterine device
  - ▶ Tampon use
  - ▶ GBS carriage in sexual partner(s)
  - ▶ Low levels of type-specific antibody
  - ▶ Diabetes
- Predisposing/risk factors for GBS infection in the neonate may include (CDC, 1996):
  - ▶ Maternal genital tract colonization with GBS
  - ▶ Maternal GBS bacteriuria
  - ▶ Premature delivery

- ▶ Prolonged rupture of membranes
- ▶ Maternal intrapartum fever
- ▶ Maternal age 20 years or less
- ▶ African-American mother
- ▶ Low levels of maternal anti-GBS capsular antibody
- ▶ Maternal history of birth of infant with GBS disease
- ▶ Low birth weight infant
- ▶ Heavy surface colonization of neonate with GBS
- ▶ Vertical, nosocomial or community acquisition of GBS (risks for late-onset disease).

NOTE: One-third of neonatal GBS infections and 10 percent of mortality occur(s) in full-term infants without risk factors (Katz, 1993).

- Symptomatology
  - ▶ Colonization is usually asymptomatic.
  - ▶ Symptoms of maternal infection (as may be seen with cystitis, pyelonephritis, chorioamnionitis, and/or endomyometritis) may include fever, chills, malaise, abdominal distention, pelvic pain, dysuria, urgency, frequency, flank pain.

Objective

- Evidence of GBS bacteriuria and/or anogenital cultures positive for GBS
- Signs of acute maternal GBS infection:
  - ▶ Elevated temperature
  - ▶ Tachycardia
  - ▶ Abdominal distention
  - ▶ Uterine/adnexal tenderness
  - ▶ Costovertebral angle tenderness
  - ▶ Elevated white blood cell (WBC) count.
- Neonatal manifestations of early-onset disease due to GBS:
  - ▶ Respiratory signs (apnea, grunting, tachypnea, cyanosis)
  - ▶ Hypotension
  - ▶ Lethargy
  - ▶ Irritability
  - ▶ Poor feeding
  - ▶ Fever or hypothermia
  - ▶ Hypoglycemia

   ▶ Jaundice

   ▶ Hyperbilirubinemia.

● Late-onset neonatal disease signs:

   ▶ Meningitis

   ▶ Localized infections of middle ears, sinuses, conjunctiva, breasts, lungs, bones, joints, and skin may also be present (Eriksen & Blanco, 1993; Gibbs & Sweet, 1994)

Assessment

● Group B streptococcus (GBS) colonization/infection

   ▶ R/O asymptomatic bacteriuria (ASB) or cystitis secondary to GBS

   ▶ R/O obstetrical/puerperal complications due to GBS

     – PROM

     – Preterm labor

     – Chorioamnionitis

     – Endomyometritis

     – Bacteremia

     – Wound infection

   ▶ Differential diagnosis of febrile illness in the parturient includes (Haft & Kasper, 1991)

     – Pelvic infection due to gram-negative or anaerobic bacteria

     – Puerperal sepsis due to *Streptococcus pyogenes*

     – Septic pelvic vein thrombophlebitis

     – Urinary tract infection (UTI)

     – Mastitis

     – Toxic shock syndrome

     – Retained products of conception

     – Viral illness

     – Drug-associated fever

   ▶ R/O neonatal GBS infection

Plan

Diagnostic Tests

● Culture is the usual method for diagnosis of GBS colonization (ACOG, 1992).

   NOTE: Culture results performed antenatally should be available at the time/place of delivery (ideally, 24-hour access to results).

- If a screening-based approach to diagnosis is used (see Figure 10.6), obtain one or two swabs of the vaginal introitus and anorectum at 35 to 37 weeks' gestation (speculum examination is not required and cervical cultures are not acceptable) (CDC, 1996). Samples should be labeled specifically "for GBS culture."

  NOTE: Combined use of lower vaginal *and* anorectal culture increases likelihood of isolation of GBS by 5 to 27 percent over vaginal culture alone. Screening cultures collected late in pregnancy have a higher predictive value for maternal colonization at delivery. Note, however, that prenatal screening cultures will not correctly identify *all* women with intrapartum GBS carriage (ACOG, 1996; CDC, 1996).

- Anogenital GBS cultures obtained earlier in gestation (i.e., before 35 weeks) are not recommended. In addition, antenatal screening of gravidas with a history of giving birth to an infant with GBS infection is not required (CDC, 1996). GBS cultures should be obtained in patients with preterm PROM (ACOG, 1996). See Chapter 6.24, *Premature Rupture of Membranes.*

- In certain settings, rapid antigen tests may be utilized to assist intrapartal clinical decision making:

  ► Immunofluorescent antibody tests

  ► Antigen detection tests

  ► Rapid (5-hour) culture

  ► Nucleic acid probes

  NOTE: Both false-positives and false-negatives exist with these tests; heavier GBS colonization increases accuracy.

- Gram stain is not recommended for screening (ACOG, 1992).

- Routine urinalysis and/or culture should be performed at initial prenatal visit to assess for pyuria/bacteriuria.

  ► Tests should be repeated after treatment for ASB or cystitis.

  ► Patients at high risk for UTI should be considered for screening more than once during pregnancy (Haft & Kasper, 1991).

- Additional tests as indicated for intrapartal febrile patients may include: complete blood count (CBC), blood cultures, amniocentesis for culture and gram stain, pelvic ultrasound, CT scan.

- See Treatment/Management.

Treatment/Management

- Standards of care vary from institution to institution. Each institution and its obstetrical team should examine their clinical resources and populations' characteristics prior to implementing a preventive management scheme (Yancy & Duff, 1994).

- CDC recommendations for the prevention of early-onset GBS neonatal disease are depicted in Figures 10.6 and 10.7 (ACOG, 1996; CDC, 1996). Strategies include

▶ A screening-based approach (i.e., anogenital culture at 35-37 weeks' gestation) as the primary risk-determinant (Figure 10.6)

OR

▶ A risk-factor approach based solely on clinical risk factors (Figure 10.7) .

● Women with GBS bacteriuria (symptomatic or asymptomatic) during pregnancy require treatment consisting of a 1-week course of ampicillin or amoxicillin at the time of diagnosis (ACOG, 1996; Haft & Kasper, 1991).

▶ Recurrent bacteriuria is an indication for antibiotic suppression; consult with physician.

▶ Intrapartal chemoprophylaxis will also be indicated as shown in the figures.

▶ See also *Asymptomatic Bacteriuria* protocol.

● Intrapartum chemoprophylactic regimens (CDC, 1996)

▶ Penicillin G, 5 million units IV initially, then 2.5 million units IV every 4 hours until delivery (recommended regimen)

OR

Ampicillin, 2 grams IV initially, then 1 gram IV every 4 hours until delivery (alternate regimen)

▶ Penicillin-allergic individuals may be treated with clindamycin 900 mg IV every 8 hours until delivery (recommended regimen) or erythromycin 500 mg IV every 6 hours until delivery (alternate regimen).

NOTE: Inpatient management will be dictated by the physician in charge of the patient's care. Ongoing antibiotic therapy will be necessary in symptomatic GBS chorioamnionitis. Further details of inpatient management are beyond the scope of this protocol.

Consultation

● Seek physician consultation for all cases of maternal GBS colonization and in the presence of risk factors for maternal/neonatal disease.

● Refer patients with recurrent GBS bacteriuria to urology.

Patient Education

● Inform the patient of her GBS status, as indicated.

▶ Discuss the etiology, transmission, and transient nature of the organism.

▶ Discuss the implications of GBS during pregnancy, the puerperium and neonatal periods.

▶ Particulars regarding treatment/management will be based upon site-specific policies and practice.

▶ Inform patients of the preventive strategies in place at the treating institution and the risks and benefits of intrapartum chemoprophylaxis.

▶ Provide patient-education materials (see Appendix 10.3a).

- Encourage use of male or female condoms during sexual intercourse to decrease the potential for sexual transmission of GBS.

- Advise patient/partner of signs/symptoms of sexually transmitted disease (STD) and need for evaluation if present.

- Educate regarding signs and symptoms of preterm labor starting at approximately 20 weeks; reinforce teaching as indicated. See Chapter 6.25, *Preterm Labor*.

Follow-up

- Prepare the mother for the possibility of intrapartum chemoprophylaxis, based on antenatal culture results or clinical risk factors.

- Routine neonatal antimicrobial prophylaxis is not recommended for infants born to mothers receiving intrapartum chemoprophylaxis. Infants suspected of having sepsis require full diagnostic evaluation and empiric therapy (CDC, 1996). Details of neonatal management are beyond the scope of this chapter. Refer to the American Academy of Pediatrics 1997 reference.

- Refer families who have a child with GBS disease or its sequelae to social services, if indicated.

- Carry out routine 6-week postpartum examination with attention to the usual particulars. See Chapter 4.3, *Postpartum Visit*.

  ▶ Signs and symptoms of ongoing infection should be assessed.

  ▶ Inquiry into status of the infant is essential and appropriate pediatric follow-up should be ensured if the infant was treated for GBS disease.

- In all cases, document GBS status (positive antenatal culture or GBS bacteriuria) and management thereof on the problem list and in progress notes. In addition, document history of previous child with GBS infection on the problem list.

Figure 10.6

Prevention strategy for early-onset group B streptococcal (GBS) disease using prenatal screening at 35-37 weeks' gestation.

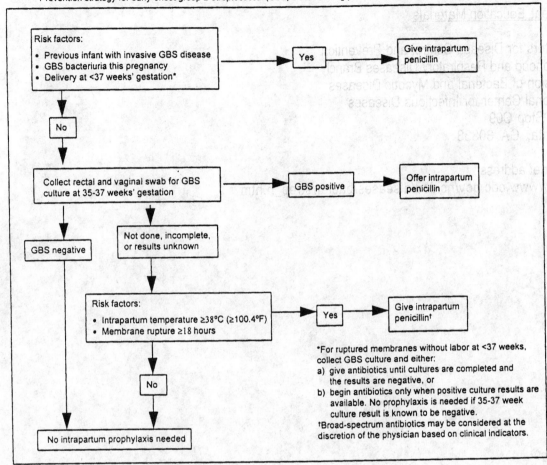

Figure 10.7

Prevention strategy for early-onset group B streptococcal (GBS) disease using risk factors.

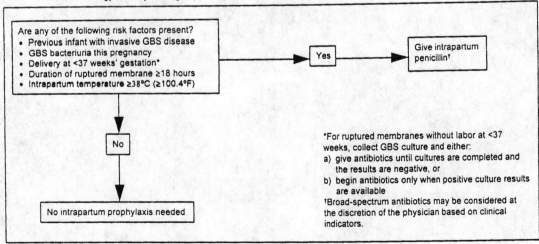

SOURCE: Centers for Disease Control and Prevention. (1996). Prevention of perinatal group B streptococcal disease: A public health perspective. *Morbidity and Mortality Weekly Report, 45*(RR-7), 1-24.

Appendix 10.3a

Patient Education Materials

Centers for Disease Control and Prevention
Childhood and Respiratory Diseases Branch
Division of Bacterial and Mycotic Diseases
National Center for Infectious Diseases
Mail Stop C09
Atlanta, GA 30333

Internet address:
http://www.cdc.gov/ncidod/diseases/bacter/strep_b.htm

REFERENCES

American Academy of Pediatrics. (1992). Guidelines for prevention of group B streptococcal infection by chemoprophylaxis. *Pediatrics, 9*, 775–779.

American College of Obstetricians and Gynecologists (ACOG). (1992). *Group B streptococcal infections in pregnancy*. (Technical Bulletin No. 170). Washington, DC: Author.

American College of Obstetricians and Gynecologists (ACOG). (1993, May). *Group B streptococcal infections in pregnancy: ACOG's recommendations*. ACOG Newsletter. Washington, DC: Author.

American College of Obstetricians and Gynecologists (ACOG). (1996). *Prevention of early-onset group B streptococcal disease in newborns*. (Committee Opinion No. 173). Washington, DC: Author.

Baker, C.J., & Edwards, M.S. (1995). Group B streptococcus infections. In J. S. Remington & J. O. Klein (Eds.), *Infectious diseases of the fetus and newborn infant* (4th ed., pp. 742–811). Philadelphia, PA: W.B. Saunders.

Boyer, K.M., & Gotoff, S.P. (1986). Prevention of early-onset neonatal group B streptococcal disease with selective intrapartum chemoprophylaxis. *New England Journal of Medicine, 314*, 1665–1669.

Boyer, K.M., & Gotoff, S.P. (1988). Antimicrobial prophylaxis of neonatal group B streptococcal sepsis. *Clinics in Perinatology, 15(4)*, 831–851.

Centers for Disease Control and Prevention (CDC). (1996). Prevention of perinatal group B streptococcal disease: A public health perspective. *Morbidity and Mortality Weekly Report, 45(RR–7)*, 1–24.

Dinsmoor, M.J. (1990). Group B streptococcus still poses a challenge. *Contemporary OB/GYN, 35(5)*, 93–104.

Eriksen, N.L., & Blanco, J.D. (1993). Group B streptococcal infection in pregnancy. *Seminars in Perinatology, 17(6)*, 432–442.

Eschenbach, D.A. (1985). Contending with the problem of chlamydial infection. *Contemporary Ob/Gyn, 25(2)*, 125–136.

Fletcher, J.L., & Gordon, R.C. (1990). Perinatal transmission of bacterial sexually transmitted diseases. Part II: Group B streptococcus and *Chlamydia trachomatis*. *The Journal of Family Practice, 30(6)*, 689–696.

Gardner, S.E., Yow, M.D., Leeds, L.J., Thompson, P.K., Mason, E.O., Jr., & Clark, D.J. (1979). Failure of penicillin to eradicate group B streptococcal colonization in the pregnant woman. A couple study. *American Journal of Obstetrics and Gynecology, 135*, 1062–1065.

Gibbs, R.S. & Sweet, R.L. (1994). Clinical disorders. In R.C. Creasy & R. Resnik (Eds.), *Maternal-fetal medicine: Principles and practice* (3rd ed., pp. 655–657). Philadelphia, PA: W.B. Saunders.

Haft, R.F., & Kasper, D.L. (1991, December 11). Group B streptococcus infection in mother and child. *Hospital Practice*, 111–134.

Institute of Medicine. National Academy of Sciences. (1985). Prospects for immunizing against streptococcus group B. In *New vaccine development: Establishing priorities* (Vol 1, pp. 424–439). Washington, DC: National Academy Press.

Katz, V.L. (1993). Management of group B streptococcal disease in pregnancy. *Clinical Obstetrics and Gynecology, 36(4)*, 832–842.

Møller, M., Thomsen, A.C., Borch, K., Dinesen, K., & Zdravkovic, M. (1984). Rupture of fetal membranes and premature delivery associated with group B streptococci in urine of pregnant women. *Lancet, 2*, 69–70.

Noya, F.J.D., & Baker, C.J. (1992). Prevention of group B streptococcal infection. *Infectious Disease Clinics of North America, 6(1)*, 41–54.

Ohlsson, A., & Myhr, T.L. (1994). Intrapartum chemoprophylaxis of perinatal group B streptococcal infections: A critical review of randomized controlled trials. *American Journal of Obstetrics and Gynecology, 170(3)*, 910–917.

Regen, J.A., Klebanoff, M.A., Nugent, R.P., and the Vaginal Infections and Prematurity Study Group. (1991). The epidemiology of group B streptococcal colonization in pregnancy. *Obstetrics & Gynecology, 77(4)*, 604–610.

Thomsen, A.C., Mørup, L., & Hansen, K.B. (1987). Antibiotic elimination of group B streptococci in urine in prevention of preterm labor. *Lancet, 1*, 591–593.

Yancy, M.K., & Duff, P. (1993). Group B streptococcal infections during pregnancy. *Current Opinion in Obstetrics and Gynecology, 5*, 508–512.

Yancy, M.K., & Duff, P. (1994). An analysis of the cost-effectiveness of selected protocols for the prevention of neonatal group B streptococcal infection. *Obstetrics & Gynecology, 83(3)*, 367–371.

Chapter 4

LISTERIA

Winifred L. Star

Listeria monocytogenes is an aerobic and facultatively anaerobic, small gram-positive rod, frequently confused with a diphtheroid. The organism is not species-specific and can be recovered from multiple sources: water, milk, soil, decayed matter, wood and other material, dust, plants, animals, and birds. Listeriosis in humans presents in both epidemic and sporadic forms; both forms are associated with contamination of food and food products (Gibbs & Sweet, 1994; Schlech III, 1991). The incubation period for foodborne transmission is 21 days (American Academy of Pediatrics, 1997).

Listeriosis is especially prone to adversely affect immunocompromised adults and fetuses with immature immune systems (Gibbs & Sweet, 1994). Infection in a nonpregnant adult may have a wide variety of manifestations, including central nervous system infection and undifferentiated sepsis and, rarely, endocarditis, pneumonia, septic arthritis, osteomyelitis, and peritonitis (*Infectious Disease Alert*, 1992). The majority of nonperinatal deaths occur in the immunocompromised, the elderly, or those with underlying medical illnesses (Sirry, George, & Whittle, 1994). A large surveillance project undertaken in the United States by the Centers for Disease Control and Prevention (CDC) between 1988 and 1990 uncovered 301 cases of listeriosis in four geographic areas. An annual incidence of 7.4 cases/million in the population was established; sixty-seven deaths were reported (23 percent of cases). Ninety-nine cases occurred among pregnant women or their newborns (33 percent of cases) (CDC, 1992).

Maternal listeriosis is a rare but significant cause of spontaneous abortion, intrauterine death, premature labor and delivery, and neonatal sepsis (Barresi, 1980). Fetal infection can occur from hematogenous transplacental spread secondary to maternal bacteremia, from fetal swallowing of contaminated amniotic fluid, or from an ascending infection of the vagina and cervix into the uterine cavity. Many infections in pregnancy are asymptomatic or present with manifestations similar to flulike, upper respiratory, or gastrointestinal disorders. Overt maternal infections are observed mostly in the second and third trimesters. Significant maternal morbidity is uncommon; however, occasionally diffuse sepsis will develop (Enockssen, Wretlind, Sterner, & Anzen, 1990; Gibbs & Sweet, 1994). Incidence of fetal death is greater when infection occurs in early pregnancy (Sirry et al., 1994). Maternal infection can occur without infection of the infant (MacGowan, Cartlidge, MacLeod, & McLauchlin, 1991; McLauchlin, 1990). Timely institution of antimicrobial therapy is critical and can be lifesaving; the organism is exquisitely sensitive to ampicillin.

Neonatal listeriosis has two distinct clinical entities: early- and late-onset disease. Early-onset disease, also called congenital listeriosis, is acquired via hematogenous spread through the placenta or through an ascending route (Enocksson et al., 1990). It manifests within the first few days of birth (up to 7 days of age) as a diffuse sepsis with multiorgan involvement including the lungs, liver, and central nervous system (Gibbs & Sweet, 1994). Respiratory distress, apnea, cyanosis, pneumonia, hepatosplenomegaly, and skin rashes are manifestations of early-onset disease (Bortolussi & Schlech III, 1995; Enocksson, 1990). Early-onset listeriosis is associated with a high stillbirth rate, and neonatal mortality rates of 15 to 50 percent have been reported, more frequently occurring in low-birth weight infants (Gibbs & Sweet, 1994; McLauchlin, 1990).

Late-onset disease, usually seen in term infants, occurs 1 to 5 weeks after delivery secondary to infection acquired through a colonized birth canal. The maternal perinatal course has been generally uneventful as the mother is usually an asymptomatic carrier (Boucher & Yonekura, 1986; Enocksson et al., 1990; Gibbs & Sweet, 1994). Babies with late-onset disease may have feeding difficulties, irritability, lethargy, and fever; meningitis is present in the vast majority of cases (Enocksson, et al., 1990). The mortality rate in late-onset disease is 10 to 20 percent (rates approaching 40 percent have been reported). Although uncommon, surviving infants may suffer from long-term sequelae including hydrocephaly and/or neurodevelopmental handicaps (Gibbs & Sweet, 1994; Bortolussi & Schlech III, 1995; McLauchlin, 1990). Late-onset postnatal disease may also occur as a result of nosocomial infection. The source of infection may be contaminated hands or fomites, or droplets from nasopharyngeal carriers among hospital personnel (Enocksson et al., 1990).

An intermediate-onset category of neonatal illness has also been described. Onset of symptoms is in 3 to 5 days and clinical illness presentations seem to overlap early- and late-onset disease types (Enocksson et al., 1990; McLauchlin, 1990).

Recurrent listeriosis in subsequent pregnancies is extremely rare. Nonpregnant individuals, however, may have recurrent episodes and chronic infection or long-term carriage may take place (McLauchlin, 1990).

Database

Subjective

- Asymptomatic genital tract or fecal carriage may occur:
  - ▶ As many as 2 to 5 percent of pregnant women may harbor listeria vaginally.
  - ▶ Transient fecal carriage may occur in 5 to 10 percent of individuals.
  - ▶ Sexual and fecal-oral transmission is possible.
- Maternal illness is usually mild and self-limited. Symptoms may include
  - ▶ Fever (usually low-grade), chills, headache
  - ▶ Malaise, myalgia, fatigue
  - ▶ Nausea, vomiting, diarrhea
  - ▶ Watery nasal discharge
  - ▶ Sore throat
  - ▶ Itching
  - ▶ Dysuria, frequency
  - ▶ Abdominal cramping/pain, back pain
  - ▶ Vaginal bleeding
  - ▶ Uterine contractions
  - ▶ Rupture of membranes
  - ▶ Malodorous/discolored amniotic fluid
  - ▶ Alternately, patient may present with symptoms of meningitis, or adult respiratory distress syndrome (ARDS).

- Obtain complete medical and habits history to identify risk factors for susceptibility to infection:
  - ▶ Significant immunocompromise
  - ▶ Malignancy
  - ▶ Diabetes
  - ▶ Hemochromatosis
  - ▶ Renal disease/failure
  - ▶ Systemic lupus erythematosus
  - ▶ Organ transplantation
  - ▶ Narcotic addiction
  - ▶ Intravenous drug use or alcoholism
  - ▶ Liver disease

Objective

- Serious illness in the mother is rare. The following clinical signs may be present:
  - ▶ Vital signs: elevated temperature
  - ▶ HEENT examination
    - – Rhinorrhea; coryza
    - – Purulent conjunctiva
    - – Injected pharynx
  - ▶ Lymph node examination: cervical adenopathy
  - ▶ Skin/mucous membranes: cutaneous purple lesions of the throat, urethra, or vagina
  - ▶ Preterm labor
  - ▶ Rupture of membranes
  - ▶ Malodorous/stained amniotic fluid (indicative of amnionitis)

Assessment

- *Listeria monocytogenes* infection, maternal and/or neonatal
  - ▶ R/O *bacillus* species infection (may mimic listeriosis)
  - ▶ R/O febrile illness secondary to other bacterial/viral infection
  - ▶ R/O maternal bacteremia
  - ▶ R/O Maternal immunocompromise (HIV infection)

Plan

Diagnostic Tests

- Diagnosis should be based on positive cultures for *L. monocytogenes* isolated from various body fluids: maternal blood, vaginal/cervical material, urine, amniotic fluid, lochia, meconium (Bortolussi & Schlech III, 1995).

  NOTE: Inform the laboratory that *Listeria* is being ruled out because there is morphologic similarity of the organism to diphtheroids.

- Antibody titers may be used for diagnosis of maternal infection (although value of serologic testing is not well-established). Peak rise occurs 2 to 4 weeks after onset of infection.

- Additional laboratory tests and their findings:

  ▶ Complete blood count shows leukocytosis or neutropenia, thrombocytopenia (in severe disease).

  ▶ C-reactive protein (CRP) is elevated.

  ▶ Complement fixation test: complement-fixing *Listeria* antibody titer greater than1:8.

- Gram's stain of gastric aspirate, cerebrospinal fluid (CSF), meconium or tissue smears from infected newborn may be performed, as indicated.

- Placental swab and placental tissue specimen for culture and histology.

Treatment/Management

- A high index of suspicion should be maintained for febrile illness due to *L. monocytogenes* (Gibbs & Sweet, 1994). Treatment for listeriosis may need to be instituted prior to availability of diagnostic tests results (K. P. Beckerman, M.D., personal communication, October 8, 1996).

- If maternal *L. monocytogenes* is identified, antibiotic treatment should be instituted.

  ▶ Optimum therapy includes a combination of

    – Ampicillin (1–2 grams IV every 4 to 6 hours)

      AND

    – An aminoglycoside (e.g., gentamicin 2 mg/kg IV every 8 hours)

    – Duration of therapy is usually 1 week (Gibbs & Sweet, 1994; Sweet & Gibbs, 1995). Physician should dictate dosage regimens.

      NOTE: Erythromycin (avoiding the estolate form) may be used in penicillin-allergic individuals (Bortolussi & Schleck III). Full details of inpatient management are beyond the scope of this chapter.

      NOTE: *Listeria* is resistant to all cephalosporins; ten percent of isolates are penicillin-resistant but ampicillin/amoxicillin-sensitive (Enocksson et al., 1990).

- If amnionitis is not present or acute symptoms of amnionitis have subsided, consider oral antibiotics.

  ▶ Amoxicillin 2 to 3 grams/day p.o. in divided doses for 14 days (Bortolussi & Schlech III, 1995)

- Preterm labor in the setting of a flulike syndrome is highly suggestive of listeriosis and antibiotic therapy should be initiated until the diagnosis is ruled out (K. P. Beckerman, M.D., personal communication, October 8, 1996). Preterm labor in a febrile mother is generally allowed to progress.

- A pediatric team should be standing by in the delivery room to assess the infant. Multiple neonatal cultures should be obtained prior to antibiotic treatment of the newborn (treatment of mother should not be delayed for the purpose of obtaining neonatal cultures). Further details on neonatal therapy are beyond the scope of this chapter. See the American Academy of Pediatrics 1997 reference.

Consultation

- Consult with a physician in all cases. Depending on site-specific practice, the client with listeriosis may be managed by a physician.

Patient Education

- Educate the client regarding the nature of the infection, possible sources of infection, transmission, perinatal implications, and treatment/management modalities. The physician in charge of the client's care may be responsible for detailing the perinatal issues.

- Educate client about the possibility of foodborne transmission. High-risk foods include raw dairy products, soft cheeses, prepacked salad, uncooked/undercooked chilled foods, raw or undercooked poultry, processed meat. See Table 10.4, Recommendations for Preventing Foodborne Listeriosis.

Follow-up

- Obtain repeat maternal cultures (blood and cervical) following antibiotic therapy.
- Continue on-going pediatric care and management of affected infant.
- Report cases of listeriosis to the appropriate public health department.
- Document maternal listeriosis diagnosis and treatment on problem list and in progress notes.

Table 10.4

Recommendations for Preventing Foodborne Listeriosis

For All Persons

- Avoid use of untreated manure on crops destined for human consumption.

- Thoroughly cook raw food from animal sources (e.g., beef, pork, and poultry).

- Thoroughly wash raw vegetables before eating.

- Keep uncooked meats separate from vegetables, cooked foods, and ready-to-eat foods.

- Avoid consumption of raw (unpasteurized) milk or food made from raw milk.

- Wash hands, knives, and cutting boards after handling uncooked foods.

Additional Recommendations for Persons at High Risk*

- Avoid soft cheeses (e.g., Mexican-style, feta, Brie, Camembert, and blue-veined cheeses). (There is no need to avoid hard cheeses, cream cheese, cottage cheese, or yogurt).

- Leftover foods or ready-to-eat foods (e.g., hot dogs) should be reheated until steaming hot before eating.

- Although the risk of listeriosis associated with foods from delicatessen counters is relatively low, pregnant women and immunosuppressed persons may choose to avoid these foods or to thoroughly reheat cold cuts before eating.

* Persons immunocompromised by illness or use of medications, pregnant women, and the elderly.

Source: Modified from Centers for Disease Control and Prevention. (1992). Update: Foodborne listeriosis—United States, 1988–1990 *Morbidity and Mortality Weekly Report, 41*(15), p. 257.

References

American Academy of Pediatrics (AAP). *1997 Red book: Report of the Committee on Infectious Diseases* (24th ed., pp. 327–329). Elk Grove Village, IL: Author.

Barresi, J.A. (1980). Listeria monocytogenes: A cause of premature labor and neonatal sepsis. *American Journal of Obstetrics and Gynecology, 136*(3), 410–411.

Bortolussi, R., & Schlech, W.F., III. (1995). Listeriosis. In J.S. Remington & J.O. Klein (Eds.), *Infectious diseases of the fetus and newborn infant* (4th ed., pp. 1055–1073). Philadelphia, PA: W.B. Saunders.

Boucher, M., & Yonekura, M. (1986). Perinatal listeriosis (Early-onset): Correlation of antenatal manifestations and neonatal outcome. *Obstetrics and Gynecology, 68*(5), 593–597.

Centers for Disease Control and Prevention (CDC). 1992. Update: Foodborne listeriosis - United States, 1988–1990. *Morbidity and Mortality Weekly Report, 41(15)*, 251–258.

Chapman, S.T. (1986). Bacterial infections in pregnancy. *Clinics in Obstetrics and Gynecology, 13*(2), 397–416.

Enocksson, E., Wretlind, B., Sterner, G., & Anzen, B. (1990). Listeriosis during pregnancy and in neonates. *Scandinavian Journal of Infectious Disease, (Suppl. 71)*, 89–94.

Gellin, B.G., Broome, C.V., Bibb, W.F., Weaver, R.E., Gaventa, S., Mascola, L., and the Listeriosis Study Group. (1991). The epidemiology of listeriosis in the United States—1986. *American Journal of Epidemiology, 133*, 392–401.

Gibbs, R.S., & Sweet, R. L. (1994). Clinical disorders. In R. K. Creasy & R. Resnik (Eds.), *Maternal-fetal medicine: Principles and practice* (3rd ed., pp. 657–658). Philadelphia, PA: W. B. Saunders.

Gray, J.W., Barrett, J.F.R., Pedler, S.J., & Lind, T. (1993). Faecal carriage of listeria during pregnancy. *British Journal of Obstetrics and Gynecology, 100*, 873–874.

Infectious Disease Alert. Listeriosis in normal and immunocompromised hosts. Volume 11, No. 16, 101–104.

Leung, T.N., Cheung, K.L., & Wong, F. (1994). Congenital listeriosis: Case reports and review of literature. *Asia-Oceania Journal of Obstetrics and Gynecology, 20*(2), 173–177.

MacGowan, A.P., Cartlidge, P.H.T., MacLeod, F., & McLauchlin, J. (1991). Maternal listeriosis in pregnancy without fetal or neonatal infection. *Journal of Infection, 22*, 53–57.

McLauchlin, J. (1990). Human listeriosis in Britain, 1967–85: A summary of 722 cases. *Epidemiological Infection, 104*, 181–189.

Schlech, W.F., III. (1991). Listeriosis: Epidemiology, virulence, and the significance of contaminated foodstuffs. *Journal of Hospital Infection, 19*, 211.

Sirry, H.W., George, R.H., & Whittle, M.J. (1994). Meningo-encephalitis due to listeria monocytogenes in pregnancy. *British Journal of Obstetrics and Gynecology, 101*, 1083–1084.

Sweet, R.L., & Gibbs, R.S. (1995). *Infectious diseases of the female genital tract* (3rd ed., pp. 502–506). Baltimore, MD: Williams & Wilkins.

Valkenburg, M.H., Essed, G., & Potters, H. (1988). Perinatal listeriosis underdiagnosed as a cause of pre-term labour? *European Journal of Obstetrics, Gynecology, & Reproductive Biology, 27,* 283–288.

Workowski, K.A., & Flaherty, J.P. (1992). Systemic *Bacillus* infection mimicking listeriosis of pregnancy. *Clinical Infectious Diseases, 14,* 694–696.

Chapter 5

MEASLES (RUBEOLA)

Winifred L. Star

Measles (rubeola) is a highly communicable childhood disease. It is caused by a paramyxovirus, which spreads via direct contact with infectious droplets that gain access to a susceptible individual via the nose, oropharynx, and conjunctival mucosa or, less commonly, by airborne spread. Incubation time is about 10 days (range 8 to 12 days) from exposure to onset of prodromal symptoms. The contagion period is from 1 to 2 days before the onset of symptoms to 4 days after the appearance of the rash. Disease patterns vary markedly with respect to age, incidence, and severity of infection in different geographic locations. Measles in pregnant women may be seen more often among individuals from rural, isolated areas (American Academy of Pediatrics [AAP], 1997; Gershon, 1995; Gibbs & Sweet, 1994; Stein & Greenspoon, 1991). Most individuals in the United States born prior to 1957 have been naturally infected with measles (and mumps) and can be considered immune (American College of Obstetricians and Gynecologists [ACOG], 1991). A live attenuated measles vaccine, which has been in use since 1963, has reduced the incidence of the disease significantly; however, from 1989 to 1991 a resurgence in measles, now under control, was reported in the United States (Atkinson, Hadler, Redd, & Orenstein, 1992).This recrudescence was mostly due to low immunization rates in urban, preschool-age children. Since 1992, the incidence of measles in the United States has been very low (less than 1,000 reported cases per year from 1993 to 1995.) (AAP, 1997)

Maternal measles is less common than either chickenpox or mumps: An incidence of 0.4 to 0.6 cases per 10,000 pregnancies (before the licensing of live measles vaccine) has been reported. Several studies have indicated that pregnant women with measles are at greater risk of serious complications and death than nonpregnant women. Mortality is most often due to bacterial pneumonia. An increased rate of premature delivery has been documented in pregnancies complicated by measles, especially with onset in late gestation. Although there is no statistically valid proof of increased risk of spontaneous abortion with maternal measles, the disease may be responsible for specific instances of fetal loss. Teratogenicity has not been proven or refuted because the condition is so rare during pregnancy; no particular constellation of abnormalities has been found in association with the sporadic instances of congenital defects reported after maternal measles (Atmar, Englund, & Hammill, 1991; Gershon, 1995; Gibbs & Sweet, 1994; Grandien & Sterner, 1990).

Measles appearing in the newborn or in the first 10 days of life is considered to be acquired transplacentally; later-onset measles is postnatally acquired. The spectrum of illness in congenital measles may range from mild to rapidly fatal; a mortality rate of 32 percent has been reported (56 percent in preterm infants) (Gibbs & Sweet, 1994; Grandien & Sterner, 1990).

Complications of measles include otitis media, croup, bacterial pneumonia, encephalitis, hepatitis, thrombocytopenic purpura, myocarditis, and subacute sclerosing panencephalitis (Atmar et al., 1992; Gibbs & Sweet, 1994). Atypical measles, a syndrome occurring in adolescents or adults who received inactivated measles vaccine or live measles vaccine before 12 months of age, has been reported. Rather than a protective immunity to measles, these individuals develop a hypersensitivity and, when infected by the measles virus, may experience severe illness which can be fatal (Hashmey & Shandera, 1996).

Measles Vaccine

Live measles vaccines are derivatives of the Edmonston B strain. The vaccine is available as a monovalent vaccine (measles only) and in polyvalent vaccines containing measles and rubella virus vaccines (MR) and measles, mumps, and rubella virus vaccines (MMR). Measles vaccine is indicated for persons susceptible to measles (unless otherwise contraindicated); it produces seroconversion in over 95 percent of recipients and prevents clinical illness in more than 90 percent of exposed susceptible persons (Gershon, 1995). Vaccine-induced antibody levels have been shown to persist for at least 13 years without substantial decline (Merck & Company, 1991). However, data is accumulating that measles antibody titers are lower in women vaccinated during childhood than in women who have had naturally-occurring measles. In addition, offspring of vaccinated women appear to lose transplacentally-acquired measles antibodies before one year of age (Gershon, 1995). See Follow-up section for further information.

Although contraindicated during pregnancy because there are theoretical concerns about fetal infection, inadvertent measles vaccination should not be an indication for pregnancy termination (CDC, 1993a).

Database

Subjective

- Symptoms of acute measles include the following (Gibbs & Sweet, 1994):

  ▶ Prodrome of fever and malaise about 10 days postexposure

  ▶ Coryza (nasal obstruction, sneezing, sore throat), conjunctivitis, and cough follows within 24 hours; the catarrhal phase is then exacerbated with marked conjunctivitis and photophobia for several days.

  ▶ Koplik's spots appear at end of prodrome about 2 days prior to rash (see Objective section).

  ▶ Maculopapular rash on head, neck, behind ears spreading to trunk, upper, then lower extremities 12 to 14 days after exposure, usually 4 days after onset of symptoms (see Objective section).

- Clients with *atypical* measles may complain of high fever, headache, arthralgias, abdominal pain, and rashes without Koplik's spots.

- Clients may have symptoms associated with measles complications (see Introduction).

- Individuals who are considered immune to measles

  ▶ Have had a documented episode of diagnosed measles

  ▶ Have laboratory evidence of measles immunity

  ▶ Were born before 1957

  OR

  ▶ Have had a documented measles immunization for inidviduals born after 1956, two doses of measles vaccine are required for evidence of immunity (AAP, 1997).

Objective

- Temperature is elevated temperature and may be as high as 104-105°F (40-40.6°C).

- HEENT examination reveals

  ▶ Observation of Koplik's spots:

    – Tiny, granular, slightly papular white lesions with erythematous halos

    – Start in the lateral buccal mucosa, may extend to lips, eyelids, inner conjunctiva (may also appear in the vagina)

    – Last for 1 to 4 days

  ▶ Additional findings may include pharyngeal edema, yellowish tonsilar exudate, central coating of tongue with red tip and margins.

- Skin examination reveals distinctive eruption of rash (Gershon, 1995; Hashmey & Shandera, 1996):

  ▶ 1 to 2 mm red macules enlarging over 2 to 3 days to irregular, blotchy maculopapular lesions larger than 1 cm

    – Rash begins on head and neck especially behind ears and on forehead

    – In severe cases rash may coalesce to form nearly uniform erythema on some body areas

  ▶ Rash progresses to trunk, then upper extremities (including palms) by the second day; lower extremities (including soles) involved by third day.

  ▶ Rash begins to fade in order of appearance by third or fourth day.

    – Slight desquamation may follow

    – Hyperpigmentation remains in the fair-complected

- Cardiorespiratory examination reveals tachycardia, tachypnea, dyspnea, rhonchi.

- Abdominal examination occasionally reveals splenomegaly.

- Lymph node examination: generalized lymphadenopathy

  NOTE: A clinical case of measles is defined by the CDC as an illness consisting of
  - A generalized rash lasting greater than or equal to 3 days,
  - Fever 38.3°C (101° F), and
  - The occurrence of cough, coryza, or conjunctivitis (Atkinson et al., 1992).
  "A confirmed case of measles is defined as one that meets the clinical case definition and is either serologically confirmed or epidemiologically linked to another clinical case" (Atkinson et al., 1992, p. 1).

- *Atypical* measles may present with high temperature, papular or hemorrhagic rash without Koplik's spots, abdominal tenderness, interstitial/nodular infiltrates, occasionally pleural effusion (Hashmey & Shandera, 1996).

- Uterine contractions may be present.

- Patients may have signs of measles complications (see introductory section).

Assessment

- Maternal exposure to measles
  - ▶ R/O measles
  - ▶ R/O atypical measles
  - ▶ R/O other infectious diseases with cutaneous lesions, such as rubella, scarlet fever, echovirus, coxsackievirus, adenovirus, enterovirus, erythema infectiosum (fifth disease), secondary syphilis, Rocky Mountain spotted fever, toxoplasmosis, mononucleosis, meningococcemia
  - ▶ R/O drug reaction, other allergies
  - ▶ R/O complications of measles, such as pneumonia, otitis media, encephalitis, hepatic dysfunction, etc.
  - ▶ R/O preterm labor

Plan

Diagnostic Tests

- The diagnosis of measles is usually made on clinical grounds (Koplik's spots are pathognomonic).

- Laboratory diagnosis of acute infection is made by observation of a substantial rise in measles-specific IgG antibody titers from acute and convalescent sera. An acute titer should be drawn shortly after appearance of the rash, a convalescent titer 2 to 4 weeks later.

- A single sample for measles-specific IgM may be obtained 2 to 5 days after rash-onset; IgM is usually undetectable 30 to 60 days later.

- During febrile phase of a measles infection, the disease can be diagnosed by viral isolation in tissue culture from nasopharyngeal secretions, conjunctiva, blood, or urine; however, this testing is technically difficult and usually is not available (AAP, 1997).

- Additional tests may include
  - ▶ Complete blood count (CBC) with differential (leukopenia usually present)
  - ▶ Urinalysis (proteinuria often present)
  - ▶ Chest x-ray (may reveal evidence of pneumonia, pleural effusion)
  - ▶ Sputum Gram stain and culture (if pneumonia present)
  - ▶ Liver function studies (may be elevated)

Treatment/Management

- Maintain respiratory isolation of client for 4 days after rash onset.

- Advise regarding symptomatic relief for uncomplicated measles (e.g., bed rest, increased fluids, acetaminophen as needed for relief of fever).

- Prescribe antibiotic therapy for otitis media or pneumonia, based on results of Gram stain and culture. Consult with physician.

- Give passive immunization to susceptible pregnant women with immune globulin (IG) 0.25 mL/kg IM, as soon as possible postexposure, ideally within 6 days (AAP, 1997; Gibbs & Sweet, 1994).

  NOTE: There is no known risk to the fetus from passive immunization. Live-virus measles, however, is *contraindicated during pregnancy* (Advisory Committee on Immunization Practices [ACIP], 1994).

- IG is also indicated for susceptible household contacts of measles patients, especially if younger than one year of age or if immunocompromised (AAP, 1997).

  ▸ Usual dose is 0.25 mL/kg of body weight IM or 0.5 mL/kg IM for the immunocompromised (maximum dose 15 mL in either case) and should be given within 6 days of exposure.

  NOTE: IG is not indicated for household contacts who have received one dose of vaccine at 12 months of age or older, unless immunocompromised (AAP), 1997). Refer to the American Academy of Pediatrics 1997 reference for additional information. Consult with physician, as indicated.

  ▸ Live-virus vaccine, if given within 72 hours of exposure to measles, will provide protection in some cases. IG and measles vaccine should not be administered simultaneously. See Follow-up section for further information on vaccination.

- Antiviral therapy with aerosolized ribavirin therapy has been used past the 20th week of gestation in a series of patients with potentially life-threatening disease (Atmar et al., 1992). Consult with infectious disease specialist. Not approved by the Federal Drug Administration (FDA) for this use.

Consultation

- Consult with a physician for all clients with measles during pregnancy.

- If complications exist, refer client to a physician for further management.

- Consultation with an infectious disease specialist may be warranted.

Patient Education

- Educate the client regarding etiology of infection, transmission, and possible complications.

- Advise the client to call her provider or return to the office immediately if signs/symptoms of complications develop.

- Offer suggestions for symptomatic relief.

- Discuss course of congenitally acquired disease in the neonate (may range from mild to rapidly fatal). Postnatally acquired infection is usually mild, thus, reassurance is in order.

- Educate the woman regarding the possible need for immunizing close contacts and/or family members (Shannon, 1995). See the Treatment/Management and Follow-up sections.

Follow-up

- Gravidas with measles should be monitored for sequelae, and if complications arise, admitted to the hospital and managed by a physician.

- Individuals who received IG after a measles exposure should receive measles vaccine (if not contraindicated) 5 months later if dose was 0.25 mL/kg or 6 months later if dose was 0.5 mL/kg, provided that the person is at least 12 months old (AAP, 1997). See also vaccination information below.

- Infants should be given IG 0.25 mL/kg IM if born to women with measles in the last few weeks of pregnancy or in the first week postpartum (Gibbs & Sweet, 1994). Guidelines for prevention of measles in the neonate should be discussed with the pediatric staff. See also Table 10.4.a

- Preconceptional testing for immunity may be in order in areas where measles outbreaks are occurring; seronegative women may then receive vaccination prior to conception. Measles vaccine may be administered alone or in combination with mumps and rubella virus vaccines (see below).

- Regarding vaccination

  ▶ In the United States, the combined measles, mumps, and rubella live vaccine (MMR) is recommended to children 12 to 15 months of age, with a second dose at 4 to 6 years of age or 11 to 12 years of age (the second dose may be administered at any visit, however, provided that at least one month has elapsed since the first dose and that both doses are administered at or after 12 months of age (American Academy of Pediatrics, Committee on Infectious Diseases, 1997).

  ▶ For prevention of sporadic measles outbreaks as the sole objective, consider revaccination with a monovalent measles vaccine. If concern also exists regarding immunity to mumps or rubella, revaccination with appropriate monovalent or polyvalent vaccines should be considered (Merck & Company, 1991).

  ▶ *All women of reproductive age should be immune to measles, mumps, and rubella.* MMR vaccine is advisable for all susceptible women (provided they are not pregnant or other contraindications exist).

      NOTE: Reasonable precautions prior to administration of MMR in women of childbearing age include
      • Asking women if they are pregnant and excluding vaccination of those that say they are
      • Explaining the theoretical risks of the vaccine to potential vaccinees
      • Advising against pregnancy for 3 months after vaccination (ACIP, 1990).

  ▶ Persons receiving MMR vaccine can shed these viruses but generally do not transmit them; thus, the vaccine can be safely administered to family members/close contacts of pregnant women (ACOG, 1991; ACIP, 1994).

  ▶ Contraindications to MMR vaccine include (but are not limited to) the following: pregnancy, history of anaphylactic reaction to eggs or neomycin, and significant immunocompromise (except HIV infection) (AAP, 1997).

      – Breastfeeding is *not* a contraindication to vaccination (CDC, 1993b).

- Refer to vaccine package insert(s) for additional information. See also Chapter 10.6, *Mumps*; Chapter 10.8, *Rubella;* Section 1 *Preconception Health Care—An Overview;* and Chapter 4.5, *Travel During Pregnancy.*

▶ "To decrease nosocomial infection, vaccination programs should be established to ensure that health care personnel who will be in contact with patients with measles are immune to the disease." (AAP, 1997, p. 347).

- Document measles diagnosis and complications thereof in progress notes and problem list. In addition, if there is non-immunity to rubella it should be noted on the problem list so that postpartum vaccination can be employed (unless contraindications exist).

Table 10.4.a
Guidelines for Preventative Measures After Exposure to Measles in Nursery/Maternity Service

Type of Exposure/Disease	Measles present (Prodrome or rash)[a]		Disposition
	Mother	Neonate	
A. Siblings at home with measles[a] when neonate & mother ready for discharge	No	No	1. Neonate: protective isolation and IG Indicated unless mother has unequivocal history of previous measles or measles vaccination.[b] 2. Mother: with history of previous measles or measles vaccination, she may either remain with neonate or return to older children. Without previous history she may remain with neonate until older siblings no longer infectious, or she may receive IG prophylactically and return to older children.
B. Mother without history of measles or vaccination exposed during measles period 6-15 days antepartum[c]	No	No	1. Exposed mother and infant: administer IG to each and send home at earliest date unless there are siblings at home with communicable measles. Test mothers for susceptibility if possible. If susceptible, administer live measles vaccine 5 months[d] after IG. 2. Other mothers and infants: same unless clear history of previous measles or measles vaccination in the mother. 3. Hospital personnel: unless clear history of previous measles or measles vaccination administer IG within 72 hours of exposure. Vaccinate 5 months[d] later.
C. Onset of maternal measles ante or postpartum[e]	Yes	Yes	1. Infected mother and infant: isolate together until clinically stable, then send home. 2. Other mothers and infants: same as B-3 except infants should be vaccinated at 12-15 months of age. 3. Hospital personnel: same as B-3.
D. Onset of maternal measles ante or postpartum[e]	Yes	No	1. Infected mother: isolate until no longer infectious[e] 2. Infected mother's infant: isolate separately from mother. Administer IG immediately. Send home when mother is no longer infectious. Alternately, observe in isolation for 18 days for modified measles,[f] especially if IG administration was delayed for >4 days. 3. Other mothers and infants: same as C-2. 4. Hospital personnel: same as B-3.

[a]Catarrhal stage or less than 72 hours after onset of exanthem.

[b]Vaccination with live attenuated measles virus.

[c]With exposure less than 6 days antepartum, mother would not be potentially infectious until at least 72 hours postpartum.

[d]Previous recommendations were 6 weeks to 3 months. High doses of IG can inhibit the immune response to measles vaccine for more than 3 months.

[e]Considered infectious from onset of prodrome until 72 hours after onset of exanthem.

[f]Incubation period for modified measles may be prolonged beyond the usual 10–14 days.

Sources: Adapted from Chickenpox, measles and mumps, by A.A. Gershon, 1995. In J.S. Remington & J.O. Klein (Eds.), *Infectious diseases of the fetus and newborn infant* (4th ed., p. 603, Table 13–12). Copyright 1995 W.B. Saunders. Reprinted with permission. Advisory Committee on Immunization Practices. (1994). *MMWR, 43(RR-1)*, pp. 9, 15–17.

References

Advisory Committee on Immunization Practices (ACIP). (1990). Rubella prevention. Recommendations of the Immunization Practices Advisory Committee (ACIP). *Morbidity and Mortality Weekly Report, 39*(RR–15), 1–18.

Advisory Committee on Immunization Practices (ACIP). (1994). General recommendations on immunization. Recommendations of the Advisory Committee on Immunization Practices. *Morbidity and Mortality Weekly Report, 43*(RR–1), 1–38.

American Academy of Pediatrics, Committee on Infectious Diseases (1997). Recommended childhood immunization schedule—United States, January–December 1997. *Pediatrics, 99*(1) 136–137.

American Academy of Pediatrics (AAP). (1997). *1997 Red book: Report of the Committee on Infectious Diseases* (24th ed., pp. 344–357). Elk Grove Village, IL: Author.

American College of Obstetricians and Gynecologists (ACOG). (1991). Immunization during pregnancy. (Technical Bulletin No. 160). Washington, DC: Author.

Atkinson, W.L., Hadler, S.C., Redd, S.B., & Orenstein, W.A. (1992). Measles surveillance - United States, 1991. *Morbidity and Mortality Weekly Report, 41*(SS–6), 1–12.

Atmar, R.L., Englund, J.A., & Hammill, H. (1992). Complications of measles during pregnancy. *Clinical Infectious Diseases, 14 (January)*, 217–226.

Centers for Disease Control and Prevention (CDC). (1990). Case definitions for public health surveillance. *Morbidity and Mortality Weekly Report, 39*(RR–13), 1–43.

Centers for Disease Control and Prevention (CDC). (1993a). Measles vaccination information. Fax document #241602. Atlanta, GA: Author

Centers for Disease Control and Prevention (CDC). (1993b). Measles vaccine normal side effects and adverse reactions. Fax document #241003. Atlanta, GA: Author

Gershon, A.A. (1995). Chickenpox, measles, and mumps. In J.S. Remington & J.O. Klein (Eds.), *Infectious diseases of the fetus and newborn infant* (4th ed., pp. 591–603). Philadelphia, PA: W.B. Saunders.

Gibbs, R.S., & Sweet, R.L. (1994). Clinical disorders. Measles. In R.K. Creasy & R. Resnik (Eds.), *Maternal-fetal medicine. Principles and practice* (3rd ed., pp. 674–675). Philadelphia, PA: W.B. Saunders.

Grandien, M., & Sterner, G. (1990). Measles in pregnancy. *Scandinavian Journal of Infectious Disease, (Suppl. 7.)*, 45–48.

Hashmey, R., & Shandera, W.X. (1996). Infectious diseases: Viral and rickettsial. In L.M. Tierney, S.J. McPhee, & M.A. Papadakis (Eds.), *Current medical diagnosis and treatment* (35th ed., pp. 1167–169). Stamford, CT: Appleton & Lange.

Merck & Company. (1991). Attenuvax® Package insert. West Point, PA: Merck, Sharp, & Dohme.

Shannon, M.T. (1995). Measles (Rubeola). In W.L. Star, L.L. Lommel, & M.T. Shannon (Eds.), *Women's primary health care: Protocols for practice* (11–46 to 11–48). Washington, DC: American Nurses.

Stein, S.J., & Greenspoon, J.S. (1991). Rubeola during pregnancy. *Obstetrics and Gynecology, 78(5, Pt. 2)*, 925–929.

Chapter 6

MUMPS

Winifred L. Star

Mumps is a viral (paramyxovirus) disease of childhood affecting the parotid and salivary glands and, less commonly, the brain, pancreas, and gonads. It is transmitted by droplets, saliva, and fomites to susceptible individuals but is not as contagious as measles or chicken pox. The incubation period is from 16 to 18 days (range 12 to 25 days). Communicability is usually 1 to 2 days (but may be as long as 7 days) before the onset of parotid swelling and lasting as long as 9 days afterward. Only 10 percent of mumps cases occur in persons older than 15 years of age. Ninety percent of adults without knowledge of past infection are immune on serologic testing. During adulthood, mumps infection is likely to be more severe. Complications of mumps are uncommon but may include aseptic meningitis, pancreatitis, mastitis, thyroiditis, myocarditis, nephritis, arthritis, migratory arthralgias, hearing impairment, oophoritis, and orchitis in males. (American Academy of Pediatrics (AAP), 1997; Gibbs & Sweet, 1994; Gershon, 1995; Hashmey & Shandera, 1996).

The incidence of mumps in pregnancy is estimated to be from 0.8 to 10 cases/10,000 pregnancies (Miller & Hager, 1992). Maternal illness is fairly benign, however, there appears to be a twofold increase in spontaneous abortion if mumps occurs during the first trimester (usually within 2 weeks of the infection). Complications of prematurity, intrauterine growth restriction, or perinatal mortality are not significant, and teratogenicity is unproven. Congenital mumps or postnatally acquired neonatal mumps is extremely rare. The major concern has been the postulation between maternal mumps infection and the later development of endocardial fibroelastosis (Gibbs & Sweet, 1994; Miller & Hager, 1992); more studies are required to support or refute this concern.

Mumps Vaccine

Mumps vaccine is a live virus vaccine prepared from the Jeryl Lynn (B level) strain of mumps virus. Since introduction of the vaccine in 1967 the incidence of reported mumps cases has decreased steadily in the United States except for a brief resurgence between 1985 and 1987 (Advisory Committee on Immunization Practices [ACIP], 1989). The vaccine is available in both monovalent (mumps only) and polyvalent (in combination with measles and rubella virus vaccines [MMR]) forms.

The vaccine is indicated for immunization against mumps in persons 12 months of age or older and is usually administered simultaneously with measles and rubella vaccines. Live attenuated mumps vaccine is about 95 percent efficacious in preventing mumps disease and induces antibodies in more than 97 percent of recipients (although a lower titer results than one from natural infection); immunity is long-lasting (more than 25 years) (AAP, 1997; ACIP, 1989; Gershon, 1995; Merck & Company, 1990).

No evidence of congenital malformation has been noted in association with live-virus mumps vaccine. The vaccine virus, however, can infect the placenta and fetus; thus, due to *theoretical* risk of fetal damage the vaccine should not be given to pregnant women and pregnancy should be avoided for 3 months following vaccination (CDC, 1995). Inadvertent vaccination during pregnancy should not be considered an indication for termination (AAP, 1997; ACIP, 1989). See the Follow-up section for further information.

Database

Subjective

- Symptoms of mumps include
    - ▶ Prodrome of fever, malaise, myalgia, anorexia
    - ▶ Pain and swelling of one or both parotid glands, usually in succession 1 to 3 days apart; onset usually within 24 hours of prodrome, resolution within 1 week.
- With complications, the following may exist:
    - ▶ Headache and lethargy (with meningitis)
    - ▶ Upper abdominal pain and nausea (with pancreatitis)

Objective

- Vital signs
    - ▶ Elevated temperature
- HEENT
    - ▶ Facial edema
    - ▶ Red, swollen Stensen's duct orifice
    - ▶ Parotid gland swelling with tenderness to palpation; obliteration of space between earlobe and angle of mandible (Gershon, 1995).

        NOTE: Parotid gland swelling should be differentiated from lymph node swelling, which is more posterior and inferior.
    - ▶ Submaxillary and sublingual gland swelling/tenderness in some cases
- Signs of mumps complications
    - ▶ Nuchal rigidity or other meningeal signs in meningitis
    - ▶ Epigastric tenderness to palpation in pancreatitis
    - ▶ Lower abdominal tenderness and ovarian enlargement in oophoritis
- Persons should be considered susceptible to mumps unless they
    - ▶ Have documentation of physician-diagnosed mumps
    - ▶ Have documentation of at least one dose of vaccine on or after the first birthday
    - ▶ Have serologic evidence of immunity
    - ▶ Were born before 1957 (AAP 1997)

Assessment

- Mumps exposure
  - ▶ R/O maternal mumps infection
  - ▶ R/O anterior cervical lymphadenitis
  - ▶ R/O recurrent idiopathic parotitis
  - ▶ R/O calculi in parotid ducts
  - ▶ R/O parotitis secondary to other causes(bacterial organisms, other viral illness, drug reaction)
  - ▶ R/O sarcoidosis
  - ▶ R/O parotid gland tumor
  - ▶ R/O complications of mumps

Plan

Diagnostic Tests

- Diagnosis can be made on clinical grounds in the presence of acute, bilateral, painful parotitis with history of recent exposure (Gershon, 1995).
- Laboratory tests for confirmation may include
  - ▶ Culture isolation of mumps virus from saliva, throat washings, urine, or cerebrospinal fluid (CSF)
  - ▶ Fourfold rise in titer of mumps-specific antibody in acute and convalescent sera
  - ▶ Mumps-specific IgM in single serum specimen
  - ▶ Enzyme immunoassay (EIA) to confirm immunity (skin tests are unreliable and should not be used for this purpose (AAP, 1997).
- Additional tests may include
  - ▶ Complete blood count (white blood cell count may be elevated, normal, or depressed and may reveal mild lymphocytosis or polymorphonuclear leukocytosis)
  - ▶ Serum amylase (may be elevated)
  - ▶ CSF analysis (pleocytosis with predominance of polymorphonuclear leukocytes; normal to low glucose)

Treatment/Management

- Maintain respiratory isolation of client until 9 days after onset of parotid swelling.
- Continue bed rest during febrile period.
- Maintain adequate hydration.

- Suggest symptomatic relief.

  ▶ Acetaminophen for analgesia

  ▶ Cold or heat applied to the parotid glands to alleviate discomfort

- Termination of pregnancy is not indicated for maternal mumps (Gibbs & Sweet, 1994), but patients with mumps complications should be hospitalized and managed by a physician.

- Live-virus mumps vaccine is contraindicated during pregnancy. Mumps immune globulin is no longer available because it was not effective for disease prevention.

- For exposed susceptible persons (e.g., close contacts, household members, hospital personnel, puerperal mothers) administration of mumps vaccine can be considered (may theoretically modify/prevent disease by inducing neutralizing antibodies before illness onset; will provide protection from subsequent exposures) (AAP, 1997; Gershon, 1995). See also Follow-up section.

  NOTE: Most individuals born prior to 1957 have been naturally infected with mumps (and measles) and can be considered immune; thus, vaccination is not advised for these persons unless proven susceptible (i.e., seronegative) (90 percent of adults with no knowledge of past infection are found to be immune upon serologic testing) (AAP, 1997; American College of Obstetricians and Gynecologists [ACOG], 1991).

- If parotitis or other manifestations of maternal mumps are present in the immediate antepartum or postpartum period, it is prudent to isolate the infected mother from other mothers and neonates (Gershon, 1995). Hospital policy will determine whether mother and baby are to be isolated from each other.

Consultation

- Consultation is advisable in all cases.

- Patients with mumps complications should be admitted to the hospital and managed by a physician.

- Consultation with an infectious disease specialist may be warranted.

Patient Education

- Discuss etiology and benign nature of the infection.

- Advise the client of potential complications and need to inform her health care provider should signs of complications occur.

- Reassure the mother regarding fetal implications.

- Educate her regarding signs and symptoms of spontaneous abortion if mumps are contracted in the first trimester.

- Offer suggestions for symptomatic relief.

- Advise regarding immunization as indicated. See the Follow-up section.

Follow-up

- Continue routine prenatal care unless complications exist.

- Observe for complications.

- Regarding vaccination:

  ▶ In the United States, the combined measles, mumps, and rubella virus vaccine (MMR) is the vaccine of choice for routine administration, to be used in all situations where recipients are likely to be susceptible to all three infections; it is routinely recommended for children 12 to 15 months of age, with a second dose at 4 to 6 years of age or 11 to 12 years of age (the second dose may be administered at any visit, however, provided that at least one month has elapsed since the first dose and that both doses are administered at or after 12 months of age (American Academy of Pediatrics, Committee on Infectious Diseases, 1997).

  ▶ *All women of reproductive age should be immune to measles, mumps, and rubella.* MMR vaccine is advisable for all susceptible women (provided they are not pregnant or other contraindications exist).

    NOTE: Reasonable precautions prior to administration of MMR in women of childbearing age include
    - Asking women if they are pregnant and excluding vaccination of those that say they are
    - Explaining the theoretical risks of the vaccine to potential vaccinees
    - Advising against pregnancy for 3 months after vaccination (ACIP, 1990).

  ▶ Persons receiving MMR vaccine can shed these viruses but generally do not transmit them; thus, the vaccine can be safely administered to family members/close contacts of pregnant women (ACIP, 1994; ACOG, 1991).

  ▶ Contraindications to MMR vaccine include (but are not limited to) the following: pregnancy, history of anaphylactic reaction to eggs or neomycin, and significant immunocompromise (except HIV infection) (AAP, 1997).

    – Breastfeeding is *not* a contraindication to vaccination.

    – Refer to vaccine package insert(s) for additional information. See also Chapter 10.5, *Measles*; Chapter 10.8, *Rubella*; Section 1, *Preconception Health Care—An Overview*; and Chapter 4.5, *Travel During Pregnancy*.

- Document mumps diagnosis and complications thereof in progress notes and problem list. In addition, if there is nonimmunity to rubella it should be noted on the problem list so that postpartum vaccination can be employed (unless contraindications exist).

References

Advisory Committee on Immunization Practices (ACIP). (1989). Recommendations of the Immunization Practices Advisory Committee. Mumps prevention. *Mortality and Morbidity Weekly Report, 38*(22), 388–400.

Advisory Committee on Immunization Practices (ACIP). (1990). Rubella prevention. Recommendations of the Immunization Practices Advisory Committee. *Morbidity and Mortality Weekly Report, 39*(RR-15), 1–18.

Advisory Committee on Immunization Practices (ACIP). (1994). General recommendations on immunization. Recommendations of the Advisory Committee on Immunization Practices. *Morbidity and Mortality Weekly Report, 43*(RR-1), 1–38.

American College of Obstetricians and Gynecologists (ACOG). (1991). Immunization during pregnancy. (Technical Bulletin No. 160). Washington, DC: Author.

American Academy of Pediatrics (AAP). (1997). *1997 Red book: Report of the Committee on Infectious Diseases* (24th ed., pp. 366–369). Elk Grove Village, IL: Author.

American Academy of Pediatrics, Committee on Infectious Diseases. (1997). Recommended childhood immunization schedule—United States, January–December 1997. *Pediatrics, 99*(1), 136–137.

Centers for Disease Control and Prevention (CDC). (1995). Mumps and pregnancy. Fax document #242002. Atlanta, GA: Author.

Gershon, A.A. (1995). Chickenpox, measles and mumps. In J. S. Remington & J. O. Klein (Eds.), *Infectious diseases of the fetus and newborn* (4th ed., pp. 603–609). Philadelphia, PA: W.B. Saunders.

Gibbs. R.S., & Sweet, R.L. (1994). Clinical disorders. In R.K. Creasy & R. Resnik (Eds.), *Maternal-fetal medicine* (3rd. ed., pp. 674–675). Philadelphia, PA: W. B. Saunders.

Hashmey, R., & Shandera, W.X. (1996). Infectious diseases: Viral and rickettsial. In L.M. Tierney, S.J. McPhee, & M.A. Papadakis (Eds.), *Current medical diagnosis and treatment* (35th ed., pp. 1169–1170). Stamford, CT: Appleton & Lange.

Merck & Company. (1990). Mumpsvax® Drug package insert. West Point, PA: Author.

Miller, R.D., & Hager, W.D. (1992). Mumps in pregnancy. *Contemporary OB/GYN, 37(2)*, 87–88.

Sterner, G., & Grandien, M. (1990). Mumps in pregnancy at term. *Scandinavian Journal of Infectious Disease, 71*, 36–38.

Chapter 7

PARVOVIRUS

Winifred L. Star

The human parvovirus B19 was discovered in 1975 and was subsequently shown to be the cause of several diseases, including the common childhood disease erythema infectiosum (fifth disease), transient aplastic crisis (TAC) in patients with chronic hemolytic anemias, a chronic rheumatoidlike arthritis, and chronic bone marrow suppression (Sahakian, Weiner, Naides, Williamson, & Scharosch, 1991). Other conditions that have an association with B19 include hemophagocytic syndrome, myocarditis, certain neurologic diseases (e.g., peripheral nerve abnormalities and sporadic cases of meningitis, encephalopathy, seizure disorders), and systemic necrotizing vasculitis (Török, 1995).

Erythema infectiosum (EI), outbreaks of which peak in winter and spring, most commonly occurs in children aged 4 to 14 years and is characterized by features similar to influenza. A "slapped cheek" rash, which spreads to the trunk and extremities in a lacelike pattern, may appear. The respiratory tract is the likely portal of entry and the incubation period is approximately 4 to 14 days (may be up to 3 weeks). Transmission may also occur vertically from mother to fetus, via contaminated blood products or needles (including tattoo needles), and possibly by fomites and environmental contamination. Transmission of the virus through breastfeeding has not been reported. Approximately 50 percent of reproductive age women are immune to parvovirus (Boley & Popek, 1993; Centers for Disease Control and Prevention [CDC], 1989).

Adverse pregnancy outcomes attributed to parvovirus include spontaneous abortion, hydrops fetalis, premature delivery, small-for-gestational-age infants, and stillbirth. However, the majority of maternal infections (at least 80 percent, possibly as high as 95 percent) are associated with normal fetal outcomes. Vertical transmission risk from mother to fetus has been estimated at 33 percent, although precise information on fetal risk and transplacental infection is lacking (Brown, 1989; Hall, 1994; Public Health Laboratory Service Working Party on Fifth Disease, 1990; Rodis et al., 1990).

Risk of fetal death attributable to parvovirus following documented maternal infection is estimated to be less than 10 percent from available prospective studies (Public Health Laboratory Service Working Party on Fifth Disease, 1990; Rodis et al., 1990). The greatest risk appears in gestations under 20 weeks, although losses may occur at any gestational age (Boley & Popek, 1993). Most fetal loss occurs within 4 weeks of maternal rash/arthropathy. Rates of loss during asymptomatic maternal infection are not known (Morey, Keeling, Porter, & Fleming, 1992). Further studies are needed to assess the risk of parvovirus at different stages of pregnancy and to evaluate the role of B19 as a causative agent in fetal death (Brown, 1989).

Nonimmune hydrops fetalis (NIHF), occurring in less than 5 percent of fetuses with parvovirus, is one of the most severe manifestations of fetal infection, occurring 3 to 5 weeks (range 1 to 12 weeks) after maternal exposure. Several pathogenic mechanisms are responsible for this complication. Since B19 has a predilection to attack erythroid progenitor cells the fetus is at risk of developing severe aplastic anemia because of the susceptibility of its immature red blood cells to the effects of the virus (Gibbs & Sweet, 1994). Chronic severe anemia, hypoxia, high-output cardiac failure, myocarditis, compromised hepatic function, and impaired albumin production may all contribute to the development of an hydropic fetus (Morey et al., 1992; Török, 1995). Hypertensive disorders of pregnancy have been reported in some women with pregnancies complicated by B19-associated hydrops. Optimum treatment for NIHF has yet to be determined, and spontaneous resolution of the condition (usually within 1 to 7 weeks) may occur without treatment (Boley & Popek, 1993). It has not been determined why some infected fetuses develop fatal hydrops and others survive (Morey et al., 1992). Intrauterine transfusion (IUT) has been successfully applied in several cases of NIHF.

There are no epidemiologic data to confirm that parvovirus is a teratogen; however, circumstantial evidence exists that suggests the infection may be a cause of birth defects in some cases (Keyserling, 1997; Török, 1995). One report has described ocular defects (similar to those seen in congenital rubella) in an 11-week abortus of a mother who had a serologically confirmed infection at 6 weeks' gestation (Hartwig, Vermeij-Keers, van Elsacker-Niele, & Fleuren, 1989). Additional rare cases have been reported that associate maternal parvovirus infection with neonatal anomalies, including cleft lip or palate, webbed joints, ocular malformations, skeletal muscle anomalies, hepatocellular damage, skeletal myositis, and myocarditis (cited in Katz, McCoy, Kuller, and Hansen, 1996). Additional studies are needed.

Optimal management of a pregnant woman who has been exposed to or infected with B19 is controversial. Further research is needed to demonstrate the efficacy of different therapeutic approaches and interventions. In addition, more information is needed on the long-term sequelae of infants infected in utero who appear normal at birth: There is an existing report describing a perinatal encephalopathy manifested by migrational abnormalities, intracranial calcifications, and severe neurological dysfunction (Conry, Török, & Andrews, 1993).

Parvoviral infection from a public health perspective requires consideration. Occupational risk factors include exposure in schools and day-care centers. During outbreaks of B19 infection in these settings and in close-contact exposures in the home, options for preventing transmission are limited because by the time symptoms develop, the period of infectiousness has passed (Cartter et al., 1991; CDC, 1989; Gillespie et al., 1990). Health care workers are at risk for nosocomial transmission of B19 from patients with TAC (these patients are infectious during the course of the illness) and immunodeficient patients with chronic B19 infection (CDC, 1989).

Database

Subjective

- There may be known exposure to household member or school-age child with fifth disease. A health care worker may also report exposure. The type of exposure determines risk of infection (see Table 10.5).

- In children, erythema infectiosum is usually mild, with the following presentation:

  ▶ Prodrome of low-grade fever, headache, malaise, myalgias, coryza, gastrointestinal "upset"

  ▶ Facial rash (7 to 10 days after prodrome) followed by a reticular trunk and extremity rash (which may be pruritic); rash may reappear for several weeks following nonspecific stimuli (e.g., temperature change, sunlight, emotional stress (CDC, 1989)

  NOTE: Once rash develops children are no longer infectious.

  ▶ Duration of illness usually 10 days or less.

  ▶ Atypical presentations may include mild respiratory symptoms without rash.

- ▶ Arthralgia, arthritis-like symptoms especially of knees (fewer than 10 percent of cases).
- ▶ Infection may be asymptomatic.
- Adult infection is usually asymptomatic, or symptoms are variable, and may include the following:
  - ▶ Fever
  - ▶ Swollen lymph glands
  - ▶ Reticular rash as described in Objective section (absence of rash is more common)
  - ▶ Symmetrical arthralgia, arthritis-like symptoms affecting hands, wrists, knees
    - – Onset of within few days rash (if present)
    - – Resolution usually within 2 weeks but may persist for months to years

      NOTE: Arthralgia may occur as sole manifestation of infection.
- Patients with TAC may complain of fever, headache, malaise, myalgias, weakness and lethargy; rash is uncommon.

Objective

- Seroprevalence of IgG antibodies to B19 is age dependent (Anderson, 1987)
  - ▶ Ages 1 to 5 years: 2 to 15 percent
  - ▶ Ages 5 to 19 years: 15 to 60 percent
  - ▶ Adults: 30 to 60 percent
- Clinical signs of erythema infectiosum
  - ▶ Vital signs may reveal elevated temperature.
  - ▶ Lymph node examination may reveal adenopathy.
  - ▶ Skin examination may reveal
    - – Erythematous maculopapular facial rash affecting cheeks ("slapped cheek" rash)
    - – Symmetrical maculopapular, reticulated rash on arms moving caudally to involve trunk, buttocks, thighs
    - – Other cutaneous manifestations (e.g., vesicular, petechial, or desquamative rashes)
  - ▶ Extremity examination may reveal
    - – Symmetrical tenderness, redness, warmth, swelling of joints
      - * In adults, metacarpophalangeal and proximal interphalangeal joints and knees most affected
      - * In children, knees most affected
- Patients with TAC may present with pallor, tachycardia, and severe weakness; rash is uncommon.

- Nonimmune hydrops fetalis characterized by
  - ▶ Ascites
  - ▶ Pericardial/pleural effusion
  - ▶ Skin edema
  - ▶ Myocarditis
  - ▶ Myositis of skeletal muscle
  - ▶ Leukoerythroblastic response of liver, spleen, kidney
  - ▶ Bone marrow aplasia and hemolysis
  - ▶ Heart failure
  - ▶ Anemia
  - ▶ Low red and white cell counts in peripheral blood (Kinney & Kumar, 1988)
  - ▶ Associated oligohydramnios, polyhydramnios
- Signs of preeclampsia may (rarely) occur as a complication of fetal hydrops. See Chapter 6.13, *Hypertensive Disorders of Pregnancy*.

Assessment

- Maternal exposure to parvovirus B19 infection
  - ▶ R/O parvovirus B19 infection
  - ▶ R/O other infectious diseases including rubella, rubeola, scarlet fever, measles
  - ▶ R/O systemic lupus erythematosus
  - ▶ R/O rheumatoid arthritis
  - ▶ R/O fibromyalgia
  - ▶ R/O fetal infection
- Nonimmune hydrops fetalis
  - ▶ R/O isoimmunization
  - ▶ R/O syphilis
  - ▶ R/O fetal anomalies (especially cardiac)
  - ▶ R/O abnormal karyotype (especially Down syndrome, Turner syndrome)

Plan

Diagnostic Tests

- Anti-B19 IgM antibodies
  - ▶ Appear just before onset of symptoms
  - ▶ Peak 2 to 3 weeks later, decline over 30 to 60 days (but can persist for up to 10 months)

▶ Most sensitive test to detect recent infection (Török, 1995).

   NOTE: False negative IgM results (10 to 20 percent) may occur depending on an individual's immune response and the variability of the incubation period (The Permanente Medical Group Perinatal Group Recommendations, 1994).

- Anti-B19 IgG antibodies

   ▶ Appear by 7 days after symptom onset

   ▶ Peak at 1 month, but persist for years/life

   ▶ Previous infection with B19 defined as presence of IgG in absence of IgM

      – Presence of IgG correlates with lower risk of subsequent infection.

      – Diagnosis via IgG alone requires acute and convalescent titers; significant rise between titers is indicative of acute infection (Boley & Popek, 1993).

   NOTE: Since laboratories may report both IgM and IgG antibody results, a single specimen obtained between 4 days and 4 weeks of symptom onset or 2 weeks postexposure may suffice to establish the serologic diagnosis of acute infection (Mead, 1989). In immunocompromised individuals with chronic B19 infection, the B19 antibody may not be detectable; thus, additional testing for B19 DNA or viral antigens may be necessary to document infection (CDC, 1989).

- Virus culture

   ▶ Practical systems for culturing the virus do not exist at this time.

   ▶ Viral DNA may be identified in respiratory secretions or serum (during prodromal illness) by DNA hybridization studies or polymerase chain reaction (PCR) assays.

- Additional laboratory tests may include

   ▶ Complete blood count (CBC)

      – Hemoglobin may be decreased 2 to 3 g/dL

      – Reticulocyte count may be decreased

      – Platelets, neutrophils, lymphocytes may be moderately decreased.

   ▶ Rheumatoid factor or antinuclear antibody (may be transiently positive)

   ▶ Other tests for autoimmune disease, such as anti-dsDNA, anti-ssDNA, antilymphocytic IgM antibodies (may be positive)

   ▶ Bone marrow studies (may show macroerythroblastic changes, large proerythroblasts)

- Serial MSAFP measurements may be performed if maternal infection diagnosed to aid in predicting fetal infection (elevated levels may precede onset of hydrops) (Bernstein & Capeless, 1989; Carrington et al., 1987)

- Serial ultrasonography (every 1 to 2 weeks for 12 weeks) may be performed to evaluate for fetal hydrops, if maternal infection diagnosed (Ghidini & Lynch, 1994)

- Fetal infection may be confirmed by the following:

   ▶ IgM or B19 DNA in fetal blood obtained via cordocentesis at 18 weeks or more

   ▶ B19 DNA in amniotic fluid obtained by amniocentesis

▶ IgM in cord or neonatal blood

▶ B19 DNA in fetal tissues

▶ Immunohistochemistry or light microscopy identification of characteristic intranuclear inclusions in cord blood or fetal tissues

▶ Anti-B19 IgG persistence (high titer) in infants blood after 1 year of age (Alger, 1997; Boley & Popek, 1993)

NOTE: A complete autopsy should be performed on stillborn infants, including serology; cultures of affected tissue, stool, and cerebrospinal fluid (CSF); and routine histology of all organs. Gross/microscopic examination of placenta should also be performed (Boley & Popek, 1993).

Treatment/Management

● Guidelines for assessment and treatment/management are controversial and may vary from institution to institution. Consult with a physician. Options listed below should be viewed with cautious regard. Also see the Diagnostic Tests section.

▶ Serum testing for maternal IgM and IgG antibodies after exposure to parvoviral infection

▶ Serial MSAFP levels following serologic confirmation of maternal infection

▶ Serial ultrasonography to assess for hydrops fetalis following serologic confirmation of maternal infection

▶ Amniocentesis, percutaneous umbilical blood sampling (PUBS) to assess for fetal B19 IgM or B19 DNA and other fetal hematologic indices of infection

▶ IUT to alleviate severe anemia if fetal hydrops is demonstrated (Bernstein & Capeless, 1989)

NOTE: Some institutions do not support significant testing, observation, or potentially morbid interventions (e.g., IUT) (The Permanente Medical Group Perinatal Group Recommendations, 1994). Some interventions can only be carried out at specialized centers.

● Therapeutic abortion has not been recommended when maternal infection is diagnosed.

● No specific antiviral therapy or vaccine is available at this time (a vaccine is under development).

▶ Parvovirus immunoglobulin is not recommended for postexposure prophylaxis in immunocompetent persons.

▶ Intravenous immunoglobulin (IVIG) has been used empirically in immunocompromised individuals with chronic B19; IVIG may be considered for prophylaxis after B19 exposure in this group and for patients with symptomatic anemia and parvoviremia (Guerina, 1994).

NOTE: The use of IVIG in treatment of hydropic fetuses requires further investigation (Alger, 1997).

● Symptomatic relief measures for acute erythema infectiosum may include:

▶ Analgesics (e.g., acetaminophen) as needed for fever, arthralgia

▶ Antihistamines (e.g., diphenhydramine) as needed for pruritus

NOTE: Adult dose 25 to 50 mg po every 6 to 8 hours as needed or at bedtime only. Antihistamines should be used sparingly during pregnancy. Warn patient about side effect of drowsiness.

- TAC requires prompt treatment; patients may require hospitalization and transfusion. Further details on management are beyond the scope of this chapter.

Consultation

- Consult with a physician for women exposed to or with suspected/confirmed parvovirus infection.
- Depending on site-specific practice, client may be managed by a obstetrician or perinatologist.
- Consult with the infection control division at the worksite, if indicated, if pregnant woman is a health care worker.

Patient Education

- Discuss the nature of the virus, its incubation/contagious period and mode of transmission.
- Explain the potential risks to exposed pregnant women.
  - ▶ Discuss the possible perinatal effects of parvovirus infection so informed decisions regarding assessment and management can take place (see introductory section and Tables 10.5 and 10.6).
  - ▶ Discuss risk in the context of other pregnancy risks and those associated with intervention (CDC, 1989).
  - ▶ Counseling may be carried out by the physician responsible for the client's care.
- If serological testing is performed, assure clients who are IgM-negative but IgG-positive that they are at little, if any, risk from parvovirus infection. Those with IgM antibodies have recently been infected and the fetus may be at risk of parvovirus-related adverse effects or fetal death (Rodis et al., 1990).
- Advise health care workers regarding nosocomial transmission of B19 from patients with TAC and immunodeficient patients with chronic B19 infection (these patients are highly contagious).
  - ▶ Preventive measures (i.e., infection-control practices) should be undertaken to reduce possible transmission (CDC, 1989).
  - ▶ Pregnant workers should not care for TAC or immunocompromised patients and should be advised regarding the potential fetal risks involved.
  - ▶ Consultation with the infection control division at the worksite may be indicated.
- Advise pregnant women that they need not be routinely excluded from working in school or day-care environments during outbreaks of fifth disease (Cartter et al., 1991)
  - ▶ Options for preventing transmission are limited in these settings (i.e., by the time symptoms develop in children, the period of infectiousness has passed).

▶ During protracted outbreaks, pregnant personnel should be advised regarding transmission and acquisition of infection; ultimately the decision to avoid the environment will be up to the individual.

▶ Good handwashing and additional hygienic measures should be followed at the workplace (CDC, 1989).

Follow-up

● Widespread serologic screening of pregnant women is not recommended at this time.

▶ Pregnant women may receive serologic testing if exposed to parvovirus in the work setting (or to an infected child at home).

▶ Pregnant women should receive counseling about maternal/fetal risk of infection as well as means to reduce future risk of infection.

● Patient should be observed for pregnancy-induced hypertension/ preeclampsia in cases where hydrops fetalis is diagnosed.

● Maintain appropriate pediatric care in cases where congenital infection is suspected. Health care workers should be aware that the infant and its body fluids/organs may be infective (Boley & Popek, 1993).

● Emotional support is important for the client/couple who has had an adverse pregnancy outcome. Refer to psychological, social, or other support services, as indicated.

● Document exposure/diagnosis of parvovirus infection of mother/fetus in the problem list and detail the specifics of assessment/management in the progress notes.

Table 10.5

Risk of Maternal Infection by Exposure

- Nonimmune household contact (with persons with TAC or EI): 50 percent risk.

- Nonimmune school staff (during epidemics): 20 percent to 30 percent risk.

- Nonimmune health care worker: 35 percent risk.

Source: Boley, T.J., & Popek, E.J. (1993). Parvovirus infection in pregnancy. *Seminars in Perinatology, 17*(6), 411.

Table 10.6

Risk of Fetal Death Due to Parvovirus in Pregnant Woman with Unknown Immune Status

Formula for Risk of Fetal Death

Rate of susceptibility of infection (50 percent for adults) x Rate of maternal infection following exposure
x Risk of fetal death following confirmed maternal infection x 100
(See Table 10.5 for risk estimates in different populations)

A 10 percent maximum fetal death rate is assumed in formula. Using these data the following risks of fetal death in mother with unknown immune status can be estimated for the following categories:

- Household contact = 2.5%
  (0.5 x 0.5 x 0.1 x 100)

- School staff = 1.5%
  (0.5 x 0.3 x 0.1 x 100)

- Health care worker = 1.75%
  (0.5 x 0.35 x 0.1 x 100)

Sources: Boley, T.J., & Popek, E.J. (1993). Parvovirus infection in pregnancy. *Seminars in Perinatology, 17*(6), 411; Centers for Disease Control (CDC). (1989). Current trends: Risks associated with human parvovirus B19 infection. *Morbidity and Mortality Weekly Report, 38*(6), 83, 85. Atlanta, GA.

References

Anderson, L.J. (1987). Role of parvovirus B19 in human disease. *Pediatric Infectious Diseases, 6*, 711-718.

Bell, L.M., Naides, S.J., Stoffman, P., Hodinka, R.L., & Plotkin, S.A. (1989). Human parvovirus B19 infection among hospital staff members after contact with infected patients. *New England Journal of Medicine, 321*, 485.

Bernstein, I.M., & Capeless, E.M. (1989). Elevated maternal serum alpha feto-protein and hydrops fetalis in association with fetal parvovirus B19 infection. *Obstetrics & Gynecology, 74*(3, II), 456-457.

Boley, T.J., & Popek, E.J. (1993). Parvovirus infection in pregnancy. *Seminars in Perinatology, 17*(6), 410-419.

Brown, K.E. (1989). What threat is human parvovirus to the fetus? A review. *British Journal of Obstetrics and Gynaecology, 96*(7), 764-767.

Carrington, D., Gilmore, D.H., Whittle, M.J., Aitken, D., Gibson, A.A. M., Patrick, W.J.A., Brown, T., Caul, E.D., Field, A.M., Clewley, J.P., & Cohen, B.J. (1987). Maternal serum alpha-fetoprotein: A marker for fetal aplastic crisis during intrauterine human parvovirus infection. *Lancet, 1*, 433-435.

Cartter, M.L., Farley, T.A., Rosengren, S., Quinn, D.L., Gillespie, S.M., Gary, G.W., & Hadler, J.L. (1991). Occupational risk factors for infection with parvovirus B19 among pregnant women. *The Journal of Infectious Diseases, 163*, 282-285.

Centers for Disease Control and Prevention (CDC). (1989). Current trends: Risks associated with human parvovirus B19 infection. *Morbidity and Mortality Weekly Report, 38*(6), 81-88, 93-97.

Chorba, T., Coccia, P., Holman, R.C., Tattersal, P., Anderson, L.J., Sudman, J., Young, N.S., Kurczynski, E., Saarinen, U.M., Moir, R., Laurence, D.N., Jason, J.M., & Evatt, B. (1986). The role of parvovirus B19 in aplastic crisis and erythema infectiosum (fifth disease). *Journal of Infectious Diseases, 154*, 74-79.

Conry, J.A., Török, T.J., & Andrews, I. (1993). Perinatal encephalopathy secondary to in utero human parvovirus B19 infection. *Neurology, 43*, A346.

Gibbs, R.S., & Sweet, R.L. (1994). Clinical disorders. In R.K. Creasy & R. Resnik (Eds.), *Maternal-fetal medicine: Principles and practice* (3rd ed., pp. 671-673). Philadelphia, PA: W.B. Saunders.

Gillespie, S.M., Cartter, M.L., Asch, S., Rokos, J.B., Gary, W., Tsou, C.J., Hall, D.B., Anderson, L.J., & Hurwitz, E.S. (1990). Occupational risk of human parvovirus B19 infection for school and day-care personnel during an outbreak of erythema infectiosum. *Journal of the American Medical Association, 263*, 2061-2065.

Guerina, N.G. (1994). Management strategies for infectious diseases in pregnancy. *Seminars in Perinatology, 18(4)*, 305-320.

Hall, C.J. (1994). Parvovirus B19 infection in pregnancy. *Archives of Diseases in Children, 71*(1 Spec. No.), F4-F5.

Hartwig, N.G., Vermeij-Keers, C., van Elsacker-Niele, A.M. W., & Fleuren, G.J. (1989). Embryonic malformations in a case of intrauterine parvovirus B19 infection. *Teratology, 39*, 295-302.

Katz, W.L., McCoy, M.C., Kuller, J.A., & Hansen, W.F. (1996). An association between fetal parovirus B19 infection and fetal anomalies: A report of two cases. *American Journal of Perinatology, 13*, 45–45.

Keyserling, H.L. (1997). Other viral agents or perinatal importance. Varicella, parovirus respiratory syncytial virus, and enterovirus. *Clinics in Perinatology, 24*(1), 193–211.

Kinney, J.S., & Kumar, M.L. (1988). Should we expand the TORCH concept? *Clinics in Perinatology, 15*(4), 727-745.

Maeda, H., Shimokawa, H., Satoh, S., Nakano, H., & Nunove, T. (1988). Nonimmune hydrops fetalis resulting from intrauterine parvovirus B19 infection: Report of two cases. *Obstetrics & Gynecology, 73*(3,II), 482-485.

Mead, M. (1989). Parvovirus B19 infection and pregnancy. *Contemporary Ob/Gyn, 34*(3), 56-69.

Morey, A.L., Keeling, J.W., Porter, H.J., & Fleming, K.A. (1992). Clinical and histopathologic features of parvovirus B19 infection in the human fetus. *British Journal of Obstetrics and Gynecology, 99*(7), 566-574.

The Permanente Medical Group Perinatal Group Recommendations. (1994). Perinatologists of the Northern California Region. *Parvovirus: A proposal for obstetrical management*. Internal document.

Plummer, F.A., Hammond, G.W., Forward, K., Sekla, L., Thompson, L.M., Jones, S.E., Kidd, I.M., & Anderson, M.J. (1985). An erythema infectiosum-like illness caused by human parvovirus infection. *New England Journal of Medicine, 313*, 74-79.

Public Health Laboratory Service Working Party on Fifth Disease. (1990). Prospective study of human parvovirus (B19) infection in pregnancy. *British Medical Journal, 300*, 1166-1170.

Rodis, J.F., Quinn, D.L., Gary, W. Jr., Anderson, L.J., Rosengren, S., Cartter, M.L., Campbell, W.A., & Vintzileos, A.M. (1990). Management and outcomes of pregnancies complicated by human B19 parvovirus infection: A prospective study. *American Journal of Obstetrics and Gynecology, 163*(No. 4, Pt. 1), 1168-1171.

Sahakian, V., Weiner, C.P., Naides, S.J., Williamson, R.A., & Scharosch, L.L. (1991). Intrauterine transfusion treatment of nonimmune hydrops fetalis secondary to human parvovirus B19 infection. *American Journal of Obstetrics and Gynecology, 164*(4), 1090-1091.

Török, T.J. (1995). Human parvovirus B19. In J.S. Remington & J.O Klein (Eds.), *Infectious diseases of the fetus and newborn infant* (4th ed., pp. 668-702). Philadelphia, PA: W.B. Saunders.

Chapter 8

RUBELLA

Winifred L. Star

Rubella infection (also known as German or 3-day measles) is a moderately communicable exanthemous disease caused by the togavirus, transmitted via direct or droplet contact with infective nasopharyngeal secretions. The infection is most common among children 5 to 9 years of age, with its peak occurrence in late winter or early spring. The incubation period is from 14 to 21 days (average 16 to 18 days). Maximal transmissibility is from a few days prior to the rash to 5 to 7 days afterward. By reproductive age, 75 to 85 percent of the population has had rubella; post-infection immunity is usually lifelong, even in subclinical cases (American Academy of Pediatrics [AAP], 1997; Gibbs & Sweet, 1994; Hashmey & Shandera, 1996). Central nervous system (CNS) complications (1/6,000 cases) and thrombocytopenia (1/3,000 cases) can occur following acute infection; the former is more likely in adults (Advisory Committee on Immunization Practices [ACIP], 1990).

The principal significance of rubella is the effect it may have on a fetus. Infection during pregnancy is associated with spontaneous abortion, stillbirth, and congenital rubella infection of the neonate. Congenital rubella syndrome (CRS) is a constellation of anomalies:

- Auditory (sensorineural deafness)

- Ophthalmic (glaucoma, cataracts, microphthalmia, chorioretinitis)

- Cardiac (atrial or ventricular septal defects, patent ductus arteriosus, pulmonary artery stenosis)

- Neurologic (mental retardation, microcephaly, meningoencephalitis)

In addition, other complications such as intrauterine growth restriction, radiolucent bone disease, hepatosplenomegaly, thrombocytopenia, jaundice, and purpura can occur (ACIP, 1990; American Academy of Pediatrics [AAP], 1997; Shannon, 1995). Defects not noticeable at birth may develop later from continued viral replication (e.g., hearing loss, ocular damage, CNS disease, and endocrinopathies) (Cooper, Preblud, & Alford, 1995; Zeichner & Plotkin, 1988).

Incidence rates of CRS in the United States are 0.7 to 1/100,000 live births (Grangeot-Keros, 1992). The risk varies according to gestational age at the time of maternal infection. Miller et al. (1982) reported a 90 percent risk of fetal defects when infection occurs before 11 weeks of gestation, 33 percent for infection between 11 and 12 weeks, 11 percent between 13 to 14 weeks, 24 percent between 15 to 16 weeks, and 0 percent after 16 weeks (Miller, Cradock-Watson, & Pollock, 1982).

Rubella Reinfection

Although rare, rubella reinfection has been seen both in individuals with a history of naturally occurring infection and in vaccinated persons (Bakshi & Cooper, 1990). Reinfection is most likely in vaccinees whose antibody titers have declined to low levels (O'Shea, Best, & Banatvala, 1983). Fetal risk from maternal reinfection is substantially lower than that following primary infection; however, there are growing numbers of documented cases of congenital infection after maternal reinfection—exact incidence is unknown (most infections are subclinical) and precise degree of fetal risk is still obscure (probably less than 5 percent) (Chen & Chu, 1993; Miller, 1990). There are no features that distinguish congenital disease secondary to reinfection from that of primary infection. CRS has not been reported after reinfection beyond 12 weeks' gestation (Robinson, Lemay, & Vaudry, 1994; Schoub, Blackburn, O'Connell, Kaplan, & Adno, 1990).

Rubella vaccine

The vaccine currently available in the United States, RA 27/3, is a live rubella virus vaccine. It is available in monovalent (rubella only) or in polyvalent (in combination with measles vaccine [MR] or with measles and mumps vaccines [MMR]) forms.

Vaccination produces seroconversion in more than 90 percent of recipients. Vaccine-induced protection is long term, probably lifelong (although vaccine-induced titers may be lower than those stimulated by natural rubella infection). In the United States, widespread use of the vaccine has resulted in dramatic declines in rates of infection as well as the number of infants born with CRS. Between 1988 and 1990, however, a moderate resurgence of rubella occurred, mostly among persons 15 years of age or older. Efforts to increase delivery of the vaccine to young adults have led to the current decline in incidence rates. Surveys indicate, however, that 6 to 11 percent of postpubertal females remain seronegative (ACIP, 1990; Centers for Disease Control and Prevention [CDC] 1993; CDC, 1997).

Risk to the fetus from live virus rubella vaccine appears to be small. Data collected by the CDC since 1979 reveal no evidence that the vaccine causes CRS (CDC, 1989). The maximal theoretical risk for congenital rubella from the vaccine is estimated to be 1.6 percent (AAP, 1997). Due to concern about fetal risk, however, women of childbearing age should receive vaccine only if nonpregnant and should be counseled to avoid pregnancy for 3 months after vaccination (ACIP, 1990). If vaccination occurs within 3 months before or after conception, the risk of CRS is so small as to be negligible; thus, inadvertent vaccination of a pregnant woman should not be a reason in itself to consider termination of pregnancy (AAP, 1997; ACIP, 1990; CDC, 1993).

Database

Subjective

- Client may report exposure to individual with rubella. Specific history should include
  - ▶ Date of contact
  - ▶ Specific symptoms and date of onset
  - ▶ Previous immunization
  - ▶ Date/results of previous antibody testing (Grangeot-Keros, 1992).
- Features of symptomatic disease include
  - ▶ Mild prodrome
    - – Malaise
    - – Low-grade fever
    - – Headache
    - – Anorexia
    - – Mild eye irritation

- Sore throat

- Cough

- Coryza

▶ Enlarged lymph nodes 5 to 10 days *prior* to rash

▶ Fine rash beginning on face, spreading to trunk and extremities, fading quickly; rash may be pruritic

▶ Transient polyarthralgia/polyarthritis (25 percent of adult cases) (Hashmey & Shandera, 1996)

NOTE: Twenty-five to 50 percent of cases may be subclinical.

Objective

● Physical examination may reveal

  ▶ Vital signs

    - Temperature slightly elevated or within normal limits

  ▶ HEENT examination

    - Posterior cervical, postauricular, and suboccipital lymphadenopathy

    - Patchy erythema of throat and palate

    - Reddened conjunctiva

  ▶ Skin examination

    - Fine, pink, maculopapular rash spreading from face, to trunk, to extremities in rapid progression (2- to 3-day period); absence of rash also common

  ▶ Extremities

    - Tender, erythematous joints

● For a CRS infant, observe fetal anomalies as described in the introduction. Clinical features of congenital rubella may be transient, permanent, or of late-onset.

● Individuals can be considered immune to rubella only if they have documentation of:

  ▶ Laboratory evidence of rubella immunity

OR

  ▶ Adequate immunization with at least one dose of rubella vaccine on or after the first birthday (ACIP, 1990).

Assessment

● Maternal exposure to rubella

  ▶ R/O rubella infection

  ▶ R/O complications of rubella infection

▶ R/O measles

▶ R/O enteroviral infection

▶ R/O adenoviral infection

▶ R/O cytomegaloviral infection

▶ R/O Epstein-Barr viral infection

▶ R/O parvoviral infection

▶ R/O roseola

▶ R/O scarlet fever

▶ R/O drug reaction

▶ R/O mycoplasma infection

▶ R/O congenital rubella infection

Plan

Diagnostic Tests

- See Figures 10.8.1 and 10.8.2

- All pregnant clients should be screened for rubella immunity as soon as possible in pregnancy. Ideally, rubella testing is done prior to conception so that nonimmune individuals may be vaccinated (see Follow-up section).

- Diagnosis of acute rubella infection based on clinical evidence alone is unreliable; serologic confirmation is essential and should include testing for both IgG and IgM antibody.

  ▶ If tests for IgM are negative or unavailable, perform testing for IgG antibody. Fourfold or greater rise in rubella IgG antibody levels from acute and convalescent sera is indicative of infection. An acute-phase specimen should be drawn as soon as possible after rash onset (ideally within 7 days) and a convalescent sample 10 to 14 days later. Specimens should be tested in parallel.

  NOTE: High IgG antibody levels may be present in up to 15 percent of the population and do not by themselves indicate acute infection; thus single specimens for IgG are not helpful. (AGOG, 1992).

  ▶ Presence of rubella IgM antibody indicates acute infection; detected from early onset of illness, reaches peak in 7 to 10 days, persists up to 4 weeks after appearance of rash (ACOG, 1992).

  NOTE: False positives may occur if the sera contains rheumatoid antibody. A negative test does not definitively prove lack of infection because of the potential for a false-negative result due to early waning of antibody (ACOG, 1992).

- In a vaccinated pregnant woman, diagnosis of rubella infection may be difficult

  ▶ Rises in IgG may occur after recent exposure, but in the absence of IgM, probably indicate a "boosting" of antibody due to reinfection rather than a primary response to infection (ACOG, 1992).

  ▶ IgM responses are low or absent in reinfection (Miller, 1990).

- IgG avidity may distinguish primary infection from reinfection (low avidity indices are seen in primary infection) (Grangeot-Keros, 1992; Hedman & Rousseau, 1989).

  ▶ Detection of maternal IgA antibodies may be sought in some cases.

- If more than 5 weeks have elapsed since exposure to rash illness or more than 4 weeks after rash onset in client whose immune status is unknown, diagnosis is difficult. Interpretation may be as follows:

  ▶ Lack of IgG means there is no evidence of recent infection, but the client is susceptible to infection.

  ▶ Presence of IgG means there is evidence of previous infection, but the date of onset and the risk to fetus is difficult to determine.

    – Low-level antibody indicates a more remote infection. Consider repeating IgG levels to evaluate rise or decline, or test for rubella IgM (ACOG, 1992).

- Diagnosis of fetal infection has been attempted via amniocentesis for viral isolation of amniotic fluid by culture or polymerase chain reaction (PCR) for viral DNA, percutaneous umbilical blood sampling (PUBS) for rubella-specific IgM, or chorionic villus biopsy for isolation of virus, antigen, or viral DNA. These techniques have serious limitations and may not reliably distinguish an infected fetus.

- Neonatal infection may be diagnosed by

  ▶ Rubella-specific IgM antibody in cord blood or infant's blood (rarely persists after 6 months of age)

  ▶ Rise in rubella-specific IgG titers

  ▶ Persistence of rubella-specific IgG for more than 8 to 12 months (in absence of rubella vaccine or postnatal exposure)

  ▶ Isolation of rubella virus from nasopharynx, conjunctiva, blood, urine or cerebrospinal fluid (CSF) of affected infant (virus may be excreted for months—years, average 6 months) (Forsgren, Sterner, Grandien, Enocksson, & Barr, 1990).

- Additional laboratory tests

  ▶ Complete blood count may reveal leukopenia or thrombocytopenia in acute maternal infection.

  ▶ Viral culture isolated from maternal blood and throat 7 to 10 days after exposure (viral shedding from throat continues for 1 week).

Treatment/Management

- Nonimmune pregnant women with exposure to rubella or a rubella-like illness should be evaluated serologically for evidence of infection (ACOG, 1992). See the Diagnostic Tests section.

- When maternal infection has been diagnosed, the client can be referred to a physician for further management.

- Immune globulin (IG) is generally not recommended for postexposure prophylaxis. IG may be considered if rubella exposure has occurred early in gestation and pregnancy termination is not be an option.

  ▶ A dose of 0.55 mL/kg may prevent/modify infection (AAP, 1997).

▶ Live-virus rubella vaccine is contraindicated in pregnancy, and it does not prevent illness in susceptible persons after exposure. It may be given to a nonpregnant, exposed person, however, because if exposure does not result in infection, immunization will provide future protection (AAP, 1997).

● Suggest analgesics and antipyretics (e.g., acetaminophen), as needed, for symptom relief in acute infection. Patient should be isolated from susceptible individuals until 1 week after rash eruption (Shannon, 1995).

● Use laboratory analyses and historical and clinical indices to determine maternal risk and guide counseling regarding possible risks to the fetus. If maternal infection is diagnosed, attempts at fetal diagnosis may be undertaken. Discussion regarding fetal risks and fetal diagnosis is generally undertaken by the physician in charge of the client's care. See the Diagnostic Tests section.

● Elective pregnancy termination is an option when maternal infection occurs in the first trimester.

▶ Termination is generally not recommended after midgestation infection or in cases of maternal reinfection given the apparent low risk of fetal sequelae (Ghidini & Lynch, 1994; Robinson et al., 1994).

▶ Discussion regarding termination is generally undertaken by the physician in charge of the client's care.

Consultation

● Seek physician consultation for nonimmune clients with suspected rubella exposure. Depending on site-specific practice, client may be managed by an obstetrician or perinatologist after maternal infection is diagnosed.

● In complicated cases, consultation with an infectious disease expert may be warranted and may be necessary for interpretation of laboratory results.

● Patient may be referred to a genetic counselor for consultation.

Patient Education

● Advise nonimmune women to avoid exposure to school-age children with rash illnesses or known rubella infection. The client should be informed that if nonimmune she will be vaccinated postpartum, usually in the hospital prior to discharge (see the Follow-up section).

● Educate all pregnant women about the nature of rubella infection: communicability, symptom-relief measures, potential fetal risks, diagnostic modalities, and possible complications.

▶ If rubella vaccination is inadvertently given to a pregnant woman or if pregnancy occurs within 3 months of immunization, counsel the woman regarding the theoretical fetal risks.

● Discussion of elective pregnancy termination is appropriate when infection has occurred in the first trimester.

Follow-up

- Nonimmune clients should receive rubella vaccine postpartum prior to hospital discharge. (Women giving birth at home should receive vaccination as soon as possible if nonimmune.)

  ▶ There is no contraindication to vaccinating a susceptible mother during breast-feeding.

  ▶ Patient should be counseled that conception should be avoided for 3 months after vaccine administration.

  NOTE: Side effects of the vaccine may include low-grade fever, rash, and lymphadenopathy; arthralgia and transient arthritis may also occur, and rarely, transient peripheral neuritic problems (ACIP, 1990).

- In cases where Rho(D) immune globulin or another blood product was required postpartum in addition to rubella vaccination (or MMR) for the nonimmune parturient, perform antibody testing at least 8 weeks later to ensure immunity. (Blood and other antibody-containing products can diminish the immune response to vaccines) (AAP, 1997).

- Regarding vaccination

  ▶ In the United States, the combined measles, mumps, and rubella live vaccine (MMR) is recommended for children 12 to 15 months of age, with a second dose at 4 to 6 years of age or 11 to 12 years of age (the second dose may be administered at any visit, however, provided that at least 1 month has elapsed since the first dose and that both doses are administered at or after 12 months of age (American Academy of Pediatrics, Committee on Infectious Diseases, 1997).

  ▶ *All women of reproductive age should be immune to measles, mumps, and rubella.* MMR vaccine is advisable for all susceptible women (provided they are not pregnant or other contraindications exist).

  NOTE: Reasonable precautions prior to administration of MMR in women of childbearing age include the following:

  - Ask women if they are pregnant and exclude vaccination of those that say they are.

  - Explain the theoretical risks of the vaccine to potential vaccines.

  - Advise against pregnancy for 3 months after vaccination (ACIP, 1990).

  ▶ Persons receiving MMR vaccine can shed these viruses but generally do not transmit them; thus, the vaccine can be safely administered to family members and close contacts of pregnant women (ACOG, 1991; ACIP, 1994).

  ▶ Contraindications to MMR vaccine include (but are not limited to)

  - Pregnancy

  - History of anaphylactic reaction to eggs or neomycin

  - Significant immunocompromise (except HIV infection) (AAP, 1997).

  - Refer to vaccine package insert(s) for additional information. See also Chapter 10.5, *Measles;* Chapter 10.6, *Mumps;* Section 1, *Preconception Health Care — An Overview;* and Chapter 4.5, *Travel During Pregnancy.*

  ▶ Breast-feeding is *not* a contraindication to vaccination (CDC, 1993).

- Newborns with possible exposure to rubella during gestation should be carefully examined and followed closely by the pediatric team.

  ▶ Specific diagnostic tests may be utilized in the neonatal period (see the Diagnostic Tests section).

  ▶ Infants with documented CRS require long-term follow-up. These children should be considered infectious for the first year of life (unless nasopharyngeal/urine cultures are repeatedly negative); thus, susceptible pregnant visitors should be advised accordingly (Cooper et al., 1995).

- Suspected cases of rubella and CRS should be reported to the local or state health department.

- "All susceptible health care personnel who may be exposed to patients with rubella should be immunized for the prevention or transmission of rubella to pregnant patients as well as for their own health" (AAP, 1997, p. 459).

- Document maternal/fetal rubella infection in problem list and progress notes. In addition, "rubella nonimmune" status should be noted on the problem list so that postpartum vaccination can be employed.

Figure 10.8.1

Diagnosis of Acute Rubella Infection in Pregnancy

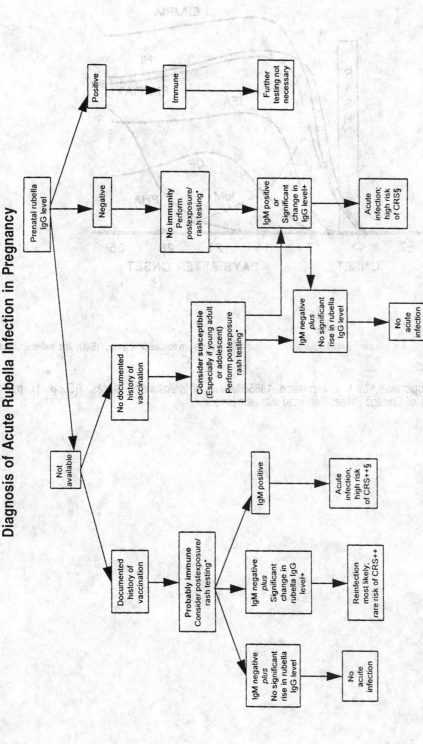

* Should include IgM and IgG testing of acute specimen and paired acute and convalescent sera for IgG levels. Acute specimens should be drawn as soon as possible after rash onset, followed by a convalescent specimen 2-3 weeks later. For exposure to rubella, acute specimens should be drawn immediately, followed by convalescent specimen 4-5 weeks later.
+ Since what constitutes a significant change in IgG level or low IgG level varies by type of assay and laboratory, interpretation of levels by laboratory is needed.
++ Consultation with clinical virologist or other expert in diagnosis of rubella is warranted.
§ If infection occured in first trimester of pregnancy.

Source: "Rubella and Pregnancy," by the American College of Obstetricians and Gynecologists (ACOG), 1992, Technical Bulletin No. 171, p. 4. Copyright 1992 by the ACOG. Reprinted with permission.

Figure 10.8.2

Immune Response in Acute Rubella Infection[1]

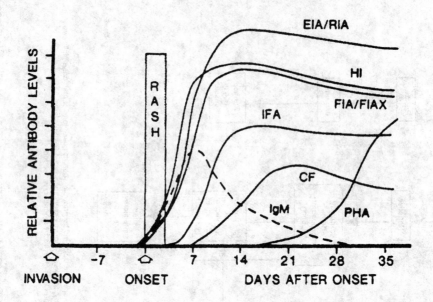

[1]Most commonly used assays for both IgG and IgM include hemagglutination inhibition (HI), enzyme immunosorbent assay (EIA), and indirect fluorescent immunoassay.

Source: "Available rubella serologic tests," by K. L. Herrmann, 1985 *Reviews of Infectious Diseases, 7*(Suppl. 1), p. S109. Copyright 1991 by the University of Chicago Press. Reprinted with permission.

References

Advisory Committee on Immunization Practices (ACIP). (1990). Rubella prevention. Recommendations of the Immunization Practices Advisory Committee (ACIP). *Morbidity and Mortality Weekly Report, 39*(No. RR-15), 1–18.

Advisory Committee on Immunization Practices (ACIP). (1994). General recommendations on immunization. Recommendations of the Advisory Committee on Immunization Practices (ACIP). *Morbidity and Mortality Weekly Report, 43*(RR 1), 1–38.

American Academy of Pediatrics (AAP). (1997). *1997 Red book: Report of the committee of infectious diseases* (24th ed., pp. 456–462). Elk Grove Village, IL: Author.

American College of Obstetricians and Gynecologists (ACOG). (1992). *Rubella and Pregnancy.* (Technical Bulletin No. 171). Washington, DC: ACOG.

Bakshi, S.S., & Cooper, L.Z. (1990). Rubella and mumps vaccine. *Pediatric Clinics of North America, 37*(3), 651–668.

Centers for Disease Control and Prevention (CDC). (1989). Rubella vaccination during pregnancy - United States, 1971–1988. *Morbidity and Mortality Weekly Report, 38*(17), 289–293.

Centers for Disease Control and Prevention (CDC). (1993). Rubella Vaccine. Fax document #243004. Atlanta, GA: Author.

Centers for Disease Control and Prevention (CDC). (1997). *CDC prevention guidelines: A guide to action.* Baltimore, MD: Williams & Wilkins.

Chen, F.P., & Chu, K.K. (1993). Subclinical rubella infection in pregnancy: Report of a case. *Journal Formos Medical Association, 92*(3), 294–295.

Cooper, L.Z., Preblud, S.R., & Alford, C.A. (1995). Rubella. In J.S. Remington & J.O. Klein (Eds.), *Infectious diseases of the fetus and newborn infant* (4th ed., pp. 268–311). Philadelphia, PA: W.B. Saunders.

Forsgren, M., Sterner, G., Grandien, M., Enocksson, E., & Barr, B. (1990). Management of women at term with pregnancy complicated by rubella. *Scandinavian Journal of Infectious Diseases, Suppl. 71,* 49–52.

Freij, B.J., South, M., & Sever, J.L. (1988). Maternal rubella and the congenital rubella syndrome. *Clinics in Perinatology, 15*(2), 247–257.

Gibbs, R.S., & Sweet, R.L. (1994). Clinical disorders. In R.K. Creasy & R. Resnik (Eds.), *Maternal-fetal medicine. Principles and practice* (3rd. ed., pp. 660–661). Philadelphia, PA: W.B. Saunders.

Ghidini, A., & Lynch, L. (1994). Management strategies for congenital infections. *The Mount Sinai Journal of Medicine, 61*(5), 376–388.

Grangeot-Keros, L. (1992). Rubella and pregnancy. *Pathologie Biologie, 40*(7), 706–710.

Hashmey, R., & Shandera, W.X. (1996). Infectious diseases: Viral and rickettsial. In L.M. Tierney Jr., S.J. McPhee, & M.A. Papadakis (Eds.), *Current medical diagnosis and treatment* (3rd ed., pp. 1172–1173). Stamford, CT: Appleton & Lange.

Hedman, K., & Rousseau, S.A, (1989). Measurement of avidity of specific IgG for verification of recent primary rubella. *Journal of Medical Virology, 27*, 288–292.

Herrmann, K.L. (1985). Available rubella serologic tests. *Reviews of Infectious Diseases, 7*(Suppl. 1), S108–S112.

Miller, E. (1990). Rubella infection. *Archives of Diseases in Children, 65*(8), 820–821.

Miller, E., Cradock-Watson, J.E., & Pollock, T.M. (1982). Consequences of confirmed maternal rubella at successive stages of pregnancy. *Lancet, 2*, 781–784.

O'Shea, S., Best, J.M., & Banatvala, J.E. (1983). Viraemia, virus excretion, and antibody responses after challenge in volunteers with low levels of antibody to rubella virus. *Journal of Infectious Diseases, 148*, 639–647.

Robinson, J., Lemay, M., & Vaudry, W.L. (1994). Congenital rubella after anticipated maternal immunity: two cases and a review of the literature. *Pediatric Infectious Disease Journal, 13*, 812–815.

Schoub, B.D., Blackburn, N.K., O'Connell, K., Kaplan, A.B., & Adno, J. (1990). Symptomatic rubella re-infection in early pregnancy and subsequent delivery of an infected but minimally involved infant. A case report. *South Africa Medical Journal, 78*, 484–485.

Shannon, M.T., (1995). Rubella. In W.L. Star, L.L. Lommel, & M.T. Shannon (Eds.), *Women's primary health care: Protocols for practice* (pp. 11–11, 11–57.) Washington, DC: American Nurses Publishing.

Zeichner, S.L., & Plotkin, S.A. (1988). Mechanisms and pathways of congenital infections. *Clinics in Perinatology, 15*(2), 163–189.

Chapter 9

TOXOPLASMOSIS

Winifred L. Star

Toxoplasma gondii is one of the most widespread protozoan parasites existing in nature; it is found in all orders of mammals and some birds. The life cycle of toxoplasma occurs in three phases: trophozoite or tachyzoite (invasive form), tissue cyst (latent form), and oocyst (found only in intestinal tract of cats and excreted in their feces). The definitive host is the cat. Cats acquire toxoplasmosis by eating food that contains viable tissue cysts, such as infected rodents or small birds or raw or inadequately cooked meat. Humans generally become infected by consuming cysts in raw or under-cooked meat of an infected animal, via contact with oocyst-contaminated water or food, or from exposure to the feces of an infected cat. Transmission of infection can also occur by transfusion with infected blood or blood products, organ transplants from seropositive donors to seronegative recipients, or transplacentally from mother to fetus (Remington, McLeod, & Desmonts, 1995). The incubation period for acquired infection is about 7 days (range 4 to 21 days). Person-to-person transmission does not occur.

Following infection by cysts or oocysts, an acute parasitemia occurs; the organism then invades the tissues of multiple organs and may remain viable for the life of the host. A healthy individual may control spread of the organism through humoral and cell-mediated immunity; however the immuno-compromised host may suffer from progressive or reactivated disease (Gibbs & Sweet, 1994; Guerina, 1994). Encephalitis, hepatitis, pneumonia, and myocarditis are common complications in the immunosuppressed (Buxton, 1990; Freij & Sever, 1996).

Seroprevalence of antitoxoplasmal antibodies among women of childbearing age as well as the incidence of infection during pregnancy varies with geographic location. Data from various United States locations indicate that 3 to 30 percent of women have serologic evidence of past infection (Freij & Sever, 1996). The incidence of acute infection during pregnancy is estimated to be 0.2 to 1 percent; congenital toxoplasmosis incidence has been estimated in the range of 1/1,000 to 1/10,000 live births (American Academy of Pediatrics [AAP], 1997; Wong & Remington, 1994).

Acute primary toxoplasmosis in pregnancy is associated with abortion, prematurity, intrauterine growth restriction, and congenital infection of the fetus (Gibbs & Sweet, 1994). It appears that successful transmission of infection from mother to fetus is dependent upon three factors: maternal parasitemia (initial or recurrent), maturity of the placenta (volume/flow of blood in the organ), and stage/competency of maternal immune response to *T. gondii* (either complete, deficient, absent) (Remington et al., 1995).

The incidence of congenital infection will depend upon the trimester in which maternal infection has occurred. The rate of fetal infection seems to be higher in the third trimester than in the first trimester (65 percent versus 17 percent); however, the severity of fetal infection is greater if maternal disease occurs in the first trimester. One-third of affected fetuses have clinically detectable illness; two-thirds have subclinical disease (i.e., serologic or cerebrospinal fluid abnormalities only) but may suffer from late sequelae, including chorioretinitis, developmental delay, and hearing loss (Freij & Sever, 1996; Gibbs & Sweet, 1994; Matsui, 1994). In affected infants, a wide spectrum of disease exists ranging from isolated abnormalities to multiple organ system involvement (Freij & Sever, 1996). Few infants with clinical disease demonstrate the classic triad of intracerebral calcifications, chorioretinitis, and hydrocephaly. More commonly, findings include chorioretinitis, abnormal spinal fluid, anemia, splenomegaly, jaundice, fever, lymphadenopathy, seizures, or vomiting (Gibbs & Sweet, 1994). Approximately 10 percent of congenitally infected infants have severe disease at birth and 10 percent of these will die; most surviving infants have major sequelae, including mental retardation, spasticity, seizures, or visual defects (Freij & Sever, 1996). With specific chemotherapy the risk of congenital infection can be significantly reduced (Bakht & Gentry, 1992). In addition, when treatment extends postnatally, the prognosis for infants is improved (Freij & Sever, 1996).

Chronic (or latent) maternal infection is not a risk for congenital infection in an otherwise healthy immunocompetent woman. The immunocompromised patient with prior infection may be capable of transmission of *T. gondii* to the fetus if she has been unable to contain or suppress chronic toxoplasma (Remington et al., 1995; Wong & Remington, 1994).

Database

Subjective

- Disease is usually subclinical.

- Clinically apparent disease may resemble the "flu" or mononucleosis and is usually mild and self-limiting. Symptoms may include

  ▶ Fever, chills

  ▶ Fatigue, malaise, myalgia

  ▶ Headache

  ▶ Sore throat

  ▶ Tender or nontender lymphadenopathy (may persist/recur for 6 months or more)

  ▶ Maculopapular rash

  ▶ Ocular symptoms (more rare), including "hazy" vision, eye pain, photophobia

- Symptom onset is generally 1 to 2 weeks after infection, subsiding over 2 weeks to several months.

Objective

- Vital signs may demonstrate an elevated temperature.

- Skin examination may reveal maculopapular rash.

- Lymph node examination may reveal diffuse lymphadenopathy (Wong & Remington, 1994).

  ▶ Nodes most commonly involved are in the posterior cervical, suboccipital, supraclavicular, axillary, and/or inguinal regions (mesenteric and mediastinal nodes may also be involved).

  ▶ Nodes are usually discrete, of variable firmness, nontender and nonsuppurative.

  ▶ Single or multiple nodes may be involved.

- Abdominal examination may reveal hepatosplenomegaly.

- Ophthalmologic examination may disclose clusters of yellow-white patches in optic fundus (Gibbs & Sweet, 1994).

- Clinical findings of congenitally infected infants are described in the introductory section.

Assessment

- Toxoplasmosis

  ► R/O mononucleosis

  ► R/O cytomegalovirus infection

  ► R/O cat-scratch disease

  ► R/O tuberculosis

  ► R/O tularemia

  ► R/O oncologic conditions such as lymphoma, leukemia

  ► R/O sarcoidosis

  ► R/O immunosuppression (e.g., HIV infection)

  ► R/O congenital toxoplasmosis

  ► R/O other congenital infections including herpes simplex virus infection, rubella and syphilis

Plan

Diagnostic Tests

- See Table 10.7, Serologic Tests for Diagnosis of Toxoplasmosis.

- Routine screening of pregnant women for toxoplasmal antibodies is not indicated (except in the presence of HIV infection) (American Academy of Pediatrics [AAP] & the American College of Obstetricians & Gynecologists [AGOG], 1997). Asymptomatic women who request screening should be thoroughly informed regarding the implications of the tests. Cat ownership is not an indication for screening (Alger, 1997).

  NOTE: Women who have been tested prior to pregnancy and demonstrate seroreactivity are immune from clinically significant reinfection during pregnancy (ACOG, 1993).

- Use serologic techniques to confirm the diagnosis of maternal toxoplasmosis when the history and signs/symptoms are suggestive of disease and serologic testing for mononucleosis is negative or when fetal malformations have been detected by ultrasound (e.g., hydrocephaly, microcephaly, intracranial calcifications, ventricular dilatation) (ACOG, 1993; Sever, 1990).

  ► Interpretation of test results can be difficult; thus, consultation is advised. It is recommended that acute infection be confirmed by a reference laboratory (Alger, 1997).

- Laboratory tests on the mother may include

▶ *Toxoplasma*-specific IgM antibodies

- – Test usually becomes positive within 1 to 2 weeks of infection

- – Antibodies peak in 1 month and persist for a few weeks to many months in acute infection (usually undetectable after 6 to 9 months)

- – High titers suggest acute infection (especially when accompanied by IgG titers >1:512).

- – Low titers are seen in patients infected several months earlier.

- – Negative test rules out recently acquired infection (unless tested too early).

- – IgM may persist in low titer for years in 5 percent of chronic infections (AAP, 1997; Freij & Sever, 1996; Remington et al., 1995; Wong & Remington, 1994).

   NOTE: Tests for specific IgM antibodies should be run by an experienced laboratory; the "test kits" used by some labs may give false-positive and false-negative results.

▶ *Toxoplasma*-specific IgG antibodies

- – Antibodies appear early (often in first week of infection) and peak in 1 to 2 months.

- – Levels gradually decline, but can remain for years–life.

- – High titer (>1:1000) in single sample is suggestive of acute infection.

- – Titer absence indicates susceptibility to infection.

   * Seronegative women should have titers repeated in 2 to 4 weeks if index of suspicion is high for infection.

   * Acute infection diagnosed by seroconversion or by a fourfold rise in titer from acute and convalescent sera (tested simultaneously). (These clients should also have IgM determinations performed.)

- – IgG may persist for years in high titer in 5 percent of chronic infections (AAP, 1997; Gibbs & Sweet, 1994; Remington et al., 1995).

▶ *Toxoplasma*-specific IgA

- – Antibodies are detected at the end of the first month of infection and are usually gone within 4 to 7 months (but may persist for 6+ months).

- – Antibodies are found in more than 95 percent of patients with acute infection.

- – IgA antibodies are rare in chronic infection (Freij & Sever, 1996).

- – IgA antibody test may need to be performed at reference laboratory.

▶ *Toxoplasma*-specific IgE antibodies

- – IgE antibodies appear around time of IgA and persist for less than 4 months (but may appear up to 8 months) (may not be commercially available).

▶ IgG-avidity testing may discriminate recent from past infection (Aedes, 1991; Lappalainen et al., 1993).

● Additional laboratory tests and their findings may include the following:

▶ Atypical lymphocytosis in peripheral blood smear

▶ Negative heterophile (1 to 5 percent of infectious mononucleosis caused by *T. gondii*)

- Immunosuppressed individuals may require confirmation of infection via direct detection of *T. gondii* or its antigens/DNA in their body fluids or tissue.

- In women with confirmed infection during pregnancy, consider prenatal fetal diagnosis. Fetal diagnosis may include the following modalities:

  ▶ Isolation of *T. gondii* via tissue culture or mouse inoculation of amniotic fluid or fetal blood (which are obtained by amniocentesis or cordocentesis, respectively, under ultrasound guidance after 18 weeks)

  ▶ Polymerase chain reaction (PCR) analysis of amniotic fluid

  ▶ Presence of *Toxoplasma*-specific IgM, IgA, and IgE in fetal blood.

  ▶ Evaluation of nonspecific indicators of infection in fetal blood (e.g., increased white blood cell and high eosinophil counts, low platelet count, elevated total IgM content, elevated hepatic enzymes)

  ▶ Fetal serum *Toxoplasma*-specific IgA and IgE antibodies

  ▶ Serial ultrasound examinations to assess for ventricular dilatation, cerebral/hepatic calcifications, ascites, hydrops, hepatomegaly, increased placental width, and pleural/pericardial effusion (Freij & Sever, 1996; Gibbs & Sweet, 1994; Jacquemard, Hohlfeld, Mirlesse, Forestier, & Daffos, 1995; Pratlong et al., 1994).

  NOTE: Certain aspects of fetal testing may only be available at specialized centers. Use of these diagnostic modalities will be determined by the physician in charge of the client's care.

- Congenital infection is confirmed by the following:

  ▶ Isolation of the organism from the placenta or infant's blood

  ▶ Detection of *Toxoplasma* antigens or DNA in infant's body fluids

  ▶ *Toxoplasma*-specific IgM, IgA or IgE antibodies in infant's serum

  ▶ Persistence of *Toxoplasma*-specific IgG beyond 12 months of age.

Treatment/Management

- Acute infection in adults is self-limited and requires no treatment.

- Therapeutic abortion may be an option when the fetus has been diagnosed with congenital infection and is severely affected.

- Maternal chemotherapy may be provided to reduce incidence/severity of fetal infection. *An obstetrician, perinatologist, or infectious disease expert must determine the drug regimens.*

- If the diagnosis of acute maternal toxoplasmosis is made the following medication should be utilized:

  ▶ Spiramycin: 1 gram p.o. every 8 hours without food, administered from diagnosis to 21 weeks' gestation

    – If the fetus is proved to be unaffected, the drug is given prophylactically at same dose until delivery (Freij & Sever, 1996; Remington et al., 1995).

NOTE: Spiramycin is effective in reducing disease transmission to fetus, but it does not alter fetal pathology if infection occurs. The drug is available only by request from the U.S. Food and Drug Administration (telephone number [301] 827-4573 or [301] 827-4420). Side effects include nausea, vomiting, diarrhea, anorexia; less frequently, vertigo, dizziness, flushing, and feelings of coolness (Wong & Remington, 1994).

- If fetal infection is confirmed after 18 weeks' gestation, additional drugs may include 3-week courses of a combination of

  ▶ Pyrimethamine: loading dose 100 mg p.o. per day in two divided doses for 2 days, then 50 mg per day

  PLUS

  ▶ Sulfadiazine: loading dose 75 mg/kg p.o. per day in two divided doses (maximum 4 grams/day) for 2 days, then 100 mg/kg p.o. per day in two divided doses (maximum 4 grams/day)

  PLUS

  ▶ Leucovorin (folinic acid): 10 to 20 mg p.o. daily (during and for one week after pyrimethamine therapy)

  Alternating with 3 weeks of

  ▶ Spiramycin: 3 grams p.o. per day until delivery (Daffos et al., 1988; Freij & Sever, 1996; Hohlfeld et al., 1989; Remington et al. 1995).

These treatment regimens must be established by the physician in charge of the case.

NOTE: Pyrimethamine is a folic acid antagonist and may cause reversible bone marrow suppression. Clients should be monitored carefully for hematologic toxicity with weekly blood counts, including platelets. Drug should be discontinued if severe anemia, granulocytopenia, or thrombocytopenia develops (may be resumed on resolution of abnormalities). Side effects include bad taste in mouth, headache, and gastrointestinal discomfort. In addition, the drug has been shown to be teratogenic in animals and is contraindicated in the first trimester. Sulfadiazine may cause skin hypersensitivity, GI discomfort, crystalluria, hematuria, and reversible acute renal failure/bone marrow suppression. Folinic acid counters the bone marrow suppressive effects of pyrimethamine and sulfadiazine (Freij & Sever, 1996).

- Serial ultrasound examination of the fetus may be undertaken at regular intervals (every 2 weeks) from the time of diagnosis of maternal infection until the end of pregnancy to assess for signs of fetal infection. See Objective section.

Consultation

- Consultation with a physician is required for all cases. Referral to an obstetrician or perinatologist may be required in some settings. Management in conjunction with an infectious disease expert may be necessary. *It is imperative in all cases that the physician consultant establish the medication regimens for maternal/fetal infection.*

- Immunocompromised women (e.g., those with HIV infection or AIDS) with acute toxoplasmosis infection should be managed by a physician.

- Consultation is advisable for interpretation of laboratory test results.

Patient Education

- Discuss the nature of the infection, means of transmission, primary prevention, implications of the disease for the fetus, and the diagnostic and treatment modalities available.

  ▶ Client education is generally carried out by the physician responsible for her care.

  ▶ See Table 10.8, Prevention Measures for Toxoplasmosis.

- Discuss adverse effects and side effects of drugs used for fetal therapy. See Treatment/ Management section; refer to *Physicians' Desk Reference* and drug package inserts for further information.

- Preconception counseling should include recommendations that a recently infected woman postpone pregnancy for at least 3 months; congenital infection, though rare, has been documented in women who have acquired the infection more than 1 month before conception (Alger, 1997; Wong & Remington, 1994).

Follow-up

- If screening has been performed early in gestation, conduct further evaluation on women found to be seropositive to exclude recent toxoplasma infection.

  ▶ Seronegative women should follow guidelines to prevent infection (see Table 10.8)

    – Retesting may be done at 20 to 22 weeks and at term. This will allow for appropriate antenatal and neonatal management decisions to be made (Bakht & Gentry, 1992; Freij & Sever, 1996).

- High-risk cases should be referred to a pediatrician prior to delivery to discuss management of the congenitally infected infant.

- Refer women/couples to psychological and/or social services, if appropriate, to assist with preparations for an affected child.

- Infants (both symptomatic and asymptomatic) with congenital toxoplasmosis are generally treated with combinations of pyrimethamine, sulfadiazine, spiramycin, and folinic acid for 1 year; corticosteroids may be added in certain cases. Treatment is individualized and baby should be followed closely by a pediatric infectious disease specialist. Details on infant drug regimens are beyond the scope of this chapter.

- Document diagnosis of maternal/fetal toxoplasma infection in the problem list and progress notes.

Table 10. 7

Serologic Tests for Diagnosis of Toxoplasmosis

Test Method	Comments
Sabin-Feldman Dye Test	Requires live parasites; cumbersome; rarely used by laboratories; usually positive within 1-2 weeks of infection; peaks by 2 months, then declines but remains positive for several years; acute infections associated with high titers, chronic infections with low titers; does not differentiate between IgG and IgM antibodies.
Indirect fluorescent antibody test	IFA used to detect Toxoplasma-specific IgG or IgM; less sensitive than enzyme immunoassays; IgM-IFA usually positive for up to 4 months after infection; IgG-IFA may persist at low levels for life; false-positive IgM-IFA may be seen in sera with antinuclear antibodies (ANA) or rheumatoid factor (RF); false-negative IgM-IFA may be due to inhibitory effect of high IgG titers in acute infection.
Enzyme-linked immunosorbent assays (ELISA)	
IgG ELISA	Absence usually indicates susceptibility.
IgM ELISA	More sensitive than IgM-IFA; possible false-positive results in sera with RF or ANA; specific IgM detectable for months-years (especially if double-sandwich IgM assay (DS-IgM-ELISA) used; about 25 percent of congenitally infected infants negative by this assay.
IgA ELISA	Useful in diagnosis of acute or congenital toxoplasmosis; antibody appearance/disappearance similar to IgM; +/- more sensitive than IgM ELISA.
IgE ELISA	Useful in diagnosis of acute or reactivated toxoplasmosis; not available commercially.
Differential agglutination test	Research tool used in adults only; helpful in discerning recent from old infection in women with both IgG and IgM.
Immunosorbent agglutination test	ISAGA used to detect Toxoplasma-specific IgM, IgA, and IgE; very sensitive; can remain positive for several months to several years.
Indirect hemagglutination test	Not useful for diagnosing infection during pregnancy; titers take several weeks before becoming positive; frequently negative in congenital infection.
Other tests	Enzyme-linked immunofiltration assays, avidity ELISA, Western blots (research tools presently).

Table 10.8

Prevention Measures for Toxoplasmosis

- A pregnant woman should avoid close contact with cats during pregnancy. Handwashing is necessary after handling cats, especially before eating. Pet owner may consider having cat tested for toxoplasmosis.

- Ideally, cats should be kept indoors. Stray/feral cats should not be allowed in the house. Kennels should be avoided to prevent contact with other cats that may be infected.

- Cats should not be fed raw meat, rather, only cooked meat or commercially prepared dried or canned food.

- Contact with cat feces should be avoided. Disposable gloves should be worn when handling cat litter boxes and while gardening. Keep hands away from the face during these activities and wash them thoroughly afterwards. Do not flush cat feces down the toilet – if available use domestic refuse bins.

- Cat litter boxes should be emptied of feces daily. Boxes may be disinfected by adding boiling water to the empty box for 5 minutes; alternately a 7 percent ammonia solution may be added to the empty box and left in place for 3 hours. Ideally, someone other than the pregnant woman should attend to the litter box.

- Children's sandboxes should be covered when not in use; if the sand becomes contaminated with cat feces, discard it. Sand and soil should not be ingested. Uncovered public sandpits should be avoided.

- Undercooked or raw meat should not be eaten (assume that all sheep, pig, and goat meat may be infected; beef, venison, and poultry are lesser risk). Meat should be cooked at >66° C (150° F), smoked, or cured in brine before eating; storage at proper temperatures is also important. Freezing meat at -20° C for >24 to 48 hours kills toxoplasma tissue cysts.

- After handling raw meat hands should not come into contact with the eyes or mouth and should be washed thoroughly.

- Utensils used for preparation of raw meat should be cleaned as soon as possible after use. Kitchen surfaces and cutting boards should also be cleaned promptly after food preparation. Ideally, separate surfaces and utensils for preparing raw and cooked foods should be used.

- Fruits and vegetables should be washed thoroughly (or peeled) prior to eating. Unpasteurized milk (especially goat's milk) and raw eggs should be avoided.

- Flies and cockroaches should be prevented from coming into contact with meats, fruits and vegetables (they are capable of carrying infected oocysts).

- Pregnant women should not help with the lambing of ewes or care of newborn lambs. Also, farrowing sows and kidding goats is risky.

Sources: Ausman, L.F. (1993, April). Toxoplasmosis and pregnancy. *The Canadian Nurse*, 31–32; Bakht, F.R., & Gentry, L.O. (1992). Toxoplasmosis in pregnancy: An emerging concern for family physicians. *American Family Physician* 45(4), 1683–1690; Buxton, D. (1990). Toxoplasmosis. *The Practitioner, 234*, 42–44.

References

Aedes, A.E. (1991). Evaluating the sensitivity and predictive value of tests of recent infection: toxoplasmosis in pregnancy. *Epidemiological Infection, 107*, 527–535.

Alger, I.S. (1997). Toxoplasmosis and parvovirus. *Infectious Disease Clinics of North America, 11*(1), 55–75.

American Academy of Pediatrics (AAP). (1997). *1997 Red Book*. Report of the Committee of Infectious Diseases (24th ed., pp. 530–535). Elk Grove Village, IL: Author.

American Academy of Pediatrics (AAP) and the American College of Obstetricians & Gynecologists (ACOG). (1997). Guidelines for perinatal care (4th ed. pp. 247–249). Elk Grove Village, IL: Author.

American College of Obstetricians and Gynecologists (ACOG). (1993). Perinatal viral and parasitic infections. (Technical Bulletin. No. 177). Washington, DC: Author.

Ausman, L.F. (1993, April). Toxoplasmosis and pregnancy. *The Canadian Nurse*, 31–32.

Bakht, F.R., & Gentry, L.O. (1992). Toxoplasmosis in pregnancy: An emerging concern for family physicians. *American Family Physician, 45*(4), 1683–1690.

Buxton, D. (1990). Toxoplasmosis. *Practitioner, 234*(1481), 42–44.

Daffos, F., Forestier, F., Capella-Pavlovsky, M., Thulliez, P., Aufrant, C., Valenti, D., & Cox, W. L. (1988). Prenatal management of 746 pregnancies at risk for congenital toxoplasmosis. *The New England Journal of Medicine, 318*(5), 271–275.

Freij, B.J., & Sever, J.L. (1996). What do we know about toxoplasmosis? *Contemporary OB/GYN, 41(2)*, 41–69.

Gibbs, R.S., & Sweet, R.L. (1994). Clinical disorders. In R.K. Creasy & R. Resnik (Eds.), *Maternal-fetal medicine* (3rd ed., pp. 690–691). Philadelphia, PA: W.B. Saunders.

Guerina, N. G. (1994). Congenital infection with *Toxoplasma gondii*. *Pediatric Annals, 23*(3), 138–151.

Guerina, N.G., Hsu, H.W., Meissner, H.C., Maguire, J.H., Lynfield, R., Stechenberg, B., Abroms, I., Pasternak, M.S., Hoff, R., Eaton, R.B., Grady, G.F., and New England Regional Toxoplasma Working Group. (1994). Neonatal serologic screening and early treatment for congenital *Toxoplasma gondii* infection. *New England Journal of Medicine, 330*, 1858–1863.

Hohlfeld, P., Daffos, F., Thulliez, P., Aufrant, C., Couvreur, J., MacAlesse, J., Descombey, D., & Forestier, F. (1989). Fetal toxoplasmosis: Outcome of pregnancy and infant follow-up after in utero treatment. *Journal of Pediatrics, 115*, 765–769.

Jacquemard, F., Hohlfeld, P., Mirlesse, V., Forestier, F., & Daffos, F. (1995). Prenatal diagnosis of fetal infections. In J.S Remington & J.O. Klein (Eds.), *Infectious diseases of the fetus and newborn infant* (4th ed., pp. 99–107). Philadelphia: W.B. Saunders.

Krick, J.A., & Remington, J.S. (1978). Toxoplasmosis in the adult – an overview. *New England Journal of Medicine, 298*(50).

Lappalainen, M., Koskela, P., Koskiniemei, M., Ammala, P., Hiilesmaa, V., Teramo, K., Raivio, K.O., Remington, J.S., & Hedman, K. (1993). Toxoplasmosis acquired during pregnancy: Improved diagnosis based on avidity of IgG. *The Journal of Infectious Diseases, 167,* 691–697.

Matsui, D. (1994). Prevention, diagnosis, and treatment of fetal toxoplasmosis. *Clinics in Perinatology, 21*(3), 675–689.

McAuley, J., Boyer, K.M., Patel, D., Mets, M., Swisher, C., Roizen, N., Wolters, C., Stein, L., Stern, M., Schey, W., Remington, J., Meier, P., Johnson, D., Heydeman, P., Holfels, E., Withers, S., Mack, D., Brown, C., Patton, D., & McLeod, R. (1994). Early and longitudinal evaluations of treated infants and children and untreated historical patients with congenital toxoplasmosis: the Chicago collaborative treatment trial. *Clinical Infectious Diseases, 18,* 38–72.

Pratlong, F., Boulot, P., Issert, E., Msika, M., Dupont, F., Bachelard, B., Sarda, P., Viala, J.L., & Jarry, D. (1994). Fetal diagnosis of toxoplasmosis in 190 women infected during pregnancy. *Prenatal Diagnosis, 14,* 191–198.

Remington, J.S., McLeod, R., & Desmonts, G. (1995). Toxoplasmosis. In J.S. Remington & J.O. Klein (Eds.), *Infectious diseases of the fetus and newborn infant* (4th ed., pp. 140–267). Philadelphia, PA: W.B. Saunders.

Sever, J.L. (1990). Toxoplasmosis. *Contemporary Ob/Gyn, 35*(3),13–17.

Sever, J.L., Ellenberg, J.H., Ley, A.C., Madden, D.L., Fuccillo, D.A., Tzan, N.R., & Edmonds, D.M. (1989). Toxoplasmosis: Maternal and pediatric findings in 23,000 pregnancies. *Pediatrics, 82,* 181–192.

Wilson, M., Ware, D.A., & Juranek, D.D. (1990). Serologic aspects of toxoplasmosis. *Journal of the American Veterinary Medical Association, 196*(2), 277–280.

Wong, S.-Y., & Remington, J.S. (1994). Toxoplasmosis in pregnancy. *Clinical Infectious Diseases, 18,* 853–862.

Patient Education Materials

U.S. Department of Health and Human Services, Public Health Service, National Institutes of Health (NIH) (1983). *Toxoplasmosis* (Publication No. 83–308). Bethesda, MD: Author.

Chapter 10

TUBERCULOSIS INFECTION

Maureen T. Shannon

Tuberculosis is an infection that is caused by *M. tuberculosis* bacilli, a member of the *Mycobacterium* genus. The majority of illness observed in humans attributed to *Mycobacterium* species are caused by *M. tuberculosis*, although *Mycobacterium bovis* and *Mycobacterium africanum* may, in rare instances, be responsible for human infections (Sepkowitz, Raffalli, Riley, Kiehn, & Armstrong, 1995).

Worldwide, tuberculosis infection is recognized as a major public health problem. It is estimated that 1.8 billion people have been infected with tuberculosis with 10 million new active cases occurring annually. It is responsible for the death of 3 million people in the world every year. In the United States, the identification and therapeutic management of individuals with *M. tuberculosis* infection resulted in a steady decline in reported cases between the 1920s through the 1970s. However, in the 1980s, a reverse in this trend began, and between 1985 and 1990 there was a 15.8 percent increase in reported cases of tuberculosis. The greatest increase has been documented among foreign-born residents, Asian-Americans, American Hispanics, women, and individuals younger than 25 and older than 44 years of age (Cantwell, Snider, Jr., Cauthen, & Onorato, 1994; Center for Disease Control and Prevention [CDC], 1993; CDC, 1998). This increase has been attributed to a number of factors:

- The increasing number of homeless individuals and individuals living in crowded conditions

- Inadequate screening of foreign-born residents, and

- The human immunodeficiency virus (HIV) epidemic (Cantwell et al., CDC, 1998; 1994; Miller & Miller, Jr., 1996; Sepkowitz et al., 1995).

Currently in the United States there are approximately 10 million to 15 million individuals with latent tuberculosis infection. During 1997, the reported new case rate was 7.4/100,000 persons; a 7 percent decrease in new cases compared to 1996 and a 26 percent decrease compared to 1992 (CDC, 1998). This decrease reflects a substantial decline in tuberculosis in U.S.-born persons. The proportion of new cases reported among foreign-born persons increased by 6 percent during this same period of time, with the case rate for foreign-born persons continuing to be four to five times higher than that reported for U.S.-born persons (CDC, 1998).

M. tuberculosis is a nonmotile, aerobic, nonspore-forming, slow-growing bacteria that is an obligate parasite. Most infections with *M. tuberculosis* result from the inhalation of small (1 to 5 μm) infectious respiratory droplet nuclei, although exposure through the ingestion of contaminated substances (e.g., milk infected with *M. bovis*) or inoculation with infectious secretions or tissue (e.g., health care worker exposures) have been associated with transmission (Sepkowitz et al., 1995). Prolonged exposure to an infectious person or environment is necessary for effective respiratory transmission to occur. In general, 30 percent of individuals exposed to an infectious person (i.e., a person with acid-fast bacilli present on a sputum smear) will become infected with tuberculosis (i.e., have a positive tuberculosis skin test develop) (Sepkowitz et al., 1995). After inhalation of infectious respiratory droplets the organism is transmitted to the terminal airspaces where it will either die or remain viable and multiply. The most common pulmonary sites of infection are the anterior segment of the upper lobes, the middle lobe, lingula, and lower division of the lower lobes. However, dissemination of the organism to extrapulmonary sites can occur, resulting in infection of the kidneys, liver, spleen, bones, bone marrow, brain, ovaries, and the endometrium.

The incubation period between acquisition of *M. tuberculosis* to the development of a positive tuberculin skin test (TST) is 2 to 12 weeks (American Academy of Pediatrics [AAP], 1997). The majority of individuals infected with tuberculosis have adequate cell-mediated immune responses to the infection and can effectively limit multiplication of the bacilli through encapsulation and calcification of the organism. However, 10 percent of infected individuals are unable to successfully contain the organism and will develop active clinical disease (either pulmonary or extrapulmonary). Of these individuals, active clinical disease will manifest within the first year of infection, while the remainder will develop active clinical disease 1 or more years after infection (CDC 1990). The prompt identification of infected individuals with latent infection can prevent the development of active tuberculosis (and prevent exposure in uninfected individuals) through the administration of prophylactic antituberculosis medications (e.g., isoniazid [INH]) for 6 to 12 months.

Complicating the treatment strategies for individuals with tuberculosis is the emergence of *multidrug-resistant tuberculosis* (MDR-TB). The majority of individuals with MDR-TB are also HIV infected. The case–fatality rate associated with this condition is extremely high, ranging from 72 percent to 89 percent (CDC, 1990). Resistance to both isoniazid (INH) and rifampin (RFM) has been reported in the majority of cases; however, resistance to other antituberculosis medications has been documented (American Thoracic Society, 1994; CDC, 1992).

Controversy exists regarding the impact of tuberculosis infection on pregnancy. It is generally agreed that untreated active tuberculosis infection during pregnancy provides a greater hazard to the pregnant woman and her fetus than the pharmacologic agents that are used to treat the disease (American Thoracic Society, 1994; Miller & Miller, Jr., 1996). Adverse perinatal outcomes have been reported in pregnant women living in other countries who have experienced active tuberculosis infection. These complications included low birth weight, prematurity, and perinatal death and were attributed to delays in diagnosis, incomplete or inadequate treatment, and advanced pulmonary lesions in this group of women (Jana, Vasishta, Jindal, Khunnu, & Ghosh, 1994). In general, tuberculosis infection has not demonstrated an adverse effect on pregnancy outcome when women are identified early in the disease process and effective therapeutic interventions are initiated (Miller & Miller, Jr., 1996). However, identification of this infection through prenatal screening of pregnant women with TST is essential so that appropriate therapy can be initiated, since studies have documented active pulmonary disease in asymptomatic pregnant women (Carter & Mates, 1994).

Congenital tuberculosis infection, although uncommon, may occur when a woman develops an active case of tuberculosis during her pregnancy, especially if she becomes bacteremic (AAP, 1997; Miller & Miller, Jr., 1996). The mortality rate in infants diagnosed with this disease was reportedly 38 percent in one study (Cantwell et al., 1994). This high mortality rate was associated with a delay in the initiation of appropriate treatment as a result of not recognizing the presence of this neonatal disease (Cantwell et al., 1994).

The diagnosis of congenital tuberculosis infection requires the recognition of specific criteria including: a proven tuberculosis lesion within the first week of life; tuberculosis infection of the maternal genital tract and/or placenta; neonatal hepatic granuloma or a primary hepatic complex; and/or exclusion of the possibility of infection through investigation of the infant's personal and hospital contacts (Miller & Miller, Jr., 1996).

Database

Subjective

A woman may be without knowledge of exposure to tuberculosis. High risk factors include the following (American Thoracic Society, 1994; Miller & Miller, Jr., 1996; Shannon, 1995; Stauffer, 1996):

- Individual history of positive TSTs (e.g., PPD)

- Member of an ethnic or socioeconomic group at risk for infection (e.g., Asian, Hispanic, or African-American ethnicity; homeless)

- Arrival in the United States from a country that is endemic for tuberculosis

- A history of medical factors associated with an increased risk of active tuberculosis:

  ▶ HIV infection

  ▶ Malignancies

  ▶ Hematological disorders

  ▶ Silicosis

  ▶ Gastrectomy

  ▶ Jejunoileal bypass

  ▶ Chronic renal failure

  ▶ Weight loss of 10 percent or more of ideal body weight

  ▶ Prolonged high-dose corticosteroid therapy and/or other immunosuppressive therapy

  ▶ Abnormal chest X-ray demonstrating fibrotic lesions consistent with healed tuberculosis

  ▶ Positive tuberculosis skin test within 2 years without assessment for preventive therapy

- Women with tuberculosis infection may be asymptomatic (latent infection) or may have a history of one or more of the following symptoms (active clinical infection) (American Thoracic Society, 1990; Miller & Miller, Jr., 1996; Shannon, 1995; Stauffer, 1996):

  ▶ Malaise

  ▶ Night sweats

  ▶ Remittent fever, occurring in the early afternoon

  ▶ Conjunctivitis or keratitis

  ▶ Erythema nodosum—painful red nodules, commonly present on the anterior aspects of the legs

  ▶ Cough that may produce mucopurulent sputum

  ▶ Hemoptysis

  ▶ Intermittent chills

  ▶ Weight loss

  ▶ Wheezing

▶ Chest pain (if involvement of the pleura, pericardium)

▶ Ulcers of the mouth and/or pharynx (rare)

▶ Hoarseness (rare, associated with laryngeal involvement)

▶ Dysphagia (rare, associated with laryngeal involvement)

▶ Enlarged, firm, tender cervical or supraclavicular lymph nodes that may soften, slough, and drain

▶ Dysuria, hematuria, and flank pain if renal involvement (70 percent of persons with renal tuberculosis report these symptoms)

▶ Pelvic pain and/or abdominal pain may be reported in women with genital tuberculosis infection

▶ Red, painful joints (usually monoarticular, weight-bearing) after a traumatic event if skeletal tuberculosis is present

▶ Central nervous system symptoms may be reported (e.g., confusion, headache, change in mentation, nuchal rigidity) if coexistent with meningitis

NOTE: In immunocompromised (e.g., HIV-infected) women, the symptoms of active tuberculosis may be subtle and atypical.

Objective

● Physical examination may be unremarkable, especially in women with latent infection, or may demonstrate one or more of the following findings depending on the extent of infection and the immune status of the woman (Miller & Miller, Jr., 1996; Sepkowitz et al., 1995):

▶ Vital signs

– Within normal limits (WNL)

– Or may reveal an elevated temperature (> 37.7 °C [100° F]), pulse, and respiratory rate depending on the status of the woman

– Weight may be less than 10th percentile of ideal body weight for height; may be less than normal for gestation of pregnancy

▶ Skin

– May be WNL

– May reveal pallor if woman has moderate to severe anemia associated with hematologic abnormalities that occur with miliary tuberculosis

– Erythematous nodules of the anterior aspect of the legs may be evident if erythema nodosum

▶ Eyes may manifest erythema and discharge associated with conjunctivitis or keratitis

▶ Mouth ulcerations may be present

▶ Lymphadenopathy

– May palpate a firm, enlarged, single, tender cervical or supraclavicular node (over time the node will soften, slough, and drain)

▶ Dullness to percussion of the chest wall (if active pulmonary disease)

▶ Palpation of chest wall may reveal tactile fremitus if pleural thickening or fluid

▶ Auscultation of the lungs may demonstrate

   – Increased tubular breath sounds and whispered pectoriloquy

   – Rubs (if there is pleural effusion)

   – Post tussive crackles (may be elicited after the woman takes several short coughs)

   – Amphoric breath sounds (distant, hollow breath sounds noted over tuberculosis cavities)

▶ Abdominal examination may reveal

   – Splenomegaly

   – Fundal height less than expected for weeks of gestation

▶ Examination of the extremities may reveal erythema nodosum

▶ Neurological examination may reveal

   – Nuchal rigidity

   – Mental confusion

   – Photosensitivity (if meningeal involvement)

▶ Pelvic examination may reveal

   – An ulcerative, granulomatous cervical mass

   – Enlarged, tender ovary

   – Tender uterus

Assessment

● Tuberculosis infection (latent, active)

  ▶ R/O MDR-TB

  ▶ R/O meningitis

  ▶ R/O pneumonia

  ▶ R/O IUGR

  ▶ R/O immune deficiency (e.g., HIV infection)

  ▶ R/O cancer

Plan

Diagnostic Tests

The following is a presentation of the tests used for screening and to confirm active disease; however, when active tuberculosis infection is suspected or confirmed, consultation with an obstetrician and infectious disease specialist is indicated. Any further diagnostic evaluations should be ordered and interpreted by the consulting physician(s).

- Tuberculin skin testing is recommended for all pregnant women. The test is an important screening tool, but does not distinguish past infection from current disease.

  NOTE: The cell-mediated effect of pregnancy on a woman's immune system does not interfere with tuberculin skin test interpretations, unless the woman has an underlying immunosuppressive condition (e.g., HIV-infection, malignancy) (Miller & Miller, Jr., 1996).

- There are two types of tuberculin skin tests:

  ▶ The multiple puncture devices (e.g., tine test).

  ▶ The Mantoux Test (the recommended screening test for tuberculosis). However, to be an effective screening test it must be properly administered and read within the recommended time interval.

  – The recommendations for the placement and interpretation of the Mantoux Test are as follows:

  * The placement of the test consists of the administration of an intradermal injection of 0.1 ml solution containing 5 tuberculin units (TU) of purified protein derivative (PPD), using a #26 or #27 needle, on the volar aspect of the woman's forearm. If the test is applied properly, an elevated, blanched wheal will occur at the site of the injection.

  * The test should be read 48 to 72 hours after placement. The site of the test should be evaluated for induration (not erythema). The transverse diameter of the area of induration should be measured in millimeters.

  * The definition of a positive skin test reaction depends on the probability of tuberculosis infection given a person's particular situation. A test is read as positive if the measured induration is within the size required for specific populations as delineated below (American Thoracic Society, 1994; Miller & Miller, Jr., 1996; Stauffer, 1996).

  - An induration of 5 mm or more is considered a positive reaction if the woman is known or suspected to be HIV-infected, has a close contact with an infectious person, or has clinical or chest radiograph evidence of tuberculosis.

  - An induration of 10 mm or more is considered a positive reaction if a woman is in one of the following at-risk groups:

    > Health care workers

    > Immigrants from a country with a high prevalence of tuberculosis

    > Intravenous drug abusers known to be HIV-seronegative

    > Members of certain ethnic groups (e.g., African-American, Hispanic, Native American)

    > Residents of prisons, shelters, or health care facilities

    > Diabetes mellitus patients

    > End-stage renal disease patients

    > Those in prolonged therapy with adrenocorticosteroids or immunosuppressive agents

    > Silicosis patients

> Post-gastrectomy or intestinal bypass patients

> Certain hematologic and/or reticuloendothelial disease patients (e.g., leukemia, Hodgkin's disease)

> Malnourished (10 percent below ideal body weight) individuals

- An induration of 15 mm or more is considered a positive reaction in a woman who is not in a high-risk category or exposed to a high-risk environment.

   > A false-positive result can occur if the woman is infected with a nontuberculous mycobacteria (Sepkowitz et al., 1995).

   > A negative PPD does not eliminate the possibility of tuberculosis infection, since it takes 2 to 12 weeks after infection for an individual to develop the tissue hypersensitivity response necessary to demonstrate a positive reaction. In addition, false negative results (i.e., anergy) are estimated to be as high as 20 percent in individuals with active tuberculosis infection, which may be a result of depressed cell-mediated immunity associated with certain conditions (e.g., HIV-infection, corticosteroid therapy, malnutrition, etc.).

NOTE: A woman who has received a *Calmette-Guerin bacillus* (BCG) vaccination may have a positive PPD response as a result of the BCG vaccination *or* tuberculosis infection. In the United States, a person with a history of receiving a BCG vaccine who does have a positive tuberculin test is considered to have tuberculosis infection and should be further evaluated to assess the presence of active tuberculosis (American Thoracic Society, 1994).

- A chest radiograph should be ordered for any woman with a positive PPD and/or signs and symptoms suggestive of tuberculosis infection.

  ▶ Ideally the chest x-ray should be ordered at the time the positive PPD is documented.

  ▶ Chest x-rays are not contraindicated in pregnant women, if clinically indicated. Whenever possible, obtain the chest x-ray after the first trimester as a precaution.

  – With shielding of the abdomen, a chest x-ray has a mean fetal dose of only 1–5 mrad (1/1000 the minimal dose implicated in teratogenicity, childhood leukemia) (Miller & Miller, Jr., 1996).

  – However, the chest x-ray with abdominal shielding may be deferred until the second trimester at the discretion of the clinician or at the request of the patient to minimize any theoretical risks to the fetus.

  ▶ The following radiograph findings suggestive of pulmonary tuberculosis may be evident (Miller, & Miller, Jr., 1996; Shannon, 1995; Stauffer, 1996):

  – Patchy, nodular infiltrates (usually evident in the apical or subapical aspects of the upper lobes or the superior segment of the lower lobes)

  – Cavitation (usually evident in the apical segment of the lower lobes)

  – Multiple, discrete infiltrates adjacent to a cavity (associated with bronchogenic spread)

  – Fibrotic scars, granulomatous and exudative lesions, and caseation

  – A pneumonic lesion with enlarged hilar lymph nodes in any region of the lung

- Miliary infiltrate(s)

- Pleural effusion (in some individuals this is the only chest x-ray finding)

- Air-fluid levels in association with lower-lobe cavitation, but are uncommon in upper-lobe infection

- Segmental or lobar atelectasis may be present

NOTE: In HIV-infected individuals, the chest x-ray findings may be subtle and atypical resulting in misdiagnosis.

- Obtain sputum specimens for acid-fast bacilli (AFB) culture and acid-fast stain to confirm active pulmonary tuberculosis.

  ▶ Sputum acid-fast stain with evidence of acid-fast bacilli is diagnostic of pulmonary infection and indicates that the woman is highly infectious. This diagnostic test is positive in 50 percent to 80 percent of individuals with pulmonary tuberculosis (American Thoracic Society, 1990).

  ▶ A positive sputum AFB culture is diagnostic of active pulmonary tuberculosis and sensitivity testing can provide information about the presence of organisms resistant to antituberculosis drugs (American Thoracic Society, 1994; Miller & Miller, Jr., 1996; Des Prez & Heim, 1990).

  NOTE: Usually three to five early morning daily specimens are collected and should be sufficient to obtain an adequate sample for culture. In individuals unable to produce enough sputum in the early morning, 24-hour sputum collection or sputum induction may be done.

  ▶ Polymerase chain reaction (PCR) tests for rapid diagnosis are approved only for smear-positive respiratory tract specimens. PCR tests are expensive, of limited availability (i.e., available in research laboratories), and should be ordered in consultation with a specialist in tuberculosis (AAP, 1997).

- Aspiration of gastric contents is rarely done because of the success of other methods to obtain AFB testing (i.e., sputum induction).

- Complete blood count (CBC) may be within normal limits (WNL) or may demonstrate a decreased hemoglobin/hematocrit, an increased leukocyte count, a decreased platelet count, and an increased monocyte count.

- Obtain a serum chemistry panel to rule out the presence of renal or hepatic involvement. Results may demonstrate

  ▶ Elevated liver function tests (ALT, AST) in association with hepatic involvement or as a result of other medical conditions (e.g., substance abuse)

  ▶ Hyponatremia (present in advanced disease)

- Urinalysis may reveal pyuria, hematuria, and albuminuria in individuals with renal involvement.

- Other specimens obtained for AFB culture (e.g., cerebrospinal fluid, tissue biopsies) may be positive.

- Computerized tomography (CT) or magnetic resonance imaging (MRI) scans may reveal the presence of focal lesions, cerebral infarctions, hydrocephalus, or basilar arachnoid meningitis in women with CNS involvement (Des Prez & Heim, 1990).

Treatment/Management

- The therapeutic interventions indicated in the care of pregnant women with tuberculosis should be determined by the physician consultant.

  ▶ Treatment guidelines are updated by the American Thoracic Society and the Centers for Disease Control and should be referred to by clinicians involved in the care of individuals with tuberculosis.

  ▶ Current therapeutic interventions recommended for pregnant women with latent and active pulmonary tuberculosis are as follows (AAP, 1997; American Thoracic Society, 1994; Miller & Miller, Jr., 1996).

    – Pregnancy does not appear to substantially increase the risk of developing active tuberculosis. Therefore, the majority of pregnant women with latent infection (PPD positive result with a normal chest x-ray) can begin prophylactic therapy with INH *after* delivery and should continue therapy for a minimum of 6 months. An asymptomatic pregnant woman with a positive TST, a negative chest x-ray, and *recent* contact with an infectious person should initiate prophylactic therapy during pregnancy and continue for 6 months. The regimen should begin after the first trimester (AAP, 1997; Miller & Miller, Jr., 1996).

      * The recommended regimen for prophylactic therapy is INH 300 mg p.o. daily and Vitamin B_6 (pyridoxine) 50 mg p.o. daily.

      NOTE: INH therapy has been proven to be more than 90 percent effective in preventing the development of active tuberculosis when taken as prescribed. However, it is associated with an increased incidence of hepatotoxicity in certain groups of individuals including pregnant women, alcoholics, and injection drug users. Transient elevations in transaminase levels have been reported in up to 20 percent of individuals receiving INH.

    – Women who may not be able to comply with daily recommended therapy should receive therapy twice a week by directly observed therapy (DOT).

      * The recommended therapy is INH 900 mg p.o and Vitamin B_6 (pyridoxine) 50 mg p.o.

    – An asymptomatic woman over 35 years of age with a positive TST and a normal chest x-ray should not receive INH prophylaxis unless it is documented that she converted (i.e., positive TST) within the past 2 years or she is HIV positive (Miller & Miller, Jr., 1996).

    – In HIV-infected pregnant women with a positive TST and negative chest x-ray, the risk of developing active pulmonary or extrapulmonary tuberculosis is increased. Therefore, INH and Vitamin B_6 therapy should be initiated during pregnancy (after the first trimester) and continued for 12 months.

    – Pregnant women with active pulmonary tuberculosis should begin treatment for the infection during the pregnancy, and should continue therapy for 6 months.

      * The recommended medications that should be initiated are INH 300 mg p.o. daily plus rifampin (RFM) 600 mg p.o. daily plus ethambutol (EMB) 2 to 2.5 gm p.o. daily plus vitamin B_6 (pyridoxine) 50 mg p.o. daily

      NOTE: Routine pyrazinamide administration is recommended by international tuberculosis organizations; however, its use in pregnant women in the United States is controversial because there is insufficient data regarding possible teratogenic effects (Miller & Miller, Jr., 1996). In general, it is not recommended for use in pregnant women in the United States (AAP, 1997).

* In some pregnant women requiring DOT to ensure compliance with therapy, the administration of the above medications at the recommended doses can be done twice a week.

* In HIV-infected pregnant women, the administration of chemotherapeutic agents for active tuberculosis should continue for a minimum of 6 months after sputum cultures are negative.

NOTE: Ethambutol is included in the initial treatment regimen as a means of preventing the development of MDR-TB in areas where primary INH resistance is increased. Ethambutol can be discontinued after 2 months of therapy if the results of drug susceptibility studies indicate that the organism is fully susceptible to INH and RFM. Ethambutol may be eliminated from the initial regimen if the woman's exposure to a primary INH-resistant strain of tuberculosis is unlikely. Information regarding the possibility of MDR-TB in an area is available through local and state public health departments.

– When evidence of organism resistance to specific chemotherapeutic agents through AFB susceptibility studies is documented, the treatment regimen and the duration of therapy should be modified. The physician managing the woman's care should consult a tuberculosis specialist to determine the most effective agents to include in the treatment regimen. As many as five to six chemotherapeutic agents may be necessary in some cases.

▶ Pregnant women with asymptomatic active tuberculosis infection should be placed on modified bedrest, and receive adequate nutrition and hydration.

▶ Hospitalization of a woman is indicated if she has evidence of miliary tuberculosis (i.e., lymphohematogenous spread), significant debilitation, cannot care for herself, or is likely to expose susceptible individuals during the infectious stage of her disease (Stauffer, 1996).

– HIV counseling and testing should be offered to any pregnant woman with tuberculosis infection and unknown HIV serostatus. This is recommended because of the high incidence of tuberculosis in HIV-infected individuals (Cantwell et al., 1994).

▶ Recommend immunization with pneumococcal vaccine for pregnant women with tuberculosis infection.

▶ Refer pregnant women with chemical dependency problems to appropriate counseling and treatment.

▶ Order serial sonograms in women with suspected or documented intrauterine growth restriction.

▶ Initiate fetal movement counts at 28 weeks gestation.

▶ Initiate antenatal testing (e.g., nonstress tests with amniotic fluid index) between 32 to 34 weeks gestation in pregnant women with active tuberculosis.

● Contacts of pregnant women diagnosed with infectious tuberculosis are at a significant risk for developing the disease. Therefore, identify and evaluate contacts for infection.

Consultation

- Consult with a physician for a woman with suspected or documented tuberculosis infection.

- Consult with a physician specializing in the evaluation and treatment of tuberculosis for a woman with suspected MDR-TB, severe symptoms, evidence of debilitating disease, symptoms of toxicity associated with chemotherapeutic agents, or suspected noncompliance with treatment regimens.

Patient Education

- Educate the woman about tuberculosis infection including the cause of the infection, clinical manifestations, clinical course, diagnostic tests, therapeutic interventions, the need for compliance with treatment recommendations, possible side effects/toxicity of the chemotherapeutic agent(s), follow-up evaluations, prognosis, and the need for testing of close contacts.

- Educate the woman with suspected or documented infectious tuberculosis about respiratory precautions including (MacDonald, 1994):

  ▶ Generally, respiratory precautions are needed during the first 2 weeks of therapy, and involve the wearing of a face mask that covers the nose and mouth.

  ▶ Ventilation of rooms is essential to reduce the number of droplet nuclei within the environment and decrease the likelihood of transmission to others.

- The physician responsible for the woman's care and/or the pediatrician who will be caring for the infant should discuss the plan of care for the infant after delivery.

  ▶ The plan should be individualized according to the status of the mother (i.e., infectious or noninfectious) and other household members; and should be in compliance with recommendations from the American Thoracic Society (1994) and the American Academy of Pediatrics (1997).

  ▶ Separation of the mother and infant should be minimized. However, separation of the infant from the woman and other household members with infectious tuberculosis is indicated until they are proven to be noncontagious.

  ▶ In addition, infants born to women with hematogenous spread of tuberculosis (e.g., miliary disease, meningitis, or bone involvement) should be evaluated for congenital tuberculosis infection (AAP, 1997; American Thoracic Society, 1994; Cantwell et al., 1994).

  NOTE: Women with latent or active, noncontagious tuberculosis infection (i.e., sputum smears and cultures are negative for AFB) who are taking antituberculosis medications may breastfeed their infants, since the small amount of these agents in breastmilk does not produce toxicity in nursing infants. However, the presence of these agents in breastmilk should not be considered effective for the treatment of disease or as a preventive treatment in nursing infants (AAP, 1997; American Thoracic Society, 1994).

- If the woman smokes cigarettes, discuss the adverse effects of smoking on her, her fetus and other household members. Provide referrals to smoking cessation programs within the community.

- Women requiring hospitalization should discuss with the physician responsible for their care the reason(s) for hospitalization.

- Women with tuberculosis with unknown HIV serostatus should be educated about the need to consider HIV testing. If a woman decides to be tested, comprehensive counseling and either confidential or anonymous testing should be arranged for her (see Chapter 14.5, *Human Innunodeficiency Virus*).

Follow-up

- Follow-up evaluations of a woman with tuberculosis should be determined by the physician(s) responsible for her care.

- If a woman is receiving INH therapy, obtain baseline and monthly transminase levels.

- If a woman has active tuberculosis infection, obtain monthly sputum evaluations until negative results are documented. This is a means of assessing the effectiveness of therapy and determining any evidence of drug resistance.

  ▶ A woman with positive sputum result after 3 months of therapy should be evaluated for possible noncompliance with treatment regimens and/or possible drug resistance.

- A woman who experiences any signs and/or symptoms of complications or adverse side effects associated with the chemotherapeutic agents should return for immediate evaluation.

- Tuberculosis is a CDC-reportable disease and notification of the local public health department is mandated by law whenever an individual is diagnosed with tuberculosis.

- Document diagnosis of tuberculosis and management thereof in progress notes and problem list.

References

American Academy of Pediatrics (AAP). (1997). *1994 Red Book: Report of the Committee on Infectious Disease* (24th ed., pp. 550–567). Elk Grove Village, IL: Author.

American Thoracic Society. (1990). Diagnostic standards and classification of tuberculosis. *American Review of Respiratory Diseases, 142,* 725–735.

American Thoracic Society. (1994). Treatment of tuberculosis and tuberculosis infection in adults and children. *American Review of Respiratory and Critical Care Medicine, 149,* 1359–1374.

Cantwell, M.F., Z.M., Costello, A.M., Sands, L., Green, W.F., Ewing, Jr., E.P., Balway, S. E., & Onorato, I.M. (1994). Brief report: Congenital tuberculosis. *New England Journal of Medicine, 330*(15), 1051–1054.

Cantwell, M.F., Snider, Jr., D.E., Cauthen, G.M., & Onorato, I.M. (1994). Epidemiology of tuberculosis in the United States, 1985 through 1992. *Journal of the American Medical Association, 272*(7), 535–539.

Carter, E.J., & Mates, S. (1994). Tuberculosis during pregnancy. The Rhode Island experience, 1987 to 1991. *Chest, 106*(5), 1466–1470.

Centers for Disease Control and Prevention (CDC). (1990). Screening for tuberculosis and tuberculosis infection in high-risk populations. Recommendations of the Advisory Committee for the Elimination of Tuberculosis. *Morbidity and Mortality Weekly Report, 39*(RR–8), 1–8.

Centers for Disease Control and Prevention (CDC). (1992). Management of persons exposed to multidrug-resistant tuberculosis. *Morbidity and Mortality Weekly Report, 41*(RR–11), 61–70.

Centers for Disease Control and Prevention (CDC). (1993). Initial therapy for tuberculosis in the era of multidrug resistance. Recommendations of the Advisory Council for the elimination of tuberculosis. *Morbidity and Mortality Weekly Report, 42*(RR–7), 1–8.

Centers for Disease Control and Prevention (CDC). (1998). Tuberculosis morbidity—United States, 1997. *Morbidity and Mortality Weekly Report, 47*(13), 253–257.

Des Prez, R.M., & Heim, C.R. (1990). Mycobacterial diseases. In G. L. Mandell, R. G. Douglas, Jr., & J. E. Bennett (Eds.), *Principles and practice of infectious diseases* (3rd ed., pp. 1877–1906). New York: Churchill Livingstone.

Jana, N., Vasishta, S.K., Jindal, S.K., Khunna, B., & Ghosh, K. (1994). Perinatal outcome in pregnancies complicated by pulmonary tuberculosis. *International Journal of Obstetrics & Gynecology, 44,* 119–124.

MacDonald, N.E. (1994). Recommendations for infection control in outpatient care for the prevention of tuberculosis. *The Pediatric Infectious Disease Journal, 13*(10), 939–940.

Miller, K. S., & Miller, Jr., J. M. (1996). Tuberculosis in pregnancy: Interactions, diagnosis, and management. *Clinical Obstetrics and Gynecology, 39*(1), 120–142.

Sepkowitz, K.A., Raffalli, J., Riley, L., Kiehn, T.E., & Armstrong, D. (1995). Tuberculosis in the AIDS era. *Clinical Microbiology Reviews, 8*(2), 180–199.

Shannon, M.T. (1995). Tuberculosis. In W.L. Star, L.L. Lommel, & M.T. Shannon (Eds.), *Women's primary health care: Protocols for practice* (pp. 5–55, 5–63). Washington, DC: American Nurses Publishing.

Stauffer, J.L. (1996). Lung. In L.M. Tierney, Jr., S.J. McPhee, & M.A. Papadakis (Eds.), *Current medical diagnosis and treatment* (35th ed., pp. 215–294). Norwalk, CT: Appleton & Lange.

Chapter 11

VARICELLA ZOSTER VIRUS

Winifred L. Star

Varicella zoster virus (VZV) is a human herpes virus that causes two distinct illnesses:

- Primary varicella zoster infection, or chickenpox, a highly contagious infection that occurs predominantly during childhood (about 95 percent of adults in the United States are immune to varicella and fewer than 2 percent of reported cases occur after age 20)

- Reactivated varicella virus infection, known as herpes zoster or shingles, which occurs as a result of reactivation of latent virus persisting in the nerve ganglia after primary disease resolution. Herpes zoster is generally associated with advancing age, immunosuppression, and certain malignancies, but also occurs in healthy individuals (Shannon, 1995).

Transmission of primary varicella infection is via aerosol spread of infected respiratory secretions or direct contact with vesicular fluid from skin lesions. The incubation period is usually 14 to 16 days (range 10 to 21 days). Contagion begins from 1 to 2 days prior to onset of the rash and may last as long as 5 days after the onset of lesions (American Academy of Pediatrics [AAP], 1997).

Adult primary varicella infection can run a more virulent course and complications are more common than in children. Pneumonia may develop in about 14 percent of maternal cases of varicella; mortality rates may reach 40 percent if antiviral therapy is not administered. Secondary bacterial infections, especially with group A beta-hemolytic streptococci are common. Neurologic complications that may occur include encephalitis, aseptic meningitis, Guillain-Barré syndrome, Reye's syndrome, stroke, and transverse myelitis. Thrombocytopenia, bleeding diathesis, conjunctivitis, arthritis, pericarditis, hepatitis, acute renal necrosis, and glomerulonephritis may also occur (Freij & Sever, 1995; Hashmey & Shandera, 1996; Shannon, 1995).

Herpes zoster infection presents as a painful eruption of cutaneous lesions along single or multiple dermatomes, usually lasting from 14 to 21 days (Shannon, 1995). Herpes zoster patients are contagious and able to transmit virus to varicella-susceptible persons, with possible resultant varicella infection in the nonimmune individual (Sterner, Forsgren, Enocksson, Grandien, & Granström, 1990). Complications of herpes zoster may include postherpetic neuralgia, cellulitis, transient motor neuropathies, ocular inflammation, vasculopathy, pneumonitis, myocarditis, pancreatitis, esophagitis, enterocolitis, and the Ramsey Hunt syndrome (Shannon, 1995).

Varicella during pregnancy is estimated to occur in 1/2,000 pregnancies; herpes zoster is less common occurring in 1/10,000 pregnancies (not of perinatal significance) (American College of Obstetricians and Gynecologists [ACOG], 1993; Ghidini & Lynch, 1993). Spontaneous abortion, prematurity, and fetal death as consequences of maternal varicella infection do not appear to be in excess. Severe maternal infection, especially if associated with pneumonia, may result in preterm labor. Fetal infection following primary maternal infection may occur in one of three forms:

1) the congenital varicella syndrome
2) late gestation infection resulting in perinatal varicella
3) congenital herpes zoster during infancy (Smego & Asperilla, 1991).

Herpes zoster infection occurring in pregnancy is unlikely to cause significant congenital malformation.

In early pregnancy (up to 20 weeks) primary maternal varicella infection may result in the fetal congenital varicella syndrome (also called varicella embryopathy), characterized by anomalies of the

- Skin (cicatricial lesions)

- Nervous system (microcephaly, cortical atrophy, paralysis, seizures, psychomotor retardation)

- Musculoskeletal system (limb hypoplasia, muscle atrophy, malformed digits)

- Ophthalmologic system (cataracts, microphthalmia, chorioretinitis, Horner's syndrome)

- Gastrointestinal system (atresia, stenosis)

- Genitourinary system (hydronephrosis) (Alkalay, Pomerance, & Rimoin, 1987; Chapman & Duff, 1993).

Atypical, incomplete manifestations of this syndrome may also occur (Gershon, 1995). Risk of vertical transmission of VZV from mother to fetus is estimated at 25 to 40 percent; however, the congenital varicella syndrome occurs only rarely—a 1.8 percent incidence if maternal varicella occurs in the first trimester and less than 1 percent incidence if maternal infection occurs later (Enders, Miller, Cradock-Watson, & Ridehalgh, 1994; Gershon, 1988; Ghidini & Lynch, 1994; Paryani & Arvin, 1986; Pastuszak et al., 1994). Malformations developing after exposure beyond 20 weeks' gestation consist mainly of skin lesions or limb defects (Brunell, 1992; Michie et al., 1992). One-third of infants with congenital varicella syndrome will succumb in the neonatal period; survivors have significant sequelae.

Severity of congenital chickenpox infection in the neonate is related to time of onset of maternal infection. If maternal varicella occurs within 5 days before delivery to 2 days after delivery, neonatal infection may occur in 25 percent of infants and the case mortality rate may be as high as 20 to 30 percent. In these cases, neonatal lesions usually appear 5 to 10 days after birth (Chapman & Duff, 1993; Freij & Sever, 1995; Gershon, 1988). Maternal infections occurring 5 to 21 days prior to delivery result in neonatal lesions in the first 4 days of life. Because the effects of maternal antibodies moderate neonatal illness in these cases, the prognosis is good and there is no risk of mortality (Freij & Sever, 1995). On occasion, herpes zoster may present in the newborn period or during early childhood, usually as a benign manifestation of intrauterine varicella exposure (Chapman & Duff, 1993; Freij & Sever, 1995). Postnatally acquired varicella has a mild course and favorable outcome (Sterner et al., 1990).

Varicella Reinfection

After a case of chickenpox, immunity to future disease is generally lifelong. It has been recognized recently, however, that waning immunity to varicella can occur after primary infection or vaccination, although this phenomena seems rare. Clinical and serologic evidence of reinfection has been documented in immune adults after exposure to chickenpox; infection is usually mild in these cases (Gershon et al., 1984). In addition, maternal reinfection during pregnancy in women with preexisting antibodies has been identified; risk of fetal infection in these cases appears to be negligible but further study is required (Gershon et al., 1984; Martin, Junker, Thomas, Van Allen, & Friedman, 1994). Clinical reinfections may be more likely to occur in immunocompromised persons (Gershon et al., 1984).

Varicella Vaccine

Varicella virus vaccine is a live attenuated preparation of the Oka/Merck strain of varicella virus. The primary indication is for active immunization of individuals 12 months of age and older. The vaccine has been shown to be effective in protecting children as well as adolescents and adults against chickenpox. The seroconversion rate (i.e., detectable antibody greater than 0.3 [gp ELISA]) in children 12 months to 12 years of age after one dose is 97 percent. In adolescents and adults 13 years of age and older, the seroconversion rate is 99 percent after two doses (Merck & Company, 1996; Kaiser Permanente Northern California, 1995). Waning of immunity in vaccine recipients has not been demonstrated (studies to date have shown no loss of immunity for up to 10 years in healthy children) (AAP, 1997; Kaiser Permanente Northern California, 1995). The vaccine is contraindicated in pregnancy, and pregnancy should be avoided for 3 months following immunization.

Database

Subjective

- History should include inquiry about past varicella infection or immunization.

- Woman may report exposure to individual with chickenpox or shingles during current pregnancy.

  NOTE: Casual contact is less likely to transmit infection than prolonged, close contact. "Significant exposure" is considered to be household or classroom contact involving 1 hour or more of close play/interaction (some experts suggest 5 minutes or more), or intimate face-to-face contact where droplets can be exchanged. Zoster infection exposure connotes direct contact with vesicle fluid (AAP, 1994; Russell, 1992).

- Symptoms of primary varicella zoster infection include the following:

  ▶ Prodrome of headache, fever, chills, malaise, myalgia, arthralgia

  ▶ Discrete pruritic rash following prodrome (see the Objective section)

  ▶ Dry cough, dyspnea, fever, hemoptysis, or pleuritic chest pain, which may develop about 1 to 6 days after rash eruption (symptoms of pneumonia)

  ▶ Headache, drowsiness, convulsions, ataxia, altered sensorium (symptoms of encephalitis)

  ▶ Bleeding from mucous membranes, unexplained bruising (secondary to severe thrombocytopenia) (Hashmey & Shandera, 1996; Russell, 1992; Shannon, 1995)

  ▶ Infection may be subclinical (unusual in primary infection)

- Symptoms of herpes zoster infection may include the following:

  ▶ Prodrome of fever, headache, malaise, dysesthesia(s) preceding appearance of rash

  ▶ Painful skin lesions resembling chickenpox in dermatomal pattern (see the Objective section)

    – Pain/paresthesia in involved dermatome may precede exanthem by 4 to 5 days.

    – Pain may occur in the absence of rash (*zoster sine herpete*).

    – Pain may continue for several weeks after lesion resolution.

  ▶ Facial weakness, peripheral motor weakness, vertigo, tinnitus, etc. (symptoms specific to nerve involvement)

▶ Visual disturbances, eye pain (symptoms of ocular complications)

▶ Dyspnea (if pneumonia exists)

▶ Symptoms secondary to central nervous system complications, such as headache, stiff neck, or coordination problems. (Hashmey & Shandera, 1996; Russell, 1992; Shannon, 1995).

Objective

● Elevated temperature may be present.

● Skin examination

  ▶ Evidence of varicella lesions

    – Macules progressing to papules, vesicles, crusts

    – Most prominent on face, scalp, trunk, and extremities (lesions may also involve the mouth, throat, conjunctiva, vulva)

    – Crusts slough in 7 to 10 days

    – Resolution usually in less than 2 weeks

    – Occasionally lesions may be bullous or hemorrhagic

    – Superinfection of skin lesions may develop

  ▶ Evidence of zoster lesions

    – Tender erythematous papules progressing to vesicles, then pustules, in a dermatomal pattern (thoracic and lumbar distributions most common)

    – Crusting in 7 to 10 days after initial eruption

    – Resolution in about 14 to 21 days

    – *Disseminated herpes zoster* is represented by more than 20 lesions outside the primary and adjacent dermatome, which appear 4 to 11 days after lesion eruption in primary dermatome (Shannon, 1995).

  ▶ Petechiae, ecchymosis may be present secondary to thrombocytopenia.

● Pulmonary examination may reveal tachypnea, crackles, wheezes, and/or cyanosis if pneumonia present.

● HEENT/neurological examination

  ▶ Conjunctivitis, keratitis may be present with ocular complications.

  ▶ Facial palsy, diminished hearing, lesions in external auditory canal/tympanic membrane may be present in Ramsey Hunt syndrome.

  ▶ Ataxia, nystagmus, nuchal rigidity may be present with encephalitis.

● Ultrasound examination may identify fetal anomalies associated with congenital varicella syndrome:

  ▶ Hepatic calcification

▶ Ascites

▶ pericardial effusions

▶ Hepatomegaly

▶ Intrauterine growth restriction

▶ Polyhydramnios (most frequent finding)

▶ Microcephaly

▶ Cerebral ventricular dilatation

▶ Fetal hydrops

▶ Hand/foot deformities

▶ Hydrocephalus (Brunell, 1992; Freij & Sever, 1995; Lécuru et al., 1994)

NOTE: Abnormalities may be detected 5 to 19 weeks after maternal infection (Freij & Sever, 1995).

- Presentation of neonatal infection will depend on the timing of maternal infection and may include

  ▶ Cutaneous lesions

  ▶ Fever

  ▶ Hemorrhagic rash

  ▶ Generalized visceral involvement

  ▶ Pneumonia

  ▶ Hepatitis

  ▶ Encephalitis (Pastuszak et al., 1994)

- Usual interval from onset of rash in mother to onset in neonate is 9 to 15 days (range 1 to 16 days) (AAP, 1997). Neonate may appear to have stigmata of congenital varicella syndrome (see Introductory section).

Assessment

- Maternal exposure to varicella

  ▶ R/O primary varicella zoster infection (chickenpox)

  ▶ R/O recurrent varicella infection

  ▶ R/O herpes zoster infection (shingles)

  ▶ R/O herpes simplex virus infection

  ▶ R/O other viral infections (e.g., atypical measles)

  ▶ R/O allergic reaction (e.g., poison oak)

  ▶ R/O complications of varicella infection

  ▶ R/O disseminated herpes zoster infection

▶ R/O immunosuppression (e.g., HIV infection)

▶ R/O fetal varicella infection

Plan

Diagnostic Tests

- Diagnosis is generally made on the basis of clinical findings; however, the following laboratory tests may be ordered:

  ▶ VZV-specific IgG

    – Fourfold or greater rise in titer from acute and convalescent sera is evidence of acute infection

    – Presence of IgG antibody (within few days of exposure) indicates prior immunity

    – Absence of IgG indicates susceptibility (Chapman & Duff, 1993)

  ▶ VZV-specific IgM

    – Presence in single serum sample suggests recent infection.

    NOTE: Serological testing must be completed within 24 to 48 hours so that varicella zoster immune globulin (VZIG) may be administered in a timely fashion. Types of tests used will depend upon laboratory capabilities (e.g., fluorescent antibody to membrane antigen [FAMA], enzyme-linked immunosorbent assay [ELISA]).

  ▶ Culture of vesicular fluid to confirm varicella zoster virus (obtained during first 3 to 4 days after eruption)

  ▶ Immunofluorescent staining of vesicular scrapings to distinguish varicella zoster from herpes simplex virus

  ▶ Tzanck smear of scrapings from vesicle bases

    – May reveal multinucleated giant cells; does not differentiate varicella zoster from herpes simplex virus. (Hashmey & Shandera, 1996).

- Additional tests may include the following:

  ▶ Complete blood count (CBC) (may reveal leukopenia)

  ▶ Platelet count (may reveal thrombocytopenia)

  ▶ Chest x-ray (may reveal patchy or diffuse nodular infiltrates—indicative of pneumonia)

  ▶ Lumbar puncture, as indicated, for patients suspected of having encephalitis (may reveal increased cell counts and/or protein concentrations) (Shannon, 1995).

- Amniocentesis, cordocentesis, and chorionic villus sampling have been utilized in an attempt to confirm fetal infection by isolating the virus from amniotic fluid, measuring varicella zoster-specific IgM in fetal blood, or isolating varicella zoster virus DNA by polymerase chain reaction (PCR); these techniques are not routinely used, however, and are not able to diagnose congenital varicella syndrome in a fetus.

- Directed ultrasound may identify findings consistent with the congenital varicella syndrome; see the Objective section.

Treatment/Management

- See Figure 10.9, Varicella Exposure In Pregnancy.

- If patient has a known history of prior infection and has been exposed in pregnancy, presume immunity; no further testing/treatment is necessary.

- If maternal exposure to varicella was *less than 96 hours ago* and patient has no prior history of chickenpox:

  ▶ Verify that contact actually has varicella; ascertain type of exposure. See Table 10.10.

  ▶ Establish varicella immunity via laboratory tests.

  ▶ If immune, no further testing/treatment is necessary.

  ▶ If nonimmune (or if testing can not be done promptly) offer passive immunization with VZIG; usual adult dose is 125 units/10 kg body weight IM (up to a total of 625 units) (AAP, 1997; AAP and the American College of Obstetricians and Gynecologists [ACOG], 1997).

  NOTE: *VZIG must be administered within 96 hours of exposure to be effective.* It will either prevent or attenuate varicella infection in susceptible gravidas; it is not known, however, whether VZIG will prevent fetal development of congenital varicella syndrome. VZIG may be available locally or can be obtained from the nearest American Red Cross or from the Centers for Disease Control and Prevention (CDC) in Atlanta, Georgia.

- If exposure was *more than 96 hours ago* and client has no known history of varicella:

  ▶ Order a varicella test of immunity.

  ▶ If immune, no further testing/treatment is necessary.

  ▶ If nonimmune, advise of incubation/communicable period.

  ▶ Advise postponement of prenatal office visits until period of communicability has passed.

  ▶ Advise regarding symptomatic relief in event of infection (see below).

  ▶ Educate regarding signs/symptoms of complications.

- If maternal infection is diagnosed, serial ultrasound may be performed after 20 weeks' gestation to assess for evidence of congenital infection. Termination of pregnancy is not routinely recommended to exposed women because of the rarity of the congenital varicella syndrome. Pregnancy termination may be a consideration when there is evidence of significant fetal abnormalities. Counseling must be individualized and is generally the responsibility of the physician in charge of the client's care.

- For women with primary varicella infection during pregnancy the following measures are indicated (Chapman & Duff, 1993; Freij & Sever, 1995; Shannon, 1995):

  ▶ Physical consultation/management

  ▶ Bed rest if febrile

  ▶ Fluids

▶ Acetaminophen, as needed, for analgesia/fever

▶ Isolation for a minimum of 5 days after onset of rash and for the duration of vesicular eruption (for hospitalized patients isolation guidelines will depend on site-specific policies)

▶ Lesions to be kept clean and dry

▶ Topical therapy for relief of pruritus (e.g., calamine lotion or 0.5 percent camphor and 0.5 percent menthol; colloidal oatmeal or cornstarch baths)

▶ Systemic antihistamines for severe pruritus (e.g., diphenhydramine 25 mg p.o. every 4 to 6 hours as needed)

NOTE: Warn client about side effect of drowsiness.

▶ Topical antibiotic for secondary bacterial infection of lesions as indicated (e.g., mupirocin 2 percent ointment t.i.d. to q.i.d.).

NOTE: If infection is extensive, oral antibiotics may be required (e.g., dicloxacillin 250 mg p.o. q.i.d. for 10 days)

▶ Observation for evidence of disseminated disease

▶ Hospitalization for serious complications; antiviral therapy for varicella pneumonia:

  – Acyclovir 10 to 15 mg/kg or 500 mg/m^2 IV 3 times daily (every 8 hours) for 7 days; equivalent oral dose is 800 mg 5 times/day (Chapman & Duff, 1993; Freij & Sever, 1995; Gibbs & Sweet, 1994; Smego & Asperilla, 1991).

  NOTE: Oral acyclovir is not routinely prescribed in the pregnant adolescent or adult with uncomplicated varicella; however, some experts will recommend its use, especially in the third trimester (AAP, 1997). An Acyclovir in Pregnancy Registry is being maintained by the Burroughs Wellcome Company in conjunction with the CDC; health care providers are encouraged to call 1(800) 722-9292, ext. 39437, to register pregnant women treated with acyclovir.

▶ Isolation of mother from infant when maternal chickenpox occurs within 5 days of delivery or immediately postpartum and no lesions are present in the neonate (newborn isolation guidelines will be determined by hospital policies).

▶ See Table 10.9 for preventive guidelines after chickenpox exposure in nursery/maternity service. Further details regarding inpatient management are beyond the scope of this protocol.

● For herpes zoster infection the following measures are indicated (Freij & Sever, 1995; Shannon, 1995):

▶ Precautions to prevent spread of virus (e.g., use of gloves when coming into contact with lesions)

▶ Gentle cleansing/drying of involved areas

▶ Pain relief measures, as needed

  – Local applications of cool/heat

  – Open, wet compresses/topical soaks with Burow's solution

  – Calamine lotion

- – Prescription analgesics may be indicated for severe pain (consult with physician, as indicated)

▶ Ophthalmologic evaluation for eye involvement

▶ Treatment of secondary bacterial infection of lesions as indicated; systemic antibiotics may be required (e.g., amoxicillin and clavulanic acid 500 mg p.o. t.i.d. for 7 to 10 days) (Shannon, 1995). (Consult with physician.)

▶ Consideration of antiviral therapy (Consult with physician.)

▶ Hospitalization for disseminated disease; patient will be managed by physician

▶ Prevention of direct contact of newborn with maternal lesions (mother and baby need not be separated)

- Susceptible persons at high risk of developing severe varicella should be given VZIG (see Table 10.10 and Table 10.11.). Administration of VZIG to healthy, nonpregnant, susceptible adults after varicella exposure is not routinely recommended (AAP, 1997).

- Infants born to mothers who develop varicella between 5 days before and 2 days after delivery should receive 125 units of VZIG IM as soon as possible after delivery (AAP, 1997).

▶ Premature neonates (i.e., born at less than 28 weeks' gestation) who are exposed to varicella postnatally should also receive 125 units of VZIG, regardless of maternal history (AAP & ACOG, 1997).

▶ Antiviral therapy with acyclovir has been employed to treat severe varicella infection in the neonate (Sterner et al., 1990). The pediatrician will dictate neonatal care.

- VZIG is not indicated for the infant of a mother with herpes zoster infection, unless zoster occurred in mother on day of delivery in which case it may be considered (Prober, Gershon, Grose, McCracken, & Nelson, 1990).

NOTE: A gravida with appearance of herpes zoster within 7 days before term is potentially contagious and precautions should be taken to prevent transmission; if zoster appears more than 7 days prior to labor and the lesions are crusted, risk for transmission is small (Sterner et al., 1996).

Consultation

- Consult with a physician in instances where mother has been exposed to varicella and is nonimmune.

- Depending on site-specific practices, patient with primary varicella or herpes zoster may be managed by an obstetrician or perinatologist.

- Eye involvement in herpes zoster requires ophthalmologic referral.

- Patients with evidence of serious complications or disseminated disease infection should be admitted to the hospital and managed by a physician.

- Refer client to a genetic counselor for consultation if exposure to varicella has occurred or if there is evidence of congenital varicella syndrome.

- Consult with facility's employee health/infection control services, if indicated, regarding prevention measures, isolation policies, and immunization practices.

Patient Education

- Counsel women who are nonimmune to varicella to avoid contact with individuals with chickenpox and direct contact with the vesicular fluid of shingles; possible exposures should be reported promptly to the health care provider.

- Discuss the nature of varicella infection, including transmission, infectivity, clinical course, complications, and treatment measures.

- Discuss the incidence of congenital varicella syndrome and emphasize that this is not a frequent complication. Client education may also be done by the physician involved in her care.

- If a nonimmune gravida has been exposed to chickenpox

  ▶ Discuss the diagnostic testing involved.

  ▶ Stress the importance of timing in administration of VZIG (within 96 hours of exposure).

  ▶ Emphasize that passive immunization does not reliably prevent infection, and that it is unknown whether VZIG will prevent development of congenital varicella syndrome; rather, VZIG administration is aimed at modifying maternal disease severity (Prober et al., 1990).

    – If an injection fee is charged, the client should be informed of the cost.

    – Advise the client of possible reactions to the injection:

      * Local pain and swelling

      * Constitutional symptoms

      * Anaphylaxis (rarely)

- See the Treatment/Management section.

Follow-up

- Monitor woman closely for evidence of complications of primary varicella or dissemination of herpes zoster infection; hospitalization is warranted in these cases for intravenous antiviral medication. Specifics regarding intravenous therapy and inpatient management are beyond the scope of this chapter. Patient will be managed by a physician.

- Refer to psychosocial, social, or other support services, if indicated, in cases where it is known that the patient will deliver an infant with congenital varicella syndrome.

- Long-term pediatric follow-up (including ophthalmologic evaluation) is indicated for the infant with evidence of congenital varicella infection.

- Infants born with abnormalities after maternal herpes zoster infection should be investigated for evidence of congenital varicella infection; other causes for the defects should also be sought (Enders et al., 1994).

- Regarding vaccine

  ▶ Varicella virus live vaccine (VARIVAX®) is indicated for active immunization against varicella virus in susceptible individuals 12 months of age and older.

  ▶ Susceptible children may receive one dose of the vaccine at any visit after the first birthday.

  ▶ Those individuals who lack a reliable history of chickenpox and were not previously vaccinated should receive a "catch-up" vaccination during the 11- to 12-year-old visit.

  ▶ Persons 13 years of age or older should receive two doses of the vaccine at least 1 month apart if they were not previously immunized or they lack a history of varicella infection (AAP, 1997; American Academy of Pediatrics, Committee on Infectious Diseases, 1997).

  NOTE: Prescreening for varicella immunity prior to administration of the vaccine in healthy adolescents and adults is optional. Vaccine is not indicated if seropositivity is determined. Simultaneous administration of varicella vaccine with other vaccines is acceptable; however, varicella vaccine should not be given for at least 5 months after administration of immune globulin (including VZIG), blood products, or plasma transfusions. See drug package insert for further information.

  ▶ The vaccine is contraindicated in pregnancy, and pregnancy should be avoided for 3 months following vaccination.

  NOTE: A VARIVAX Pregnancy Registry has been established to monitor maternal-fetal outcomes of women inadvertently given the vaccine 3 months before or during pregnancy. Report cases to 1-800-986-8999.

- Follow-up of VZIG recipients for varicella immunity should be undertaken by the individual's primary health care provider.

- Susceptible staff members exposed to patients with chickenpox or shingles should consult with their facility's employee health/infection control services immediately. See also Table 10.9.

- Document exposure to varicella during pregnancy and status of varicella immunity on problem list and in progress notes. Note administration of VZIG, as indicated. Also document presence of maternal/fetal varicella infection clearly.

Table 10.9

Guidelines for Preventive Measures After Exposure to Chickenpox in Nursery/Maternity Service

Type of Exposure/Disease	Chickenpox lesions present Mother	Neonate	Disposition
A. Siblings at home have active chickenpox when neonate & mother ready for discharge	No	No	1. Mother: if hx of chickenpox, may return home. If no hx she should be tested for VZV antibody.[a] If test positive, may go home; if test negative VZIG[b] is given and she is discharged home. 2. Neonate: may be sent home with mother if mother has hx of varicella or is VZV antibody-positive. If mother susceptible, give VZIG to infant and send home or place in protective isolation.
B. Mother with no history of chickenpox; exposed during period 6–20 days antepartum[d]	No	No	1. Exposed mother and infant: send home at earliest date unless siblings at home have communicable chickenpox.[c] If so, may give VZIG and discharge home as above. 2. Other mothers and infants: no special management indicated. 3. Hospital personnel: no precautions indicated if there is hx of previous chickenpox/zoster. In absence of hx, immediate serologic testing is indicated to determine immune status.[a] Nonimmune personnel should be excluded from pt. contact until 21 days after an exposure. 4. If mother develops varicella 1–2 days postpartum, infant should be given VZIG.
C. Onset of maternal chickenpox ante or postpartum[d]	Yes	No	1. Infected mother: isolate until no longer clinically infectious. If seriously ill, treat with acyclovir (see text). 2. Infected mother's infant: give VZIG[b] to neonates born to mothers with onset of chickenpox < 5 days before delivery and isolate separately from mother. **Send home with mother if no lesions develop by the time mother is noninfectious.** 3. Other mothers and infants: send home at earliest date. VZIG may be given to exposed neonates. 4. Hospital personnel: same as B-3.
D. Onset of maternal chickenpox antepartum[c]			1. Mother: isolation unnecessary. 2. Infant: isolate from other infants but not from mother. 3. Other mothers and infants: same as C-3 (if exposed). 4. Hospital personnel: same as B-3 (if exposed).
E. Congenital chickenpox	No	Yes	1. Infected infant and its mother: same as D-1 and 2. 2. Other mothers and infants: same as C-3. 3. Hospital personnel: same as B-3.

[a] Send serum to virus diagnostic laboratory for determination of antibodies to VZV by a sensitive technique such as FAMA, LA, or ELISA. Personnel may continue to work for 8 days after exposure pending serologic results because they are not potentially infectious during this period. Antibodies to VZV >1:4 probably are indicative of immunity.

[b] VZIG is available through the American Red Cross. The dose for a newborn is 1.25 mL (1 vial). The dose for a pregnant woman is conventionally 6.25 mL (5 vials).

[c] Considered noninfectious when no new vesicles have appeared for 72 hours and all lesions have crusted.

[d] If exposure occurred < 6 days antepartum, mother would not be potentially infectious until at least 72 hours postpartum.

Source: From "Chickenpox, measles and mumps," by A. A. Gershon. In J.S. Remington & J.O. Klein (Eds.), *Infectious diseases of the fetus and newborn infant* (4th ed., p. 590). Copyright 1995 by W.B. Saunders. Adapted with permission.

Table 10.10
Types of Exposure to Varicella or Zoster for Which VZIG is Indicated[*,†]

- Household: Residing in the same household.

- Playmate: Face-to-face[‡] indoor play.

- Hospital:
  Varicella:
  a) In same 2- to 4-bed room, or adjacent beds in a large ward,
  b) Face-to-face[‡] contact with an infectious staff member or patient, or
  c) Visit by a person deemed contagious.

  Zoster: Intimate contact (e.g., touching or hugging) with a person deemed contagious.

- Newborn infant: Onset of varicella in the mother 5 days or less before delivery or within 48 hours after delivery. VZIG is not indicated if the mother has zoster.

[*] Patients should meet criteria of both significant exposure and candidacy for receiving VZIG, as given in Table 10.11.
[†] VZIG should be administered within 96 hours (preferable sooner) after exposure.
[‡] Experts differ in the duration of face-to-face contact that warrants the administration of VZIG. However, the contact should be nontransient. Some experts suggest a contact of 5 or more minutes as constituting significant exposure for this purpose; others define close contact as more than 1 hour.

Table 10.11

Candidates for VZIG, Provided Significant Exposure[*] Has Occurred

- Immunocompromised children without history of chickenpox.[†]

- Susceptible, pregnant women.

- Newborn infant whose mother had onset of chickenpox within the 5 days before delivery or within the 48 hours after delivery.

- Hospitalized premature infant ($\geq$28 weeks' gestation) whose mother has no history of chickenpox.

- Hospitalized premature infants (<28 weeks' gestation or $\leq$1000 grams), regardless of maternal history.

[*]   See Table 10.10

[†] Immunocompromised adolescents and adults are likely to be immune, but if susceptible, they should also receive VZIG.

Source: From "Varicella-zoster infections," by the American Academy of Pediatrics, Committee on Infectious Diseases. *1994 Red book: Report of the Committee on Infectious Diseases* (23rd ed., pp. 514–515), Copyright 1994 by the American Academy of Pediatrics. Reprinted with permission.

Figure 10.9

Varicella Exposure in Pregnancy

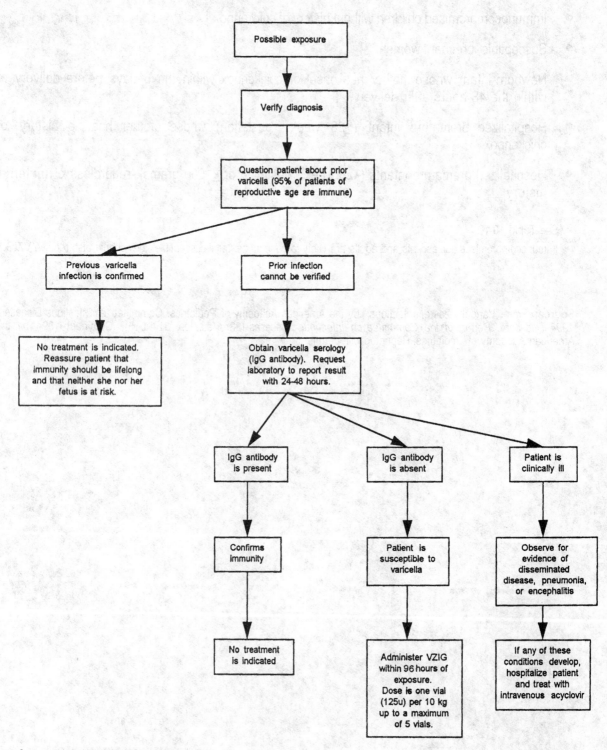

References

Alkalay, A L., Pomerance, J.J., & Rimoin, D.L. (1987). Fetal varicella syndrome. *Journal of Pediatrics, 111*, 320–323.

American Academy of Pediatrics (AAP). (1994). *1994 Red book: Report of the Committee on Infectious Diseases* (23rd ed., pp. 511–517). Elk Grove, IL: Author.

American Academy of Pediatrics (AAP). (1997). *1997 Red book: Report of the Committee on Infectious Diseases* (24th ed., pp. 573–585). Elk Grove, IL: Author.

American Academy of Pediatrics, Committee on Infectious Diseases. (1997). Recommended childhood immunization schedule—United States, January–December 1997. *Pediatrics, 99*(1), 136–137.

American Academy of Pediatrics (AAP) and the American College of Obstetricians and Gynecologists (ACOG). (1997). *Guidelines for perinatal care* (4th ed.; pp. 226–227). Elk Grove, IL: Author.

American College of Obstetricians and Gynecologists (ACOG). (1993). *Perinatal viral and parasitic infections.* (Technical Bulletin No. 177). Washington, DC: Author.

Brunell, P.A. (1992). Varicella in pregnancy, the fetus, and the newborn: Problems in management. *The Journal of Infectious Diseases, 166*(Suppl. 1), S42–S47.

Chapman, C., & Duff, P. (1993). Varicella in pregnancy. *Seminars in Perinatology, 17*(6), 401–409.

Enders, G., Miller, E., Cradock-Watson, J., & Ridehalgh, M. (1994). Consequences of varicella and herpes zoster in pregnancy: prospective study of 1,739 cases. *The Lancet, 343*, 1547–1550.

Freij, B.J., & Sever, J.L. (1995). Chickenpox and shingles susceptibility. *Contemporary OB/GYN, 40*(4), 66–74.

Gershon, A.A. (1988). Chickenpox: How dangerous is it? *Contemporary Ob/Gyn, 31*(3), 41–56.

Gershon, A.A. (1995). Chickenpox, measles and mumps. In J.S. Remington & J.O. Klein (Eds.), *Infectious diseases of the fetus and newborn infant* (4th ed., pp. 565–618). Philadelphia, PA: W.B. Saunders.

Gershon, A.A., Steinberg, S., Gelb, S., and the National Institute of Allergy and Infectious Diseases Collaborative Varicella Vaccine Study Group. (1984). Clinical reinfection with varicella zoster virus. *Journal of Infectious Diseases, 149*(2), 137–142.

Gibbs, R.S., & Sweet, R.L. (1994). Clinical disorders. In R.K. Creasy & R. Resnik (Eds.), *Maternal-fetal medicine. Principles and practice* (3rd ed., pp. 664–666). Philadelphia, PA: W.B. Saunders.

Ghidini, A., & Lynch, L. (1993). Prenatal diagnosis and significance of fetal infections. *Western Journal of Medicine, 159*, 366–373.

Hashmey, R., & Shandera, W.X. (1996). Infectious diseases: Viral and rickettsial. In L.M. Tierney, Jr., S.J. McPhee, & M.A. Papadakis (Eds.), *Current medical diagnosis and treatment* (35th ed., pp. 1161–1163). Stamford, CT: Appleton & Lange.

Kaiser Permanente Northern California. *New Drug Briefs*. (1995). Internal Document.

Lécuru, F., Taurelle, R., Bernard, J.-P., Parrat, S., Lafay-pillet, M.-C., Rozenberg, F., Lebon, P., & Dommergues, M. (1994). Varicella zoster virus infection during pregnancy: the limits of prenatal diagnosis. *European Journal of Obstetrics & Gynecology, 56*, 67–68.

Martin, K.A., Junker, A.K., Thomas, E. E., Van Allen, M.I., & Friedman, J.M. (1994). *The Journal of Infectious Diseases, 170*, 991–995.

Merck & Company. (1996). *Varivax®* [Varicella virus vaccine live (Oka/Merck)]. Drug package insert. West Point, PA: Merck Vaccine Division.

Michie, C.A., Acolet, D., Charlton, R., Stevens, J.P., Happerfield, L.C., Bobrow, L.G., Kangro, H., Gau, G., & Modi, N. (1992). Varicella-zoster contracted in the second trimester of pregnancy. *Pediatric Infectious Disease Journal, 11*, 1050–1053.

Northern California Kaiser Permanente Varicella Vaccine Consensus Guidelines. (1995). As contained in *New Drug Briefs*. Kaiser Permanente Northern California. Internal document.

Paryani, S.G., & Arvin, A.M. (1986). Intrauterine infection with varicella-zoster virus after maternal varicella. *New England Journal of Medicine, 314*, 1542–1546.

Pastuszak, A.L., Levy, M., Schick, B., Zuber, C., Feldkamp, M., Gladstone, J., Bar-Levy, F., Jackson, E., Donnenfeld, A., Meschino, W., & Koren, G. (1994). Outcome after maternal varicella infection in the first 20 weeks of pregnancy. *New England Journal of Medicine, 330*, 901–905.

Prober, C.G., Gershon, A.A., Grose, C., McCracken, G.H., & Nelson, J.D. (1990). Consensus: Varicella-zoster infections in pregnancy and the perinatal period. *Pediatric Infectious Disease Journal, 9*(12), 865–869.

Russell, L.K. (1992). Management of varicella-zoster virus infection during pregnancy and the peripartum. *Journal of Nurse-Midwifery, 37*(1), 17–24.

Shannon, M.T. (1995). Varicella zoster virus. In W.L. Star, L.L. Lommel, & M.T. Shannon (Eds.), *Women's primary health care: Protocols for practice* (pp. 11–58, 11–63. Washington, DC: American Nurses Publishing.

Smego, R.A., & Asperilla, M.O. (1991). Use of acyclovir for varicella pneumonia during pregnancy. *Obstetrics & Gynecology, 78*(6), 1112–1116.

Sterner, G., Forsgren, M., Enockkson, E., Grandien, & Granström, G. (1990). Varicella-zoster infections in late pregnancy. *Scandinavian Journal of Infectious Diseases, Suppl. 71*, 30–35.

SECTION 11

RESPIRATORY CONDITIONS

Chapter 1

ASTHMA

Maureen T. Shannon

Asthma is a chronic inflammatory disorder of the airways that causes recurrent episodes of airway obstruction in response to a variety of inhaled irritants, including allergens, respiratory viruses, and some occupational exposures. The episodes are usually associated with airflow obstruction that often reverses either spontaneously or with treatment (National Institutes of Health [NIH], 1997). Some individuals experience symptoms principally following exercise (exercise induced bronchospasm). Others experience the majority of symptoms during sleep (nocturnal asthma). Asthma occurs in individuals with genetic predispositions; many individuals have family members with asthma or other atopic disorders, such as allergic rhinitis or eczema.

An asthma exacerbation occurs when the individual's airway is exposed to a triggering agent or antigen. This trigger causes an inflammatory response involving mast cells, eosinophils, T-lymphocytes, macrophages, neutrophils, and epithelial cells. Histamine and leukotrienes from the mast cell produce bronchoconstriction of smooth muscle. The above inflammatory sequence results in smooth muscle contraction (bronchospasm), edema, and excess mucus production and plugging of the airways. The narrowing of small airways can then lead to air trapping, hypoxemia, carbon dioxide (CO_2) retention, increasing pulmonary vascular resistance, and negative pleural pressure (American College of Obstetricians and Gynecologists (ACOG), 1996; Mabie, 1996; NIH, 1991). These physiologic processes are responsible for the clinical symptoms commonly observed in individuals with asthma, specifically wheezing, chest tightness, shortness of breath and coughing, and can lead to progressive use of accessory muscles, pulsus paradoxus, and respiratory failure.

Asthma is currently classified as one of four types: mild intermittent, mild persistent, moderate persistent, and severe persistent. Clinical characteristics and lung function measurements are used to determine an individual's classification, which in turn determines a specific type of therapy. The current classification system is described in Figures 11.1 through 11.4.

In 1991, there were over 8.8 million office visits for asthma making it the tenth ranking medical diagnosis in the United States (Schappert, 1993); it currently affects over 14 million persons in the United States, with death rates highest for 15- to 24-year-old African-Americans (NIH, 1997). Although asthma mortality has increased during the past decade, it is still uncommon (Weiss & Wagener, 1990) with 5,000 deaths annually (NIH, 1997). Asthma-related deaths may, in fact, be a result of underestimation of the severity of the disease on the part of the affected individual and the clinician, causing a delay in the initiation of or an underutilization of appropriate therapy. In addition, certain risk factors have been associated with an increased possibility of death due to asthma:

- Age (increased rates are observed in 5 to 34 year olds)

- Ethnicity (blacks are twice as likely to die as Caucasians)

- History of previous life-threatening acute asthma exacerbation (e.g., intubation, respiratory failure)

- History of hospital admission for asthma during the past year

- Inadequate medical treatment for the severity of disease

- Lack of access to medical care

- Psychological/psychosocial problems (Clark, et al., 1993)

Up to 4 percent of pregnancies are complicated by asthma; but the actual incidence may be higher, since 10 percent of the U.S. population has nonspecific airway hyperresponsiveness. The effect of pregnancy on the course of asthma varies among women; 30 percent of women experience an increase in severity, 30 percent a decrease in severity, and the rest no change in disease symptoms (ACOG, 1996; NIH, 1991). The time when symptoms are most severe during pregnancy is between 29 and 36 weeks' gestation; symptoms are noticeably less severe during the last 4 weeks of pregnancy. During intrapartum, approximately 10 percent of women with asthma experience wheezing; however, the majority of women respond to inhalation treatment with a bronchodilator (NIH, 1991). By 3 months postpartum, a woman's symptoms usually return to her prepregnancy level of severity (NIH, 1991).

In general, well-controlled asthma during pregnancy is not associated with adverse perinatal outcomes. However, pregnant women with poorly controlled asthma have an increased incidence of prematurity, low birth weight (LBW), preeclampsia, and perinatal mortality (ACOG, 1996). Exacerbation of asthma during pregnancy can result in a reduction in maternal partial pressure of oxygen (PO_2) leading to maternal hypoxia, hypercapnia and alkalosis. Such a decrease in maternal pulmonary function has been correlated with decreased fetal oxygenation and the development of fetal hypoxia. Asymmetrical fetal growth restriction has also been reported in infants born to women with severe asthma (Clark et al, 1993). Therefore, close monitoring of maternal pulmonary function and response to treatment is necessary to prevent adverse fetal consequences. Treatment strategies include the following:

- Objective evaluation of maternal pulmonary function and fetal well-being

- Avoidance or control of environmental precipitation factors

- Pharmacologic interventions

- Patient education (Clark et al., 1993; NIH, 1991)

Because asthma is such a widespread chronic disease with acute exacerbations that cause considerable patient dysfunction and extensive use of health care services, the National Heart, Lung and Blood Institute of the NIH created the National Asthma Education Program (NAEP) that has developed Guidelines for the Diagnosis and Management of Asthma (NIH, 1997). Many of the guidelines have been incorporated into this chapter, which presents the care plan for pregnant women with mild intermittent, persistent, and moderate persistent asthma. The care of a pregnant woman with severe asthma or disease that is unresponsive to appropriate therapy is beyond the scope of this text. A pregnant woman with severe asthma should be referred to a physician for evaluation and treatment.

Database

Subjective

- The woman may report any of the following predisposing factors (NIH, 1991, 1997):
  ▶ Family or personal history of asthma, allergic rhinitis, eczema
  ▶ History of other allergic disorders (e.g., allergic rhinitis, sinusitis, atopic dermatitis, nasal polyposis)
  ▶ History of lower respiratory infections in childhood (e.g., bronchitis, pneumonia)

- ▶ Passive exposure to smoke (tobacco or wood)

- ▶ Smoking

- ▶ Environmental/occupational exposure to allergens, pets, house dust mites, mold

- ▶ Environmental/occupational exposure to chemicals/pollutants/irritants (e.g., aerosols, perfumes, detergents, construction, fumigation)

- ▶ Medications (i.e., history of use of drugs associated with asthma, such as aspirin, nonsteroidal anti-inflammatory [NSAID] agents, beta-blockers)

- ▶ Food/beverage additives (e.g., sulfites)

- ▶ Weather (temperature) change

- ▶ History of exacerbation of symptoms with exercise or at night

- ▶ Endocrine factors (e.g., thyroid disease)

- ▶ Age of initial diagnosis of asthma

- ▶ Symptoms occurring or worsening during menses

- ▶ Symptoms occurring or worsening during strong emotional expression (laughing, crying)

- ● The woman may report one or more of the following symptoms (Clark et. al, 1993; Mabie, 1996; NIH, 1991, 1997; Shannon, 1995):

- ▶ Wheezing

- ▶ Chest tightness

- ▶ Shortness of breath

- ▶ Daytime cough

- ▶ Nighttime cough

- ▶ Sputum production (usually clear; may be scant to copious in amount)

- ▶ Activity limitation

- ▶ Fever

- ▶ Chest pain

- ▶ Lethargy

- ▶ Anxiety

- ▶ Confusion

- ▶ Palpitations

NOTE: When assessing the woman's symptoms, it is important to determine the following: onset of symptoms, duration of symptoms, pattern of symptoms (e.g., episodic, continuous symptoms with intermittent exacerbations), course of disease, treatment(s) that relieved symptoms, aggravating factors or seasonal variations, and any use of medical services (e.g., hospital, emergency room, or urgent care clinic).

Objective

- During an exacerbation, the physical examination may reveal the following (Mays & Leiner, 1995; NIH, 1991; NIH, 1997; Shannon, 1995):
  - ▶ Vital signs
    - Temperature elevation may be present (if coexistent pulmonary infection).
    - Increased pulse and respirations may be observed.
    - Blood pressure may reveal pulsus paradoxus (i.e., a fall of more than 12 mm Hg in the systolic pressure during inspiration. This is usually observed during severe asthma exacerbations).
  - ▶ General appearance
    - The woman may appear fatigued, lethargic, disoriented, and/or breathless when attempting to talk (indicates severe asthma with respiratory arrest imminent) (Mays & Leiner, 1995).
    - Use of accessory muscles of respiration (e.g., chest, neck abdomen) may be observed.
    - The woman may be in a hunched posture while breathing.
    - Neck vein distention may be evident.
  - ▶ Skin examination
    - Cyanosis
    - Evidence of eczema/atopic dermatitis or other allergic manifestation
  - ▶ HEENT examination
    - Nasal erythema, edema (if coexistent rhinitis)
    - Purulent nasal discharge (if coexistent sinusitis)
    - Nasal polyp(s)
  - ▶ Physical examination of the chest
    - Stridor
    - Pigeon chest or hyperexpansion of the thorax
    - Hollowness to chest wall percussion.
  - ▶ Auscultation of chest
    - Decreased intensity of breath sounds
    - Prolonged phase of forced expiration (typical for airflow obstruction)
    - Wheezing (this finding is not a reliable indicator of severity of disease [NIH, 1997])
    - Inspiratory crackles
    - Inspiratory or expiratory rhonchi

▶ Auscultation of the heart

   – Cardiac gallop

   – Increased P_2

▶ Abdominal examination may reveal fundal height less than expected for dates (if coexistent intrauterine growth restriction [IUGR]).

Assessment

● Asthma

  ▶ R/O chronic bronchitis

  ▶ R/O emphysema

  ▶ R/O laryngeal or vocal cord dysfunction

  ▶ R/O congestive heart failure

  ▶ R/O imminent respiratory failure

  ▶ R/O Drug reaction (e.g., beta-blockers)

  ▶ R/O IUGR

  ▶ R/O acute inhalation of irritating substance

  ▶ R/O mechanical obstruction of airway

  ▶ R/O pulmonary embolism

  ▶ R/O pulmonary infiltration with eosinophilia

  ▶ R/O cough secondary to drugs (angiotensin-converting enzyme [ACE] inhibitors)

Plan

Diagnostic Tests

● Perform objective measures of lung function on all women to establish a diagnosis, monitor progress, and judge severity during acute exacerbations of asthma.

NOTE: It is important to use objective measures of lung function because a woman's history and physical examination findings may not correlate with the severity of air flow obstruction (Clark et. al, 1993; NIH, 1997; Rivo & Malveaux, 1992).

● Order the following tests to ascertain the pulmonary function of the woman (See Table 11.1, Normal Pulmonary Values in Pregnant and Nonpregnant Women):

  ▶ Spirometry. Spirometry is widely utilized, although this type of equipment is not frequently found in most primary care offices. Airway obstruction impacts flow rates and produces changes in the forced vital capacity (FVC), forced expiratory volume in one second (FEV_1), and the maximum midexpiratory flow rate (MMEF). In asthma, an obstructive pattern will be demonstrated.

▶ Peak Expiratory Flow Rate (PEFR). Peak expiratory flow rate meters are widely available as small office equipment or inexpensive (approximately $30) plastic, portable models. These meters measure PEFR, which correlates well with FEV_1. Asthma reduces PEFR and FEV_1. PEFR values determine early signs of exacerbation, assess response to therapy, and document circadian variation in the disease.

NOTE: Predicted values are between 380 and 550 L/minute for women, and these values do not change as a result of pregnancy. However, a "personal best" is determined for each individual at a time when asthma has been well controlled. Adjustments in asthma therapy are based on the percent of the woman's personal best (NIH, 1997). In moderate to severe asthma, PEFR should be obtained twice a day (12 hours apart). The best value is usually observed at night after the woman has had treatment(s) during the day (Clark et al., 1993). Reversibility of hyperresponsiveness is defined as a minimum of 15 percent increase in PEFR or FEV_1 after two puffs of a $beta_2$ agonist inhaler (Mabie, 1996).

● Depending on clinical history and physical examination, the following additional tests may be ordered:

▶ Chest x-ray. A chest x-ray should be ordered to rule out pneumonia in a febrile woman, if other obstructive phenomena are suspected, to assess other cardiopulmonary disease, or to assess the presence of pneumothorax or atelectasis in an acutely ill woman.

▶ Sputum for gram stain. Stain may demonstrate the presence of eosinophils (characteristic of asthma), or neutrophils (if coexistent bronchitis).

▶ Sputum specimen for culture and sensitivity. Culture may reveal organisms indicative of pneumonia (if there is coexistent pulmonary infection).

▶ Complete blood count (CBC). CBC may reveal eosinophilia (indicative of an allergic component) or leukocytosis (if a coexistent pulmonary infection).

▶ Skin testing to determine hypersensitivity to specific allergens. Skin test may be positive for a particular antigen.

▶ Nasal secretions smear. Smear may demonstrate eosinophils (indicative of an allergic component) or neutrophils (if there is coexistent sinusitis).

▶ Serum theophylline level. This is used as a baseline or to evaluate therapeutic levels in a woman using theophylline for symptom relief.

NOTE: The therapeutic range for a theophylline level during pregnancy is 8–12 μg/mL.

● In acute exacerbations of asthma with moderate to severe symptoms the following tests may be ordered after consultation with a physician (ACOG, 1996; Mabie, 1996; Mays & Leiner, 1995; NIH, 1991):

▶ Oxygen saturation (will be decreased)

NOTE: A pregnant woman with an oxygen saturation of 95 percent or less needs intensive, stepped-up therapy and may require hospitalization for observation to assess response to treatment.

▶ Blood gases

− The normal blood gas values for a pregnant women are a pH 7.4, a PO_2 of 100–105 mm Hg, and a PCO_2 of 30 mm Hg (ACOG, 1996).

- Partial pressure of oxygen (PO_2) will be decreased (if the PO_2 is less than 70 mm Hg hospitalization is indicated).

- Partial pressure of carbon dioxide (PCO_2) will be increased in severe asthma episodes (i.e., *more than* 35 mm Hg); normal or low in mild to moderate asthma (because of hyperventilation).

- pH will be reduced.

NOTE : Although some sources recommend arterial blood gas measurement (NIH, 1991), this test is technically difficult outside the hospital setting and is accompanied by more complications than using transcutaneous oxygen saturation with a digital pulse oximeter (Holmgren & Sixt, 1992). Elevations in PCO_2 will also be lower than corresponding arterial values (Holmgren & Sixt, 1992).

- Obtain obstetrical ultrasound in all asthmatic women to accurately determine gestational age, or in a woman with fundal height that is less than expected for weeks of gestation to rule out IUGR. Obtain serial ultrasounds (every 2 to 4 weeks) if IUGR is documented.

Treatment/Management

- A wide variety of treatment strategies are available to control asthma. The more severe, frequent or disabling the symptoms, the greater the combination and dosages of medications. Tailoring the medication regimen to allow maximum functioning with the minimum of symptoms and medication side effects for the woman is the goal of individualized management (see Figures 11.1 through 11.5).

- The following are *general* guidelines for environmental control approached in a "stepwise" fashion for asthma therapy (Clark et al., 1993, Mabie, 1996; Mays & Leiner, 1995; NIH, 1997; Shannon, 1995). See Table 11.2.

  ▶ Environmental control should be individualized and based on the woman's history of allergic/irritant exposure.

    - Outdoor measures

      * Avoid unnecessarily heavy exposure to outdoor allergens (e.g., pollens, ragweed, molds).

      * Avoid activities that may increase symptoms (e.g., mowing the lawn).

    - Indoor measures

      * Keep the house as clean as possible, especially the bedroom.

      * Wear a mask when vacuuming and use special vacuums with HEPA filters.

      * Pets should sleep outdoors, or if not possible, in areas where the woman has limited exposure to animal hair, fur, and dander.

      * Maintain low humidity to inhibit growth of mold and mildew.

      * Encase mattresses and pillows in plastic covers.

      * Wash bedding every week in water with a temperature of *at least* 130°F.

* Limitation of exposure to rugs, upholstered furniture, and stuffed animals especially in the bedroom.

* Remove carpets on concrete if possible.

● The following are general guidelines for pharmacologic interventions approached in a stepwise fashion (Clark et al., 1993, Mabie, 1996; Mays & Leiner, 1995; NIH, 1997; Shannon, 1995).

NOTE: The risks associated with uncontrolled asthma during pregnancy (especially placental hypoxemia) require that aggressive pharmacologic therapies are initiated and adjusted to attain optimal maternal pulmonary function. Limited studies have not reported an increased incidence of congenital anomalies in association with the use of inhaled anti-inflammatory agents, or inhaled beta-adrenergic agonists (NIH, 1991).

▶ In general, the drugs that should be avoided during pregnancy include alpha adrenergic agents, epinephrine, quinolones, tetracyclines, and sulfonamides (Mabie, 1996). Refer to Figures 11.1, 11.2, 11.3, 11.4, and 11.5 for the treatment algorithms, Tables 11.4 and 11.5 for the classification of pharmacologic agents, and Table 11.6 for the doses used in pregnancy.

NOTE: Any woman exhibiting severe symptoms, a PEFR less than 60 percent of baseline, or symptoms that persist after appropriate therapy needs an immediate evaluation by an asthma specialist.

– Exercise-induced asthma (EIB)

* Use two puffs of short acting $beta_2$ agonist immediately prior to exercise; repeat p.r.n. if exercise continues for 2 hours or more (to prevent symptom development).

* If symptoms are experienced during exercise after the above regimen, then administer two puffs of $beta_2$ agonist. Future preexercise treatment should then include four puffs of a $beta_2$ agonist or cromolyn sodium, *or* two puffs of a $beta_2$ agonist plus two puffs of cromolyn sodium.

* Using salmeterol has been shown to prevent EIB for 10 to 12 hours.

* Cromolyn and nedocromil (2 puffs), shortly before exercise also prevent EIB.

– Nocturnal asthma

* Two puffs of inhaled $beta_2$ agonist (e.g., albuterol) at bedtime may relieve symptoms (Jenne, 1984).

* Sustained release theophylline 200 mg p.o. taken between 6:00 PM and 8:00 PM may also relieve symptoms (Arkinstall, 1987; Clark et al., 1993). The dose of theophylline should be adjusted to attain serum levels between 8 to 12 μg/mL (ACOG, 1996).

NOTE: In a woman with primarily nocturnal symptoms, consider an evaluation to rule out the possibility of gastroesophageal reflux. Women with symptoms ≤ twice weekly, with nighttime symptoms ≤ twice monthly, who are asymptomatic between exacerbations and have FEV, or PEF ≥ 80 percent predicted are classified with mild intermittent asthma. No daily medication is needed; only treatment for quick relief.

- Mild intermittent asthma

  * The use of beta$_2$ agonists alone is recommended because these agents have a faster onset of action, fewer adverse side effects, and achieve desired results at lower doses than oral medications.

  * If the symptoms resolve and pulmonary function tests (i.e., PEFR) normalize with the use of these medications, the woman may use this therapy indefinitely for the treatment of mild intermittent exacerbations (ACOG, 1996; Clark et. al., 1993; Mabie, 1996; Rivo & Malveaux, 1992). The use of more than one canister in 1 month indicates inadequate control and a need to alter therapy (NIH, 1997).

  * One of the following short-acting beta$_2$-agonists may be prescribed as two puffs prior to trigger exposure and/or t.i.d.-q.i.d. as needed during the acute exacerbation:

    • Albuterol

    • Albuterol hfa

    • Bitolterol

    • Pirbuterol

    • Terbutaline

    NOTE: The need to use an inhaler 3 or more times a week necessitates further evaluation to eliminate the possibility of worsening disease. Additional therapy may be required based on this evaluation (ACOG, 1996; Clark et al, 1993; Mabie, 1996).

- Mild persistent asthma.

  * Women with symptoms more than twice but less than seven times weekly or more than twice monthly nighttime symptoms or PEF variability of 20 to 30 percent with PEF $\geq$ 80 percent predicted are classified with mild persistent asthma. These women should be prescribed daily anti-inflammatory medicine (NIH, 1997) for long-term control.

    • Beclomethasone (42 mcg/puff) 1 to 3 puffs, t.i.d. to q.i.d.

    • Budesonide turbuhaler one to two inhalations daily

    • Flunisolide two to four puffs daily

    • Fluticasone (six inhaled preparations available) two to six inhalations daily (preparation dependent)

    • Triamcinolone four to ten puffs daily

       or

    Cromolyn two to four puffs t.i.d.-q.i.d.

    • Nedocromil two to four puffs b.i.d.-q.i.d

  * Other alternative, but not preferred therapies include theopylline, zafirlukast, zileuton (NIH, 1997) or the newly FDA-approved (1998) montelukast.

    – <u>Moderate persistent asthma</u>

        * Women with daily symptoms, limited activity, or nighttime symptoms or PEF between 60–80 percent of normal are classified as having moderate persistent asthma.

        * Inhaled anti-inflammatory agents are the primary therapy for the treatment of moderate asthma. Inhaled anti-inflammatory agents inhibit several of the mediators of inflammation and may enhance response to inhaled bronchodilators.

        * The following anti-inflammatory agents may be used in pregnant women in moderate doses and added to the use of an inhaled beta$_2$ agonist (prescribed every 6 to 8 hours with total number of doses not to exceed three to four doses a day) (ACOG, 1996; Mabie, 1996):

          • Twelve to twenty puffs of beclomethasone (42 µg/puff) daily

             or

          Ten to twenty puffs of triamcinolone acetonide (100µg/puff) daily

             or

          Two to three inhalations of budesonide (200 µg/dose) daily

             or

          Four to eight puffs of flunisolide (250 µg/puff) daily

             or

          Two to six puffs of fluticasone (110 µg/puff) daily

          • If needed, a long acting inhaled beta$_2$ agonist, (salmeterol (21 µg/puff), 2 puffs every 12 hours, can be added

             or

          Sustained release theophylline 200 mg p.o. between 6:00 PM and 8:00 PM to control nocturnal symptoms. Adjust dose to attain serum level of 8 to 12 µg/mL (ACOG, 1996; Mabie, 1996).

        NOTE: A 4- to 6-week trial of these agents is necessary before effectiveness of the therapy can be determined. Beclomethasone is the preferred agent during pregnancy because there has been more human experience with this agent (Mabie, 1996). Side effects associated with the use of these medications include occasional coughing, dysphonia, and oral candidiasis. The use of a spacer device reduces the incidence of systemic effects and oral candidiasis, and enhances pulmonary tract penetration (Clark et al., 1993; Mabie, 1996; NIH, 1991).

▶ For women with inadequate responses to therapy (based on FEV$_1$ or PEFR measurements or persistence of symptoms) after using maximum dosages of inhaled beta$_2$ agonists (e.g., >20 putts beclomethasone [42 µg]), sustained release theophylline, and anti-inflammatory agents, a short course of oral corticosteroids should be prescribed. In such instances, consult with a physician prior to initiating the following short course regimen:

    – Prednisolone 40 mg/day (single or divided dose) for 7 days, then taper by decreasing dose by 5 mg/day (ACOG, 1996)

► Influenza immunization is recommended annually for pregnant women with moderate to severe asthma and should be administered after the first trimester whenever possible. (See Chapter 11.3, *Influenza*).

- The following are additional measures to be taken when a woman has asthma.

  ► Initiate fetal movement counts beginning at 28 weeks' gestation in all women

  ► Initiate antenatal fetal surveillance (e.g., nonstress tests [NSTs], amniotic fluid index [AFI], biophysical profile [BPP], contraction stress test [CST]) between 32 weeks' gestation in women with severe asthma and suspected or documented IUGR (ACOG, 1996; Mabie, 1996).

  ► If a woman smokes, advise her to stop. If she is exposed to passive smoke, discuss ways to eliminate this trigger (e. g., ventilation of room, request no smoking inside the home).

  ► Refer women exhibiting significant signs or symptoms of depression, anxiety, or other psychological sequelae associated with chronic disease to psychological evaluation and/or counseling, if indicated.

Consultation

- Consult with a physician if a woman exhibits moderate persistent to severe persistent asthma symptoms, has significant side effects associated with medications, or has documented or suspected IUGR.

- Consult with a physician if a woman has a history of multiple emergency room/hospital visits, symptoms that are atypical and raise questions about other diagnostic possibilities, less than optimal response to therapeutic interventions, complicating factors that require special care (e.g., nasal polyps), or other significant complications (e.g., pneumonia, suspected tension pneumothorax).

- Refer to an asthma specialist and transfer care to a perinatologist, if a woman has severe persistent asthma, moderate persistent asthma that is not responding adequately to therapy, or a history that places her at an increased risk of asthma associated mortality.

- Consult, as needed, for prescriptions.

Patient Education

- Educate the woman about asthma including the cause(s), clinical course, preventive measures, treatment options, possible complications, side effects of medications, and when and where to seek *immediate* medical care if/when asthma worsens.

- Educate the woman about the need to avoid triggering agents and prevent exacerbations or asthma.

- If the woman smokes, discuss the adverse maternal-fetal effects and the need to stop smoking. Refer the woman to community programs that are available for smoking cessation.

- Instruct the woman in the proper use of metered-dose inhalers (MDIs) and spacer devices for inhaled medications. Review the following instructions for the use MDIs with her (Rivo & Malveaux, 1992; Shannon, 1995)

  ▶ Make sure there is enough medicine in the canister. An easy way to determine this is to place the canister in a container of water: If it sinks to the bottom it is full, if it floats on the surface (sideways) it is empty.

  ▶ To use an inhaler refer to Figure 11.6.

- Educate the woman about the importance of adequate therapy to control her asthma. Provide information about medications, their proper use, possible side effects (maternal and fetal), and when to notify health care providers after initiating therapy (e.g., if expected response does not occur or for significant side effects).

- Reinforce the routine use of peak flow meters for the monitoring of pulmonary function.

- Educate the woman and her family regarding emergency measures that should be implemented (e.g., contacting emergency care providers if woman does not respond to therapy).

- Discuss the reason(s) for diagnostic tests that are being ordered (e.g., chest x-ray, obstetrical ultrasound, NST). Once results from tests are obtained, review these with the woman.

- Educate the woman about signs and symptoms of depression, anxiety or other emotional/psychological sequelae associated with chronic disease.

- If a woman is planning to breast-feed, discuss the effect(s) that taking medication(s) might have on her infant. Inhaled pharmacologic agents have low maternal serum levels and, therefore, the infant is exposed to insignificant amounts if breast-fed.

NOTE: Theophylline concentration in breast milk is approximately 1 percent of the maternal dose, a level substantially less than the standard dose that is prescribed for infants (NIH, 1991). Systemic corticosteroids are present in low concentrations in breast milk; however, infants born to women on corticosteroid therapy should be evaluated for adrenal insufficiency (Briggs, Freeman & Yaffe, 1994, NIH, 1991).

Follow-up

- See women with mild intermittent asthma every 3 to 4 weeks for prenatal care and review of pulmonary function measurements (e.g., PEFR values).

- See women with mild intermittent asthma as soon as possible for an evaluation if they experience persistent symptoms, that place her in the mild persistent category.

- Women with moderate persistent or severe persistent asthma should return for prenatal and pulmonary function evaluations per the recommendations of the consulting physician (perinatologist or asthma specialist).

- Women with an acute, severe exacerbation, or whose PEFR 70 percent or less of baseline should be seen immediately by the consulting physician or emergency department (i.e., labor and delivery or emergency room) for evaluation and treatment. Follow-up evaluations will be determined by the physician responsible for her care.

- Document the diagnosis of asthma and management thereof in the problem list and progress notes.

Table 11.1

Normal Pulmonary Values in Pregnant and Nonpregnant Women

Term	Definition	Values		Clinical Significance in Pregnancy
		Nonpregnant	**Pregnant**	
Tidal volume (V_T)	The amount of air moved in one normal respiratory cycle	450 mL	600 mL (increases up to 40%)	
Respiratory rate (RR)	Number of respirations per minute	16/min	Changes very little	
Minute ventilation	The volume of air moved per minute; product of RR and V_T	7.2 L	9.6 L (increased up to 40% because of the increase in V_T)	Increase oxygen available for the fetus
Forced expiratory volume in one second (FEV_1)		Approximately 80–85% of the vital capacity	Unchanged	Valuable to measure because there is no change due to pregnancy
Peak expiratory flow rate (PEFR)			Unchanged	Valuable to measure because there is no change due to pregnancy
Forced vital capacity (FVC)	The maximum amount of air that can be moved from maximum inspiration to maximum expiration	3.5 L	Unchanged	If over 1 L, pregnancy is usually well tolerated.
Residual volume (RV)	The amount of air that remains in the lung at the end of a maximal expiration	1,00 mL	Decreases by around 200 mL to around 800 mL	Improves gas transfer from alveoli to blood

Source: American College of Obstetricians and Gynecologists (1996). Pulmonary disease in pregnancy. *ACOG technical bulletin No. 224* (p.2). Washington, D.C.: the Author. Reprinted with permission

Table 11.2

Stepwise Approach for Managing Asthma in Adults and Children Older Than 5 Years of Age

Treatment		Preferred treatments are in bold print.	
	Long-term Control	Quick Relief	Education
STEP 4 **Severe** **Persistent**	Daily medications: • **Anti-inflammatory: inhaled cortico-steroid (high dose), AND** • Long-acting bronchodilator: either **long-acting inhaled beta$_2$-agonist**, sustained-release theophylline, or long-acting beta$_2$-agonist tablets, AND • Corticosteroid tables or syrup long term (2 mg/kg/day, generally do not exceed 60 mg per day).	• Short-acting bronchodilator: **inhaled beta$_2$-agonist** as needed for symptoms. • Intensity of treatment will depend on severity of exacerbation. • Use of a short-acting inhaled beta$_2$-agonist on a daily basis, or increasing use, indicates the need for additional long-term-control therapy.	Steps 2 and 3 actions plus: • Refer to individual education/counseling
STEP 3 **Moderate** **Persistent**	Daily medications: • Either Anti-inflammatory: **inhaled cortico-steroid (high dose), OR** Inhaled **corticosteroid (low-medium dose)** and add a long-acting bronchodilator, especially for nighttime symptoms: either **long-acting inhaled beta$_2$-agonist,** sustained-release theophylline, or long-acting beta$_2$-agonist tablets. • If needed Anti-inflammatory: **inhaled cortico-steroid (medium dose), AND** **Long-acting bronchodilator,** especially for nighttime symptoms: either **long-acting inhaled beta$_2$-agonist,** sustained-release theophylline, or long-acting beta$_2$-agonist tablets.	• Short-acting bronchodilator: **inhaled beta$_2$-agonist** as needed for symptoms. • Intensity of treatment will depend on severity of exacerbation: see component 3-Managing Exacerbations. • Use of a short-acting inhaled beta$_2$-agonist on a daily basis, or increasing use, indicates the need for additional long-term-control therapy.	
STEP 2 **Mild** **Persistent**	One daily medications: • **Anti-inflammatory:** either **inhaled cor-ticosteroid (low dose),** or **cromolyn or nedocromil.** • Sustained-release theophylline to serum concentration of 5-15 mcg/mL is an alternative, but not preferred, therapy. Zafirlukast or zileuton may also be considered for patients ≥12 years of age, although their position in therapy is not fully established.	• Short-acting bronchodilator: **inhaled beta$_2$-agonist** as needed for symptoms. • Intensity of treatment will depend on severity of exacerbation. • Use of a short-acting inhaled beta$_2$-agonist on a daily basis, or increasing use, indicates the need for additional long-term-control therapy.	Step 1 actions plus: • Teach self-monitoring • Refer to group education if available • Review and update self-management plan
STEP 1 **Mild** **Intermittent**	• No daily medication needed	• Short-acting bronchodilator: **inhaled beta$_2$-agonist** as needed for symptoms. • Intensity of treatment will depend on severity of exacerbation. • Use of a short-acting inhaled beta$_2$-agonist on a daily basis, or increasing use, indicates the need for additional long-term-control therapy.	• Teach basic facts about asthma • Teach inhaler/spacer/holding chamber techniques • Discuss roles of medication • Develop self-management plan • Develop action plan for when and how to take rescue actions, especially for patients with a history of severe exacerbations • Discuss appropriate environmental control measures to avoid exposure to know allergens and irritants

↓ **STEP DOWN:** Review treatment every 1 to 6 months; a gradual stepwise reduction in treatment may be possible.

↑ **STEP UP:** If control is not maintained, consider step up. First, review patient medication technique, adherence, and environmental control (avoidance of allergens or other factors that contribute to asthma severity).

NOTE:
• **The stepwise approach presents general guidelines to assist clinical decisionmaking; it is not intended to be a specific prescription. Asthma is highly variable; clinicians should tailor specific medication plans to the needs and circumstances of individual patients.**
• Gain control as quickly as possible; then decrease treatment to the least medication necessary to maintain control. Gaining control may be accomplished by either starting treatment at the step most appropriate to the initial severity of the condition or starting at a higher level of therapy (e.g., a course of systemic corticosteroids or higher dose of inhaled corticosteroids).
• A rescue course of systemic corticosteroids may be needed at any time and at any step.
• Some patients with intermittent asthma experience severe and life-threatening exacerbations separated by long periods of normal lung function and no symptoms. This may be especially common with exacerbations provoked by respiratory infections. A short course of systematic corticosteroids is recommended.
• At each step, patients should control their environment to avoid or control factors that make their asthma worse (e.g., allergens, irritants); this requires specific diagnosis and education.
• Referral to an asthma specialist for consultation or comanagment is recommended if there are difficulties achieving or maintaining control of asthma or if the patient requires step 4 care. Referral may be considered if the patient requires step 3 care (see also 1-Initial Assessment and Diagnosis).

Source: Adapted from the National Heart, Lung, and Blood Institute's National Asthma Education and Prevention Program's Asthma Management Report: Diagnosis and Management of Asthma."

Table 11.3

Types of Medications for Treatment of Asthma

Medication–Generic Chemical Name	Product Name	Preps Available	Mechanism	Uses/Advantages	Disadvantages
Beta-adrenergic agonist			Relax smooth muscles, and may modulate mast cell release of mediators	Efficacious; rapid onset of action; can be easily delivered to airways via nebulizer or metered dose inhaler. Primary drugs for use in exercise-induced, nocturnal, or mild asthma. Can be used in conjunction with inhaled corticosteriods in moderate/severe asthma to help decrease symptoms of an exacerbation.	Can produce tachyphylaxis, cardiac arrhythmias, and paradoxical bronchoconstriciton.
Albuterol	Ventolin® Proventil®	Oral/Inhaled Nebulized			
Metaproterenol sulfate	Alupent® Metaprel®	Oral/Inhaled			
Pirbuterol acetate	Maxair™	Oral/Inhaled			
Bitolterol mesylate Isoetharine	Tornalate®	Oral/Inhaled			
Epinephrine		Inhaled Subcutaneous			High alpha adrenergic component seldom indicated
Terbutaline sulfate	Bretnaire® Bricanyl®	Oral/Sub q			
Methylxanthine Theophylline (Currently prolonged release most useful.)	Elixophyllin® SR Slo-bid™ Slo-Phyllin® Theo-Dur®	Oral Oral Oral Oral	Bronchodilator; may have some anti-inflammatory response	Mainstay for decades but highest rate of side effects. Sustained release useful for nighttime asthma. Can be added to ß-agonists as 2nd line drug; serum level must be monitored (desired level during pregnancy is 5-12 Mg/ml	Significant ß and some adrenergic side effects, CV, muscle tremor, abdominal pain
Anticholinergics Ipratropium	Atrovent®	Inhaled Inhaled	Reduce vagal tone to airway	Effective in status asthmaticus in conjunction with beta-agonists	Limited use outside of ER

Table 11.3 (cont.)

Types of Medications for Treatment of Asthma

Medication–Generic Chemical Name	Product Name	Preps Available	Mechanism	Uses/Advantages	Disadvantages
Mast-cell Stabilizer Cromolyn sodium Nedocromil	Intal® Tilade®	Inhaled	Stabilize mast cells; inhibit release of mediators of inflammation	Minimal, if any, side effects; localize to lungs; used for exercise-induced asthma, or in combination regimens for moderate asthma.	Less effective than inhaled corticosteriods.
Corticosteroids: Prednisone Solucortef, solumedrol		Oral Intravenous	Interrupt development and terminate ongoing inflammatory response	Earlier treatment of severe asthma attack.	Prolonged oral and parenteral administration associated with fluid retention, weight gain, mood alteration, increase BP, diabetes mellitus, immune suppression, adrenal atrophy, aseptic necrosis of femoral head, and decreased birthweight (300–400 gm).
Beclomethasone Triamcinolone Flunisolide	Beclovent, Vanceril Azmacort AeroBid	Inhaled		Effective in controlling airway inflammation and safer than systematic agents. Primary drug in moderate/severe asthma in adults.	

Copyright M. Shannon

Table 11.4

Usual Dosages for Quick-Relief Medications

Medication	Dosage Form	Adult Dose	Child Dose	Comments
Short-Acting Inhaled Beta₂-Agonist				
Albuterol Albuterol HFA Bitolterol Pirbuterol Terbutaline	**MDIs** 90 mcg/puff, 200 puffs 90 mcg/puff, 200 puffs 370 mcg/puff, 300 puffs 200 mcg/puff, 400 puffs 200 mcg/puff, 300 puffs	• 2 puffs, q 5 minutes prior to exercise • 2 puffs tid-qid prn	• 1-2 puffs 5 minutes prior to exercise • 2 puffs tid-qid prn	• An increasing use or lack of expected effect indicates diminished control of asthma. • Not generally recommended for long-term treatment. Regular use on a daily basis indicates the need for additional long-term-control therapy. • Differences in potency exist so that all products are essentially equipotent on a per puff basis. • May double usual dose for mild exacerbation. • Nonselective agents (i.e., epinephine, isoproterenol, metaproterenol) are not recommended due to their potential for excessive cardiac stimulation, especially in high doses.
Albuterol Rotahaler	**DPI** 200 mcg/capsule	1-2 capsules q 4-6 hours as needed and prior to exercise	1 capsule q 4-6 hours as needed and prior to exercise	
Albuterol	**Nebulizer solution** 5 mg/mL (0.5%)	1.25-5 mg (.25-1 cc) in 2-3 cc of saline q 4-8 hours	0.05 mg/kg (min 1.25 mg, max 2.5 mg) in 2-3 cc of saline q 4-6 hours	May mix with cromolyn or ipratropium nebulizer solutions. May double dose for mild exacerbations.
Bitolterol	2 mg/mL (0.2%)	.05-3.5 mg (.25-1 cc) in 2-3 cc of saline q 4-8 hours	Not established	May not mix with other nebulizer solutions.
Anticholinergics	**MDI** 18 mcg/puff, 200 puffs	2-3 puffs q 6 hours	1-2 puffs q 6 hours	Evidence is lacking for anticholinergics producing added benefit to beta₂-agonists in long-term asthma therapy.
Ipratropium	**Nebulizer solution** .25 mg/mL (0.025%)	0.25-0.5 mg q 6 hours	0.25 mg q 6 hours	
Systemic Corticosteroids				
Methylprednisolone	2, 4, 8, 16, 32 mg tablets	• Short course "burst": 40-60 mg/day as single or 2 divided doses for 3-10 days	• Short course "burst": 1-2 mg/kg/day, maximum 60 mg/day, for 3-10 days	• Short course "bursts" are effective for establishing control when initiating therapy or during a period of gradual deterioration. • The burst should be continued until patient achieves 80% PEF personal best or symptoms resolve. This usually requires 3-10 days but may require longer. There is no evidence that tapering the dose following improvement prevents relapse.
Prednisolone	5 mg tabs, 5 mg/5 cc, 1 5 mg/5 cc,			
Prednisone	1, 2.5, 5, 10, 20, 25 mg tablets; 5 mg/cc, 5 mg/5 cc			

Source: Asthma Education and Prevention Program's Asthma Management Report "Guidelines for the Diagnosis and Management of Asthma." NIH Publication No. 97-4051. April 1997.

Table 11.5

Usual Dosages for Long-Term-Control Medications

Medication	Dosage Form	Adult Dose	Child Dose	Comments
Inhaled Corticosteroids (see also figures 3-5b and 3-5c)				
Systemic Corticosteroids			(Applies to all three systemic corticosteroids)	
Methylprednisolone	2, 4, 8, 16, 32 mg tablets	■ 7.5-60 mg daily in a single dose or qid as needed for control ■ Short-course "burst": 40-60 mg per day as single or 2 divided doses for 3-10 days	■ 0.25-2 mg/kg daily in single dose or qid as needed for control ■ Short course "burst": 1-2 mg/kg/day, maximum 60 mg/day, for 3-10 days	■ For long-term treatment of severe persistent asthma, administer single dose in a.m. either daily or on alternate days (alternate-day therapy may produce less adrenal suppression). If daily doses are required, one study suggests improved efficacy and no increase in adrenal suppression when administered at 3:00 p.m. (Beam et al. 1992). ■ Short courses or "bursts" are effective for establishing control when initiating therapy or during a period of gradual deterioration. The burst should be continued until patient achieves 80% PEF personal best or symptoms resolve. This usually requires 3-10 days but may require longer. There is no evidence that tapering the dose following improvement prevents relapse.
Prednisolone	5 mg tablets, 5 mg/cc, 15 mg/cc			
Prednisone	1, 2.5, 5, 10, 20, 25 mg tablets; 5 mg/cc solution			
Cromolyn and Nedocromil				
Cromolyn	MDI 1 mg/puff Nebulizer solution 20 mg/ampule	2-4 puffs tid-qid 1 ampule tid-qid	1-2 puffs tid-qid 1 ampule tid-qid	■ One dose prior to exercise or allergen exposure provides effective prophylaxis for 1-2 hours.
Nedocromil	MDI 1.75 mg/puff	2-4 puffs bid-qid	1-2 puffs bid-qid	■ See cromolyn above.
Long-Acting Beta$_2$-Agonists				
Salmeterol	**Inhaled** MDI 21 mcg/puff, 60 or 120 puffs DPI 50 mcg/blister	2 puffs q 12 hours 1 blister q 12 hours	1-2 puffs q 12 hours 1 blister q 12 hours	■ May use one dose nightly for symptoms. **Should not be used for symptom relief or for exacerbations.**
Sustained-Release Albuterol	**Tablet** 4 mg tablet	4 mg q 12 hours	0.3-0.6 mg/kg/day, not to exceed 8 mg/day	
Methylxanthines				
Theophylline	Liquids, sustained-release tablets, and capsules	Starting dose 10 mg/kg/day up to 300 mg max; usual max 800 mg/day	Starting dose 10 mg/kg/day; usual max: ■ <1 year of age: 0.2 (age in weeks) + 5 = mg/kg/day ■ ≥1 year of age: 16 mg/kg/day	■ Adjust dosage to achieve serum concentration of 5-15 mcg/mL at steady-state (at least 48 hours on same dosage). ■ Due to wide interpatient variability in theophylline metabolic clearance, routine serum theophylline level monitoring is important. ■ See factors below that can affect levels.

Table 11.5 (Con't)

Usual Dosages for Long-Term-Control Medications

	Factors Affecting Serum Theophylline Concentrations*		
Factor	Decreases Theophylline Concentrations	Increases Theophylline Concentrations	Recommended Action
Food	↓ or delays absorption of some sustained-release theophylline (SRT) products	↑ rate of absorption (fatty foods) products	Select theophylline preparation that is not affected by food.
Diet		↓ metabolism (high protein)	Inform patients that major changes in diet are not recommended while taking theophylline.
	↓ metabolism (high carbohydrate)		
Systemic, febrile viral illness (e.g., influenza)	↓ metabolism		Decrease theophylline dose according to serum concentration level. Decrease dose by 50 percent if serum concentration measurement is not available
Hypoxia, cor pulmonale, and decompensated congestive heart failure, cirrhosis	↓ metabolism		Decrease dose according to serum concentration level
Age	↑ metabolism (1 to 9 years)	↓ metabolism (<6 months, elderly)	Adjust dose according to serum concentration level.
Phenobarbital, phenytoin, carbamazepine	↑ metabolism		Increase dose according to serum concentration level.
Cimetidine		↓ metabolism	Use alternative H₂ blocker (e.g., famotidine or ranitidine).
Macrolides: TAO, erythromycin, clarithromycin		↓ metabolism	Use alternative antibiotic or adjust theophylline dose.
Quinolones: ciprofloxacin, enoxacin, pefloxacin		↓ metabolism	Use alternative antibiotic or adjust theophylline dose. Circumvent with ofloxacin if quinolone therapy is required.
Rifampin	↑ metabolism		Increase dose according to serum concentration level.
Ticlopidine		↓ metabolism	Decrease dose according to serum concentration level
Smoking	↑ metabolism		Advise patient to stop smoking; increase dose according to serum concentration level.

Leukotriene Modifiers

Zafirlukast	20 mg tablet	40 mg daily (1 tablet bid)	■ For zafirlukast, administration with meals decreases bioavailability; take at least 1 hour before or 2 hours after meals.
Zileuton	300 mg tablet 600 mg tablet	2,400 mg daily (two 300 mg tablets or one 600 mg tablet, qid)	■ For zileuton, monitor hepatic enzymes (ALT).
Montelukast	5 mg chewable 10 mg tablet	one 10 mg tablet daily in evening	

* This list is not all inclusive; for discussion of other factors, see package inserts.

Table 11.6

Dosages of Medications for Asthma During Pregnancy*

Drug Class	Medication (generic name)	Dosage
	Acute Exacerbation	
Beta-Agonists Inhaled	Albuterol *or* Metaproterenol	2.5 mg (0.5 mL of a 0.5% solution, diluted with 2-3 mL of normal saline)
Subcutaneous	Terbutaline	0.25 mg
Corticosteroids Intravenous	Methylprednisolone *or*	60-80 mg IV bolus every 6-8 hours
	Hydrocortisone *or*	2.0 mg/kg IV bolus every 4 hours
	Hydrocortisone	2.0 mg/kg IV bolus, then 0.5 mg/kg/h continuous intravenous infusion
Oral	A typical oral regimen that may be used as a substitute for IV corticosteroids might be prednisone or methylprednisolone	60 mg given immediately, the 60-120 mg/d in divided doses, tapered over several days at the discretion of the physician
With improvement in the patient's condition (e.g., stabilized PEFR), corticosteroids are usually tapered to a single daily dose of oral prednisone or methylprednisolone (e.g., 60 mg/d) or divided dose (e.g., 20 mg three times daily), then gradually further reduced over 7-14 days.
If the patient requires a prolonged course of oral corticosteroids, side effects may be minimized by a single morning dose given on alternate days.
	Ambulatory Management of Chronic Asthma	
Anti-inflammatory	Cromolyn sodium	2 puffs q.i.d. (inhalation)

2 sprays in each nostril b.i.d.-q.i.d. (intranasally for nasal symptoms) |
| | Beclomethasone | 2-5 puffs b.i.d.-q.i.d. (inhalation)

2 sprays in each nostril b.i.d. (intranasally for allergic rhinitis) |
| | Prednisone | Burst for active symptoms: 40 mg/d, single or divided dose for 1 week, then taper for 1 week.
If prolonged course is required, single morning dose on alternate days may minimize adverse effects. |
| Bronchodilator | Inhaled beta$_2$-agonist | 2 puffs every 4 hours as needed |
| | Theophylline | Oral: Dose needed to reach serum concentration level of 8–12 &g/mL |

* Abbreviations: IV, intravenous: PEFR, peak expiratory flow rate: q.i.d., four times daily; b.i.d., two times daily.

National Asthma Education Program. Report of the working Group on Asthma in Pregnancy. Management of asthma during pregnancy. Bethesda, Maryland: Department of Health and Human Services, 1993:29, 41; NIH publication no. 93-3279.

Source: American College of Obstetricians and Gynecologists (1996). Pulmonary disease in pregnancy. *ACOG technical bulletin No. 224* (p.2). Washington, DC: Author. Reprinted with permission

Figure 11.1

Exercise-Induced Asthma

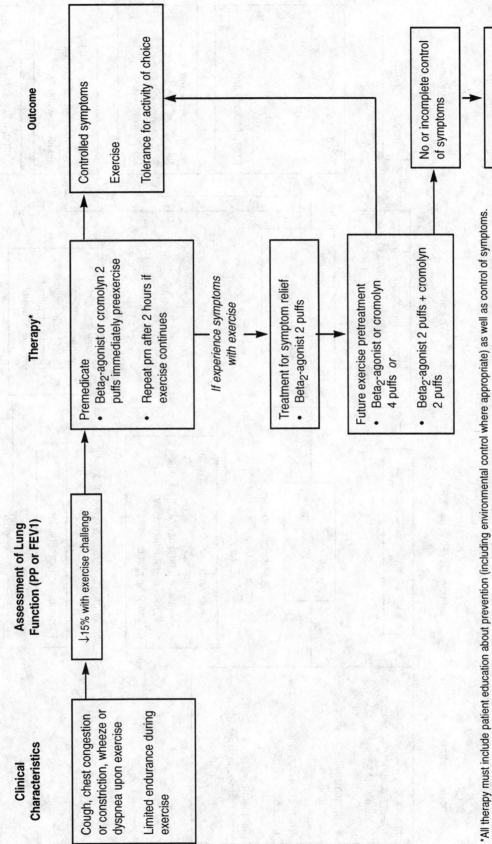

Clinical Characteristics

Cough, chest congestion or constriction, wheeze or dyspnea upon exercise

Limited endurance during exercise

Assessment of Lung Function (PP or FEV1)

↓15% with exercise challenge

Therapy*

Premedicate
- Beta$_2$-agonist or cromolyn 2 puffs immediately preexercise
- Repeat prn after 2 hours if exercise continues

If experience symptoms with exercise

Treatment for symptom relief
- Beta$_2$-agonist 2 puffs

Future exercise pretreatment
- Beta$_2$-agonist or cromolyn 4 puffs *or*
- Beta$_2$-agonist 2 puffs + cromolyn 2 puffs

Outcome

Controlled symptoms

Exercise

Tolerance for activity of choice

No or incomplete control of symptoms

Refer to specialist

*All therapy must include patient education about prevention (including environmental control where appropriate) as well as control of symptoms.

Note: From Guidelines for the diagnosis and management of asthma. Executive Summary. National Asthma Education Program. National Institutes of Health. Publication no. 91-3042A. June 1991. Reprinted by permission.

Figure 11.2

Management of Chronic Mild Asthma During Pregnancy

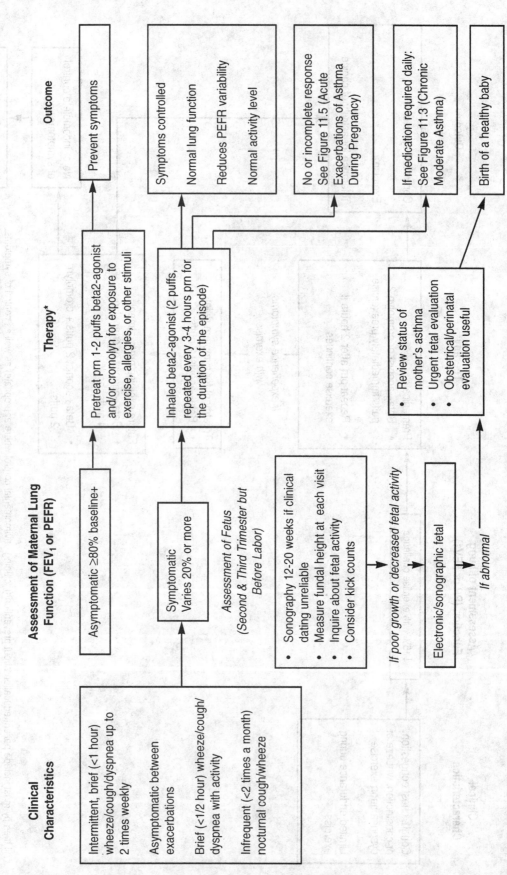

| Clinical Characteristics | Assessment of Maternal Lung Function (FEV₁ or PEFR) | Therapy* | Outcome |

Clinical Characteristics

Intermittent, brief (<1 hour) wheeze/cough/dyspnea up to 2 times weekly

Asymptomatic between exacerbations

Brief (<1/2 hour) wheeze/cough/dyspnea with activity

Infrequent (<2 times a month) nocturnal cough/wheeze

Assessment of Maternal Lung Function (FEV₁ or PEFR)

Asymptomatic ≥80% baseline+

Symptomatic Varies 20% or more

Assessment of Fetus (Second & Third Trimester but Before Labor)

- Sonography 12-20 weeks if clinical dating unreliable
- Measure fundal height at each visit
- Inquire about fetal activity
- Consider kick counts

If poor growth or decreased fetal activity

Electronic/sonographic fetal

If abnormal

Therapy*

Pretreat prn 1-2 puffs beta2-agonist and/or cromolyn for exposure to exercise, allergies, or other stimuli

Inhaled beta2-agonist (2 puffs, repeated every 3-4 hours prn for the duration of the episode)

- Review status of mother's asthma
- Urgent fetal evaluation
- Obstetrical/perinatal evaluation useful

Outcome

Prevent symptoms

Symptoms controlled

Normal lung function

Reduces PEFR variability

Normal activity level

No or incomplete response See Figure 11.5 (Acute Exacerbations of Asthma During Pregnancy)

If medication required daily: See Figure 11.3 (Chronic Moderate Asthma)

Birth of a healthy baby

* All therapy must include patient education about prevention (including environmental control where appropriate) as well as control of symptoms.

+ PEFR percent baseline refers to the norm for the individual, established by the clinician. This may be percent predicted based on standardized norms or percent of patient personal best.

Source: Reprinted with permission from W.C. Mabie, Asthma in pregnancy. Clinical Obstetrics and Gynecology. 39(1), 1996, p.59.

Figure 11.3

Management of Chronic Moderate Asthma During Pregnancy

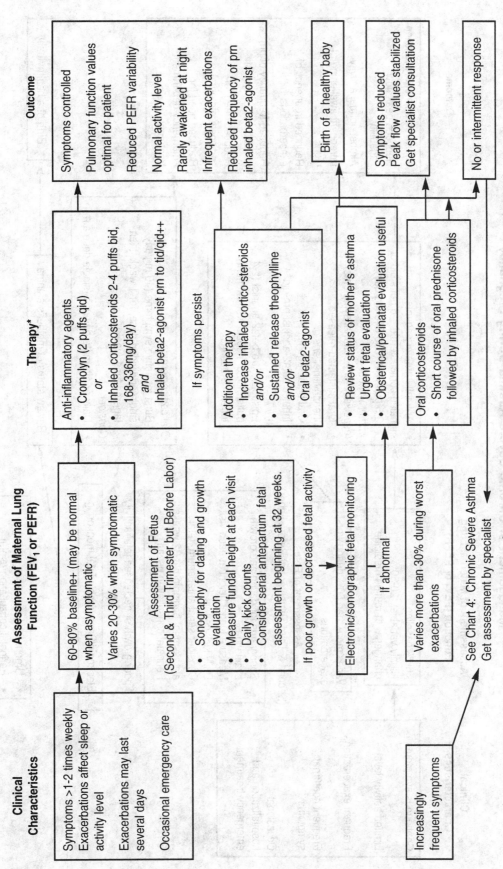

| Clinical Characteristics | Assessment of Maternal Lung Function (FEV₁ or PEFR) | Therapy* | Outcome |

Figure content:

Clinical Characteristics

Symptoms >1-2 times weekly
Exacerbations affect sleep or activity level

Exacerbations may last several days

Occasional emergency care

Increasingly frequent symptoms

Assessment of Maternal Lung Function (FEV₁ or PEFR)

60-80% baseline+ (may be normal when asymptomatic)

Varies 20-30% when symptomatic

Assessment of Fetus (Second & Third Trimester but Before Labor)

- Sonography for dating and growth evaluation
- Measure fundal height at each visit
- Daily kick counts
- Consider serial antepartum fetal assessment beginning at 32 weeks.

If poor growth or decreased fetal activity

Electronic/sonographic fetal monitoring

If abnormal

Varies more than 30% during worst exacerbations

See Chart 4: Chronic Severe Asthma
Get assessment by specialist

Therapy*

Anti-inflammatory agents
- Cromolyn (2 puffs qid)
  or
- Inhaled corticosteroids 2-4 puffs bid, 168-336mg/day)
  and
  Inhaled beta2-agonist prn to tid/qid++

If symptoms persist

Additional therapy
- Increase inhaled cortico-steroids
  and/or
- Sustained release theophylline
  and/or
- Oral beta2-agonist

- Review status of mother's asthma
- Urgent fetal evaluation
- Obstetrical/perinatal evaluation useful

Oral corticosteroids
- Short course of oral prednisone followed by inhaled corticosteroids

Outcome

Symptoms controlled
Pulmonary function values optimal for patient
Reduced PEFR variability
Normal activity level
Rarely awakened at night
Infrequent exacerbations
Reduced frequency of prn inhaled beta2-agonist

Birth of a healthy baby

Symptoms reduced
Peak flow values stabilized
Get specialist consultation

No or intermittent response

---

* All therapy must include patient education about prevention (including environmental control where appropriate) as well as control of symptoms.

\+ PEFR percent baseline refers to the norm for the individual, established by the clinician. This may be percent predicted based on standardized norms or percent of patient personal best.

\++ If exceed 3-4 doses a day, consider additional therapy other than inhaled beta2-agonist.

Source: Reprinted with permission from W.C. Mabie, Asthma in pregnancy. Clinical Obstetrics and Gynecology. 39(1), 1996, p.59.

Figure 11.4

Management of Chronic Severe Asthma During Pregnancy

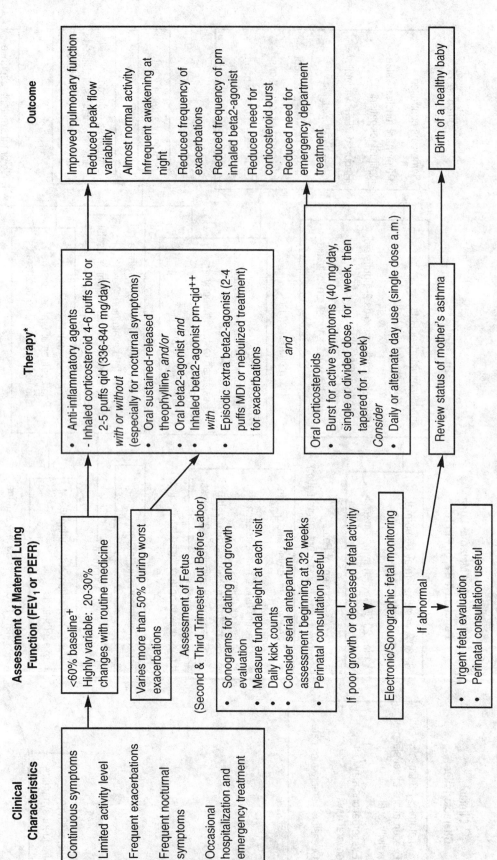

| Clinical Characteristics | Assessment of Maternal Lung Function (FEV₁ or PEFR) | Therapy* | Outcome |

Clinical Characteristics
- Continuous symptoms
- Limited activity level
- Frequent exacerbations
- Frequent nocturnal symptoms
- Occasional hospitalization and emergency treatment

Assessment of Maternal Lung Function (FEV_1 or PEFR)
- <60% baseline⁺
- Highly variable: 20-30% changes with routine medicine
- Varies more than 50% during worst exacerbations

Assessment of Fetus
(Second & Third Trimester but Before Labor)
- Sonograms for dating and growth evaluation
- Measure fundal height at each visit
- Daily kick counts
- Consider serial antepartum fetal assessment beginning at 32 weeks
- Perinatal consultation useful

If poor growth or decreased fetal activity

Electronic/Sonographic fetal monitoring

If abnormal

- Urgent fetal evaluation
- Perinatal consultation useful

Therapy*
- Anti-inflammatory agents
  - Inhaled corticosteroid 4-6 puffs bid or 2-5 puffs qid (336-840 mg/day)
  with or without
  (especially for nocturnal symptoms)
- Oral sustained-released theophylline, *and/or*
- Oral beta2-agonist *and*
- Inhaled beta2-agonist prn-qid⁺⁺
  with
- Episodic extra beta2-agonist (2-4 puffs MDI or nebulized treatment) for exacerbations

and

Oral corticosteroids
- Burst for active symptoms (40 mg/day, single or divided dose, for 1 week, then tapered for 1 week)
  Consider
- Daily or alternate day use (single dose a.m.)

Review status of mother's asthma

Outcome
- Improved pulmonary function
- Reduced peak flow variability
- Almost normal activity
- Infrequent awakening at night
- Reduced frequency of exacerbations
- Reduced frequency of prn inhaled beta2-agonist
- Reduced need for corticosteroid burst
- Reduced need for emergency department treatment

Birth of a healthy baby

* All therapy must include patient education about prevention (including environmental control where appropriate) as well as control of symptoms.

+ PEFR percent baseline refers to the norm for the individual, established by the clinician. This may be percent predicted based on standardized norms or percent of patient personal best.

++ If exceed 3-4 doses a day, consider additional therapy other than inhaled beta2-agonist.

Source: Reprinted with permission from W.C. Mabie, Asthma in pregnancy. Clinical Obstetrics and Gynecology. 39(1), 1996, p.59.

Figure 11.5

Home Management of Acute Exacerbations of Asthma During Pregnancy

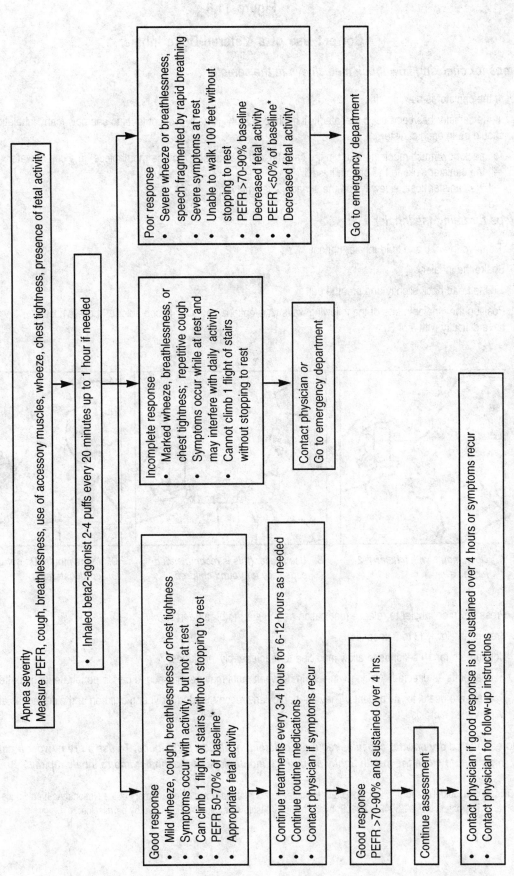

Apnea severity
Measure PEFR, cough, breathlessness, use of accessory muscles, wheeze, chest tightness, presence of fetal activity

- Inhaled beta2-agonist 2-4 puffs every 20 minutes up to 1 hour if needed

Good response
- Mild wheeze, cough, breathlessness *or* chest tightness
- Symptoms occur with activity, but not at rest
- Can climb 1 flight of stairs without stopping to rest
- PEFR 50-70% of baseline*
- Appropriate fetal activity

- Continue treatments every 3-4 hours for 6-12 hours as needed
- Continue routine medications
- Contact physician if symptoms recur

Good response
PEFR >70-90% and sustained over 4 hrs.

Continue assessment

- Contact physician if good response is not sustained over 4 hours or symptoms recur
- Contact physician for follow-up instructions

Incomplete response
- Marked wheeze, breathlessness, or chest tightness; repetitive cough
- Symptoms occur while at rest and may interfere with daily activity
- Cannot climb 1 flight of stairs without stopping to rest

Contact physician *or*
Go to emergency department

Poor response
- Severe wheeze or breathlessness, speech fragmented by rapid breathing
- Severe symptoms at rest
- Unable to walk 100 feet without stopping to rest
- PEFR >70-90% baseline
- Decreased fetal activity
- PEFR <50% of baseline*
- Decreased fetal activity

Go to emergency department

* PEFR percent baseline refers to the norm for the individual, established by the clinician. This may be percent predicted based on standardized norms or percent of patient's personal best.

Source: Reprinted with permission from W.C. Mabie, Asthma in pregnancy. Clinical Obstetrics and Gynecology, 39(1), 1996, p.66.

Figure 11.6

Correct Use of a Metered-Dose Inhaler

Steps for checking how much medicine is in the canister

1. If the canister is new, it is full

2. If the canister has been used repeatedly, it might be empty. (Check product label to see how many inhalations should be in each canister.)

    To check how much medicine is left in the canister, put the canister (not the mouthpiece) in a cup of water.
    —If the canister sinks to the bottom it is full
    —If the canister floats sideways on the surface, it is empty.

Steps for using the inhaler

1. Remove the cap and hold inhaler upright.

2. Shake the inhaler.

3. Tilt the head back slightly and breathe out.

4. Position the inhaler in one of the following ways (A is optional, but C is acceptable for those who have difficulty with A or B):

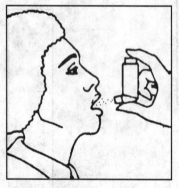 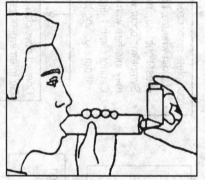 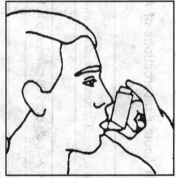

A. *Open mouth with inhaler 1–2 inches away* B. *Use spacer (this is recommended especially for young children* C. *In the mouth. Do not use for corticosteroids*

5. Press down on inhaler to release medication as you start to breathe in slowly.

6. Breathe in slowly (3 to 5 seconds).

7. Hold breath for 10 seconds to allow medicine to reach deeply into lungs.

8. Repeat puffs as directed. Waiting 1 minute in between puffs may permit second puff to penetrate lungs better.

9. Spacers are useful for all patients. They are particularly recommended for young children and older adults and for use with inhaled steroids.

*Note: Inhaled dry powder capsules require a different inhalation techniques. To use a dry powder inhaler, it is important to close the mouth tightly around the mouthpiece of the inhaler and to inhale rapidly.

Source: From Guidelines for the Diagnosis and Management of Asthma. Executive Summary of the National Asthma Education Program. Publication NO. 91-3042A, (p.109) by the National Institutes of Health. Reprinted by permission.

References

American College of Obstetricians and Gynecologists (ACOG). (1996). Pulmonary disease in pregnancy. *ACOG Technical Bulletin No. 224* .Washington, DC: Author.

Arkinstall, W.W. (1987). Once-daily sustained-release theophylline reduces clinical variation in spirometry and symptomatology in adult asthmatics. *American Review of Respiratory Diseases, 135*, 316–321.

Briggs, G.G., Freeman, R.K., & Yaffe, S.J. (1994). *Drugs in pregnancy and lactation* (4th ed.). Baltimore, MD: Williams & Wilkins.

Clark, S.L. & the National Asthma Education Program Working Group on Asthma and Pregnancy of the National Institutes of Health (NIH) and the National Heart, Lung and Blood Institute. (1993). Asthma in pregnancy. *Obstetrics and Gynecology, 82*(6), 1036–1040.

Holmgren, D. & Sixt, R. (1992). Transcutaneous and arterial blood gas monitoring during acute asthmatic symptoms in older children. *Pediatric Pulmonary, 14*(2), 80–84.

Jenne, J.W. (1984). Theophylline use in asthma: Some current issues. *Clinics in Chest Medicine, 5*, 645–658.

Mabie, W.C. (1996). Asthma in pregnancy. *Clinical Obstetrics and Gynecology, 39*(1), 56–69.

Mays, M., & Leiner, S. (1995). Asthma: A comprehensive review. *Journal of Nurse-Midwifery, 40(3)*, 256–268.

National Institutes of Health (NIH). (1991). *Guidelines for the diagnosis and management of asthma. Executive Summary of the National Asthma Education Program.* Publication No. 91-3042A. June, 1991.

National Institutes of Health (NIH). (1997). *Guidelines for the diagnosis and management of asthma. Executive Summary of the National Asthma Education Program.* Publication No. 97-4051. April, 1997.

Rivo, M.L., & Malveaux, F.J. (1992). Outpatient management of asthma in adults. *American Family Physician, 45*(5), 2105–2113.

Schappert, S.M. (1993). *National ambulatory medical care survey: 1991 summary. Advance data from vital and health statistics, No. 230.* Hyattsville, MD: National Center for Health Statistics.

Shannon, M.T. (1995). Asthma. In W.L. Star, L.L. Lommel, & M.T. Shannon (Eds.), *Women's primary health care: Protocols for practice* (pp. 5–3, 5–11). Washington, DC: American Nurses Publishing.

Stauffer, J.L. (1996). Pulmonary diseases. In L.M. Tierney, Jr., S.J. McPhee, M.A. Papadakis, & S. A. Schroeder (Eds.), *Current medical diagnosis and treatment* (32nd ed., pp. 214–294). Norwalk, CT: Appleton & Lange.

Weiss, K.B. & Wagener, D.K. (1990). Changing patterns of asthma mortality: Identifying target populations at high risk. *Journal of American Medical Association, 264*, 1683–1687.

Wooley, M. (1990). Duration of protective effect of terbutaline sulfate and cromolyn sodium alone and in combination on exercise-induced asthma. *Chest ⁀7*, 39–45.

Chapter 2

BRONCHITIS—ACUTE

Maureen T. Shannon

Acute bronchitis is an inflammation of the trachea and the bronchial wall. It results from infection with a virus, mycoplasma, or bacteria or from exposure to an irritant (e.g., smoke, dust, or pollen) (Marchese & Diamond, 1995; Mays & Leiner, 1996).

The primary symptom associated with acute bronchitis is a cough that persists for several weeks. Usually there is a history of a recent upper respiratory infection (URI). In the majority of women, the episode is self-limited, lasting approximately 2 weeks, and requiring only symptomatic treatment. However, in women with a history of chronic obstructive pulmonary disease (COPD), acute bronchitis may require more pharmacological management (e.g., antibiotic therapy). Use of antibiotics for acute bronchitis in healthy individuals without a history of COPD is not recommended, especially since this practice may result in the development of drug resistant strains of bacteria. However, inhalation therapy with bronchodilators may have beneficial effects in some individuals (Mainous, Zoorob, & Hueston, 1996; Mays & Leiner, 1996; Orr, Scherer, MacDonald, & Moffat, 1993).

The development of acute bronchitis during pregnancy has not been associated with any adverse maternal or perinatal complications. However, in pregnant women with COPD or asthma, the development of acute bronchitis may lead to pulmonary complications (e.g., pneumonia). A woman presenting with a history of a chronic cough should be evaluated for other pathology (e.g., chronic reflux esophagitis, asthma, tuberculosis, pertussis) in addition to acute bronchitis.

Database

Subjective

- The woman may report a history of predisposing factors associated with bronchitis including (Shannon, 1995)

  ▶ Smoking

  ▶ Recent URI

  ▶ Recent influenza infection

  ▶ COPD

  ▶ Asthma

- The woman may report one or more of the following symptoms (Shannon, 1995):

  ▶ Productive cough (mucoid to purulent)

  ▶ Substernal chest discomfort

  ▶ Low-grade fever

▶ URI symptoms:

  – Malaise

  – Rhinorrhea

  – Sore throat

  – Headache

Objective

● Physical examination may reveal

  ▶ A normal or mildly elevated temperature

  ▶ Pharyngeal hyperemia

  ▶ Auscultation of the lungs demonstrates rhonchi, wheezing, or crackles without consolidation

Assessment

● Acute bronchitis

  ▶ R/O asthmatic bronchitis

  ▶ R/O pneumonia

  ▶ R/O URI

  ▶ R/O influenza

  ▶ R/O group A streptococcal pharyngitis

  ▶ R/O allergic rhinitis

  ▶ R/O chronic sinusitis

  ▶ R/O COPD

  ▶ R/O tuberculosis

  ▶ R/O pertussis

  ▶ R/O chronic reflux esophagitis

Plan

Diagnostic Tests

The diagnosis of acute bronchitis is usually based upon the history, clinical presentation, and physical examination findings. However, the following tests may be ordered for women with severe symptoms, a history of pulmonary conditions, or when other pathology is suspected.

- Chest x-ray —usually within normal limits (WNL)

- Sputum cultures and/or smears—may demonstrate a specific pathogen (usually common oropharyngeal contaminants are recovered and are of unknown significance)

- Tuberculosis skin test—if placed should be read in 48 to 72 hours and should not demonstrate any induration (see Chapter 10.10, *Tuberculosis*)

Treatment/Management

- Symptomatic treatment of a woman with acute bronchitis includes rest, increased fluid intake, and the use of acetaminophen, 650 mg p.o. every 4 hours, as needed (for relief of associated symptoms of headache, fever).

- Cough suppression can be attempted through the use of medications containing dextromethorphan. The usual dose is 15 mg p.o. every 6 hours. Advise the woman to ask the pharmacist for a nonalcohol containing preparation.

- Consider the use of an inhaled bronchodilator in a woman with diffuse abnormal breath sounds (e.g., wheezing).

  ▶ The usual dose is albuterol one to two puffs every 4 hours

- Antimicrobial therapy is not indicated in the treatment of acute bronchitis in healthy women. However, in women with a history of preexisting pulmonary disease (e.g., COPD), the use of antibiotics may be beneficial. The following agents may be considered for use:

  ▶ Erythromycin 250 mg p.o. q.i.d. for 7 to 10 days

    NOTE: Avoid the use of erythromycin estolate, which has been documented to induce hepatotoxicity in pregnant women (Briggs, Freeman, & Yaffe, 1994). Erythromycin provides a wide spectrum of coverage for limited cost.

  ▶ Amoxicillin 500 mg p.o. t.i.d. for 7 to 10 days

- If the woman is suspected of having influenza type A infection and she is at an increased risk of complications associated with this disease, amantadine hydrochloride may be prescribed after consultation with a physician (see Chapter 11.3, *Influenza*).

- If pertussis is suspected, consultation with a physician. The antibiotic therapy recommended for pertussis is erythromycin or trimethoprim-sulfamethoxazole for 14 days.

Consultation

- Consult with a physician, as indicated, for pregnant women with COPD, severe respiratory symptoms, significant underlying medical conditions, or when inadequate response to treatment is suspected or documented.

Patient Education

- Educate the woman about acute broncitis, the cause(s), treatment, signs and symptoms of complications, and any plans for follow-up evaluations.

- Reassure the woman that acute bronchitis has not been associated with any adverse fetal/neonatal consequences.

- If the woman requires pharmacological therapy, educate her about the reason for a recommended medication, proper administration of the medication, and the possible side effects.

- If the woman smokes, educate her about the adverse maternal and fetal consequences of smoking, and ways to reduce or stop smoking. If possible, refer her to smoking cessation programs with ongoing support groups. Such programs have been documented to prevent relapses (Schwartz, 1992).

Follow-Up

- If physician consultation is indicated, follow-up per recommendation of the physician.

- Evaluate women who have been prescribed antibiotics 1 to 2 weeks after the initiation of therapy.

- Document diagnosis of acute bronchitis and management thereof in progress notes and problem list.

References

Briggs, G.G., Freeman, R.K., & Yaffe, S.J. (1994). *Drugs in pregnancy and lactation* (4th ed.). Baltimore: Williams & Wilkins.

Mainous, A.G., Zoorob, R.J., & Hueston, W. J. (1996). Current management of acute bronchitis in ambulatory care: The use of antibiotics and bronchodilators. *Archives of Family Medicine, 5*(2), 79–83.

Marchese, T.W., & Diamond, F.B. (1995). Primary care for women. Comprehensive assessment of the respiratory system. *Journal of Nurse-Midwifery, 40*(2), 150–162.

Mays, M., & Leiner, S. (1996). Primary care for women. Management of common respiratory problems. *Journal of Nurse-Midwifery, 41*(2), 139–154.

Orr, P.H., Scherer, K., MacDonald, A., & Moffatt, M.E. (1993). Randomized placebo-controlled trials of antibiotics for acute bronchitis: A critical review of the literature. *Journal of Family Practice, 36*(5), 507–512.

Schwartz, J.L. (1992). Methods of smoking cessation. *Medical Clinics of North America, 76*(2), 451–476.

Shannon, M.T. (1995). Bronchitis–acute. In W. L. Star, L.L. Lommel, & M.T. Shannon (Eds.), *Women's primary health care: Protocols for practice* (pp. 5–15, 5–16). Washington, DC: American Nurses Publishing.

Chapter 3

INFLUENZA INFECTION

Maureen T. Shannon

Influenza is a systemic illness that is caused by one of the orthomyxoviruses—type A, B, or C (LaForce, Nichol, & Cox, 1994; Nicholson, 1992). Influenza virus types A and B are usually responsible for the epidemics that occur in the fall or winter. The clinical presentation of infections caused by types A and B are similar, while type C influenza infection is associated with less severe symptoms. Influenza viruses are capable of antigenic variation, a characteristic that results in the development of viral strains to which populations may have little or no immunity (LaForce, Nichol, & Cox, 1994; Nicholson, 1992). Consequently, persons previously immunized or infected with a specific type of influenza virus may again be susceptible to the effects of the virus in subsequent epidemics (Centers for Disease Control and Prevention [CDC], 1997; LaForce, Nichol, & Cox, 1994).

Influenza virus transmission occurs via infected respiratory droplets; the survival of airborne virus is enhanced by low environmental temperature and low humidity (Nicholson, 1992). Individuals are most infectious 24 hours prior to the onset of symptoms. Cessation of viral shedding in nasal secretions occurs within 7 days after the onset of symptoms. The incubation period ranges from 1 to 7 days, although it is commonly between 2 to 3 days (Nicholson, 1992). Clinical manifestations of infection usually last from 4 to 7 days after the onset of symptoms. Complications associated with influenza may include otitis media, sinusitis, myositis, bronchitis, primary viral pneumonia, secondary bacterial pneumonia, and rarely, encephalitis, pericarditis, myocarditis, and thrombophlebitis. The mortality rate associated with influenza is reportedly between 1 and 4 percent with the highest rates associated with persons 65 years of age or older (CDC, 1992; CDC, 1997).

Disproportionately increased death rates observed in pregnant women during the influenza pandemics of 1889, 1918, and 1957 have led to concern regarding influenza infection during pregnancy. However, it is unclear during these epidemics whether pregnant women were more likely to have developed influenza infection or more susceptible to the development of influenza-associated pneumonia. Currently, there is evidence that pregnant women with influenza during the second and third trimesters are more likely to have a severe form of the infection and a higher likelihood of experiencing complications requiring hospitalization (Amstey, 1996; CDC, 1997; Gibbs & Sweet, 1994; Nicholson, 1992). Therefore, it is recommended that pregnant women who will be beyond the first trimester (i.e., equal to or greater than 14 weeks' gestation) during the influenza season receive the influenza vaccine (CDC, 1997).

The effects of influenza infection during pregnancy on spontaneous abortion rates, congenital anomalies, and prematurity are controversial, especially since there are no well-controlled studies investigating this issue and because variations in the virus from epidemic to epidemic make analysis difficult (Gibbs & Sweet, 1994). Although influenza virus has been cultured from amniotic fluid and congenitally acquired influenza infection has been documented, convincing evidence that links maternal influenza infection with adverse perinatal outcomes is lacking (e.g., spontaneous abortion, congenital anomalies, prematurity, stillbirth) (Amstey, 1996; Gibbs & Sweet, 1994; Nicholson, 1992).

Database

Subjective

- The woman may report one or more of the following symptoms with symptoms ranging from mild to severe (Amstey, 1996; LaForce et al., 1994; Nicholson, 1992; Shannon, 1995).

  ▶ Sudden onset of fever

  ▶ Chills and/or rigors

  ▶ Malaise

  ▶ Myalgia (usually affecting the back and limbs)

  ▶ Headache

  ▶ Cough (initially nonproductive but may become productive if bacterial superinfection)

  ▶ Nasal congestion

  ▶ Rhinorrhea

  ▶ Sore throat

  ▶ Conjunctivitis

  ▶ Photophobia

  ▶ Substernal discomfort or soreness

  ▶ Dyspnea or shortness of breath (if associated pneumonia, pericarditis, or myocarditis)

  ▶ Abdominal pain

  ▶ Anorexia

  ▶ Nausea

  ▶ Vomiting

  ▶ Diarrhea

Objective

- Physical examination may reveal the following (Amstey, 1996; LaForce, Nichol, & Cox, 1994; Nicholson, 1992; Shannon, 1995):

  ▶ Elevated temperature (usually between 38° and 40° C [100.4°–104° F])

  ▶ Weight loss (if severe nausea and vomiting)

  ▶ Hot or moist skin with flushed appearance

  ▶ Tachypnea (if associated pneumonia)

  ▶ Tachycardia (if there is significant fever, dehydration, or associated pneumonia, or pericarditis)

  ▶ Nasal hyperemia, with or without clear discharge

  ▶ Pharyngeal hyperemia

▶ Conjunctival erythema and/or discharge

▶ Tender enlarged cervical lymph nodes

▶ Basilar crackles or rhonchi upon auscultation of the lungs, if there is bronchitis or pneumonia

▶ A rub, upon auscultation of the heart if there is pericarditis

▶ Abdominal examination within normal limits (WNL), usually, including normal fundal height for gestation

▶ A change in mental status (may be observed in patients with central nervous system [CNS] complications)

Assessment

- Influenza (type A, B, or C)
  - ▶ R/O dehydration
  - ▶ R/O upper respiratory infection (URI)
  - ▶ R/O group A streptococcal pharyngitis
  - ▶ R/O *Mycoplasma* infection
  - ▶ R/O rubeola (prodromal phase)
  - ▶ R/O otitis media
  - ▶ R/O bronchitis
  - ▶ R/O pneumonia
  - ▶ R/O pericarditis
  - ▶ R/O myocarditis
  - ▶ R/O encephalitis
  - ▶ R/O pyelonephritis

Plan

Diagnostic Tests

- The following tests may be ordered if complications associated with influenza are suspected:
  - Complete blood count (CBC)—may be WNL or demonstrate leukopenia
  - Chest x-ray—may reveal evidence of bronchitis, pneumonia, pericarditis, or myocarditis in women experiencing these complications
  - Influenza virus culture—may be isolated from the throat or nasopharynx

  NOTE: Specimens for culture should be obtained within 72 hours of illness because of the rapid decline in quantity of virus after this time. A minimum of 24 hours is required to demonstrate virus, and an additional 24 to 48 hours to determine the virus type (LaForce et al., 1994).

- Immunofluorescence of nasopharyngeal specimens for influenza antigen—may be positive (sensitivity is variable)

- Acute and convalescent titers (either complement fixation or hemagglutination inhibition tests) of serum—will reveal a fourfold increase in titers

Treatment/Management

- Symptomatic treatment includes rest, increased fluid intake, and the use of acetaminophen 650 mg p.o. every 4 hours to reduce fever and help relieve myalgia.

  NOTE: Advise pregnant women to avoid the use of aspirin because of its associated maternal and neonatal hemostasis problems. In addition, adolescents (as well as children) should not receive aspirin during viral illnesses because of the associated risk of developing Reye's syndrome.

- Severely ill women may require hospitalization, especially if significant dehydration or medical complications are suspected. Consult with a physician and transfer care for any pregnant woman with significant illness.

- In severely ill women or women with medical complications, consider amantadine and prescribe after consultation with a physician. Amantadine is an antiviral medication with a 50 percent efficacy rate in reducing severe symptoms in individuals infected with influenza type A (it has no effect on symptoms associated with influenza type B). Treatment should begin within 48 hours of symptom development.

  ▶ The usual dose is amantadine hydrochloride 100 mg p.o. b.i.d. for 3 to 5 days

  NOTE: The development of viral resistance to amantadine has been documented in persons receiving 5 to 7 days of therapy. In addition, transmission of resistant virus is possible. Therefore, the duration of amantadine therapy should be limited to 3 to 5 days, or discontinued 24 to 48 hours after resolution of signs and symptoms of infection (CDC, 1997).

  ▶ In women with renal disease, the dose of amantadine may need to be reduced depending upon the results of creatinine clearance levels.

  NOTE: There is limited data available regarding possible adverse effects of amantadine during pregnancy. However, in animals it has demonstrated embryotoxic and teratogenic effects when given in high doses. Limited data regarding use during the first trimester have demonstrated an increased incidence of congenital defects; however, the number of early pregnancy exposures is too small for definitive conclusions to be drawn. As a result, the risks versus the possible benefits of this intervention must be evaluated on an individual basis. In addition, the manufacturer recommends that women taking amantadine should not breast-feed, although concentrations of the medication in breast milk are low (Briggs, Freeman, & Yaffe, 1994). The potential side effects associated with amantadine use include CNS symptoms (e.g., confusion, inability to concentrate, depression, hallucinations, jitteriness, insomnia, tremors) and nausea.

- Antenatal testing during the third trimester (e.g., nonstress test with an amniotic fluid index) may be indicated in women with severe illness or influenza associated complications.

- Immunization with polyvalent influenza virus vaccine (one 0.5 mL IM injection) during the fall provides partial immunity for up to 1 year.

  ▶ Annual immunization is necessary since the antigenic configuration of the virus changes yearly. Annual immunization recommendations may change, and therefore it is important to review current CDC guidelines on a yearly basis (CDC Influenza Update Voice Information System is 404/332-4551).

▶ Currently, the vaccine is advised for pregnant women who will be equal to or greater than 14 weeks' gestation during the influenza season (CDC, 1997).

▶ Influenza vaccination should not be administered to women with a known anaphylactic hypersensitivity to eggs or other components of the influenza vaccine (CDC, 1997).

NOTE: Influenza vaccine is an inactivated virus. Whenever possible, administration of the vaccine after the first trimester is a reasonable precaution.

Consultation

● Consult with a physician for any woman with severe illness, suspected/diagnosed complications associated with influenza, or for any woman being considered for amantadine therapy.

● Transfer care of any women requiring hospitalization to the consulting physician.

● Consult, as necessary, for prescription medications.

Patient Education

● Educate the woman about influenza, including the cause, clinical course, diagnostic tests that may be necessary, treatment options, possible complications, and any indicated follow-up.

● When transfer of care to a physician is indicated, discuss the reason(s) for this plan. The physician responsible for care should explain interventions to women needing hospitalization and/or amantadine therapy.

● Reassure the woman that maternal influenza infection has generally not been associated with any adverse outcome in the infant.

● Educate women about preventative measures that may be taken to avoid future influenza infection (e.g., influenza vaccination, proper handwashing).

Follow-up

● If consultation with a physician was necessary, follow-up per physician recommendation.

● If any symptoms of complications develop, the woman should return for reevaluation.

● Document influenza infection and treatment in progress notes and problem list.

References

Amstey, M.S. (1996). Influenza complications. *Contemporary OB/GYN, 41*(1), 15–19.

Briggs, G.G., Freeman, R.K., Yaffe, S.J. (1994). *Drugs in pregnancy and lactation* (4th ed.). Baltimore, MD: Williams & Wilkins.

Centers for Disease Control and Prevention (CDC). (1992). Influenza surveillance—United States, 1991–1992. *Morbidity and Mortality Weekly Report, 41*(SS-5), 35–46.

Centers for Disease Control and Prevention (CDC). (1997). Prevention and control of influenza. Recommendations of the Advisory Committee on Immunization Practices (ACIP). *Morbidity and Mortality Weekly Report, 46*(RR-9), 1–25.

Gibbs, R.S., & Sweet, R.L. (1994). Clinical disorders. In R.K. Creasy & R. Resnik (Eds.), *Maternal-fetal medicine. Principles and practice* (3rd ed., pp. 639–703). Philadelphia, PA: W.B. Saunders.

LaForce, F.M., Nichol, K.L., & Cox, N.J. (1994). Influenza: Virology, epidemiology, disease, and prevention. *American Journal of Preventive Medicine, 10*(Suppl), 31–44.

Nicholson, K.G. (1992). Clinical features of influenza. *Seminars in Respiratory Infections, 7*(1), 26-37.

Shannon, M.T. (1995). Influenza. In W.L. Star, L.L. Lommel, & M.T. Shannon (Eds.), *Women's primary health care. Protocols for practice* (pp. 5–27, 5–30). Washington, DC: American Nurses Publishing.

Chapter 4

PNEUMONIA

Maureen T. Shannon

Pneumonia is an infection of the lung that is caused by various pathogens, including bacteria, viruses, and fungi. Individuals may be exposed to the infecting organism by transmission from colonization in the upper respiratory tract, through hematogenous spread, or by inhaling infected droplets. The clinical manifestations observed with pneumonia have traditionally been categorized into "pyogenic" or "atypical" presentations. Pneumonias resulting from infection with a pyogenic organism (e.g., *Streptococcus pneumoniae*) typically have an abrupt onset of illness, are associated with significant morbidity, and require prompt identification and treatment if serious sequelae are to be avoided. Atypical pneumonias (e.g., *Mycoplasma pneumoniae*) reportedly have a more gradual onset and often resolve without therapy (Mays & Leiner, 1996). However, exceptions to these definitions exist.

Some investigators have proposed that the hormonal, anatomic, and physiologic changes induced by pregnancy enhance a woman's susceptibility to pneumonia. Immunologic changes associated with gestation (e.g., decreases in natural killer-cell activity, lymphocyte proliferative responses, and number of T-helper cells) alter the woman's cell-mediated responses to certain infections, especially viral and fungal pathogens responsible for pneumonia. In addition, the increased oxygen consumption and decreased functional residual capacity observed during normal gestation, especially during the third trimester, further diminish a woman's ability to tolerate even limited periods of hypoxia that may result from pneumonia and its complications (Rigby & Pastorek, 1996; Rodrigues & Niederman, 1992). These physiologic dynamics may be responsible for the increased morbidity and mortality reported in pregnant women diagnosed with viral or fungal pneumonias.

The increased risk of pneumonia-associated complications during pregnancy reportedly correlates with several maternal factors, including

- The presence of underlying maternal disease (e.g., pulmonary disease, human immunodeficiency virus [HIV] infection)

- Maternal health status at the time clinical manifestations develop

- How early in the illness therapeutic interventions are initiated (Berkowitz & LaSala, 1990; Rigby & Pastorek, 1996; Rodrigues & Niederman, 1992).

Although pneumonia during pregnancy has an overall mortality rate of 1 percent, it is the most common nonobstetric cause of maternal death (Rigby & Pastorek, 1996). In addition, an association between maternal pneumonia and an increased incidence of preterm labor, small for gestational age infants, intrauterine fetal deaths, and neonatal deaths has been reported (Benedetti, Valle, & Ledger, 1982; Berkowitz & LaSala, 1990; Madinger, Greenspoon, & Eilrodt, 1989).

The pathogen(s) responsible for the majority of community-acquired pneumonias observed in adult populations are often not identified in individual cases. However, when identification of pneumonia pathogens has been accomplished, those observed in pregnant women are similar to those identified in nonpregnant populations. The most frequently reported bacterial organisms identified in pregnant women are *Streptococcus pneumoniae (S. pneumoniae)*, followed by *Haemophilus influenzae (H. influenzae)*, *Mycoplasma pneumoniae (M. pneumoniae)*, *Legionella pneumophila (L. pneumophila)*, *Chlamydia pneumoniae (C. pneumoniae* [TWAR]), and *Moraxella catarrhalis (M. catarrhalis)* (Rigby & Pasternak, 1996; Rodrigues & Niederman, 1992). Viral pathogens associated with pneumonia during pregnancy include influenza A, varicella virus, para-influenza viruses, adenovirus, respiratory syncytial virus, and other viruses associated with exanthems (e.g., measles). Pneumonia resulting from fungi (e.g., *Pneumocystis carinii, Aspergillus fumigatus*) are rarely seen in individuals with competent immune systems but are of concern in immunocompromised women (e.g., HIV-infected women). However, in certain regions of the United States, fungal pneumonias (e.g., *Coccidioides immitis)* are observed more commonly. Dissemination of these fungal pathogens can result in significant maternal morbidity and/or death (Peterson, Schuppert, Kelly, & Pappagianis, 1993; Rigby & Pastorek, 1996).

Nosocomial acquisition of pneumonia organisms also can occur. Pathogens frequently, although not exclusively, associated with nosocomial infection include *Staphylococcus aureus (S. aureus), Klebsiella pneumoniae (K. pneumoniae), Escherichia coli (E. coli), Pseudomonas aeruginosa (P. aeruginosa)*, as well as influenza viruses type A and B. Finally, pneumonia can develop in women who experience aspiration during the intrapartum period. This is usually associated with the administration of general anesthesia or as a result of endotracheal intubation. A woman may aspirate oropharyngeal bacteria or liquid and/or particulate matter from the stomach (including gastric acid) (Rodrigues & Niederman, 1992).

An in-depth presentation inclusive of all pathogens, clinical manifestations, and treatment modalities for the various types of pneumonia is beyond the scope of this chapter. This chapter presents information about selected common pathogens associated with pneumonia, their clinical manifestations, and current treatment recommendations.

Database

Subjective

Predisposing Factors

- The woman may report one or more of the following (Rigby & Pastorek, 1996; Shannon, 1995):
    - ▶ Cigarette use
    - ▶ History of underlying pulmonary or cardiac disease
    - ▶ History of splenectomy
    - ▶ History of chronic medical illness (e.g., kidney disease)
    - ▶ History of substance use (e.g., alcohol abuse, injection drug use)
    - ▶ History of immune deficiency (e.g., HIV infection, receipt of immunosuppressive medications)
    - ▶ History of anemia
    - ▶ History of recent upper respiratory infection (URI), influenza, or viral exanthem (e.g., rubeola, varicella)
    - ▶ History of recent hospitalization
    - ▶ Recent immigration

Symptoms

The symptoms reported by pregnant women with pneumonia are similar to those reported by nonpregnant adults. The intensity of the symptoms will vary depending upon the pathogen causing the pneumonia, as well as the woman's baseline health status.

- Bacterial pneumonia: The woman will report the abrupt onset of several of the following symptoms (Mays & Leiner, 1996; Rigby & Pastorek, 1996; Rodrigues & Niederman, 1992; Shannon, 1995):

  ▶ Fever often greater than 38° C (100.4° F) (especially in women with pneumococcal pneumonia)

  ▶ Cough producing copious amounts of thick, purulent, and/or blood-tinged mucous.

  ▶ Chills

  ▶ Chest pain

  ▶ Dyspnea

  ▶ Malaise

  ▶ Headache (rare)

  ▶ Myalgia

  ▶ Change in mental status (often noted in *L. pneumophila*)

  ▶ Nausea, vomiting, diarrhea (usually in association with *L. pneumophila*)

- Viral pneumonia: The symptoms associated with viral pneumonia are similar to those noted by women with bacterial pneumonias. However, the following may be reported as a result of the woman's underlying viral illness (Rigby & Pastorek, 1996; Shannon, 1995):

  ▶ History of a viral exanthem that may indicate recent rubeola or varicella virus infection (see Chapter 10.5, *Measles [Rubeola]*, and Chapter 10.11, *Varicella Zoster Virus*).

  ▶ History of symptoms that may indicate recent influenza infection (see Chapter 11.3, *Influenza*).

- Atypical pneumonia: The woman with *M. pneumoniae* or *C. pneumoniae* (TWAR) pneumonia may report a gradual onset of the following symptoms (Mays & Leiner, 1996; Shannon, 1995):

  ▶ Headache

  ▶ Malaise

  ▶ Low-grade fever

  ▶ Sore throat

  ▶ Enlarged cervical lymph glands (if *M. pneumoniae*)

  ▶ Persistent, nonproductive cough (especially if *M. pneumoniae*)

  ▶ Chest muscle discomfort (not pleuritic pain)

  ▶ Symptoms associated with sinusitis

    − Headache

    − Purulent nasal discharge

- Fever

- Periorbital discomfort/ache

► Central nervous system (CNS) symptoms, including stiff neck, problems with coordination, and diminished hearing (occurs in up to 7 percent of patients with *M. pneumoniae* pneumonia)

Objective

The following physical findings may be noted in pregnant women with pneumonia (Rigby & Pastorek, 1996; Rodrigues & Niederman, 1992):

● General

► May appear anxious, apprehensive, agitated, or confused, depending upon level of hypoxia and/or coexistent morbidity (e.g., meningitis).

● Vital signs

► Temperature may be elevated or normal.

► Blood pressure may be normal or decreased (if shock or significant dehydration).

► Pulse may be increased.

► Respiratory rate may be normal or increased; orthopnea may be evident.

● Skin

► Color may be normal, or grayish-to-cyanotic depending upon the woman's oxygen perfusion.

► Poor tissue turgor may be evident if the woman is dehydrated.

► Rash may be evident in women with a concomitant viral or fungal (e.g., *Coccidioides immitis*) infection.

● Chest

► Upon examination, diminished excursion of the thorax may be observed if significant chest pain/discomfort.

► Palpation of the chest wall

- Tenderness to palpation of intercostal muscles may be noted.

- Increased tactile fremitus may be noted in area(s) of consolidation.

► Percussion of chest may reveal

- Decreased diaphragmatic excursion on affected side, if there is accumulation of pleural fluid at the lung bases

- Dullness in area(s) of consolidation

► Auscultation of the lungs may reveal

- Crackles

- Bronchial or tubular breath sounds (if consolidation)

- Pleural friction rub (if pleural effusion)

- Diminished or absent vesicular breath sounds (if pleural effusion)

- Increased bronchophony, egophony, and whispered pectoriloquy (if consolidation or pleural effusion)

  ▶ Auscultation of the heart may reveal a systolic murmur (if endocarditis).

- Abdominal examination may reveal

  ▶ Diffuse tenderness to palpation

  NOTE: During pregnancy a woman with pneumonia may present with minimal pulmonary/respiratory complaints, but will report abdominal discomfort or pain.

  ▶ Fundal height less than normal for weeks of gestation may be noted (if intrauterine growth restriction [IUGR])

- Neurological examination may reveal nuchal rigidity and/or altered mentation (if CNS involvement).

Assessment

- Pneumonia (bacterial, viral, atypical, fungal)

  ▶ R/O bacteremia

  ▶ R/O meningitis

  ▶ R/O cardiac disease

  ▶ R/O influenza infection

  ▶ R/O tuberculosis

  ▶ R/O adult respiratory distress syndrome

  ▶ R/O pulmonary embolism and infarction

  ▶ R/O neoplasm

  ▶ R/O immune deficiency

  ▶ R/O pertussis

  ▶ R/O IUGR

Plan

Diagnostic Tests

- A number of the following diagnostic tests may be ordered after consultation with a physician. Results from the tests will vary depending upon the type and severity of the pneumonia.

  ▶ Complete blood count (CBC) may reveal

  - Bacterial pneumonias (especially *S. pneumoniae*) will usually demonstrate a leukocytosis with a left shift present. However, up to 25 percent of patients may have a WBC within normal limits (WNL) (Musher, 1991).

- Hemoglobin/hematocrit (Hgb/Hct) may be elevated if the woman is dehydrated or decreased if she has coexistent anemia.

- Decreased platelets may be noted when *L. pneumophila* infection is present (Nguyen, Stout, & Yu, 1991).

▶ Serum chemistry panel may reveal

- Elevated transaminases (ALT, AST) and decreased serum sodium (less than 130 mEq/L) in *L. pneumophila* infection (Nguyen et al., 1991)

- Increased serum bilirubin (at least 3 to 4 mg/dL) and lactate dehydrogenase (less than 250 U/L) is often noted in *S. pneumoniae* infection (Musher, 1991).

▶ Gram stain of sputum may reveal the organism if an adequate sputum specimen is obtained. A reliable sputum specimen (evaluated on low magnification) must contain a minimum of 25 polymorphonuclear (PMN) cells/field and 5 or more squamous epithelial cells to minimize the possibility of contamination from upper airway organisms (Hampson, Woolf & Springmeyer, 1991; Mays & Leiner, 1996).

▶ Specimens for culture

- Sputum culture to identify a specific organism may be positive if adequate sputum specimen has been obtained. If the patient is unable to produce an adequate specimen, sputum induction may be necessary.

- In women presenting with significant symptoms, blood or pleural fluid specimens should be obtained for culture. A positive result is considered diagnostic for the causative organism (e.g., *S. pneumoniae*, *H. influenzae*, influenza virus type A).

- Cultures from urine and stool specimens may be obtained to identify possible pathogens (e.g., *Coccidioides immitis*, cytomegalovirus [CMV]).

▶ Pulse oximetry may demonstrate a decreased PaO_2 (e.g., less than or equal to 95 percent) indicating hypoxia.

▶ Blood gases may demonstrate hypoxia.

NOTE: The normal blood gas values for a pregnant woman are pH = 7.4, PO_2 = 100 to 105 mm Hg, PCO_2 = 30 mm Hg.

▶ Chest radiographs may demonstrate local or diffuse changes including infiltration, consolidation, pleural effusion, and abscess formation (rarely). In women with HIV infection the chest x-ray findings may be subtle

▶ Serum antibody titer(s).

- Acute and convalescent serum antibody titers for a viral pathogen, when suspected, may demonstrate a four-fold rise in titer indicating recent infection.

- IgM titer rise may indicate acute infection with viral or fungal pathogen.

- Cold agglutinin titer greater or equal to 1:64 is suggestive of *M. pneumoniae* infection (50 percent of patients with *M. pneumoniae* infection demonstrate such a rise in titer) (Martin & Bates, 1991).

Treatment/Management

- Treat and manage a pregnant woman with pneumonia in collaboration with a physician.

- A pregnant woman with moderate to severe symptoms, evidence of hypoxia, a history of underlying medical conditions which may impair immune response, or in whom a particularly virulent organism is suspected should be hospitalized.

- In uncomplicated community-acquired pneumonia, outpatient therapy is possible. Empiric antibiotic therapy for suspected bacterial pneumonia should cover the most common pathogens associated with community-acquired disease (i.e., *S. pneumoniae*, *H. influenzae*) such as one of the following agents:

  - ▶ Amoxicillin and clavulanate 500 mg p.o. t.i.d. for 10 days

  - ▶ Cefuroxime 250 to 500 mg p.o. b.i.d. for 10 days

  - ▶ Trimethoprim/sulfamethoxazole DS 1 tablet p.o. b.i.d. for 10 days

- If an atypical pathogen (e.g., *M. pneumoniae*) is suspected, then a macrolide antibiotic is advised, such as erythromycin 250–500 mg p.o. q.i.d. for 14 days.

- Clinical care of a pregnant woman suspected of having pneumonia as a result of influenza virus type A infection should be managed by the consulting physician. In such instances, the use of amantadine hydrochloride should be considered (see Chapter 11.3, *Influenza*).

- Care of a pregnant woman suspected of having varicella pneumonia should be managed by the consulting physician. In such instances, the use of intravenous acyclovir is indicated (see Chapter 10.11, *Varicella Zoster Virus*).

- A pregnant woman suspected or documented to have a fungal pneumonia should be managed by the consulting physician. Discussion of the therapeutic agents for the various fungal pneumonias is beyond the scope of this chapter.

- A woman diagnosed with *Pneumocystis carinii* pneumonia (PCP) is presumed to be HIV-infected. If documentation of the woman's HIV serostatus is lacking, counsel her about HIV infection and obtain voluntary consent for testing (see the Chapter 14.5, *Human Immunodeficiency Virus*, for the implications of HIV infection during pregnancy and for the neonate).

- Symptomatic treatment of pneumonia includes rest, increased fluid intake, adequate protein and carbohydrate intake, and the use of acetaminophen 650 mg p.o. every 4 hours as needed to relieve fever and discomfort.

- If the woman smokes, advise her to stop to prevent exacerbation of symptoms, further damage to her lung tissue, and adverse effects on her fetus. If the woman does not smoke but lives in an environment in which she is exposed to secondary smoke, advise her to limit her exposure as much as possible.

- Initiate antenatal testing (e.g., nonstress tests [NSTs], amniotic fluid index [AFIs]) between 32 and 34 weeks' gestation in a woman with IUGR, or who has a history of moderate to severe pneumonia during her pregnancy.

- Obtain serial obstetrical ultrasounds every 3 to 4 weeks in women with IUGR to assess fetal growth.

- Pneumococcal vaccination is recommended for women who are (Centers for Disease Control and Prevention [CDC], 1997)

  ▶ Immune competent but have chronic illnesses (e.g., diabetes mellitus, cardiovascular disease, pulmonary disease, alcoholism, cirrhosis or cerebrospinal fluid leaks)

  ▶ Immunocompromised (e.g., chronic renal failure, nephrotic syndrome, splenic dysfunction or anatomic asplenia, Hodgkin's disease, lymphoma, multiple myeloma, or conditions such as organ transplantation)

  ▶ HIV-infected (both asymptomatic and symptomatic) (see Chapter 14.5, *Human Immunodeficiency Virus,* for additional information)

  ▶ Living in environments or social settings with an identified increased risk of pneumococcal disease and its complications (e.g., certain Native American tribes)

- Pneumococcal polyvalent vaccine 0.5 mL IM affords protection against 23 strains of *S. pneumoniae* in immunocompetent individuals.

  NOTE: The duration of immunity is unknown; however, it is estimated to be protective for 5 to 10 years (CDC, 1997). Pneumococcal vaccine is a killed-bacteria vaccine, with the risk to the fetus unknown. Ideally, this vaccine should be administered prior to pregnancy or after the first trimester of pregnancy.

- Influenza vaccination should be administered annually to women who will be equal to or greater than 14 weeks' gestation during influenza season (see Chapter 11.3, *Influenza*).

  NOTE: Pneumococcal and influenza vaccines reportedly can be given at the same time at different sites without an increased incidence of side effects (CDC, 1997).

Consultation

- Consult with a physician for any pregnant woman with suspected or documented pneumonia.

- Transfer the care of women with moderate to severe symptoms, evidence of hypoxia, a history of an underlying medical condition that may impair immune response, complications of pneumonia, or poor response to initial therapy to the physician for management.

Patient Education

- Educate the woman about pneumonia, including the probable cause, clinical course, diagnostic tests indicated, treatment options, possible maternal and fetal complications, and need for follow-up.

- Educate the woman regarding signs and symptoms of possible complications associated with pneumonia and the need for immediate evaluation if any occur.

- If the woman's condition requires hospitalization for treatment, the physician responsible for her care should discuss the treatment options and need for hospitalization with her.

- Educate the woman about the need for compliance with treatment regimens to facilitate resolution of the pneumonia and prevent the development of resistant strains of bacteria.

- If the woman smokes, advise her to stop smoking and provide her with information regarding smoking cessation programs and community resources available to her.

- Educate the woman about the need for immunizations as indicated (e.g., influenza, pneumococcal).

- Pregnant women without evidence of HIV counseling and voluntary testing should be offered these options with provision of confidentiality regarding results if testing is performed.

Follow-Up

- If the woman is hospitalized, schedule follow-up visits as recommended by the physician responsible for her care.

- Follow-up evaluation is indicated in any woman who develops persistent symptoms after initiation of appropriate therapy, who may be noncompliant with treatment regimens, or who develops symptoms of complications.

- Women responding to outpatient treatment and without evidence of obstetrical problems should return for routine obstetrical assessments per institution-specific protocols.

- Women with evidence of obstetrical complications (e.g., IUGR) should have follow-up appointments for clinical assessments and fetal surveillance (e.g., NSTs, serial ultrasounds) as indicated (see Treatment and Management sections of this chapter; see also Chapter 6.15, *Intrauterine Growth Restriction/Small for Gestational Age*).

- Document diagnosis of pneumonia and treatment thereof in progress notes and problem list.

References

Benedetti, T.J., Valle, R., & Ledger, W.J. (1982). Antepartum pneumonia in pregnancy. *Obstetrics and Gynecology, 144*(4), 413–417.

Berkowitz, K., & LaSala, A. (1990). Risk factors associated with the increasing prevalence of pneumonia during pregnancy. *American Journal of Obstetrics and Gynecology, 163*(3), 981–985.

Centers for Disease Control and Prevention (CDC). (1997). Prevention of pneumococcal disease: Recommendations of the Immunization Practices Advisory Committee (ACIP). *Morbidity and Mortality Weekly Report, 46*(RR–8), 1–24.

Hampson, N.B., Woolf, R.A., & Springmeyer, S.C. (1991). Oral antibiotics for pneumonia. *Clinics in Chest Medicine, 12*(2), 395–407.

Madinger, N.E., Greenspoon, J.S., & Eilrodt, A.G. (1989). Pneumonia during pregnancy: Has modern technology improved maternal and fetal outcome? *American Journal of Obstetrics and Gynecology, 161*(3), 657–662.

Martin, R.E., & Bates, J.H. (1991). Atypical pneumonia. *Infectious Disease Clinics of North America, 5*(3), 585–601.

Mays, M., & Leiner, S. (1996). Primary care for women. Management of common respiratory problems. *Journal of Nurse-Midwifery, 41*(2), 139–154.

Musher, D.M. (1991). Pneumococcal pneumonia including diagnosis and therapy of infection caused by penicillin-resistant strains. *Infectious Disease Clinics of North America, 5*(3), 509–521.

Nguyen, M H., Stout, J.E., & Yu, V.L. (1991). Legionellosis. *Infectious Disease Clinics of North America, 5*(3), 561–584.

Peterson, C.M., Schuppert, K., Kelly, P.C., & Pappagianis D. (1993). Coccidioidomycosis and pregnancy. *Obstetrical and Gynecological Survey, 48*(3), 149–156.

Rigby, F.B., & Pastorek, J.G. (1996). Pneumonia during pregnancy. *Clinical Obstetrics and Gynecology, 39*(1), 107–119.

Rodrigues, J., & Niederman, M.S. (1992). Pneumonia complicating pregnancy. *Clinics in Chest Medicine, 13*(4), 679–691.

Shannon, M.T. (1995). Pneumonia. In W. Star, L.L. Lommel, & M.T. Shannon (Eds.), *Women's primary health care: Protocols for practice* (pp. 5–38, 5–44). Washington, DC: American Nurses Publishing.

Chapter 5

UPPER RESPIRATORY INFECTION

Maureen T. Shannon

Lucy Newmark Sammons

An upper respiratory infection (URI) is defined as an infectious disease process involving the nasal passages, pharynx, and/or bronchi. URIs are the most common illnesses in adults. A variety of viruses cause URIs including coronavirus, rhinovirus, adenovirus, respiratory syncitial virus, parainfluenza virus, and influenza types A, B, and C (Beckmann et al., 1995; Rabinowitz, 1990). The virus is transmitted by close contact and enters the body via the ciliated epithelium of the nose. This exposure results in edema and hyperemia of the nasal mucosa with a subsequent increase in the secretion of the mucous glands responsible for the production of serous and mucinous fluid. The narrowing of the nasal passages as a result of nasal mucosal edema causes the nasal obstructive symptoms associated with an URI (Shannon, 1995).

Although URIs are considered to be benign infections, there are complications that may occur, including acute otitis media, acute sinusitis, acute or chronic bronchitis, or pneumonia. Often these complications develop after a secondary bacterial infection is superimposed on the original viral infection. Women at an increased risk of developing complications usually have a history of smoking, recurrent sinusitis, cardiac or pulmonary disease, chronic anemia, or an altered immune response. Pregnancy does not alter the progress of URIs, and there is no increased incidence of complications reported in association with pregnancy alone. Since viremia does not occur with this infection, adverse fetal effects are extremely rare (Beckmann et al., 1995).

Database

Subjective

Woman will report the following:

- Rhinorrhea—usually clear but may be purulent if secondary bacterial infection
- Nasal congestion
- Sneezing
- Postnasal drainage
- Nonproductive cough
- "Scratchy" sore throat
- Headache
- Fever
- Malaise
- Hoarseness

Objective

Physical examination will demonstrate the following:

- Normal or mildly elevated temperature
- Respiratory rate within normal limits (WNL)
- Nasal turbinates may be pale, boggy, or erythematous
- Presence of vesicles on oropharynx
- Pharyngeal mucosa may be erythematous
- Tonsillar pillars may be slightly edematous with or without exudate
- Enlarged tonsillar and/or cervical lymph nodes may be palpated
- Auscultation of the lungs demonstrates normal breath sounds
- No evidence of bacterial complications or more severe pathology, including

  ▶ Temperature of 103° F or more (≥ 39.5° C.)

  ▶ Tachypnea

  ▶ Pain on percussion over frontal or maxillary sinuses

  ▶ Mucopurulent nasal discharge

  ▶ Pharyngeal mucosa erythematous, edematous, with petichiae; presence of yellow or white exudate or follicles

  ▶ Opaque maxillary or frontal sinuses on transillumination

  ▶ Other abnormalities of ears, eyes, cranial nerves, nose, mouth, throat, neck, pharnyx, lungs, or generalized disease signs suggesting more serious pathology

Assessment

- Upper respiratory infection (URI)

  ▶ R/O rhinitis (allergic, vasomotor, pregnancy associated, medicamentosa)

  ▶ R/O acute sinusitis

  ▶ R/O group A streptococcal pharyngitis

  ▶ R/O acute otitis media

  ▶ R/O bronchitis

  ▶ R/O pneumonia

  ▶ R/O influenza

  ▶ R/O infectious mononucleosis

  ▶ R/O measles, mumps

  ▶ R/O cytomegalovirus (CMV)

Plan

Diagnostic Tests

- There are no specific diagnostic tests indicated. However, one or more of the following tests may be ordered to eliminate or document the presence of other pathologic conditions.

  ▶ Throat culture for group A streptococcus will be negative.

  ▶ Monospot test will be negative for infectious mononucleosis.

  ▶ Nasal smear may demonstrate greater than 4 percent eosinophils, indicating allergic rhinitis.

  ▶ CMV IgM titer will be negative for acute CMV infection.

  ▶ Chest x-ray will be within normal limits (WNL).

  ▶ Radiographs of sinuses will be WNL.

Treatment/Management

- There is no specific treatment that has been found to be effective in shortening or eliminating the symptoms of an URI.

- Advise rest, increased hydration (especially with warm liquids), and diet as tolerated.

- Symptomatic treatment with home remedies may include

  ▶ Saline gargles ($^1/_4$ teaspoon of salt in 8 ounces of warm water) t.i.d. for relief of sore throat.

  ▶ Buffered saline nose spray to reduce nasal dryness, bleeding, and vascular congestion.

  ▶ Steam vaporizer to help liquefy secretions.

  NOTE: Warn the woman about the placement of a steam vaporizer in areas where small children or other household members may be harmed if the liquid is spilled.

  ▶ Camphor/menthol ointment (Vicks®) may provide relief of head and chest cold symptoms when applied topically or in vaporizer.

- Advise the woman that she may use acetaminophen 650 mg p.o. every 4 hrs p.r.n. to relieve fever or generalized discomfort.

  NOTE: Aspirin should not be used during pregnancy because of its effects on maternal and neonatal hemostasis mechanisms resulting in an increased risk of hemorrhage (Briggs, Freeman, & Yaffe, 1994). In addition, in adolescents, as well as young children, its use has been associated with the development of Reye syndrome.

- The use of a decongestant may be necessary to relieve nasal congestion. Over-the-counter (OTC) preparations are available but the woman should be advised to take only those decongestant preparations recommended by her clinician, such as pseudoephedrine HCL 30 mg to 60 mg p.o. every 4 to 6 hours, as needed (maximum 24 hour dose ≤ 240 mg).

- The use of antihistamines to relieve rhinorrhea and sneezing may be necessary. There are several OTC preparations of antihistamines but the woman should be advised to take only those recommended by her clinician. Some of the preparations available include

▶ Chlorpheniramine 4 mg to 8 mg p.o. b.i.d. or t.i.d.

▶ Diphenhydramine 25 mg p.o. b.i.d. or t.i.d.

NOTE: The use of antihistamines in general during the last 2 weeks of pregnancy has reportedly been associated with retrolentel fibroplasia in premature infants (Briggs et al., 1994). Women using antihistamine preparations should be advised to avoid activities requiring concentration (e.g., operating a motor vehicle) because of the associated central nervous system effects (e.g., drowsiness).

- Prescribing antibiotics is unnecessary because they are ineffective in the treatment of this viral infection and will not prevent the development of associated complications.

- Initiate antibiotics in women who develop secondary bacterial infections (e.g., acute otitis media, acute sinusitis, pneumonia).

- Influenza vaccine may be given to women who will be equal to or more than 14 weeks pregnant during the influenza season (Centers for Disease Control and Prevention [CDC], 1997).

- In pregnant women at high risk for complications associated with epidemic influenza A who are suspected of this respiratory infection, amantadine therapy may be considered after evaluating the perinatal risks versus the benefits of this medication (CDC, 1997).

Consultation

- Consult with a physician for evaluation and management of suspected pathology beyond scope of practice.

- Consult with a perinatalogist whenever use of amantadine is being considered (see Chapter 11.3, *Influenza*).

Patient Education

- Explain the causes of symptoms, the mechanism of infection, and rationale for recommended treatments.

- Discuss environmental factors that may increase symptoms and advise the woman to reduce exposure to irritants (e.g., chemicals, smoke).

- Educate the woman about the use of OTC medications and advise her not to use any OTC medication unless she has contacted her provider.

- Educate the woman to contact her provider if the treatment approach is not successful, or if she develops symptoms of complications.

- Educate the woman who smokes about the adverse maternal and fetal effects associated with nicotine use. Refer her to smoking cessation programs.

Follow-up

- Educate the woman to contact her provider if any signs or symptoms of secondary bacterial infection occurs (e.g., URI symptoms beyond 10 to 14 days, persistent or rising fever after initial 2 to 3 days, nasal discharge or sputum becomes increasingly mucopurulent, sinuses become tender), other evidence of systemic disease develops, or if inadequate relief from discomfort obtained.

- If mild symptoms without complications, reevaluate degree of symptoms and effectiveness of therapeutics on following visit.

- Document diagnosis of URI and management thereof in progress notes and problem list.

References

Beckmann, C.R.B., Ling, F.W., Barzansky, B.M., Bates, G.W., Herbert, W. N. P., Laube, D.W., & Smith, R.P. (1995). *Obstetrics and gynecology* (2nd ed., pp. 84–85). Baltimore, MD: Williams & Wilkins.

Briggs, G,G., Freeman, R.K., Yaffe, S.J. (1994). *Drugs in pregnancy and lactation* (4th ed.). Baltimore, MD: Williams & Wilkins.

Centers for Disease Control and Prevention (CDC). (1997). Prevention and control of influenza. Recommendations of the Immunization Practices Advisory Committee (ACIP). *Morbidity and Mortality Weekly Report, 46*(RR-9), 1–25.

Rabinowitz, H.K. (1990). Upper respiratory tract infection. *Primary Care, 17*(4), 793–809.

Shannon, M.T. (1995). Rhinitis. In W.L. Star, L.L. Lommel, & M.T. Shannon (Eds.), *Women's primary health care. Protocols for practice* (pp. 5–45, 5–49). Washington, DC: American Nurses Publishing.

SECTION 12

THYROID CONDITIONS

Chapter 1

EUTHYROID OF PREGNANCY

Maureen T. Shannon

Euthyroid of pregnancy is a term used to describe the normal enlargement of the thyroid gland often observed during pregnancy. This enlargement is attributed to increased vascularity and glandular hyperplasia that occurs in response to the effects of pregnancy hormones on thyroid regulation and secretion. Specifically, the hyperestrogenemia of pregnancy results in three separate but interrelated stimuli: an increase in the level of circulating thyroxine binding globulin (TBG), an increase in the level of circulating human chorionic gonadotropin (hCG), and a decrease in the availability of iodine due to increased iodine clearance by the kidneys(American College of Obstetricians & Gynecologists [ACOG], 1993; Brent, 1997; Hall, 1995; Hall, Richards, & Lazarus, 1993; Seely & Burrow, 1994). The interpretation of thyroid function tests (TFTs) during pregnancy requires an understanding of these interrelationships and their effects on specific TFT results (see Table 11.1, Effects of Pregnancy on Laboratory Tests Commonly Used to Evaluate Thyroid Function).

The enlargement observed with euthyroid is diffuse, nontender, and not more than twice the expected size for a normal thyroid gland. In addition, the woman does not report any signs or symptoms that may be associated with thyroid disease. Although euthyroid of pregnancy is a very common physical finding, the possibility of hypothyroidism or hyperthyroidism should not be overlooked when evaluating any enlargement of the thyroid gland. In general, a third generation thyroid stimulating hormone (TSH) level (with improved sensitivity for low values), a free T4 (FT4) concentration, and the free thyroxine index (FTI) are the laboratory tests used to evaluate the majority of thyroid function abnormalities during pregnancy (Brent, 1997; Fischbach, 1996; Seely & Burrow, 1994).

Database

Subjective

- No personal or family history of thyroid disease
- No symptoms associated with thyroid disease

Objective

- Blood pressure within normal limits (WNL)
- Pulse WNL
- Thyroid gland palpation may reveal diffuse, soft, nontender enlargement not more than twice normal size without nodules
- Other components of physical examination WNL

Assessment

- Euthyroid of pregnancy
  - ▶ R/O hypothyroidism
  - ▶ R/O hyperthyroidism
  - ▶ R/O thyroid mass

Plan

Diagnostic Tests (see Table 11.1)

- Thyroid stimulating hormone (TSH) level (will be WNL)
- Total thyroxine (T4) (increased)
- Triiodothyronine (T_3) resin uptake (decreased)
- Free T4 (FT4) WNL (unchanged from nonpregnant levels)
- Free thyroxine index (FTI) WNL

Treatment/Management

- No treatment is indicated in euthyroid of pregnancy.

Consultation

- Physician consultation is indicated in women who are being evaluated for thyroid disease.

Patient Education

- Educate the woman regarding the tests that are being ordered.
- Discuss laboratory test results when they are obtained.
- Reassure the woman that this physical finding is very common during pregnancy and that it does not have any associated adverse effects on her or her infant.

Follow-up

- Routine prenatal follow-up visits are indicated unless thyroid disease is diagnosed.
- Document findings of thyroid gland enlargement in physical examination section of chart and progress notes.

Table 12.1

Effects of Pregnancy on Laboratory Tests Commonly Used to Evaluate Thyroid Function

Test	Normal Pregnancy	Hyperthyroidism	Hypothyroidism (Primary)
TSH	No change	Normal to decreased	Increased
TBG	Increased	Increased	Increased
Total T4	Increased	Increased	Decreased
FT4	No change	Increased	Decreased
FTI	No change	Increased	Decreased
Total T_3	Slightly increased	Increased	Normal to slightly decreased
T_3RU	Decreased	Increased	Decreased
TSAb	Negative	Often positive	Negative

TSH = thyroid stimulating hormone
TBG = thyroid-binding globulin
T4 = thyroxine
T_3 = triiodothyronine

FT4 = free T4
FTI = free thyroxine index
T_3RU = T3 resin uptake
TSAb = thyroid stimulating antibody

Source: Adapted with permission from Beckman, C.R.B., Ling, F.W., Barzansky, B.M., Bates, G.W., Herbert, W.N.P., Laube, D.W., & Smith, R.P. (1995). *Obstetrics and gynecology* (2nd. ed., p. 96). Baltimore, MD: Williams & Wilkins.

References

American College of Obstetricians & Gynecologists (ACOG) (1993). *Thyroid disease in pregnancy.* (Technical bulletin no. 181). Washington, DC: Author.

Beckman, C. R. B., Ling, F. W., Barzansky, B. M., Bates, G. W., Herbert, W. N. P., Laube, D. W., & Smithe, R. P. (1995). *Obstetrics and gynecology* (2nd ed., pp. 95-96). Baltimore, MD: Williams & Wilkins.

Brent, G.A. (1997). Maternal thyroid function: Interpretation of thyroid function tests in pregnancy. *Clinical Obstetrics and Gynecology, 40*(1), 3–15.

Fischbach, F. (1996). *A manual of laboratory and diagnostic tests* (5th ed., pp. 423-439). Philadelphia, PA: Lippincott.

Hall, R. (1995). Pregnancy and autoimmune endocrine disease. *Baillière's Clinical Endocrinology and Metabolism, 9*(1), 137-155.

Hall, R., Richards, C. J., & Lazarus, J. H. (1993). The thyroid and pregnancy. *British Journal of Obstetrics and Gynaecology, 100*, 512-515.

Seely, B. L., & Burrow, G. N. (1994). Thyroid disease and pregnancy. In R. K. Creasy & R. Resnik (Eds.), *Maternal-fetal medicine. Principles and practice* (3rd ed., pp. 979-1003). Philadelphia, PA: W. B. Saunders.

Sipes, S. L., & Malee, M. P. (1992). Endocrine disorders in pregnancy. *Obstetrics and Gynecologic Clinics of North America, 19*(4), 655-677.

Chapter 2

HYPERTHYROIDISM

Maureen T. Shannon

Hyperthyroidism is a disorder that occurs when there has been a chronic elevation of free thyroid hormone levels resulting in overstimulation of the basal metabolism. This clinical syndrome is usually evident before a woman becomes pregnant, but initial episodes can occur during pregnancy. The reported incidence of this disorder during pregnancy is 0.2 percent (American College of Obstetricians & Gynecologists [ACOG], 1993; Mestman, 1997; Mestman, Goodwin, & Montoro, 1995). The most common cause of hyperthyroidism during pregnancy is Grave's disease, an autoimmune disorder associated with thyroid-stimulating antibody production (ACOG, 1993; Mestman, 1997; Mestman et al., 1995). Other less common etiologies include toxic adenoma, multinodular toxic goiter, viral thyroiditis, gestational trophoblastic disease (GTD), iodine-induced hyperthyroidism, iatrogenic hyperthyroidism, and hyperthyroxemia due to hyperemesis gravidarum.

Hyperthyroidism unresponsive to therapy during pregnancy has been associated with an increased incidence of preeclampsia, congestive heart failure, thyrotoxicosis, intrauterine growth retardation (IUGR), preterm labor and delivery, low birth weight infants, and stillbirths (ACOG, 1993; Mestman, 1997; Mestman et al., 1995). Neonatal hypothyroidism and goiter can result if large doses of antithyroid medications plus iodine therapy are used to treat maternal hyperthyroidism (ACOG, 1993). Careful monitoring of maternal thyroid function tests (TFTs) and minimal doses of antithyroid medications have decreased the incidence of neonatal hypothyroidism. Monitoring of maternal TFTs should continue during the postpartum period, because there is an increased risk of thyroid storm occurring after delivery (ACOG, 1993).

Database

Subjective

- May report a personal or family history of thyroid disease
- May report one or more of the following:
  - ▶ Unintentional weight loss
  - ▶ Palpitations
  - ▶ Anxiety
  - ▶ Fatigue
  - ▶ Excessive perspiration
  - ▶ Heat intolerance
  - ▶ Diarrhea
  - ▶ Muscle weakness
  - ▶ Difficulty concentrating

► Neck mass

► Hyperemesis

Objective

- Weight may be significantly less than expected for height and reported dietary intake

- Pulse greater than 100 beats per minute at rest and will not decrease with a Valsalva maneuver

- Thyroid gland palpation may reveal a diffusely enlarged (two to five times normal size), firm, non-tender thyroid

- Auscultation over thyroid gland may reveal a bruit

- Exopthalmopathy

- Hyperreflexia

- Pretibial edema

- Hair may feel fine and appear to be thinning

- Plummer's nails (onycholysis)—loosening/detachment of the nails from the nail beds may be observed.

- Skin may be warm and dry

- Periorbital skin may appear yellow

- Speech may be rapid and/or excited

- Fundal height measurement may be less than expected for weeks of gestation

- Fine tremors of fingers may be observed

Assessment

- Enlarged thyroid—probable hyperthyroidism
  - ► R/O Grave's disease
  - ► R/O thyrotoxicosis
  - ► R/O thyroid cancer
  - ► R/O hyperemesis gravidarum
  - ► R/O GTD
  - ► R/O IUGR

Plan

Diagnostic Tests

The usual biochemical tests to confirm hyperthyroidism during pregnancy include the TSH and free T 4 (FT4), although other diagnostic tests may be ordered as indicated (Mestman, 1997; Mestman et al., 1995; Seely & Burrow, 1994):

- TSH may be within normal limits (WNL) or decreased.

- Free T4 increased.

- Total T_3 increased.

- Total T4 increased.

- Thyroid binding globulins (TBG) WNL for pregnancy.

- Free thyroxine index (FTI) increased.

- Thyroid-stimulating antibodies (TSAb)—Antithyroid peroxidase (anti-TPO) and thyroid stimulating hormone receptor bodies (TSHRAb) are present in Grave's disease (Mestman, 1997).

  NOTE: An increased maternal TSHRAb titer (greater than 30 percent) during the third trimester is associated with an increased risk of neonatal hyperthyroidism and, possibly, neonatal thyrotoxicosis as a result of transplacental transfer of maternal TSAbs (Mestman, 1997). The perinatal mortality rate for neonatal thyrotoxicosis is reportedly 30 to 50 percent (ACOG, 1993; Mestman et al., 1995).

- Ultrasonography may reveal IUGR or fetal goiter (due to excessive doses of maternal antithyroid medications).

- White blood cell (WBC) count may reveal mild leukopenia.

- Liver transaminases (ALT [SGPT], AST [SGOT]) may be slightly elevated

- Alkaline phosphatase may be increased above the usual elevation expected during pregnancy.

- Serum calcium may be elevated (observed in less than 10 to 27 percent of individuals with hyperthyroidism).

Treatment/Management

- Physician consultation is indicated in women who are being evaluated for thyroid disease. Women who are diagnosed with hyperthyroidism may be co-managed with a physician in some clinical settings.

- Treatment options for the woman with hyperthyroidism will be determined by the consulting physician.

  ▶ The goal of treatment is to restore and maintain a euthyroid state, and prevent fetal thyroid dysfunction using minimum amounts of antithyroid medications.

  ▶ Initial pharmacological therapy usually includes:

    – Propylthiouracil (PTU) 100 to 150 mg p.o. t.i.d. (or 200 to 300 mg p.o. t.i.d. in women with severe clinical manifestations)

        OR

    – Methimazole 10 to 20 mg p.o. b.i.d. (or 30 mg p.o. b.i.d. in women with severe clinical manifestations)

  NOTE: As soon as a woman's clinical symptoms resolve and TFTs are within the upper third of normal, the dose of antithyroid medication is reduced to half the initial dose (usually this requires 2 to 6 weeks of therapy at the initial higher doses). Adjustments in antithyroid medication continue every

1 to 2 weeks, as needed, to maintain minimal clinical symptomatology and laboratory values that are within an acceptable range (Mestman, 1997; Mestman et al., 1995; Seely & Burrow, 1994). Approximately 30 percent of women will remain euthyroid on small doses of antithyroid medications (e.g., 50 to 100 mg PTU or 5 to 10 mg methimazole) and may discontinue therapy after 32 weeks' gestation (Mestman, 1997).

- Beta blockers may be used in women manifesting severe hypermetabolic symptoms and may be continued for a few weeks or until acceptable TFT results are obtained (Seely & Burrow, 1994; Mestman et al., 1995). Adjust the dose of these medications to maintain a maternal resting pulse rate between 70 and 90 beats per minute (Mestman, 1997). Beta blockers that can be prescribed include

  ▶ Propranolol 20 to 40 mg p.o. t.i.d. or q.i.d.

    OR

  ▶ Atenolol 25 to 50 mg p.o. b.i.d.

    NOTE: These drugs are not considered teratogenic but fetal and neonatal toxicities may be observed. Both drugs are excreted in breastmilk; however, propranolol can be considered for use in women who are nursing their infants. Close observation of these infants for manifestations of ß-blockade is indicated (Briggs, Freeman, & Yaffe, 1994).

- Initiate serial ultrasonography every 3 to 4 weeks in women with suspected/documented IUGR to assess interval growth.

- Initiate daily fetal movement counts in women beginning at 28 weeks' gestation.

- Weekly antenatal fetal surveillance (e.g., nonstress test [NST], amniotic fluid index [AFI], or biophysical profile [BPP]) should be initiated at 32 weeks' gestation in women with poor response to therapy, women with Grave's disease with high TSAb levels or if IUGR is suspected/documented (Mestman, 1997; Mestman et al., 1995).

Consultation

- Consultation with a physician is mandatory in all suspected cases of hyperthyroidism.

Patient Education

- Education of the woman should include information regarding the possible cause(s) of the enlarged thyroid, the diagnostic tests that have been ordered and their results, the reason for fetal surveillance tests (if ordered), and the reason for consultation/referral to physician care.

- Discuss treatment options, risks, side effects, and possible fetal/neonatal effects with woman.

- The pediatrician who will be caring for the infant after birth should present the indications for neonatal thyroid function testing.

- Present information regarding the signs and symptoms of thyroid storm and the possibility of its occurrence postpartum.

- Breast-feeding is not contraindicated in a woman receiving antithyroid medication if the daily dose does not exceed 150 mg a day of PTU or 10 mg a day of methimazole. The concentration of either medication in breast milk is low. However, because there is a higher concentration of methimazole in breast milk compared to PTU, some authorities recommend that breast-feeding women receive PTU instead of methimazole (Mestman, 1997). The total daily dose should be divided and administered after the woman has breast-fed her infant. The infant should be monitored with TFTs at intervals determined by the infant's clinician (Mestman et al., 1995).

Follow-up

- Follow-up evaluations should be determined by the consulting physician. In general, clinical response to initial pharmacologic interventions can be expected within 2 to 6 weeks; tapering of antithyroid medications should begin once a response to therapy has been documented. Therefore, repeat TFTs are usually obtained 2 to 3 weeks after initiation of or changes in antithyroid medications (Mestman, 1997).

- Document diagnosis of hyperthyroidism and treatment thereof in problem list and progress notes.

References

American College of Obstetricians & Gynecologists (ACOG) (1993). *Thyroid disease in pregnancy.* (Technical bulletin no. 181.) Washington, DC: Author.

Briggs, G.G., Freeman, R.K., & Yaffe, S.J. (1994). *Drugs in pregnancy and lactation* (4th ed.). Baltimore, MD: Williams & Wilkins.

Mestman, J.H. (1997). Hyperthyroidism in pregnancy

Mestman, J.H., Goodwin, T.M., & Montoro, M.M. (1995). Thyroid disorders of pregnancy. *Endocrinology and Metabolism Clinics of North America, 24*(1), 41-71.

Seely, B.L., & Burrow, G.N. (1994). Thyroid disease and pregnancy. In R. K. Creasy & R. Resnik (Eds.), *Maternal-fetal medicine: Principles and practice* (3rd ed., pp. 979-1003). Philadelphia, PA: W.B. Saunders.

Chapter 3

HYPOTHYROIDISM

Maureen T. Shannon

Hypothyroidism is a deficiency in thyroid secretion resulting in a decreased basal metabolic rate. During pregnancy, primary hypothyroidism is diagnosed if there is an elevation in the level of thyroid stimulating hormone (TSH) and a lack of expected increase in the circulating levels of thyroxin (T4) (American College of Obstetricians & Gynecologists [ACOG], 1993). Secondary or pituitary hypothyroidism occurs when the TSH is elevated but the free T4 (FT4) level is normal. Secondary hypothyroidism is diagnosed as a result of laboratory findings, since women with this condition are usually asymptomatic (Seely & Burrow, 1994). In the United States, the most common cause of hypothyroidism during pregnancy is Hashimoto's thyroiditis, an autoimmune disorder characterized by the presence of antimicrosomal and antithyroglobulin antibodies. It has a reported incidence of 8 to 10 percent in women of reproductive age (Seely & Burrow, 1994). Other causes of hypothyroidism include iodine deficiency, medications (including iodide, lithium, amiodarone, and antithyroid drugs), destruction of the gland (due to surgery or radioactive iodine), and, rarely, idiopathic thyroid atrophy (Mestman, Goodwin, & Montoro, 1995; Montoro, 1997; Seely & Burrow, 1994).

Hypothyroidism complicating pregnancy is uncommon, since this disorder is associated with an increased incidence of infertility (ACOG, 1993). However, the presence of hypothyroidism does not absolutely preclude the possibility of conception. When pregnancy does occur the perinatal complications associated with uncorrected hypothyroidism include pregnancy-induced hypertension, preeclampsia, postpartum hemorrhage, anemia, abruptio placenta, and stillbirths (ACOG, 1993; Davis, Leveno, & Cunningham, 1988; Mestman et al., 1995, Montoro, 1997). In general, maternal hypothyroidism does not cause fetal hypothyroidism since the fetus begins producing thyroid hormone after 12 weeks' gestation (ACOG, 1993; Sipes & Malee, 1992). However, cretinism has been reported in infants born to hypothyroid women in iodine deficient regions of the United States (Seely & Burrow, 1994). Congenital hypothyroidism has an incidence of approximately 1 in 7,000 births in the United States and can be detected at birth through abnormal thyroid function tests (TFTs), specifically T4 and TSH. Once diagnosed, the prompt initiation of adequate therapy in these situation can prevent the adverse sequelae associated with congenital hypothyroidism (ACOG, 1993; Seely & Burrow, 1994).

Database

Subjective (Montoro, 1997)

- May report a personal or family history of thyroid disease
- May report a history of thyroidectomy or radioactive iodine therapy for Grave's disease
- May report history of type I diabetes mellitus
- May be asymptomatic
- May report one or more of the following:
  - ▶ Fatigue
  - ▶ Obesity

  ▶ Thinning of eyebrows/hair

  ▶ Facial or periorbital edema

  ▶ Thickened or coarse skin

  ▶ Numbness, tingling of fingers

  ▶ Cold intolerance

  ▶ Constipation

  ▶ Muscle cramps

  ▶ Depression

Objective

The physical examination will reveal one or more of the following (Montoro, 1997):

- Excessive weight gain

- Temperature may reveal hypothermia

- Decreased pulse

- Blood pressure may be increased if coexistent pregnancy-induced hypertension (PIH)

- Dry skin (xerosis)

- Loss of hair from outer third of the eyebrows

- Examination of the eyes may reveal exopthalmosis, lid lag

- Palpation of the thyroid may reveal thyromegaly

- Deep-tendon reflexes exhibit delayed relaxation phase

- Dry, coarse-feeling hair

- Neurological examination may reveal slow speech, somnolence, poor concentration, cerebellar ataxia

- Examination of extremities may reveal edema of the hands, ankles, and face

Assessment

- Possible hypothyroidism

  ▶ R/O euthyroid of pregnancy

  ▶ R/O Hashimoto's thyroiditis

  ▶ R/O thyroid mass (e.g., tumor, cancer)

  ▶ R/O PIH

  ▶ R/O preeclampsia

- Xerosis

Plan

Diagnostic Tests

The usual biochemical tests that are ordered to confirm the diagnosis of hypothyroidism during pregnancy are TSH, free T4 (FT4), and free thyroxine index (FTI); however, other diagnostic tests may be ordered, as indicated:

- TSH increased

- Free T4 (FT4) decreased

- Free thyroxine index (FTI) decreased

- Liver transaminases (ALT [SGPT], AST [SGOT]) may be slightly increased

- Hemoglobin and hematocrit may be decreased (up to 40 percent of patients may have anemia) (Montoro, 1997)

- Serum cholesterol may be elevated

- Creatine phosphokinase (CPK) may be elevated.

- Antimicrosomal and antithyroglobulin antibodies will show elevated titers in women with Hashimoto's thyroiditis.

- Ultrasonography may reveal IUGR, fetal goiter, or fetal bradycardia (if fetal hypothyroidism is present)

Treatment/Management

- Consult with a physician when evaluating a woman for thyroid disease. Once diagnosed, co-management of a woman's thyroid disease is warranted.

- Thyroid replacement therapy should be determined by the physician consultant.

  ▶ The goal of thyroid replacement therapy is to maintain a normal TSH concentration at a minimum level of medication.

  ▶ If a woman with preexisting hypothyroidism becomes pregnant, TSH levels should be obtained at 6 to 8, 16 to 20, and 28 to 32 weeks' gestation. The general consensus is to adjust the thyroxine replacement levothyroxine sodium as follows (Montoro, 1997):

    − If TSH is elevated but less than 10 mU/mL, add 50 mcg/day.

    − If TSH is less than 10 but more than 20 mU/mL, add 75 mcg/day.

    − If TSH is more than 20 mU/mL, add 100 mcg/day.

  ▶ Newly diagnosed women should begin therapy with levothyroxine sodium 2μg/kg/day or 150 mcg/day p.o. with an increase in the dose every 4 to 8 weeks until the TSH returns to the lowest limits of normal (Montoro, 1997; Seely & Burrow, 1994).

  NOTE: Levothyroxine sodium is secreted in low concentrations in the breast milk at levels that apparently do not interfere with neonatal thyroid screening tests. In addition, the concentrations are too low to protect hypothyroid infants from the disease (Briggs, Freeman, & Yaffe, 1994). Usually 8 weeks of thyroxine replacement is required before changes in TSH levels can be observed. Therefore, serial measurements of free T4 and TSH concentrations every 4 weeks are necessary to monitor the adequacy of replacement therapy (Hall, 1995; Montoro, 1997). Once the patient attains a euthyroid state, laboratory evaluations can occur at less frequent intervals (Montoro, 1997).

- Serial ultrasonography should be obtained every 3 to 4 weeks in women with suspected/documented IUGR.

- The woman should begin fetal movement counts at 28 weeks' gestation.

- Weekly antenatal fetal surveillance (e.g., NST, AFI, BPP) should be initiated at 32 to 34 weeks.

- Co-management of women responding to thyroid replacement therapy is possible.

Consultation

- Consultation with a physician is mandatory in all women with suspected or documented hypothyroidism.

Patient Education

- Education of the woman should include information regarding the possible diagnosis, the diagnostic tests ordered and their results, and the reason for consultation with a physician. Explain the need for repeat TFTs once thyroid replacement therapy has started.

- Educate the woman about the therapeutic interventions indicated, the risks, side effects, and any possible fetal/neonatal effects.

- The clinician who will be caring for the infant after birth should present the indications for neonatal thyroid function testing.

Follow-up

Routine prenatal visits can continue as long as the woman is responding to thyroid replacement therapy.

- Follow-up evaluations and repeat TFTs to monitor thyroid replacement therapy should be determined by the consulting physician (see Treatment/Management section).

- Document diagnosis of hypothyroidism and treatment thereof in problem list and progress notes.

References

American College of Obstetricians & Gynecologists (ACOG) (1993). *Thyroid disease in pregnancy.* (Technical bulletin no. 181.) Washington, DC: Author.

Briggs, G.G., Freeman, R.K., & Yaffe, S.J. (1994). *Drugs in pregnancy and lactation* (4th ed.). Baltimore, MD: Williams & Wilkins.

Davis, L.E., Leveno, K.J., & Cunningham, F.G. (1988). Hypothyroidism complicating pregnancy. *Obstetrics & Gynecology, 72,* 108-112.

Hall, R. (1995). Pregnancy and autoimmune endocrine disease. *Baillière's Clinical Endocrinology and Metabolism, 9*(1), 137-155.

Mestman, J.H., Goodwin, T.M., & Montoro, M.M. (1995). Thyroid disorders of pregnancy. *Endocrinology and Metabolism Clinics of North America, 24*(1), 41-71.

Montoro, M.N. (1997). Management of hypothyroidism during pregnancy. *Clinical Obstetrics and Gynecology, 40*(1), 65–80.

Seely, B.L., & Burrow, G.N. (1994). Thyroid disease and pregnancy. In R. K. Creasy & R. Resnik (Eds.), *Maternal-fetal medicine. Principles and practice* (3rd ed., pp. 979-1003). Philadelphia, PA: W.B. Saunders.

Sipes, S.L., & Malee, M.P. (1992). Endocrine disorders in pregnancy. *Obstetrics and Gynecologic Clinics of North America, 19*(4), 655-677.

Chapter 4

TRANSIENT POSTPARTUM THYROID DYSFUNCTION (POSTPARTUM THYROIDITIS)

Maureen T. Shannon

Transient postpartum thyroid dysfunction (postpartum thyroiditis) is an autoimmune disorder occurring in 5 to 10 percent of pregnancies (Novy, 1994; Seely & Burrow, 1994). It is characterized by the presence of antimicrosomal antibodies in the majority of women in whom it is diagnosed (Browne-Martin & Emerson, 1997). This finding supports the hypothesis that the women affected by this disorder probably have a preexisting subclinical autoimmune thyroiditis during pregnancy (Novy, 1994). In addition, the levels of these antibodies during the first trimester of pregnancy have been predictive of the development of postpartum thyroiditis in women at risk for thyroid disease (e.g., women with a family history of thyroid disease).

Transient postpartum thyroid dysfunction can be overlooked because its symptoms are often dismissed as being the expected manifestations of a woman's psychological and physiologic adjustments during the initial postpartum months. It has a biphasic pattern characterized by the development of hyperthyroid symptoms approximately 2 to 3 months after birth that continue for up to 4 months. This is followed by a hypothyroid phase lasting from 1 to 3 months. However, not all women with postpartum thyroid dysfunction will have documentation of this biphasic pattern because the diagnosis of this disorder may not occur until several months after delivery when the hyperthyroid phase has subsided (Mestman, Goodwin, & Montoro, 1995). The disorder spontaneously regresses in 70 to 90 percent of patients, but may recur with a more protracted course in subsequent pregnancies. In 10 to 30 percent of women, permanent hypothyroidism is documented (American College of Obstetricians & Gynecologists [ACOG], 1993; Browne-Martin & Emerson, 1997; Hall, 1994; Seely & Burrow, 1994). In addition, there are reports of an association between transient postpartum thyroid dysfunction and depression; however, this association is difficult to confirm given the 10 percent background prevalence for postpartum depression (Hall, 1995; Seely & Burrow, 1994). Pharmacologic therapy may be indicated in women with clinical symptoms and laboratory evidence of hypothyroidism.

Database

Subjective

- Hyperthyroid phase (see also the Subjective section of Chapter 12.2, *Hyperthyroidism*). The most common symptoms reported by women during this phase include

  - ▶ Fatigue

  - ▶ Palpitations

  - ▶ Emotional lability

  - ▶ Thyroid enlargement that may be painful

- Hypothyroid phase (see also the Subjective section of the Chapter 12.3, *Hypothyroidism*). Women are often asymptomatic during this phase (Hall, Richards, Lazarus, 1993). However, the most common symptoms reported by women during this phase may include

▶ Depression

▶ Thyroid enlargement that may be painful

▶ Problems with memory and concentration

Objective

● Hyperthyroid phase (see also Objective section of Chapter 12.2, *Hyperthyroidism*).

▶ Palpation of the thyroid may reveal a normal size or slightly enlarged gland (ACOG,1993).

● Hypothyroid phase (see also Objective section of Chapter 12.3, *Hypothyroidism*).

▶ Palpation of the thyroid gland usually reveals a diffuse enlargement of the gland.

Assessment

● Transient postpartum thyroid dysfunction (postpartum thyroiditis)

▶ R/O hyperthyroidism

▶ R/O Grave's disease

▶ R/O Hashimoto's thyroiditis

▶ R/O hypothyroidism

▶ R/O postpartum depression

▶ R/O Sheehan's syndrome

Plan

Diagnostic Tests

● Hyperthyroid phase (see Diagnostic Tests section listed in Chapter 12.2, *Hyperthyroidism*)

▶ Total T4 is increased.

▶ Thyroid antimicrosomal antibody is present in titers greater than 1:100.

▶ Thyroid uptake of radioiodine or technetium is low.

● Hypothyroid phase (see Diagnostic Tests section in Chapter 12.3, *Hypothyroidism*)

▶ Thyroid antimicrosomal antibody present in titers greater than 1:100.

▶ TSH is increased.

▶ Free T4 is decreased.

Treatment/Management

● Consult with a physician when a women is suspected of having transient postpartum thyroid dysfunction.

- The physician consultant determines the pharmacologic therapy of a woman, and it is usually based on the severity of symptoms present.

  ► During the hyperthyroid phase, pharmacologic treatment should be limited to the use of beta blockers for a few weeks to reduce the hypermetabolic symptoms (see Chapter 12.2, *Hyperthyroidism*). The use of propylthiouracil (PTU) is contraindicated because it is ineffective for this type of hyperthyroidism, and it may facilitate the development of the hypothyroid phase of this disorder (ACOG, 1993).

  ► During the hypothyroid phase, women manifesting hypothyroid symptoms may benefit from a low dose of levothyroxine sodium (.050 to 0.075 µg per day) (Browne-Martin & Emerson, 1997). This therapy may continue for 12 to 18 months, with a gradual reduction in the dose and eventual discontinuation of the medication (ACOG, 1993; Seely & Burrow, 1994).

- Repeat thyroid function tests (TFTs) should be done at appropriate intervals, determined by the physician consultant (see Treatment/Management sections of Chapter 12.2, *Hyperthyroidism,* and Chapter 12.3, *Hypothyroidism*).

- Women with significant psychological symptoms (e.g., depression, anxiety) should be referred for an appropriate evaluation.

Consultation

- Consult with a physician for all women who are suspected of having transient postpartum thyroid dysfunction.

- Co-management of women diagnosed with this condition is possible in some clinical settings and is determined by institution-specific policies and procedures.

Patient Education

- Education of the woman should include information regarding the possible cause(s) of her symptoms, the diagnostic tests ordered, and their results (when available).

- When the diagnosis of transient postpartum thyroiditis has been made, educate the woman regarding the course of the disorder, possible therapeutic interventions, the likelihood of spontaneous regression, possible recurrence following future births, and the need to continue with follow-up evaluations so that monitoring for evidence of permanent hypothyroidism can occur.

- Reassure the woman regarding the validity of her symptoms.

Follow-up

- Long-term follow-up evaluations of women diagnosed with this disorder is essential and should be determined by the physician consultant (see Treatment/Management sections of Chapter 12.2, *Hyperthyroidism,* and Chapter 12.3, *Hypothyroidism*).

- Document history of postpartum thyroid dysfunction and its management in problem list and progress notes.

References

American College of Obstetricians & Gynecologists (ACOG) (1993). *Thyroid disease in pregnancy.* (Technical bulletin no. 181.) Washington, DC: Author.

SmithBrowne-Martin, K., & Emerson, C.H. (1997). Postpartum thyroid dysfunction. *Clinical Obstetrics and Gynecology, 40*(1), 90–101.

Hall, R. (1995). Pregnancy and autoimmune endocrine disease. *Baillière's Clinical Endocrinology and Metabolism, 9*(1), 137-155.

Hall, R., Richards, C.J., & Lazarus, J.H. (1993). The thyroid and pregnancy. *British Journal of Obstetrics and Gynaecology, 100*, 512-515.

Mestman, J.H., Goodwin, T.M., & Montoro, M.M. (1995). Thyroid disorders of pregnancy. *Endocrinology and Metabolism Clinics of North America, 24*(1), 41-71.

Novy, M.J. (1994). The normal puerperium. In A. H. DeCherney & M. L. Pernoll (Eds.), *Current obstetric & gynecologic diagnosis & treatment* (8th ed., pp. 253-254). Norwalk, CT: Appleton & Lange

Seely, B.L., & Burrow, G.N. (1994). Thyroid disease and pregnancy. In R. K. Creasy & R. Resnik (Eds.), *Maternal-fetal medicine. Principles and practice* (3rd ed., pp. 979-1003). Philadelphia, PA: W.B. Saunders.

SECTION 13

URINARY TRACT CONDITIONS

Chapter 1

ASYMPTOMATIC BACTERIURIA

Winifred L. Star

Asymptomatic bacteriuria (ASB) is defined as the presence of 100,000 or more colony-forming units of a single uropathogen per milliliter of urine on two consecutive clean-catch midstream-voided specimens in the absence of signs or symptoms of urinary tract infection (UTI) (Gibbs & Sweet, 1994; Kass, 1956). The bacteria responsible for 60 to 90 percent of asymptomatic infections is *Escherichia coli*. Other common pathogens include *Proteus mirabilis, Klebsiella pneumoniae*, the enterococci, and Group B beta-hemolytic streptococci (Gibbs & Sweet, 1994). Recently, *Staphylococcus saprophyticus* has been noted to be an important pathogen in UTIs, but its role in ASB of pregnancy is less clear (Sweet & Gibbs, 1995). In addition, *Ureaplasma urealyticum* and *Gardnerella vaginalis* can be found in the bladder during pregnancy but may not have significant pathogenic roles (Andriole, 1992).

The prevalence of asymptomatic bacteriuria in pregnancy ranges from 2 to 11 percent (the majority of studies indicate the range is between 4 and 7 percent). Bacteriuria during pregnancy is a manifestation of lifelong susceptibility to urinary tract infection, and in many cases ASB predates pregnancy (Fowler, 1989; Sweet & Gibbs, 1995). Of women without bacteriuria at initial screening, only 1 to 2 percent will acquire it later in pregnancy; however, recurrence of ASB during the same pregnancy has been noted to occur in 16 to 33 percent of cases (Andriole & Patterson, 1991; Sweet & Gibbs, 1995; U.S. Preventive Services Task Force, 1996).

The significance of asymptomatic bacteriuria lies in its potential to cause acute pyelonephritis. Studies indicate that 13 to 65 percent of women with untreated ASB go on to develop pyelonephritis during pregnancy. When bacteriuria is treated the incidence of acute pyelonephritis is lowered to 5 percent or less (average 2.9 percent). Therefore, recognition and prompt treatment of asymptomatic infection is warranted and may prevent 70 to 80 percent of cases of pyelonephritis (Gibbs & Sweet, 1994; Lucas & Cunningham, 1993; Sweet & Gibbs, 1995). ASB rarely resolves spontaneously.

Asymptomatic bacteriuria has been implicated as a risk factor for preterm delivery and low birth weight infants. Additional, unproven claims link ASB with anemia, preeclampsia, chronic renal disease, amnionitis, and endometritis: There is controversy in these areas. Clearly, the overriding concern is the risk of developing pyelonephritis with its attendant increased maternal and fetal morbidity and mortality rates (Gibbs & Sweet, 1994; Sweet & Gibbs, 1995).

It has been estimated that 10 to 15 percent of women with bacteriuria in pregnancy have evidence of chronic pyelonephritis 10 to 12 years after delivery; renal failure develops in one in 3,000. Thus, women with ASB of pregnancy should have long-term follow-up to detect urinary tract abnormalities (Sweet & Gibbs, 1995).

Database

Subjective

- Predisposing factors

  ▶ History of UTIs, reflux nephropathy

  NOTE: Of pregnant women with ASB, 25 to 50 percent may have renal tissue involvement and silent pyelonephritis—a group at high risk for symptomatic pyelonephritis during pregnancy (Sweet & Gibbs, 1995).

  ▶ Lower socioeconomic status

  ▶ Sexual activity

  ▶ Increased age

  ▶ Increased parity

  ▶ Sickle cell trait/disease

  ▶ Diabetes mellitus

  ▶ Catheterization

- Symptomatology

  ▶ None for ASB

  ▶ Client may report signs or symptoms of vaginitis or sexually transmitted disease (STD) if there is concomitant infection.

Objective

- Physical examination is within normal limits (WNL).

- Urine pH may be elevated (normal pH is 5.0–6.0).

- Urine dipstick may be positive for protein, leukocyte esterase, nitrites, and/or blood.

- Microscopic urinalysis may reveal white blood cells (WBCs), red blood cells (RBCs), or bacteria.

- Gram stain of uncentrifuged urine or sediment may show gram-negative bacilli or gram-positive cocci.

- Quantitative culture of a clean-catch midstream-voided urine specimen reveals 10^5 or more colony-forming units per milliliter (cfu/mL) of a uropathogenic organism.

NOTE: In *asymptomatic* women, lower colony counts (less than 10^4) suggest periurethral contamination and rarely persist on reculture. Presence of multiple organisms in similar quantities and predominance of lactobacilli and diphtheroids increases probability of a contaminated specimen (Hooten, 1990). (In catheter specimens, colony counts from 10^2 to 10^5 have been used to represent significant bacteriuria; *any quantity* of organisms isolated from bladder aspirate specimens represents true bladder bacteriuria [although a slight risk of contamination exists in such specimens]) (Hooten, 1990).

- Squamous epithelial cells in large numbers (more than 10 per low-power field) on microscopic urinalysis often represents vaginal or perineal contamination; a few squamous cells are seen in most urine specimens and have little clinical significance (Ravel, 1995; Ringsrud & Linné, 1995).

- Pyuria without bacteriuria may be present in association with chlamydial or gonococcal urethritis/cervicitis. Pelvic examination and wet mounts of vaginal discharge may show signs of concomitant infection. See Section 14, *Vaginitis and Sexually Transmitted Diseases*.

Assessment

- Asymptomatic bacteriuria

  ▶ R/O cystitis

  ▶ R/O urethral syndrome

  ▶ R/O vaginitis

  ▶ R/O STDs

  ▶ R/O obstetrical complication(s)

  ▶ R/O acute/chronic, concomitant medical problem(s)

Plan

Diagnostic Tests

- Perform culture of clean-catch, midstream-voided urine specimen on all gravidas at entry to care. (The U.S. Preventive Services Task Force [1996] recommends culture at 12 to 16 weeks' gestation.)

  NOTE: Routine screening for ASB in pregnancy with nitrite and leukocyte esterase testing or other rapid screening tests is not recommended because poor test characteristics (sensitivity of only 50 percent for dipstick testing) compared to urine culture has been reported among pregnant women (Millar & Cox, 1997; U.S. Preventive Services Task Force, 1996). If nonculture methods detect evidence of pyuria or bacteriuria a urine specimen for culture and susceptibility testing should be obtained prior to treatment (McNeeley Jr., 1993). Urine should be planted on culture media within 20 minutes to avoid erroneously high colony counts (bacteria will multiply if left at room temperature); if it cannot be cultured within this time, refrigerate urine (Sox Jr., 1995).

- Avoid catheterization during pregnancy; however, it may be indicated in certain circumstances to assess true bladder bacteriuria (e.g., if clean-catch specimens are repeatedly contaminated) (Andriole & Patterson, 1991; Millar & Cox, 1997). Direct bladder aspiration is rarely performed in pregnancy. Consult with a physician if these modalities are being considered.

- Consider screening individuals of African and Mediterranean descent for G6PD deficiency when nitrofurantoin or sulfonamides are used for treatment. See Chapter 9.5, *Glucose-6-Phosphate Dehydrogenase Deficiency*. All blacks should be routinely screened for sickle cell trait. See Chapter 9.7, *Hemoglobin S and Sickle Cell Trait*.

- Additional tests may include (but are not limited to)
  - ▶ Vaginal wet mounts
  - ▶ Testing for *Neisseria gonorrhoeae* and *Chlamydia trachomatis*
  - ▶ Renal function studies and/or ultrasound
- See the Objective section.

Treatment/Management

The goal of treatment is to maintain a sterile urine for the remainder of pregnancy (Levine, 1993). Treatment should be guided by antimicrobial susceptibilities.

- Antibiotic regimens may include (but are not limited to) the following (Cunningham et al., 1997; Gibbs & Sweet, 1994; Kiningham, 1993; McNeeley Jr., 1993):
  - ▶ Ampicillin 250-500 mg p.o. every 6 hours for 3, 7, or 10 days
  - ▶ Amoxicillin 250-500 mg p.o. every 8 hours for 3, 7, or 10 days
  - ▶ Cephalexin 250-500 mg p.o. every 6 hours for 3, 7, or 10 days
  - ▶ Cephradine 250-500 mg p.o. every 6 hours for 3, 7, or 10 days
  - ▶ Nitrofurantoin 50-100 mg p.o. every 6 hours for 3, 7, or 10 days
  - ▶ Sulfisoxazole 500 mg p.o. every 6 hours for 3, 7, or 10 days
- Single-dose regimens have also been used (Cunningham et al., 1997; Millar & Cox, 1997):
  - ▶ Ampicillin 2 grams p.o.
  - ▶ Amoxicillin 3 grams p.o.
  - ▶ Cephalexin 2 grams p.o.
  - ▶ Nitrofurantoin 200 mg p.o.
  - ▶ Sulfisoxazole 2 grams p.o.

NOTE: Length of treatment may vary depending on prescribing practices of the clinical setting and characteristics of the client (e.g., gestational age at time of diagnosis, immunosuppressive states, urogynecologic factors, other complicating factors). Confer with physician regarding duration of therapy.

- In many areas of the United States there is high prevalence of *E. coli* resistance to ampicillin/amoxicillin and related penicillins. Thus, these drugs should not be used as first-line therapy on an empiric basis; rather, their use should be guided by the sensitivities. If the percentage of resistance is low in a given locale (this can be ascertained by communication with the local bacteriology laboratory) initial therapy with these agents may be appropriate while sensitivity tests are pending.

- Do not prescribe sulfonamides to women near term because there is a risk of neonatal hyperbilirubinemia and kernicterus. For women with G6PD deficiency, do not prescribe nitrofurantoin or sulfonamides because there is a risk of hemolysis (Briggs, Freeman, &

Yaffe, 1994; Sweet & Gibbs, 1994). See *Physicians' Desk Reference* or Briggs et al. (1994) for further information.

- Clinically, a single positive culture of $\geq 10^5$ colonies/mL of a uropathogen is sufficient for starting therapy (Levine, 1993); however, in an *asymptomatic* woman, an initial abnormal screening culture may be repeated, and if again positive, treatment prescribed (Zinner, 1992). In addition, single isolates at lower concentrations may be significant and treatment may be also be considered in these cases (Lucas & Cunningham, 1993).

- Treat vaginitis and STDs as indicated. Partner treatment is also indicated for any identified STDs in client. Refer to Section 14, *Vaginitis and Sexually Transmitted Diseases.*

- See Follow-up section.

Consultation

- Consult with a physician when considering catheterization.

- Consult with a physician for women with recurrent asymptomatic bacteriuria and when suppressive therapy is being considered. Consult with a urologist for refractory cases.

- Consult for any obstetrical complications, as indicated.

Patient Education

- Discuss normal anatomic changes of the urinary tract in pregnancy and the etiology of asymptomatic bacteriuria.

- Stress the importance of completing the medication despite absence of symptoms.

- Advise client that untreated bacteriuria may lead to pyelonephritis, which is associated with an increased risk of premature labor and delivery.

  ▸ Alert client to the signs and symptoms of acute cystitis and pyelonephritis; See Chapters 13.2 and 13.3, *Cystitis* and *Pyelonephritis* respectively.

  ▸ Discuss preterm birth prevention routinely at 20 to 24 weeks of pregnancy and as indicated. See Chapter 6.25, *Preterm Labor.*

- Encourage adequate fluid intake throughout pregnancy. Client need not force fluids when on antibiotics; rather, she should drink to satisfy thirst (Pollen, 1995).

  NOTE: There is evidence that cranberry juice has bacteriostatic properties but no controlled trials have been performed in pregnancy assessing its ability to decrease the prevalence of AS or incidence of pyelonephritis (Millar & Cox, 1997).

- Teach or review personal hygiene techniques, as necessary.

- Recommend voiding prior to and following intercourse.

Follow-up

- Subsequent urine cultures are not required during pregnancy for women who initially have sterile urine (unless client is symptomatic or has evidence of pyuria/bacteriuria on dipstick at routine prenatal visits) (Kiningham, 1993). Repeat urine culture in the beginning of the third trimester for clients at high risk for bacteriuria (Andriole & Patterson, 1991).

- If the client *is* treated for asymptomatic bacteriuria, order urine culture on a clean-catch, midstream-voided specimen after completion of drug therapy and then periodically until delivery (some experts recommend every 4 to 6 weeks) (Bint & Hill, 1994; Cox, Crombleholme, Hooten, & Mead, 1993).

  NOTE: After documenting that culture shows a clearing of bacteriuria with treatment, some sites may opt to perform periodic screening via dipstick testing (leukocyte esterase and nitrites), with follow-up microscopic urinalysis or culture as indicated (Cox et al., 1993). Clinicians may wish to discuss the frequency of screening and the modalities utilized with the physician-consultant.

- If infection was not eradicated, as evidenced by follow-up culture, client should be retreated for 7 to 14 days according to the sensitivities (a different antibiotic from the first is advisable) (Andriole & Patterson, 1991; Kiningham, 1993; Millar & Cox, 1997). Consult with the physician.

- Suppressive therapy (begun immediately following a course of antibiotics while urine is sterile) should be considered for those clients with persistent relapse (growth of same organism within 2 weeks of therapy cessation) or reinfection (recurrence of infection with different species/strain more than 2 weeks after cessation of therapy) (Kiningham, 1993). Consult with a physician.

  ▶ Therapy can be effected with (but may not be limited to) the following regimens (Andriole & Patterson, 1991; Kiningham, 1993; McNeeley Jr., 1993; Sweet & Gibbs, 1995):

    – Amoxicillin 250 mg p.o. at bedtime

    – Ampicillin 250 mg p.o. b.i.d.

    – Cephalexin 250-500 mg p.o. b.i.d.

    – Nitrofurantoin 50-100 mg p.o. at bedtime or 50 mg p.o. b.i.d.

  ▶ Continue medication for the remainder of pregnancy—some experts recommend up to 2 to 6 weeks postpartum (consult with a physician) (Cox et al., 1993; Sweet & Gibbs, 1995).

  ▶ Follow-up cultures should be performed periodically for the remainder of pregnancy to detect the possibility of reinfection by a resistant organism (Andriole & Patterson, 1991). Consult with a physician regarding frequency of screening and alternate screening modalities.

  NOTE: A reasonable alternative to suppressive therapy in a woman who has had a *single* relapse or reinfection would be a repeat course of antibiotics then close surveillance with follow-up cultures (or other screening modalities) throughout pregnancy (Kiningham, 1993). Consult with a physician.

- At each prenatal visit, women treated for ASB should have a careful dipstick assessment for protein, nitrites, and leukocyte esterase on a clean-catch, midstream urine specimen. Positive findings warrant further evaluation with urine culture.

- Obtain follow-up cultures after delivery for women with recurrent or persistent bacteriuria during pregnancy and refer them for complete urologic evaluation (usually performed 3 to 6 months postpartum) (Andriole & Patterson, 1991).

- Document presence of ASB and treatment thereof in progress list and progress notes. Note on the problem list the presence of group B streptococcus as indicated. Document the presence of an STD as indicated.

REFERENCES

Andriole, V.T. (1992). Urinary tract infections in the 90s: Pathogenesis and management. *Infection, 20*(Suppl. 4), S251–S256.

Andriole, V.T., & Patterson, T.F. (1991). Epidemiology, natural history, and management of urinary tract infections in pregnancy. *Medical Clinics of North America, 75*(2), 359–373.

Bint, A.J., & Hill, D. (1994). Bacteriuria of pregnancy – an update on significance, diagnosis, and management. *Journal of Antimicrobial Chemotherapy, 33*(Suppl. A), 93–97.

Briggs, G.G., Freeman, R.K., & Yaffe, S.J. (1994). *Drugs in pregnancy and lactation* (4th ed.). Baltimore, MD: Williams & Wilkins.

Cox, S., Crombleholme, W., Hooten, T, & Mead, P. (1993). Urinary tract infection: Is it reinfection or recurrence? *Contemporary OB/GYN, 38*(2), 84–108.

Cunningham, F.G., MacDonald, P.C., Gant, N.F., Levano, K.J., Gilstrap, L.C. III, Hankins, G.D.V., & Clark, S.L. (1997). Renal and urinary tract disorders. Williams obstetrics (20th ed.; pp. 1125–1144). Stamford, CT: Appleton & Lange.

Fowler, J.E. (1989). *Urinary tract infection and inflammation.* Chicago: Year Book Medical Publishers.

Gibbs, R.S., & Sweet, R.L. (1994). Maternal and fetal infections. In R.K. Creasy & R. Resnik (Eds.), *Maternal-fetal medicine: Principles and practice* (3rd ed., pp. 639–644). Philadelphia, PA: W.B. Saunders.

Hooten, T.M. (1990). The epidemiology of urinary tract infection and the concept of significant bacteriuria. *Infection, 18*(Suppl. 2), 540–542.

Kass, E.H. (1956). Asymptomatic infections of the urinary tract. *Transactions of the Association of American Physicians, 69*, 56–64.

Kiningham, R.B. (1993). Asymptomatic bacteriuria in pregnancy. *American Family Physician, 47*(5), 1232–1238.

Levine, M.G. (1993, August). The diagnosis of urinary tract infections during pregnancy. *Nebraska Medical Journal*, 282–285.

Lucas, M.J., & Cunningham, F.G. (1993). Urinary tract infection in pregnancy. *Clinical Obstetrics and Gynecology, 36*(4), 855–868.

McNeeley, S.G., Jr. (1993). Lower urinary tract infections in pregnancy. *Contemporary OB/GYN, 38*(3), 99–104.

Millar, L.K., & Cox, S.M. (1997). Urinary tract infections complicating pregnancy. *Infectious Disease Clinics of North America, 11*(1), 13–26.

Pollen, J.J. (1995). Short-term course for uncomplicated cystitis. *Contemporary Nurse Practitioner, 1*(4), 21–30.

Ravel, R. (1995). *Clinical laboratory medicine: Clinical applications of laboratory data* (pp. 147–158). St. Louis, MO: Mosby.

Ringsrud, K.M., & Linné, J.J. (1995). *Urinalysis and body fluids: A color text* (pp. 104–105). St. Louis, MO: Mosby.

Sox, H.C., Jr. (1995). *Common diagnostic tests: Use and interpretation* (2nd ed., pp. 286–301). St. Louis, MO: Mosby.

Sweet, R.L., & Gibbs, R.S. (1995). *Infectious diseases of the female genital tract* (3rd ed., pp. 429–464). Baltimore, MD: Williams & Wilkins.

U.S. Preventive Services Task Force. (1996). Screening for asymptomatic bacteriuria. *Guide to clinical preventive services* (2nd ed., pp. 347–359). Baltimore, MD: Williams & Wilkins.

Zinner, S.H. (1992). Management of urinary tract infections in pregnancy: A review with comments on single dose therapy. *Infection, 20*(Suppl. 4), S280–S285.

Chapter 2

CYSTITIS

Winifred L. Star

Lower urinary tract infection (UTI), or acute cystitis, occurs in about 1 percent of pregnant women, of whom about 60 percent have had negative urine cultures on initial screening; most cases tend to occur in the second trimester (Sweet & Gibbs, 1995). Lower UTI also occurs in approximately 2 to 4 percent of postpartum patients (Clark, 1995). Pregnancy itself does not predispose a woman to the development of lower UTI and the frequency of acute cystitis is not substantially increased during this time (only 17 percent of patients develop recurrence during pregnancy) (Sweet & Gibbs, 1995).

In young adult women, uncomplicated infections are caused by *Escherichia coli* in 80 to 90 percent of cases; 10 to 20 percent of infections are due to *Staphylococcus saprophyticus*. Other gram-negative organisms, such as *Klebsiella, Enterobacter, Proteus*, and *Pseudomonas* species, and gram-positive organisms, such as the enterococci and group B streptococci, may also be implicated (Davison & Lindheimer, 1989; Lucas & Cunningham, 1993; Sweet & Gibbs, 1995). In addition, regional or local variations in bacterial organisms may exist (Powers, 1991). The clean-catch, midstream-voided urine specimen in a client with acute cystitis usually reveals 10^5 or more colonies of a bacterial organism per milliliter of urine, although lesser colony counts may exist in active infection.

The primary risk of acute cystitis during pregnancy is the development of acute pyelonephritis with its attendant risk for preterm labor and delivery. Pregnancy-related anatomic, physiologic, and hormonal changes predispose a woman to the development of upper urinary tract infection. Thus, women with acute cystitis should receive immediate therapy (see the Treatment/Management section).

Database

Subjective

- Predisposing factors
  - ▶ Increased receptivity of uroepithelial, periurethral, and vaginal cells for uropathic bacteria
  - ▶ Pathogenic factors of bacteria: fimbriae or pili, K antigen, hemolysin, antimicrobial resistance (Sweet & Gibbs, 1995)
  - ▶ History of UTIs
  - ▶ Urinary tract obstruction, stasis, vesicoureteral reflux, urinary retention
  - ▶ Sexual activity
  - ▶ Diaphragm-spermicide use
  - ▶ Recent catheterization/instrumentation of urinary tract; indwelling catheter
  - ▶ Diabetes mellitus
  - ▶ Sickle cell trait/disease
  - ▶ Lewis blood-group nonsecretor (Le[a+b-]) and recessive (Le[a-b-]) phenotypes (Andriole, 1992)
  - ▶ Lower socioeconomic status

▶ Risk for postpartum infection may be increased by (Clark, 1995)

- Bladder hypotonia
- Urinary stasis
- Catheterization
- Frequent pelvic examinations
- Epidural/conduction anesthesia
- Genital tract injury
- Bacteriuria during pregnancy
- Operative delivery, anatomic disorders

● Symptomatology

▶ Symptoms of acute infection may include

- Urinary urgency, frequency, dysuria, nocturia
- Hesitancy, difficulty starting stream, urinary retention
- Incomplete emptying, dribbling
- Suprapubic pain or tenderness
- Tenesmus
- Hematuria; cloudy, malodorous urine

▶ Increased frequency of urination normally present in pregnancy may mimic symptoms of cystitis.

▶ Vulvovaginal infections and sexually transmitted diseases (STDs) may produce symptoms that mimic those of cystitis.

▶ Nausea, vomiting, fever, chills, flank pain/tenderness are usually absent in lower UTI.

Objective

● Vital signs usually within normal limits (WNL).

● Abdominal examination may reveal tenderness in the suprapubic area; costovertebral angle tenderness (CVAT) is generally absent in uncomplicated lower UTIs.

● Gross inspection of urine may reveal hematuria; urine may be cloudy and/or malodorous.

● Urine pH may be elevated (normal pH is 5.0 to 6.0).

● Urine dipstick may be positive for nitrites, leukocyte esterase, protein, and/or blood.

● Microscopic urinalysis may reveal white blood cells (WBCs), red blood cells (RBCs), and/or bacteria.

● Gram stain of uncentrifuged urine or sediment may show gram-negative bacilli or gram-positive cocci.

- Quantitative culture of clean-catch midstream-voided urine reveals 10^5 colonies/mL or more of a uropathogenic bacterial organism.

  NOTE: Lesser degrees of bacteriuria (i.e., 10^2 to 10^4 colonies/mL) may be present in acutely symptomatic women (Andriole, 1992). Presence of multiple organisms in similar quantities and predominance of lactobacilli and diphtheroids on culture increase probability of a contaminated specimen (Hooten, 1990). (In catheter specimens, colony counts from 10^2 to 10^5 have been used to represent significant bacteriuria; any quantity of organisms from bladder aspirate specimen represents true bladder bacteriuria [although a slight risk of contamination exists in such specimens]) (Hooten, 1990).

- Squamous epithelial cells in large numbers (more than 10 per low-power field) on microscopic urinalysis represent vaginal or perineal contamination; a few squamous cells are seen in most urine specimens and have little clinical significance (Ravel, 1995; Ringsrud & Linné, 1995).

- Pyuria without bacteriuria may be present in association with chlamydial or gonococcal urethritis/cervicitis. Pelvic examination and wet mounts of vaginal discharge may show evidence of concomitant infection. See Section 14, *Vaginitis and Sexually Transmitted Diseases.*

Assessment

- Acute cystitis

  ▶ R/O urethral syndrome

  ▶ R/O pyelonephritis

  ▶ R/O appendicitis

  ▶ R/O vaginitis

  ▶ R/O STDs

  ▶ R/O obstetrical complications

  ▶ R/O acute/chronic, concomitant medical problem(s)

Plan

Diagnostic Tests

- Perform quantitative culture and antimicrobial susceptibility testing on a clean-catch, midstream-voided urine specimen. If nonculture methods detect evidence of bacteriuria, obtain a specimen for culture and sensitivities prior to treatment (McNeeley Jr., 1993).

  NOTE: Urine should be planted on culture media within 20 minutes to avoid erroneously high colony counts (bacteria will multiply if left at room temperature); if it cannot be cultured within this time, refrigerate urine (Sox Jr., 1995).

- Repeat a culture to ascertain the presence of a dominant pathogen when the sample is contaminated; in addition, the findings may be correlated with the results of a microscopic urinalysis.

- Avoid catheterization during pregnancy; however, it may be indicated in certain circumstances to assess true bladder bacteriuria (e.g., if clean-catch specimens are repeatedly contaminated)

(Andriole & Patterson, 1992; Millar & Cox, 1997). Direct bladder aspiration is rarely performed in pregnancy. Consult with a physician if these modalities are being considered.

- Consider screening individuals of African and Mediterranean descent for G6PD when nitrofurantoin or sulfonamides are used for treatment. See Chapter 9.5, *Glucose-6-Phosphate Dehydrogenase Deficiency.* All blacks should be routinely screened for sickle cell trait. See Chapter 9.7, *Hemoglobin S and Sickle Cell Trait.*

- Additional tests may include (but are not limited to)
  - ▶ Vaginal wet mounts
  - ▶ Testing for *Neisseria gonorrhoeae, Chlamydia trachomatis,* and herpes simplex virus
  - ▶ Renal function studies and/or ultrasound, as indicated.

- See the Objective section.

Treatment/Management

- Begin treatment immediately in a pregnant woman with acute cystitis.

- Drugs of choice may include (but are not limited to) the following (Cunningham et al., 1997; McNeeley Jr., 1993; Millar & Cox, 1997; Sweet & Gibbs, 1995):
  - ▶ Amoxicillin 250–500 mg p.o. every 8 hours for 3, 7, or 10 days
  - ▶ Cephalexin 250–500 mg p.o. every 6 hours for 3, 7, or 10 days
  - ▶ Nitrofurantoin 50–100 mg p.o. every 6 hours for 3, 7, or 10 days
  - ▶ Sulfisoxazole 500 mg p.o. every 6 hours for 3, 7, or 10 days

- Single-dose therapies have also been used (pyeloneparitis must be ruled out) (Cunningham et al., 1997):
  - ▶ Amoxicillin 3 grams p.o.
  - ▶ Ampicillin 2 grams p.o.
  - ▶ Cephalosporin 2 grams p.o.
  - ▶ Nitrofurantoin 2 grams p.o.
  - ▶ Sulfonamide 2 grams p.o.

NOTE: Length of treatment may vary depending on prescribing practices of the clinical setting and characteristics of the client (e.g., gestational age at time of diagnosis, immunosuppressive states, urogynecologic factors, other complicating factors). Confer with physician regarding duration of therapy. Change of drug may be necessary after sensitivities are reviewed.

- In many areas of the United States there is high prevalence of *E. coli* resistance to ampicillin/amoxicillin and related penicillins. Thus, these drugs should not be used as first-line therapy on an empiric basis; rather their use should be guided by the sensitivities. If the percentage of resistance is low in a given locale (this can be ascertained by communication with the local bacteriology laboratory) initial therapy with these agents may be appropriate while sensitivities are pending.

- Do not prescribe sulfonamides near term because there is a risk of neonatal hyperbilirubinemia and kernicterus. For women with G6PD deficiency, do not prescribe sulfonamides or nitrofurantoin because there is a risk of hemolysis (Briggs, Freeman, & Yaffe, 1994; Sweet & Gibbs, 1995).

- Treat vaginitis and STDs as indicated. Partner treatment is indicated for any identified STDs in client—provide referrals as necessary. See Section 14, *Vaginitis and Sexually Transmitted Diseases.*

- See the Follow-up section.

Consultation

- Consult with a physician when considering catheterization.

- Consult with a physician for women with repeated episodes of cystitis for which suppressive therapy is being considered. Consult with a urologist for refractory cases.

- If acute pyelonephritis is suspected or diagnosed, refer client to physician.

Patient Education

- Discuss normal anatomical and hormonal changes of the urinary tract in pregnancy and the etiology of acute cystitis.

- Explain that cystitis symptoms should abate in 48 hours after initiation of drug therapy. Stress the importance of finishing the complete course of medication.

- Advise regarding the risks and signs/symptoms of pyelonephritis and preterm labor. See Chapter 13.3, *Pyelonephritis* and Chapter 6.25, *Preterm Labor.*

- Encourage adequate fluid intake throughout pregnancy. Client need not force fluids while on antibiotics; rather, she should drink to satisfy thirst (Pollen, 1995).

  ▶ Recommend avoidance of caffeinated and carbonated beverages.

  ▶ Acidification of the urine may be aided by the ingestion of cranberry, plum, prune, or apricot juice (Clark, 1995).

- Teach or review personal hygiene practices, as indicated.

- Recommend voiding prior to and following intercourse.

- Provide education on STDs and safer sex, as indicated.

Follow-up

- Order urine culture after completion of drug therapy and if acute cystitis symptoms reappear later in pregnancy.

- At each prenatal visit, women treated for cystitis should have a careful dipstick assessment for protein, nitrites, and leukocyte esterase on a clean-catch midstream-voided urine specimen. Positive findings warrant follow-up culture.

- Suppressive antibiotic therapy for the remainder of pregnancy may be considered for women with recurrent cystitis. Consult with a physician.

  ▶ Therapy may be effected with (but is not limited to) the following regimens (Andriole & Patterson, 1991; McNeeley Jr., 1993; Sweet & Gibbs, 1995):

    – Amoxicillin 250 mg p.o. at bedtime

    – Cephalexin 250–500 mg p.o. b.i.d.

    – Nitrofurantoin 50–100 mg p.o. at bedtime or 50 mg p.o. b.i.d.

- Postcoital antibiotic prophylaxis for women with a history of recurrent UTI is also effective in reducing recurrences during pregnancy (Lucas & Cunningham, 1993). Nitrofurantoin 50 mg p.o. or cephalexin 250 mg p.o. after intercourse may be used (Pfau & Sacks, 1992; Sweet & Gibbs, 1995). Consult with a physician.

- Refer clients with repeated episodes of cystitis during pregnancy for postpartum urologic evaluation (usually performed 3 to 6 months after delivery).

- Document diagnosis of cystitis and treatment thereof in progress notes and problem list. Note on problem list the presence of group B streptococcus, as indicated. Document the presence of an STD, as indicated.

References

Andriole, V.T. (1992). Urinary tract infections in the 90s: Pathogenesis and management. *Infection, 20*(Suppl. 2), S251–S256.

Andriole, V.T., & Patterson, T.F. (1991). Epidemiology, natural history, and management of urinary tract infections in pregnancy. *Medical Clinics of North America, 75*(2), 359–373.

Briggs, G.G., Freeman, R.K., & Yaffe, S.J. (1994). *Drugs in pregnancy and lactation* (4th ed.). Baltimore, MD: Williams & Wilkins.

Clark, R.A. (1995). Infections during the postpartum period. *Journal of Obstetric, Gynecologic, and Neonatal Nursing, 24*(6), 542–548.

Cox, S., Crombleholme, W., Hooton, T., & Mead, P. (1993). Urinary tract infection: Is it reinfection or recurrence? *Contemporary OB/GYN, 38*(2), 84–108.

Cunningham, F.G., MacDonald, P.C., Grant, N.F., Levano, K.J., Gilstrap, L.C. III, Hankins, G.D.V., & Clark, S.L. (1997). Renal and urinary tract disorders. Williams obstetrics (20th ed.; pp. 1125–1144). Stamford, CT: Appleton & Lange.

Davison, J. M., & Lindheimer, M. D. (1989). Renal disorders. In R.K. Creasy & R. Resnik (Eds.), *Maternal-fetal medicine: Principles and practice* (2nd ed., pp. 824–827). Philadelphia, PA: W.B. Saunders.

Hooten, T.M. (1990). The epidemiology of urinary tract infection and the concept of significant bacteriuria. *Infection, 18*(Suppl. 2), 540–542.

Kiningham, R.B. (1993). Asymptomatic bacteriuria in pregnancy. *American Family Physician, 47*(5), 1232–1238.

Lucas, M. J., & Cunningham, F.G. (1993). Urinary infection in pregnancy. *Clinical Obstetrics and Gynecology, 36*(4), 855–868.

McNeeley, S.G., Jr. (1993). Lower urinary tract infections in pregnancy. *Contemporary OB/GYN, 38*(3), 99–104.

Millar, L.K., & Cox, S.M. (1997). Urinary tract infections complicating pregnancy. *Infectious Disease Clinics of North America, 11*(1), 13–26.

Pfau, A., & Sacks, T.G. (1992). Effective prophylaxis for recurrent urinary tract infections during pregnancy. *Clinical Infectious Diseases, 14*, 810–814.

Pollen, J.J. (1995). Short-term course for uncomplicated cystitis. *Contemporary Nurse Practitioner, 1*(4), 21–30.

Powers, R.D. (1991). New directions in the diagnosis and therapy of urinary tract infections. *American Journal of Obstetrics and Gynecology, 164*(No. 5, Pt. 2), 1387–1389.

Ravel, R. (1995). *Clinical laboratory medicine: Clinical applications of laboratory data* (pp. 147–158). St. Louis, MO: Mosby.

Ringsrud, K.M., & Linné, J.J. (1995). *Urinalysis and body fluids: A color text and atlas* (pp. 104–105). St. Louis, MO: Mosby.

Shortliffe, L.M.D. (1992). UTI during pregnancy: It's not the same. *Contemporary OB/GYN, 37*(10), 69–82.

Sox, H.C., Jr. (1990). *Common diagnostic tests: Use and interpretation* (2nd ed., pp. 287–301). Philadelphia, PA: American College of Physicians.

Sweet, R.L., & Gibbs, R.S. (1995). *Infectious diseases of the female genital tract* (3rd ed., pp. 429–464). Baltimore, MD: Williams & Wilkins.

Chapter 3

PYELONEPHRITIS

Winifred L. Star

Acute pyelonephritis is the most common serious urinary tract complication affecting pregnancy, with an incidence of 1 to 2.5 percent. *Escherichia coli* causes about 80 percent of infections. Other common pathogens include *Klebsiella-Enterobacter*, *Proteus* species, and *Staphylococcus aureus*. The enterococcus and group B streptococcus are being increasingly recognized as pathogens in acute pyelonephritis (Cox, 1992; Sweet & Gibbs, 1995).

The presence of asymptomatic bacteriuria is a major risk factor for the development of pyelonephritis; 13 to 65 percent of untreated pregnant women with asymptomatic bacteriuria go on to develop this complication. Early detection and treatment of bacteriuria reduces the incidence of pyelonephritis by 70 to 80 percent. Recurrence rates of pyelonephritis in pregnancy are about 10 to 18 percent (Gibbs & Sweet, 1994; Sweet & Gibbs, 1995).

Several pregnancy-related factors predispose to the development of acute pyelonephritis. Anatomical and hormonal changes encourage dilatation and relaxation of the collecting system of the kidney leading to stasis of urine and facilitation of bacterial migration. Glycosuria, common in normal pregnancy, favors bacterial overgrowth. Estrogen may enhance growth of *E. coli*. The cumulative effects of these physiological changes is an increased risk that infection, which may begin in the bladder, will ascend to the kidneys (Gibbs & Sweet, 1989).

The most significant complication of pyelonephritis is preterm labor and delivery. Other reported complications include hemolytic anemia, thrombocytopenia, hypertension, pulmonary insufficiency, adult respiratory distress syndrome, transient renal insufficiency, chronic renal failure, renal/perinephric abscess, and recurrent pyelonephritis (Plattner, 1994; MacMillan & Grimes, 1991). Maternal sepsis may develop in 10 percent of pyelonephritis cases; septic shock may ensue in these women (McNeeley, 1988; Sweet & Gibbs, 1995).

Database

Subjective

- Predisposing factors
  - ▶ Physiologic changes of pregnancy
  - ▶ Asymptomatic bacteriuria
  - ▶ Cystitis
  - ▶ Ureteral or renal/calculi
  - ▶ Obstructive/neurologic disorders of the urinary tract
  - ▶ History of renal anomaly or pyelonephritis
  - ▶ Presence of adhesions on bacterial surface

- Symptoms (generally have a rapid onset)
  - ▶ Fever (usually spiking)
  - ▶ Shaking chills
  - ▶ Nausea with or without vomiting, anorexia
  - ▶ Flank or back pain (more commonly on the right)
  - ▶ Urinary urgency, frequency, dysuria may be present
  - ▶ Headache may be present
  - ▶ Lower abdominal pain may be present
  - ▶ Respiratory insufficiency symptoms, including dyspnea and tachypnea, may be present

Objective

- Woman appears ill; signs of dehydration may be present.

- Fever, a universal sign, is present and may reach 40° C (104° F).

- Tachycardia and hypotension may be present.

- Client exhibits costovertebral angle tenderness (CVAT), usually on the right.

- Lower abdominal tenderness may be present.

- Respiratory signs, including dyspnea, tachypnea, and hypoxemia, may be present if respiratory insufficiency develops; chest x-ray may be consistent with pulmonary edema.

- Gross hematuria may be present; urine may be cloudy or malodorous.

- Urine dipstick is positive for nitrites, leukocyte esterase, protein, and/or blood.

- Microscopic urinalysis reveals presence of white blood cells (WBCs), red blood cells (RBCs), bacteria, and/or white blood cell casts.

- Gram stain of uncentrifuged urine or sediment shows gram-negative bacilli or gram-positive cocci.

- Quantitative urine culture shows >100,000 colonies/mL of a pathogenic organism.

  NOTE: Lesser bacterial counts may be present or cultures may be negative if antibiotic therapy has been initiated prior to the onset of pyelonephritis. Colony counts of less than 10^5 in a client with clinical findings of acute pyelonephritis (and no other obvious explanation, such as use of antimicrobials) suggests urinary tract obstruction, perinephric abscess, or nonurinary tract abdominopelvic disorders (Sox Jr., 1990).

- Urine immunofluorescence test (if done) may be positive for antibody-coated bacteria.

- Blood cultures are positive in about 10 to 15 percent of cases.

- Elevations in serum creatinine or drops in creatinine clearance of 50 percent or more may occur.

- Squamous epithelial cells in large numbers (more than 10 per low-power field) on microscopic urinalysis represent vaginal or perineal contamination; a few squamous cells are seen in most urine specimens and have little clinical significance (Ravel, 1995; Ringsrud & Linné, 1995).

- Pyuria without bacteriuria may be present in association with chlamydial or gonococcal urethritis/cervicitis. Pelvic examination and wet mounts of vaginal discharge may show evidence of concomitant infection. See Section 14, *Vaginitis and Sexually Transmitted Diseases*.

- Perform pelvic examination, as indicated, to assess for cervical effacement and dilatation.

Assessment

- Pyelonephritis
  - ▶ R/O appendicitis
  - ▶ R/O nephrolithiasis
  - ▶ R/O perinephric abscess
  - ▶ R/O vaginitis
  - ▶ R/O STDs
  - ▶ R/O complications of pyelonephritis during hospitalization (responsibility of physician); see Introductory section
  - ▶ R/O acute/chronic concomitant medical problem(s)

Plan

Diagnostic tests

- Perform quantitative culture and antimicrobial susceptibility testing on a clean-catch midstream-voided urine specimen.
- Additional tests may include (but are not limited to) the following:
  - ▶ Complete blood count (CBC)
  - ▶ Serum creatinine and other renal function tests
  - ▶ Electrolytes
  - ▶ Blood cultures
  - ▶ Testing for *Neisseria gonorrhoeae*, *Chlamydia trachomatis*, group B streptococcus
  - ▶ X-ray
  - ▶ Intravenous pyelogram
  - ▶ Ultrasonography
- See the Objective section.

Treatment/Management

- Woman should be hospitalized and managed by a physician.

NOTE: Outpatient therapy has been undertaken in selected cases. Strict inclusion criteria and formal treatment regimens are mandatory. Further studies are needed to document the safety of outpatient management. (See Angel et al., 1990; Brooks & Garite, 1995; Garite & Walker, 1997; Millar, Wing, Paul, & Grimes, 1995; and Sanchez-Ramos et al., 1997).

- Therapeutic interventions include

  - ▶ Broad spectrum intravenous antibiotics (e.g., combination of ampicillin or cephalosporin with an aminoglycoside)

  - ▶ Intravenous hydration

  - ▶ Lowering of temperature

  - ▶ Balancing electrolytes

  - ▶ Monitoring of renal function, intake and output assessment

  - ▶ Support of respiratory function

  - ▶ Observation for shock and other complications. The details of inpatient management are beyond the scope of this protocol.

- On hospital discharge, a 7- to 14-day course of oral antibiotics is generally prescribed (Millar & Cox, 1997; Plattner, 1994); suppressive therapy for the remainder of pregnancy may also be undertaken. See the Follow-up section.

- Treat vaginitis or identified STDs as indicated. See Section 14, *Vaginitis and Sexually Transmitted Diseases.* Provide partner referrals for treatment of STDs as necessary.

Consultation

- Woman should be hospitalized and managed by a physician after diagnosis is established.

- Consult with physician regarding ongoing suppressive therapy after hospital discharge.

- If considering *surveillance* for urinary tract infection rather than suppressive therapy (see the Follow-up section), consult with a physician.

Patient Education

- Discuss the etiology of pyelonephritis, signs of complications, and the need for hospitalization.

- Discuss the importance of antibiotic therapy and compliance with outpatient medication regimen after hospital discharge.

- Educate the client regarding health maintenance and prevention measures for urinary tract infection. See Chapter 13.2, *Cystitis.*

- Discuss preterm labor signs and symptoms. See Chapter 6.25, *Preterm Labor.*

- Provide education on STDs and safer sex, as indicated.

Follow-up

- Obtain post-treatment urine culture. If positive, an appropriate antibiotic should be initiated based upon the sensitivities (Plattner, 1994).

- Women with pyelonephritis are usually given suppressive antibiotic therapy for the duration of pregnancy. (Some sites may continue drug treatment for up to 6 weeks postpartum.) Consult with a physician.

  ▶ Drugs may include (but are not limited to) (Gibbs & Sweet, 1994; Millar & Cox, 1997; Plattner, 1994; Sandberg & Brorson, 1991)

  – Amoxicillin 250 mg p.o. at bedtime

  – Nitrofurantoin 50–100 mg p.o. at bedtime

  – Cephalexin 250 mg p.o. at bedtime

  NOTE: Nitrofurantoin should not be prescribed to women with G6PD deficiency because of the risk of hemolysis (Briggs, Freeman, & Yaffe, 1994).

- An alternative to suppressive therapy is monthly evaluation of urine cultures for the remainder of pregnancy with prompt antibiotic treatment if bacteriuria identified (Cox, Crombleholme, Hooton, & Mead, 1993; Gibbs & Sweet, 1994; Millar & Cox, 1997; Sweet & Gibbs, 1995). Consult with physician.

  NOTE: Some sites may opt to use the dipstick nitrite and leukocyte esterase tests for screening with follow-up urine cultures, if positive, and then treat accordingly (Cox et al., 1993). Consult with a physician.

- Urine culture should be performed 6 to 8 weeks postpartum to rule out asymptomatic infection (Cox, 1992).

- Patients with repeated urinary tract infection/pyelonephritis in pregnancy should be referred for postpartum urologic evaluation (usually performed 3 to 6 months after delivery).

- Document diagnosis of pyelonephritis, management thereof, and any associated complications in the progress notes and problem list. Note on the problem list the presence of group B streptococcus as indicated. Document presence of an STD as indicated.

References

Angel, J.L., O'Brien, W.F., Finan, M.A., Morales, W.J., Lake, M. & Knuppel, R.A. (1990). Acute pyelonephritis in pregnancy: A prospective study of oral versus intravenous antibiotic therapy. *Obstetrics and Gynecology, 76*, 28–32.

Briggs, G.G., Freeman, R.K., & Yaffe, S.J. (1994). *Drugs in pregnancy and lactation* (4th ed.). Baltimore, MD: Williams & Wilkins.

Brooks, A.M., & Garite, T.J. (1995). Clinical trial of the outpatient management of pyelonephritis in pregnancy. *Infectious Diseases in Obstetrics and Gynecology, 3*, 50–55.

Cox, S.M. (1992). Pyelonephritis. *Contemporary OB/GYN, 37*(5), 117–123.

Cox, S., Crombleholme, W., Hooton, T., & Mead, P. (1993). Urinary tract infection: Is it recurrence or reinfection? *Contemporary OB/GYN, 38*(2), 84–108.

Garite, T.J., & Walker, C. (1997). Outpatient management of pyelonephritis: A reasonable option during pregnancy? *Contemporary OB/GYN, 42*(5), 57–77.

Gibbs, R.S. & Sweet, R.L. (1989). Maternal and fetal infections. Clinical disorders. In R. K. Creasy & R. Resnik (Eds.), *Maternal-fetal medicine: Principles and practice* (2nd ed., pp. 662–667). Philadelphia, PA: W. B. Saunders.

Gibbs, R.S. & Sweet, R.L. (1994). Maternal and fetal infections. Clinical disorders. In R. K. Creasy & R. Resnik (Eds.), *Maternal-fetal medicine: Principles and practice* (3rd ed., pp. 639–644) Philadelphia, PA: W. B. Saunders.

MacMillan, M.C., & Grimes, D.A. (1991). The limited usefulness of urine and blood cultures in treating pyelonephritis in pregnancy. *Obstetrics and Gynecology, 78*(5, Pt. 1), 745–748.

McNeeley, S.G. (1988). Treatment of urinary tract infections during pregnancy. *Clinical Obstetrics and Gynecology, 31*(2), 480–487.

Millar, L.K., & Cox, S.M. (1997). Urinary tract infections complicating pregnancy. *Infectious Disease Clinics of North America, 11*(1), 13–26.

Millar, L.K., Wing, D.A., Paul, R.H., & Grimes, D.A. (1995). Outpatient treatment of pyelonephritis in pregnancy: A randomized controlled trial. *Obstetrics and Gynecology, 86*, 560–564.

Plattner, M.S. (1994). Pyelonephritis in pregnancy. *Journal of Neonatal Nursing, 8*(1), 20–27.

Ravel, R. (1995). *Clinical laboratory medicine: Clinical applications of laboratory data* (pp. 147–158). St. Louis, MO: Mosby.

Ringsrud, K.M., & Linné, J.J. (1995). *Urinalysis and body fluids. A color text* (pp. 104–105). St. Louis, MO: Mosby.

Sanchez-Ramos, L., McAlpine, K.J., Adair, C.D., Kaunitz, A.M., Delke, I., & Briones, D.K. (1995). Pyelonephritis in pregnancy: Once-a-day ceftriaxone vs. multiple doses of cephazolin. *American Journal of Obstetrics and Gynecology, 172*, 129–133.

Sandberg, T. & Brorson, J.-E. (1991). Efficacy of long-term antimicrobial prophylaxis after acute pyelonephritis in pregnancy. *Scandinavian Journal of Infectious Disease, 23*, 221–223.

Sox, H.C. Jr. (1990). *Common diagnostic tests. Use and interpretation* (2nd ed.). Philadelphia, PA: American College of Physicians.

Sweet, R.L., & Gibbs, R.S. (1995). *Infectious diseases of the female genital tract* (3rd ed., pp. 429–464). Baltimore, MD: Williams & Wilkins.

SECTION 14

VAGINITIS AND SEXUALLY TRANSMITTED DISEASES

Chapter 1

CHLAMYDIA TRACHOMATIS

Winifred L. Star

Chlamydial infection is the most common bacterial sexually transmitted disease (STD) in the United States, affecting an estimated 4 million persons per year (U.S. Preventive Services Task Force, 1996). The chlamydiae are a group of obligate intracellular bacteria differentiated from other microorganisms by a unique developmental cycle. *Chlamydia trachomatis* is one of three species within the genus (the others are *Chlamydia psittaci* and *Chlamydia pneumoniae*). There are fifteen serotypes of *C. trachomatis*, including the agents which cause trachoma (A, B, Ba, C), those causing lymphogranuloma venereum (LGV) (L-1, L-2, L-3), and the sexually transmitted disease strains (D through K) (Schachter, 1990).

Chlamydia, similar to gonorrhea, is responsible for a variety of clinical syndromes in women, including urethritis, cervicitis, endometritis, Bartholinitis, and proctitis. In the female, the primary site of chlamydial infection is the endocervix. The incubation period for *C. trachomatis* is 6 to 14 days, but the organism may be harbored in the female reproductive tract for extended periods of time (Sweet & Gibbs, 1995). Approximately two-thirds of women with cervical infection are asymptomatic; however, one-third of these women will have clinical evidence of infection (Sweet & Gibbs, 1995). The most serious complication of chlamydial infection is salpingitis, or pelvic inflammatory disease (PID). In turn, ectopic pregnancy, tubal factor infertility and chronic pelvic pain are significant sequelae of PID. In men, chlamydia is responsible for nongonococcal urethritis, epididymitis, prostatitis, proctitis, and Reiter's syndrome. There is evidence that *C. trachomatis* can be isolated from the cervix of 60 to 70 percent of female sex partners of men with chlamydial urethritis. Of persons with genital chlamydial infection, 20 to 40 percent of men and 40 to 60 percent of women have concurrent gonococcal disease (Graham & Blanco, 1990; Handsfield & Pollock, 1990; McGregor & French, 1991). Infection with chlamydia (as well as other inflammatory or ulcerative sexually transmitted diseases [STDs]) may facilitate human immunodeficiency virus (HIV) transmission (U.S. Preventive Services Task Force, 1996; Woolf, Jonas, & Lawrence, 1996).

The prevalence of chlamydia in pregnancy ranges from 2 to 37 percent depending upon the population studied. Women with *C. trachomatis* cervical infection at the time of elective abortion are at increased risk for postabortal endometritis (McGregor & French, 1991). Whether chlamydial infection is associated with adverse perinatal outcome remains controversial (Gibbs & Sweet, 1994; Wendel & Wendel, Jr., 1993). Some studies have demonstrated a link between cervical chlamydial infection and preterm premature rupture of membranes, preterm labor and delivery, low birth weight infants, increased perinatal mortality, and/or late-onset postpartum endometritis. Other studies have failed to demonstrate such associations (Gibbs & Sweet, 1994). Thus, the final assessment regarding the role of chlamydia on perinatal morbidity and mortality awaits further large-scale prospective research.

In the newborn, *C. trachomatis* may cause inclusion conjunctivitis and pneumonia. Transmission occurs at the time of birth via contact with infected secretions in the birth canal. Twenty to 50 percent of exposed infants develop conjunctivitis in the first month of life and 10 to 20 percent develop pneumonia between the fourth and eleventh weeks (Gibbs & Sweet, 1994; Schachter & Grossman, 1995). Clinical manifestations consist of ocular discharge, conjunctival erythema, and eyelid edema (Martin, 1990). In the majority of infants, conjunctivitis resolves spontaneously; however, corneal scarring may occur in some untreated cases. The course of chlamydial pneumonia is generally benign but there is a risk to the infant of developing chronic respiratory problems. Symptoms include staccatolike cough, tachypnea, and nasal congestion, usually without fever (Schachter & Grossman, 1995). In children beyond infancy, chlamydial infection should arouse suspicion for sexual abuse (American Academy of Pediatrics [AAP], 1997).

Database

Subjective

Risk factors

- Young age (i.e., under 25 years of age; highest prevalence among 15 to 19 year olds)
- New or multiple sexual partners in past 3 months
- Sexual partner that has had other partners in past 3 months
- Partner(s) with nongonococcal urethritis (NGU)
- Coinfection or previous infection with gonorrhea
- Inconsistent use of barrier contraceptives
- Cervical eversion
- Oral contraceptives (may induce cervical eversion)
- Single marital status
- Black race
- Lower socioeconomic status
- Inner-city dweller

Symptomatology

- Two-thirds of women with chlamydial infection of the cervix are asymptomatic (Sweet & Gibbs, 1995).
- Symptomatic clients may report the following:
  - ▶ Eye irritation, redness (if conjunctivitis present; presumed route of infection via autoinoculation from infected genital secretions)
  - ▶ Labial swelling; swollen inguinal lymph nodes
  - ▶ Abnormal vaginal discharge
  - ▶ Postcoital or intermenstrual vaginal bleeding or spotting
  - ▶ Urgency, frequency, dysuria
  - ▶ Dyspareunia
  - ▶ Dysmenorrhea
  - ▶ Abdominal/pelvic pain

> ► Anorectal complaints including
>> – Anal irritation
>> – Rectal pain
>> – Mucoid or purulent rectal discharge
>> – Painful defecation, hematochezia, tenesmus, diarrhea, or constipation (if proctitis present)

- Patients with PID or late-onset postpartum endometritis may present with the following symptoms:
  - ► Fever
  - ► Chills
  - ► Malaise
  - ► Nausea/vomiting
  - ► Abdominal/pelvic pain

NOTE: Symptoms of chlamydial PID are usually less severe than seen in gonococcal PID; PID is rare in pregnancy, especially after 12 weeks' gestation.

- Partner(s) may have the following symptoms:
  - ► Urethral discharge
  - ► Dysuria
  - ► Epididymal pain/swelling
  - ► Rectal pain/discharge and/or pain during defecation (in men engaging in receptive anal intercourse)
  - ► Inguinal adenopathy

History

- Obtain a complete health history:
  - ► Menstruation
  - ► Sexual history, such as sexual orientation/practices, date(s) of last sexual contact(s), number of partners in past 3 months
  - ► Client and partner(s) STD history and presence of signs/symptoms of STD in client/partner(s)
  - ► Obstetrical and gynecological history
  - ► Medical history including medication and allergies
  - ► Habits
  - ► Psychosocial history

Objective

- A thorough STD examination includes the following assessments (Centers for Disease Control and Prevention, 1991):

  ▶ Vital signs, as indicated

  ▶ General skin inspection of face, trunk, forearms, palms, soles for lesions, rashes, or discoloration

  ▶ Inspection of pharynx/oral cavity for erythema, injection, lesions, or discoloration

  ▶ Abdominal inspection and palpation for masses, tenderness, or rebound tenderness

  ▶ Inspection of pubic hair for lice and nits

  ▶ Inspection of external genitalia for discharge, masses, or lesions; inspection and palpation of Bartholin's, urethral, and Skene's (BUS) glands for discharge, or masses

  ▶ Inspection of vagina for blood, discharge, or lesions

  ▶ Inspection of cervix for lesions, discharge, eversion, erythema, edema, or friability; assessment for cervical motion tenderness

  ▶ Uterine assessment for size, shape, consistency, mobility, and tenderness

  ▶ Palpation of adnexa for masses or tenderness

  ▶ Inspection of anus for lesions, bleeding, or discharge

    – Rectal exam, as indicated

  ▶ Assessment for presence or absence of associated cervical and linguinal lymphadenopathy

- Physical examination of the woman with chlamydia may be within normal limits (WNL) Assessments/findings may include

  ▶ Vital signs (elevated temperature may be present)

  ▶ Eyes (red conjunctiva or watery to mucopurulent discharge [in chlamydial conjunctivitis])

  ▶ Lymph nodes (inguinal lymphadenopathy may be present)

  ▶ Abdomen (assess for inguinal adenopathy, tenderness, and/or rebound tenderness)

  ▶ Genitalia and pelvis

    – BUS glands (purulent or mucoid exudate may be expressed from ducts; swelling, abscess formation may be present)

    – External genitalia (erythema, edema, abnormal discharge, or excoriation may be present)

    – Vagina (mucopurulent discharge or blood may be present)

    – Cervix (mucopurulent discharge and edema, erythema, or friability in zone of eversion may be present [for so-called mucopurulent cervicitis or MPC see below]; assess for cervical motion tenderness)

    – Uterus (assess size, shape, consistency, mobility, and presence of tenderness)

    – Adnexa (assess for presence of masses and/or tenderness)

- Anus and rectum (erythema or mucopurulent discharge may be present—an uncommon presentation)

- Mucopurulent cervicitis, if present, may be caused by chlamydial (or gonococcal) infection; however, in most cases neither organism can be isolated. Criteria for presumptive diagnosis includes the following:

  ▶ Mucopurulent or purulent exudate visible in the endocervical canal or on an endocervical swab specimen

  ▶ Easily induced cervical bleeding

  ▶ Increased number of polymorphonuclear leukocytes (PMNs) on endocervical Gram-stain (low positive predictive value) (CDC, 1998)

Assessment

- Chlamydia trachomatis

  ▶ R/O chlamydia trachomatis

  ▶ R/O gonorrhea

  ▶ R/O syphilis

  ▶ R/O vaginitis (i.e., trichomoniasis, bacterial vaginosis, candidiasis)

  ▶ R/O urinary tract infection

  ▶ R/O MPC due to nonmicrobiologic determinant (e.g., inflammation in an ectropion)

  ▶ R/O urethral syndrome

  ▶ R/O chlamydial conjunctivitis

  ▶ R/O appendicitis

  ▶ R/O septic abortion

  ▶ R/O PID

  ▶ R/O tubo-ovarian abscess

  ▶ R/O adnexal torsion

  ▶ R/O ectopic pregnancy

  ▶ R/O Fitz-Hugh-Curtis syndrome (perihepatitis)

  ▶ R/O Reiter's syndrome

  ▶ R/O squamous intraepithelial lesion (SIL)

  ▶ R/O HIV infection

Diagnostic Tests

- Laboratory diagnosis is mandatory.

  ▶ The most specific test for screening in asymptomatic persons is culture (U.S. Preventive Services Task Force, 1996).

▶ For screening during pregnancy, samples are generally obtained from the endocervix, but specimens from other sources may be obtained, as indicated (e.g., some nucleic acid amplification tests can be done on specimens from the vaginal introitus or urine but this may not be routine practice in an obstetrical setting). See Table 14.2, Directions for Obtaining GC or CT Samples from Selected Sites of Infection, in Chapter 14.4, *Gonorrhea.*

▶ Nonculture tests may include antigen detection methods (direct fluorescent antibody [DFA], and enzyme immunoassays [EIA]), and nucleic acid detection methods (polymerase chain reaction [PCR], DNA hybridization probe, and ligase chain reaction [LCR]).

NOTE: Nonculture tests are less specific and may produce false-positive results. Confirmation of positive results from some nonculture tests may be necessary in low-risk patients (e.g., those involved in monogamous relationships, no history of STD, member of low-prevalence [less than 5 percent] population) or for whom misdiagnosis may lead to psychological/social distress (CDC, 1993). (For further information on laboratory diagnosis of chlamydia see Black, 1997.)

● Perform serologic test for syphilis (VDRL or RPR).

● Offer HIV testing (pretest and posttest counseling and informed consent is necessary).

● Other laboratory tests used to aid diagnosis may include (but are not limited to) the following:

▶ Microscopic evaluation of saline wet mount of vaginal discharge (may show excess numbers of white blood cells [WBCs])

NOTE: *C. trachomatis* does not cause vaginitis; increased WBCs found in a wet mount are secondary to endocervical inflammation, characterized by leukocytic and lymphocytic infiltration.

▶ Pap smear (may reveal inflammatory atypia and/or dyskaryotic changes, dysplasia) (Sweet & Gibbs, 1995)

▶ Complete blood count (CBC) (leukocytosis may be seen in patients with PID)

▶ Erythrocyte sedimentation rate (ESR) (may be elevated in PID)

▶ C-reactive protein (may be elevated in PID)

● Additional tests may include urinalysis/urine culture, hepatitis B and C testing.

● Perform additional prenatal laboratory tests per site-specific protocol.

● IgG and IgM antibody testing has little value for routine diagnosis of acute genital tract chlamydial infection; however, chlamydia serology is useful for persons with symptoms consistent with LGV (Black, 1997; CDC, 1993).

Treatment/Management

Treatment/Management

General Considerations

● Pregnant women may be tested for chlamydia at the first prenatal visit, based on history, risk factors, and physical examination findings.

▶ Screening of high-risk women for *C. trachomatis* (rather than routine testing of all women) is recommended by the American College of Obstetricians and Gynecologists (ACOG) 1994).

▶ Repeat testing in the third trimester if woman is at risk for STDs.

NOTE: The following criteria may assist in identifying women who should be screened for chlamydia:

- Age under 25
- New or multiple concurrent sex partners
- Inner-city residence
- Unmarried status
- History or presence of other STDs
- Little or no prenatal care (American Academy of Pediatrics [AAP] and ACOG, 1997)

Note: Consult with local health authorities, if indicated, to help identify additional high-risk populations.

- Perform a serologic test for syphilis on all women at the first prenatal visit, in the third trimester if at high risk for STD, and prior to leaving the hospital after delivery. See Chapter 14.6, *Syphilis*.

- Screen all women who present with preterm labor (especially if membranes have ruptured) for the presence of chlamydia and gonorrhea (as well as for bacterial vaginosis, trichomoniasis, and group B streptococcus).

- Treat HIV-infected persons with the same drug regimens as for those without HIV.

- Treatment/management of complicated cases will generally be undertaken by a physician. Refer patients with chlamydial conjunctivitis to an ophthalmologist.

Drug Regimens

Recommended Regimens

- Erythromycin base 500 mg p.o. q.i.d. for 7 days

> OR

- Amoxicillin 500 mg p.o. t.i.d. for 7 days (CDC, 1998)

Alternative Regimens

- Erythromycin base 250 mg p.o. q.i.d. for 14 days

> OR

- Erythromycin ethylsuccinate 800 mg p.o. q.i.d. for 7 days

> OR

- Erythromycin ethylsuccinate 400 mg p.o. q.i.d. for 14 days

> OR

- Azithromycin 1 gram p.o. in a single dose (preliminary data indicate that this drug may be safe and effective but data are insufficient to recommend routine use in pregnant women (CDC, 1998).

NOTE: Doxycycline, tetracycline, erythromycin estolate, and the quinolones are contraindicated in pregnant persons.

Mucopurulent Cervicitis

- Ideally, treatment is based on laboratory test results. If there is a high likelihood of infection with GC and/or chlamydia or the client is not likely to return for follow-up care, treat empirically for either or both infections (refer to CDC, 1998 for additional information).

Partner Therapy

- Evaluate, test, and treat for chlamydia all sexual partners if their last sexual contact was during the 60 days preceding onset of the client's symptoms or diagnosis of chlamydia. The client's most recent sex partner should be treated if intercourse took place prior to the aforementioned time period. Drug regimens include the following.

Recommended Regimens

- Azithromycin 1 gram p.o. b.i.d. in a single dose

  OR

- Doxycycline 100 mg p.o. b.i.d. for 7 days (CDC, 1998)

Alternative Regimens

- Erythromycin base 500 mg p.o. q.i.d. for 7 days

  OR

- Erythromycin ethylsuccinate 800 mg p.o. q.i.d. for 7 days

  OR

- Ofloxacin 300 mg p.o. b.i.d. for 7 days (CDC, 1998)

  NOTE: Erythromycin is less efficacious than azithromycin or doxycycline (CDC, 1998).

Consultation

- Physician consultation is indicated for complications of chlamydial infections (e.g., PID, tubo-ovarian abscess, Fitz-Hugh-Curtis syndrome). Complicated cases may require consultation with an infectious disease expert.

- Consult with local health authorities, if indicated, to identify high-risk groups.

- Refer clients with chlamydial conjunctivitis to an ophthalmologist.

- Refer for psychosocial support services, if indicated.

Patient Education

- Discuss cause of infection, mode of transmission, incubation period, risk factors, symptoms, potential perinatal and neonatal complications, and treatment modalities. Alert client to possible side effects of medication.

- Stress compliance with treatment regimen and importance of partner evaluation and therapy. Refer partner to STD clinic or other source of health care as indicated.

- Discuss candidiasis prophylaxis, especially for patients prone to *Candida* infection secondary to antibiotics (see Chapter 14.7, *Vaginitis*).

- Advise abstinence from intercourse until both client and partner have completed treatment (i.e., 7 days after single-dose regimen or after completion of a 7-day regimen). Advise prompt follow-up should signs and symptoms of infection persist or recur.

- Address STD prevention.

    ▶ Provide guidelines for safer sex practices.

    ▶ Encourage careful "screening" of sex partners and committed use of condoms

    ▶ Educate regarding signs/symptoms of STDs and advise abstinence from sexual activity if these signs develop.

    NOTE: Clients should be advised to always have condoms (male and/or female) available and use them correctly and consistently, especially if having intercourse with new, multiple, or nonmonogamous partners and partners whose HIV status and risk status are unknown (Woolf, Jonas, & Lawrence, 1996). Ideally, both partners should be tested for STDs (including HIV) before initiating intercourse (CDC, 1998). See Table 14.1, Safer Sex Recommendations.

- Assist woman in understanding how specific sexual behaviors relate to STD acquisition. Advise against use of drugs and alcohol because these substances impair judgment and may lead to unsafe sex (Woolf et al., 1996). Tailor prevention measures to injection-drug users and/or their sexual partners.

- Allow patient to ventilate her emotions regarding the diagnosis of an STD. Provide literature on STDs as available. See Appendix 14.1a, Patient Education Resources for Sexually Transmitted Disease.

Follow-up

- In pregnancy, retesting for chlamydia (preferably by culture) is recommended 3 weeks after completion of treatment (CDC, 1998).

- If client reports ongoing or recurring signs or symptoms of infection, inquire about compliance with medication, drug reaction or side effects, partner therapy, sexual exposure and use of condoms, and whether reinfection is likely. Discuss the need for improved client-partner compliance with STD prevention measures, as indicated.

- Reevaluate clients with persistent signs/symptoms for *C. trachomatis* and *N. gonorrhoeae*. Perform wet mounts to rule out the presence of vaginitis.

- Repeat *C. trachomatis* and *N. gonorrhoeae* testing in the third trimester if at risk for STD.

- Perform serologic test for syphilis at about 28 weeks' gestation and again at delivery.

- If initially negative, repeat HBsAg testing in late pregnancy for all high-risk women (e.g., injecting-drug users, women with STDs) (CDC, 1998).

- HIV-testing may be repeated in 3 months.

- Follow up on all positive laboratory tests.

  ▶ Counsel HIV-positive women appropriately and refer them for early intervention services. See Chapter 14.5, *Human Immunodeficiency Virus*, for further information and for additional lab tests that may be necessary.

  ▶ Give Hepatitis B antigen-positive women appropriate counseling and advise them of the need for immunoprophylaxis of their offspring, their sex partner(s), and all household members. See Chapter 10.2, *Hepatitis A, B, C, D, and E,* for further information and for additional lab tests that may be ordered.

  ▶ Treat concomitant STDs and other conditions, as indicated.

  ▶ Refer clients with abnormal Pap smears for colposcopy, as indicated. See Chapter 6.1, *Abnormal Cervical Cytology.*

- Ongoing psychosocial support is important for the woman in gaining control over her sexual situation and to enable her to successfully prevent future STDs.

- Address substance abuse issues and other high-risk behaviors. Refer to support services (e.g., public health nursing, drug treatment programs, psychological/social services), as indicated.

- Contraceptive counseling for postpartum women should include strategies to reduce future exposure to STDs.

- All newborns should receive topical ophthalmic prophylaxis for gonococcal ophthalmia shortly after birth (required by law in most states). (See Chapter 14.4, *Gonorrhea.*) Topical prophylaxis with silver nitrate, erythromycin, or tetracycline will not, however, reliably prevent *chlamydial* conjunctivitis (AAP, 1997).

- Systemic treatment is indicated for neonatal conjunctival infections and pneumonia. Details on neonatal drug regimens are beyond the scope of this protocol. Close follow-up of neonates is necessary (AAP, 1997; Hess, 1993).

- Chlamydia cases should be reported to the local public health department within 7 calendar days from the time of identification.

- Document history of chlamydia and/or other STDs and treatment thereof in progress notes and problem list. A history of abnormal cervical cytology should also be noted. Behaviors that place the patient at high risk for STDs may be noted on the problem list as appropriate.

Table 14.1

Safer Sex Recommendations

Safer sex: Extremely low- or no-risk practices
Abstention from sexual contact
Self-masturbation
Touching, massaging, hugging, caressing
Social (dry) kissing

Probably safe: Very low-risk practices (small theoretic risk)
French (wet) kissing
Mutual masturbation (if no cuts on hands, or ulcers or lesions on genitals of either partner)
Vaginal sex with a male or female condom (put latex or polyurethane condom in place before any penetration)
Fellatio with condom (place latex condom on partner's penis before oral contact)
Cunnilingus with dental dam (place latex dam over partner's vaginal area before oral contact)
Anilingus (rimming) with dental dam (place latex dam over anus before oral contact)
Contact with urine (water sports; only with intact skin, avoid contact with mouth)
Using one's own sex toys (no sharing of any toys which contact body fluids)
Anal sex with condom (place latex condom on penis prior to penetration; probably safer with use of ample water-based lubrication
Mutually monogamous sex between two persons who have no HIV risk factors and who are known to be uninfected

Possibly unsafe: No strong proof, but some evidence that transmission can occur
Fellatio (sucking partner's penis and swallowing semen)
Cunnilingus (oral contact with partner's genital area and vaginal secretions)
Anilingus without a latex dam

Unsafe sex: High risk of transmitting HIV
Anal intercourse without a latex condom (highest risk is to the receptive partner)
Anal penetration with the hand (fisting) or other rectal trauma without a latex glove or fisting followed by anal intercourse
Anal douching in combination with anal sex
Vaginal intercourse without a male or female condom
Sex with numerous partners

Source: Palacio. H. (1994). Safer sex. In P.T. Cohen, M.A. Sande, & P.A. Volberding (Eds), *The AIDS knowledge base* (2nd ed., p 10.6–10.12). Boston, MA: Little, Brown and Company. Reprinted with permission.

References

Advances in sexually transmitted diseases. (1996). Course presented by the San Francisco STD/HIV Training Center. April 18 & 19, 1996. San Francisco, CA.

Alexander, L.L. (1992). Sexually transmitted diseases: Perspectives on this growing epidemic. *Nurse Practitioner, 17*(10), 31–42.

American Academy of Pediatrics (AAP). (1997). *1997 Red book: Report of the Committee on Infectious Diseases* (24th ed., pp. 170–174). ELk Grove Village, IL: Author.

American Academy of Pediatrics (AAP) and the American College of Obstetricians and Gynecologists (ACOG). (1997). *Guidelines for perinatal care* (4th ed., pp. 236–237). Elk Grove Village, IL: Authors

American College of Obstetricians and Gynecologists (ACOG). (1994). *Gonorrhea and chlamydial infections.* Technical Bulletin No. 190. Washington, DC: Author.

Black, C.M. (1997). Current methods of laboratory diagnosis of *Chlamydia trachomatis* infections. *Clinical Microbiology Reviews, 10*(1), 160–184.

Centers for Disease Control and Prevention (CDC). (1985). *Chlamydia trachomatis* infections: policy guidelines for prevention and control. *Morbidity and Mortality Weekly Report 34*(Suppl. 3S), 53S–74S.

Centers for Disease Control and Prevention (CDC). (1991). *Sexually transmitted diseases: Clinical practice guidelines.* Atlanta, GA: CDC.

Centers for Disease Control and Prevention (CDC). (1993). Recommendations for the prevention and management of *Chlamydia trachomatis* infections, 1993. *Morbidity and Mortality Weekly Report, 42*(RR–12), 1–39.

Centers for Disease Control and Prevention (CDC). (1998). 1998 Sexually transmitted diseases treatment guidelines. *Morbidity and Mortality Weekly Report, 47*(No. RR–1), 52–59.

Cohen, I., Veille, C., & Calkins, B.M. (1990). Improved pregnancy outcome following successful treatment of chlamydial infection. *Journal of the American Medical Association, 263*, 3160–3168.

Gibbs, R.S., & Sweet, R.L. (1994). Clinical disorders. In R.K. Creasy & R. Resnik (Eds.), *Maternal-fetal medicine: Principles and practice* (3rd ed., pp. 682–686). Philadelphia, PA: W.B. Saunders.

Graham, J.M., & Blanco, J.D. (1990). Chlamydial infections. *Primary Care, 17*(1), 85–93.

Handsfield, H.H., & Pollock, P.S. (1990). Arthritis associated with sexually transmitted diseases. In K.K. Holmes, P.-A. Mårdh, P. F. Sparling, P.J. Wiesner W. Cates, Jr., S.M. Lemon, & W.E. Stamm (Eds.), *Sexually transmitted diseases* (2nd ed., pp. 737–751). New York: McGraw-Hill.

Hess, D.L. (1993). Chlamydia in the neonate. *Neonatal Network, 12*(3), 9–12.

Martin, D.H. (1990). Chlamydial infections. *Medical Clinics of North America, 74*(6), 1367–1387.

McGregor, J.A., & French, J.I. (1991). *Chlamydia trachomatis* infection during pregnancy. *American Journal of Obstetrics and Gynecology, 164*(No. 6, Pt. 2), 1782–1788.

Palacio, H. (1994). Safer sex. In P.T. Cohen, M. A. Sande, & P.A. Volberding (Eds.), *The AIDS knowledge base* (2nd ed., p. 10.6–10.12). Boston, MA: Little, Brown, and Company.

Ryan, G.M., Abdella, T.N., & McNeely, S.G. (1990). *Chlamydia trachomatis* infection in pregnancy and effect of treatment on outcome. *American Journal of Obstetrics and Gynecology, 162,* 34–39.

Schachter, J. (1990). Biology of *Chlamydia trachomatis.* In K K. Holmes, P.-A. Mårdh, P.F. Sparling, P.J. Wiesner W. Cates, Jr., S.M. Lemon, & W.E. Stamm (Eds.), *Sexually transmitted diseases* (2nd ed., pp. 167). New York: McGraw-Hill.

Schachter, J., & Grossman, M. (1995). Chlamydia. In J.S. Remington & J.O. Klein (Eds.), *Infectious diseases of the fetus and newborn infant* (4th ed., pp. 657–667). Philadelphia, PA: W.B. Saunders.

Ståmm, W.E., & Holmes, K.K. (1990). *Chlamydia trachomatis* infections of the adult. In K.K. Holmes, P.-A. Mårdh, P.F. Sparling, P.J. Wiesner W. Cates, Jr., S.M. Lemon, & W.E. Stamm (Eds.), *Sexually transmitted diseases* (2nd ed., pp. 181–193). New York: McGraw-Hill.

Sweet, R.L., & Gibbs, R.S. (1995). *Infectious diseases of the female genital tract* (3rd ed, pp. 64–110). Baltimore, MD: Williams & Wilkins.

U.S. Preventive Services Task Force. (1996). *Guide to clinical preventive services* (2nd ed.). Baltimore. MD: Williams & Wilkins.

Wendel, P.J., & Wendel, G.D., Jr. (1993). Sexually transmitted diseases in pregnancy. *Seminars in Perinatology, 17*(6), 443–451.

Woolf, S.H., Jonas, S., & Lawrence, R.S. (1996). *Health promotion and disease prevention in clinical practice.* Baltimore, MD: Williams & Wilkins.

Appendix 14.1a

Patient Education Resources for Sexually Transmitted Diseases

National STD Hotline
1 (800) 227-8922

Agency for Health Care Policy and Research
Publications Clearinghouse
P.O. Box 8547
Silver Spring, MD 20907
1 (800) 358-9295

American Academy of Family Physicians
8880 Ward Parkway
Kansas City, MO 64114-2797
1 (800) 944-0000

American Social Health Association
P.O. Box 13827
Research Triangle Park, NC 27709
(919) 361-8400

Centers for Disease Control and Prevention
AIDS and HIV Hotline
1 (800) 342-2437
1 (800) 344-7432 (Spanish)
1 (800) 243-7889 (TTY)

CDC Treatment Guidelines
(888) 232-3228 [toll free] (press options 2, 5, 1, 1 to order)

Channing L. Bete Co., Inc.
200 State Road
South Deerfield, MA 01373-0200

Krames Communication
1100 Grundy Lane
San Bruno, CA 94066-3030

National Institute of Allergy and Infectious Diseases
MSC 2520
Building 31, Room 7A50
31 Center Drive
Bethesda, MD 20892
(301) 496-5717

Chapter 2

CONDYLOMATA ACUMINATA

Lisa L. Lommel

Condylomata acuminata, also known as genital or venereal warts, is primarily a sexually transmitted disease (STD) caused by the human papillomavirus (HPV). This double-stranded DNA virus belongs to the papovavirus family and has the ability to remain latent. There are over 70 known serotypes of HPV to date that cause a variety of clinical wart syndromes. Human papillomavirus serotypes 6, 11, 42, 43, 44, and 53–55 are responsible for the majority of benign anogenital disease and usually present as papillary condylomas and, less frequently, as flat condylomas. Serotypes 16, 18, 45, and 56 usually result in flat condylomas and have been associated with premalignant and malignant anogenital disease. More than 90 percent of cervical neoplasia has been strongly associated with these latter serotypes (American College of Obstetricians and Gynecologists [ACOG], 1994; Wood, 1991). There are three classifications of genital HPV infection: 1) latent infections that have no visible lesions and are detected by DNA hybridization, 2) subclinical lesions identified by application of 5 percent acetic acid and inspection under magnification, and 3) clinical lesions identified without aid of magnification (ACOG, 1994). Co-factors such as immunosuppression, herpes simplex virus, smoking, other sexually transmitted infections, and long-term oral contraceptive use are thought to contribute to HPV-related neoplasias (Schaffer & Philput, 1992). Human-papillomavirus–related neoplasia can also occur on the penis, anus, and vulva (Fletcher, 1991) Other complications of condylomata acuminata include ulceration, hemorrhage, secondary infection, and giant condylomas. In pregnancy, presence of HPV infection was found to be associated with poor healing of episiotomy repairs (dehiscence), especially in smokers (Snyder, Hammond, & Hankins, 1990).

Genital HPV infections are one of the most common sexually transmitted diseases in the United States. Occurrence rates are highest in the sexually active, young-adult population age 15 to 25 years. The incubation period for subclinical warts or the clinical appearance of warts may range from 1 month to several years, with the average range of 2 to 3 months. Transmission rates are difficult to establish because of the latent nature of the disease. It is thought that up to 85 percent of women whose partners have condylomata will develop the lesion . The incidence, prevalence, and replication of HPV in pregnant women is higher than nonpregnant women. The relative state of immunosuppression and hormonal influences during pregnancy greatly contribute to these factors (Vogel, 1992). Condylomata in pregnancy may become large enough to impede delivery necessitating cesarean section. Premature rupture of membranes (PROM) or chorioamnionitis due to secondary infection of condylomas by vaginal and rectal bacteria may occur.

The primary goal of treatment is to remove symptomatic genital lesions, although genital warts are often asymptomatic. Treatment may induce wart-free periods but will not affect the natural history of HPV infection. If not treated, visible genital warts may resolve on their own, remain unchanged, or increase in size or number. There is no evidence to show that treatment of visible warts will affect the development of cervical cancer (CDC, 1998).

Treatment of HPV infection includes a variety of local, destructive, and immunotherapies. Recurrence of clinical lesions are common after destructive therapy because HPV-associated lesions can be surrounded by a diffuse area of subclinical infection. Repeated treatments are often needed to achieve stable remission. Spontaneous regression of genital lesions may occur because of host immune responses. Lasting clinical remission has been achieved by localized destruction of obvious lesions and the body's cellular immune response.

Perinatal transmission of HPV occurs during delivery as infants are exposed to the affected genital tract of their mothers. Infected infants may develop respiratory papillomatosis and/or genital lesions, with serotypes 6 and 11 causing the vast majority of disease. Transmission usually follows vaginal delivery but has also been reported after cesarean section (Fletcher, 1991). It is estimated that approximately one infant case of juvenile laryngeal papillomata (JLP) occurs for every 1,000 infected mothers. Juvenile laryngeal papillomatosis has been shown to be rarely associated with mortality, although significant long-term morbidity is common. Typical presentation of hoarseness and respiratory distress can begin at age 2 years through adolescence. The larynx, trachea, and pulmonary tree may all be affected, requiring multiple surgical interventions. External anogenital and conjunctival lesions have been reported in children born to affected mothers, although such lesions are rare (Fletcher, 1991). Aggressive treatment of maternal condylomata has been suggested but not proven to reduce the risk for juvenile laryngeal papillomas or genital infections (Wood, 1991). Cesarean section is not recommended to reduce transmission of virus to the neonate (Patsner, Baker & Orr, 1990). Congenital genital lesions have also been reported (Fletcher, 1991).

Routine viral screening and typing for detection of HPV is not yet standard practice. Evaluation for signs and symptoms of HPV infection can be accomplished for women by history, Pap smear, and physical examination. Further evaluation will be limited by practice-site availability of laboratory techniques, colposcopy, and experienced clinicians. The only definitive diagnostic test for presence of HPV is by histologic evaluation of a biopsy.

Database

Subjective

- Majority of patients are asymptomatic
- Presence of vulvar lesion on self or lesion on sexual partner
- Vulvar pruritus, burning, and/or bleeding
- Dyspareunia
- Profuse vaginal discharge and/or pruritus
- Accompanying signs and symptoms of vaginitis
- History of abnormal or suspicious Pap smear
- Risk factors for developing cervical cancer may include (Cothran & White, 1995)
  - ▶ Multiple sexual partners
  - ▶ Cigarette smoking
  - ▶ Immunosuppressed state
  - ▶ Pregnancy
  - ▶ Oral contraceptive use

Objective

- Latent disease is defined by absence of morphologic abnormalities.

- Subclinical infection usually appears as flat condylomata, which most often affect the cervix, followed by the vulva, vagina, and anal epithelium in site frequency. Flat condylomata appear as 1-to-4-mm-in-diameter, flat-topped papules. They are usually not seen without the application of acetic acid to produce acetowhitening and the use of magnification.

- Clinically apparent lesions appear as flat condylomata or acuminata. Acuminata present as small 2 to 3 mm in diameter, soft, papillary growths occurring singly or in clusters. Older and larger lesions may have a cauliflower-like appearance.

- Vagina and introitus usually present with multiple, fine, fingerlike projections.

- Squared-off keratotic papules may be seen on nonmucosal dry areas of the groin.

- Lesions of varying presentation may be seen in the mouth, larynx, or conjunctivae.

- Bleeding and/or excoriation of the lesions may be present due to irritation from clothing or scratching.

- Signs of concomitant vaginitis or STD may be present

Assessment

- Condylomata acuminata

  - ▶ R/O condylomata lata of secondary syphilis

  - ▶ R/O molluscum contagiosum

  - ▶ R/O folliculitis

  - ▶ R/O vaginitis

  - ▶ R/O concomitant STD

  - ▶ R/O squamous intraepithelial lesion (SIL)

  - ▶ R/O seborrheic keratosis

  - ▶ Acetowhitening may be due to

    - – HPV infection

    - – Variation of normal epithelium

    - – Tissue inflammation secondary to vaginitis

    - – Allergic or contact dermatitis

    - – Microtrauma

    - – Post-treatment areas (up to 6 months)

    - – Lichen sclerosis and atrophicus

    - – Pantyhose or tight pants

    - – Hyperkeratosis

Plan

Diagnostic Tests

- Examination of genital tissue is facilitated by applying liberal amounts of 5 percent acetic acid (ordinary white vinegar) with large cotton swabs.

    ▶ Acetic acid causes the larger nuclei of proliferating epithelium to appear opaque (acetowhitening) because it causes the cytoplasm of the cells to shrink.

    ▶ Flat lesions not ordinarily seen and papillary lesions will be enhanced after 1 to 5 minutes of exposure to acetic acid.

    ▶ Magnification (with magnifying glass or colposcope) will further aid in evaluation.

    NOTE: Acetowhitening is *not* diagnostic of HPV infection (see Assessment for differential diagnosis)–it serves to increase the index of suspicion in an otherwise unsuspicious area. Further evaluation is necessary for all suspicious lesions.

- A Pap smear of the cervical transformation zone is used as a screening technique. Because of the prevalence of false negatives, a negative Pap does not indicate absence of disease. The Pap smear should not be the only technique for cervical evaluation where there is evidence of disease elsewhere or if the cervix does not appear normal. The presence of koilocytes (halo cells) on Pap smear is indicative of HPV infection.

- A colposcopy and directed biopsy can confirm HPV infection in acetowhitened, suspicious lesions and rule out SIL. Biopsy for diagnosis is required in all cases except the most obvious classical condylomata acuminata (ACOG, 1994). The colposcopy and/or biopsy is performed by a trained health care provider.

- The digene hybrid capture HPV DNA assay is the most current comprehensive HPV test available for clinical use. It identifies the presence of the fourteen common anogenital HPV types. The assay distinguishes low-risk HPV types (6, 11, 42, 43, and 44) from intermediate and high-risk HPV types (16, 18, 31, 33, 35, 45, 51, 52, and 56) (Richart, Meijer, Greenberg, Schiffman, & Cox, 1995). However, it is not yet a standard test in clinical practice.

- Prepare wet mounts for presence of vaginitis, as indicated.

- Obtain VDRL/RPR, HIV, gonorrhea, and chlamydia cultures, as indicated.

- With grossly visible lesions, consider glucose screening to rule out diabetes.

- Perform additional cultures, as indicated (e.g., herpes simplex virus).

Treatment

- There are numerous modalities available for the treatment of cervical, vaginal, vulvar, perineal and anal HPV lesions. No one treatment is satisfactory for all circumstances

    ▶ A small-to-moderate number of condylomata may initially receive chemical treatment (Luchtenfeld, 1994).

       – Trichloracetic acid in concentrations of at least 85 to 90 percent in ethanol solution (70 percent) may safely treat *noncervical* individual lesions in pregnancy.

    *   Under controlled magnification, the solution is applied with a small cotton tipped or pointed wooden applicator to the surface of the wart lesions and a small amount of surrounding skin. Allow to dry, at which time a white "frosting" develops.

    *   The acid does not need to be washed off after application. A moderate to intense burning sensation may be felt by the patient for 5 to 10 minutes after application. Powder with talc or sodium bicarbonate to remove unreacted acid if an excess amount is applied.

    *   Applications may be repeated every 7 to 14 days depending upon individual healing time.

    –   Liquid nitrogen (–196°C) applied by freezing the cotton tip of a swab and then touched on a noncervical lesion can be used in pregnancy. This technique requires repeated applications and causes significant localized discomfort, tissue necrosis, and occasional bleeding (Ferenczy, 1995).

    –   Podophyllin 0.5 percent podofilox solution and 5 percent 5-fluorouracil in cream (Efudex®) should *not* be used in pregnancy because they may be absorbed into the vascular system and cause serious complications in the mother; they are also teratogenic to the fetus (ACOG, 1994).

    –   Patient-applied therapies, podofilox, and imiquimod, should *not* be used in pregnancy (CDC, 1998).

▶   Recurrent lesions, large lesions, or extensive disease respond better to ablative (CO$_2$ laser, surgical excision, and/or electrocautery) therapy (Luchtenfeld, 1994).

    –   Electrocautery, loop electrosurgical excision procedure (LEEP), large loop excision of the transformation zone (LEETZ), cryocautery, and laser therapy are the therapies of choice for resistant or extensive lesions in pregnancy. These techniques are performed by the physician when appropriate.

● Treatment of the cervix should be conducted by those with specific training in colposcopy and cervical treatment methods. High-grade intraepithelial lesions (SIL) must be excluded before treatment is begun.

● Interferon therapy should *not* be used in pregnancy because it may interfere with normal liver, bone marrow, and immune functions (ACOG, 1994).

● Treat concomitant vaginal infection or STD, as appropriate.

● Active treatment of clinically obvious vulvar condylomata acuminata in the area of a potential episiotomy site is recommended because there is a risk of dehiscence (Snyder et al., 1990).

● Treat visible lesions to reduce risk of further growth in size and number (Ferenczy, 1995).

● Treatment is not recommended for clinically negative, HPV-DNA-positive women. Follow-up at regular intervals is advised for these women (see Follow-up section) (Ferenczy, 1995).

● Spontaneous regression of clinically visible lesions has been documented. The incidence of regression in a given patient is unknown. Regression cannot be predicted.

Consultation

- Consult with a physician as necessary.

- Refer to a trained health-care provider for colposcopy and directed biopsy.

- Refer for treatment of the cervix and electrocautery, cryocautery, or laser therapy.

Patient Education

- Explain about the virus, its transmission, and consequences.

- Discuss the link with cervical cancer and the need for follow-up.

- Explain that warts can be cured, especially when treatment of the patient and partner occur simultaneously.

- Explain that although the warts are curable, recurrences are common because the virus can live in normal-appearing cells.

- Inform patient prior to treatment regarding post-treatment pain associated with specific therapies.

- Advise client to call her health care provider if signs of infection appear, such as redness, increased pain, or presence of pus.

- Advise client that sexual partner(s) should undergo self-examination for presence of HPV or other STDs. Provide referrals to a source of health care if necessary.

- Explain that condoms decrease risk of viral transmission to an uninfected partner or reinfecting an already infected partner with a new subtype. Condoms are still of undetermined long-term benefit in a monogamous relationship and have been found not to affect treatment success rate in the female (CDC, 1998). They do, however, decrease the risk of other sexually transmitted diseases.

- Advise the patient to keep the vulva clean and dry; a damp environment enhances growth of the warts.

- Advise the patient to wear cotton underwear and loose fitting clothing.

- Advise maintenance of a healthy lifestyle to aid the immune system including diet, rest, stress reduction, and exercise.

- Explain importance of proper thorough treatment of concomitant vaginitis or STD.

- Discuss feelings that the patient may have regarding her experiences with this infection.

Follow-up

- Self-examination and semi-annual or annual health exams are recommended to assess disease recurrence.

- Follow-up Pap smear schedules will vary between sites. It is suggested that if the cervix is treated, a Pap smear should be done every 3 months for 2 years, then every 6 months for 3 years, and then annually if screen results are negative (Kelley, Galbraith, & Vermund, 1992).

- Pap smears should be obtained on a yearly basis, at least, from women who have been treated for HPV infection or SIL after initial treatment. See Chapter 6.1, *Abnormal Cervical Cytology*.

- Document HPV/SIL diagnosis and management thereof in problem list and progress notes.

References

American College of Obstetricians and Gynecologists (ACOG). (1994). Genital human papillomavirus infections (Technical Bulletin No. 193). Washington, DC: Author.

Centers for Disease Control and Prevention (1998). 1998 guidelines for treatment of sexually transmitted diseases, *Morbidity and Mortality Weekly Report, 47*(1).

Cothran, M.M. & White, J.E. (1995). Update on human papillomavirus. *Journal of American Academy of Nurse Practitioners, 7* (12), 583–589.

Ferenczy, A. (1995). Epidemiology and clinical pathophysiology of condylomata acuminata. *American Journal of Obstetrics and Gynecology, 172* (4), 1331–1339.

Fletcher, J.L. (1991). Perinatal transmission of human papillomavirus. *AFP, 43*(1), 143–148.

Kelley, K.F., Galbraith, M.A., & Vermund, S.H. (1992). Genital human papillomavirus infection in women. *Journal of Obstetric, Gynecologic, and Neonatal Nursing, 21*(6), 503–515.

Kling, A. (1992). Genital Warts—Therapy. Seminars in Dermatology, *11*(3), 247–255.

Luchtenfeld, M.A. (1994). Perianal condylomata acuminata. *Surgical Clinics of North America, 74* (6), 1327–1338.

Patsner, B., Baker, D.A., & Orr, J.W. (1990). Human papillomavirus genital tract infections during pregnancy. *Clinical Obstetrics and Gynecology, 33*(2), 258–267.

Richart, R. M., Meijer, C., Greenberg, M.D. Schiffman, M.H. & Cox, J. T. (1995). HPV DNA testing comes of age. *Contemporary Ob/Gyn, June,* 79–99.

Schaffer, S.D., & Philput, C.B. (1992). Predictors of abnormal cervical cytology: Statistical analysis of human papillomavirus and cofactors. *Nurse Practitioner, 17*(3), 46–50.

Snyder, R. R., Hammond, T.L., & Hankins, G.D.V. (1990). Human papillomavirus associated with poor healing of episiotomy repairs. *Obstetrics and Gynecology, 76*(4), 664–667.

Vogel, L.N. (1992). Epidemiology of human papilloma virus infection. *Seminars in Dermatology, 11*(3), 226–228.

Wood, C.L. (1991). Laryngeal papillomas in infants and children: Relationship to maternal disease. *Journal of Nurse-Midwifery, 36*(5), 297–302.

Chapter 3

GENITAL HERPES SIMPLEX VIRAL INFECTIONS

Maureen T. Shannon

Genital herpes simplex virus infection is a common sexually transmitted disease. There are two types of herpes simplex virus (HSV) that are responsible for infection: type 1 (HSV-1), which is associated with the majority of oral infections and infections that occur above the waist, and type 2 (HSV-2), which is responsible for the majority of the infections observed in the genitalia (Gibbs & Sweet, 1994; Murphy, 1995). Although approximately 90 percent of clinical presentations follow this pattern, either type of HSV may be responsible for an infection (Gibbs & Sweet, 1994). There is no cure for HSV infections; however, recurrent genital HSV infections in immunocompetent individuals usually become milder and less frequent over time.

Four genital HSV clinical presentations in adults have been observed. First-episode primary genital herpes occurs when a woman *without* antibodies to either HSV-1 or HSV-2 becomes infected and develops systemic and local symptoms. The clinical manifestations associated with this syndrome usually include systemic flu-like symptoms (i.e., fever, headache, chills, malaise) and severe local symptoms (i.e., painful ulcerative lesions, inguinal adenopathy, pelvic pain, vaginal discharge). The local symptoms may persist for up to 4 weeks. During pregnancy, the major risk factor associated with the development of primary HSV infection is serologic discordance between the woman and her partner (Brown, 1995).

First-episode nonprimary HSV infection occurs when a woman *with* antibodies to HSV-1 or HSV-2 experiences an initial clinical episode. Unlike first-episode primary genital herpes, there are no systemic symptoms reported, and the clinical manifestations observed are similar to recurrent genital HSV infection (i.e., local symptoms of varying severity).

The third clinical presentation is recurrent genital HSV infection. These recurrent clinical episodes are associated with milder local symptoms of shorter duration. Viral shedding during recurrent episodes usually lasts from 3 to 5 days (Gibbs & Sweet, 1994).

Finally, asymptomatic HSV infection has been observed in women without a history of HSV symptoms or clinical manifestations who have demonstrated serologic evidence of antibodies to HSV. The rate of asymptomatic HSV infection in pregnant women has been reported to be between 32 and 66 percent in various studies (Frenkel et al., 1993; Kalhanjian et al., 1992; Prober et al., 1988).

In pregnancy, maternal genital infection with HSV can have adverse effects on both the mother and the fetus. Pregnant women rarely have disseminated primary HSV-2 infection. When dissemination does occur, it usually happens during the latter half of pregnancy (Brown, 1995). Clinical manifestations of disseminated HSV-2 infection in the mother include pneumonitis, endometritis, hepatitis with or without coagulopathy, thrombocytopenia, leukopenia, and/or encephalitis (Brown, 1995; Stagno & Whitley, 1985). The observed mortality rate among pregnant women affected by dissemination of primary HSV-2 infection has been reported to be as much as 50 percent, with a fetal wastage rate of 50 percent (although the fetal deaths were not always associated with maternal deaths) (Stagno & Whitley, 1985). Although rare, transplacental transmission of HSV has been reported. Fetal sequelae of HSV infection includes congenital malformations (e.g., cutaneous, ocular, neurological), chorioretinitis, retinal dysplasia, microophthalmia, and microcephaly (Hutto et al., 1987; Mann & Grossman III, 1996). A spontaneous abortion rate of 25 to 30 percent has been observed in women who contract a primary HSV-2 infection before the 20th week of pregnancy (Stagno & Whitley, 1985).

Primary genital infection, symptomatic, recurrent local infections, and asymptomatic viral shedding of HSV-2 by pregnant women near term have been associated with viral transmission to the fetus or newborn during the peripartum period. A risk of HSV infection in excess of 50 percent has been noted in neonates whose mothers deliver when early stages of a primary genital HSV infection are occurring (in the third trimester) (Arvin, 1991; Brown, Berry, & Vontver, 1986; Brown et al., 1987). However, in pregnant women with recurrent genital HSV infection who have asymptomatic shedding of the virus at the onset of labor, the risk of neonatal herpes infection has been estimated to be less than 5 percent (American Academy of Pediatrics [AAP], 1997; Arvin, 1991; Boucher et al., 1990; Brown et al., 1986; Centers for Disease Control and Prevention [CDC], 1998). Multiple factors appear to influence an infant's risk of developing HSV infection including prematurity, low birth weight, the use of invasive fetal monitoring devices, the amount of inoculum present, and the level of maternal neutralizing antibodies present in the fetus/neonate (Arvin, 1991; Brown, 1995; Brown et al., 1986; Overall, 1994; Prober et al., 1987). The most severe sequelae of neonatal HSV infections include dissemination of infection with involvement of the central nervous system and visceral organs resulting in severe disability and/or death in 50 percent of affected infants (Arvin, 1991; Stagno & Whitley, 1985).

Up to 80 percent of infected infants are born to women who have no history of HSV exposure and who are asymptomatic during the peripartum period (AAP, 1997; Maccato, 1993). As a result, clinicians have been faced with the challenge of developing strategies to prevent neonatal infections in this population of women. Previously, weekly HSV cultures beginning at 34 to 36 weeks gestation in women with a history of recurrent genital HSV were recommended as a means of screening for asymptomatic HSV shedding near term. However, it has been documented that this practice does not predict whether asymptomatic reactivation of HSV infection will occur at the time of delivery (Arvin et al., 1986). Additionally, it was determined that many women were undergoing cesarean sections, with the associated morbidity and mortality, for questionable benefits. Therefore, it is now recommended that weekly antepartum cultures of patients with a history of recurrent HSV infection be discontinued and that the method of delivery for these patients be determined by the presence or absence of suspicious genital lesions at the time of labor (American College of Obstetricians and Gynecologists [ACOG], 1988; U.S. Preventive Services Task Force, 1996). Cesarean sections should be performed when women in labor present with suspicious genital lesions. However, women without symptoms of HSV infection (i.e., prodromal symptoms) or suspicious lesions may attempt a vaginal delivery (ACOG, 1988; CDC, 1993; Maslow & Bobitt, 1988; Gibbs & Sweet, 1994).

Although weekly HSV cultures from pregnant women with a history of HSV are no longer recommended, HSV cultures should be obtained from women who have suspicious lesions at the time of labor and delivery, and their infants. This may be an important means of identifying infants who have been exposed to HSV during the intrapartum period. Documentation of a positive culture result will definitively diagnose neonatal herpes infection and may expedite the initiation of antiviral therapy in infants affected by this disease.

The use of antiviral agents, specifically acyclovir, is recommended for pregnant women experiencing severe first-episode primary HSV infection or for those with disseminated disease (ACOG, 1988). Furthermore, it has been documented that this agent prophylactically suppresses recurrent episodes of genital HSV after a primary episode during pregnancy, preventing the need for surgical intervention in women (i.e., cesarean section delivery) and HSV infection in neonates (Frenkel et al., 1991; Scott, Sanchez, Jackson, Zeray, & Wendel, 1996). In one study, prophylactic acyclovir did not increase asymptomatic viral shedding in the women or demonstrate adverse effects on the fetus/neonate (Scott et al., 1996). Similar studies are under way and may provide additional information regarding options for prophylactic treatment of HSV in pregnant women.

Database

Subjective

- With first-episode primary infection women may report the following (Murphy, 1995):
  - ▶ Exposure to an infected person
  - ▶ Systemic symptoms associated with viremia
    - – Elevated temperature
    - – Chills
    - – Headache
    - – Myalgia
    - – Malaise
    - – Generalized lymphadenopathy
  - ▶ Itching, tingling and/or burning at the site of the infection
  - ▶ Painful genital lesions including erythematous papules, vesicles, ulcerations, and/or pustules with crusts
  - ▶ Inguinal lymphadenopathy
  - ▶ Dyspareunia
  - ▶ Leukorrhea
  - ▶ Dysuria, urinary retention
  - ▶ Rectal pain/discomfort (if anal or perianal lesions)
  - ▶ Symptoms usually resolve within 2 to 4 weeks

  NOTE: Approximately 32 percent of women have acquired HSV asymptomatically (Frenkel et al., 1993).

- With first-episode non-primary or recurrent infection women may report the following (Murphy, 1995):
  - ▶ History of previous episode(s)
  - ▶ Hyperesthesia of the area where the lesion(s) will develop
  - ▶ Itching and/or burning of the affected site
  - ▶ Painful genital, anal, perianal, buttock, or thigh lesion(s)
  - ▶ Leukorrhea

▶ Dysuria, urinary retention

▶ Dyspareunia

▶ Symptoms resolve within 7 days

NOTE: Asymptomatic viral shedding by pregnant patients with recurrent genital HSV-2 infections has been observed to be between 3 to 15 percent (CDC, 1998; Osborne & Adelson, 1990; Stagno & Whitley, 1985).

Objective (Murphy, 1995)

● Elevated temperature (primary HSV-2)

● Inguinal and generalized lymphadenopathy (primary HSV-2)

● Splenomegaly (primary HSV-2)

● Hepatomegaly (primary HSV-2)

● Painful lesions of the vulva, vagina, perianal area, buttocks, and/or thighs (may be papules, vesicles, ulcerations, pustules or crusts)

● Vaginal lesion(s) may resemble mucous patches, bleeding lesions with central necrosis and elevated borders, or ulcers

● Cervical involvement may be observed resembling generalized cervicitis (e.g., erythema, cervical discharge), superficial ulcerations, or a necrotic mass (less common)

● Atypical lymphocytosis (primary HSV-2)

● Altered fetal growth by fundal measurements and obstetrical ultrasound (intrauterine growth restriction [IUGR]) can occur in pregnant women with primary HSV infections; see Chapter 6.15, *Intrauterine Growth Restriction*).

● Giant multinucleated cells with inclusion bodies in Pap smear of vesicular fluid may be revealed (indicates a viral infection but is not *diagnostic* of HSV).

● Elevation in serologic study titers (not specific for genital infections).

● HSV culture of the base of the lesion or cervix may be positive (diagnostic of HSV infection or shedding).

● Syphilis serology (i.e., RPR, VDRL) and gonorrhea (GC) and chlamydia (CT) testing (may be positive if concomitant infection)

Assessment

● Genital HSV infection (either primary, first episode nonprimary, or recurrent)

▶ R/O disseminated HSV infection

▶ R/O herpes zoster

▶ R/O allergic reaction

▶ R/O other sexually transmitted diseases (STDs) (e.g., chancroid, syphilis, human immunodeficiency virus [HIV] infection)

▶ R/O other causes of cervicitis (e.g., other STDs, carcinoma)

▶ R/O urinary tract infection (UTI)

Plan

Diagnostic Tests

● HSV culture of suspicious lesions

▶ A positive result is definitive of HSV infection and can distinguish between HSV-1 and HSV-2

▶ However, a negative culture does not eliminate the possibility of HSV infection (Roussis, Campbell, & Cox, 1994).

NOTE: The success of obtaining an accurate HSV culture result is directly related to the technique used to obtain the specimen. Use cotton- or dacron-tipped swabs to obtain the sample from the base of the lesion(s) to maximize the viral burden. Do not use calcium alginate swabs since use of these swabs may inactivate HSV. As soon as possible, place the sample in the culture medium and send it to the laboratory for processing. Results from a culture will be available in 1 to 3 days (AAP, 1997; Maccato, 1993).

● Pap smear

▶ Test may reveal giant multinucleated cells with inclusion bodies suggesting HSV infection.

▶ The Pap smear has a low sensitivity for HSV (Hensleigh, 1994; Maccato, 1993).

● Tzanck smear

▶ Test may reveal cellular changes associated with HSV infection.

▶ However, the test has a low sensitivity for HSV and cannot differentiate between HSV-1, HSV-2, or varicella zoster virus (Hensleigh, 1994; Maccato, 1993).

● HSV serology tests (i.e., IgM, IgG titers)

▶ Serology tests can be ordered to document seroconversion after a primary infection and as a possible screening test for evidence of past infection.

▶ A fourfold increase or greater in acute and convalescent IgG antibody titers indicates seroconversion

NOTE: Most commercial assays cannot distinguish between HSV-1 and HSV-2 types.

▶ Current research methods involve the use of Western blot or immunoassays that can detect the HSV-2 glycoprotein G (gG) and differentiate between HSV-1 and HSV-2. These methods are not currently available outside of research settings (Hensleigh, 1994).

● HSV antigen testing

▶ Rapid assay tests for the detection of HSV antigens are being evaluated in research settings and have reportedly been sensitive and specific when lesions are present. However, these tests have not proven to be as effective in the detection of asymptomatic shedding (Hensleigh, 1994).

- DNA hybridization (e.g., polymerase chain reaction)
  - ▶ These methods are currently being used in research settings for diagnostic purposes (AAP, 1997; Maccato, 1993).
- Syphilis serology (e.g., RPR or VDRL)
  - ▶ These tests may be reactive if coexistent syphilis infection is present.
- Cervical tests for *N. gonorrhoeae* and *C. trachomatis*
  - ▶ Cultures may be positive if coexistent gonococcal or chlamydial cervicitis
- Obstetrical ultrasound
  - ▶ Ultrasound may reveal IUGR, which may occur with disseminated primary HSV infection.

Treatment/Management

- There is no cure for HSV infection.
- Consider initiation of acyclovir for the treatment of acute HSV infection since this therapy may decrease the severity and duration of the episode.
  - ▶ The recommended dose is (CDC, 1998)
    - – Acyclovir 200 mg p.o. five times a day for 5 days

      OR
    - – Acyclovir 400 mg p.o. t.i.d. for 5 days

      OR
    - – Acyclovir 800 mg p.o. b.i.d. for 5 days
  - ▶ Once the acute episode has resolved, consider chronic suppressive therapy, especially after 36 weeks' gestation, as a means of preventing lesions at the time of labor and, thus, the need for a cesarean section (Frenkel et al., 1993; Scott et al., 1996).
    - – However, this approach is still regarded as experimental by some authorities (Mann & Grossman III, 1996).
    - – The recommended dose for HSV prophylaxis is acyclovir 400 mg p.o. b.i.d (CDC, 1998).

  NOTE: As of this writing, the use of acyclovir during pregnancy has not been associated with an increased incidence of congenital anomalies or a clustering of anomalies (Briggs, Freeman, & Yaffe, 1994; CDC, 1998). Women who receive acyclovir during pregnancy should be registered in the Acyclovir Registry. The registry collects anonymous information about the incidence of congenital anomalies observed in infants born to women receiving acyclovir during pregnancy. Women can be registered by calling 1 (800) 722-9292, extension 39437.

  - ▶ Women with disseminated HSV infection require hospitalization and intravenous administration of acyclovir. Refer them to an obstetrician or perinatologist for evaluation and treatment.

- HSV lesions should be kept dry and clean. The use of topical therapies (e.g., compresses of cold milk, colloidal oatmeal, or Domeboro solution) may be beneficial and should be applied to the lesions every 2 to 4 hours.

- Symptomatic relief measures may include the following:
  - ▶ Acetaminophen 650 mg p.o. every 4 hours for fever and pain relief
  - ▶ Topical xylocaine may be applied to site of lesions for local pain relief
- If no genital lesions are present and the woman is not reporting symptoms associated with HSV prodrome at the time of labor, a vaginal delivery may be attempted.
- A cesarean section is indicated if HSV lesions are present or the women reports symptoms associated with HSV prodrome at the time of labor.
  - ▶ A culture should be taken of any suspicious lesions when the woman is examined.
  - ▶ Cultures of the infant should also be obtained to rule out HSV infection.
- Breastfeeding is not contraindicated unless there are lesions present on the breast (AAP, 1997).

Consultation

- Consult with a physician (required) if a pregnant woman experiences primary HSV infection whether or not she exhibits signs and symptoms of disseminated disease.
- Refer women experiencing primary HSV infection to a genetics counselor for a discussion about perinatal complications associated with congenital HSV infection.

Patient Education

- Educate the woman about HSV infection and the plan of care specific to her clinical situation (e.g., diagnostic tests, symptomatic treatment, risk of neonatal infection, perinatal/neonatal clinical care).
- Teach symptomatic treatment of HSV lesions.
- Teach/review perineal hygiene and proper handwashing technique. Educate the woman about the possibility of autoinoculation and the need for proper hygiene to prevent this from occurring.
- Discuss ways to reduce factors that may stimulate an HSV outbreak including fatigue, stress, poor nutrition, irritation/friction, intercourse, and excessive exposure to sun or heat.
- Educate the patient about the importance of abstaining from oral/genital sexual contact when she is experiencing HSV prodromal symptoms and during active infections. Advise the use of condoms to prevent transmission of HSV and other sexually transmitted diseases. Discuss HIV infection and offer testing as indicated.
- Explain the importance of immediately going to the hospital if she thinks she is in labor or may have experienced rupture of membranes.
- Educate the woman and family members or friends about the importance of handwashing before touching the infant.
  - ▶ Educate the woman and any family member who may have oral HSV infection about the need to prevent neonatal contact with any suspicious lesions.
  - ▶ In addition, individuals should be educated to avoid close contact (e.g., kissing, nuzzling) with the infant if they are experiencing symptoms of HSV prodrome.

▶ A mask should be worn if oral HSV lesions or prodromal symptoms are evident (AAP, 1997).

▶ Women with nipple lesions suspicious for HSV should be advised not to breast-feed (AAP, 1997).

- Arrange for the woman and the father of the baby to meet the clinician who will be responsible for their infant's care so they can establish rapport and have the opportunity to have their concerns addressed before delivery.

Follow-up

- Continue routine prenatal follow-up unless complications develop.
- Document history of HSV infection in the woman and management thereof in progress notes and problem list.

References

American Academy of Pediatrics (AAP). (1997). *1994 Red book: Report of the Committee on Infectious Diseases* (24th ed., pp. 266–276). Elk Grove Village, IL: Author.

American College of Obstetricians and Gynecologists (ACOG). (1988). *Perinatal herpes simplex virus infections.* ACOG technical bulletin no. 122. Washington, DC: Author.

Arvin, A.M. (1991). Relationships between maternal immunity to herpes simplex virus and the risk of neonatal herpesvirus infection. *Reviews of Infectious Diseases, 13*(Suppl.), S953–S956.

Arvin, A.M., Hensleigh, P.A., Prober, C.G., Au, D.S., Yasukawa, L.L., Wittek, A.E., Palumbo, P.E., Paryani, S.G., & Yeager, A.S. (1986). Failure of antepartum maternal cultures to predict the infant's risk of exposure to herpes simplex virus at delivery. *New England Journal of Medicine, 315*(13), 796–800.

Briggs, G.G., Freeman, R.K., & Yaffe, S.J. (1994). *Drugs in pregnancy and lactation* (4th ed.). Baltimore, MD: Williams & Wilkins.

Boucher, F.D., Yasukawa, L.L., Bronzan, R.N., Hensleigh, P.A., Arvin, A.M., & Prober, C.G. (1990). A prospective evaluation of primary genital herpes simplex virus type 2 infections acquired during pregnancy. *Pediatric Infectious Disease Journal, 9*(7), 499–504.

Brown, Z.A. (1995). Preventing vertical transmission of herpes simplex. *Contemporary OB/GYN, 40*(7), 27–40.

Brown, Z.A., Berry, S., & Vontver, L.A. (1986). Genital herpes virus infections complicating pregnancy: Natural history and peripartum management. *The Journal of Reproductive Medicine, 31*(5), 420–425.

Brown, Z.A., Vontver, L.A., Benedetti, J., Critchlow, C.W., Sells, C.J., Berry S., & Corey, L. (1987). Effects on infants of a first episode of genital herpes during pregnancy. *New England Journal of Medicine, 317*(20), 1246–1251.

Centers for Disease Control and Prevention (CDC). (1998). 1998 Guidelines for treatment of sexually transmitted diseases. *Morbidity and Mortality Weekly Report, 47*(RR-11), 20–26.

Frenkel, L.M., Brown, Z.A., Bryson, Y.J., Corey, L., Unadkat, J.D., Hensleigh, P.A., Arvin, A.M., Prober, C.G., & Connor, J.D. (1991). Pharmacokinetics of acyclovir in the term human pregnancy and neonate. *American Journal of Obstetrics and Gynecology, 164*(2), 569–576.

Frenkel, L.M., Garratty, E.M., Shen, J.P., Wheeler, N., Clark, O., & Bryson, Y.J. (1993). Clinical reactivation of herpes simplex virus type 2 infection in seropositive pregnant women with no history of genital herpes. *Annals of Internal Medicine, 118*(6), 414–418.

Gibbs, R.S., & Sweet, R.L. (1994). Maternal and fetal infections. In R.K. Creasy & R. Resnik (Eds.), *Maternal-fetal medicine. Principles and practice* (3rd ed., pp. 639–703). Philadelphia, PA: W.B. Saunders.

Hensleigh, P.A. (1994). Herpes in pregnancy—it's especially serious for the neonate. *Contemporary OB/GYN, 39*(10), 25–40.

Hutto, C., Arvin, A., Jacobs, A., Steele, R., Stagno, S., Lyrene, R., Willett, L., Powell, D., Anderson, R., & Werthammer, J. (1987). Intrauterine herpes simplex virus infections. *Journal of Pediatrics, 110*(1), 97–101.

Kalhanjian, J.A., Soroush, V., Au, D.S., Bronzan, R.N., Yasukawa, L.L., Weylman, L.E., Arvin, A.M., & Prober, C.G. (1992). Identification of women at unsuspected risk of primary infection with herpes simplex virus type 2 during pregnancy. *New England Journal of Medicine, 326*(14), 916–920.

Maccato, M. (1993). Herpes in pregnancy. *Clinical Obstetrics and Gynecology, 36(4)*, 869–877.

Mann, M., & Grossman, III, J.H. (1996). Herpes simplex. In J.T. Queenan & J.C. Hobbins (Eds.), *Protocols for high-risk pregnancies* (3rd ed., pp. 336–345). Cambridge, MA: Blackwell Scientific.

Maslow, A.S., & Bobitt, J.R., (1988). Herpes in pregnancy: Exploring clinical options. *Contemporary OB/GYN, 32*(4), 44–61.

Murphy, J.M. (1995). Genital herpes simplex virus. In W.L. Star, L.L. Lommel, & M.T. Shannon (Eds.), *Women's primary health care: Protocols for practice.* Washington, DC: American Nurses Publishing.

Osborne, N.G., & Adelson, M.D. (1990). Herpes simplex and human papilloma genital infections: Controversy over obstetric management. *Clinical Obstetrics and Gynecology, 33*(4), 801–811.

Overall, Jr., J.C. (1994). Herpes simplex virus infection of the fetus and newborn. *Pediatric Annals, 23*(3), 131–136.

Prober, C.G., Hensleigh, P.A., Boucher, F.D., Yasukawa, L.L., Au, D.S., & Arvin, A.M. (1988). Use of routine viral cultures at delivery to identify neonates exposed to herpes simplex virus. *New England Journal of Medicine, 318*(14), 887–891.

Prober, C.G., Sullender, W.M., Yasukawa, L.L., Au, D.S., Yeager, A.S., & Arvin, A.M. (1987). Low risk of herpes simplex virus infection in neonates exposed to the virus at the time of vaginal delivery to mothers with recurrent genital herpes simplex virus infections. *New England Journal of Medicine, 316*(5), 240–244.

Roussis, P., Campbell, B.A., & Cox, S.M. (1994). Viral infections. In G.D. Willett (Ed.), *Laboratory testing in OB/GYN* (pp. 23–30). Boston: Blackwell Scientific Publications.

Scott, L.L., Sanchez, P.J., Jackson, G.L., Zeray, F., & Wendel, Jr., G.D. (1996). Acyclovir suppression to prevent cesarean delivery after first-episode genital herpes. *Obstetrics and Gynecology, 87*(1), 69–73.

Stagno, S., & Whitley, R.J. (1985). Herpes virus infections of pregnancy. *New England Journal of Medicine, 313*(21), 1327–1330.

U.S. Preventative Services Task Force (1996). *Guide to clinical preventive services* (2nd ed., pp. 335–345). Alexandria, VA: International Medical Publishing, Inc.

Chapter 4

GONORRHEA

Winifred L. Star

Gonorrhea (also known as GC), caused by *Neisseria gonorrhoeae*, a gram-negative diplococcus, the most commonly reported communicable disease. Since 1975, the overall incidence of reported gonorrhea has decreased steadily in the United States; however, among developed countries, the United States has the highest gonorrhea rates, with an estimated 600,000 new infections occurring annually. Over 60 percent of gonococcal infections occur in persons under age 25, with female adolescents ages 15 to 19 having the highest rates (Centers for Disease Control and Prevention [CDC], 1995a, 1995b, 1998; U.S. Preventive Services Task Force, 1996). Gonococcal infection may be asymptomatic or may cause urethritis, cervicitis, proctitis, pharyngitis, Bartholinitis, conjunctivitis, pelvic inflammatory disease (PID), or disseminated infection (Hook III & Handsfield, 1990).

The majority of cases of gonorrhea occur as a result of sexual transmission. The incubation period is usually 2 to 7 days. Females are at greater risk of infection than males because of retention of infected ejaculate within the vagina (Hook III & Handsfield, 1990). After a single sexual encounter, the risk of transmission from an infected male to an exposed female is estimated to be 50 to 90 percent; risk to a male from an infected female is 20 to 25 percent (Sweet & Gibbs, 1995). Of patients with gonorrhea, coinfection with *Chlamydia trachomatis* occurs in 20 to 50 percent of women and 15 to 35 percent of men (Gibbs & Sweet, 1994; Stamm & Holmes, 1990). The major sequelae of gonococcal infection in nonpregnant women is acute salpingitis or PID, which increases risk for tubal infertility and ectopic pregnancy. Infection with gonorrhea (as well other inflammatory or ulcerative sexually transmitted diseases [STDs]) may facilitate human immunodeficiency virus (HIV) transmission (Wasserheit, 1992).

The incidence of gonorrhea in pregnancy has been reported to be between 0.5 and 7 percent (Gibbs & Sweet, 1994). In early pregnancy, women with untreated gonococcal infections are at risk for spontaneous septic abortion; endometritis after an elective abortion or chorionic villus sampling procedure may also occur (Morales, 1992; Wendel, 1990). Acute salpingitis is rare during pregnancy but is associated with substantial fetal wastage (usually during the first trimester). In addition, tubo-ovarian abscess may occur as result of reactivation of prior salpingitis (Morales, 1992; Roberts, 1992). Perinatal complications of gonococcal infection may include premature rupture of membranes (PROM), preterm delivery, intrauterine growth restriction (IUGR), chorioamnionitis, and postpartum endometritis or sepsis (Gibbs & Sweet, 1994). Vertical transmission of gonorrhea to the neonate results in conjunctivitis in 30 to 40 percent of cases (Morales, 1992). Another form of gonococcal infection in pregnancy, the amniotic infection syndrome, may manifest as placental, fetal membrane, and umbilical cord inflammation occurring after premature rupture of membranes and is associated with infected oral or gastric aspirate, leukocytosis, neonatal infection, and maternal fever (Gibbs & Sweet, 1994).

The most common clinical presentation of gonorrhea in pregnancy is disseminated gonococcal infection (DGI). DGI occurs in 0.5 to 3 percent of all patients and can be mild or lead to chronic disability or death (Wilson, 1988). Risk for disseminated infection increases in the second and third trimesters. Two stages of DGI are recognized. The first is an early bacteremic phase characterized by chills, fever, and skin lesions. The second stage is heralded by septic arthritis with characteristic synovial effusions, most commonly of the knees, ankles, and wrists (Gibbs & Sweet, 1994). Bacteremia associated with disseminated infection may occasionally lead to perihepatitis and rarely to endocarditis, pericarditis, or meningitis (CDC 1998, Morales, 1992).

Neonatal complications of maternal gonococcal infection include ophthalmia neonatorum, plus a variety of other syndromes: systemic gonococcal disease, localized mucosal disease, neonatal sepsis and abscess formation (Gutman, 1995). Thirty to 50 percent of infants exposed to gonococci will develop ophthalmia; if left untreated corneal scarring, abscess, eye perforation, and permanent blindness may result (O'Hara, 1993) Routine ocular prophylaxis in the newborn period has significantly reduced ophthalmic complications. Septic arthritis is the most common manifestation of systemic infection and usually occurs from 1 to 4 weeks after delivery; natural history of this condition is uncertain. Localized mucosal infection may present as vaginitis, rhinitis, urethritis, funisitis, and anorectal infection. Abscesses (scalp, gingiva, umbilical stump) and neonatal sepsis have been directly or indirectly related to maternal *N. gonorrhoeae* infection (Gutman, 1995). Gonococcal infection in children beyond the newborn period is a strong indicator of sexual abuse; thus, all cases must be carefully investigated.

Antibiotic Resistance

In recent years treatment for gonorrhea has been complicated by antibiotic-resistant strains. Resistance can be of two types: 1) plasmid-mediated resistances to penicillin, tetracycline, and fluroquinolones and 2) chromosomally mediated resistance to *N. gonorrhoeae* (CMRNG). Strains with resistance to penicillin (penicillinase-producing *N. gonorrhoeae* [PPNG], also called beta-lactamase-producing *N. gonorrhoeae*) are gonococcal strains that have acquired an extra chromosomal element that encodes for beta-lactamase, an enzyme that destroys the beta-lactam ring of penicillin (CDC, 1987, 1991a). Cases of PPNG have been reported in most states. Strains with tetracycline resistance are called TRNG; strains with resistance to both penicillin and tetracycline are called PPNG/TRNG. It is now estimated that 32 percent of gonococcal isolates in the United States are penicillin or tetracycline resistant (Gorwitz, Nakashima, & Moran, 1993). Quinolone-resistant *N. gonorrhoeae* (QRNG) has been reported sporadically from many parts of the world; however, it is still rare in the United States. Provided the QRNG strains comprise less than 1 percent of all *N. gonorrhoeae* strains isolated, fluroquinolone regimens can be used with confidence (although this class of drug is contraindicated in pregnancy) (CDC, 1998). CMRNG can include resistance to penicillin, tetracycline, spectinomycin, cefoxitin, and related antimicrobials. Ten to 15 percent of all gonococci in this country have chromosomally mediated resistance (Zenilman, 1993).

Database

Subjective

Risk factors

- Young age

- Early onset of sexual activity

- Unmarried

- Black or other minority race

- Urban residence or residence in communities with high prevalences of STDs (GC rates highest in rural Southeast)

- Lower socioeconomic status

- Illicit drug use

- Trading sex for drugs or money
- Prostitution
- New, multiple sexual partner(s)
- Partner with STD
- Prior history of gonorrhea, other STD
- Concomitant STD
- Exposure to core group transmitters (i.e., persons with repeated gonorrhea episodes, those engaging in high-risk behaviors and having sex despite symptoms)
- Limited access to health care
- History of PID
- Non-use of barrier contraception
- Cervical eversion
- Oral contraceptives (due to influence on cervical eversion)
- Deficiency in complement components C5, C6, C7, C8 (risk for recurrent DGI)

Symptomatology

- Client may be asymptomatic (up to 80 percent of women) or may complain of the following:
  - ▶ Copious, purulent discharge from eye (in gonococcal conjunctivitis, rare in adults; usually due to autoinoculation from anogenital infection)
  - ▶ Sore throat (in pharyngeal gonorrhea, more prevalent in pregnant women; usually coexists with infection at another site)
  - ▶ Lymph node swelling (cervical, inguinal area)
  - ▶ Vulvar pruritus, irritation; swelling of labia
  - ▶ Abnormal vaginal discharge (with or without odor)
  - ▶ Abnormal menstrual cycles; intermenstrual spotting or bleeding, postcoital bleeding
  - ▶ Urinary urgency, frequency, dysuria
  - ▶ Dyspareunia
  - ▶ History of dysmenorrhea
  - ▶ Lower abdominal/pelvic pain or low backache
  - ▶ Anal irritation, pruritus; rectal fullness, pressure, burning, stinging pain, tenesmus, constipation
  - ▶ Mucopurulent rectal discharge, hematochezia

  NOTE: Rectal mucosa is infected in 35 to 50 percent of women with GC cervicitis usually due to perineal contamination with cervicovaginal exudate; the rectum is the sole site of infection in 5 percent of women with GC, but patients are usually asymptomatic (Hook III & Handsfield, 1990, Wexner, 1990).

- Clients with DGI may complain of
  - ▶ Joint pain in single or multiple joints (most commonly wrists, knees, small joints of hands, or ankles)
  - ▶ Skin lesions, predominantly on extremities (Handsfield & Pollock, 1990)
- Women with PID may present with fever, chills, malaise, nausea, vomiting, abdominal/pelvic pain.

  NOTE: PID is uncommon in pregnancy especially after 12 weeks' gestation.

- Client may report that partner(s) have symptoms of urethral/rectal discharge, dysuria, frequency, redness of urethral meatus, epididymal pain/swelling, lower abdominal pain, rectal pain, tenesmus, pus/blood in stool.

History

- Obtain complete health history:
  - ▶ Menstruation
  - ▶ Past STDs of client and partner
  - ▶ Sexual orientation/practices
    - – Date(s) of last sexual contact(s)
    - – Number of partners in past 3 months
  - ▶ Presence of signs, symptoms of STD in client and partner(s)
  - ▶ Client and/or partner(s) drug injection activities
  - ▶ Obstetrical
  - ▶ Gynecological
  - ▶ Medical (including medication and allergies)
  - ▶ Habits
  - ▶ Psychosocial

Objective

- A *thorough* STD examination includes the following assessments (CDC, 1991):
  - ▶ Vital signs, as indicated
  - ▶ General skin inspection of face, trunk, forearms, palms, and soles for lesions, rashes, or discoloration
  - ▶ Inspection of pharynx/oral cavity for erythema, injection, lesions, or discoloration
  - ▶ Abdominal inspection and palpation for masses, tenderness, or rebound tenderness
  - ▶ Inspection of pubic hair for lice and nits
  - ▶ Inspection of external genitalia for discharge, masses, or lesions; inspection and palpation of Bartholin's, urethral, and Skene's (BUS) glands for discharge, or masses

▶ Inspection of vagina for blood, discharge, or lesions

▶ Inspection of cervix for lesions, discharge, eversion, erythema, edema, or friability; assessment for cervical motion tenderness

▶ Uterine assessment for size, shape, consistency, mobility, and tenderness.

▶ Palpation of adnexa for masses, or tenderness

▶ Inspection of perianus, anus, and rectum for lesions, bleeding, or discharge

▶ Rectal exam, as indicated

▶ Assessment for presence or absence of associated cervical or inguinal lymphadenopathy

● Physical examination of the patient with gonorrhea may be within normal limits (WNL). Assessments/findings may include

▶ Vital signs (elevated temperature in PID and DGI)

▶ Eyes (copious, purulent discharge; red conjunctiva with edema; possible keratitis, corneal ulceration [in gonococcal conjunctivitis])

▶ Pharynx (may be injected; cervical lymphadenopathy may be present in pharyngeal gonorrhea)

▶ Lymph nodes (cervical lymphadenopathy may be present [in pharyngeal gonorrhea]; inguinal lymphadenopathy may also be present)

▶ Skin (assess volar aspect of arms, hands, and fingers for cutaneous manifestations of DGI)

  – A classic lesion will be a tender, necrotic pustule on an erythematous base.

  – Lesions may also present as macules, papules, pustules, bullae, or ecchymoses.

  – Lesions are usually 1 to 2 mm (to 1 cm) in diameter, generally on distal portion of extremity, with an average of five to thirty lesions (Hook III & Handsfield, 1990).

▶ Extremities (assess hands, wrists, knees, and ankles for manifestations of DGI)

  – Tenderness, swelling, erythema, joint effusion

  – Pus may be aspirated from affected joints

▶ Abdomen (assess for masses, tenderness and/or rebound tenderness; assess for inguinal adenopathy)

▶ Genitalia and pelvis

  – BUS glands (purulent or mucoid exudate may be expressed from ducts; swelling or abscess formation may be present)

  – External genitalia (erythema, edema, abnormal discharge, or excoriation may be present)

  – Vagina (mucopurulent discharge or blood may be present)

  – Cervix (mucopurulent discharge and edema, erythema, friability in zone of eversion may be present; for so-called mucopurulent cervicitis or MPC, see below; assess for cervical motion tenderness [CMT])

  – Uterus (assess size, shape, consistency, mobility, and presence of tenderness)

  – Adnexa (assess for presence of masses, and/or tenderness)

    – Anus and rectum (assess for erythema or mucopurulent discharge and, on endoscopic rectal examination, friability, erythema, mucoid/purulent discharge, and ulceration

    NOTE: Anoscopy is not usually performed unless symptoms of proctitis are present.

- Mucopurulent cervicitis, if present, may be caused by gonococcal or chlamydial infection; however, in most cases neither organism can be isolated. Criteria for presumptive diagnosis includes the following:

  ▶ Mucopurulent or purulent exudate visible in the endocervical canal or on an endocervical swab specimen

  ▶ Easily induced cervical bleeding

  ▶ Increased number of polymorphonuclear leukocytes (PMNs) on endocervical Gram-stain (low positive predictive value) (CDC, 1998)

Assessment

- Gonorrhea (indicate site of infection)

  ▶ R/O gonorrhea

  ▶ R/O DGI

  NOTE: DGI must be distinguished from other polyarticular dermatitis-tenosynovitis syndromes and the monarticular arthritides (e.g., Reiter's syndrome, meningococcemia, acute rheumatoid arthritis, other septic arthritides, immune-complex arthritides caused by hepatitis B or HIV, and Lyme disease) (Knapp & Thompson, 1990).

  ▶ R/O *Chlamydia trachomatis* infection

  ▶ R/O herpes simplex virus infection

  ▶ R/O syphilis

  ▶ R/O vaginitis (i.e., trichomoniasis, bacterial vaginosis, candidiasis)

  ▶ R/O MPC due to nonmicrobiologic determinant (e.g., inflammation in an ectropion)

  ▶ R/O gonococcal conjunctivitis

  ▶ R/O gonococcal, group A beta-hemolytic streptococcal pharyngitis

  ▶ R/O urinary tract infection (UTI)

  ▶ R/O urethral syndrome

  ▶ R/O PID

  ▶ R/O Tubo-ovarian abscess

  ▶ R/O Adnexal torsion

  ▶ R/O Appendicitis

  ▶ R/O Ectopic pregnancy

  ▶ R/O Septic abortion

  ▶ R/O Squamous intraepithelial neoplasia (SIL)

▶ R/O Endocarditis, meningitis

▶ R/O HIV infection

Plan

Diagnostic Tests

● Laboratory diagnosis is mandatory.

▶ Direct culture from the site(s) of exposure is the most sensitive and specific test for detecting gonococcal infection in asymptomatic persons (U.S. Preventive Services Task Force, 1996).

▶ For screening during pregnancy, samples are generally obtained from the endocervix, but additional potential sites of infection should be cultured, as indicated (e.g., conjunctiva, pharynx, urethra, rectum, accessory gland ducts, synovia). See Table 14.2, 1, Directions for Obtaining GC or CT Samples from Selected Sites of Infection.

● Nonculture diagnostic tests such as nucleic acid amplification tests and enzyme immunoassays (EIA) are also available.

NOTE: If these tests are used for screening, verification of positive results may be necessary. Nonculture tests do not provide information on antibiotic susceptibility (U.S. Preventive Services Task Force, 1996).

● Gram-stained smear from endocervical secretions may show gram-negative intracellular diplococci.

NOTE: In women, test is only 50 to 70 percent sensitive. A smear should be performed only by trained individuals and must be followed by culture. Gram's stain should not be used for pharyngeal specimens but may be a useful adjunct to culture diagnosis of GC in conjunctiva, skin, or joint fluids.

● In clients with suspected DGI

▶ Obtain cultures from the following sources (Mårdh & Danielsson, 1990):

– Endocervix

– Oropharynx

– Rectum

– Blood

– Joint fluid

– Skin lesions

NOTE: All isolates should be screened for antimicrobial resistance.

▶ Acute and convalescent antibody titers may be obtained.

▶ Synovial fluid leukocyte counts may be obtained (counts may be more than 20,000 to 40,000 WBCs per cubic millimeter).

▶ DGI is diagnosed as follows:

    – Proven DGI—positive cultures from joints, blood, skin lesions

    – Probable DGI—positive cultures from primary mucosal site, negative cultures from blood or other sterile site in client with arthritis, dermatitis syndrome

    – Possible DGI—negative cultures but positive response to treatment in client with an arthritis or dermatitis syndrome (Hook & Handsfield, 1990)

● Perform serological test for syphilis (VDRL or RPR).

● Offer HIV testing (pretest and posttest counseling and informed consent is necessary).

● Other laboratory tests used to aid diagnosis may include (but are not limited to) the following:

▶ Microscopic evaluation of saline wet mount of vaginal discharge (may show excess number of white blood cells [WBCs] per high power field)

▶ Complete blood count (CBC) (leukocytosis may be seen in patients with DGI or PID)

▶ Erythrocyte sedimentation rate (ESR) (may be elevated in PID)

▶ C-reactive protein (may be elevated in PID)

▶ Screening for complement deficiency (may be considered in cases of recurrent systemic gonococcal infection) (Hook III & Handsfield, 1990)

● Additional tests may include Pap smear, urinalysis, urine culture, hepatitis B and C testing.

● Perform additional prenatal laboratory tests per site-specific protocol.

Treatment/Management

General Considerations

● Test pregnant women for gonorrhea at the first prenatal visit based on history, risk factors, and physical examination findings.

▶ Repeat testing in the third trimester of pregnancy for high-risk women (American Academy of Pediatrics [AAP] and American College of Obstetricians and Gynecologists [ACOG], 1998; ACOG, 1994).

    – High-risk groups include young women (age under 25) with two or more sex partners in the last year, persons with history of repeated episodes of gonorrhea, commercial sex workers, and women living in a high-prevalence area for *N. gonorrhoeae*.

    NOTE: Consult with local health authorities, if indicated, to help identify additional high-risk populations (CDC, 1998; U.S. Preventive Services Task Force, 1996).

● Perform a serologic test for syphilis for all women at the first prenatal visit, in the third trimester (i.e., 28 weeks' gestation) if at high risk for STD, and prior to leaving the hospital after delivery. See Chapter 14.6, *Syphilis*.

● Clients with suspected gonorrhea should be tested simultaneously for chlamydia. See also Chapter 14.1, *Chlamydia*.

- Screen all women who present with preterm labor for the presence of gonorrhea and chlamydia (as well as for bacterial vaginosis, trichomoniasis, and group B streptococcus).

- Recognition of the signs and symptoms of endocarditis and meningitis is essential. Prompt referral to a physician is warranted in these cases. Refer clients with ophthalmia for ophthalmologic assessment (including slit-lamp examination).

- Treat HIV-infected persons with the same drug regimens as for those without HIV.

Drug Regimens

Uncomplicated Cervical, Urethral, or Rectal Infection

Recommended Regimens

- Cefixime 400 mg p.o. in a single dose

    OR

- Ceftriaxone 125 mg IM in a single dose

    PLUS

- Erythromycin base 500 mg p.o. q.i.d. for 7 days

    OR

- Amoxicillin 500 mg p.o. t.i.d. for 7 days (to cover coexisting chlamydia) (CDC, 1998).

    ▶ Alternatives to erythromycin (above) include

    – Erythromycin base 250 mg p.o. q.i.d. for 14 days, *or*

    – Erythromycin ethylsuccinate 800 mg p.o. q.i.d. for 7 days, *or*

    – Erythromycin ethylsuccinate 400 mg p.o. q.i.d. for 14 days *or*

    – Azithromycin 1 gram p.o. in a single dose (CDC, 1998)

    NOTE: After administration of IM medication observe all clients for at least 20 to 30 minutes for evidence of untoward drug reaction. Cross-reactivity of third-generation cephalosporins and penicillin in penicillin-allergic individuals is rare. Ceftriaxone should be withheld in persons with a history of anaphylactic or histamine response to penicillin (City and County of San Francisco, Department of Public Health, 1989). Preliminary data indicate azithromycin may be safe and effective in pregnancy; however, data are insufficient to recommend routine use (CDC, 1998). Pregnant women should not be treated with quinolones, doxycycline or tetracycline.

Alternative Regimens

- Ceftizoxime 500 mg IM in a single dose

    OR

- Cefotaxime 500 mg IM in a single dose

    OR

- Cefotetan 1 gram IM in a single dose

  OR

- Cefoxitin 2 grams IM in a single dose *with* probenecid 1 gram p.o. (CDC, 1993).

  NOTE: None of these injectable cephalosporins offers any advantage compared with ceftriaxone and clinical experience with these regimens is limited (CDC, 1998). Alternate regimens should be followed by a regimen to cover presumptive or diagnosed chlamydia.

- For individuals who cannot tolerate a cephalosporin give spectinomycin 2.0 grams IM in a single dose (followed by regimen to cover presumptive or diagnosed chlamydia) (CDC, 1998).

  NOTE: This regimen is *not* reliable for pharyngeal infection.

Pharyngeal Infection

- Ceftriaxone 125 mg IM in single dose (followed by regimen to cover presumptive or diagnosed chlamydia) (CDC, 1998).

  NOTE: Chlamydial coinfection of the pharynx is unusual but coinfection at genital sites can occur; therefore treatment for both GC and chlamydia is suggested (CDC, 1998).

Conjunctivitis

- Ceftriaxone 1 gram IM in a single dose.
- Lavage infected eye with saline solution once (CDC, 1998).

Disseminated Gonococcal Infection (DGI)

- Hospitalization is recommended. Evaluate the patient for evidence of endocarditis and meningitis. Case will be managed by a physician.

Recommended initial drug regimen

- Ceftriaxone 1 gram IM or IV every 24 hours (CDC, 1998).

Alternative Initial Regimens

- Cefotaxime 1 gram IV every 8 hours

  OR

- Ceftizoxime 1 gram IV every 8 hours (CDC, 1998).
- Pregnant patients allergic to beta-lactam drugs should receive spectinomycin 2 grams IM every 12 hours (CDC, 1998).

  NOTE: All regimens are continued for 24 to 48 hours after improvement begins; then therapy may be switched to the following regimen: cefixime 400 mg p.o. b.i.d. for 7 days (CDC, 1998).

- All DGI patients should be treated presumptively for chlamydia unless testing has ruled out this infection. Refer the client's partner for evaluation and treatment (CDC, 1998).

Mucopurulent Cervicitis

- Ideally, treatment is based on laboratory test results. If there is a high likelihood of infection with GC and/or chlamydia or the client is not likely to return for follow-up care, treat empirically for either or both infections (refer to CDC, 1998 for additional information).

Partner Therapy

- Evaluate and treat for both gonorrhea and chlamydia all sexual partners of clients with gonorrhea if their last sexual contact was within 60 days before the onset of the client's symptoms or diagnosis.

- The client's most recent sexual partner should be treated if intercourse was more than 60 days prior to the client's diagnosis or onset of symptoms.

- Regimens include any of the aforementioned recommended or alternative drugs listed under uncomplicated cervical, urethral, or rectal infection, as well as those that follow.

  ▶ Ciprofloxacin 500 mg p.o. in a single dose

  ▶ Ofloxacin 400 mg p.o. in a single dose

  ▶ Enoxacin 400 mg p.o. in a single dose

  ▶ Lomefloxacin 400 mg p.o. in a single dose

  ▶ Norfloxacin 800 mg p.o. in a single dose

  NOTE: Single-dose quinolones appear to be safe and effective but data on their use are limited (CDC, 1998).

- For pharyngeal infection

  ▶ Ceftriaxone 125 mg IM in a single dose

  OR

  ▶ Ciprofloxacin 500 mg in a single dose

  OR

  ▶ Ofloxacin 400 mg p.o. in a single dose

  NOTE: All regimens should include therapy for possible coinfection with chlamydia, such as azithromycin 1 gram p.o. in a single dose *or* doxycycline 100 mg p.o. b.i.d. for 7 days (CDC, 1998).

Consultation

- Physician management is required for patients with PID, DGI, endocarditis, and/or meningitis. Complicated cases should be managed in consultation with an infectious disease expert.

- Consult local health authorities for guidance in identifying groups at high risk for gonorrhea.

- Refer adult clients with ophthalmia for ophthalmologic assessment (including slit-lamp examination).

- Refer to psychosocial support services, if indicated.

Patient Education

- Discuss cause of infection, mode of transmission, incubation period, risk factors, symptoms, potential perinatal and neonatal complications, and treatment modalities. Alert client to possible side effects of medication.

- Stress compliance with treatment regimen and importance of partner evaluation and therapy. Refer partner to STD clinic or other source of health care as indicated.

- Discuss candidiasis prophylaxis, especially for women prone to *Candida* infections secondary to antibiotics.

- Advise abstinence from intercourse until both client and partner have completed therapy and symptoms (if present) have abated. Advise prompt follow-up should signs and symptoms of infection persist or recur.

- Address STD prevention.

  - ▶ Provide guidelines for safer sex practices

  - ▶ Encourage careful "screening" of sex partners and committed use of condoms

  - ▶ Educate regarding signs/symptoms of STDs and advise abstinence from sexual activity if these signs develop.

  NOTE: Clients should be advised to always have condoms (male and/or female) available and use them correctly and consistently, especially if having intercourse with new, multiple, or nonmonogamous partners or partners whose HIV status and risk status are unknown (Woolf, Jonas, & Lawrence, 1996). Ideally, both partners should be tested for STDs (including HIV) before initiating intercourse (CDC, 1998). See Table 14.1, Safer Sex Recommendations, in Chapter 14.1, *Chlamydia*.

- Assist client in understanding how specific sexual behaviors relate to STD acquisition. Advise against use of drugs and alcohol, because these substances impair judgment and may lead to unsafe sex (Woolf at al., 1996). Tailor prevention messages to injection-drug users and/or their sexual partners.

- Allow woman to ventilate her emotions regarding the diagnosis of an STD. Provide literature on STDs as available. See Appendix 14.1a, Patient Education Resources, in Chapter 14.1.

Follow-up

- Perform test-of-cure after treatment is completed.

- If patient reports ongoing or recurring signs/symptoms, inquire about compliance with medication, drug reaction or side effects, partner therapy, sexual exposure and use of condoms, and whether reinfection is likely. Discuss the need for improved compliance with STD prevention measures and partner treatment, as indicated.

- Clients with persistent symptoms should be cultured for *N. gonorrhoeae* with isolates tested for antimicrobial susceptibility. Also, rule out infection with other organisms (e.g., *C. trachomatis*). In addition, perform a wet mount to rule out the presence of vaginitis.

- For clients treated with spectinomycin, perform a pharyngeal culture 3 to 5 days after treatment if pharyngeal infection was suspected or diagnosed.

- Repeat *N. gonorrhoeae* and *C. trachomatis* testing in the third trimester if at risk for STD.

- Perform a serologic test for syphilis at about 28 weeks' gestation and again at delivery

- If initially negative, repeat HBsAg testing in late pregnancy for all high-risk women (e.g., injecting-drug users, women with STDs) (CDC, 1998).

- HIV-testing may be repeated in 3 months.

- Follow up on all positive laboratory tests.

  ▶ Counsel HIV-positive women appropriately and refer them for early intervention services. See Chapter 14.5, *Human Immunodeficiency Virus*, for further information and for additional lab tests that may be necessary.

  ▶ Give hepatitis B antigen-positive women appropriate counseling and advise them of the need for immunoprophylaxis of their offspring, their sex partner(s), and all household members. See Chapter 10.2, *Hepatitis A, B, C, D, and E*, for further information and for additional lab tests that may be ordered.

  ▶ Treat concomitant STDs and other conditions, as indicated.

  ▶ Refer clients with abnormal Pap smears for colposcopy, as indicated. See Chapter 6.1, *Abnormal Cervical Cytology*.

- Ongoing psychosocial support is important for the woman in gaining control over her sexual situation and to enable her to successfully prevent future STDs.

- Address substance abuse issues and other high-risk behaviors. Refer to support services (e.g., public health nursing, drug treatment programs, psychological, social services), as indicated.

- Contraceptive counseling for postpartum women should include strategies to reduce future exposure to STDs.

- For prophylaxis for gonococcal ophthalmia neonatorum, all newborns should receive either 0.5 percent erythromycin or 1 percent tetracycline ophthalmic ointment or 1 percent silver nitrate solution as a single application shortly after birth (may be delayed for up to one hour) without subsequent irrigation. Silver nitrate causes more chemical conjunctivitis but appears to be the best agent in areas with applicable PPNG incidence) (American Academy of Pediatrics, 1997).

  NOTE: Ophthalmic prophylaxis is required by law in most states.

- Infants with evidence of ophthalmia neonatorum, scalp abscess, or disseminated infections should be hospitalized, cultured appropriately, and receive systemic treatment. Details on neonatal drug therapy are beyond the scope of this guideline.

- Cases of gonorrhea must be reported to the local public health department within 7 calendar days of identification.

- Document history of gonorrhea and/or other STDs and treatment thereof in progress notes and problem list. A history of abnormal cervical cytology should also be noted. Behaviors that place the client at high risk for STDs may be noted on the problem list as appropriate.

Table 14.2

Directions for Obtaining GC* or CT* Samples from Selected Sites of Infection

UNIVERSAL PRECAUTIONS SHOULD BE APPLIED WHEN OBTAINING ALL SAMPLES

- **Endocervical sample:** Bacteriostatic lubricant should not be used in the vagina prior to obtaining sample. First, cleanse the cervix of external exudate and/or vaginal secretions. Next, obtain an endocervical specimen with sampling swab inserted 1–2 cm into the endocervical canal and rotate gently for 10–30 seconds; then place in appropriate transport media. Endocervical cells are necessary for chlamydia specimens. (A cytobrush provides an excellent sampling device; swabs with plastic or wire shafts and cotton, rayon, dacron or calcium alginate tips can also be used; chlamydia samples should be obtained after those for gonorrhea.) For nonculture tests, use swab provided and follow manufacturers directions. (When cervical samples are being collected for STD diagnostic purposes they may be obtained prior to the Pap smear if it is also being performed.)

- **Urethral samples (women):** Strip the urethra towards its orifice to express exudate for sample. Alternately, gently insert urogenital swab 1–2 cm into urethra; rotate in one direction for at least one revolution (about 5 seconds). Place in appropriate transport media.

- **Rectal samples:** Blindly pass a sampling swab 2–4 cm into the anal canal using lateral pressure to avoid feces. Allow 15–30 seconds for secretions to absorb. Discard swab with gross fecal contamination; try again. Place in appropriate transport media.

  Direct anoscopy should be employed for sample collection in patients with symptoms of proctitis.

- **Pharynx:** Obtain samples of the throat by swabbing the tonsillar crypts and behind the uvula (posterior pharynx). Place in appropriate transport media.

- **Conjunctiva:** Clear eye of mucus/discharge with sterile cotton ball. Rub sampling device across the conjunctiva, sampling the less affected areas first to reduce further contamination of the eye. Place in appropriate transport media.

- **Joint fluid:** Aspirate fluid from infected joints using sterile needle attached to syringe. Transport to laboratory in capped syringe or place specimen into a sterile tube or blood culture bottle. (Gram stain and culture should be performed.)

- **Skin lesions:** Scrape off skin material with sterile lancet or scalpel and smear specimen onto glass slide. Send to laboratory for examination with fluorescent antibody techniques.

NOTE: When plating GC sample onto culture media, use a "Z" stroke and a "cross-streak" pattern; alternately, place swab into special transport kit provided. Don't use wooden Q-tips for sampling swabs if transporting specimens in nonnutritive media. GC culture plates should be at room temperature at time of inoculation. Within 15 minutes of sample collection, cultures for gonococcal isolation should be placed in a CO_2-enriched atmosphere (e.g., candle-extinction jar or container with CO_2-generating tablet). Specimens should be incubated within 1–2 hours at 35°–37° C. Chlamydia cultures should be refrigerated as soon as possible after collection. For nonculture tests, follow manufacturers instructions. For chlamydia cultures, special transport media must be used and culture temperature/storage requirements are stringent — refer to laboratory.

Isolates from pharynx, eye, or sites other than anogenital area that are presumptively identified as *N. gonorrhoeae* must be definitively identified by additional testing. Positive nonculture chlamydia tests may need to be verified by culture or second nonculture test. Refer to the laboratory for further information on direct fluorescent antibody (DFA) tests, enzyme immunoassay tests (EIA), nucleic acid hybridization tests (DNA probe), rapid chlamydia tests, and leukocyte esterase tests (LET).

*GC = gonorrhea; CT = chlamydia

Sources: "Gonococcal infections in the adult," by E.W. Hook III & H.H. Handsfield, "*Neisseria gonorrhoeae*," by P.-A. Mårdh & D. Danielsson, and "Chlamydia trachomatis", by W.E Stamm & P. -A. Mårdh, 1990, in K.K. Holmes et al. (Eds.), 1990, *Sexually transmitted diseases* (2nd ed., pp. 157–157, 904–906, 919–920). New York: McGraw-Hill; "Laboratory methods," STD Intensive for Clinicians, 1994, San Francisco STD, HIV Prevention Training Center; "Guide for the diagnosis of gonorrhea using culture and gram stain," by the Centers for Disease Control, 1991, Atlanta: CDC; "*Clinicians handbook of preventive services*," 1994, by the U.S. Department of Health and Human Services, Washington, DC: U.S. Government Printing Office; "Recommendations for the prevention and management of Chlamydia trachomatis infection," 1993 by the Centers for Disease Control and Prevention, *MMWR, 42*(RR to 12), p. 1–39.

References

Alexander, L.L. (1992). Sexually transmitted diseases: Perspectives on this growing epidemic. *Nurse Practitioner, 17*(10), 31–42.

American Academy of Pediatrics (AAP). (1997). Antimicrobial prophylaxis. *1997 Red book: Report of the Committee on Infectious Diseases* (24th ed. pp. 212–219, 601–602). Elk Grove Village, IL: Author.

American Academy of Pediatrics (AAP) and American College of Obstetricians and Gynecologists (ACOG). (1997). Guidelines for perinatal care (4th ed; pp. 235–236). Elk Grove Village, IL: Author.

American College of Obstetricians and Gynecologists (ACOG). (1994). *Gonorrhea and chlamydial infections* (Technical Bulletin No. 190). Washington, DC: Author.

Centers for Disease Control and Prevention (CDC). (1985). *Chlamydia trachomatis* infections. Policy guidelines for prevention and control. *Morbidity and Mortality Weekly Report, 34*(Suppl. 3S), 53S–74S.

Centers for Disease Control and Prevention (CDC). (1987). Antibiotic to resistant strains of Neisseria gonorrhoeae. *Morbidity and Mortality Weekly Report, 36*(Suppl. 5S), 1S–18S.

Centers for Disease Control and Prevention (CDC). (1991a). *Guide for the diagnosis of gonorrhea using culture and Gram-stained smear.* Atlanta, GA: Author.

Centers for Disease Control and Prevention (CDC). (1991b). *Sexually transmitted diseases. Clinical practice guidelines.* Atlanta, GA: Author.

Centers for Disease Control and Prevention (CDC). (1998). 1998 sexually transmitted diseases treatment guidelines. *Morbidity and Mortality Weekly Report, 47*(No. RR-1), 52–53, 59–69.

Centers for Disease Control and Prevention (CDC), Division of STD/HIV Prevention. (1995a). *Sexually transmitted disease surveillance, 1994.* Atlanta, GA: Author.

Centers for Disease Control and Prevention (CDC). (1995b). Increasing incidence of gonorrhea. *Morbidity and Mortality Weekly Report, 44*(14), 282–285.

City and County of San Francisco, Department of Public Health. (1989). *Medical Alert—PPNG in San Francisco.* San Francisco: Department of Public Health.

Gibbs, R.S. & Sweet, R. (1994). Clinical disorders. In R. K. Creasy & R. Resnik (Eds.), *Maternal-fetal medicine: Principles and practice* (3rd ed., pp. 678–681). Philadelphia, PA: W.B. Saunders.

Gorwitz, R.J., Nakashima, A.K., & Moran, J.S. (1993). Sentinel surveillance for antimicrobial resistance in *Neisseria gonorrhoeae*—United States, 1988–1991. In: CDC surveillance summaries, August 13, 1993, *Morbidity and Mortality Weekly Report, 42*, 29–39.

Gutman, L.T. (1995). Gonococcal infection. In J.S. Remington & J. O. Klein (Eds.), *Infectious diseases of the fetus and newborn infant* (4th ed., pp. 1087–1104). Philadelphia, PA: W.B. Saunders.

Handsfield, H.H., & Pollock, P. S. (1990). Arthritis associated with sexually transmitted diseases. In K.K. Holmes, P.-A. Mårdh, P.F. Sparling, P.J. Wiesner, W. Cates, Jr., S.M. Lemon, & W.E. Stamm (Eds.), *Sexually transmitted diseases* (2nd ed., pp. 737–751). New York: McGraw–Hill.

Hook III, E.W., & Handsfield, H.H. (1990). Gonococcal infections in the adult. In K.K. Holmes, P.-A. Mårdh, P.F. Sparling, P.J. Wiesner, W. Cates, Jr., S.M. Lemon, & W.E. Stamm (Eds.), *Sexually transmitted diseases* (2nd ed., pp. 149–165). New York: McGraw–Hill.

Knapp, J.S., & Thompson, S.E. (1990). Gonorrhea. Reprinted by the U.S. Department of Health and Human Services. Public Health Service. Centers for Disease Control from *Atlas of Sexually Transmitted Diseases* (pp. 5.1–5.22).

Mårdh, P-A., & Danielsson, D. (1990). *Neisseria gonorrhoeae*. In K. K. Holmes, P.-A. Mårdh, P.F. Sparling, P.J. Wiesner, W. Cates, Jr., S.M. Lemon, & W.E. Stamm (Eds.), *Sexually transmitted diseases* (2nd ed., pp. 903–916). New York: McGraw–Hill.

Morales, W.J. (1992). Gonococcal infections in pregnancy. *Contemporary OB, GYN, 27*(7), 92–96.

O'Hara, M.A. (1993). Ophthalmia neonatorum. *Pediatric Clinics of North America, 40*, 715–725.

Roberts, R. (1992). Sexually transmitted diseases in pregnancy. *British Journal of Hospital Medicine, 47*(9), 674–679.

San Francisco STD/HIV Prevention Training Center. (1994). *Laboratory methods*. STD Intensive for Clinicians, November 11–14, 1994. San Francisco, CA.

Stamm, W.E., & Holmes, K.K. (1990). *Chlamydia trachomatis* infections of the adult. In K.K. Holmes, P.-A. Mårdh, P.F. Sparling, P. J. Wiesner, W. Cates, Jr., S.M. Lemon, & W.E. Stamm (Eds.), *Sexually transmitted diseases* (2nd ed., pp. 181–193). New York: McGraw–Hill.

Star, W.L. (1995). Gonorrhea. In W.L. Star, L L. Lommel, & M.T. Shannon (Eds.), *Women's primary health care: Protocols for practice* (pp. 13–17, 13–25). Washington, DC: American Nurses.

Sweet, R.L., & Gibbs, R.S. (1995). *Infectious diseases of the female genital tract* (3rd ed., pp. 134–146). Baltimore, MD: Williams & Wilkins.

U. S. Department of Health and Human Services. (1994). *Clinician's handbook of preventive services*. Washington, DC: U. S. Government Printing Office.

U. S. Preventive Services Task Force. (1996). Screening for gonorrhea – including ocular prophylaxis in newborns. *Guide to clinical preventive services. Report of the U. S. Preventive Services Task Force* (2nd ed., pp. 293–302). Baltimore, MD: Williams & Wilkins.

Wasserheit, J.N. (1992). Epidemiological synergy: interrelationships between human immunodeficiency virus infection and other sexually transmitted diseases. *Sexually transmitted diseases, 19*(2), 61–77.

Wendel, G.D., JR. (1990). Sexually transmitted diseases in pregnancy. *Seminars in Perinatology, 14*(2), 171–178.

Wexner, S.D. (1990). Sexually transmitted diseases, of the colon, rectum, and anus. *Sexually Transmitted Diseases, 32*(12), 1048–1062.

Wilson, D. (1998). An overview of sexually transmissible diseases in the perinatal period. *Journal of Nurse-Midwifery, 33*(33), 115–128.

Woolf, S.H., Jonas, S., & Lawrence, R.S. (1996). *Health promotion and disease prevention in clinical practice*. Baltimore, MD: Williams & Wilkins.

Zenilman, J.M. (1993). Gonorrhea: Clinical and public health issues. *Hospital Practice, 28*(2A), 29–50.

Chapter 5

HUMAN IMMUNODEFICIENCY VIRUS

Maureen T. Shannon

In 1981, the first cases of acquired immunodeficiency syndrome (AIDS) in the United States were reported to the Centers for Disease Control and Prevention (CDC, 1981). During the early years of this epidemic, the actual pathogen responsible for the disease was unknown. In 1983 the human immunodeficiency virus (HIV) was discovered. Within 2 years of the identification of HIV, antibody testing was developed to screen for this infection. Several studies investigating HIV transmission have documented that HIV can be transmitted through contact with infected bodily secretions or tissues, through sharing of contaminated needles, or from an infected woman to her fetus/neonate during pregnancy, labor and delivery, or through breast-feeding (CDC, 1982; Des Jarlais & Friedman, 1988; European Collaborative Study, 1988; Padian et al., 1987).

As of June 1997, 612,078 cases of AIDS have been reported in the United States (CDC, 1997a). Of these, 92,242 cases (15 percent) are women. However, 20 percent of the AIDS cases reported between July 1996 and June 1997 occurred in women (CDC, 1997b). Analysis of risk factors reported in women diagnosed with AIDS between July 1996 and June 1997 reveals that 33 percent had a history of injection drug use (IDU), 40 percent had heterosexual contact with a person at risk for HIV infection (31 percent of these partners had a history of IDU), 2 percent received a blood transfusion/product, and 25 percent did not report or identify a risk factor. Of women under the age of 25 with an AIDS diagnosis reported during this time, 54 percent reported acquiring HIV through heterosexual contact compared to 29 percent reporting a history of IDU (CDC, 1997a). This observed trend in heterosexual transmission of HIV is projected to continue (CDC, 1995a).

AIDS is the third leading cause of death for women between the ages of 25 and 44 and the leading cause of death for black women in this age group. Women of color continue to be disproportionately represented in this epidemic, with black and Hispanic women accounting for 75 percent of reported AIDS cases in women. In 1994, the death rate attributed to HIV infection in black women between 25 and 44 years of age surpassed that of white men in the same age group (CDC, 1995a; Gwinn & Wortley, 1996). Furthermore, during 1996, a significant decline in AIDS-associated deaths was observed in white males in the United States, while the AIDS mortality rate in women increased by 3 percent (CDC, 1997b).

Seroprevalence estimates indicate that approximately one million individuals in the United States are infected with HIV. Included in this estimate are 80,000 women of reproductive age (Gwinn & Wortley, 1996; Minkoff, 1991). Anonymous seroprevalence studies of neonates have revealed that between 6,500 to 7,000 HIV-infected women give birth annually in the U.S with the highest number of cases reported in New York, New Jersey, Florida, California and Texas (Gwinn & Wortley, 1996). Of infants born to these women, approximately 25 percent will be infected as a result of perinatal exposure to HIV (Smith & Rogers, 1996). Currently in the United States, an estimated 20,000 children are HIV infected; 7,902 children (less than 13 years of age) have been diagnosed with AIDS. Perinatal transmission of HIV is responsible for more than 90 percent of pediatric AIDS cases in the United States (CDC, 1997a).

A woman can transmit HIV to her infant during pregnancy, labor and delivery, and through breast-feeding (Cotton & Watts, 1995; European Collaborative Study, 1992; Goedert, Duliege, Amos,

Felton, & Biggar, 1991; Minkoff, 1995; Orloff, Simonds, Steketee, & St. Louis, 1996; Peckham & Gibbs, 1995). The exact mechanisms by which HIV is transmitted perinatally are unknown; however, it is theorized that more than 50 percent of transmission occurs during the peripartum period. Various studies have reported a number of factors associated with increased perinatal transmission rates including high maternal viral load, low maternal CD4 cell counts, increased maternal CD8 cell counts, duration of rupture of membranes, vaginal bleeding, maternal infections, placental membrane inflammation, preterm birth, neonatal skin abrasions, maternal drug use, and birth order among twins (i.e., first-born twins have a higher infection rate than second-born twins) (Blanche, 1994; Burns et al., 1994; Dickover, et al., 1995; European Collaborative Study, 1992; Goedert et al., 1991; Orloff et al., 1996; Thomas et al., 1994).

The use of zidovudine (abbreviated ZDV or AZT) by HIV-infected pregnant women has been shown to decrease perinatal transmission (Boyer et al., 1994; CDC, 1994; Connor et al., 1994; Matheson et al., 1994; Sperling et al., 1996). In February 1994 results of AIDS Clinical Trials Group (ACTG) Protocol 076 were reported. This National Institutes of Health (NIH)-sponsored study investigated the safety and efficacy of maternal and neonatal ZDV administration to reduce the risk of perinatal HIV infection. This double-blinded, randomized, placebo-controlled clinical trial studied asymptomatic HIV-infected pregnant women with CD4 counts greater that 200 who had not previously received ZDV or any other antiretroviral (see Table 14.3, ACTG Protocol 076 Regimen). The women in the treatment group (who received ZDV) had a perinatal transmission rate of 8.3 percent compared to the placebo group who had a transmission rate of 25 percent. This was a 67 percent reduction in perinatal transmission (CDC, 1994). Less dramatic but nonetheless significant decreases in perinatal transmission rates have been reported in HIV-infected pregnant women in more advanced stages of disease (e.g., with a CD4 count of less than 200) who received ZDV during their pregnancies compared to women who did not receive ZDV therapy during pregnancy (Boyer et al., 1994; Matheson et al., 1994).

Further evidence of decreased perinatal transmission of HIV in association with ZDV administration during late antepartum (i.e., 36 weeks' gestation or more) and intrapartum periods was documented in a study conducted in Thailand. In this investigation, HIV-infected pregnant women were randomized to receive either ZDV or a placebo beginning at 36 weeks gestation. The dose of ZDV was 300 mg orally twice a day during pregnancy and 300 mg orally every 3 hours during labor. There was no administration of ZDV to infants in this study. The results demonstrated a 51 percent decrease in perinatal transmission risk in the infants born to women who received ZDV (CDC, 1998a).

A recent study found a lower rate of perinatal transmission in women taking ZDV who had an elective cesarean section (1.5 percent) compared with women taking ZDV who had vaginal deliveries (6 percent) or non-scheduled cesarean sections (11 percent) (Mandelbrot, Le Chenadac, Berrebi, Bongain, Benifla, Delfraissy, et al., 1998). However, in the absence of other confirmatory studies, no recommendations have been developed regarding the role of elective cesarean sections for reduction of perinatal transmission.

HIV Pathogenesis

HIV infection is a complex chronic infectious disease that is caused by a retrovirus. Over time, the majority of infected individuals usually demonstrate severe immune suppression and dysfunction, and eventually develop acquired immunodeficiency syndrome (AIDS), a condition associated with significant morbidity and mortality.

When an individual becomes infected with HIV, the virus must seek out and attach to CD4-positive receptor sites present on the surface of certain cells in the human body. These CD4 cells include T lymphocytes (specifically, CD4-positive [CD4+] lymphocytes), monocytes, macrophages, microglial cells, and follicular dendritic cells (Smith & Rogers, 1996). Once the virus has attached to the host cell's receptor site, it can enter the cell and begin the process of encoding its genomic information within the nucleus, a process that requires an enzyme called reverse transcriptase. Once the encoding of the virus gene has occurred, the virus can replicate and produce several viral particles, which emerge from the infected cell (Smith & Rogers, 1996). HIV's rapid replication results in the production of up to a billion new viral particles every 24 hours. The infected individual's immune system responds by producing similar levels of CD4 lymphocytes in an attempt to rid the body of HIV (Ho, Neumann, Perelson, Chen, & Leonard, 1995). Over time, CD4 cells progressively decline and immune function deteriorates.

The clinical manifestations of HIV vary depending upon the level of immune dysfunction of an individual. Approximately 2 to 4 weeks after infection, 70 percent of individuals manifest systemic symptoms of the acute HIV retroviral syndrome. Once this acute syndrome resolves, individuals usually remain asymptomatic for an average of 10 years (El-Sadr et al., 1994; Smith & Rogers, 1996). Although there may be no evidence of active disease during this time, investigators have demonstrated evidence of viral replication within lymphoid tissues and blood (Ho et al., 1995; Panteleo et al., 1993). Investigators have correlated a more rapid progression to AIDS-defining conditions and death in individuals with baseline viral load measurements of greater than 10,190 copies/mL (Mellors et al., 1996). In addition, higher levels of replication are known to produce viral strains that are resistant to some antiretroviral agents.

A decline in an individual's CD4 cell count provides laboratory evidence of this destructive process on the immune system. The average CD4 cell count in a noninfected individual is greater than 800 cells/mm^3. However, infected individuals will usually have a decline of 50 to 80 cells/mm^3 annually. Eventually this decline in CD4 cells results in an advanced state of immunocompromise and immune system dysfunction, which allows the development of opportunistic infections (OIs) (e.g., cytomegalovirus [CMV], toxoplasmosis, *Pneumocystis carinii* pneumonia [PCP]), neoplasias (e.g., lymphoma, cervical cancer), or debilitating conditions (e.g., wasting syndrome, dementia) (Casey, Cohen, & Hughes, 1996; El-Sadr et al., 1994; Mellors et al., 1996; Smith & Rogers, 1996). See Table 14.5, 1993 Revised Classification System for HIV Infection and Expanded AIDS Surveillance Case Definition for Adolescents ($\geq$ 13 years) and Adults, and Table 14.6, Clinical Categories of HIV Infection.

Gender-specific manifestations of HIV disease progression have been observed. Gynecologic complications associated with HIV infection have been reported in a number of studies. As HIV disease progresses, women are at an increased risk for the development of recalcitrant, recurrent vaginal candidiasis (which usually precedes the development of oral candidiasis); cervical dysplasia (with an estimated eight- to elevenfold increase compared to noninfected women); chronic herpes simplex virus (HSV) infection; and pelvic inflammatory disease (PID) (Anastos & Greenblatt, 1994; Bardequez, 1996; Carpenter et al., 1991; Clark, Brandon, Dumestre, & Pindaro, 1993; Imam et al., 1990; Maiman et al., 1990; Marte, Cohen, Fruchter, & Kelly, 1990; Minkoff, 1991; Rhoads, Wright, Redfield, & Burke, 1987). In 1992, the CDC included these conditions in the classification of advanced HIV infection, and added invasive cervical cancer to the list of AIDS-defining conditions (CDC, 1992).

Pregnancy is associated with a decline in cell-mediated immunity in both HIV-infected and noninfected women, although this decline is not considered substantial enough to render women significantly immunocompromised (Minkoff, 1995). Serial measurements of CD4 cell lymphocytes reveal a decline in levels observed to begin in the first trimester of pregnancy and continue until just prior to delivery. A rebound to pregravid levels is reported in noninfected women and the majority of infected women. Natural history studies have not documented acceleration of HIV disease progression in asymptomatic HIV-infected pregnant women. However, women in more advanced stages of disease (e.g., CD4 cell counts less than 300) have been documented to be at a significantly increased risk for the development of serious infections during pregnancy, (Bardequez, 1996; Cotton & Watts, 1995; Minkoff et al., 1990; Minkoff, 1995).

The effect of pregnancy on a woman's viral load is unknown. Studies investigating viral load measurements in HIV-infected pregnant women have demonstrated an increased risk of perinatal transmission associated with high maternal viral load late in gestation or during labor (Dickover et al., 1995; Fang et al., 1994; Weiser, et al., 1994). However, there does not seem to be a level at which the risk of perinatal transmission is nonexistent (i.e., women have transmitted HIV to their fetuses and newborns even though their viral load measurements were low) (Sperling et al., 1996).

In response to data that correlates high viral load with an increased risk of progression to AIDS and death (Mellors et al., 1996), an expert panel convened to evaluate antiretroviral therapy strategies. In 1997, this panel published guidelines for the use of antiretroviral drugs in adults. The panel recommended that combination antiretroviral therapy, ideally using three drugs, be initiated in HIV-infected adults with symptomatic disease or in those with asymptomatic disease who have high viral titers and/or low CD4+ T cell counts (see Table 14.8, Indications for the Initiation of Antiretroviral Therapy) (Carpenter et al., 1997). The panel also concluded that treatment of HIV infection with a single agent is contraindicated, since the use of a single drug rapidly results in viral resistance.

As a result of these guidelines, the Public Health Service (PHS) convened a task force to address the use of antiretrovirals, including ZDV monotherapy and combination antiretroviral therapy, during pregnancy. In 1998, the PHS published its own set of guidelines for the use of antiretroviral therapy in pregnant women to reduce perinatal transmission and address the need to offer appropriate therapeutic interventions to improve maternal health (see Table 14.9 Clinical Scenarios and Recommendations for the Use of Antiretroviral Drugs to Reduce the Risk of Perinatal Transmission) (CDC, 1998). The PHS document acknowledges the importance of evaluating and treating maternal health with appropriate therapeutic interventions (e.g., combination antiretroviral treatment strategies), as well as utilizing ZDV to reduce the risk of perinatal transmission. It emphasizes that ZDV is the only antiretroviral that has demonstrated a significant reduction in the risk of perinatal HIV transmission. It reiterates that there are limited data available about the unknown long-term effects on children exposed to these drugs in-utero. Finally, the guidelines recognize that the decision whether or not to initiate a particular antiretroviral therapy during pregnancy or neonatal period remains that of the mother and, as such, should be respected.

Since the recognition of HIV infection, clinicians and researchers have developed various therapies to prevent or treat the associated conditions. Although some of these therapeutic interventions, especially antiretroviral medications, have been documented to improve the quality of life and prolong survival time for many individuals (see Table 14.11 Antiretroviral Medications, Dosages, Possible Side Effects, and Drug Interactions), as of this writing there remains no cure for HIV infection.

Database

Subjective

- The woman may report one or more of the following risk factors associated with HIV infection:
  - ▶ History of injection drug use (IDU) and needle sharing
  - ▶ History of sexual contact with a person at risk for HIV infection with any of the following:
    - – History of IDU
    - – History of bisexuality
    - – Diagnosed with or symptomatic of HIV infection or AIDS
    - – Hemophiliac
    - – Lives or lived in an area where HIV/AIDS is endemic
    - – Recipient of a blood product or tissue between mid-1970s to June 1985
    - – Sexual partner(s) at risk for HIV infection
    - – Sexual partner(s) with unknown serostatus
  - ▶ Received tissue or a blood product between the mid-1970s and June 1985
  - ▶ Lived in an area where HIV infection is endemic
  - ▶ Has child(ren) diagnosed with HIV infection or AIDS
  - ▶ Had an unscreened artificial insemination
  - ▶ Had occupational exposure to human blood or body fluids/tissue
  - ▶ Has clinical signs/symptoms associated with HIV infection
  - ▶ Other risk factors associated with HIV exposure:
    - – History of sexually transmitted disease(s) (STDs)
    - – Drug use
    - – Multiple sexual partners
    - – Exchanging sex for money, drugs, food, shelter
    - – Sexual partner with a history of incarceration
- The woman may be asymptomatic or report any of the following symptoms depending upon the stage of HIV infection (Casey et al., 1996; Shannon, 1995).
  - ▶ Acute HIV retroviral syndrome
    - – Fever
    - – Sweating
    - – Malaise
    - – Sore throat
    - – Rigors

- Gastrointestinal symptoms including nausea, vomiting, diarrhea, and anorexia
- Generalized rash
- Enlarged lymph nodes
- Muscle aches
- Headaches
- Photophobia
- Stiff neck
- Altered mental status

▶ Progressive HIV infection

- HIV-infected individuals may remain asymptomatic for an average of 10 years after seroconversion. The following symptoms may be reported as HIV disease progresses (Casey et al., 1996; Shannon, 1995):

  * Some generalized symptoms

    • Enlarged lymph nodes

    • Fatigue

    • Night sweats

    • Intermittent low-grade fever(s)

    • Weight loss

  * Some dermatologic manifestations

    • Generalized dry skin

    • Erythematous, scaly skin of the scalp, eyebrows, nasolabial folds, trunk, groin

    • Scaly patches with areas of central clearing

    • Grouped vesicles of the lips, genitalia, or perianal region(s) that are usually painful and recurrent

    • Painful eruption(s) of vesicles in a wide distribution (dermatomal pattern) usually unilateral and occurring on the trunk, head, or neck

    • Thick, erythematous plaques with well-defined margins; intermittently pruritic; often reported at the site of trauma

    • Erythematous papular or pustular lesions at hair follicles of the face, trunk; may be tender and pruritic

    • Oval nodules that become reddish-purple in color; are 1–2 cm in diameter; reported on the face, trunk, legs, and hard palate

      NOTE: These are rarely reported in HIV-infected women.

    • Petechiae, unexplained ecchymosis

* Some ophthalmic symptoms

  • Abrupt onset of "floaters" (small floating spots in field of vision)

  • Intermittent or persistent blurred vision

  • Intermittent episodes of flashes of light

  • Photophobia

  • Loss of vision

* Some oral symptoms

  • Canker sores of tongue and buccal mucosa

  • Grouped vesicles or ulcers of lips or buccal mucosa

  • White patches on buccal mucosa and/or tongue that may or may not scrape off

  • Erythema, edema, bleeding of gums

  • Nodules that are reddish-purple in color (usually noted on the hard palate)

* Some respiratory symptoms

  • Dyspnea that may be mild to severe depending upon the underlying condition

  • Shortness of breath (may be mild to severe)

  • A persistent dry, hacking cough (often noted in PCP)

  • Abrupt onset of productive cough with minimal to copious amounts of purulent mucous (see Chapter 11.4, *Pneumonia*)

* Some gastrointestinal symptoms

  • Chronic, intermittent diarrhea with or without bloating

  • Odynophagia

  • Dysphagia

  • Jaundice

  • Anorexia

  • Hematemesis, melena (rare)

* Some neurological symptoms

  • Memory lapses, mental confusion, inability to think clearly, or flat affect

  • Frequent or persistent headaches with or without fever(s)

  • Dysesthesia of extremities

  • Problems with coordination or balance

  • Seizures

* Some gynecological manifestations

- Erythema and/or pruritis of vulvovaginal and/or perianal areas

- Vaginal discharge that is indicative of candidiasis, trichomoniasis, bacterial vaginosis, chlamydia, or gonorrhea (see specific chapters in Section 14, *Vaginitis and Sexually Transmitted Diseases*)

- Recurrent, painful blister(s), ulcer(s), or lesions in the vulvovaginal and/or perianal regions (may be indicative of herpes simplex virus [HSV] infection)

- Verruciform lesions of the vulvovaginal, perineal, or anal regions that may be recurrent (may be indicative of human papilloma virus [HPV] infection)

- A history or documented evidence of cervical intraepithelial neoplasia (CIN) or cervical cancer

Objective

- The physical examination may be within normal limits (WNL) or demonstrate significant pathologic findings, depending upon the immune status of the woman and any coexisting conditions that may be present. The following clinical manifestations may be evident (Casey et al., 1996; Shannon, 1995).

  ▶ General examination may reveal a thin, wasted body type, and/or a flat affect.

  ▶ Vital signs are usually WNL but will change depending upon any underlying illness (e.g., bacterial pneumonia) that may coexist.

  ▶ Examination of the skin may reveal the following conditions:

    – Xerosis (generalized dry skin)

    – Seborrheic dermatitis (erythematous scaly skin of the scalp, eyebrows, nasolabial folds, trunk, groin)

    – Folliculitis (erythematous papular or pustular lesions of hair follicles of the face, trunk; may be tender to palpation)

    – Psoriasis (thick, erythematous plaques with well-defined margins)

    – Tinea corporis (erythematous, papulosquamous, circumscribed, raised scaling lesions with areas of central clearing; usually affects smooth, non-hairy portions of skin)

    – HSV infection (usually a single vesicle or grouped vesicles of the lips, genitalia, or perianal region(s) that are painful to palpation)

    – Herpes zoster (vesicular eruption in a dermatomal pattern (usually unilateral); most frequently noted on the trunk, head, or neck; painful to palpation; a disseminated pattern may be noted)

    – Molluscum contagiousum (discrete, umbilicated, pearly white, smooth papules; usually noted in the pubic and genital areas, but may be evident on the face, neck and trunk)

    – Kaposi's sarcoma (KS) (flat or elevated reddish-purple nodule(s) or plaques varying in size from 1 to 2 cm in diameter may be observed [rare in women])

  ▶ Examination of the eyes (including funduscopic) may reveal the following:

    – Cotton wool patches with or without evidence of hemorrhage (this finding is not necessarily associated with a specific disease process) (Shin & Avers, 1988)

- Dry, granular, white retinal opacification with hemorrhage (evidence of retinopathy)

- Bright red subconjunctival hemorrhage (may indicate KS)

- Visual field defects, optic atrophy, pupillary abnormalities, cranial nerve palsies (may indicate neuro-ophthalmic signs of intracranial disease or other conditions)

▶ Examination of the oropharynx may reveal the following:

- Erythema, edema, hypertrophy of gingiva (gingivitis)

- Smooth, erythematous patches of the hard or soft palate, mucosa or dorsum of the tongue (atrophic candidiasis)

- Raised, white patches on tongue or buccal mucosa that scrape off with tongue blade; patches may be on an erythematous base (candidiasis)

- White or whitish-gray, raised irregularly shaped lesions with vertical folds or corrugations of the lateral (often posterior, inferior) tongue that do not scrape off (hairy leukoplakia)

- Small erythematous, eroded, or fissured lesions at corners of mouth (angular chelitis)

- Reddish-purple-blue–colored, flat or elevated, single or multiple lesions of the mouth (may indicate KS)

- Small vesicular or ulcerated painful lesions of the lips palate or gingiva (may indicate HSV infection)

- Single or multiple verruciform lesions that may be cauliflower-like or flat (may indicate HPV infection)

▶ Examination of the lungs will reveal findings consistent with any coexisting pulmonary disease (see specific Respiratory infection protocols).

NOTE: Pulmonary problems in HIV-infected individuals (e.g., PCP, bacterial pneumonia) often present with subtle physical examination findings, such as tachypnea, rales, and diminished breath sounds.

▶ Cardiac examination is usually WNL. If significant cardiac disease coexists (e.g., endocarditis associated with injection drug use, cardiomyopathy) the following symptoms may be evident:

- Increased pulse rate

- Murmur

- S_3 gallop

▶ Abdominal examination may reveal the following:

- Enlarged liver

- Enlarged spleen

- Fundal height less than expected for gestational age if intrauterine growth restriction (IUGR) present

▶ Palpation of lymph nodes may reveal the following:

- Enlarged, soft, mobile node(s) with or without tenderness

- Single or multiple hard, enlarged node(s) (may be indicative of lymphoma)

▶ Neurological examination may reveal the following:

- Flat affect

- Diminished recent memory

- Decreased fine and gross motor movements

- Decreased proprioception

- Abnormal, symmetric or asymmetric deep tendon reflexes

- Paraparesis

- Ataxia

▶ Musculoskeletal examination may reveal may reveal the following:

- Decreased muscle tone

- Decreased muscle strength

▶ Pelvic examination may reveal physical findings consistent with vaginitis, cervicitis, condyloma acuminata, molluscum contagiousum, HSV infection, other sexually transmitted diseases, vulvar/vaginal/cervical/anal intraepithelial neoplasia (see specific chapters for descriptions of physical findings).

Assessment

● Human immunodeficiency virus (HIV) infection

▶ R/O acquired immunodeficiency syndrome (AIDS)

▶ R/O minor opportunistic infections (e.g., oral candidiasis)

▶ R/O immune dysfunction from other causes (e.g., neoplasms, autoimmune disorders)

▶ R/O sexually transmitted diseases (STDs)

▶ R/O IUGR

▶ R/O psychological disorders associated with chronic disease (e.g., depression)

● Assess factors associated with increased risk of HIV infection

Plan

Diagnostic Tests

● In August 1995, the CDC published guidelines for the *universal counseling* and *voluntary* HIV testing of all pregnant women in the United States (CDC, 1995b).

▶ The CDC guidelines clearly state that *mandatory* HIV testing of women or infants is not recommended.

▶ The guidelines also endorse HIV testing within the context of primary health care.

▶ For women such counseling, testing and access to care should occur prior to conception whenever possible (CDC, 1995b).

▶ **NOTE:** Interpretation and implementation of these guidelines varies among states.

● If a pregnant woman discloses that she is HIV-infected, verification of her serostatus is essential (either by obtaining a copy of previous test results or repeat testing of the woman) prior to the initiation of any pharmacologic interventions. (See Patient Education for information regarding informed consent and disclosure of HIV test results).

● The testing available to identify HIV infection involves indirect and direct methods.

▶ The indirect methods are HIV antibody tests and include the enzyme-linked immunosorbent assay (ELISA), Western Blot, and immunofluorescence assay (IFA).

– HIV antibody tests: A woman will usually demonstrate a positive result 6 to 12 weeks after infection with the virus. However, in rare instances, some individuals may not have detectable antibodies until 6 months after infection. The following tests can be ordered:

* The enzyme-linked immunosorbent assay (ELISA) test is a very sensitive but less specific antibody test used as an initial screening test for the presence of HIV antibodies. If the initial test is positive the test is usually repeated at least once on the same specimen. If the repeat ELISA test is positive, a confirmatory antibody test is done (e.g., Western blot, IFA).

* Immunofluorescence assay (IFA) can be done to confirm the initial ELISA test result and involves a process that attaches a fluoresein label to the HIV antibodies present in a specimen. This specimen is then evaluated under an ultraviolet microscope; the presence of bright spots of fluorescence indicates a positive test.

* The Western blot is a confirmatory test that involves direct evaluation of the specimen for the presence of antibodies to specific HIV antigens. It is a very sensitive and specific antibody test. Strict guidelines are used for the interpretation of findings, and it is the preferred test for confirmation of positive ELISA results. A fully reactive Western blot test confirms HIV seropositive ELISA results.

NOTE: When both the ELISA and Western blot test results are positive, the sensitivity and specificity are each greater than 99 percent (Grady & Vogel, 1993). An infected woman may have a negative result if she is in the "window period," during which time she is not producing a measurable level of antibodies. An indeterminate result (i.e., a positive ELISA with an indeterminate Western blot) can occur in a woman who is in the process of seroconverting. In such instances, perform a repeat antibody test at an interval appropriate to her last known HIV exposure (i.e., 6 to 12 weeks after last exposure). In addition, consider a viral test (e.g., DNA PCR, p24 antigen assay), since these tests can determine serostatus sooner than waiting for several weeks to repeat an antibody test.

▶ The direct methods are viral tests and include HIV culture, qualitative DNA polymerase chain reaction (PCR), and p24 antigen assays. In adults, the most common testing performed is HIV antibody testing. The following tests may be ordered to document the HIV status of a woman after she has received pretest counseling and after consent for HIV testing has been obtained (Casey et al., 1996; Grady & Vogel, 1993):

– The HIV antigen (p24 antigen) assay measures the presence of HIV core protein in a specimen. When HIV replication is active (e.g., during seroconversion) there is an increased concentration of p24 antigen. However, this test has a low sensitivity in asymptomatic HIV-infected individuals with CD4 cell counts greater than 200. This test is not used to determine HIV serostatus in the general population.

- The ICDp24 antigen assay dissociates the antigen and antibody complex so that a more accurate measurement of the p24 antigen level can be obtained. This test is used primarily in research settings.

- HIV cultures can be performed on a number of body fluids and tissues and may be positive depending upon the concentration of the virus in the specimen. HIV cultures are expensive, the virus is difficult to grow, and meticulous laboratory procedures are essential to ensure accurate results. Erratic results have been associated with a number of factors, including contamination of specimens and low concentration of virus in specimens. For these reasons, this process is not commonly used to determine HIV status in adult populations.

- The qualitative DNA polymerase chain reaction (PCR) amplifies the DNA of specimen cells to determine the presence of HIV in the cell. It is very sensitive and specific, and results are available within a few days. However, this test is expensive and requires an experienced laboratory staff with meticulous technique to perform it. False-positive results are possible since any trace of a DNA sequencing pattern similar to HIV may be interpreted as positive.

● Order a complete T-lymphocyte count, which may reveal the following (Casey et al., 1996):

▸ Decreased T-helper cell (CD4) count (normal count is greater than 800 cells/mm^3)

▸ Increased T-suppressor cell (CD8) count

▸ Inversion of T-helper to T-suppressor cell ratio (normal ratio 2:1)

NOTE: There is considerable circadian, intralaboratory, and interlaboratory variation in T-lymphocyte levels. Ideally, tests should be obtained at the same laboratory and at approximately the same time of day as previous samples to maintain some consistency in values. Samples should not be obtained until 2 to 3 weeks after recovering from an illness, since intercurrent illness can effect values (Grady & Vogel, 1993).

▸ Viral load measurements in HIV-infected adults are being used as surrogate markers to assess an individual's risk for disease progression, determine when to initiate antiretroviral therapy, and monitor clinical response to therapeutic interventions. The types of viral load assays that are commercially available include the following (Casey et al., 1996):

- The branched-chain DNA signal amplification assay (bDNA) is a qualitative measure of HIV RNA in plasma with a detection limit of 5,000 virions/mL. This test can quantitate HIV RNA in up to 90 percent of HIV-infected adults with CD4 cell counts less than 500/mm^3.

- The quantitative competitive polymerase chain reaction (QC-PCR) quantitatively measures HIV RNA viral load in HIV-infected individuals with as few as 50 virions/mL.

NOTE: Although these assays both measure viral load, comparison of values obtained from different assays is not recommended. Use the same assay consistently to monitor response to therapy and risk of disease progression for each individual. Base treatment decisions on a sustained change in viral load measurement and not on a single value. In addition, acute illness and immunizations are associated with significant transient elevations in levels. Therefore, samples should not be obtained until 4 to 6 weeks *after* an illness and/or administration of an immunization. The following schedule has been suggested for obtaining viral load measurements in adults (CDC, 1998b; Saag et al., 1996):

- Baseline value: Average of two samples obtained 2 to 4 weeks apart.

- Repeat level: Every 3 to 4 months, prior to initiating or changing antiretroviral therapy, and 4 weeks after initiating or changing antiretroviral therapy

- Obtain a complete blood count (CBC), differential, and platelet count, which may be WNL or reveal the following (Casey et al., 1996; Shannon, 1995):

  ▶ Leukopenia

  ▶ Lymphocytopenia

  ▶ Decreased red blood cells (RBCs), hematocrit (Hct), or hemoglobin (Hgb)

  ▶ Increased MCV between l05 to 110 in women taking ZDV

  ▶ Thrombocytopenia

- Perform a chemistry panel, which may be WNL or reveal the following in the presence of concomitant disease(s) (Casey et al., 1996):

  ▶ Elevated alanine transaminase (ALT, SGPT) or aspartate transaminase level (AST, SGOT) (in presence of hepatitic disease)

  ▶ Elevated lactate dehydrogenase (LDH) (may be evidence of PCP if CD4 count is less than $200/mm^3$)

  ▶ Decreased serum cholesterol (may be depleted because of chronic disease state with wasting)

- Obtain a syphilis serology (e.g., VDRL or RPR).

- Screen for hepatitis, including hepatitis B surface antigen and antibody, and antibody C antibody (see Chapter 10.2, *Hepatitis A, B, C, D, and E*).

- Do toxoplasmosis serology (IgG) to determine the woman's immune status. This documentation is helpful should symptoms of encephalitis develop and a diagnosis of CNS toxoplasmosis is being considered.

NOTE: Approximately 15 percent of HIV-infected individuals with toxoplasmosis may have false negative serology results (Lawlor, Fischer, & Adelman, 1995).

- Obtain a glucose-6-phosphate dehydrogenase (G6PD) level, since women with a deficiency of this enzyme develop a hemolytic anemia when placed on some of the therapeutic agents that are frequently used during the course of HIV disease (e.g., dapsone, sulfonamides, primaquine) (Cosby & Stringari, 1991).

- Perform a tuberculin skin testing with PPD. Induration of 5 mm or more at the site of the PPD is considered to be a positive tuberculin skin test in HIV-infected individuals. Obtain a chest x-ray, if possible, after the first trimester.

NOTE: The placement of control skin tests to make sure an HIV-infected person is not anergic is no longer recommended for a variety of reasons, including problems with standardization and reproducibility of these agents (CDC, 1997c).

- Obtain cervical cytology all HIV-infected pregnant women as part of their initial prenatal visit. The following national guidelines regarding the frequency of Pap smears have been proposed for HIV-infected women:

  ▶ A woman with no history of any abnormal cervical cytology should have Pap smears obtained 6 months apart. If both results are benign and the smears are both adequate (i.e., endocervical cells are present), then annual Pap smear testing can be continued (Caschetta, 1992; El Sadr et al., 1994).

  NOTE: A pregnant woman within this category should have a Pap smear obtained during her initial prenatal visit and may have the second Pap smear obtained during the postpartum visit (even though this may delay obtaining the second Pap smear a few months beyond the recommended 6 months).

  ▶ Women without a history of abnormal cervical cytology who have a CD4 count of less than 500 should have Pap smear testing every 6 months (ACOG, 1992; Baker, 1994; Minkoff & DeHovitz, 1991).

  ▶ Women with cervical cytology results indicating atypical squamous cells of undetermined significance (ASCUS) or any higher grade abnormality should be referred for colposcopy with repeat evaluation(s) and Pap smears per recommendation of the colposcopist (ACOG, 1992; Baker, 1994; Minkoff & DeHovitz, 1991).

- Conduct appropriate testing to rule out the presence of sexually transmitted diseases (STDs) (e.g., chlamydia, gonorrhea).

- Obtain a wet mount of vaginal secretions to evaluate for the presence of vaginal/cervical pathogens requiring treatment (e.g., candidiasis, trichomoniasis, bacterial vaginosis).

- Obtain obstetrical ultrasound for obstetrical indications, *not* on the basis of the HIV infection of the woman.

- Amniocentesis, chorionic villus sampling (CVS), and cordocentesis are invasive diagnostic tests which pose a theoretical risk of increased fetal exposure to maternal infectious cells. As of this writing, there are no data available regarding the effect of these procedures on perinatal transmission rates (Bardequez, 1996; Cotton & Watts, 1995; Minkoff, 1995). Cordocentesis and CVS are associated with a greater risk of a maternal-fetal bleed (Cullen, Sanches-Ramos, & Delke, 1992) and, therefore, are not recommended by some authorities for use in HIV-infected women (Bardequez, 1996). An HIV-infected pregnant woman considering amniocentesis (e.g., a woman over age 35) must be counseled about the theoretical risk(s) versus the benefits of the information gained from undergoing this procedure.

- Offer and obtain triple marker screening between 15 to 20 weeks' gestation (see Chapter 3.3, *Triple Marker Prenatal Screening*).

- Obtain a 50-gram 1-hour glucose screen for gestational diabetes between 24 to 28 weeks' gestation (see Chapter 6.11, *Gestational Diabetes Mellitus*).

- Do not routinely order obstetrical ultrasounds, nonstress tests (NSTs), biophysical profiles (BPPs), or contraction stress tests (CSTs) an for HIV-infected woman unless there is an obstetrical or medical indication for such evaluations.

- Order routine follow-up tests of an HIV-positive woman based upon symptoms of HIV disease progression, therapeutic interventions that have been initiated, and institution-specific protocols.

Most authorities recommend the following tests be obtained every trimester unless there is evidence of disease progression and/or concern that prophylactic therapy may be needed to prevent the development of OIs (Bardequez, 1996; Cotton & Watts, 1995; Minkoff, 1995):

▶ For CD4 cell counts

- Greater than 500/mm^3: repeat every trimester

- 200 to 300/mm^3: repeat every 6 to 8 weeks (to monitor for decline to a level less than 200/mm^3, at which time initiation of prophylactic regimens should begin)

- Less than 200/mm^3 repeat 1 week after obtaining an initial value of less than 200/mm^3 (to confirm the level and determine need for the initiation of prophylactic regimens)

NOTE: Changes in the CD4+ T-cell count during pregnancy may reflect physiologic blood volume and/or hemodynamic alterations associated with pregnancy. The CD4+ percentage is a more stable laboratory marker during pregnancy and may be a more accurate measure of immune status during pregnancy (CDC, 1998b).

▶ Viral load measurements may be obtained per institution-specific protocols.

▶ Repeat CBC, as clinically indicated. A woman beginning ZDV therapy should have a CBC done prior to initiation of ZDV and after 2 weeks of ZDV therapy. If these results are normal, a CBC should be done every 3 months unless there is evidence of hematological side effects (Casey et al., 1996).

NOTE: Some investigators suggest monthly CBC testing after the initiation of ZDV in pregnant women (Minkoff, 1995).

▶ Repeat transaminase levels, as indicated. A woman taking ZDV should have repeat transaminase levels evaluated every trimester.

NOTE: Some investigators suggest monthly chemistry panels during pregnancy for a woman taking ZDV (Minkoff, 1995).

▶ Repeat VDRL or RPR, as indicated, based on the woman's history of unprotected sexual activity. In areas of high seroprevalence for syphilis, consider repeating a syphilis serology during the third trimester.

▶ Repeat chlamydia testing, gonorrhea cultures, and vaginal/cervical wet mounts, as indicated, based on the woman's history of unprotected sexual activity. In areas of high prevalence for chlamydia and gonorrhea or if a woman has been treated for an STD during early pregnancy, consider repeat testing during the third trimester.

▶ Obtain serial obstetrical ultrasounds every 3 to 4 weeks in a woman suspected of or documented to have IUGR (see Chapter 6.15, *Intrauterine Growth Restriction*).

Treatment/Management

The rapid changes in treatment options and the complexity of some of these therapies necessitates a multidisciplinary approach to the clinical care of an HIV-infected pregnant woman; collaboration with perinatologists, HIV specialists, gynecologists, and pediatric infectious disease specialists is essential. The plan of care is based upon her stage of HIV disease. As HIV disease progresses to advanced immune dysfunction (CD4 cell count of less than 200/mm^3), the risk of developing a major OI or other condition associated with an AIDS diagnosis increases significantly, and prophylactic administration of a number of pharmacologic agents may be indicated. The management of a pregnant woman who has progressed to this stage of HIV infection, who has a major OI or other AIDS defining condition, or who has an elevated viral load measurement and decreased CD4+ cell count is beyond the scope of this protocol. The following therapeutic interventions are recommended for HIV-infected pregnant women who are asymptomatic with a high CD4+ cell count and an undetectable viral load measurement.

- Counsel a woman with a normal CD4+ T-cell count and an undetectable viral load measurement about the use of antiretroviral therapy, per ACTG Protocol 076, to reduce the risk of perinatal transmission (see Table 14.4, ACTG Protocol 076: Components of Counseling for HIV-Infected Pregnant Women) (CDC, 1995c) and the use of combination antiretroviral therapy for maternal health as determined by clinical and laboratory parameters (see Table 14.8, Clinical Scenarios and Recommendations for the Use of Antiretroviral Drugs to Reduce the Risk of Perinatal HIV Transmission) (CDC, 1998b).

  ▶ The following regimen may be initiated after the first trimester in a woman desiring ZDV monotherapy to reduce the risk of perinatal transmission:

    – Zidovudine 200 mg p.o. t.i.d.

  NOTE: Side effects associated with ZDV include bone marrow suppression with the development of anemia, granulocytopenia, and elevated liver transaminase levels. Interruption or permanent discontinuation of therapy is indicated in a woman with evidence of severe anemia (Hgb less than 9 g/dL), an absolute neutrophil count (ANC) of less than 1,000/mm^3, a platelet count less than 100,000, or an ALT or AST level greater than five times the upper limits of normal (Minkoff, 1995).

  Two potentially fatal, albeit rare, side effects reported with ZDV use include lactic acidosis and severe hepatomegaly with steatosis. The majority of these cases have occurred in moderately obese, nonpregnant women. The causal relationship between these conditions and ZDV is unknown at this time. Close monitoring of transaminase levels in a woman with history of liver disease or hepatomegaly is advised.

- Counsel women requiring combination antiretroviral therapy for health (i.e., with evidence of clinical disease progression and/or surrogate marker evidence of increased risk for disease progression) regarding the options, including the use of ZDV per the ACTG Protocol 076 regimen (see Table 14.8, Clinical Scenarios and Recommendations for the Use of Antiretroviral Drugs to Reduce the Risk of Perinatal HIV Transmission) (CDC, 1998b).

  ▶ Initiation of or a change in antiretroviral therapy (e.g., ZDV monotherapy or combination therapy) should be per the recommendation of the consulting perinatologist and HIV specialist.

  ▶ Data regarding the perinatal or neonatal effects of antiretrovirals other than ZDV are extremely limited and have not been obtained through randomized controlled clinical trials (see Table 14.9, Antiretrovirals in Pregnant Women, Neonates and Children). A presentation of the current data regarding antiretrovirals other than ZDV should be provided by the consulting perinatologist and HIV specialist.

  NOTE: It is recommended that clinicians enroll pregnant women taking antiretrovirals in the Antiretroviral Pregnancy Registry at (800) 722-9292, extension 38465. This registry is compiling perinatal outcomes associated with the use of antiretrovirals during pregnancy. Women can be enrolled anonymously.

- Initiate PCP primary prophylaxis in women with an absolute CD4 cell count of less than 200/mm³ or less than 14 percent of total lymphocytes (CDC, 1995d).

  ▶ Systemic agents are preferred since extrapulmonary PCP has been documented with the use of aerosolized pentamidine.

  ▶ The following medications have *not* been associated with any increased incidence of adverse maternal, fetal, or neonatal outcomes (including kernicterus) in HIV-infected pregnant women who require PCP prophylaxis, and can be initiated if there is no medical contraindication (e.g., allergy) for its use (Bardequez, 1996; Cotton & Watts, 1995; Minkoff, 1995).

    – Trimethoprim (TMP)/sulfamethoxazole (SMX)160 mg/800 mg one tablet p.o. three times a week

      OR

    – TMP/SMX 160/800 mg one tablet p.o. q.d.

  ▶ If the woman has an allergy to TMP/SMX then the following medication may be prescribed as follows (Bardequez, 1996; Cotton & Watts, 1995):

    – Dapsone 50 mg b.i.d.

      OR

    – Dapsone 100 mg p.o. q.d.

- Women with contraindications to systemic agents for primary PCP prophylaxis should begin aerosolized pentamidine treatments if there are no contraindications (e.g., pulmonary disease).

  NOTE: Aerosolized pentamidine is localized to the lung with little, if any, extrapulmonary distribution, and poses no adverse risk to the fetus. However, there is an increased risk of extrapulmonary and breakthrough pulmonary PCP associated with this therapy (Bardequez, 1996; Cotton & Watts, 1995; Minkoff, 1995).

  ▶ The following regimen is recommended and may be initiated during the first trimester if indicated:

    – Aerosolized pentamidine 300 mg/month delivered by Respirgard II® or Ultra Vent® Nebulizers

- Women with a CD4 cell count less than 75/mm³ should initiate prophylaxis against *Mycobacterium avium* complex (MAC) per recommendation of the perinatologist and HIV specialist.

- Treat women with evidence of oral candidiasis and no clinical evidence of esophagitis (e.g., dysphagia, odynophagia, retrosternal pain when swallowing) with one of the following medications (Cotton & Watts, 1995):

  ▶ Clotrimazole oral troches: one troche five times a day for 7 to 10 days (advise the patient to suck, not swallow, the troche until it completely dissolves)

  ▶ Nystatin 500,000 units (5 mL) swish and swallow five times a day for 7 to 10 days

  NOTE: Reserve the use of systemic therapy for esophagitis and prescribe only after consultation with a perinatologist and HIV specialist.

- Treat women with evidence of vaginitis, cervicitis, or other STDs, as indicated (see other specific chapters in Section 14).

- Women with a positive tuberculin skin test (i.e., at least 5 mm induration) and a negative chest X-ray should begin tuberculosis prophylaxis:

  ▶ Isoniazid 300 mg p.o. q.d. and vitamin B_6 50 mg p.o. q.d.

  NOTE: In HIV-infected pregnant women, the initiation of this regimen should not be postponed until after delivery (Bardequez, 1996; Cotton & Watts, 1995).

- Refer women with a cervical cytology report indicating ASCUS or any higher grade lesion(s) to an experienced colposcopist for evaluation and indicated treatment.

- Pneumococcal, diphtheria-tetanus, and influenza immunizations have been associated with a transient (i.e., 4-week) increase of viral load in HIV-infected adults (O'Brien, 1996). The administration of these immunizations during pregnancy is controversial because there is a potentially increased risk of HIV transmission to the embryo/fetus from the increased maternal viral load. Review institution-specific protocols and consult with a perinatologist regarding the administration of these immunizations to HIV-infected pregnant women.

- Nonstress testing should be initiated at 34 weeks' gestation in any woman receiving combination antiretroviral therapy, since the fetal effects of such agents used in combination are unknown (CDC, 1998).

- Unless clinically indicated, avoid invasive procedures (e.g., amniotomy, fetal scalp sampling, etc.) during the intrapartum period as a means of reducing fetal exposure to infectious maternal secretions. As soon as possible after birth, wipe maternal secretions off the infant; and completely bathe the infant once thermoregulation is stable.

Consultation

- Consult with a physician for any woman suspected of being HIV-positive or with documented evidence of HIV-seropositive status with or without symptomatic disease.

- Consult with a physician for any HIV-infected woman with evidence of a major opportunistic infection or AIDS-defining condition, lack of response to therapeutic interventions, serious side effect or suspected toxicity to a medication, who is being considered for prophylactic therapy (e.g., TMP/SMX for PCP prophylaxis), or who is currently taking or considering the initiation of combination antiretroviral therapy.

- Consult with a physician regarding current guidelines for mode of delivery and risk of perinatal transmission for all women.

- The complex and often rapidly evolving nature of the clinical care of HIV infected individuals has resulted in the establishment of national and regional consultation services for clinicians. See Appendix 14.5a, Support for Clinicians and HIV-infected Persons.

- Psychological or psychiatric consultation is indicated for women with evidence of moderate-to-severe psychiatric symptoms (e.g., anxiety, depression) or who may be exhibiting neuropsychiatric manifestations of HIV (e.g., HIV dementia).

- Arrange a consultation with a pediatric HIV specialist for a woman during her pregnancy so she can discuss plans for her infant's care. During this appointment, the specialist should provide information about the HIV testing of her infant (e.g., types of tests used, when testing is done), current recommended prophylactic therapies (e.g., neonatal ZDV per ACTG Protocol 076 regimen,

TMP/SMX prophylaxis to prevent PCP), and the current treatment(s) available if an infant is determined to be infected.

- Consult, as needed, for prescriptions

Patient Education

- Educate women about HIV infection, including the modes of transmission, clinical course (especially the chronicity of the disease), indicated diagnostic tests, available therapeutic options, prevention of further exposure to HIV and other STDs in sexually active women (see Table 14.1 Safe Sex Guidelines), symptoms of complications requiring immediate evaluation, and indicated follow-up.

- Present current information about the effects of pregnancy on HIV disease progression, the effects of HIV infection on pregnancy outcome, perinatal transmission rates, therapeutic interventions for women during pregnancy, care of a perinatally exposed infants, and clinical trials available to the woman and her infant should be presented in a nonjudgmental manner.

- Recommend that women not breast-feed their infants because of the possibility of transmitting HIV through breast milk.

- A detailed presentation of the care for a perinatally exposed infant is beyond the scope of this protocol and should be provided by the pediatric HIV specialist. However, women should understand that a term infant born to an HIV-infected mother will have a positive result to HIV antibody testing because of the transplacental passage of maternal HIV IgG antibodies. This result reflects *maternal* infection and indicates the infant is *at risk* of exposure/infection. Viral load tests (e.g., HIV culture, HIV DNA PCR, ICDp24 antigen) are used to determine the HIV serostatus of infants less than 18 months of age (Nesheim, 1996). For additional information about the diagnosis of HIV infection in infants the reader is referred to Nesheim (1996).

- Discuss the reason for any referrals that are being made and the importance of keeping such appointments. Such referrals may include appointments with a perinatologist, HIV specialist, and pediatric HIV specialist.

- Discuss the need for testing individuals who may have had exposure through sexual contact or needle sharing activities. If a woman has other children, assess the possible need for testing of her children based upon the woman's history of exposure, date of first positive test result, and ages of her children.

- Educate women who continue to use drugs/alcohol about the adverse effects on her health and the health of the fetus, the need to consider drug treatment, and, if she is an active IDU, the importance of avoiding sharing needles to prevent transmission of HIV and other infectious diseases (e.g., hepatitis B and C).

- Prior to obtaining a woman's medical records, discuss the need for confirmation of her HIV status and how this can be obtained.

  ▶ In many locations a special consent for disclosure of HIV test results must be signed in addition to standard medical record release forms. Furthermore, informed consent of a woman (in some states this is written consent) regarding HIV testing is required prior to obtaining such tests.

  ▶ Disclosure of HIV test results should involve only the woman and the provider or counselor who obtained the test. Ideally, the woman should return to the provider or counselor to receive her results in person and to receive follow-up counseling regarding implication(s) of the results (including repeat testing based on continued high-risk behaviors).

- Educate women regarding any potential short- or long-term side effects associated with medications and when they should seek an immediate evaluation (e.g., symptoms of an allergic reaction).

- Advise women not to donate blood products or consent to organ donation.

- Advise women not to share personal hygiene implements that could be contaminated with blood (e.g., toothbrushes, razors).

- Educate women who are toxoplasmosis IgG-negative about ways to reduce the risk of becoming infected with toxoplasmosis (see Chapter 10.9, *Toxoplasmosis*).

- Educate women about contraceptive options available to them after delivery. Currently, limited data is available regarding the various contraceptive methods and the impact on HIV disease and/or transmission.

  ▶ Most methods are acceptable when combined with effective STD prevention strategies.

  ▶ Intrauterine devices are not recommended because of the risk of uterine infections associated with their use (Minkoff, 1995; Rompalo, Anderson, & Quinn, 1992).

  ▶ Some protease inhibitors reduce serum concentrations of ethinyl estradiol.

  ▶ When hormonal contraceptives are being considered for a woman receiving combination antiretroviral therapy, consult a clinical pharmacist or HIV specialist to obtain current information about potential drug interactions.

- Advise women regarding the need to disclose their HIV status to other medical providers so that appropriate therapy for any illness or condition can be prescribed.

- Educate women about community resources available to them for psychosocial support (e.g., HIV-specific woman's groups, legal counseling, financial aid, etc.). See Appendix 14.5a for resources that may be helpful for some women.

Follow-up

- See the Consultation section.

- See Diagnostic Tests and Treatment/Management sections for recommendations for follow-up evaluations of asymptomatic HIV-infected pregnant women.

- See women with symptoms that suggest a possible opportunistic infection or complication immediately for an evaluation.

- An AIDS diagnosis *is* a reportable condition with notification of the local public health department mandated by law. In some states, HIV infection is a reportable condition. Contact the local public health department for the appropriate forms and the procedure(s) to follow.

- Document in progress notes and problem list (as appropriate and without breaching confidentiality).

Table 14.3

ACTG Protocol 076 Zidovudine Regimen

Antepartum

100 mg orally five times a day

(begin after the 13th week of gestation)

Intrapartum

Loading dose: 2 mg/kg IV for 1 hour

followed by

Maintenance dose: 1 mg/kg IV until the cord is clamped

Neonatal

2 mg/kg p.o. every 6 hours

or

1.5 mg/kg IV every 6 hours if the infant is n.p.o.

(begin within 8 hours after birth and continue until 6 weeks of age)

Source: Centers for Disease Control and Prevention (CDC) (1994). Zidovudine for the prevention of HIV transmission from mother to infant. *Morbidity and Mortality Weekly Report, 43*(16), 285–286.

Table 14.4

ACTG Protocol 076: Components of Counseling for HIV-Infected Pregnant Women

Explain overall perinatal transmission rate <u>without</u> ACTG Protocol 076 Regimen:
- 25% of infants

Explain elements of ACTG Protocol 076 study:
- antepartum & intrapartum & neonatal ZDV administration
- placebo and study drug arms
- asymptomatic HIV-infected pregnant women with CD4 > 200/mm3
- initiation of maternal treatment between 14 to 34 gestational weeks

Review results of study:
- placebo arm = 25% of infants infected
- study drug arm = 8.3% of infants infected
  <u>NOTE:</u> <u>8.3% perinatal transmission rate still occurred in ZDV group.</u>

Reported results of study:
- Maternal: minimal side effects in both placebo and study group including mild transient headache, fatigue, anemia
- Infant: transient mild anemia that resolved without treatment in infants with in-utero and neonatal exposure to ZDV

Safety:
- Short-term: No adverse maternal, perinatal, neonatal outcomes associated with ZDV. No increased incidence of congenital anomalies in ZDV group compared to placebo group and general population. No clustering of congenital anomalies observed.
- Long-term: Theoretical but unknown
  Possible maternal risks:
  – alteration of HIV disease
  – development of viral resistance
  Possible infant risks:
  – reports of mutagenic/carcinogenic effects in rodents exposed in-utero to extremely high doses
- NOTE: Long-term follow-up of infants/children participating in this study will continue until they are 21 years old. Women who participated in the study are being followed for three years after completion of the protocol.

Limitations of study:
- Unknown efficacy of regimen in pregnant women with symptomatic disease, CD4 count less than 200/mm^3, or high viral loads.
- Unknown efficacy in women with history of prior use of ZDV or other antiretroviral medication.
- Unknown efficacy in women initiating ZDV treatment later than 34 gestational weeks, during labor, or in infants without maternal use of ZDV during pregnancy and/or labor.

Source: Centers for Disease Control & Prevention (CDC). (1995). Recommendations of the U.S. Public Health Service Task Force on the use of zidovudine to reduce perinatal transmission of human immunodeficiency virus. *Morbidity and Mortality Weekly Report, 43*(RR-11), 1–20.

Table 14.5

1993 Revised Classification System for HIV Infection and Expanded AIDS Surveillance Case Definition for Adolescents (≥ 13 years) and Adults

	Clinical Categories		
CD4 + Lymphocyte Categories	(A) Asymptomatic, acute (primary) HIV, or persistent generalized lymphadenopathy (PGL)	(B) Symptomatic, not (A) or (C) conditions	(C) **AIDS-indicator conditions**
1. ≥ 500/μl	A1	B1	**C1**
2. 200 - 499/μl	A2	B2	**C2**
3. <200/μl (AIDS indicator T-cell count)	**A3**	**B3**	**C3**

* **AIDS-defining categories are represented in bold letters and numbers.**

Source: Centers for Disease Control & Prevention (CDC). (1992). 1993 Revised classification system for HIV infection and expanded surveillance case definition for AIDS among adolescents and adults. *Morbidity and Mortality Weekly Report, 41*(RR-17), p. 4.

Table 14.6

Clinical Categories and Conditions of HIV Infection

Category A Conditions	Category B Conditions	Category C Conditions
Asymptomatic HIV infection	Bacillary angiomatosis	Candidiasis of trachea, bronchi, or lungs
Persistent generalized lymphadenopathy	Oropharyngeal candidiasis (thrush)	Esophageal candidiasis
Acute (primary) HIV infection	Vulvovaginal candidiasis - persistent, frequent, or poorly responsive to treatment	Coccidioidomycosis - extrapulmonary or disseminated
	Cervical dysplasia (moderate - severe), carcinoma-in-situ	Cervical cancer, invasive
	Constitutional symptoms (e.g., fever [>38.5° C/101°F] or diarrhea lasting >1 month	Cryptococcosis, extrapulmonary
	Hairy leukoplakia, oral	Cryptosporidiosis, chronic intestinal of > 1 month's duration
	Herpes zoster - 2 distinct episodes, or involving more than 1 dermatome	Cytomegalovirus (CMV) disease (other than nodes, spleen, or liver)
	Idiopathic thrombocytopenia purpura	CMV retinitis (with loss of vision)
	Listeriosis	HIV-related encephalopathy
	Pelvic inflammatory disease (especially if complicated by tubo-ovarian abscess)	Herpes simplex - chronic ulcer(s) (> 1 month's duration); or bronchitis, pneumonitis, esophagitis
	Peripheral neuropathy	Histoplasmosis, extrapulmonary or disseminated
		Isosporiasis, chronic intestinal (> 1 month's duration)
		Kaposi's sarcoma
		Lymphoma, Burkitt's
		Mycobacterium avium complex or *M. kansasii* (disseminated or extrapulmonary)
		Mycobacterium tuberculosis (any site)
		Mycobacterium, other species or unidentified species, extrapulmonary or disseminated
		Pneumocystis carinii pneumonia
		Pneumonia, recurrent
		Progressive multifocal leukoencephalopathy
		Salmonella septicemia
		Toxoplasmosis of brain
		HIV wasting syndrome

Source: Centers for Disease Control & Prevention (CDC). (1992). 1993 Revised classification system for HIV infection and expanded surveillance case definition for AIDS among adolescents and adults. *Morbidity and Mortality Weekly Report, 41*(RR-17), 1–19.

Table 14.7

Indications for the Initiation of Antiretroviral Therapy

Clinical Category	CD4+ T Cell Count and HIV RNA	Recommendation
Symptomatic (e.g., AIDS, thrush, unexplained fever)	Any value	Treat
Asymptomatic	CD4+ T cells < 500/mm^3 or HIV RNA >10,000 (bDNA) or >20, 000 (RT-PCR)	Treatment should be offered. Strength of recommendation is based on prognosis for disease-free survival and willingness of the patient to accept therapy.
Asymptomatic	CD4+T cells > 500/mm3 and HIV RNA <10,000 (bDNA) or < 20,000 (RT-PCR)	Many experts would delay therapy and observe; however, some experts would treat.

*Some experts would observe patients with CD4+ T-cell counts between 350 and 500/mm^3 and HIV RNA levels <10,000 (bDNA) or <20,000 (RT-PCR)

Source: Carpenter, C. C., Fischl, M. A., Hammer, S. M., Hirsch, M. S., Jacobsen, D. M., Katzenstein, D. A., et al. (1997). Antiretroviral therapy for HIV infection in 1997. Updated recommendations of the International AIDS Society - USA Panel. *Journal of the American Medical Association, 277* (24), 1962-1969.

Table 14.8

Clinical Scenarios and Recommendations for the Use of Antiretroviral Drugs to Reduce the Risk of Perinatal HIV Transmission

1. **HIV-infected pregnant woman without previous antiretroviral (ARV) therapy.**	• HIV-infected pregnant woman must receive standard clinical, immunologic, and virologic evaluation. Recommendations for initiation and choice of ARV therapy should be based on the same parameters used for persons who are not pregnant. However, discussion of the unknown risks and benefits of a particular therapy during pregnancy must occur.
	• The three-part ZDV regimen should be recommended for all HIV-infected pregnant women to reduce the risk of perinatal transmission.
	• The combination of the ZDV regimen with additional ARV drugs for the treatment of HIV infection should be:
	  a. discussed with the woman
	  b. recommended for women whose clinical, immunologic, virologic status indicated the need for this therapy
	  c. offered to other infected women
	• Women who are in the first trimester of pregnancy may consider delaying initiation of therapy until after 10-12 weeks' gestation

2. **HIV-infected women receiving ARV therapy during the current pregnancy.**	• Women receiving ARV therapy in whom pregnancy is identified after the 1st trimester should continue therapy. • Women receiving ARV therapy in whom pregnancy is identified during the 1st trimester should be counseled regarding the benefits and potential risks of ARV administration during this period, and continuation of therapy should be considered. • If ARV therapy is discontinued during the 1st trimester, ALL drugs should be stopped simultaneously to avoid the development of resistance. • If the current maternal therapy regimen does not include ZDV, the addition of ZDV or substitution of ZDV with another nucleoside analogue ARV after 14 weeks' gestation is recommended. • ZDV administration during the intrapartum period and for the newborn is recommended.
3. **HIV-infected woman in labor who has had no prior ARV therapy.**	• Administration of intrapartum I.V. ZDV should be recommended along with the 6-week ZDV regimen for the infant. • Appropriate assessment of the woman during the immediate postpartum period should occur to determine whether ARV therapy is needed for her own health.

(Continued)

Table 14.8 (continued)

Clinical Scenarios and Recommendations for the Use of Antiretroviral Drugs to Reduce the Risk of Perinatal HIV Transmission

4. Infants born to HIV-infected mothers who have received no ARV therapy during pregnancy or during the intrapartum period.	• The 6-week neonatal ZDV component of the regimen should be discussed with the mother and offered for the newborn. • Neonatal ZDV should be initiated as soon as possible after birth—preferably within 12-24 hours after birth. • Some clinicians may choose to use ZDV in combination with other ARV drugs, particularly if the mother is known or suspected to have ZDV-resistant virus. However, the efficacy of this approach for prevention of transmission is unknown, and appropriate dosing regimens for neonates are incompletely defined. • Appropriate assessment of the woman during the immediate postpartum period should occur to determine whether ARV therapy is needed for her own health.

NOTE: Discussion of treatment options and recommendations should be noncoercive, and the final decision regarding the use of ARV drugs is the responsibility of the woman. A decision to not accept treatment with ZDV or other drugs should not result in punitive action or denial of care. Use of ZDV should not be denied to a woman who wishes to minimize exposure of the fetus to other ARV drugs and who therefore chooses to receive only ZDV during pregnancy to reduce the risk for perinatal transmission.

Source: Centers for Disease Control & Prevention (1998b). Public Health Service Task Force recommendations for the use of antiretroviral drugs in pregnant women infected with HIV-1 for maternal health and for reducing perinatal HIV-1 transmission in the United States. *Morbidity and Mortality Weekly Report, 47*(RR-2), 1–30.

Table 14.9

Antiretrovirals in Pregnant Women, Neonates, and Children

Antiretroviral Agent	FDA Approved			FDA Pregnancy Category	Placental Passage	Long-term Animal Carcinogenic Studies
	For Prevention of Perinatal Transmission	In Neonates	In Children			
NRTIs						
Didanosine (ddI, VIdex)	No	Yes	Yes	B	Yes (human)	Negative (no tumors, lifetime rodent study)
Lamivudine (3TC, Epivir)	No	No	Yes (> 4 mo)	C	Yes (human)	Negative (no tumors, lifetime rodent study)
Stavudine (d4T, Zerit)	No	No	Yes (> 1 mo)	C	Yes (rhesus)	Not completed
Zalcitabine (ddC, Hivid)	No	No	No	C	Yes (rhesus)	Positive (rodent, thymic lymphomas)
Zidovudine (AZT, ZDV, Retrovir)	Yes	Yes	Yes	C	Yes (human)	Positive (rodent, noninvasive vaginal epithelial tumors)
nNRTIs:						
Delavirdine (Rescriptor)	No	No	No	C	Unknown	Not completed
Nevirapine (Viramune)	No*	No	No	C	Yes (human)	Not completed
Protease Inhibitors:						
Indinavir (Crixivan)	No**	No**	No	C	Yes (rats)	Not completed
Nelfinavir (Viracept)	No**	No**	Yes (>2 mo)	B	Unknown	Not completed
Ritonavir (Norvir)	No**	No**	Yes (>2 mo)	B	Yes (rats)	Not completed
Saquinavir (Invirase)	No**	No**	No	B	Unknown	Not completed

NRTI: nucleoside reverse transcriptase inhibitor
nNRTI: nonnucleoside reverse transcriptase inhibitor

* Phase II/III perinatal study investigating the safety and efficacy of nevirapine administered to pregnant women and newborns is under way through the AIDS Clinical Trials Group (ACTG).

** Phase I perinatal studies investigating safety and pharmacokinetics of protease inhibitor administered to pregnant women and newborns are under way through the ACTG.

Adapted from Pitt, J., & Cotton, D. (1997). Treating the HIV-infected pregnant woman and her child. *AIDS Clinical Care, 9*(12), 91-93, 95. CDC, (1998b). Public Health Service Task Force recommendations for the use of antiretroviral drugs in pregnant women infected with HIV-1 for maternal health and for reducing perinatal HIV-1 transmission In the United States. *Morbidity and Mortality Weekly Report, 47*(RR-2), 1-30.

Table 14.10

Antiretroviral Medications, Dosages, Possible Side Effects, and Drug Interactions

Antiretroviral Medication	Dose	Possible Side Effects	Drug Interactions
Nucleoside Reverse Transcriptase Inhibitors (NRTI's)			
Zidovudine (AZT, ZDV, Retrovir)	200 mg. p.o. t.i.d. or 300 mg. p.o. b.i.d.	Malaise, nausea, headache, insomnia, myalgias, anemia, granulocytopenia, thrombocytopenia, seizures, toxic myopathy, lactic acidosis, hepatomegaly with steatosis, elevated aminotransferase levels; macrocytosis (expected effect that does not require intervention)	Probenecid may increase ZDV levels. Use of other myelosuppressive drugs (e.g., trimethoprim-sulfamethoxazole, ganciclovir) with ZDV requires careful monitoring.
Didanosine (ddI, Videx)	For patients > 60 kg: 200 mg. p.o. b.i.d. (as 2 100 mg. tablets)or 250 mg. p.o. b.i.d. powder For patients <60 kg: 125 mg. (tablet) p.o. b.i.d. or 167 mg. (powder) p.o. b.i.d.	Pancreatitis, painful peripheral neuropathy (dose related, reversible), nausea, abdominal cramping, diarrhea (related to antacid in formulation) diarrhea, hyperglycemia, hyperuricemia, headache, insomnia, seizures, elevated triglyceride & amylase levels, thrombocytopenia, retinal atrophy	Antacids & H_2 antagonists can increase ddI levels; avoid pancreatic toxins (e.g., alcohol, systemic pentamidine); avoid neurotoxic drugs (e.g., ddC, d4T, ganciclovir, vinca alkaloids). Drugs with impaired absorption due to coadministration with buffered products (e.g., ketoconazole, indinavir) will have decreased absorption when used with ddI (due to buffer in formulation of ddI). **NOTE:** Administer ddI on an empty stomach 2 hours apart from antacids, drugs whose absorption is impaired by buffered products, or H_2 antagonists.
Zalcitabine (ddC, Hivid)	0.75 mg. p.o. t.i.d. For patients <30 kg: 0.375 mg. p.o. t.i.d.	Peripheral neuropathy (dose related, reversible); stomatitis, aphthous ulcers, esophageal ulcers; rash; pancreatitis; elevated aminotransferase levels; cardiomyopathy	Avoid concomitant neurotoxic drugs (e.g., ddI, d4T, INH) and alcohol/other pancreatic toxins.

(Continued)

Table 14.10 (continued)

Antiretroviral Medications, Dosages, Possible Side Effects, and Drug Interactions

Antiretroviral Medication	Dose	Possible Side Effects	Drug Interactions
Stavudine (d4T, Zerit)	40 mg. p.o. b.i.d. For patients 40-60 kg: 30 mg. p.o. b.i.d. **NOTE:** Lower doses of this drug have been shown to be efficacious with less incidence of peripheral neuropathy. These doses are: 20 mg. p.o. b.i.d.; and for patients 40-60 kg: 15 mg. p.o. b.i.d.	Peripheral neuropathy; aminotransferase elevations; anemia, macrocytosis; insomnia, anxiety	Avoid concomitant use of neurotoxic or pancreatic toxic drugs.
Lamivudine (3TC, Epivir)	150 mg. p.o. b.i.d. For patients <50 kg: 2 mg/kg p.o. b.i.d.	Infrequent reports of nausea, headache, fatigue, insomnia, peripheral neuropathy, myalgia, rash; rare reports of neutropenia, thrombocytopenia	

(Continued)

Table 14.10 (continued)

Antiretroviral Medications, Dosages, Possible Side Effects, and Drug Interactions

Antiretroviral Medication	Dose	Possible Side Effects	Drug Interactions
Non-Nucleoside Reverse Transcriptase Inhibitors (nNRTIs)			
Nevirapine (Viramune)	200 mg. p.o. daily for 14 days; if no side effects (i.e., rash) then begin 200 mg. p.o. b.i.d.	Rash - maculopapular, can develop Stevens-Johnson syndrome; nausea, vomiting; fatigue; aminotransferase elevations; fever, headache	Induces the P-450 enzyme; therefore, avoid concomitant use of protease inhibitors, rifampin, rifabutin.
Delavirdine (Rescriptor)	200 mg. p.o. t.i.d. for 14 days; if no side effects (e.g., rash) then begin 400 mg. p.o. t.i.d.	See under Nevirapine	Inhibits P-450 enzyme; therefore, avoid concomitant use of rifampin, rifabutin, phenytoin, astemizole, carbamazepine. Increased levels of delavirdine when used concomitantly with ketoconazole, fluconazole, clarithromycin, and fluoxetine. Delavirdine increases levels of saquinavir and indinavir; therefore reductions in these protease inhibitor doses are indicated.
Protease Inhibitors (PI's)			
Saquinavir (Invirase)	600 mg. p.o. t.i.d.	Headache; nausea, abdominal pain, diarrhea; fever	Increased levels of saquinavir with concomitant use of ritonavir, delavirdine, ketoconazole, grapefruit juice. Avoid concomitant use of saquinavir with rifampin, rifabutin, phenobarbital, phenytoin, nevirapine, and other p-450 enzyme inducers. NOTE: Administer saquinavir within 2 hours of a high-fat meal to increase absorption. Saquinavir has poor bioavailability (i.e., 4%); however, concomitant use with ritonavir can enhance bioavailability. A more bioavailable preparation of saquinavir (Fortovase®) is being evaluated for use.

(Continued)

Table 14.10 (continued)

Antiretroviral Medications, Dosages, Possible Side Effects, and Drug Interactions

Antiretroviral Medication	Dose	Possible Side Effects	Drug Interactions
Ritonavir (Norvir)	300 mg. p.o. b.i.d. increasing to 600 mg. p.o. b.i.d. over 4 - 6 days (to reduce GI side effects); then 600 mg. p.o. b.i.d..	Nausea, vomiting, diarrhea, anorexia; fatigue, headache, circumoral paresthesia, dizziness; increased aminotransferase, triglycerides, cholesterol, creatine phosphokinase levels	Multiple drug interactions due to ritonavir's potent P-450 enzyme inhibition. Avoid concomitant use of rifabutin, rifampin, terfenadine, astemizole, cisapride, and some benzodiazepine derivatives. Dosages of some antidepressants and narcotics need to be adjusted when used with ritonavir. Combination of ritonavir and saquinavir (with adjustment in doses for both drugs) can be initiated in patients with increased viral load measurements. NOTE: Ritonavir capsules must be refrigerated. Liquid preparation stable at room temperature for up to 30 days.
Indinavir (Crixivan)	800 mg. p.o. every 8 hours Dose reduced to 600 mg. p.o. every 8 hours for patients with hepatic disease	Nephrolithiasis; asymptomatic hyperbilirubinemia; elevated aminotransferase levels; nausea, vomiting, diarrhea, abdominal pain; headache; rash; physical changes including increased abdominal girth, decreased upper extremity mass, "buffalo hump" of upper back	Avoid concomitant use of rifampin, astemizole, cisapride, triazolam, terfenadine, midazolam. Decrease rifabutin dosage if used with indinavir. Decrease indinavir dosage when used with ketoconazole. Increase indinavir dose if given with nevirapine. NOTE: Patients must drink at least six 8-ounce glasses of noncaffeinated beverages daily (to reduce likelihood of nephrolithiasis). Indinavir must be taken on an empty stomach or with milk, juice, coffee, tea. Indinavir and ddI must be administered at least 1 hour apart.
Nelfinavir (Viracept)	750 mg. p.o. t.i.d. For patients having difficulty with adherence to t.i.d. dosing, some clinicians will prescribe Nelfinavir at 1250 mg. p.o. b.i.d	Loose stools, diarrhea	Inhibitor of P-450 enzyme; therefore, avoid concomitant use with rifampin, rifabutin, astemizole, terfenadine, cisapride.

Sources: Goldschmidt, R. H., & Dong, B. J. (1997). Treatment of AIDS and HIV-related conditions1997. *Journal of American Board of Family Practice, 10*(2), 144 - 167.
Sanford, J. P., Gilbert, D. N., Moellering, Jr., R. C., & Sande, M. A. (1997). *The Sanford guide to HIV/AIDS therapy* (6th ed.). Vienna, VA: Antimicrobial Therapy, Inc.

Appendix 14.5a

Support for Clinicians and HIV-infected Persons

Free telephone consultation for clinicians
The HIV Warmline
Monday through Friday, 7:30 AM to 5 PM (Pacific Standard Time)
1 (800) 933-3413
This service is provided by the AIDS Education Training Center (AETC) Program at San Francisco General Hospital.

Information about clinical research trials
The AIDS Clinical Trials Information Service
1 (800) 874-2572

Information about HIV treatment
The American Foundation for AIDS Research
1 (800) 392-6327

Information about antiretroviral therapy during pregnancy and perinatal outcomes
Antiretroviral Pregnancy Registry
1 (800) 722-9292, extension 38465

Information about post-exposure prophylaxis (PEP)
Centers for Disease Control and Prevention Registry
(888) 737-4448 or (888) HIV-4PEP

Women Organized Against Life-Threatening Disease (WORLD)
P.O. Box 11535
Oakland, CA 94611
Telephone: (510) 658-6930
Provides information and support to women with HIV infection.

National AIDS HOTLINE
1-800-342-2437
Provides consumer information about HIV.
1 (800) 874-2572

References

American College of Obstetricians and Gynecologists (ACOG). (1992). Human immunodeficiency virus infection. *ACOG Technical Bulletin no. 165.* Washington, DC: the Author.

Anastos, K., & Greenblatt, R. (1994). Epidemiology and natural history of HIV infection among women. *HIV Advances in Research and Therapy, 4*(2), 11-20.

Baker, D. (1994). Management of the female HIV-infected patient. *AIDS Research and Human Retroviruses, 10*(8), 935-938.

Bardequez, A. D.(1996). Management of HIV infection for the childbearing age woman. *Clinical Obstetrics and Gynecology, 39*(2), 344-360.

Blanche, S. (1994). HIV in infants and children: Transmission and progression. *HIV Advances in Research and Therapy, 4*(3), 9-13.

Boyer, P., Dillon, M., Navaie, M., Deveikis, A., Keller, M., O'Rourke, S. et al. (1994). Factors predictive of maternal-fetal transmission of HIV-1. Preliminary analysis of zidovudine given during pregnancy and/or delivery. *Journal of the American Medical Association, 271*(24), 1925-1930.

Burns, D. N., Landesman, S., Muenz, L. R., Nugent, R. P., Goedert, J. J., Minkoff, H. et al. (1994). Cigarette smoking, premature rupture of membranes, and vertical transmission of HIV-1 among women with low CD4+ levels. *Journal of Acquired Immune Deficiency Syndromes, 7*(7), 718-726.

Carpenter, C. C. J., Mayer, K. H., Stein, M. D., Leibman, B. D., Fisher, A., & Fiore, T. C. (1991). Human immunodeficiency virus infection in North American women: Experience with 200 cases and a review of the literature. *Medicine, 70*(5), 307-325.

Carpenter, C. C. J., Fischl, M. A., Hammer, S. M., Hirsch, M. S., Jacobsen, D. M., Katzenstein, D. A., et al. (1996). Consensus statement. Antiretroviral therapy for HIV infection in 1996. Recommendation of an International Panel. *Journal of the American Medical Association, 276*(2), 146-154.

Casey, C. M., Cohen F., & Hughes A. (1996). *ANAC's core curriculum for HIV/AIDS nursing.* Philadelphia: Nursecom.

Caschetta, M. B. (1992). A review of reports on women and HIV. *Treatment Issues, 6*(10), 2-6.

Centers for Disease Control & Prevention (CDC). (1981). Kaposi's sarcoma and *Pneumocystis* pneumonia among homosexual men—New York City and California. *Morbidity and Mortality Weekly Report, 30,* 305-308.

CDC. (1982). Possible transfusion-associated acquired immune deficiency syndrome (AIDS)—California. *Morbidity and Mortality Weekly Report, 31,* 652-654.

CDC. (1992). 1993 Revised classification system for HIV infection and expanded surveillance case definition for AIDS among adolescents and adults. *Morbidity and Mortality Weekly Report, 41*(RR-17), 1-19.

CDC. (1994). Zidovudine for the prevention of HIV transmission from mother to infant. *Morbidity and Mortality Weekly Report, 43*(16), 285-287.

CDC. (1995a). Update: Mortality attributable to HIV infection among persons ages 25-44 years—United States, 1994. *Morbidity and Mortality Weekly Report, 45*(6), 121-125.

CDC. (1995b). U.S. Public Health Service recommendations for human immunodeficiency virus counseling and voluntary testing for pregnant women. *Morbidity and Mortality Weekly Report, 44*(RR-7), 1-13.

CDC. (1995c). Recommendations of the U. S. Public Health Service Task Force on the use of zidovudine to reduce perinatal transmission of human immunodeficiency virus. *Morbidity and Mortality Weekly Report, 43*(RR-11), 1-20.

CDC. (1995d). USPHS/IDSA guidelines for the prevention of opportunistic infections in persons infected with human immunodeficiency virus: A summary. *Morbidity and Mortality Weekly Report, 44*(RR-8), 1-34.

CDC. (1997a). *HIV/AIDS surveillance report* (June, pp. 3-37). Atlanta: U.S. Department of Health and Human Services, Public Health Service.

CDC. (1997b). Update: Trends in AIDS incidence, deaths, and prevalence - United States, 1996. *Morbidity and Mortality Weekly Report, 46*(8), 165-173.

CDC. (1997c). Anergy skin testing and preventive therapy for HIV-infected persons: Revised recommendations. *Morbidity and Mortality Weekly Report, 46*(RR-15), 1-10.

CDC. (1998a). Administration of zidovudine during late pregnancy and delivery to prevent perinatal HIV transmission - Thailand, 1996-1997. *Morbidity and Mortality Weekly Report, 47*(8), 151-154.

CDC. (1998b). Public Health Service Task Force recommendations for the use of antiretroviral drugs in pregnant women infected with HIV-1 for maternal health and for reducing perinatal HIV-1 transmission in the United States. *Morbidity and Mortality Weekly Report, 47*(RR-2), 1-30.

Clark, R. A., Brandon, W., Dumestre, J., & Pindaro, C. (1993). Clinical manifestations of infection with the human immunodeficiency virus in women in Louisiana. *Clinical Infectious Diseases, 17*(August), 165-172.

Conner, E. M., Sperling, R. S., Gelber, R., Kiselev, P., Scott, G., O'Sullivan, M. J. et al. (1994). Reduction of maternal-infant transmission of human immunodeficiency virus type 1 with zidovudine treatment. Pediatric AIDS Clinical Trials Group Protocol 076 Study Group. *The New England Journal of Medicine, 331*(18), 1173-1180.

Cosby, C. D., & Stringari, S. E. (1991). Primary care for the HIV-seropositive adult: Nurse practitioners prepare for the challenge of the 1990s. *Nurse Practitioner Forum, 2*(2), 116-125.

Cotton, D., & Watts, H. (1995). Management of HIV infection during pregnancy: New options, new questions. *AIDS Clinical Care, 7*(6), 45-49.

Cullen, M. T., Sanches-Ramos, L., & Delke, I. (1992). Prenatal diagnosis of HIV infection: The use of cordocentesis, polymerase chain reaction, and p24 antigen assay (abstract). *American Journal of Obstetrics and Gynecology, 168*, 386.

Des Jarlais, D. C., & Friedman, S. R. (1988). HIV infection among persons who inject illicit drugs: Problems and perspectives. *Journal of Acquired Immunodeficiency Syndromes, 1*, 267-272.

Dickover, R. E., Garratty, E. M., Herman, S. A., Sim, M. S., Plaeger, S., Boyer, P. J., et al. (1995). Identification of levels of maternal HIV-1 RNA associated with risk of perinatal transmission. *Journal of the American Medical Association, 275*(8), 599-605.

Dunn, D. T., Newell, M. L., Ades, A. E., & Peckham, C. S. (1992). Risk of human immunodeficiency virus type 1 transmission through breast-feeding. *Lancet, 340*, 585-588.

El-Sadr, W., Oleske, J. M., Agins, B. D., Bauman, K., Brosgart, C., et al. (1994). Evaluation and management of early HIV infection. *Clinical practice guideline No. 7*, AHCPR Publication No. 94-0572. Rockville, MD: Agency for Health Care Policy and Research, Public Health Service, U. S. Department of Health and Human Services.

European Collaborative Study (1992). Risk factors for mother-to-child transmission of HIV-1. *Lancet, 339*, 1001-1012.

Fang, G., Burger, H., Grimson, R., Tropper, P., Nachman, S., Mayer, D. et al. (1994). Maternal plasma human immunodeficiency virus type 1 RNA level: A determinant and projected threshold for mother-to-child transmission. *Proceedings of the National Academy of Science, 92*, 12100-12104.

Goedert, J. J., Duliege, A. M., Amos, C. I., Felton, S., & Biggar, R. J. (1991). International register of HIV-exposed twins. High risk of infection with human immunodeficiency virus type 1 for first-born, vaginally delivered twins. *Lancet, 338*, 1471-1475.

Goldschmidt, R. H., & Dong, B. J. (1997). Treatment of AIDS and HIV-related conditions—1997. *Journal of the American Board of Family Practice, 10*(2), 144-167.

Grady, C., & Vogel, S. (1993). Laboratory methods for diagnosing and monitoring HIV infection. *Journal of the American Association of Nurses in AIDS Care, 4*(2), 11-21.

Gwinn, M., & Wortley, P. M. (1996). Epidemiology of HIV infection in women and newborns. *Clinical Obstetrics and Gynecology, 39*(2), 292-304.

Ho, D., Neumann, A. U., Perelson, A. S., Chen, W., & Leonard, J. M. (1995). Rapid turnover of plasma virions and CD4 lymphocytes in HIV-1 infection. *Nature, 373*, 123-126.

Imam, N., Carpenter, C. C. J., Mayer, K. H., Fisher, A., Stein, M., & Danforth, S. B. (1990). Hierarchical pattern of mucosal candida infection in HIV-seropositive women. *The American Journal of Medicine, 89*, 142-146.

Lawlor, G., Fischer, T., & Adelman, D. (1995). *Manual of allergy and immunology* (3rd ed.). Boston: Little, Brown.

Maiman, M., Fruchter, R. G., Serur, E., Remy, J. C., Feuer, G., & Boyce, J. (1990). Human immunodeficiency virus infection and cervical neoplasia. *Gynecologic Oncology, 38*, 377-382.

Mandelbrot, L., Le Chenadec, J., Berrebi, A., Bongain, A., Benifla, J.L., Delfraissy, J.F., Blanche, S., Mayaux, M. Jeanne (1998). Perinatal HIV-1 transmission. Interaction between zidovudine prophylaxis and mode of delivery in the French Perinatal Cohort. Journal of the American Medical Association, *280*(1), 55-60.

Marte, C., Cohen, M., Fruchter, R., & Kelly P. (1992). Pap test and STD findings in HIV-positive women at ambulatory care sites. *American Journal of Obstetrics and Gynecology, 166*(4), 1232-1237.

Matheson, P. B., Abrams, E. J., Thomas, P. A., Hernan, M. A., Thea, D. M., Lambert, G., et al. (1994). Efficacy of antenatal zidovudine in reducing perinatal transmission of human immunodeficiency virus type 1. *Journal of Infectious Disease, 172*(August), 353-358.

Mellors, J. W., Rinaldo, Jr., C. R., Gupta, P., White, R. M., Todd, J. R., & Kingsley, L. A. (1996). Prognosis in HIV-1 infection predicted by the quantity of virus in plasma. *Science, 272*(5265), 1167-1170.

Minkoff, H. L. (1991). Gynecologic care of HIV-infected women. *Contemporary OB/Gyn, 35*(9), 46-60.

Minkoff, H. L. (1995). Pregnancy and HIV infection. In H. Minkoff, J. A. DeHovitz, & A. Duerr (Eds.), *HIV infection in women* (pp. 173-188). New York: Raven Press.

Minkoff, H., & DeHovitz, J. A. (1991). HIV infection in women. *AIDS Clinical Care, 3*(5), 33-35.

Minkoff, H. L., Willoughby, A., Mendez, H. et al. (1990). Serious infections during pregnancy among women with advanced human immunodeficiency virus infection. *American Journal of Obstetrics and Gynecology, 162*, 30-34.

Nesheim, S. R. (1996). The diagnosis and management of perinatal HIV infection. *Clinical Obstetrics and Gynecology, 39*(2), 396-410.

O'Brien, W. A. (1996). Vaccinations for patients with HIV: Weighing risks and benefits. *HIV Advances in Research and Therapy, 6*(2), 22-27.

Orloff, S. L., Simonds, R. J., Steketee R. W., & St. Louis, M. E. (1996). Determinants of perinatal HIV-1 transmission. *Clinical Obstetrics and Gynecology, 39*(2), 386-395.

Padian, N., Marquis, L., Francis, D. P., Anderson, R. E., Rutherford, G. W., O'Malley, P. M. et al. (1987). Male-to-female transmission of human immunodeficiency virus. *Journal of the American Medical Association, 258*, 788-790.

Panteleo, G., Graziosi, C., Demarest, J. F., Butini, L., Montroni, M., Fox, C. H., Orenstein, J. M., Kotler, D. P., & Fauci, A. S. (1993). HIV infection is active and progressive in lymphoid tissue during the clinically latent stage of disease. *Nature, 362*(6418), 355-358.

Peckham, C., & Gibbs, D. (1995). Mother-to-child transmission of the human immunodeficiency virus. *The New England Journal of Medicine, 333*(5), 298-302.

Pitt, J., & Cotton, D. (1997). Treating the HIV-infected pregnant woman and her child. *AIDS Clinical Care, 9*(12), 91-93, 95.

Rhoads, J. L., Wright, C., Redfield, R. R., & Burke, D. (1987). Chronic vaginal candidiasis in women with human immunodeficiency virus infection. *Journal of the American Medical Association, 257*(22), 3105-3107.

Rompalo, A. M., Anderson, J. R., & Quinn, T. C. (1992). Reproductive tract infections and their management in women infected with the human immunodeficiency virus. *Infectious Diseases in Clinical Practice, 1*(5), 277-286.

Saag, M. S., Holodniy, M., Kuritzkes, D. R., O'Brien, W. A., Coombs, R. W., Poscher, M. E., et al. (1996). HIV viral load markers in clinical practice. *Nature Medicine, 2*(6), 625-629.

Sanford, J. P., Gilbert, D. N., Moellering, Jr., R. C., & Sande, M. A. (1997). *The Sanford guide to HIV/AIDS therapy* (6th ed.). Vienna, VA: Antimicrobial Therapy, Inc.

Shannon, M. T. (1995). Human immunodeficiency virus (HIV). In W. L. Star, L. L. Lommel, & M. T. Shannon (Eds.), *Women's primary health care: Protocols for practice* (pp. 11-25 - 11-38). Washington, DC: American Nurses Publishing.

Shin, D. M., & Avers, J. (1988). *AIDS/HIV reference guide for medical professionals* (3rd ed). Los Angeles: Regents of the University of California.

Smith, D. K., & Rogers, M. F. (1996). Immunopathogenesis and detection of HIV infection in women and newborns. *Clinical Obstetrics and Gynecology, 39*(2), 277-291.

Sperling, R. S., Shapiro, D. E., Coombs, R. W., Todd, J. A., Herman, S. A., McSherry, G. D., O'Sullivan, M. J., Van Dyke, R. B., Jimenez, E., Rouzioux, C., Flynn, P. M., & Sullivan, J. L. (1996). Maternal viral load, zidovudine treatment, and the risk of transmission of human immunodeficiency virus type 1 from mother to infant. *New England Journal of Medicine, 335*(22), 1621-1629.

Thomas, P. A., Weedon, J., Krasinski, K., Abrams, E., Shaffer, N., Matheson, P., et al. (1994). Maternal predictors of perinatal human immunodeficiency virus transmission. *Pediatric Infectious Disease Journal, 13*(6), 489-495.

Weiser, B., Nachman, S., Tropper, P., Viscosi, K. H., Grimson, R., Baxter, G., et al. (1994). Quantitation of human immunodeficiency virus type 1 during pregnancy: Relationship of viral titer to mother-to-child transmission and stability of viral load. *Proceedings of the National Academy of Science, 91*, 8037-8041.

Chapter 6

SYPHILIS

Winifred L. Star

Stages of Disease

Syphilis is a chronic infectious disease caused by the *Treponema pallidum*, a motile spirochete. Transmission is predominantly via sexual contact or can occur transplacentally from mother to fetus. Occasionally, syphilis is transmitted by blood transfusion.

Sexual exposure to a person with active mucocutaneous syphilis carries up to a 60 percent risk of acquiring the disease (Thin, 1990). The organism often enters the host through disrupted epithelium at sites of minor trauma incurred during sexual activity (Hook III & Marra, 1992). Following exposure, the incubation period is approximately 21 days with a range of 10 to 90 days. After this time, the hallmark of primary syphilis—the chancre—develops at the site of inoculation. Associated regional lymphadenopathy is also present in 60 to 80 percent of these cases. When untreated, the chancre resolves spontaneously in 2 to 6 weeks (Chapel, 1984; Gibbs & Sweet, 1994; Thin, 1990).

Secondary syphilis appears from between 3 to 6 weeks and 6 months after primary inoculation; however primary and secondary syphilis may overlap (about 30 percent of cases have a healing chancre at the onset of secondary infection) (McPhee, 1984). The secondary stage is characterized by a widespread maculopapular skin rash, mucous membrane lesions, condylomata lata, and generalized lymphadenopathy. The skin lesions of secondary syphilis usually resolve in 2 to 6 weeks with or without treatment. Additional findings of secondary syphilis may include meningitis and hepatitis; renal, bone, and/or joint involvement resulting in cranial nerve palsies; jaundice; nephrotic syndrome; and arthritis and/or periostitis (Goens, Janniger, & De Wolf, 1994; Jacobs, 1996; Thin, 1990). Cutaneous lesions of secondary syphilis will resolve with or without treatment. Untreated persons will enter a latent stage, which for the majority of individuals, is asymptomatic.

The latent stage is divided into two phases: *early latent* (i.e., less than 1 year duration) and *late latent* (i.e., greater than 1 year duration). About 25 percent of individuals in the early latent phase experience an exacerbation of the mucocutaneous lesions of secondary syphilis. The latent stage is infectious only if lesions are present or, during pregnancy, when the spirochete may be transmitted transplacentally. About one third of persons with latent disease may remain in this phase for life; another one-third will develop late or *tertiary syphilis* (Centers for Disease Control and Prevention [CDC], 1991; Gibbs & Sweet, 1994; Jacobs, 1996).

Tertiary syphilis is noncontagious and includes neurosyphilis, which may also occur at any stage; cardiovascular syphilis; and gummatous (i.e., benign tertiary) syphilis. The onset of this late stage may occur from 1 to 20 years after the initial infection. The lesions of tertiary syphilis can be extremely destructive and permanently disabling (CDC, 1991; Jacobs, 1996). As previously mentioned, neurosyphilis is not limited to the tertiary stage of syphilis; rather, this condition encompasses a variety of syndromes spanning all stages of syphilis (e.g., meningitis, meningovascular syphilis, general paresis, and tabes dorsalis). There has been recent evidence of disease shift—away from the more traditional, symptomatic forms of neurosyphilis—to asymptomatic central nervous system (CNS) involvement (i.e., asymptomatic neurosyphilis), comprising subtler, less well-defined syndromes (Hook III & Marra, 1992; Lukehart et al., 1988).

Human Immunodeficiency Virus (HIV) and Syphilis

Genital ulcerative diseases are associated with a threefold to fivefold increased risk for the acquisition of human immunodeficiency virus (HIV) in exposed individuals (Hook III, 1996). Coinfection of syphilis with HIV is common. HIV-infected persons may display atypical presentations of syphilis, are more likely to present with secondary syphilis, and are at increased risk of syphilis reactivation. In addition, they may have altered serological responses, increased complication rates, inadequate responses to therapy, and/or more rapid progression to neurosyphilis or tertiary syphilis (Goens et al., 1994; Hollander & Katz, 1996; Jacoby & Steinberg, 1996; Jacobs, 1996). The immune dysfunction associated with HIV infection may allow greater treponemal proliferation during pregnancy and increase the rate of fetal infection (Ingall, Sánchez, & Musher, 1995).

Congenital Infection

Transmission of *T. pallidum* to a fetus may occur at any time during gestation; the magnitude of risk is directly related to the stage of maternal infection. Pregnant women with primary or secondary syphilis are more likely to transmit the infection (50 percent risk) than those in the early latent or late latent phase of disease (40 percent and 10 percent risk respectively). Infection may also occur at the time of delivery via fetal contact with an infectious genital lesion. Untreated syphilis during pregnancy may result in spontaneous abortion, preterm labor and delivery, stillbirth, nonimmune hydrops, or neonatal death. (Gibbs & Sweet, 1994; Sánchez & Wendel, 1997).

Congenital infection may manifest as either early or late congenital syphilis in the offspring. Early congenital infection refers to manifestations that appear within the first 2 years of life: maculopapular rash; rhinitis or "snuffles"; oropharyngeal mucous patches; hepatosplenomegaly; jaundice; lymphadenopathy; skeletal abnormalities (e.g., osteochondritis, periostitis); CNS involvement (e.g., syphilitic leptomeningitis, meningovascular syphilis); ocular abnormalities (e.g., chorioretinitis, glaucoma, uveitis); and renal dysfunction. Most infants with early congenital syphilis are asymptomatic at birth; active disease may not become evident until 3 to 8 weeks of life. If left untreated, or incompletely treated, manifestations of late congenital syphilis will appear, such as Hutchinson's teeth, mulberry molars, interstitial keratitis, eighth nerve deafness, "saddle nose," rhagades, frontal bossing, saber shins, and CNS sequelae (Berry & Dajani, 1992; Gibbs & Sweet, 1994; Ingall, Sánchez, & Musher, 1995; Sánchez, 1992). It is critical that CDC guidelines for the evaluation and treatment of infants with suspected congenital syphilis are strictly followed.

Epidemiology

An epidemic of syphilis occurred in the United States between 1986 and 1990, with the greatest incidence occurring among heterosexual black and Hispanic Americans in urban areas. At the peak in 1990, syphilis rates were reported at 20.3 cases per 100,000 people. Causes for the epidemic were attributed to crack cocaine use, the exchange of sex for money or drugs, reduction in resources for syphilis-control programs, rising poverty rates, the disenfranchisement of minority groups, and the use of spectinomycin for treatment of penicillinase-producing *Neisseria gonorrhoeae* (Nakashima, Rolfs, Flock, Kilmarx, & Greenspan, 1996; Sánchez & Wendel, 1997). In 1991 the number of reported cases of primary and secondary syphilis declined for the first time since 1985. In l994, the rate of infection was 7 to 8 cases per 100,000 persons (Gilstrap & Wendel, 1996). Incidence continues to be high in minority populations especially in the South. The male: female disease ratio for primary and secondary syphilis has decreased steadily, reflecting the larger incidence percentage among females during the epidemic period; the ratio is now 1:1 (Nakashima et al., 1996). Trends in congenital syphilis cases parallel these same rates for women. In 1992, cases of congenital syphilis decreased for the first time since 1980. The majority of cases are seen in young, unmarried women of lower socioeconomic background receiving inadequate or no prenatal care (Ingall, Sánchez, & Musher, 1995). The age distribution for syphilis differs from that of patients presenting with other bacterial STDs. Syphilis persists in both sexes into their early 30s, as opposed to other STDs, which affect mostly teens and adults under 24 years of age (Nakashima et al., 1996).

The sections to follow will address features of primary, secondary, and latent stages of syphilis as well as selected aspects of neurosyphilis and congenital syphilis. Late (i.e., tertiary) syphilis and management of syphilis in HIV-infected women will not be discussed in detail; the reader is directed to a current textbook for further information. The CDC publication on treatment guidelines for STDs will be valuable in augmenting this chapter (see CDC, 1998).

Database

Subjective

Risk/Predisposing Factors

- Positive sexual contact
- Concomitant STD, HIV infection
- Multiple sexual partners
- Commercial sex work (i.e., prostitution)
- Nonuse of barrier contraception
- Use of illicit drugs, especially crack cocaine
- Exchange of sex for drugs or money
- Urban dweller
- Limited access to health care
- Low socioeconomic status
- Lack of prenatal care (risk for congenital syphilis)
- African- and Latin-American minority groups (mainly in large urban areas of New York, California, Florida, Texas, and Michigan) (Sánchez & Wendel, 1997)

Symptomatology

Primary Syphilis

- May be asymptomatic (i.e., primary lesion may go unnoticed)
- Client may report
    - ▶ Genital or nongenital lesion (usually solitary, raised, ulcerated, painless; heals within 6 weeks)
    - ▶ Nontender regional lymph node enlargement

- Associated symptoms may include vaginal/urethral discharge, rectal pain on defecation, rectal bleeding, mucoid or blood-tinged stool

Secondary Syphilis

- Influenza-like symptoms (sore throat, malaise, headache, fever, anorexia, fatigue, weight loss, myalgia, arthralgia)

- Maculopapular skin rash involving face, trunk, extremities including palms and soles; may be pruritic

- Large, raised wartlike lesions on vulva, anus, or other warm, moist body areas

- Mucosal ulcers affecting various mucous membranes

- Generalized nontender swelling of lymph glands

- Persistence of chancre of primary syphilis (30 percent of cases)

- Additional symptoms may include, but are not limited to, patchy hair loss, joint/bone pain, abdominal pain, or symptoms of meningitis later described

  NOTE: Pregnancy has little effect on the manifestations of early (i.e., primary or secondary) syphilis (Wendel, 1990).

Latent Syphilis

- Client may note that lesions of secondary stage have healed.

- Early latent stage: Secondary syphilis relapses may occur if disease escaped diagnosis/ treatment. Neurologic relapse may be fulminating; death may ensue.

- Late latent stage: Asymptomatic—client may report history of syphilis with inadequate treatment.

Neurosyphilis

Asymptomatic Neurosyphilis

- No presenting complaints.

Syphilitic Meningitis

- Incubation period less than 1 year; most common in young adults.

- Client may complain of rash, headache, fever, stiff neck, photophobia, nausea and/or vomiting.

- Additional symptoms may include tinnitus, hearing loss, facial weakness, visual disturbances, seizures, aphagia, hemiplegia, confusion, and delirium.

Meningovascular Syphilis

- Most persons are over 30 years of age, and cases usually occur 5 to 12 years after initial infection.

- Client may report headache, dizziness, insomnia, memory loss, mood disturbances, personality or behavioral changes, slowing of mentation/speech, hemiparesis, aphasia, seizures.

<u>General Paresis and Tabes Dorsalis</u>

- This condition is not commonly found in an ambulatory obstetric population; consequently, further details will not be included here.

Tertiary (Late) Syphilis

- Refer to current textbook for further information.

History

- A *complete* medical history should be obtained with particular focus on
  - ▶ Signs/symptoms of STDs in client and partners(s)
  - ▶ Previous STDs (i.e., date, type, treatment) of client and partner(s)
  - ▶ Sexual history including
    - – Sex with men/women/both
    - – Date of last sexual encounter
    - – Number of partners in past month [3 months, 6 months, year]
    - – Type(s) of sexual practice(s)
    - – Drug injection activities of client and/or partner(s)
    - – History of laboratory tests for syphilis, HIV, hepatitis
    - – Other risk factors
- Review of systems pertinent to signs/symptoms of syphilis, other STDs

Objective

- A *thorough* STD examination includes the following assessments:
  - ▶ Vital signs, as indicated
  - ▶ General skin inspection of face, trunk, forearms, palms, and soles for lesions, rashes, or discoloration
  - ▶ Inspection of pharynx/oral cavity for erythema, injection, lesions, or discoloration
  - ▶ Abdominal inspection/palpation for masses, tenderness, or rebound tenderness
  - ▶ Inspection of pubic hair for lice/nits
  - ▶ Inspection of external genitalia for discharge, masses, or lesions; inspection, palpation of Bartholin's/urethral/Skene's glands for discharge or masses
  - ▶ Inspection of vagina for blood, discharge, or lesions
  - ▶ Inspection of cervix for lesions, discharge, eversion, erythema, edema, or friability; assessment for cervical motion tenderness
  - ▶ Uterine assessment for size, shape, consistency, mobility, and tenderness

- ▶ Palpation of adnexa for masses or tenderness

- ▶ Inspection of perianus/anus/rectum for lesions, bleeding, or discharge

- ▶ Rectal examination, as indicated, for masses or tenderness

- ▶ Assessment of presence or absence of associated cervical and inguinal lymphadenopathy (CDC, 1991)

Stages of Disease

Primary Syphilis

- Physical examination findings may reveal

  - ▶ Genital lesion

    - Usually solitary, nontender

    - Progresses from 5 to 10 mm dull red macule to papule to ulcer (i.e., chancre)

      * Clean red base with yellow-gray exudate

      * Indurated margin (stippled hemorrhage/dilated capillaries may encircle margin)

    - Chancre may occur at urethral meatus (1 to 3 percent of cases), in vagina (less than 1 percent of cases), or at cervix (5 to 44 percent of cases)

  - ▶ Nongenital lesions (5 percent of chancres)

    - May appear on lips (which is the most common site), tongue; tonsils, gingiva (rare), finger, eyelid, breast, nipple, or anus.

    - May have atypical appearance.

      NOTE: Anal chancres can be very painful, and often mistaken for herpes simplex lesions or anal fissures. Indications of chancre are a more peripheral location, irregular configuration, and mirror image (i.e., "kissing" configuration) (Celum, 1996).

  - ▶ Regional lymphadenopathy—nontender, small to moderate-sized rubbery, nonsuppurative nodes

Secondary Syphilis

- Physical examination findings may reveal

  - ▶ Elevated temperature; weight loss

  - ▶ Persistence of chancre

  - ▶ Macular eruption: 5 to 10 mm pink, rounded macular lesions initially presenting on trunk, upper extremities; blanch on palpation; appear vascular; may persist 1 to 2 months

  - ▶ Papular eruption: Follows macular eruption; reddish-copper, firm, scaling papular lesions involving trunk, face, and extremities including palms and soles. Variations may include

    - Split papules—eroded, fissured papules affecting intertriginous areas (e.g., mouth angles, nasal folds, behind ears)

- Condylomata lata—raised, lobulated, or smooth papules with moist eroded surfaces in intertriginous or other warm, moist areas (e.g., vulva, anus).

  NOTE: Highly infectious lesion; resembles condylomata acuminata but more moist

- Atypical lesions—pustular, psoriatic, papulonodular

▶ Mucosal lesions

- "Syphilitic sore throat"—most common mucosal lesion; diffuse inflammation of pharynx/tonsils.

- "Mucous patch"—7 to 10 mm slightly raised, erythematous papule with central erosion and gray/pearly membrane; may affect any mucous membrane. **NOTE:** Highly infectious lesion

▶ Alopecia: Patchy loss on scalp, eyelashes, eyebrows; diffuse thinning of hair may also occur.

▶ Lymphadenopathy: discrete, nontender, moderately enlarged, rubbery nodes in inguinal, suboccipital, posterior cervical, axillary, epitrochlear areas.

▶ Additional findings as discussed in the introduction

● Neurological examination to be performed as indicated. It may include, but not be limited to hearing assessment, assessment for extraocular movements, and other cranial nerve tests.

Latent Syphilis

● Physical examination findings may reveal

▶ Healed lesions of secondary stage; clinical findings are usually limited to positive nontreponemal and treponemal tests

▶ Relapse of secondary signs in 25 percent of cases

Neurosyphilis

Asymptomatic Neurosyphilis

● Absence of neurological findings

● Presence of abnormalities in cerebrospinal fluid (CSF) (see *Diagnostic Tests*)

Syphilitic Meningitis

● Physical examination findings may include elevated temperature; rash of secondary syphilis; nuchal rigidity; positive Kernig's sign; papilledema; third, sixth, seventh, and eighth cranial nerve deficits; or higher frequency hearing loss (Swartz, 1990) (see Diagnostic Tests section).

Meningovascular Syphilis

● Neurological findings will vary depending on the area of the brain that is affected.

● Prominent features may include, but are not limited to the following: aphasia, hemiplegia, hemianesthesia, homonymous hemianopia, choreoathetoid movements, loss of pain/temperature sense, hoarseness, palatal paralysis, diminished gag reflex, nystagmus, and hiccup (Swartz, 1990). Refer to a current textbook for further information.

Tertiary (Late) Syphilis

- Refer to a current textbook for further information.

Congenital Syphilis

- See the introduction.
- Antenatal sonography may reveal placentomegaly, hepatosplenomegaly, intrauterine growth restriction, fetal edema, ascites, hydrops.
- See Table 14.7, Congenital Syphilis Definition, for CDC case definition of congenital syphilis.

Assessment

- Syphilis (note stage)
  - ▶ R/O syphilis
  - ▶ R/O other STDs, such as herpes simplex virus infection, human papillomavirus infection, chancroid, lymphogranuloma venereum, granuloma inguinale, scabies, human immunodeficiency virus infection
  - ▶ R/O Behçet's syndrome
  - ▶ R/O aphthous ulcers
  - ▶ R/O neoplasm
  - ▶ R/O fixed drug eruption
  - ▶ R/O psoriasis
  - ▶ R/O tinea versicolor
  - ▶ R/O mononucleosis
  - ▶ R/O congenital syphilis

Plan

Diagnostic Criteria

- See Tables 14.8, 14.9, and 14.10.

Stages of Disease

Primary Syphilis

<u>Laboratory Criteria</u>

- Identification of *T. pallidum* via darkfield examination of specimen from the chancre or regional lymph node.

- *T. pallidum* can also be detected through direct fluorescent antibody testing (DFA-TP) or equivalent methods (CDC, 1996).

  NOTE: Fluorescent antibody testing has replaced darkfield microscopy in many health departments and laboratories. Specimens from mouth lesions require direct fluorescent antibody techniques for diagnosis. *Failure to demonstrate T. pallidum does not exclude the possibility of syphilis.*

<u>Case Classification</u>

- Probable case

  ▶ Clinically compatible case with one or more chancres

  ▶ Reactive serologic test (CDC, 1996)

  NOTE: The most commonly used nontreponemal tests (i.e., reagin tests) include the venereal disease research laboratory (VDRL) and rapid plasma reagin (RPR). Common treponemal tests include the fluorescent treponemal antibody absorbed (FTA-ABS) and the microhemagglutination assay for antibody to *T. pallidum* (MHA-TP).

- Confirmed case

  ▶ Clinically compatible case that is laboratory confirmed (CDC, 1996)

Secondary Syphilis

<u>Laboratory Criteria</u>

  ▶ Identification of T. pallidum from clinical specimens (e.g., chancre, skin/mucous membrane lesions, or lymph node aspirate) via darkfield microscopy, DFA-TP, *or* equivalent methods (CDC, 1996)

<u>Case Classification</u>

- Probable case

  ▶ Clinically compatible case with nontreponemal titer greater than or equal to 1:4 (CDC, 1996)

- Confirmed Case

  ▶ Clinically compatible case that is laboratory confirmed (CDC, 1996)

Latent Syphilis

Case Classification

- Probable case
  - ▶ Absence of clinical signs and symptoms and the presence of one of the following:
    - – No past diagnosis of syphilis, a reactive nontreponemal test, and a reactive treponemal test
    - – Past history of syphilis therapy and current nontreponemal test titer demonstrating fourfold or greater increase from the last nontreponemal test titer (CDC, 1996).

      NOTE: Less than 2 percent of individuals are reported to have a nonreactive nontreponemal test due to the *prozone phenomenon* (i.e., higher than optimal amount of antibody in the tested sera, preventing the flocculation reaction typical of a positive test). Request the lab to dilute the sera and continue titration (Berkowitz, Baxi, & Fox, 1990; Larsen et al., 1990; San Francisco City Clinic, 1992).

Early Latent Syphilis

Case Classification

- Probable case
  - ▶ Latent syphilis (see above) in person who has evidence of having acquired the infection within the previous 12 months based on one or more of the following:
    - – Documented seroconversion or fourfold or greater increase in nontreponemal test titer during the previous 12 months
    - – History of symptoms consistent with primary or secondary syphilis during the previous 12 months
    - – History of sexual exposure to partner who had confirmed or probable primary or secondary syphilis or early latent syphilis (documented independently as duration less than 1 year) (CDC, 1991)
    - – Reactive nontreponemal and treponemal tests from person whose only possible exposure occurred within the preceding 12 months (CDC, 1996)

Late Latent Syphilis

Case Classification

- Probable case
  - ▶ Latent syphilis in a person who has no evidence of having acquired the infection within the preceding 12 months and whose age and titer do not meet the criteria for latent syphilis of unknown duration (CDC, 1996)

    NOTE: Nontreponemal titers are usually higher during early latent syphilis than late latent syphilis, but the two types cannot be reliably distinguished on this basis (CDC, 1996).

Latent Syphilis of Unknown Duration

Case Classification

- Probable case

  ▶ Latent syphilis that does not meet the criteria for early latent syphilis

  ▶ Person is age 13 to 35 years with nontreponemal titer greater than or equal to 1:32 (CDC, 1996)

Neurosyphilis

Laboratory Criteria

- Reactive serologic test for syphilis and reactive VDRL in CSF (VDRL-CSF) (CDC, 1996)

Case Classification

- Probable case

  ▶ Syphilis of any stage, negative VDRL-CSF and both of the following:

    - Elevated CSF protein or leukocyte count in absence of other known causes of these abnormalities

    - Clinical signs or symptoms consistent with neurosyphilis without other known causes for these clinical abnormalities (CDC, 1996)

  NOTE: The VDRL-CSF is the standard serologic test for neurosyphilis. Some experts recommend an FTA-ABS of CSF (may be less specific than the VDRL-CSF but is highly sensitive); when nonreactive it provides strong evidence against neurosyphilis. CSF leukocyte is usually greater than 5 WBC/mm^3 when neurosyphilis is present. (CDC, 1991; 1998).

- Confirmed case

  ▶ Syphilis of any stage that meets laboratory criteria for neurosyphilis (CDC, 1996)

Congenital Syphilis

- Presence of one or more clinical manifestations (see introduction), along with laboratory findings, leads to diagnosis (see Table 14.7, Congenital Syphilis Case Definition, and Congenital Syphilis in the Follow-Up section).

Additional Testing

- Clients with syphilis should be tested for HIV; pretest and posttest counseling and informed consent is necessary (CDC, 1995, 1998).

- Additional laboratory tests may include, but are not limited to, Pap smear, screening for chlamydia and gonorrhea, herpes simplex virus cultures, Tzanck stain, wet mounts, hepatitis B and C testing, liver function studies, tests for autoimmune disease, complete blood count with differential, platelet count, and T-lymphocyte counts—CD4, CD8, and CD4:CD8 ratio (if client is HIV positive).

- Tuberculin skin testing may be considered.

- See Chapter 6.2, *Antiphospholipid Syndrome.*

Treatment/Management

General Considerations

- All women should have syphilis screening with a RPR or VDRL at entry to care, along with the standard prenatal laboratory tests. The RPR or VDRL should be repeated in the third trimester (i.e., 28 weeks' gestation) if at high risk for STD, and again at delivery.

  NOTE: The VDRL and RPR (i.e., nontreponemal tests) should not be used interchangeably. That is, the same test as employed initially should be ordered for the repeat testing.

- Seropositive, sexually active women should have a pelvic examination prior to syphilis staging to evaluate for internal mucosal lesions (CDC, 1998).

- Seropositive pregnant women should be considered infected until proven otherwise (i.e., treatment has been clearly documented in medical record and sequential nontreponemal titers have declined appropriately) (CDC, 1998). When there is any doubt about previous treatment, *every pregnant woman* with a reactive serologic test for syphilis should be considered infected and a candidate for treatment. The usual medical and epidemiologic follow-up can be performed later to confirm the diagnosis.

- Clients with typical lesions of primary syphilis should have a nontreponemal (i.e., reagin) test and, ideally, a darkfield examination. If the reagin test is reactive, the client should be treated for syphilis even if direct examinations for spirochetes are negative. Treponemal tests are not recommended if the reagin tests are negative, regardless of the type of lesion. Repeat nonreactive reagin tests at 1 week, 1 month, and 3 months from the initial test; nonreactive reagin tests over 3 months effectively rule out syphilis as the cause of suspicious lesions (CDC, n.d.). Suspicious mucocutaneous lesions should be evaluated with darkfield examination or DFA-TP if serologic tests are negative.

- All clients with suspected secondary syphilis should undergo nontreponemal testing. Clients with atypical findings should have a confirmatory treponemal test (CDC, n.d.).

  NOTE: If the woman has had a previous nontreponemal test, the state/local surveillance agency may be contacted to obtain the results.

- If the VDRL or RPR is reactive, but the FTA-ABS or MHA-TP is negative and the client is without clinical signs of disease, repeat the VDRL or RPR *and* FTA-ABS or MHA-TP in 4 to 6 weeks. If the treponemal tests are still negative, the results indicate a biological false-positive test for syphilis. (see Table 14.10, Potential Causes of False-positive Tests for Syphilis, and Chapter 6.2, *Antiphospholipid Syndrome.*

- Alternative diagnostic tests (e.g., biopsy and direct microscopy) should be considered for HIV-infected clients when the serologic test results do not fit the clinical picture.

- Lumbar puncture for CSF examination is not recommended for routine evaluation of clients with primary or secondary syphilis; however, if clinical signs of neurologic involvement are present (e.g., auditory, cranial nerve, meningeal, or ophthalmic manifestations), lumbar puncture and ocular slit-lamp examination should be performed. Refer the client to a physician.

- Clients with latent syphilis should be evaluated for clinical manifestations of tertiary syphilis (e.g., aortitis, neurosyphilis, gumma, and iritis). CSF examination is recommended before treatment when any of the following criteria are present:

  ▶ Neurologic or ophthalmic manifestations

  ▶ Evidence of active tertiary syphilis (e.g., aortitis, gumma, iritis)

  ▶ Treatment failure

  ▶ HIV infection with late latent syphilis or syphilis of unknown duration (CDC, 1998)

  NOTE: CSF examination may be performed for persons not meeting these criteria if dictated by additional circumstances and client preferences (CDC, 1998). If CSF evaluation is performed and abnormalities are present that are consistent with CNS syphilis, the client should be treated for neurosyphilis (CDC, 1998).

- CNS disease (i.e., neurosyphilis) can occur at any stage; any client with clinical evidence of neurologic involvement (e.g., ophthalmic or auditory symptoms, cranial nerve palsies, or signs/symptoms of meningitis) should have a CSF examination. (CDC, 1998).

  NOTE: Experts recommend that clients with evidence of auditory disease be treated in the same manner as for neurosyphilis, regardless of CSF findings. In addition, persons with syphilitic eye disease should be treated according to neurosyphilis guidelines (CDC, 1998).

Drug Regimens

Parenteral penicillin G is the preferred drug for syphilis therapy and is the only drug with documented efficacy for pregnant women with syphilis and for individuals with neurosyphilis. Preparations used (e.g., benzathine, aqueous procaine, or aqueous crystalline), dosage, and length of treatment will depend upon the stage/clinical manifestations of disease. Pregnant, penicillin-allergic persons should be treated with penicillin after desensitization, if necessary (refer to CDC, 1998 guidelines). Tetracycline and doxycycline are contraindicated during pregnancy. Erythromycin is unreliable in curing an affected fetus (CDC, 1998). Data are insufficient to recommend azithromycin or ceftriaxone (CDC, 1998).

Primary and Secondary Syphilis

- Benzathine penicillin G, 2.4 million units IM in a single dose

Early Latent Syphilis

- Benzathine penicillin G, 2.4 million units IM in a single dose (CDC, 1998)

  NOTE: Additional therapy (i.e., second dose of benzathine penicillin 2.4 million units IM 1 week after the initial dose) has been recommended by some experts for women who have primary, secondary, or early latent syphilis (CDC, 1998).

Late Latent Syphilis or Latent Syphilis of Unknown Duration

- Benzathine penicillin G, 7.2 million units total, administered as three doses of 2.4 million units IM each at 1-week intervals (CDC, 1998)

  NOTE: Serum levels are present for up to 2 weeks; thus, if client is late for injection, the treatment series need not be restarted (Hook III, 1996).

Neurosyphilis

- Client should be managed by a physician.

- Aqueous crystalline penicillin G, 18 to 24 million units daily, administered as 3 to 4 million units IV every 4 hours for 10 to 14 days.

- Alternative regimen if compliance can be assured: procaine penicillin 2.4 million units IM daily; plus probenecid, 500 mg p.o. q.i.d., both for 10 to 14 days (CDC, 1998).

- Some experts recommend benzathine penicillin 2.4 million units IM, after completion of either of the above regimens (CDC, 1998).

Partner Therapy

- All sex partners of clients with syphilis should be fully evaluated (i.e., clinically and serologically). Provide referrals to an STD clinic or other source of health care as necessary.

- Individuals exposed to a person with primary, secondary, or early latent syphilis (i.e., <1 year's duration) within the preceding 90 days should be treated presumptively, even if seronegative (CDC, 1998).

- Those exposed to a person with primary, secondary, or early latent syphilis more than 90 days prior to diagnosis should be treated presumptively if serological tests are not available immediately and follow-up can not be ensured (CDC, 1998).

- For partner notification purposes and presumptive treatment of exposed sex partners, clients who have syphilis of unknown duration and nontreponemal titers equal to or greater than 1:32 may be considered to have early syphilis (CDC, 1998).

- Long-term partners of persons with late syphilis should be evaluated clinically and serologically and treated on the basis of those findings (CDC, 1998).

- Use the following time periods before treatment to identify at-risk sex partners (CDC, 1998):

  ▶ 3 months plus duration of symptoms for primary syphilis

  ▶ 6 months plus duration of symptoms for secondary syphilis

  ▶ 1 year for early latent syphilis

Other Drug Regimens

- Nonpregnant, penicillin-allergic individuals with primary or secondary syphilis should be treated with the following:

- ▶ Doxycycline, 100 mg p.o. b.i.d. for 2 weeks

    OR

- ▶ Tetracycline, 500 mg p.o. q.i.d. for 2 weeks

    - – An alternative regimen for nonpregnant, penicillin-allergic persons whose follow-up can be ensured is erythromycin, 500 mg p.o. q.i.d. for 2 weeks (less effective regimen) (CDC, 1998).

- Nonpregnant, penicillin-allergic individuals with latent syphilis should be treated with the following regimens:

    - ▶ Doxycycline, 100 mg p.o. b.i.d.

        OR

    - ▶ Tetracycline, 500 mg p.o. q.i.d.

    Drugs are administered for 2 weeks if duration of infection less than 1 year, otherwise for 4 weeks (CDC, 1998).

    NOTE: Close follow-up is essential when any of these drug regimens are used.

Additional Considerations

- Local treatment of mucocutaneous lesions is usually not necessary. Antiseptics should not be applied to lesions prior to obtaining specimens for microscopy examination.

Consultation

- Consultation is advised for all cases, especially if complicated or client does not respond to treatment appropriately. Consultation with an infectious disease expert may be warranted.

- Pregnant women who are coinfected with HIV should be referred to a physician for treatment and management.

- Procedures such as lumbar puncture and slit-lamp evaluation will be performed by a physician, as indicated.

Patient Education

- Discuss cause of infection, mode of transmission, incubation period, course of disease, risk factors, association with HIV infection, symptoms, potential perinatal and neonatal complications, and treatment modalities. Advise the woman that breastfeeding does not result in transmission of syphilis unless there is an infectious lesion on the breast, in which case breast feeding is contraindicated.

- Stress compliance with treatment regimen and importance of partner evaluation and therapy. Refer partner to STD clinic or other source of health care, as indicated.

- Advise abstinence from intercourse until both client and partner are treated/cured. If known sexual contact with a contagious syphilitic lesion has occurred, the exposed partner should wash the contact area as soon as possible with soap and water.

- Stress that close follow-up is *extremely important*. Impress upon client the need for long-term serologic testing to ensure adequacy of therapy. If symptoms persist/recur, client and partner should be instructed to seek care promptly. Suggest to the client that she keep a diary of the VDRL or RPR results to facilitate future management.

- Address STD prevention.

  ▶ Provide guidelines for safer sex practices.

  ▶ Encourage careful "screening" of sex partners and committed use of condoms.

  ▶ Educate regarding the signs/symptoms of STDs and abstinence from sexual activity if these signs develop. See Table 14.1, Safer Sex Recommendations, and Appendix 14.1a, Patient Education Resources for STDs, in Chapter 14.1, *Chlamydia Trachomatis*.

  NOTE: Clients should be advised to always have condoms (male and/or female) available and to use them consistently, especially if having intercourse with new, multiple, and/or nonmonogamous partners and partners whose HIV status and risk status are unknown (Woolf, Jonas, & Lawrence, 1996). Ideally, both partners should be tested for STDs (including HIV) before initiating intercourse (CDC, 1998) (see Table 14.1, Safer Sex Recommendations in Chapter 14.1, *Chlamydia Trachomatis*).

- Assist client in understanding how specific sexual behaviors relate to STD acquisition. Advise against the use of drugs and alcohol as these substances impair judgment and may lead to unsafe sex (Woolf at al., 1996). Tailor prevention messages to injection-drug uses and/or their partners.

- Allow client to ventilate her emotions regarding the STD diagnosis. Provide available literature on STDs (see Appendix 14.1a, Patient Education Resources for STDs, in Chapter 14.1).

- **IMPORTANT NOTE:** Alert client to the *Jarisch-Herxheimer reaction*. This is a self-limited, acute systemic reaction that may occur within 24 hours following treatment and last for 12 to 24 hours. It has been ascribed to the release of toxins from the destruction of spirochetes, but the exact cause of the reaction remains obscure; it should not be confused with penicillin hypersensitivity or procaine reactions (Rosen, Rubin, Ellner, Tschen, & Cochran, 1989; Thin, 1990).

  ▶ Signs and symptoms include fever, headache, malaise, myalgia, pharyngitis, nausea, flushing, hyperventilation, tachycardia, and hypotension. In addition, the chancre may swell or secondary syphilitic lesions may appear for the first time. Antipyretics (e.g., acetaminophen) may be taken as needed.

  ▶ Women in the second trimester of pregnancy whose treatment precipitates this reaction are at risk for premature labor and/or fetal distress. Client education should include information on signs and symptoms of the reaction, as well as those of preterm labor. Instruction should also be given on fetal movement counts, and the woman should be advised to seek care if fetal movement decreases (Rodriguez, Meyer, & Watrobka, 1996).

- Alert patient to other possible side effects of medication utilized for treatment.

Follow-up

- See Table 14.9, Important Points in the Interpretation of Syphilis Tests.

General Considerations

- The importance of follow-up should be stressed. It is especially important in a woman of reproductive age because if inadequately treated, congenital syphilis may complicate an ensuing pregnancy.

- History collected during follow-up should include symptom status, medication compliance, drug reaction or side effects, partner therapy, sexual exposure, and use of condoms.

- Serologic titers should be repeated in the third trimester and at delivery. Titers may be checked monthly for the remainder of pregnancy in women at high risk for reinfection or in high-prevalence geographic areas (CDC, 1998). Another titer should be done at the 6-week postpartum visit, and thereafter according to the follow-up schedule for nonpregnant persons by stage of disease.

Stages of Disease

Primary and Secondary Syphilis

- Clinical and serological evaluation at 6 and 12 months following treatment; more frequent evaluation may be undertaken, as indicated.

- If signs/symptoms persist/recur or there is a sustained fourfold increase in nontreponemal titer when compared with a baseline or subsequent result, consider treatment failure or reinfection. Evaluate for HIV infection. Refer the client for lumbar puncture unless reinfection is the likely scenario. Re-treat with three weekly injections of benzathine penicillin G, 2.4 million units IM, unless neurosyphilis is disclosed by the CSF examination (CDC, 1998). Consult with a physician.

  NOTE: Clients are at risk for treatment failure when nontreponemal titers fail to decline fourfold within 6 months after therapy. Evaluate for HIV infection and provide additional clinical and serologic follow-up. Re-treat if proper follow-up can not be ensured; a CSF examination may also be indicated (CDC, 1998). Consult with a physician.

Latent Syphilis

- Nontreponemal tests should be repeated at 6, 12, and 24 months following treatment.

- If titers increase fourfold or an initially high titer (≥1:32) fails to decline at least fourfold within 12 to 24 months or signs/symptoms of syphilis develop, the client should be evaluated for neurosyphilis and re-treated appropriately (CDC, 1998). Consult with a physician.

Neurosyphilis

- CSF examination should be repeated every 6 months until the cell count is normal if pleocytosis was initially present. In cases where the cell count has not decreased after 6 months, or if the CSF is not completely normal after 2 years, re-treatment should be considered (CDC, 1998). The client should be followed by a physician.

Congenital Syphilis

- See Table 14.7, Congenital Syphilis Case Definition.

- Serologic testing should be performed at 28 weeks' gestation and at delivery in communities and populations at risk for congenital syphilis. The CDC states that "no infant should leave the hospital without the maternal serologic status having been determined at least once during pregnancy" (CDC, 1998, p. 40).

- Routine screening of umbilical cord blood or newborn sera is not recommended (serologic tests on infant serum can be nonreactive if the mother's serology is of low titer or if the mother was infected late in pregnancy). Evaluate, however, infant's serum with a nontreponemal test, if born to a seropositive mother (CDC, 1998).

- Infants born to seropositive mothers should have appropriate clinical and laboratory evaluation for congenital syphilis. Treat for presumed congenital syphilis if any of the following criteria are met:

  ▶ Mother had untreated syphilis at delivery

  ▶ Mother had serologic evidence of relapse or reinfection after treatment

  ▶ Mother was treated for syphilis during pregnancy with erythromycin or other nonpenicillin regimen

  ▶ Mother was treated for syphilis 1 month or less before delivery

  ▶ Mother was treated for syphilis during pregnancy with appropriate penicillin regimen, but nontreponemal titers failed to decrease at least fourfold

  ▶ Mother does not have well-documented history of syphilis treatment

  ▶ Mother was treated appropriately prior to pregnancy but had insufficient serologic follow-up to ensure adequate treatment response and lack of current infection (CDC, 1998)

- Congenital syphilis cases should be managed by a pediatrician. Details of inpatient therapy and follow-up for the infant are beyond the scope of this chapter.

Additional Considerations

- A woman who delivers a stillborn infant after 20 weeks' gestation should be tested for syphilis (CDC, 1993).

- Clients with primary syphilis who reside in a high HIV-prevalence area should be retested for HIV 3 months following treatment (CDC, 1998).

- Follow-up should be conducted on all positive laboratory tests.

  ▶ HIV-positive results should be conveyed face-to-face and by a provider who has received training in the complexities of test disclosure. Counsel HIV-positive individuals appropriately and refer them to the appropriate provider/agency for early intervention services. Refer to Chapter 14.5, *Human Immunodeficiency Virus,* for further information and for additional laboratory tests that may be indicated.

  ▶ Hepatitis B antigen-positive women should receive counseling regarding the implications of their positive status and need for immunoprophylaxis of their offspring, their sex partner(s), and all household members. See Chapter 10.2, *Hepatitis A, B, C, D, and E,* for further information and for additional laboratory tests that may be indicated.

  NOTE: If HBsAg was initially negative, repeat testing in late pregnancy for all high-risk women (e.g., injecting-drug users, women with STDs) (CDC, 1998).

  ▶ Treat all other concomitant STDs/identified conditions.

- The client's partner should be encouraged to follow up appropriately with the primary care provider.

- Continue to encourage safer sex practices. Ongoing psychosocial support is important in enabling the woman to gain control over her sexual situation and successfully prevent future STDs.

- Address substance abuse issues and other high-risk behaviors. Refer to support services (e.g., public health nursing, drug treatment programs, psychological/social services), as indicated.

- Syphilis cases must be reported to the local health department within 1 working day of identification or suspected case.

- Document syphilis diagnosis and treatment thereof in the progress notes and problem list. As appropriate, note on the problem list high-risk behaviors that indicate possible risk of syphilis infection or other STD.

Table 14.7

Congenital Syphilis Case Definition

Confirmed Case

- Infant in whom *Treponema pallidum* is identified by darkfield microscopy, fluorescent antibody, or other specific stains in specimens from lesions, placenta, umbilical cord, or autopsy material.

Presumptive Case

- Any infant whose mother had untreated or inadequately treated* syphilis at delivery, regardless of findings in the infant; or

- Any infant or child who has a reactive treponemal test for syphilis and any one of the following:

  ▶ Evidence of congenital syphilis on physical examination**

    OR

  ▶ Evidence of congenital syphilis on long-bone radiograph

    OR

  ▶ Reactive CSF VDRL***

    OR

  ▶ Elevated CSF cell count or protein (without other cause)***

    OR

  ▶ Quantitative nontreponemal serologic titers that are fourfold higher than the mother's (both drawn at birth)

    OR

  ▶ Reactive test for FTA-ABS-19S-IgM antibody***

Syphilitic Stillbirth

- Fetal death in which the mother had untreated or inadequately treated syphilis at delivery of a fetus after a 20-week gestation or of a fetus weighing >500 grams.

---

* Inadequate treatment consists of any nonpenicillin therapy or penicillin given less than 30 days prior to delivery.

** Signs in an infant (< 2 years of age) may include hepatosplenomegaly, characteristic skin rash, condyloma lata, snuffles, jaundice (syphilitic hepatitis), pseudoparalysis, or edema (nephrotic syndrome). Stigmata in an older child may include interstitial keratitis, nerve deafness, anterior bowing of shins, frontal bossing, mulberry molars, Hutchinson's teeth, saddle nose, rhagades, or Clutton's joints.

*** It may be difficult to distinguish between congenital and acquired syphilis in a seropositive child after infancy. Signs may not be obvious and stigmata may not yet have developed. Abnormal values for CSF VDRL, cell count, and protein, as well as IgM antibodies, may be found in either congenital or acquired syphilis. Findings on long-bone radiographs may help, since these would indicate congenital syphilis. The decision may ultimately be based on maternal history and clinical judgment; the possibility of sexual abuse must also be considered.

Source: Adapted from: "Congenital syphilis - New York City, 1986–1988," by the Centers for Disease Control, 1989, *Morbidity and Mortality Weekly Report, 38* (48), p. 828.

Table 14.8

Specimen Collection Procedure for Darkfield Microscopy

- Ensure laboratory capabilities for darkfield microscopy.
- Obtain necessary equipment:
  - ▶ 2 clean microscope slides and 2 coverslips
  - ▶ Sterile saline without bactericidal additives
  - ▶ Several sterile 4 x 4 gauze pads
  - ▶ Syringe with 20-gauge sterile needle
- Wash lesion with small amount of sterile saline on gauze pad to remove purulent matter, scab, or epithelium.

  NOTE: Use universal precautions; lesions are highly infectious.

- Gently abrade lesion with gauze pad to enhance serous fluid production.

- Apply pressure at base of lesion to well-up serum. Blot off grossly bloody serum; continue to apply pressure to obtain clear specimen.

  NOTE: Gentle suction with syringe can be used to bring up serum to surface.

- Press glass slide onto the exudate. A few drops of saline may be added to the specimen to prevent drying. Cover with coverslip.

  NOTE: To avoid false-negative result, 2 specimens should be collected from solitary lesion or 2 distinct lesions.

- Transport specimen directly to the laboratory for darkfield microscopy.

- Diagnostic material may also be obtained from enlarged regional lymph node. Prep skin with saline solution as above. Inject 0.1–0.2 mL of sterile saline into node via 20-gauge needle attached to syringe. Gently manipulate the needle tip within the node to dislodge the tissue, then aspirate a specimen. Place specimen on glass slide, apply coverslip and transport to lab.

  NOTE: If patients have been applying topical solutions to their lesions the darkfield may be negative; therefore, the test should be repeated in 1–2 days after discontinuing the use of these preparations.

- Mouth lesions must be cleansed very well and walled off completely to prevent contamination by normal oral spirochetes. Interpret results carefully.

Sources: Adapted from "The Diagnosis and Management of Maternal and Congenital Syphilis," by M.J. Crane, 1992, *Journal of Nurse-Midwifery, 37*(1), p. 16. Copyright 1992 by the American College of Nurse-Midwives. Modified with permission. Also adapted from *Sexually transmitted diseases. Clinical practice guidelines.* (pp. III–36), by the Centers for Disease Control and Prevention, (1991). Atlanta: Author; and *Criteria and Techniques for the Diagnosis of Early Syphilis* (Document No. 98–376, pp. 1–2), by the Centers for Disease Control and Prevention, n.d., Atlanta: Author.

Table 14.9

Important Points in the Interpretation of Syphilis Tests

Nontreponemal Tests (Reagin Tests)

- More than a reactive VDRL or RPR is needed to justify the diagnosis of syphilis.

- Nontreponemal tests should be used for screening and to follow response to treatment (should not be used interchangeably for sequential testing).

- Nontreponemal tests are reported as reactive or nonreactive with quantitative results reported as a dilution (i.e., 1:4) or as a reciprocal of the dilution (i.e., 4 dilutions). A fourfold titer change is equivalent to a change of two dilutions (e.g., from 1:16 to 1:4 or from 1:8 to 1:32).

- Rising titers indicate infection, reinfection, or treatment failure. A sustained 2-tube rise in titer (e.g., 1:2 to 1:8) performed by the same laboratory is minimal evidence of the need for re-treatment. The only exception is the adequately treated congenital syphilitic whose titer may fluctuate without any particular significance.

- Tests become reactive 4 to 8 weeks after infection acquired and several days to 3 weeks after chancre appearance (Jacobs, 1996; Sánchez & Musher, 1997). False negative results may occur when client receives antibiotics for another type of infection (Crane, 1992). Approximately 20 percent (range 13 to 41 percent) of clients have nonreactive tests in primary syphilis (Hook III, 1996).

- Initial nonreactive nontreponemal tests should be repeated in 1 week, 1 month, and 3 months if there is a lesion indicating syphilis. Nonreactive reagin tests over 3 months exclude syphilis as the cause of such lesions.

- In secondary and early latent syphilis >99 percent of tests will be reactive with titers usually ≥ 1:8.

- If the client with secondary syphilis develops a very high titer, the VDRL or RPR could remain nonreactive due to the *prozone phenomenon*. Thus, in all cases where suspicious lesions are present, request that the laboratory dilute the negative serum and continue titration.

- Nonreactive tests may occur in a patient with late symptomatic syphilis—either acquired or congenital. A negative nontreponemal test does not rule out syphilis.

- Reactive VDRL, performed on a sample of cerebrospinal fluid, always represents syphilis unless proved otherwise. Central nervous system involvement (except in cases of tabes dorsalis) also is indicated by elevations of spinal fluid blood cell count and total protein.

- If a VDRL or RPR performed on the cord blood of a newborn is reactive, it may be due to passive transfer of reagin from the mother. A VDRL or RPR should be performed every month for 3 months to determine whether the titer is rising or falling. If the titer falls rapidly or becomes nonreactive, then passive transfer—not congenital syphilis—is confirmed.

(Continued)

Table 14.9 (continued)

- With adequate therapy of primary and secondary syphilis titers should decline fourfold in 6 months. In primary syphilis, nontreponemal tests are usually nonreactive 1 year after treatment and in secondary syphilis, 2 years after treatment (Jacobs, 1996; Thin, 1990). For early latent syphilis, a fourfold decline in titer occurs in 12–24 months and nontreponemal tests should be nonreactive by 2 to 3 years after adequate therapy. In late latent syphilis, decreases in titers are variable after treatment is completed (Bolan, 1994; Jacobs, 1996).

- Factors associated with slower decline in test titers after treatment are prior infection, more advanced disease, and higher initial titers (Hook III, 1996).

- In some individuals after treatment, nontreponemal antibodies may remain positive in the low titer range for life (serofast state).

- A reactive VDRL or RPR in the absence of syphilis is called a biologic false positive (BFP), occurring in 1 to 2 percent of cases. Titers are usually low or weakly reactive ($\leq$ 1:4). Syphilis must always be ruled out in the occurrence of BFPs (see also Table 14.10, Potential Causes of False-positive Tests for Syphilis). Certain other spirochete infections (e.g., yaws, pinta, bejel) produce positive reactions but this should not be considered *false* positive.

Treponemal Tests

- *Do not* use treponemal tests for screening, to assess response to treatment, or as reliable markers for previous infection. Proper use would be for confirmation of nontreponemal tests and for persons with symptoms of late syphilis (Larsen et al., 1990).

- FTA-ABS is 90 to 95 percent sensitive (first to become reactive), MHA-TP is 80 to 85 percent sensitive (reactive about same time as reagin tests) (CDC, 1991).

- Treponemal tests are not recommended in the absence of reactive reagin test, regardless of the nature of the lesion (CDC, n.d.; Larsen et al., 1990).

- A reactive test indicates past or present infection.

- False positive tests may occur in $\leq$ 1 percent of the general population. See also Table 14.10, Potential Causes of False-positive Tests for Syphilis.

- Most patients with reactive treponemal tests will continue to have reactive tests for life; however, 15 to 25 percent of patients treated during the primary stage of syphilis might revert to nonreactive tests after 2 to 3 years (CDC, 1998).

Source: Adapted from *Women's Primary Health Care: Protocols for Practice* (pp. 13-55–13-56), by W.L. Star, L. L. Lommel, and M.T. Shannon, 1995, Washington DC: American Nurses. Copyright 1995 by the American Nurses Association. Adapted with permission.

Table 14.10

Potential Causes of False-positive Tests for Syphilis

Nontreponemal Tests

Infectious Causes

Pneumococcal or mycoplasmal pneumonia
Scarlet fever
Leprosy
Lymphogranuloma venereum (LGV)
Relapsing fever
Bacterial endocarditis
Malaria
Rickettsial disease
Psittacosis
Leptospirosis
Chancroid
Tuberculosis
Trypanosomiasis
Vaccina (vaccination)
Chickenpox
HIV infection
Measles
Infectious mononucleosis
Mumps
Viral hepatitis

Noninfectious Causes

Pregnancy
Chronic liver disease
Advanced cancer
Intravenous drug use
Multiple myeloma
Advancing age
Connective tissue disease
Multiple blood transfusions

Treponemal Tests

Infectious Causes

Lyme disease
Leprosy
Malaria
Infectious mononucleosis
Relapsing fever
Leptospirosis

Noninfectious Causes

Systemic lupus erythematosus

Adapted from Hook III, E.W., & Marra, C.M. (1992). Acquired syphilis in adults. *New England Journal of Medicine, 326,* 1062. ©1992 by The Massachusetts Medical Society. Reprinted with permission.

REFERENCES

Berkowitz, K., Baxi, L., & Fox, H.E. (1990). False-negative syphilis screening: The prozone phenomenon, nonimmune hydrops, and diagnosis of syphilis during pregnancy. *American Journal of Obstetrics and Gynecology, 163(3)*, 975–977.

Berry, M.C., & Dajani, A.S. (1992). Resurgence of congenital syphilis. *Infectious Disease Clinics of North America, 6(1)*, 19–29.

Bolan, G. (1994). *Syphilis.* STD Clinical Course. San Francisco: San Francisco STD/HIV Prevention Training Center.

Celum, C. (1996, April). *Rectal STDs.* Lecture and outline presented at Advances in Sexually Transmitted Diseases conference. Sponsored by the San Francisco STD/HIV Prevention Training Center, San Francisco, CA.

Centers for Disease Control and Prevention. (n.d.). *Criteria and techniques for the diagnosis of early syphilis* (Document #98-376). Atlanta, GA: Author.

Centers for Disease Control and Prevention (CDC). (1989). Congenital syphilis—New York City, 1986–1988. *Morbidity and Mortality Weekly Report, 38(48)*, 825–829.

Centers for Disease Control and Prevention (CDC). (1991). *Sexually transmitted diseases. Clinical practice guidelines.* Atlanta, GA: Author.

Centers for Disease Control and Prevention (CDC). (1995). U.S. Public Health Service recommendations for human immunodeficiency virus counseling and voluntary testing for pregnant women. *Morbidity and Mortality Weekly Report, 44(RR-7)*, 1–15.

Centers for Disease Control and Prevention (CDC). (1996). *Syphilis.* http://www.cdc.gov/epo/mmwr/other/case_def/syphil97.html.

Centers for Disease Control and Prevention (CDC). (1998). 1998 Sexually transmitted diseases. Treatment guidelines. *Morbidity and Mortality Weekly Report, 47(RR-1)*, 28–46.

Chapel, T. A. (1984). Primary and secondary syphilis. *Cutis, 33(1)*, 4–9.

City and County of San Francisco, Department of Public Health. (1992). *Macro-vue RPR card test, 18 mm circle qualitative.* San Francisco: Author.

Crane, M.J. (1992). The diagnosis and management of maternal and congenital syphilis. *Journal of Nurse-Midwifery, 37(1)*, 4–16.

Gibbs, R.S., & Sweet, R.L. (1994). Clinical disorders. In R.K. Creasy & R. Resnik (Eds.), *Maternal-fetal medicine. Principles and practice* (3rd ed., pp. 675–678). Philadelphia, PA: W.B. Saunders.

Gilstrap, L.C.III, & Wendel, G.D. (1996). Maternal syphilis. *Contemporary OB/Gyn, 41(6)*, 16–25.

Goens, J.L., Janniger, C.K., & De Wolf, K. (1994). Dermatologic and systemic manifestations of syphilis. *American Family Physician, 50(5)*, 1013–1020.

Hart, G. (1986). Syphilis tests in diagnostic and therapeutic decision making. *Annals of Internal Medicine, 104,* 368–376.

Hollander, H., & Katz, M.H. (1996). HIV infection. In L.M. Tierney, Jr., S.J. McPhee, & M.A. Papadakis (Eds.), *Current medical diagnosis and treatment* (35th ed., pp. 1235–1157). Stamford, CT: Appleton & Lange.

Hook III, E.W. (1996, April). *Diagnosis and management of syphilis in the HIV era: Principles and pitfalls.* Lecture and outline presented at Advances in Sexually Transmitted Diseases conference. Sponsored by the San Francisco STD/HIV Prevention Training Center, San Francisco, CA.

Hook III, E.W., & Marra, C.M. (1992). Acquired syphilis in adults. *New England Journal of Medicine, 326,* 1060–1069.

Ingall, D., Sánchez, P.J., & Musher, D.M. (1995). Syphilis. In J.S. Remington & J.O. Klein (Eds.), *Infectious diseases of the fetus and newborn infant* (4th ed., pp. 529–564). Philadelphia, PA: W.B. Saunders.

Jacobs, R.A. (1996). Infectious diseases: Spirochetal. In L.M. Tierney, Jr., S.J. McPhee, & M.A. Papadakis (Eds.), *Current medical diagnosis and treatment* (35th ed., pp. 1227–1237). Stamford, CT: Appleton & Lange.

Jacoby, H.M., & Steinberg, J.L. (1996). Syphilis. In H. Libman & R.A. Witzburg (Eds.). *HIV infection. A primary care manual* (3rd ed., pp. 349–361). Boston: Little, Brown and Company.

Jaffe, H.W., & Musher, D.M. (1990). Management of the reactive syphilis serology. In K.K. Holmes, P.A. Mårdh, F. Sparling, P.J. Wiesner, W. Cates, Jr., S.M. Lemon, & W.A. Stamm (Eds.), *Sexually transmitted diseases* (2nd., ed. pp. 935–939). New York: McGraw-Hill.

Larsen, S.A., Hunter, E F., & Creighton, E.T. (1990). Syphilis. In K.K. Holmes, P.-A. Mårdh, F. Sparling, P.J. Wiesner, W. Cates, Jr., S.M. Lemon, & W.A. Stamm (Eds.), *Sexually transmitted diseases* (2nd., ed. pp. 927–934). New York: McGraw-Hill.

Lukehart, S.A., Hook III, E.W., Baker-Zander, S.A., Collier, A.C., Critchlow, C.W., & Handsfield, H.H. (1988). Invasion of the central nervous system by *Treponema pallidum*: Implications for diagnosis and treatment. *Annals of Internal Medicine, 109*(11), 855–862.

McPhee, S.J. (1984). Secondary syphilis: Uncommon manifestations of a common disease. *The Western Journal of Medicine, 140*(1), 10–20.

Moore, J.E. (1949). *The diagnosis of syphilis by the general practitioner* (Publication No. 426, pp. 1–68). Washington, DC: Public Health Service Printing Office.

Nakashima, A.K., Rolfs, R.T., Flock, M.L., Kilmarx, P. & Greenspan, J.R. (1996). Epidemiology of syphilis in the United States, 1941–1993. *Sexually Transmitted Diseases, 23*(1), 16–23.

Rodriguez, A.C., Meyer, W.J., & Watrobka, T. (1996). The Jarisch-Herxheimer reaction in pregnancy: A nursing perspective. *JOGNN, 25*(5), 383–386.

Rosen, T., Rubin, H., Ellner, K., Tschen, J., & Cochran, R. (1989). Vesicular Jarisch-Herxheimer reaction. *Archives of Dermatology, 125,* 77–81.

Sánchez, P.J. (1992). Congenital syphilis. *Advances in Pediatric Infections, 7,* 161–180.

Sánchez, P.J., & Wendel, G.D. (1997). Syphilis in pregnancy. *Clinics in Perinatology, 24*(1), 71–90.

San Francisco City Clinic. 1992. *Important points in interpretation of the VDRL.* Internal document.

San Francisco Department of Public Health. (1994). *Case definition for STDs: STD Clinical Course Manual.* San Francisco: San Francisco STD/HIV Prevention Training Center.

Shannon, M. (1996, April). *Update on perinatal HIV: Current research findings and clinical interventions.* Presented at the Contemporary Forums Perinatal Nursing Conference, San Francisco, CA.

Swartz, M.M. (1990). Neurosyphilis. In K.K. Holmes, P.-A. Mårdh, F. Sparling, P.J. Wiesner, W. Cates, Jr., S.M. Lemon, & W.A. Stamm (Eds.), *Sexually transmitted diseases* (2nd ed., pp. 231–246). New York: McGraw-Hill.

Thin, R.N. (1990). Early syphilis in the adult. In K.K. Holmes, P.-A. Mårdh, F. Sparling, P.J. Wiesner, W. Cates, Jr., S.M. Lemon, & W.A. Stamm (Eds.), *Sexually transmitted diseases* (2nd ed., pp. 221–230). New York: McGraw-Hill.

Wendel, G.D. (1990). Sexually transmitted diseases in pregnancy. *Seminars in Perinatology, 14*(2), 171–178.

Woolf, S.J., Jonas, S., & Lawrence, R.S. (1996). Health promotion and disease prevention in clinical practice. Baltimore, MD: Williams & Wilkins.

Chapter 7

VAGINITIS

Winifred L. Star

Vaginitis or vaginosis may result from alterations in the vaginal ecosystem due to events or processes that disturb the normal physiology, impact the status of the epithelium, or affect the normal vaginal microflora. This protocol will cover *bacterial vaginosis*, *candidiasis*, *trichomoniasis*, and *postpartum atrophic vaginitis*.

Bacterial Vaginosis

Bacterial vaginosis (BV) is the most common vaginal infection among women of childbearing age accounting for 30 to 35 percent of cases of vaginitis (Schlict, 1994; Sobel, 1990). BV is not caused by a single infectious agent; rather, it is a clinical syndrome characterized by polymicrobial overgrowth, decrease in peroxidase-producing lactobacilli, and altered vaginal pH (Lossick, 1990). The pathogenesis of the syndrome is thought to include the elimination or reduction of antibacterial activity of the indigenous vaginal lactobacilli (Redondo-Lopez, Cook, & Sobel, 1990). The bacteria commonly associated with BV include *Gardnerella vaginalis*, anaerobes (e.g., *Prevotella* [*Bacteroides*] spp., *Mobiluncus* spp., *Peptostreptococcus*), and the genital mycoplasmas (Hillier & Holmes, 1990). Among women with BV, these organisms are present in 100- to 1000-fold greater concentrations. BV may also occur with *Candida albicans* and *Trichomonas vaginalis* infections.

BV occurs in 12 to 61 percent of gynecological patients, depending upon the population studied, and 10 to 30 percent of pregnant women (Sweet & Gibbs, 1995). BV is not considered to be exclusively an STD (sexually transmitted disease), rather a "sexually associated" one, with prevalence higher among sexually active women. Virginal females may also be affected (Bump & Buesching, 1988).

In pregnancy, BV has been associated with postabortal pelvic infection, chorioamnionitis, amniotic fluid infection, preterm labor, premature rupture of membranes (PROM), low birth weight, postpartum endometritis and bacteremia (Gravett et al., 1986; Holst, Goffeng, & Andersch, 1994; Martius & Eschenbach, 1990; McCoy, Katz, Kuller, Killam, & Livengood, 1995; Watts, Eschenbach, & Kenney, 1989; Watts, Krohn, Hillier, & Eschenbach, 1990). The rate of infection with BV during pregnancy does not change markedly with advancing gestation and spontaneous resolution may occur (Duff et al., 1991; Kurki, Sivonen, Renkonen, Savia, & Ylikorkala, 1992). The results of several studies indicate that treatment of pregnant women with BV who are at high risk for preterm delivery might reduce their risk for prematurity (Centers for Disease Control and Prevention [CDC], 1998; Hauth, Goldenberg, Andrews, DuBard, & Copper, 1995; Morales, Schoor, & Albritton, 1994). A large National Institutes of Health–funded randomized clinical trial (Maternal-Fetal Network Prospective Randomized Treatment Trial) is currently under way to assess treatment for asymptomatic BV during pregnancy. Results of this investigation should clarify the benefits of treating BV in women at both low and high risk for preterm delivery (CDC, 1958; Mead, Hillier, McDonald, McGregor, & Sweet, 1997).

Nonpregnant women with BV may be predisposed to pelvic inflammatory disease, urinary tract infection, pelvic abscesses, and cuff cellulitis following hysterectomy (Hooten, Finn, Johnson, Roberts, & Stamm, 1989; Soper, 1993; Soper, Bump, & Hurt, 1990). Additional infections that have been associated with mixed BV flora include wound infections, neonatal scalp abscesses, and nonpuerperal breast abscesses (Glupczynski et al., 1984; McGregor & French, 1988; Sturm, 1989).

Candidiasis

Candidiasis accounts for 20 to 25 percent of vaginal infections and is second to bacterial vaginosis as a cause of vaginitis (Sobel, 1990). *Candida albicans* is the fungal agent responsible for over 90 percent of infections (Ernest, 1992). Other species include *Candida glabrata* (*Torulopsis glabrata)*, and *Candida tropicalis*. Concomitant infection with *Trichomonas vaginalis* or bacterial vaginosis may exist. Recurrent infection (defined three or more clinically proven infections in 1 year) occurs in about 5 percent of women. Many factors have been implicated to explain recurrences: intestinal reservoir, sexual transmission, mucosal persistence, virulence and resistance of the organism, type and length of therapy, therapeutic compliance, repeated courses of systemic or topical antibiotics, zinc deficiency, endocrinopathies, corticosteroid use, and immunosuppression. As yet, there is limited understanding of this problem and in most cases no underlying or predisposing factors can be clearly identified (refer to the references for further information) (Sobel, 1990; Sweet & Gibbs, 1995).

During pregnancy there is increased susceptibility to candidal infection due to the hormonal environment and suppression of cell-mediated immunity; greatest incidence occurs in the third trimester. Although *Candida* is not usually associated with obstetric complications, in rare cases the organism can cause septicemia from mucosal infections, or can ascend from the maternal vagina or cervix resulting in intrauterine infection (usually limited to funisitis and chorioamnionitis) (Berry, Olson, Wen, Belfort, &, Moise, 1997; Wiesinger, Mayerhofer, Wenisch, Breyer, & Graninger, 1996). Individuals at increased risk for more extensive candidal disease or invasive intrauterine infection may include those with immunocompromised states, malignancy, sickle cell anemia, or high serum glucose levels; the presence of an intrauterine contraceptive device may also predispose to intrauterine *Candida* infection, which can lead to late abortion or premature birth (Donders, Moerman, Caudron, & Van Assche, 1990; Gibbs & Sweet, 1994). Congenital candidiasis (also rare) resulting from an ascending maternal infection or via direct contact during delivery from an infected vagina can manifest as either cutaneous or systemic neonatal disease (Schwartz & Reef, 1990). Intrauterine (but not vulvovaginal) *C. albicans* has also been identified in association with preterm rupture of membranes and premature labor (Donders et al., 1990; Mazor, Chaim, Shinwell, & Glezerman, 1993).

Trichomoniasis

Trichomonas vaginalis is a unicellular motile protozoan, which can infect the vagina, cervix, and lower urinary tract. Trichomoniasis is an STD associated with about 10 percent of vaginal infections and is third behind bacterial vaginosis and candidiasis as major causes of vaginitis (Kaufman & Faro, 1994; Sobel, 1990). *T. vaginalis* can be found in 14 to 60 percent of the male sexual partners of infected women and in 67 to 100 percent of the female partners of infected men. The incubation period is between 3 and 28 days (Heine & McGregor, 1993; Moldwin, 1992). Concomitant infection with gonorrhea may occur in 20 to 50 percent of women with trichomoniasis and approximately 35 percent of women have concomitant BV. Some experts believe that pathogenic organisms can adhere to motile trichomonads and be carried to the upper genital tract, resulting in tubal disease and subsequent infertility (Kaufman & Faro, 1994). Nonsexual transmission of trichomoniasis has been reported but is rare.

The relationship of *T. vaginalis* to pregnancy complications is a subject of debate. Complications may include PROM preterm labor, and low birth weight (Sweet & Gibbs, 1995). Perinatal transmission has been reported to occur in about 5 percent of female infants born to women with trichomoniasis; neonatal infection is transient (Goode, Grauer, & Gums, 1994; Moldwin, 1992).

Postpartum Atrophic Vaginitis

Postpartum breastfeeding women often suppress endogenous estrogen production, which leads to an atrophic condition in the vagina. In this state, the normal acidogenic vaginal flora may be replaced by mixed flora. The vaginal mucosa is thinned and the epithelium becomes susceptible to infection and trauma. Once normal menstrual cycles are resumed the vagina should return to a healthy state. The symptoms associated with this condition may be mistaken for candidiasis (Barclay, 1991; Kaufman & Faro, 1994).

Database

Subjective

Predisposing Factors

Bacterial vaginosis

- Lack of hydrogen peroxide-producing *Lactobacillus* spp.
- Sexual activity
- Sexual partner harboring BV organisms
- New/multiple sexual partners
- Intestinal reservoir of *Mobiluncus* spp.
- Intrauterine device (IUD) use
- Non-use of barrier contraception
- Concomitant STD
- Lower redox potential of vaginal epithelium
- Other factors that may alter normal vaginal flora or pH
  - ▶ Antibiotics
  - ▶ Douches
  - ▶ Foreign bodies
  - ▶ Semen
  - ▶ Menstrual blood
  - ▶ Tampons
  - ▶ Contraceptive agents
  - ▶ Stress

Candidiasis

- Pregnancy
- Glycosuria
- Diabetes mellitus (especially if poorly-controlled)
- Obesity
- Antibiotics (most commonly ampicillin, tetracycline, cephalosporins)
- Corticosteroids, immunosuppressants
- Oral contraceptives (controversial)
- Immunosuppressive states (e.g., HIV infection, AIDS)
- Retained IUD or cervical cerclage (risk factors for intrauterine *Candida* infection) (Chaim, Mazor, & Wiznitzer, 1992)
- Other possible factors contributing to candidiasis
  - ▶ Gastrointestinal (GI) tract colonization
  - ▶ Diet
  - ▶ Poor hygiene
  - ▶ Tight clothing
  - ▶ Cloth types
  - ▶ Types of sanitary products
  - ▶ Commercial products
  - ▶ Chemicals
  - ▶ Sexual practices
  - ▶ Hypothyroidism
  - ▶ Zinc/iron deficiency
  - ▶ Hypersensitivity to *Candida* organisms
  - ▶ Humoral/cellular immunity factors (Kaufman & Faro, 1994; Reed, 1992)

Trichomoniasis

- New/multiple sexual partners
- Partner with trichomoniasis
- Coexistent STD
- Non-use of barrier contraception
- Indirect or fomite exposure (rare) (e.g., toilet seats, swimming pools, bath tubs, washcloths)
- Perinatal transmission (risk for transitory neonatal infection)

Postpartum Atrophic Vaginitis

- Suppression of endogenous estrogen associated with breastfeeding

Symptomatology

Bacterial Vaginosis

- Fifty percent of women asymptomatic
- Client's chief symptom is malodorous vaginal discharge ("fishy" smelling, especially after [unprotected] intercourse or during menses)
- Complaints of vulvar pruritus, burning, irritation
- Other complaints may include low backache, postcoital spotting, irregular bleeding episodes

Candidiasis

- Ten to fifty percent of women harbor *Candida* in the vagina as harmless commensal organisms and are thus asymptomatic.
- Client may complain of vulvar pruritus, burning, soreness, abnormal discharge, external dysuria, urinary urgency/frequency, dyspareunia. Symptoms may be worse premenstrually and improve with onset of menstrual flow.
- Client may report partner has symptoms of penile "rash," itching, burning after intercourse.

Trichomoniasis

- Client may be asymptomatic (20 to 50 percent of cases).
- Client may complain of
  ▶ Increased vaginal discharge (may be malodorous)
  ▶ Vulvovaginal pruritus
  ▶ Irritation, soreness, or tenderness
  ▶ Spotting
  ▶ Dysuria, urinary frequency, or nocturia
  ▶ Dyspareunia
  ▶ Lower abdominal pain
  ▶ Tender inguinal adenopathy

  NOTE: Symptoms may appear or be exacerbated after menses or during pregnancy.
- Client may report partner has mucopurulent urethral discharge, mild urethral irritation, mild dysuria, postvoid burning.

Postpartum Atrophic Vaginitis

- Client is usually breastfeeding.
- Client may complain of vaginal soreness, dryness, burning, itching, spotting, dysuria, dyspareunia.

History

- Description of symptoms (quality of discharge [color, odor, consistency], onset, duration, course, aggravating and alleviating factors, etc.)
- Associated symptoms
- Current self-treatment measures or medications used
- History of exposure to irritants (see Table 14.12, Common Vulvovaginal Irritants)
- Partner symptomatology
- Complete medical, sexual, contraceptive, STD, OB/GYN, and habits history
- Psychosocial inquiry in chronic cases

Objective

General Assessment

- Vital signs, as indicated
- Abdominal examination (including lymph nodes), as indicated
- Uterine, adnexal, and rectovaginal examinations, as indicated and appropriate to weeks of gestation
- See below for features associated with the specific vaginitides. Refer to STD protocols throughout Section 14 for description of thorough STD examination.

Features

Bacterial Vaginosis

- White-gray, homogeneous discharge adherent to vaginal walls (may also be visible at introitus)
- Release of amine odor from vaginal discharge when mixed with 10 percent potassium hydroxide (KOH)
- Presence of clue cells on saline wet mount of vaginal discharge (at least 20 percent of vaginal epithelial cells).
- pH of vaginal fluid more than 4.5

  NOTE: Three of the above should be present to make the diagnosis.

- Additional findings may include the following:

  ▶ Lack of/little vulvovaginal inflammation

  ▶ "Bubbles" in vaginal discharge

  ▶ Microflora (coccobacilli, curved/comma-shaped bacilli with twitching motion) in intercellular background of vaginal fluid on saline wet mount

  ▶ Decreased/absent lactobacilli, few white blood cells (WBCs) on saline wet mount of vaginal discharge

    NOTE: If large numbers of WBCs are present, rule out a combined infection.

  ▶ Gram stain of vaginal discharge showing *Gardnerella* plus other bacterial morphotype and fewer than five *Lactobacillus* spp. (Spiegel, Amsel, & Holmes, 1983)

  ▶ Pap smear with BV-assiociated flora (Spiegel, 1991)

  ▶ Vaginal culture with *Gardnerella vaginalis* or anaerobes (not reliable predictor of BV; routine use is not advised) (Thomason, Gelbart, & Scaglione, 1991).

Candidiasis

- Introital and vulvar erythema, edema, excoriation, fissures, occasional pustules or erythematous nodules ("satellite lesions")

- Vaginal erythema

- Scant-to-moderate nonodorous adherent vaginal discharge, normal-appearing or thick/curdy that is white or yellow in color; pseudomembrane ("thrush" patches) may cover vaginal walls

- Saline wet mount of vaginal discharge with budding yeasts, mycelia, pseudohyphae, spores, +/- WBCs, lactobacilli

  NOTE: Do not confuse hyphal filaments with cotton fibers, rolled edges of epithelial cells, *Leptothrix*, or scratches on slide. Also, do not confuse spores with nuclei of epithelial/pus cells, powder granules, bubbles of emulsified creams, or other artifacts (Kaufman & Faro, 1994).

- KOH preparation of vaginal discharge with budding yeasts, mycelia, pseudohyphae, spores, other fungal structures; negative for amine odor.

- pH of vaginal fluid 4.0 to 4.5.

- Laboratory findings may include *Candida* on Pap smear and a vaginal culture positive for candidal organisms.

Trichomoniasis

- Erythema of vestibule and/or labia minora; vulvar edema (usually of labia minora); excoriations, abrasions in interlabial sulci, perineum (from scratching); intertrigo of outer labia majora, crural folds, inner thighs in severe cases; long-standing irritation may lead to thickening of skin and/or pigment changes.

- Abnormal discharge from urethra and/or Skene's ducts may be present.

- Vaginal discharge that is profuse, homogeneous, creamy, purulent, thin, watery, or frothy with a color of yellow, gray or green; discharge may be malodorous.

- Vaginal walls with erythema, edema, ecchymoses, petechiae, papules; vagina may feel granular; thin, gray pseudomembranes may be present (can not be wiped off).

- Cervix may be friable or erythematous with punctate hemorrhages ("strawberry cervix"; 2 to 3 percent of cases).

- Saline wet mount of discharge reveals motile trichomonads, increased WBCs, and decreased lactobacilli; red blood cells (RBCs) and microflora in intercellular background may be present.

  NOTE: Specimen should be kept warm and viewed as soon as possible in order to see motility of organism.

- KOH preparation of discharge may emit amine odor (due to presence of anaerobes)

- pH of vaginal fluid is 5 or greater.

- Laboratory findings may include trichomonads on Pap smear (low specificity), a positive vaginal culture, and urinalysis with trichomonads, or pyuria.

Postpartum Atrophic Vaginitis

- Vagina with

  ▶ Absence of rugal folds

  ▶ Pale pink, red, or whitish epithelium

  ▶ Thin, watery-yellow or slightly bloody discharge

  ▶ Petechiae or ecchymoses in severe cases

- Saline wet mount of vaginal discharge shows predominance of parabasal cells, absence of mature squamous epithelium, increased WBCs, and absence of lactobacilli.

- Vaginal fluid has a pH 5.5–7.0.

- Gram stain (if done) shows mixed flora of gram-negative rods.

- Maturation index on Pap smear (if performed) shows less than 40 percent superficial cells; parabasal cells exceed 20 percent.

Assessment

- Bacterial vaginosis

- Candidiasis

- Trichomoniasis

  OR

- Postpartum atrophic vaginitis

  ▶ R/O mixed vaginal infection

  ▶ R/O physiologic leukorrhea

▶ R/O cervicitis/STDs

▶ R/O vaginal foreign body

▶ R/O allergic/irritant vulvovaginitis

▶ R/O desquamative inflammatory vaginitis

▶ R/O cytolytic vaginosis (Döderlein cytolysis)

▶ R/O vulvar vestibulitis

▶ R/O squamous intraepithelial lesion (SIL)

▶ R/O urinary tract infection (UTI)

▶ R/O immunodeficiency (e.g., HIV infection)

▶ R/O underlying medical disorder

▶ R/O psychosomatic vaginitis

▶ R/O obstetrical/postpartum complications that may be vaginitis-associated

Plan

Diagnostic Tests

- Do not rely on client symptoms for diagnosis.

- The mainstay of clinical diagnosis is microscopy examination of the saline wet mount and KOH preparation under low (x100) and high (x400) power. Ideally, client should not have douched or used an intravaginal medication for 2 to 5 days prior to examination (Quan, 1990).

  ▶ On a saline wet mount the following may be observed: WBCs, RBCs, epithelial cells, motile trichomonads, clue cells, lactobacilli, budding yeasts, mycelia, pseudohyphae, other bacteria, other material (sperm, cotton fibers, etc.).

  ▶ In a KOH preparation the following may be observed: budding cells, mycelia, pseudohyphae, spores or other fungal structures. Assess the presence of amine odor (positive "whiff" test).

  NOTE: Physiologic secretions reveal squamous epithelial cells, lactobacilli, and occasional WBCs (not exceeding the number of epithelial cells); amine odor is not present (Chantigian, 1988).

- pH testing of vaginal fluid from lateral or posterior fornix may be used as an adjunct to diagnosis.

  NOTE: Vaginal pH can be altered by water, lubricants, semen, cervical mucus, amniotic fluid, blood.

- Gram stain may be used as an alternative method of diagnosing BV (when capabilities exist). Gram stain is classified as normal if 5 or more *Lactobacillus* morphotypes are present alone or in combination only with *Gardnerella* morphotypes. See also the Objective section.

- Routine vaginal cultures are not usually necessary to diagnose acute infections. In women with a history of persistent/recurrent vaginitis or repeatedly negative wet mounts with suspicion of candidiasis or trichomoniasis, perform cultures.

- Perform the "swab test" to assess for mucopurulent cervicitis (MPC). A positive test is one with the presence of purulent or mucopurulent cervical discharge that appears yellow when obtained on a white cotton swab; screening for *N. gonorrhoeae* and *C. trachomatis* should be carried out. See the STD protocols throughout Section 14.

- Additional laboratory evaluation of vaginitis/cervicitis may include (but are not limited to) tests for the following:

  ▶ Chlamydia trachomatis and Neisseria gonorrhoeae

  ▶ Herpes simplex viral culture

  ▶ Syphilis (serology)

  ▶ HIV and hepatitis B antibody

  ▶ Urinalysis/urine culture

  ▶ Maturation index (on Pap smear)

  ▶ Amniocentesis (may be necessary for bacteriological assessment of amniotic cavity in cases of PROM)

- Other laboratory diagnostic tests

  ▶ BV

    – Gas-liquid or thin-layer chromatography

    – Proline aminopeptidase test

  ▶ Trichomoniasis

    – Enzyme-linked immunosorbent assay (ELISA)

    – Rapid latex agglutination test

    – Direct immunofluorescence assay (DFA).

  NOTE: Tests may not be available in certain settings.

- Colposcopy may be indicated for further evaluation of an abnormal Pap smear.

Treatment/Management

General Considerations

- Evaluate patients for vaginitis when symptoms are present. Refer partner(s) to source of health care for evaluation and treatment as necessary.

- Exclude chlamydia and gonorrhea as sources of infection in the following circumstances, including but not limited to

  ▶ Woman at risk for STDs

  ▶ Presence of excess WBCs on saline wet mount

  ▶ Presence of MPC (see STD protocols)

- ▶ Recurrent/persistent vaginitis

- ▶ Etiology of vaginal symptoms cannot be determined

    NOTE: HIV infection should also be ruled out as appropriate.

- Treatment of physiologic leukorrhea should be avoided.

- *Candida* prophylaxis may be indicated during treatment with antibiotics for BV or trichomoniasis.

- Psychosocial assessments should be made in cases of recurrent STD or chronic unconfirmed vulvovaginitis (Stewart, Whelan, Fong, & Tessler, 1990).

- Routine screening for/treatment of BV in *asymptomatic* women is controversial. For patients at high risk for preterm birth, clinical evaluation and treatment has been recommended (preferably within the first 24 weeks of pregnancy) (American College of Obstetricians and Gynecologists [ACOG], 1998; Mead et al., 1997; Mead & Eschenbach, 1998).

    NOTE: Pap smears and vaginal cultures are not reliable for diagnosis; treatment should not be undertaken based on the results of these tests alone.

- Evaluate patients with signs/symptoms of preterm labor for the presence of BV and other vaginal infections/STDs and treat accordingly. See also Chapter 6.25, *Preterm Labor*, Chapter 6.24, *Preterm Rupture of Membranes,* and other STD chapters in Section 14.

- Consider screening and treatment for BV in women undergoing certain OB/GYN procedures (e.g., transvaginal chorionic villus sampling [CVS], cerclage, IUD placement, endometrial biopsy, hysteroscopy, hysterosalpingography, D&C, therapeutic abortion) or if the client is having vaginal or abdominal surgery (Thomason et al., 1991).

- Routine partner treatment is not recommended for women with BV (CDC, 1998). Abstinence from intercourse is a practical measure while the woman is being treated; advise condoms for BV prevention.

    NOTE: Male partner treatment has not been beneficial in preventing recurrent BV in the female (CDC, 1998).

- Persons with HIV should be treated with the same regimens for vaginitis as those without HIV infection (CDC, 1998).

Treatment Regimens

Bacterial Vaginosis

Recommended Regimen

- Metronidazole 250 mg p.o. t.i.d. for 7 days (CDC, 1998)

Alternative Regimens

- Metronidazole 2 grams p.o. b.i.d. in a single dose *or*
- Clindamycin 300 mg p.o. b.i.d. for 7 days (CDC, 1998)

Low-risk pregnant women may be treated with any of the above recommended or alternative regimens *or* with metronidazole gel 0.75 percent, one full applicator (5g) intravaginally b.i.d. for 5 days.

> **NOTE:** Some experts prefer systemic therapy even for low-risk women to treat possible subclinical upper genital tract infections (CDC, 1998). Vaginal treatment appears to be less effective in preventing preterm labor (ACOG, 1998). Regarding safety of metronidazole, a recent meta-analysis does not indicate teratogenicity in humans from use of this drug (CDC, 1998). During lactation, if oral metronidazole is employed, use the 2-gram dose and discontinue breastfeeding for 24 hours to allow excretion of the drug (breasts should be pumped and milk discarded) (American Academy of Pediatrics [AAP], 1997; Briggs, Freeman, & Yaffe, 1994).

Candidiasis

- Self-medication with over-the-counter (OTC) products should be attempted only if a woman has had a previously diagnosed candida infection and symptomatology is the same. Nonresolution of symptoms after treatment or symptom-recurrence within 2 months should prompt clinical diagnosis (CDC, 1998).

- Evidence of fungal elements on a Pap smear or culture is not an indication for treatment in an asymptomatic client (10 to 20 percent of women harbor *Candida* spp. and other yeasts as harmless commensal organisms in the vagina).

- Symptomatic partners of women with candidal infections (i.e., those with balanitis, penile dermatitis) should be treated with a topical antifungal agent. Refer to source of health care, as indicated.

- Evaluate women with recurrent candidiasis for predisposing conditions and, if possible, eliminate or control them. Management may include (but is not limited to):

    ▶ Use of "vaginitis diary" to identify possible precipitants

    ▶ Confirmation of infection with vaginal culture (mouth and ejaculate of partner may also be cultured) (Kaufman & Faro, 1994)

    ▶ Evaluation for HIV infection and diabetes, as appropriate

    ▶ Treatment of sexual partner(s), as indicated (see above)

    ▶ See also Table 14.13, Vulvovaginitis Prevention Strategies

Recommended Regimens (CDC, 1998)

- Choice of one of the following (where * is an oil-based preparation that can weaken latex condoms and diaphragms and § is an over-the-counter product):

    ▶ Butoconazole 2 percent cream, 5g intravaginally for 3 days*§

    ▶ Clotrimazole 1 percent cream, 5g intravaginally for 7 to 14 days*§

    ▶ Clotrimazole 100 mg vaginal tablet for 7 days*

    ▶ Clotrimazole 100 mg vaginal tablet, two tablets for 3 days*

    ▶ Clotrimazole 500 mg vaginal tablet in a single application*

▶ Miconazole 2 percent cream, 5g intravaginally for 7 days[*§]

▶ Miconazole 200 mg vaginal suppository, one suppository for 3 days[*§]

▶ Miconazole 100 mg vaginal suppository, one suppository for 7 days[*§]

▶ Tioconazole 6.5 percent ointment, 5g intravaginally in a single application[*§]

▶ Terconazole 0.4 percent cream, 5g intravaginally for 7 days[*]

▶ Terconazole 0.8 percent cream, 5g intravaginally for 3 days[*]

▶ Terconazole 80 mg suppository, one suppository for 3 days[*]

NOTE: Medication is usually applied at bedtime. Experts recommend 7 days of therapy during pregnancy (single- and/or three-day therapies may not be as effective during pregnancy or in severe/recurrent cases). The most effective regimens that have been studied for use during pregnancy are clotrimazole, miconazole, butoconazole, and terconazole (CDC, 1998). Refer to the *Physicians' Desk Reference* (PDR) for further information.

▶ For Candida-associated vulvar pruritus/inflammation

- Small amount antifungal cream to affected vulvar area q.d. to b.i.d. for up to 7 days as needed

and/or

- Low-potency corticosteroid cream/ointment to vulvar area sparingly b.i.d to t.i.d. for up to 7 days (e.g., hydrocortisone 1 to 2.5 percent).

NOTE: AVOID the use of *fluorinated* steroids.

Recurrent Candidiasis

- Confirm all cases by culture prior to treatment.

- Evaluate for predisposing conditions.

- Optimal treatment for recurrent infection during pregnancy has not been established.

- Alternation of the type of topical azole and use of longer regimens (10 to 14 days), followed by biweekly maintenance regimens may be tried; consult with a physician or clinical pharmacist.

  NOTE: Non-*albicans* species are more resistant to azoles (Mead & Eschenbach, 1998).

- Oral antifungal agents are not used during pregnancy for the treatment of vulvovaginal candidiasis. Refer to the *PDR* and/or to Briggs, Freeman, and Yaffe (1994) for further information regarding these agents. Refer to the CDC's 1998 STD treatment guidelines for further information on therapy for nonpregnant women.

Trichomoniasis

- Evaluate client for the presence of other STDs.

- Evaluate high-risk women for the presence of *T. vaginalis* on entry to prenatal care and prior to obstetric procedures (e.g., transvaginal CVS, cerclage) or gynecologic procedures (e.g., dilatation and curettage, hysterectomy) (Heine & McGregor, 1993).

- Treat all sexual partners of women with trichomoniasis appropriately. Evaluation for the presence of other STDs is also important; refer to source of health care, as indicated.

- Address fomite transmission, as appropriate to the case.

- It is preferable to not treat a woman solely on the basis of a Pap smear indicating *T. vaginalis*. Ideally, reevaluate the patient for infection (which may include historical questioning, vaginal examination, wet mount, culture) and treat accordingly (Weinberger & Harger, 1993).

Recommended Regimen

- Metronidazole 2 grams p.o. in a single dose (CDC, 1998)

  NOTE: Regarding the safety of metronidazole, a recent meta-analysis does not indicate teratogenicity in humans from use of the drug (CDC, 1998). If failure occurs with the metronidazole regimen above, consult with an infectious disease expert. See the Lossick & Kent (1991) reference for discussion on metronidazole treatment of refractory trichomoniasis. During lactation a 2-gram dose may be used; breastfeeding should be discontinued for 24 hours to allow excretion of the drug (breasts should be pumped and milk discarded) (Briggs et al.,1994).

Postpartum Atrophic Vaginitis

- Estrogen cream, one-half to a full applicator intravaginally daily for 7 days, followed by maintenance dose of one-half to a full applicator per week continued throughout the breastfeeding period (Kaufman & Faro, 1994). This dose will not affect lactation or the infant. Contraindications are the same as for oral estrogen—refer to the PDR.

- Vaginal lubricants may be used when estrogen is contraindicated.

Consultation

- Consult with an infectious disease expert, if necessary, in recalcitrant cases.

Patient Education

- See Table 14.13, Vulvovaginitis Prevention Strategies.

- Discuss physiologic leukorrhea, abnormal vaginal discharge, causes of vaginal infection, transmissibility, lifestyle behaviors that put client at risk of infection, and methods to reduce risk and spread of infection.

- If examination is within normal limits, reassure client. Advise that self-treatment of physiologic leukorrhea should be avoided.

- Stress importance of completing full course of prescribed medication for a diagnosed infection. If symptoms are unresolved client should return for reevaluation.

- Advise regarding abstinence during course of treatment for infection.

- Advise of possibility of candidiasis secondary to oral antibiotics and discuss indications for prophylactic therapy.

- Provide guidelines on safer sex practices; encourage condom use with new, multiple, or non-monogamous partners. See Table 14.1, Safer Sex Recommendations, in Chapter 14.1, *Chlamydia*.

- Recommend lubricants during intercourse to reduce discomfort associated with postpartum vaginal atrophy. Reassure patient that after breastfeeding with resumption of menstrual cycles the vagina will return to its normal state. Vaginal hormone therapy does not have adverse effects on the breastfed infant (Kaufman & Faro, 1994).

- Discuss vulvovaginal and general health and hygiene maintenance along with prophylactic measures to prevent recurrent infection. See Table 14.13, Vulvovaginitis Prevention Strategies.

- Advise regarding possible adverse effects of medications.

  ▶ Topical antifungal agents: vaginal itching, burning, irritation; flu-like symptoms (rare)

  ▶ Metronidazole: GI symptoms (e.g., nausea, vomiting, anorexia, diarrhea, constipation), headache, dizziness, metallic taste in mouth; seizures, peripheral neuropathy; reversible neutropenia. Warn against alcohol ingestion during treatment and for 24 hours thereafter (due to disulfiram-like effects).

  ▶ Clindamycin: severe diarrhea, abdominal cramps, passage of blood/mucus (due to pseudomembranous colitis).

NOTE: Refer to PDR or clinical pharmacist for further information. Be aware of concomitant medications and their interactions.

Follow-up

- Provide routine prenatal care.

- Have client return for reevaluation if symptoms do not improve with treatment. Query her regarding the taking of medication and if partner's therapy was completed, as indicated. Avoid over-the-phone diagnosis.

- In patients with recurrent infection, manage in consultation with an infectious disease specialist, as indicated.

- Consider reevaluation for BV in high-risk asymptomatic women one month after therapy to evaluate treatment efficacy.

- In patients refractory to treatment for trichomoniasis, consider metronidazole resistance. Cultures and susceptibility-testing can be performed. Consult with an infectious disease expert.

- Conduct appropriate follow-up of positive STD screening and other abnormal laboratory tests. All identified concomitant STDs must be treated. Discuss importance of partner evaluation and treatment in these situations; refer to source of health care, as indicated. See specific STD chapters throughout Section 14.

- Document diagnosis of vaginitis/STDs and treatment thereof in progress notes and problem list.

Table 14.12

Common Vulvovaginal Irritants

CHEMICAL

Bath gels/oils
Bubble baths
Condom lubricants
Chemically treated permanent-press clothing
Chemically treated water in hot tubs, swimming pools, whirlpool baths
Deodorant soaps/sprays/douches/tampons
Hair conditioners
Hair dyes
Home remedies (e.g., yogurt douches)
Laundry detergent (especially enzyme-activated "cold-water" formulas)
Over-the-counter drugs (e.g., local anesthetic ointments)
Perfumes
Shampoos
Spermicides
Sanitary napkins with deodorant, plastic shields, self adhesive panels
Talcum powder
Toilet paper, perfume-treated or dyed
Vaginal deodorants/spermicides

MECHANICAL

Cervical cap
Condom
Diaphragm
Dildos, vibrators
Exercise bicycles
Foreign bodies
Frequent masturbation
Horseback riding
Occlusive nonporous undergarments
Rowing machines
Tampons, especially with plastic applicators
Tight-fitting jeans, slacks

OTHER

Allergies to food, pet hair, yeast, molds, fungi, saliva
Excessive vaginal transudate, cervical mucus

Source: Burnhill, M.S. (1990) Clinician's guide to counseling patients with chronic vaginitis. *Contemporary OB/GYN, 35*(1), 39. Copyright 1990 by Medical Economics. Adapted with permission.

Table 14.13

Vulvovaginitis Prevention Strategies

- Use cotton underwear and loose-fitting clothing
  - ▶ Avoidance of panty hose and synthetic, elasticized garments
- Prevent fecal contamination of vagina:
  - ▶ Proper wiping technique (i.e., "front to back")
  - ▶ Masturbation with clean fingers
  - ▶ Avoidance of anal-to-vaginal intercourse or fingers into anal, then vaginal area
  - ▶ Curtailment of oral-genital sexual activity as necessary
- Reduce chemical/mechanical irritation
- Avoid douching
- Use proper vulvovaginal hygiene
  - ▶ Water only for cleansing of area; to dry, use low-setting hair dryer or "pat-dry"
  - ▶ Nonperfumed, nontalcum dusting powder may be used in crural folds for excessive sweating
  - ▶ Avoidance of feminine hygiene deodorant products
- Wash undergarments in mild detergent with good rinsing; line-dry
  - ▶ Freshly washed underclothing may be "sterilized" in the microwave 5 minutes on high
  - ▶ Alternately, panties may be boiled or soaked in bleach overnight
- Change tampons frequently during menstruation
  - ▶ Avoid tampons for 3–6 months in cases of recurrent infection
- Avoid unnecessary antibiotics
- Employ proper nutrition
  - ▶ Avoid excessive simple sugars/dairy products, artificial sweeteners, alcohol
- Prevent constipation
- Get exercise and adequate sleep
- Reduce stress
- Long-term condom use, as indicated
- Periodically soak diaphragm/cervical cap in dilute povidone-iodine solution

Sources: Burnhill, M.S. (1990). Clinician's guide to counseling patients with chronic vaginitis. *Contemporary OB/GYN,* *35*(1), 37–44; Star, W.L. (1995). *Candida* vaginitis. In W.L. Star, L.L. Lommel, & M.T. Shannon (Eds.), *Women's primary health care: Protocols for practice.* Washington, DC: American Nurses; Kaufman, R.H., & Faro, S. (1994). Candida. h R.H. Kaufman & S. Faro (Eds.), 1994, *Benign diseases of the vulva and vagina* (4th ed., pp. 321–337), St. Louis, MO: Mosby.

References

American Academy of Pediatrics (AAP). (1997). *1997 Red book. Report of the Committee on Infectious Diseases* (24th ed., pp. 77–79). Elk Grove Village, IL: Author.

American College of Obstetricians and Gynecologists (ACOG). (1996). *Vaginitis.* (Technical Bulletin No. 226). Washington, DC: ACOG.

American College of Obstetricians and Gynecologists (ACOG). (1998). Bacterial vaginosis screening for prevention of preterm delivery. (Committee Opinion No. 198). Washington, DC: ACOG.

Barclay, D.L. (1991). Benign disorders of the vulva and vagina. In M.L. Pernoll (Ed.), *Current obstetric and gynecologic diagnosis and treatment* (7th ed., pp. 692–718). Norwalk, CT: Appleton & Lange.

Berry, D.L., Olson, G.L., Wen, T.S., Belfort, M.A., & Moise, K.J. (1997). *Candida* chorioamnionitis: A report of two cases. *The Journal of Maternal-Fetal Medicine, 6*, 151–154.

Briggs, G.G., Freeman, R.K., & Yaffe, S.J. (1994). Drugs in pregnancy and lactation (4th ed.) Baltimore, MD: Williams & Wilkins.

Bump, R.C., & Buesching, W. J. (1988). Bacterial vaginosis in virginal and sexually active adolescent females: Evidence against exclusive sexual transmission. *American Journal of Obstetrics and Gynecology, 158*(4), 935–939.

Burnhill, M.S. (1990). Clinician's guide to counseling patients with chronic vaginitis. *Contemporary OB/GYN, 35*(1), 37–44.

Centers for Disease Control and Prevention (CDC). (1998). 1998 Sexually transmitted diseases treatment guidelines. *Morbidity and Mortality Weekly Report, 47* RR-1, 70–78.

Chaim, W., Mazor, M., & Wiznitzer, A. (1992). The prevalence and clinical significance of intraamniotic infection with *Candida* species in women with preterm labor. *Archives of Gynecology and Obstetrics, 251*, 9–15.

Chantigian, P.D.M. (1988). Vaginitis: A common malady. *Primary Care, 15*(3), 517–547.

Donders, G.G.G., Moerman, P., Caudron, J., & Van Assche, F.A. (1990). Intra-uterine *Candida* infection: A report of four infected fetuses from two mothers. *European Journal of Obstetrics and Gynecology and Reproductive Biology, 38*, 233–238.

Duff, P., Lee, M.L., Hillier, S.L., Herd, L.M., Krohn, M.A., & Eschenbach, D. A. (1991). Amoxicillin treatment of bacterial vaginosis during pregnancy. *Obstetrics and Gynecology, 77*(3), 431–435.

Ernest, J.M. (1992). Topical antifungal agents. *Obstetrics and Gynecology Clinics of North America, 19*(3), 587–607.

Gibbs, R.S., & Sweet, R.L. (1994). Clinical disorders. In R.K. Creasy & R. Resnik (Eds.), *Maternal-fetal medicine. Principles and practice* (3rd ed.). Philadelphia, PA: W.B. Saunders.

Glupczynski, Y.M., Labbé, M., Cokaert, F., Pepersack, P., van der Auwera, P., & Yourassowsky, E. (1984). Isolation of *Mobiluncus* in four cases of extragenital infections in adult women. *European Journal of Clinical Microbiology, 3*, 433–435.

Goode, M.A., Grauer, K., & Gums, J.G., Infectious vaginitis. *Postgraduate Medicine, 96*(6), 85–98.

Gravett, M.G., Nelson, H.P., DeRouen, C., Critchlow, C. Eschenbach, D.A., & Holmes, K.K. (1986). Independent associations of bacterial vaginosis and *Chlamydia trachomatis* infection with adverse pregnancy outcome. *Journal of the American Medical Association, 256*, 1899–1903.

Hauth, J.C., Goldenberg, R.L., Andrews, W.W., DuBard, M.B., & Copper, R.L. (1995). Reduced incidence of preterm delivery with metroidazole and erythromycin in women with bacterial vaginosis. *New England Journal of Medicine, 333*, 1732–1736.

Heine, P., & McGregor, J. A. (1993). *Trichomonas vaginalis*: A reemerging pathogen. *Clinical Obstetrics and Gynecology, 36*(1), 137–144.

Hillier, S., & Holmes, K.K. (1990). Bacterial vaginosis. In K.K. Holmes, P.-A. Mårdh, P.F. Sparling, P.J. Wiesner, W. Cates, Jr., S.M. Lemon, & W.E. Stamm (Eds.), *Sexually transmitted diseases* (2nd ed., 547–559). New York: McGraw-Hill.

Holst, E., & Brandberg, A. (1990). Treatment of bacterial vaginosis in pregnancy with a lactate gel. *Scandinavian Journal of Infectious Disease, 22*, 625–626.

Holst, E., Goffeng, A.R., & Andersch, B. (1994). Bacterial vaginosis and vaginal microorganisms in idiopathic premature labor and association with pregnancy outcome. *Journal of Clinical Microbiology, 32*(1), 176–186.

Hooten, T.M., Finn, S.D., Johnson, C., Roberts, P.L., & Stamm, W.E. (1989). Association between bacterial vaginosis and acute cystitis in women using diaphragms. *Annals of Internal Medicine, 149*, 1932–1936.

Lossick, J.G. (1990). Treatment of sexually transmitted vaginosis/vaginitis. *Reviews of Infectious Diseases, 12*(Suppl. 6), S665–S681.

Lossick, J.G., & Kent, H.L. (1991). Trichomoniasis: Trends in diagnosis and management. *American Journal of Obstetrics and Gynecology, 165*(4, Pt. 2), 1217–1222.

Kaufman, R.H., & Faro, S. (1994). *Benign diseases of the vulva and vagina* (4th ed.). St. Louis, MO: Mosby.

Kurki, T., Sivonen, A., Renkonen, O.-V., Savia, E., & Ylikorkala, O. Bacterial vaginosis in early pregnancy and pregnancy outcome. *Obstetrics and Gynecology, 80*(2), 173–177.

Martius, J., & Eschenbach, D.A. (1990). The role of bacterial vaginosis as a cause of amniotic fluid infection, chorioamnionitis and prematurity - a review. *Archives of Gynecology and Obstetrics, 247*, 1–13.

Mazor, M., Shinwell, E.S., & Glezerman, M. (1993). Asymptomatic amniotic fluid invasion with *Candida albicans* in preterm premature rupture of membranes. *Acta Obstetrica and Gynecologica Scandinavica, 72*, 52–54.

McCoy, M.C., Katz, V.L., Kuller, J.A., Killam, A.P., & Livengood, C.H. (1995). Bacterial vaginosis in pregnancy: An approach for the 1990s. *Obstetrical and Gynecological Survey, 50*(6), 482–488.

McGregor, J.A., & French, J.I. (1988). Are neonatal scalp abscesses another complication of bacterial vaginosis? *Pediatric Infectious Diseases, 7*, 437–438.

Mead, P.B., & Eschenbach, D.A. (1986). New ways to treat problem vaginitis. *Contemporary OB/GYN, 41*(4), 86–104.

Mead, P.B., & Eschenbach, D.A. (1998). Vaginitis 1998: Update and Guidelines. *Contemporary OB/GYN, 43*(1), 116–132.

Mead, P.B., Hillier, S., McDonald, H., McGregor, J.A., & Sweet, R. (1997). Screening for lower genital tract pathogens in the OB patient. *Contemporary OB/GYN, 42*(5), 126–145.

Moldwin, R.M. (1992). Sexually transmitted protozoal infections. *Urologic Clinics of North America, 19*(1), 93–101.

Morales, W.J., Schoor, S., & Albritton, J. (1994). Effect of metronidazole in patients with preterm birth in preceding pregnancy and bacterial vaginosis: A placebo-controlled, double-blind study. *American Journal of Obstetrics and Gynecology, 17*(2), 345–349.

Quan, M. (1990). Diagnosis and management of infectious vaginitis. *Journal of the American Board of Family Practice, 3*, 195–205.

Redondo-Lopez, V., , Cook, R.L., & Sobel, J.D. (1990). Emerging role of lactobacilli in the control and maintenance of the vaginal bacterial microflora. *Reviews of Infectious Diseases, 19*(5), 856–872.

Reed, B.D. (1992). Risk factors for candida vulvovaginitis. *Obstetrical and Gynecological Survey, 47*(8), 551–560.

Rein, M.F., & Müller, M. (1990). *Trichomoniasis vaginalis* and trichomoniasis. In K.K. Holmes, P.-A. Mårdh, P.F. Sparling, P.J. Wiesner, W. Cates, Jr., S.M. Lemon, & W.E. Stamm (Eds.), *Sexually transmitted diseases* (2nd ed., 481–492). New York: McGraw-Hill.

Schlict, J.R. (1994). Treatment of bacterial vaginosis. *The Annals of Pharmacotherapy, 28*, 483–486.

Schwartz, D.A., & Reef, S. (1990). *Candida albicans* placentitis and funisitis: Early diagnosis of congenital candidemia by histopathologic examination of umbilical cord vessels. *Pediatric Infectious Disease Journal, 9*(9), 661–665.

Sobel, J.D. (1990). Vaginal infections in adult women. *Sexually transmitted diseases, 74*(6), 1573–1601.

Sobel, J.D. (1995). Treating resistant vaginal infections. *The Female Patient, 20*, 32–46.

Soper, D.E. (1993). Bacterial vaginosis and postoperative infections. *American Journal of Obstetrics and Gynecology, 169*(2, Pt. 2), 467–469.

Soper, D.E., Bump, R.C., & Hurt, W.G. (1990). Bacterial vaginosis and trichomoniasis vaginitis are risk factors for cuff cellulitis after abdominal hysterectomy. *American Journal of Obstetrics and Gynecology, 163*, 1016–1023.

Spiegel, C.A. (1991). Bacterial vaginosis. *Clinical Microbiology Reviews, 4*(4), 485–502.

Spiegel, C.A., Amsel, R., & Holmes, K.K. (1983). Diagnosis of bacterial vaginosis by direct Gram stain of vaginal fluid. *Journal of Clinical Microbiology, 18*, 120–177.

Star, W.L. (1995). *Candida* vaginitis. In W.L. Star, L.L. Lommel, & M.T. Shannon (Eds.), *Women's primary health care: Protocols for practice* (12.149–12.201). Washington, DC: American Nurses.

Stewart, D.A., Whelan, C.I., Fong, I., & Tessler, K.M. (1990). Psychosocial aspects of chronic, clinically unconfirmed vulvovaginitis. *Obstetrics and Gynecology, 76*(5, Pt. 1), 852–856.

Sturm, A.W. (1989). *Mobiluncus* species and other anaerobic bacteria in non-puerperal breast abscesses. *European Journal of Clinical Microbiology and Infectious Diseases, 8,* 789–792.

Sweet, R.L., & Gibbs, R.S. (1995). *Infectious diseases of the female genital tract* (3rd ed.). Baltimore, MD: Williams & Wilkins.

Thomason, J.L., Gelbart, S.M., & Scaglione, N.J. (1991). Bacterial vaginosis: Current review with indications for asymptomatic therapy. *American Journal of Obstetrics and Gynecology, 165*(4, Pt. 2), 1210–1217.

Watts, D.H., Eschenbach, D.A., & Kenney, G.E., (1989). Early postpartum endometritis: the role of bacteria, genital mycoplasmas, and *Chlamydia trachomatis. Obstetrics and Gynecology, 73,* 52–60.

Watts, D.H., Krohn, M.A., Hillier, S.L., & Eschenbach, D.A. (1990). Bacterial vaginosis as a risk factor for post-cesarean endometritis. *Obstetrics and Gynecology, 75,* 52–58.

Weinberger, M.W., & Harger, J.H., (1993). Accuracy of the Papanicolaou smear in the diagnosis of asymptomatic infection with *Trichomonas vaginalis. Obstetrics and Gynecology, 82*(3), 425–429.

Wiesinger, E.C., Mayerhofer, S., Wenisch, C., Breyer, S., & Graninger, W. (1996). Fluconazole in *Candida Albicans* sepsis during pregnancy: Case report and review of the literature. *Infection, 24,* 263–266.

SECTION 15

PREGNANCY AND OCCUPATIONAL HEALTH

Section 15

PREGNANCY AND OCCUPATIONAL HEALTH

Barbara J. Burgel

Occupational health issues are of paramount importance during reproduction and pregnancy. The goal is to safeguard the health of both mother and fetus during pregnancy and upon return to work. The full magnitude of reproductive health hazards is not well characterized because of limited epidemiological and toxicological data (American College of Occupational and Environmental Medicine [ACOEM], 1996).

Reproductive toxicity is the occurrence of adverse effects on the reproductive system resulting from exposure to environmental or occupational agents. Developmental toxicity is the occurrence of adverse effects on a developing organism resulting from either parent's exposure to a hazard before conception, exposure of the fetus during prenatal development, or postnatal exposure (up to the time of sexual maturation). Developmental toxic outcomes can include fetal death, birth defects, and altered growth (ACOEM, 1996; Office of Technology Assessment, 1985).

Recent legislative initiatives have highlighted the importance of occupational health to pregnancy, specifically the Family Medical Leave Act enacted in 1993 and the 1991 Supreme Court Decision on Johnson Controls (See Appendix 15a, Legal and Ethical Issues Affecting Pregnancy and Work). The National Institute of Occupational Safety and Health (NIOSH) identified fertility and pregnancy abnormalities as a top priority for the National Occupational Research Agenda (U.S. Department of Health and Human Services [USDHHS], 1996). The U.S. Department of Health and Human Services (1991) *Healthy People 2000* objectives for maternal and infant health focus on the reduction of infant and maternal mortality and morbidity (USDHHS, 1991). Additionally, there are goals to support more breast-feeding, abstinence from tobacco use, increased prenatal care in the first trimester and preconception care and counseling, all of which may be health promotion activities at the work site to meet the health needs of childbearing women.

The objectives for occupational safety and health are relevant to the childbearing population, specifically those directed toward decreased lead exposure, prevention of hepatitis B infection, and back injury rehabilitation (USDHHS, 1991). This chapter targets three critical periods where occupational and environmental exposures interact with reproduction: preconception, pregnancy, and the postpartum periods.

One of the most important occupational safety and health objectives reinforces the priority of preconception counseling; that goal is to "increase to at least 75 percent the proportion of primary care providers who routinely elicit occupational health exposures as a part of patient history and provide relevant counseling" (USDHHS, 1991).

Preconception counseling is recommended to ensure that women are healthy prior to pregnancy (See Section 1, *Preconceptional Health Care*). Not only is this the ideal time to review work processes, explore potential reproductive hazards, and educate the client regarding ways to decrease exposure, but it is an opportunity to reinforce smoking cessation, reduction of alcohol intake, and avoidance of illicit drugs. Exposures to potential reproductive hazards and physical demands of work should be periodically assessed throughout pregnancy, and any work accommodations to maintain the health of both the mother and fetus should be made. Postpartum assessment includes return-to-work plans and an assessment of any potential chemical exposure that could be absorbed by the mother and excreted during lactation.

The health and safety of both the pregnant working woman and the fetus are vital and should include an employer-based comprehensive program aimed at recognizing and controlling reproductive hazards. Both women and men need to be educated about occupational and environmental exposures that could adversely affect reproduction. Most pregnant women employed in light industry are able to work until their date of delivery with minimal accommodation. Those jobs involving chemical exposure and/or increased physical demands require more aggressive work modification. Determining work accommodation for pregnant women is an interdisciplinary activity involving a clear understanding of the physiology of pregnancy and the nature of the specific work tasks, including the potential for chemical exposures and the physical and emotional requirements of the job. Consultation between the prenatal health provider with occupational and environmental health and safety experts is valuable to determine any needed work preclusions.

Database

Subjective

- A comprehensive preconception history should include an occupational, exposure, and environmental assessment, in addition to a thorough reproductive history (Keleher, 1991; USDHHS, 1992; ACOEM, 1996) Questions may include but are not limited to those found in Appendix 15b:

  ▶ Describe the client's work (job tasks and work environment). (See Table 15.1, Selected Occupations and Potential Exposures Relevant to Pregnancy.)

  ▶ Note hours, rotating shifts, amount of overtime.

  ▶ Note any exposure in the last 6 months to chemicals in work, home, hobbies, neighborhood.

  ▶ List any exposures to infectious agents in the past 6 months.

  ▶ Identify psychological work demands.

  ▶ List ergonomic work demands.

    – Lifting requirements (note weight limit and number of times per hour per day)

    – Standing (note number of hours per day)

    – Climbing ladders (note number of times per hour per day)

    – Any other ergonomic exposures

  ▶ List physical hazards.

    – Radiation

    – Heat

    – Noise

    – Any pressurized work activity or enclosure, such as diving

  ▶ Identify whether and in what circumstances the client wears protective equipment (e.g., gloves, respirator, hearing protection).

▶ Ask whether any household members come in contact with any of the above exposures.

   – Specifically assess past or present exposures of the father of the child.

▶ List any symptoms or conditions related to the client's work.

   – Do symptoms get better or worse on days off or on vacations?

   – Has there been any recent change in work practices that appear to coincide with symptoms?

▶ Have any coworkers had problems related to work?

▶ Obtain a pregnancy history, and note any miscarriages, fetal deaths, birth defects, premature deliveries, or other unusual outcomes.

▶ Identify other known reproductive risk factors (e.g., alcohol intake, illicit or prescribed medications, smoking [active or passive exposure]).

▶ Find out if the employer has a required or recommended pregnancy notification policy.

▶ Determine the client's drinking water source both at home and at work.

- A comprehensive, postconception history will include many of the questions listed above. Based on the exposure history and the current work responsibilities, the focus is to prevent current exposure and limit work activities which could harm the mother and fetus. Questions for the pregnant woman may include but are not limited to those found in Appendix 15b.

- Describe current work duties.

  ▶ Note any changes since the preconception interview.

  ▶ Assess for exposures. (See Appendix 15b.)

  ▶ Note any modifications that have occurred because of the pregnancy.

- Determine whether there are any current symptoms related to work.

- Does the client think there are any work accommodations needed at this time of her pregnancy?

- Has the client told her employer of her pregnancy?

  ▶ Has she been informed of any specific pregnancy-related hazards associated with work?

  ▶ Assess employer reaction to the pregnancy.

  ▶ Discuss specific plans for time off work and current return-to-work plans.

  ▶ Begin to plan for available benefits for time off work.

  ▶ Identify employer-based resources (e.g., an occupational health nurse, an exercise physiologist, an on-site lactation room).

  ▶ Assess the status of the pregnancy (e.g., the presence of bleeding, contractions, or other critical variables such as nutrition, alcohol use, passive or active tobacco exposure, or prescribed, over-the-counter, or illicit drug use).

- A comprehensive postpartum history specifically addresses return to work, lactation plans, and aims to prevent exposures to those substances that may be excreted through breast milk. See Appendix 15b.

▶ Discuss whether the client plans to breast-feed after the baby is born.

▶ Discuss specific return-to-work plans.

  – Note hours, shifts, any anticipated overtime

  – Describe anticipated work duties

▶ Determine whether there will be any exposure to the following substances:

  – Polychlorinated compounds (e.g., polychlorinated biphenyls [PCBs], persistent organochlorine pesticides)

  – Polycyclic aromatic hydrocarbons (PAH)

  – Nitrates, nitrites, nitrosamines

  – Nicotine, caffeine, or ethanol

  – Drugs

  – Other chemical exposures to solvents, metals, or pesticides

▶ Identify employer-based resources.

  – Is there a breast-feeding policy at work?

  – Is the client aware of any chemicals that could be excreted in your breast milk?

  – Discuss the availability of an on-site lactation room with pumps and refrigeration options at work.

  – Discuss availability of hand washing and shower facilities.

  – On-site child care facilities?

  – Any employer flex-time options?

▶ If the client does not plan on breast-feeding but is planning to return to work, assess the risk of work-to-home exposure to protect a developing fetus or a developing infant or child.

  – Does the employer have end of shift hand washing and shower facilities?

  – Does the employer launder work clothes?

  – Can housekeeping at the workplace be improved?

Objective

● Perform complete physical examination.

● If there is exposure, document the route (i.e., inhalation, skin, ingestion) and dosage.

● Document the toxicology of the exposure; match the toxicology to the symptom and/or target organ effect.

● Evaluate the potential occupational health impact of the physiological changes associated with pregnancy (see Table 15.2. Hypothesized Occupational Health Impact of Physiologic Changes in Pregnancy).

- Assess for those agents associated with adverse female reproductive or developmental effects (see Table 15.3, Agents Associated with Adverse Female Reproductive Capacity or Developmental Effects in Human and Animal Studies), including known teratogens (see Table 15.4, Known or Suspected Human Teratogens).

- Assess for exposures associated with male reproductive dysfunction (see Table 15.5, Exposures Associated with Male Reproductive Dysfunction).

- Table 15.6, Milk-to-Maternal Plasma Ratios in Exposed Women, lists those chemicals that have been found in breast milk.

- Document applicable Occupational Safety and Health Administration (OSHA) standards, and/or Environmental Protection Agency (EPA) regulations, including permissible exposure levels. See Appendix 15c, Occupational Health and Safety Resources, for information on how to research applicable standards.

- Document baseline/past medical surveillance data.

  ▶ Determine whether there is environmental monitoring data (e.g., air sampling for lead dust levels.)

  ▶ Determine whether there has been biological monitoring (e.g., tests for blood lead levels).

  NOTE: Workers have a legal right to this information from the employer, if sampling has been done.

- Document the applicable information from material safety data sheets (MSDS), which describe the toxicology and health hazards for specific hazardous substances. All workers have a legal right to MSDS information through the Hazard Communication standard.

- Request job analysis data from the employer to verify the extent of potential reproductive risk factors in current employment.

Assessment

- Pregnancy needing no work accommodations.

- Occupational exposure (maternal or paternal) that could adversely affect the ability to conceive, the health of the mother and/or the health of the developing fetus.

- Environmental exposure that could adversely affect the ability to conceive, the health of the mother and/or the health of the developing fetus.

  NOTE: Rule out nonoccupational exposures that could adversely affect the ability to conceive or affect the health of the mother and/or developing fetus.

Plan

Diagnostic Tests

- Preconception, prenatal, and postpartum laboratory evaluation depends on the specific occupational and/or environmental exposures and may include but are not limited to

  ▶ Blood lead level and sperm analysis (for lead exposure)

- ▶ Blood and urine cadmium levels (for cadmium exposure)
- ▶ Carboxyhemoglobin levels (for carbon monoxide exposure)
- ▶ Methemoglobin levels (for nitrate exposure)
- ▶ Varicella and rubella titers to assess for antibody presence (for hospital workers)
- ▶ Analysis of radiation dosimeter badge

- Consult with experts regarding other needed biological monitoring indices.

- Conduct a worksite evaluation. Worksite evaluation is an additional diagnostic tool. A visit to observe the work processes, or a videotape of the specific work process can be very helpful for work modification if there are additional questions after reviewing the job analysis.

  NOTE: Worksite evaluation is usually done by an occupational health and safety specialist, hired by the employer or by the workers compensation insurance carrier.

- Measurement of specific exposures at the worksite is done by personal breathing zone sampling of the employee.

  NOTE: An industrial hygienist, hired either by the employer or by the workers compensation insurance carrier, collects these environmental samples and evaluates control measures, such as ventilation systems.

Treatment/Management

- Occupational and environmental health exposures are managed by a hierarchy of controls, including substitution, engineering controls, administrative controls, and personal protective equipment.

  - ▶ Substitution involves using a less hazardous substance in place of the hazardous agent (e.g., use of nonleaded pigments in ceramic work).

  - ▶ Engineering controls correct hazard problems by "engineering" them out (e.g., installing a local ventilation system over the gas sterilizer to limit ethylene oxide exposure).

  - ▶ Administrative controls focus on reducing the exposure to one person by sharing the risk amongst several employees (e.g., limit ladder climbing to 2 hours per shift for each employee).

    - – Temporary modified duty is often used during the preconception period if a couple is attempting pregnancy and/or during the prenatal and postpartum periods.

  - ▶ Personal protective equipment prevents exposure by placing an individual barrier between the worker and the hazard (e.g., respirators, gloves, hearing protection, and safety glasses).

    NOTE: Ideally, personal protective equipment is used until engineering controls are implemented, if feasible.

- Determining the need for job accommodation for a pregnant employee is an individual case-by-case decision, based on the following variables:

  - ▶ Knowledge of the physical and emotional requirements of the job

- ▶ Presence of potential worksite reproductive hazards, including dose-response data, environmental sampling data

- ▶ Preconception health status of the employee

- ▶ Perspective of the pregnant employee regarding pregnancy status

- ▶ Extent of disability benefits

- ▶ Consultation with the employer based occupational health and safety resources

- The American College of Obstetrics and Gynecology (ACOG) and NIOSH (1978) note that "the normal woman with an uncomplicated pregnancy and a normal fetus in a job that presents no greater potential hazards than those encountered in normal daily life in the community may continue to work without interruption until the onset of labor and may resume working several weeks after an uncomplicated delivery."

- ACOG and NIOSH (1978) present an algorithm to facilitate decision making by the health care provider to determine if

  - ▶ The woman may continue to work without change.

  - ▶ The woman may continue to work but with certain modifications of environment or activity with either a desirable modification or an essential modification.

  - ▶ The woman should not work.

- The American Medical Association (AMA) Council on Scientific Affairs (1984a) presents guidelines for continuation of specific job functions based on week of gestation (see Table 15.7, Guidelines for Continuation of Various Levels of Work During Pregnancy).

- Physical demands, specifically prolonged standing and/or walking, appear to increase the risk of preterm delivery (Ahlborg, 1995).

  - ▶ Women should therefore avoid extremely heavy physical exertion (close to the individual's maximum capacity) in the first trimester of pregnancy, and reduce physical work load and add more frequent rest periods in the second and third trimesters (Ahlborg, 1995).

  - ▶ Decreasing maximum lifting to 20 to 25 percent during the third trimester has also been recommended (LaDou, 1990).

  - ▶ Using a rest bar, and alternating sitting, standing and walking are prudent recommendations during late in pregnancy.

- There are specific health conditions that have a strong likelihood for pregnancy complications and that may preclude work until after childbirth (Keleher, 1991; AMA, 1984b).

  - ▶ Conditions that may warrant time off work during pregnancy:

    - – A past history of an incompetent cervix

    - – Uncontrolled insulin-dependent diabetes with retinopathy

    - – Cardiac status greater than class 2

  - ▶ Decisions about time off during pregnancy are made on a case-by-case basis.

- When planning return to work, 6 weeks postvaginal delivery and 8 weeks postcesarean delivery are the expected rates of recovery for those women without major childbirth complications (AMA, 1984b).

- A return-to-work/fitness-for-duty evaluation is necessary to insure that the postpartum employee has the physical and emotional capacities to do the job.

- Potential chemical exposure via breast milk needs to be considered in job assignment postdelivery, specifically exploring those lipophilic (i.e., absorbed in fat) and low-molecular weight substances that can easily contaminate breast milk, for example, polychlorinated biphenyls (PCB's) (USDHHS, 1993). See Table 15.6, Milk-to-Maternal Plasma Ratios in Exposed Women.

- Appendix 15a, Legal and Ethical Issues Affecting Pregnancy and Work, summarizes the pertinent legal and ethical considerations affecting pregnancy and work.

Note: The Family Medical Leave Act provides up to 12 weeks of unpaid, job protected leave for pregnancy, but is limited to employees who have worked at least 12 months for employers with more than 50 employees.

- Check the state and federal reporting requirements.

  ▶ The Doctor's First Report of Occupational Injury (or other state-required form) documents the presence of a work-related condition. If there is a workers compensation claim, additional forms need completion.

  ▶ Each state has a listing of those infectious and occupational diseases which must be reported to the local health department (Mandatory Reporting of Occupational Diseases by Clinicians).

  ▶ There may be additional state required reporting requirements; for example, in California, reporting of an actual or suspected pesticide exposure is mandated.

Consultation

- Consult with occupational nursing or medicine experts, either through local health departments, poison control centers, university based occupational medicine clinics and/or through the client's employer.

- Consult with the employer of the pregnant employee, after gaining permission to do so, to request job analysis data or to design work accommodations.

- If there is a workers compensation claim, contact the workers compensation claims adjuster to request specific services, for example, environmental monitoring data.

- Federal and state Occupational Safety and Health Administration (OSHA) programs offer free consultation to employers and free technical assistance. The Environmental Protection Agency (EPA), the Agency for Toxic Substances and Disease Registry, and NIOSH, a division of the Centers for Disease Control and Prevention, all offer technical assistance.

- Computer databases include Med-line (National Library of Medicine), Reprotox (Reproductive Toxicology Center), TERIS (Teratogen Information System), and the Toxicology Information Program (National Library of Medicine) (ACOEM, 1996).

Patient Education

- Explain to the client that she has legal rights to a safe and healthy workplace, including prevention of pregnancy related discrimination (see Appendix 15a, Legal and Ethical Issues Affecting Pregnancy and Work).

- Discuss the relationship between exposure and symptoms, and explain ways to prevent future exposure.

- Outline limitations of disability benefits and facilitate good problem solving when planning work decisions.

- Refer the client to the employer's human resources department regarding the specifics of disability coverage in the company.

- Flex-time work options, breast-feeding support, and on-site child care may be offered by the employer. Advocate a self-care approach so that the pregnant employee seeks out every avenue to have a successful pregnancy.

- Refer to Appendix 15c, Occupational Health and Safety Resources, to obtain a sample handout that can be used for working women considering pregnancy.

Follow-up

- Closely follow up any continuing or new occupational and/ or environmental exposures.

- Evaluate progress of any work accommodations.

- Document in progress notes and problem list any needed time off for temporary disability based on an exposure assessment, a dose-response evaluation, the physical and emotional requirements of the job, and the status of the pregnancy. Document additional occupational health issues affecting pregnancy, as indicated.

Table 15.1

Selected Occupations and Potential Exposures Relevant to Pregnancy

Selected Occupations	Potential Exposures Relevant to Pregnancy
Agricultural workers (including gardeners and horticulture, nursery, and farm workers)	Pesticides Heat Lifting, stooping, standing
Computer chip manufacturing	Glycol ethers, and other solvents
Battery manufacturing workers	Lead Cadmium Solvents
Parking lot attendants, bridge toll workers	Carbon monoxide
Furniture stripping	Methylene chloride is metabolized to carbon monoxide
Ceramics	Lead pigment in glazes and paints
Hospital workers	Ethylene oxide (central supply) Anesthetic gases (operating room/recovery room) Chemotherapeutic agents Biological hazards Radiation Lifting

Table 15.2

Hypothesized Occupational Health Impact of Physiologic Changes in Pregnancy

Some Known Physiologic Changes	Agent or Condition	Example of Possible Impact	Suggested Job Accommodations
I. General			
↑Fatigue or stress	Inflexible hours Shift work	↑May be aggravated	Scheduling flexibility Frequent rest breaks
↑Nausea	Ketones or acrylates Exhaust fumes	↑Sensitivity to chemicals with strong, unpleasant odors	Improve ventilation Provide respiratory protection
↑Metabolic rate	Carbon tetrachloride	↑Hepatotoxicity (especially if metabolically activated)	Minimize exposure
	Protective gear	↑Discomfort or heat intolerance	
II. Cardiovascular			
↑Uteroplacental flow	Hemolytic agents (e.g., Arsine)	↓Maternal oxygen carrying capacity	Minimize exposure
	Asphyxiants (e.g., carbon monoxide, or agents that metabolize to carbon monoxide, like methylene chloride)	↓Fetal oxygenation leading to hypoxia	
↑Myocardial irritability	Chlorinated hydrocarbons (e.g., TCE)	↑Arrhythmias or MIs	Minimize exposure
↑Autonomic control of vasomotor tone	Anesthetic agents Organic solvents	↑Arterial pressure Preeclampsia	Minimize exposure
↑ Renal blood flow	Cadmium	↑Renal toxicity	Minimize exposure
III. Respiratory			
↑Respiratory rate ↑Tidal volume	All airborne chemicals	↑Absorbed dose per unit time	Minimize exposure
↑Hyperemic engorgement, capillary dilatation	Formaldehyde Sulfur dioxide	↑Sensitivity to irritants and allergens	Minimize exposure
IV. Musculoskeletal			
↑Lower back pain ↑Lumbar lordosis, symphyseal and sacroiliac loosening Shifted center of gravity	Heavy lifting Ergonomically poor chairs and work stations	↑Difficulty lifting ↑Pain	Provide mobility for postural changes Decrease maximum lifting by 20–25% in last trimester Provide well-designed chairs and work stations

Source: LaDou, J. (Ed.) (1990). *Occupational Medicine*, Norwalk, CT: Appleton & Lange. Used by permission.

Table 15.3

Agents Associated with Adverse Female Reproductive Capacity or Developmental Effects in Human And Animal Studies*

Agent	Human Outcomes	Strength of Association in Humans*	Animal Outcomes	Strength of Association in Animals*
Anesthetic gases¶	Reduced fertility, spontaneous abortion	1,3	Birth defects	1,3
Arsenic	Spontaneous abortion, low birth weight	1	Birth defects, fetal loss	2
Benzo(a)pyrene	None	NA†	Birth defects	1
Cadmium	None	NA	Fetal loss, birth defects	2
Carbon disulfide	Menstrual disorders, spontaneous abortion	1	Birth defects	1
Carbon monoxide	Low birth weight, fetal death (high doses)	1	Birth defects, neonatal mortality, fetal loss	2
Chlordecone	None	NA	Fetal loss	2,3
Chloroform	None	NA	Birth defects	1
Chloroprene	None	NA	Birth defects	2,3
Ethylene glycol ethers	Spontaneous abortion	1	Fetal loss	2
Ethylene oxide	Spontaneous abortion	1	Fetal loss, birth defects	1
Formamides	None	NA		2
Inorganic mercury¶	Menstrual disorders, spontaneous abortion	1	Fetal loss, birth defects	1
Lead¶	Spontaneous abortion, prematurity, neurologic dysfunction in child	2	Birth defects, fetal loss	2
Organic mercury	CNS malformation, cerebral palsy	2	Birth defects, fetal loss	2

(continued)

Table 15.3

Agents Associated with Adverse Female Reproductive Capacity or Developmental Effects in Human And Animal Studies* (continued)

Agent	Human Outcomes	Strength of Association in Humans*	Animal Outcomes	Strength of Association in Animals*
Physical stress	Prematurity	2		NA
Polybrominated biphenyls (PBBs)	None	NA	Fetal loss	2
Polychlorinated biphenyls (PCBs)	Neonatal PCB syndrome (low birth weight, hyperpigmentation, eye abnormalities)	2	Low birth weight, fetal loss	2
Radiation, ionizing	Menstrual disorders, CNS defects, skeletal & eye abnormalities, mental retardation, childhood cancer	2	Fetal loss, birth defects	2
Selenium	Spontaneous abortion	3	Low birth weight, birth defects	2
Tellurium	None	NA	Birth defects	2
2,4 dichlorophen-oxyacetic acid (2,4-D)	Skeletal defects	4	Birth defects	1
2,4,5 trichlorophen-oxyacetic acid (2,4,5-T)	Skeletal defects	4	Birth defects	1
Video display terminals	Spontaneous abortion	4	Birth defects	1
Vinyl chloride¶	CNS defects	1	Birth defects	1,4
Xylene	Menstrual disorders, fetal loss	1	Fetal loss, birth defects	1

§ Major studies of the reproductive health effects of exposure to dioxin are currently in progress.

* 1 = limited positive data; 2 = strong positive data; 3 = limited negative data; 4 = strong negative data

† Not applicable because no adverse outcomes were observed.

¶ Agents that may have male-mediated effects.

Source: United States Department of Health and Human Services. (1993). *Case studies in environmental medicine: Reproductive and developmental hazards.* Atlanta, GA: Agency for Toxic Substances and Disease Registry.

Table 15.4

Known or Suspected Human Teratogens

Chemicals/Drugs

> Aminopterin
> Androgenic hormones
> Antithyroid drugs
> Busulfan
> Chlorobiphenyls
> Coumarin anticoagulants
> Cyclophosphamide
> Diethylstilbestrol
> Diphenylhydantoin
> Lithium
> Mercury, organic
> Methimazole
> 13-cis-Retinoic acid
> Tetracyclines
> Trimethadione

Radiation

> Atomic weapons
> Radioiodine
> Radiotherapy

Infectious agents

> Cytomegalovirus
> Hepatitis B virus
> Herpes simplex virus
> Rubella virus
> Treponema pallidum (syphilis)
> Toxoplasma gondii
> Varicella virus (chicken pox)
> Venezuelan equine encephalitis virus

Source: United States Department of Health and Human Services. (1993). *Case studies in environmental medicine: Reproductive and developmental hazards.* Atlanta, GA: Agency for Toxic Substances and Disease Registry.

Table 15.5

Exposures Associated with Male Reproductive Dysfunction.

Agent	Human Outcomes	Strength of Association in Humans*	Animal Outcomes	Strength of Association in Animals*
Boron	Decreased sperm count	1	Testicular damage	2
Benzene	None	NA†	Decreased sperm motility, testicular damage	1
Beno(a)pyrene	None	NA	Testicular damage	1
Cadmium	Reduced fertility	1	Testicular damage	2
Carbon disulfide	Decreased sperm count, decreased sperm motility	2,3	Testicular damage	1
Carbon monoxide	None	NA	Testicular damage	1
Carbon tetrachloride	None	NA	Testicular damage	1
Carbaryl	Abnormal sperm morphology	1	Testicular damage	1
Chlordecone	Decreased sperm count, decreased sperm motility	2	Testicular damage	2
Chloroprene	Abnormal sperm morphology, decreased sperm motility, decreased libido	2	Testicular damage	1
Dibromochloro-propane (DBCP)	Decreased sperm count, azoospermia, hormonal changes	2	Testicular damage	2
Dimethyl dichloro-vinyl phosphate (DDVP)	None	NA	Decreased sperm count	2
Epichlorohydrin	None	NA	Testicular damage	2,3
Estrogens	Decreased sperm count	2	Decreased sperm count	2

(continued)

Table 15.5

Exposures Associated with Male Reproductive Dysfunction (continued)

Agent	Human Outcomes	Strength of Association in Humans*	Animal Outcomes	Strength of Association in Animals*
Ethylene oxide	None	NA	Testicular damage	1
Ethylene dibromide (EDB)	Abnormal sperm motility	1	Testicular damage	2,3
Ethylene glycol ethers	Decreased sperm count	1	Testicular damage	2
Heat	Decreased sperm count	2	Decreased sperm count	2
Lead	Decreased sperm count	2	Testicular damage, decreased sperm count, decreased sperm motility, abnormal morphology	2
Manganese	Decreased libido, impotence	1	Testicular damage	1,3
Polybrominated biphenyls (PBBs)	None	NA	Testicular damage	1
Polychlorinated biphenyls (PCBs)	None	NA	Testicular damage	1
Radiation, ionizing	Decreased sperm count	2	Testicular damage	2

* 1 = limited positive data; 2 = strong positive data; 3 = limited negative data; 4 = strong negative data

† Not applicable because no adverse outcomes were observed.

Source: United States Department of Health and Human Services. (1993). *Case studies in environmental medicine: Reproductive and developmental hazards.* Atlanta, GA: Agency for Toxic Substances and Disease Registry.

Table 15.6

Milk-to-Maternal-Plasma Ratios in Exposed Women

Chemical	Milk/Plasma Ratio
Mercury, inorganic and organic	0.9
Lead	≤ 1.0
Tetrachloroethylene	3.0
Polybrominated biphenyls (PBBs)	3.0
Polychlorinated biphenyls (PCBs)	4.0–10.0
Dieldrin	6.0
o,p-Dichlorodiphenyltrichloroethane (DDT) residues	6.0–7.0

Source: United States Department of Health and Human Services. (1993). *Case studies in environmental medicine: Reproductive and developmental hazards.* Atlanta, GA: Agency for Toxic Substances and Disease Registry.

Table 15.7
Guidelines for Continuation of Various Levels of Work During Pregnancy

Job Function	Week of Gestation
Secretarial and light clerical	40
Professional and managerial	40
Sitting with light tasks	
Prolonged (> 4 hr)	40
Intermittent	40
Standing	
Prolonged (> 4 hr)	24
Intermittent	
(> 30 min/hr)	32
(< 30 min/hr)	40
Stooping and bending below knee level	
Repetitive (> 10 times/hr)	20
Intermittent	
(< 10 to > 2 times/hr)	28
(< 2 times/hr)	40
Climbing	
Vertical ladders and poles	
Repetitive ($\geq$ 4 times/8-hr shift)	20
Intermittent (< 4 times/8-hr shift)	28
Stairs	
Repetitive ($\geq$ 4 times/8-hr shift)	28
Intermittent (< 4 times/8-hr shift)	40
Lifting	
Repetitive	
> 23 kg	20
< 23 >11 kg	24
< 11 kg	40
Intermittent	
> 23 kg	30
< 23 >11 kg	40
< 11 kg	40

Source: American Medical Association Council on Scientific Affairs. (1984). Effects of pregnancy on work performance. *JAMA, 251*,1995–1997. Used by permission.

Appendix 15a

Legal and Ethical Issues Affecting Pregnancy and Work

1. Title VII of the Civil Rights Act of 1964 prohibits discrimination based on sex. In 1978, the Pregnancy Discrimination Act, an amendment to Title VII, was passed which specifically forbids discrimination on the basis of pregnancy, childbirth, or related medical conditions. This amendment requires that women affected by these conditions be treated the same, for all employment purposes, as others not so affected but similar in their ability or inability to work (Kaczmarczyk & Paul, 1996; Rayburn & Yorker, 1991).

2. The Occupational Safety and Health Act of 1970 mandates that the employer provide a safe and healthy workplace for employees. One of the requirements of the Occupational Safety and Health Administration (OSHA) is the Hazard Communication Standard. This requires employers to provide employees with education about all hazardous materials they may come in contact with during their job duties. The provision of Material Safety Data Sheets is the cornerstone of this standard. Additional agent-specific standards outline further requirements for a reproductive health policy. For example, there is a specific OSHA standard for lead, which is a known reproductive hazard to both women and men.

3. The 1991 Supreme Court ruling in the case of the International Union, United Automobile, Aerospace and Agricultural Implements Workers of America vs. Johnson Controls Inc. reiterates that restriction of a woman's employment rights may only occur when her gender or her pregnancy interferes with actual job performance. Furthermore, the court places decision-making responsibility with the woman who is or plans to become pregnant. Employer responsibility is detailed to insure that the work site meets established health and safety standards and that employers provide employees with timely and accurate information about specific occupational reproductive hazards (Kaczmarczyk & Paul, 1996; Rayburn & Yorker, 1991).

4. The federal Family Medical Leave Act of 1993 provides job protection and an unpaid leave for up to 12 weeks for those employees experiencing the following health circumstances: a) the birth of the employee's child; b) the adoption or foster placement of a child with the employee; c) when the employee is needed to care for a parent, spouse, or child with a serious health condition; d) when the employee is unable to perform his or her job functions because of a serious health condition (cited in AAOHN, 1995). The employer must have fifty or more employees and the employee must have worked for at least one year (AAOHN, 1995).

5. In addition to the above federal laws and the Johnson Controls Supreme Court ruling, there are other state-specific laws governing pregnancy and work. Disability laws, unemployment laws, workers compensation, and pregnancy-leave policies vary from state to state. These laws will influence counseling of the pregnant employee about benefit coverage and return to work options. Consultation and coordination with human resources/personnel is often necessary.

6. Ethical dilemmas arise in the area of pregnancy and employment. As outlined above, it is imperative that employees be educated regarding the risks to a future or current pregnancy so they may act autonomously to make informed and voluntary choices. The principle of beneficence, which requires avoiding harm to others, includes three relationships: employers' duty to workers, workers' duty to offspring and employers' duty to offspring, (Office of Technology Assessment, 1985). This involves not only maintaining a safe and healthy workplace but additionally not discriminating against women because of pregnancy. Regarding rights of the fetus, a balance must be maintained in doing no harm; for example, the risk of a mildly hazardous work situation versus the benefits of having adequate finances to provide adequate prenatal nutrition may be the ethical conflict.

Appendix 15b

A Sample Occupational and Environmental Exposure Assessment
for Reproductive Health

Work Place Exposure Assessment

Work Description

Do you work outside the home?

 If yes, what is your job title?
 - How long have you been doing this type of work?
 - How long have you been at this job?
 - Describe your work (job tasks and work environment) and note the hours, amount of overtime, and whether you work rotating shifts.

 If no, detail home and volunteer activities, including hobbies and sports.

In the past 6 months, have you had any exposure to the following chemicals in your work place?
 - Metals, such as lead, cadmium, or mercury
 - Aerosolized medications, such as ribavirin or others
 - Hospital sterilizing agents, such as ethylene oxide or others
 - Pesticides (list which ones, if you know)
 - Carbon monoxide
 - Solvents, such as xylene or others
 - Any other chemical exposures
 - Hospital exposures (for example, anesthetic agents, chemotherapeutic agents, infectious diseases, or other)

Have you had any exposures to the following infectious agents in the past 6 months:
 - Rubella
 - Varicella
 - Cytomegalovirus
 - Hepatitis
 - HIV
 - Tuberculosis
 - Toxoplasmosis
 - Any other infectious exposures

Are you experiencing any of the following:
 - Stress
 - Rotating shifts
 - Overtime
 - Other psychological exposures

Are you required to do any of the following:
 - Lift heavy objects (if yes, note the maximum weight and number of times per hour per day)
 - Standing (if yes, note number of hours per day)
 - Climb ladders (if yes, note number of times per hour, per day)
 - Any other physical requirements

(continued)

Appendix 15b

A Sample Occupational and Environmental Exposure Assessment for Reproductive Health (continued)

Are you exposed to any of the following:
- Radiation
- Heat
- Noise
- Any pressurized work activity or enclosure, such as diving

Do you wear protective equipment (for example, gloves, respirator, hearing protection) and under what circumstances?

List any symptoms or conditions you have that you think are related to your work,
- Do your symptoms get better or worse on days off or on vacations?
- Has there been any recent change in your work practices that coincide with your symptoms? If yes, please list them.

Have any of your coworkers had problems related to work?

Minimizing Work-to-Home Hazard Transfer for Those Who Work Outside the Home:

Does your employer provide end-of-shift hand washing and shower facilities?

Does your employer launder the employees' work clothes or provide laundry facilities?

Is your work site generally kept clean with hazardous materials properly stored?

Assessment Work Place Pregnancy

Does your employer have a required or recommended pregnancy notification policy?

Have you told your employer of your planned or existing pregnancy?
How did your employer react?
Were you informed of any specific pregnancy-related hazards associated with your work? If yes, which ones?
Has your work been modified because you are pregnant? Do you think any work accommodation is needed at this time of your pregnancy?

If you have just had a baby:

Do you plan to breast-feed after the baby is born?

Do you have specific return-to-work plans?
- Do you know what hours or shifts you will be working?
- Do you anticipate having to work overtime?
- Do you know what your work duties will be when you return? (If yes, please describe.)

Will you have any exposure to the following substances:
- Polychlorinated compounds, for example, polychlorinated biphenyls (PCBs), persistent organochlorine pesticides, or other products
- Polycyclic aromatic hydrocarbons (PAH)
- Nitrates, nitrites, nitrosamines
- Nicotine, caffeine, and ethanol
- Drugs (list which ones)
- Other chemical exposures to solvents, metals, pesticides
- Are you aware of any chemicals that could be excreted in your breast milk?

(continued)

Appendix 15b

A Sample Occupational and Environmental Exposure Assessment for Reproductive Health (continued)

If you are returning to work outside the home, does your employer have policies or resources that could help you with your new baby?
- Is there a breast-feeding policy at your work?
- Is there an on-site lactation room with pumps available?
- Is there a place to refrigerate breast milk at the work site?
- Are there hand washing and shower facilities available?
- Does your employer have on-site child care facilities?
- Does your employer provide flex-time options?

Assessment of Other Environmental Exposures

What is your drinking water source?
- If the water source is private well, has it been assessed for nitrate levels?

Do any of your household members have any of the exposures listed in the Work Place Exposure Assessment section above? Which ones?

Does the potential father of your baby have or has he ever had any of the exposures listed in the Work Place Exposure Assessment section above? Which ones and when?

How many pregnancies have you had?
- How many children do you have?
- Have you had any miscarriages, fetal deaths, birth defects, premature deliveries, or other outcomes you think were unusual.

Do you drink alcohol?

Do you use prescribed medications?

Do you use other drugs?

Do you smoke or are you exposed to the cigarette smoke of others on a regular basis?

Appendix 15c

Occupational Health and Safety Resources

Information and Copies of OSHA Standards

Occupational Safety and Health Administration
U.S. Department of Labor
200 Constitution Avenue, NW
Washington DC 20210
(Or check state government listings for nearest regional offices)
Offers copies of standards, permissible workplace exposure levels and free technical information

Information on Environmental Regulations and Community Right-to-Know Laws

Environmental Protection Agency
Public Information Center
PM-211B,
401 M Street SW
Washington DC 20460
(Or check state government listings for nearest regional offices)

Agency for Toxic Substances and Disease Registry
ATSDR-Chamblee
1600 Clifton Road NE
Atlanta, GA 30333

Information about Occupational Health Research, Professional Education for Occupational Health and Safety, and Free Technical Information

National Institute for Occupational Safety and Health (NIOSH)
1600 Clifton Road NE
Atlanta, GA 30333

Toxic Info Line: (800)233-3360

Patient Education Materials

"If I'm Pregnant, Can the Chemicals I Work with Harm My Baby?"
California Occupational Health Program
California Department of Health Services
1515 Clay Street
Oakland, CA 94612

A Few Key Web Sites:

Occupational Safety and Health Administration	http://www.osha.gov
National Institute of Occupational Safety and Health	http://www.cdc.gov/niosh/homepage.html
Centers for Disease Control and Prevention	http://www.cdc.gov/cdc.html
Agency for Toxic Substances and Disease Registry	http://www.atsdrl.atsdr.cdc.gov:8080/atsdrhome.html

References

Ahlborg, G. (1995). Physical work load and pregnancy outcome. *Journal of Occupational and Environmental Medicine, 37*(8), 941–944.

American Association of Occupational Health Nurses (AAOHN). (1995). The family medical leave act: Advisory. *AAOHN Journal, 34*(10), 508A.

American College of Occupational and Environmental Medicine (ACOEM). (1996). ACOEM reproductive hazard management guidelines. *Journal of Occupational and Environmental Medicine, 38*(1), 83–90.

American College of Obstetrics and Gynecology and NIOSH. (1978). *Guidelines on pregnancy and work.* U.S. Department of Health, Education and Welfare (DHEW[NIOSH] Pub. No. 78–118). Washington, DC: U.S. Government Printing Office.

American Medical Association (AMA) Council on Scientific Affairs. (1984a). Effects of physical forces on the reproductive cycle. *Journal of the American Medical Association, 251*(2), 247–250.

American Medical Association (AMA) Council on Scientific Affairs. (1984b). Effects of pregnancy on work performance. *Journal of the American Medical Association, 251*(15), 1995–1997.

American Medical Association (AMA) Council on Scientific Affairs. (1985). Effects of toxic chemicals on the reproductive system. *Journal of the American Medical Association, 253*(23), 3431–3437.

Kaczmarczyk, J.M, & Paul, M.E. (1996). Reproductive health hazards in the workplace: Guidelines for policy development and implementation. *Occupational and Environmental Health, 2*(1), 48–58.

Keleher, K.C. (1991). Occupational health: How work environments can affect reproductive capacity and outcome. *The Nurse Practitioner: The American Journal of Primary Health Care, 16*(1), 23–37.

LaDou, J. (Ed.) (1990). *Occupational medicine.* Norwalk, CT: Appleton & Lange.

Office of Technology Assessment. (1985). *Reproductive health hazards in the workplace: Summary.* (OTA-BA-267). Washington, DC: U.S. Government Printing Office.

Rayburn, S.K. & Yorker, B.A.(1991). Maternal rights in the workplace. *AAOHN Journal, 39*(11), 534–536.

U.S. Department of Health and Human Services. (1991). *Healthy people 2000: National health promotion and disease prevention objectives* (DHHS Pub. No. [PHS]91–50212). Washington, DC: U.S. Government Printing Office.

U.S. Department of Health and Human Services. (1992). *Case studies in environmental medicine: Taking an exposure history.* Atlanta, GA: Agency for Toxic Substances and Disease Registry.

U.S. Department of Health and Human Services. (1993). *Case studies in environmental medicine: Reproductive and developmental hazards.* Atlanta, GA: Agency for Toxic Substances and Disease Registry.

U.S. Department of Health and Human Services. (1996). *National occupational research agenda.* Washington, DC: National Institute of Occupational Safety and Health.

SECTION 16

LACTATION

Section 16

LACTATION

Fritzi Drosten

Breast-feeding provides optimal nutrition for the human infant during the first year of life. During the last 40 to 50 years, breast-feeding was, in large part, replaced by formula feeding because of cultural influences in the United States and other western countries. Thus, many mothers of today did not see women breast-feeding during childhood and adolescence. In addition, many health providers have received little training in basic management of breast-feeding. Consequently, mothers often have difficulties establishing breast-feeding. Although an increasing number of scientific studies demonstrate the tremendous health benefits of breast-feeding, many health providers give outdated advice and often recommend formula feeding or supplementation when clients experience breast-feeding difficulties.

The breasts begin to develop in puberty with tissue and ductal growth. During pregnancy the ductal tree grows and proliferates, and during the second half of pregnancy these changes are accompanied by secretory activity and colostrum synthesis. The milk-secreting cells cluster in alveoli, which are grouped together like grapes. These clusters are connected by ductules that lead to larger ducts (similar to branches on trees), which in turn, connect to fifteen to twenty ducts that widen just behind the nipple. The larger ducts, called the lactiferous sinuses, then narrow and exit on the face of the nipple through the nipple pores (see Figure 16.1). Mammary tissue can extend into the apex of the axilla, into the epigastrium, or across the body's midline. During pregnancy, the areola darkens and the Montgomery glands, believed to protect the skin by secreting an oily substance that inhibits bacterial growth and lubricates the areolar surface, enlarge.

The delivery of the placenta causes a fall in progesterone levels and a rise in prolactin levels, which stimulates lactogenesis (milk production). During breast-feeding, the prolactin released from the anterior pituitary stimulates milk production. At the same time, oxytocin, released from the posterior pituitary gland, causes milk ejection reflex (let-down). As breast-feeding continues over time, the milk supply is regulated by supply and demand, that is, the infant "controls" milk supply by varying the strength and frequency of feeding and degree of milk removal. A newborn infant feeds more frequently while an older infant may obtain a large volume of milk in a few feedings a day.

In the first 24 hours of breast-feeding, the baby receives a small amount of colostrum (about 1.5 ounces). This first secretion is high in protein, low in fat, and rich in immunoglobulins. It helps establish nonpathogenic bacterial flora in the newborn intestinal tract and stimulate passage of meconium. Volume begins to increase in the first few days of breast-feeding: By the second day it has usually doubled in volume, and by the third day has increased eightfold. Colostrum secretion continues for about 7 days; however, the increase in volume of this early milk is so dramatic that mothers say that the "milk is in" at this time. Concurrently with increased colostrum production, varying degrees of engorgement (tissue swelling) may occur. Transitional milk, a combination of colostrum and true milk, is produced until 1 and 2 weeks' postpartum.

To feed, the neonate latches on to or grasps the nipple and sufficient areolar tissue in the mouth to massage milk from the lactiferous sinuses. The mother breast-feeds by holding the infant to the breast and assists the infant in attaining the latch. Milk flows as sucking stimulates prolactin and oxytocin release. Problems may occur if the mother who is learning how to breast-feed fails to recognize an incorrect latch; this can result in sore nipples. Soreness may deter breast-feeding efforts and inhibit the milk ejection reflex. If incorrect latching and resulting soreness are allowed to continue, the breasts become more engorged and uncomfortable as milk remains in the breast and volume increases. Unrelieved engorgement may suppress supply severely. The milk ejection reflex, stimulated by oxytocin, can be inhibited by tension, fear, and pain (Lawrence, 1994). As milk supply increases over the first week, the infant may continue with incorrect patterns and may experience symptoms of insufficient milk intake (i.e., dehydration, jaundice, or irritability).

Mothers and infants may experience problems during any stage of breast-feeding; difficulties can include mastitis, sore nipples, supply problems, plugged ducts, etc. As infants develop and grow, mothers may have problems in adjusting to different feeding patterns and behavior at the breast (e.g., biting with teething, distractibility of older infants, or transient breast refusal).

Infants may begin receiving additional solids during the second half of the first year, but should continue breast-feeding or formula feeding throughout the first year. Breast-feeding well into the second year of life is common throughout the world and is recommended by the World Health Organization (WHO, 1989).

Engorgement

Engorgement of the breasts is a common postpartum complication. The problem often is made more severe if breast-feeding is mismanaged by restricting or limiting early feedings. The swelling of the breast tissue combined with milk stasis in the alveoli and areas causes milk congestion and inhibition of the milk ejection reflex, resulting in edema and erythema. The infant, therefore, may have difficulty in draining the breast and may develop faulty sucking habits, thus causing sore nipples and further inadequate drainage (Lawrence, 1994).

Database

Subjective

- Client may complain of any of the following:
  - ▶ Full, painful, throbbing, aching warm breasts
  - ▶ Pain that extends to the axilla (may be due to tension on Cooper's ligaments) (Lawrence, 1994)
  - ▶ Breasts seem full although little milk expressible
  - ▶ Numbness or tingling in hands or arms if swelling is severe

Objective

- Breasts swollen, warm, firm, or even hard
- Low-grade fever may be present
- Engorgement (may be primarily areolar, making nipple particularly difficult for infant to grasp)
- Nodules may be present in breasts, extending into the axillae

Assessment

- Engorgement
  - ▶ R/O mastitis
  - ▶ R/O breast mass

Plan

Diagnostic Tests

- None indicated

Treatment/Management

- Use warm compresses for 10 minutes before feeing to soften breast and facilitate milk removal.

- Massage breasts gently.

- Hand express or use a pump to relieve engorgement prior to feeding.

- Maintain drainage via frequent effective nursing to empty the breasts well (Evans, Evans, & Simmer, 1995; Thomsen, Espersen, & Maigaard, 1983).

- Use cold compresses after feeding for comfort.

- Use relaxation techniques. Neck and back massage is often helpful.

- Use over-the-counter(OTC) analgesics.

  - ▶ Acetaminophen 325 mg, one to two tablets p.o. every 4 hours, as needed.

  - ▶ Ibuprofen 200 mg, one to two tablets p.o. every 4 hours, as needed (Lawrence, 1994; Townsend et al., 1984).

    NOTE: Clients who have ulcers or who are sensitive to aspirin should not take ibuprofen. Advise clients to take ibuprofen with food.

  - ▶ Salicylates (e.g., aspirin 235 to 500 mg, one to two tablets p.o. every 4 hours, as needed) are acceptable for occasional use, although there is a potential for antiplatelet effect in the infant. It is best to wait 1 or 2 hours after a dose to breast-feed (Anderson, 1991).

  NOTE: These over-the-counter analgesics are absorbed in minimal amounts in milk and generally have no effect on the infant except where stated.

- Combing of breast with a hair comb prior to expressing milk or breast-feeding may be soothing and facilitate milk removal.

- Avoid long intervals between feedings.

- For the non–breast-feeding mother, occasional warm, brief showers followed by gentle massage may relieve some of the fullness and provide comfort. Cold compresses at any time may also provide relief. Use of lactation suppressants is not recommended (Auerbach & Riordan, 1993).

- Use a bra that fits well.

Consultation

- Consult with a physician for fever above 101.6° F (38.7° C) with concurrent flulike symptoms.

- Refer to lactation consultant/specialist for further education if client has prolonged engorgement.

Patient Education

- Review the basics of correct latch and subsequent milk transfer.

- Instruct the client regarding methods of soaking breasts in warm water or devising moist compresses that stay warm for several minutes and cover entire breasts (Auerbach & Riordan, 1993).

- Instruct the client to drain each breast well.

  ▶ Do not remove infant too early.

  ▶ Breast-feeding should occur on both breasts at each feeding.

  ▶ Start feeding with the side that ended the last feeding, drain that breast well before moving the infant to the other side (Evans et al., 1995; Thomsen et al., 1983).

- Reassure client that engorgement usually lasts 48 to 72 hours.

- Reassure client regarding the presence of a milk supply when milk ejection reflex is inhibited during severe engorgement.

- Advise client to wear a well-fitted bra.

- If breast pump use is considered, inform client regarding effective pump types to relieve engorgement. Many widely available pumps are difficult to use and/or ineffective. (Lactation specialists can assist in procuring an effective pump.)

- Mother should have the ability to assess adequacy of infant feedings and provide supplemental feeding if necessary. Adequacy of feedings include the following:

  ▶ Infant swallows audibly during feeding.

  ▶ Infant feeds vigorously for several minutes every 1 to 4 hours.

  ▶ Client's breasts feel somewhat softer after a feeding.

  ▶ Infant is content or behaves as if satiated after a feeding.

  ▶ Infant voids frequently.

    NOTE: During the first few days of life, the voids will be few but will increase so that by day 5 or 6 there will be six to eight wet diapers.

  ▶ Infant begins having yellow stools by the end of the first week; during the first month, most infants will have more than one stool a day.

- Discuss use of hot or cold compresses. Excess heat may increase swelling and edema. Use of cold compresses may help to decrease swelling and relieve discomfort.

  NOTE: Cold compresses may be made by tying together plastic bags of ice to form a sort of "flower" around the breast. Cabbage leaves cooled in the refrigerator or freezer can be a comfortable compress; place in the bra until leaves are wilted, (around 20 minutes) (Lawrence, 1994).

Follow-up

- Fever that measures 101.6° F (38.7° C) or above, two times, 4 hours apart requires consideration of other etiology, such as mastitis or an infection at another site.
- Client should contact provider 24 to 48 hours after initial visit to discuss progress.
- Document in progress notes and problem list.

Inverted or Flat Nipples

Inverted nipples do not protrude outward. They may either appear inverted upon inspection or invert when the tissue behind the nipple is "pinched." This condition makes grasp of the nipple by the newborn infant difficult. Inverted nipples are caused by a persistence of the original invagination of the mammary dimple and may have adhesions that draw the nipple tissue inward. Inverted nipples may resolve during pregnancy.

Flat nipples appear flat, yet when they are grasped or pinched, they will protrude outward. Infants may have difficulty making teats out of flat of nipples, but their function is usually normal.

Database

Subjective

- Nipples do not evert.
- Client may experience sore nipples, nipple erosion, or may have mastitis.
- Client may be unable to latch infant to the breast.

Objective

- With the "pinch test," very little tissue is graspable with the fingers on the areolar tissue, or the tissue actually inverts
- Infant may have difficulty locating milk openings or removing milk from the breast

Assessment

- Flat or inverted nipples
  - ▶ R/O engorgement
  - ▶ R/O previous breast surgery
  - ▶ R/O nonfunctional nipple

Plan

Diagnostic Tests

- Perform the pinch test by compressing the breast with thumb and forefinger behind nipple.
  - ▶ Some nipples that appear everted will invert with this test.
  - ▶ Some inverted nipples will evert with pinch.

Treatment/Management

- If there are adhesions, Hoffman's exercise, prenatally initiated and practiced a few times daily, may help to loosen them (Hoffman, 1953).

  NOTE: There is controversy over whether or not these exercises work, and research is lacking. Women at risk for preterm labor should not perform these exercises. See the Patient Education section.

- Breast shells worn in the last trimester of pregnancy or before breast-feeding have traditionally been recommended to bring the nipple out (Multicentre Randomised Controlled Trial of Alternative Treatments for Inverted and Non-Protractile Nipples in Pregnancy Trial Collaborative Group [MAIN], 1994; Alexander, Grant & Campbell, 1992).

  NOTE: Prenatal use of breast shells is controversial. Recent studies have not demonstrated their effectiveness, but many lactation experts feel that they benefit some clients.

- Rolling and stretching the nipple between the thumb and forefinger may help make the nipple graspable (Cadwell, 1981).
  - ▶ Can be performed as a prenatal exercise
  - ▶ Can be performed just before the infant is put to the breast

  NOTE: Women at risk for preterm labor should not perform these exercises.

- A breast pump may be used to pull the nipple out before feedings.

- If the nipple cannot be grasped, use of a breast pump or performing manual expression may be necessary to initiate and establish milk supply while infant is learning how to feed at the breast. Expression should be done as frequently as a newborn is expected to feed, and infant should be fed milk that is expressed.

- Side-sitting or side-lying feeding may help infant to grasp nipple.

- Position and support infant to maximize *infant's* efforts to learn to shape and grasp nipple.

- Avoid giving the infant bottles or pacifiers, if possible.

Consultation

- Prenatally, refer any client with severely inverted or flat nipples to discuss options and plans for remediation to a lactation consultant.

- If client continues to have difficulty with latching the infant to the breast, has persistent nipple soreness, or wishes to learn alternate feeding methods while infant learns to breast-feed, refer her to lactation consultant for further education and assistance.

- Consider prenatal referral of any client with severely inverted nipples to a surgeon (Hauben & Mahler, 1983).

Patient Education

- Instruct the client in Hoffman's exercise: On a vertical plane, stretch the areolar tissue above and below the nipple, then on a horizontal plane stretch the nipple to the side. Exercise should be performed several times in a row, several times a day (Auerbach & Riordan, 1993; Hoffman, 1953).

- Prenatally, instruct client to wear breast shells daily, beginning in the third trimester of pregnancy. Start with an hour a day and work up to wearing them throughout the day. Inform the client that the use of the shells *may* help but if they are not comfortable their use should be discontinued.

  ▶ If postpartum, instruct client to wear breast shells for at least 30 minutes before breast-feeding.

  NOTE: Breast shells are plastic dome-shaped devices worn inside the bra. There are several types and sizes of shells available. Some have air holes around the nipples to promote circulation, while others may be solid (Lawrence, 1994; Alexander et al., 1992; MAIN, 1994).

- Discuss the nipple-rolling technique, as described in the Treatment/Management section.

- Recommend that client learn about breast-feeding through classes and reading before baby is born. Allow time to discuss issues and concerns.

- Recommend to client that she begin breast-feeding in the delivery room, if possible, after the infant is born.

- Advise client to present breast to infant with a hand shaping upper and lower portions of areolar tissue so that infant may draw in nipple at the center of the mouth.

- Instruct client in proper positioning of infant and breast to facilitate grasp of sufficient tissue for milk transfer.

- Advise client regarding early, effective treatment of sore nipples and recognition of signs and symptoms of mastitis. See the section on sore nipples in this chapter, and Chapter 6.18, *Mastitis*.

Follow-up

- Discuss breast-feeding at prenatal visits, including initiating use of Hoffman's exercises and/or breast shells during last trimester and offer support.

- Provide postpartum follow-up/availability for counseling should problems occur.

- Document in progress notes and problem list.

Milk Supply Problems

Milk supply problems are a major concern for many breast-feeding mothers. The ability to provide adequate nourishment for their infants is usually seen by mothers as part of their necessary mothering abilities, and the inability to do so is seen as a failure on their part. A common reason for discontinuing breast-feeding at any point is either a perceived or an actual insufficient milk supply. Milk oversupply can cause discomfort for both the mother and infant and is not well recognized.

Low milk supply may result from maternal causes, such as insufficient fluid intake, fatigue, and medication, infant causes, such as infrequent feedings, insufficient time at the breast, improper latch, or any combination of these. The practitioner must be aware of the interplay of factors involved in milk supply and the importance of early identification of problems. When the infant has an inability to obtain or stimulate the milk supply, the mother must stimulate and sustain the supply until the infant is able to feed unassisted. If the mother's condition is the cause of the inadequate milk supply, the infant must be sustained using breast-milk alternatives until the mother is able to meet the infant's needs.

Milk oversupply appears to be caused by feeding techniques and schedules. Feeding difficulties such as choking and gulping at the breast can result, which in turn can lead to early weaning. The following protocol is divided into two sections, low milk supply and overabundant milk supply.

Low Milk Supply

Database

Subjective

- Client may complain of
  - ▶ Infant being hungry all of the time
  - ▶ Low milk supply at a certain time of day, usually in the evening
  - ▶ Soft breasts with no milk
  - ▶ Being unable to meet infant's demands of milk supply for any reason
- Client may not have experienced any breast changes during pregnancy.
- Client may have prolonged intervals between breast-feeding or expressing of milk.
- Client may have a history of unrelieved engorgement, which may have contributed to a dramatic drop in milk supply.
- Client may have a history of breast surgery.

Objective

- Breasts may appear soft, not full.
- Client unable to express milk.
- Few swallows are heard as infant breast-feeds.
- Infant's weight gain is below normal for age.
- Infant may have signs of insufficient milk intake, such as infrequent voiding, infrequent stool, or unusual sleepiness.

Assessment

- Low milk supply, actual or perceived
  - ▶ R/O dehydration
  - ▶ R/O mastitis
  - ▶ R/O maternal exhaustion
  - ▶ R/O poor release of milk
  - ▶ R/O maternal hypothyroid condition
  - ▶ R/O inappropriate dieting
  - ▶ R/O medication/drug side effect (e.g., antihistamine, smoking)
  - ▶ R/O infant sucking problem
  - ▶ R/O infant medical condition or illness
  - ▶ R/O maternal illness (e.g., anemia, infection)
  - ▶ R/O retained placental fragments
  - ▶ R/O insufficient glandular tissue
  - ▶ R/O pregnancy
  - ▶ R/O use of nipple shields
  - ▶ R/O excessive pacifier use
  - ▶ R/O emotional disturbances of mother
  - ▶ R/O pituitary tumor in mother

Plan

Diagnostic tests

- Prolactin levels have not been shown to be useful in the diagnosis of low milk supply
- Order a complete blood count if infection or anemia are suspected.
- Conduct thyroid function tests of mother if indicated (Lawrence, 1994)

Treatment/Management

- Allow infant access to breast. Infant should be brought to the breast frequently to stimulate milk production.
- Allow infant increased frequency of breast-feeding if appetite spurt is suspected.

  NOTE: Typical appetite or growth spurts occur at the ages of 2 weeks, 1 month, 3 months, and 6 months, although they can also occur at any age. Milk supply usually increases within 48 to 72 hours.

- Assess use of formula supplements and decrease if infant's lack of appetite may be minimizing active suckling at breast.

- Observe infant at the breast and look for adequate grasp of lactiferous sinuses, swallowing, and strength and coordination of suck.

- Increase maternal caloric intake, if low.

- Increase maternal fluids if intake marginal. Mother should be instructed to drink to satisfy thirst.

- Metoclopramide has been shown to increase milk supply when other factors have been unsuccessful (Anderson & Valdéz, 1993; Budd, Erdman, & Long, 1993).

  ▶ Recommended dosage is 10 mg p.o. t.i.d. for 1 to 3 weeks.

  NOTE: Small amounts of metoclopramide appear in the mother's milk, which are minimal compared to those used in therapy of reflux for pediatric patients. The peak levels occur 2 to 3 hours post dose. Avoid feeding during this time (Hale, 1997).

- Treat sore nipples or engorgement. See the appropriate guidelines in this chapter.

- See also the Patient Education section.

- Increase numbers of milk expression sessions if mother is separated from infant, either totally, as with an ill infant, or partially, as with a working mother. Pumping should be no longer than about 15 to 20 minutes. Pumping with a double system for both breasts simultaneously can save time yet provide adequate stimulation.

  ▶ Assess type of breast pump if one is in use. Large hospital-grade breast pumps are much more efficient than small, hand-held battery or electric pumps. Mothers with large breasts may require additional consultation regarding adequate type of breast pump.

  ▶ Hand-expression, when done correctly, may be as effective as mechanical pumping, or it may augment pumping and increase milk yield.

Consultation

- Consult with a physician, as indicated, if mastitis is suspected.

- Consult with a physician, as indicated, if thyroid problem suspected.

- Refer to lactation consultant, as indicated, for complicated problems, for infant sucking problems, or to procure a breast pump or feeding device, if needed.

- Refer to or consult with a pediatrician if an infant health problem is suspected.

Patient Education

- Explain that a small amount of milk available to the infant in the first 3 days of life is to be expected.

- Explain the supply-and-demand concept: More milk is made in response to more demand from the infant. Two to three days (sometimes longer) is usually required before the milk supply increases to meet the infant's demand.

- Discuss milk volume cycles and normal infant behavior, including fussy periods in late afternoon and evening.

  ▶ Milk volume is low late in the day but fat content is high. Mother may perceive supply to be insufficient, yet it may be adequate.

  ▶ Include coping strategies for this stressful time (e.g., afternoon walks, napping with infant, getting help with household chores, minimizing other obligations, etc.).

- Explain the position of the lactiferous sinuses and the importance of the infant's ability to empty them efficiently during breast-feeding.

- Instruct in breast massage to aid in response of milk ejection reflex (Marmet, 1992).

- Discourage strict time limitations at breast. During the last portion of feeding, infant obtains hind milk (contains higher fat content), which may help infant become more satiated (Woolridge, Ingram, & Baum, 1990).

- Encourage rest and stress reduction during first month postpartum and during infant's appetite/growth spurts.

- Suggest adequate rest during the day, particularly with history of a difficult labor, if infant is breast-feeding during the night or there are many family demands on mother.

- Explain the need for adequate maternal caloric intake during breast-feeding and periods of increased demand for mother's milk.

- Instruct client to hand express or use large effective pump after feedings to remove remaining milk to stimulate additional milk production (Daly & Hartman, 1995).

- Advise against smoking , since it may impair the milk-ejection reflex and inhibit prolactin release (Anderson, 1982; Hopkinson, Schanler, Fraley, & Garza, 1992).

Follow-up

- Client should contact provider if methods used do not increase the milk supply within 48 to 72 hours.

- Client should keep log of feedings.

- Document in progress note and problem list.

- Support all efforts at increasing milk supply. Advise client to provide supplemental breast milk alternatives for infant,as necessary. Some clients with low milk supply (e.g., breast surgery, breast trauma, inadequate glandular tissue) may never be able to exclusively breast-feed.

Overabundant Milk Supply or Overactive Let-down

Database

Subjective

- Client may report that

  ▶ Infant has a lot of gas or is colicky

  ▶ Breasts are full all of the time

> ▶ Infant gags, or almost chokes on the milk with initial milk ejection reflex

> ▶ Infant will not breast-feed for long periods

> ▶ There are persistent plugged ducts

- Client may have history of repeated bouts of mastitis.

- Infant has a history of excessive weight gain.

Objective

- Infant at breast is observed to swallow seemingly large amounts of milk, perhaps combined with air upon initial milk-ejection reflex

- Breasts appear large and full

Assessment

- Overabundant milk supply, and/or overactive milk ejection reflex

  > ▶ R/O mastitis

  > ▶ R/O suck-swallow coordination problem in infant

  > ▶ R/O normally enlarged breasts of the first 6 weeks postpartum

  > ▶ R/O normal "leaky" breasts

Plan

Diagnostic Tests

- None indicated

Treatment/Management

- Observe the infant at the breast.

  > ▶ Correct positioning difficulties.

  > ▶ Assist with positions that allow the greatest control of milk swallowing without gulping, such as the sitting position, or relaxed cradle position (Auerbach & Riordan, 1993).

- Assess for proper bra fit that allows support without constriction.

- Hand express the initial milk ejection (may help the infant avoid the fastest milk flow).

- Offer only one breast at a feeding to avoid infant experiencing overfeeding discomfort. Mother may hand express a small amount of milk from the other breast for comfort, as needed.

- Down-regulate milk supply by offering infant only one breast at a feeding, draining one breast completely before offering the other breast, or using one breast for 3 to 4 hours before using other breast.

Consultation

- Consult with a physician, as indicated, if mastitis suspected.
- Refer to lactation consultant, as indicated, for complicated problems, for infant sucking problems, or persistent oversupply.

Patient Education

- Explain the supply-and-demand concept of milk supply with emphasis on how to down-regulate supply
- Advise client to allow infant to regulate milk supply. Some infants may receive adequate feeding with just a few minutes of breast-feeding (Daly & Hartman, 1995).
- Explain how the offering of only one breast at a feeding might provide the infant with more of the hind milk, which may make the infant more comfortable (Woolridge, et al., 1990).
- Demonstrate positioning that may decrease air swallowing (e.g., with infant positioned superior to breast or infant more upright, or cradle position)(Auerbach & Riordan, 1993).
- Instruct client in identification of air swallowing and how to burp the infant frequently when it occurs.

Follow-up

- Client should contact provider if problems persist beyond 72 hours after initiation of treatment.
- Document in progress note and problem list.

Plugged Ducts

Plugging of the ducts may also be called caked breasts, noninfectious milk stasis, or clogged ducts. Milk drainage to the ducts is obstructed or impaired, with the resultant symptoms and conditions described below. Contributing factors may be obstruction by physical conditions (e.g., restrictive or poorly fitted bras or infant carrier straps), persistent poor drainage (e.g., positioning of infant or infant breast-feeding style that doesn't allow adequate drainage), fatigue, or, possibly, nutritional factors (Lawrence, 1994).

Database

Subjective

- Client complains of tender, painful area or lump in breast, which may be red or warm.
- Client may also complain of painful nipple pore on affected breast (may indicate plugging at skin surface).

Objective

- Red or warm area in affected breast
- Lump may be palpated in affected breast
- Plug at nipple tip may appear as white spot (Auerbach & Riordan, 1993)

Assessment

- Plugged duct
  - ▶ R/O constrictive bra or infant front carrier as causative factors
  - ▶ R/O improper positioning
  - ▶ R/O infant related causes (e.g., Incomplete emptying)
  - ▶ R/O chronic milk oversupply
  - ▶ R/O breast mass
  - ▶ R/O galactocele
  - ▶ R/O mastitis

Plan

Diagnostic tests

- Microscopic or microbiologic laboratory analysis of milk is rarely necessary. If infectious mastitis is suspected, milk analysis will most likely demonstrate more than 10^3 bacterial colonies/mL and more than 10^6 white blood cells. Common organisms implicated are *Staphylococcus aureus*, *Escherichia coli*, and, rarely, ß hemolytic *Streptococcus* spp. (Lawrence, 1994).

Treatment/Management

- Apply moist, warm heat to affected area for several minutes prior to feeding (at least 4 times a day). Sometimes, the client may find it more comfortable to lean over and soak breasts in a sink or basin filled with warm water.
- Gently massage affected area down towards nipple.
- Hand expression may relieve a plugged duct.
- Breast-feed to drain breast as much as possible several times a day (Thomsen et al., 1983).
- Assess client for constrictive bra or activity that might restrict milk flow.
- Consider infant-related causes, such as incomplete emptying of the breast.
- Assess for positioning that limits draining affected areas of breast.
- Use over-the-counter analgesics:
  - ▶ Acetaminophen 325 mg, one to two tablets p.o. every 4 hours, as needed
  - ▶ Ibuprofen 200 mg, one to two tablets p.o. every 4 to 6 hours, as needed (Lawrence, 1994; Townsend et al., 1984).

    NOTE: Clients who have ulcers or who are sensitive to aspirin should not take ibuprofen. Advise clients to take ibuprofen with food.
  - ▶ Salicylates (e.g., aspirin 325 to 500 mg, one to two tablets p.o. every 4 hours, as needed) are

acceptable for occasional use, although there is a potential for antiplatelet effect in the infant. It is best to wait 1 or 2 hours after a dose to breast-feed (Anderson, 1991)

NOTE: These over-the-counter analgesics are absorbed in milk and generally have no effect on infant except where stated.

- See the Patient Education section.

Consultation

- Consult with a lactation consultant for persistent or repeatedly plugged ducts, or as needed for expanded patient education.

- Consult with a physician for suspected breast abscess or pathology, as needed.

Patient Education

- Instruct client to breast-feed on affected side with baby's nose and chin pointing towards affected area.

  ▶ Direct client to breast-feed with the breast in a position that utilizes gravity during the feeding, such as breast-feeding on hands and knees. Also, she can change position of infant during feedings.

- Advise client to breast-feed frequently and avoid long intervals between feedings.

- Instruct client to breast-feed so the entire breast is drained during the feeding or to try to drain the plugged duct several times a day until condition subsides.

  NOTE: If baby begins to breast-feed often and quits as milk begins flowing, attempt snuggling frequently rather than offering the breast.

- If necessary, use pump or hand expression to relieve fullness.

- Direct client to wear a well-fitted bra. Nonsupport bras and those with an underwire may contribute to plugged ducts.

- Advise client to pay attention to those activities that might contribute to milk stasis and circulation compromise, such as infant front carriers, strenuous exercising, and work-related repetitive movements.

- Encourage client to rest more when experiencing plugged ducts. Plugged ducts tend to occur more frequently when the mother is fatigued.

- Instruct client to maintain adequate fluid intake. Client should drink to satisfy thirst.

Follow-up

- Client should contact provider if she experiences fever or symptoms persist.

- Document in progress notes and problem list.

Sore Nipples

Sore nipples, one of the most common problems experienced by the lactating mother, is a common reason why breast-feeding is discontinued. The problem may develop at any time during lactation, but most frequently occurs in the first 2 weeks postpartum. The mother's anatomical variations in nipple size, shape and skin type, the infant's suckle or anatomical variations in the infant's mouth, the position and timing of the infant at the breast, or engorgement can be factors. Sore nipples can become a painful postpartum complication and may be a contributing factor to the development of mastitis.

Database

Subjective

Predisposing Factors

- Faulty positioning

- Faulty infant sucking patterns

- Improper nipple care (e.g., use of soaps or vigorous washing of the nipples)

- Poorly designed or improperly set-up breast pumps

- *Candida albicans* (e.g., in client with history of vaginal yeast infection or antibiotic treatment; infant with thrush)

- Breast engorgement in first 2 weeks postpartum

- Older infant with new teeth; biting of the breasts

- Use of strong detergents on bras

Symptomatology

- Client describes painful nipples.

- Nipple sensitivity present with the birth of infant; increases and peaks around the third postpartum day.

- Client may note cracks and sucking bruises in the first few days (often result of faulty positioning).

- Client may describe burning or itching sensation (may be due to *Candida albicans*).

- Pain may be most intense when mother observes white or purple nipple tip, normal color returns when pain subsides.

- Pain descriptors may include

  ▶ Dull

  ▶ Throbbing

  ▶ Sharp

  ▶ Pain during initial sucks, then subsiding

▶ Pain after a few minutes of feeding

▶ Pain after end of feeding

Objective

- Nipples may appear red, cracked, scabbed, or bleeding.

- Nipples may appear pink.

- Nipples and areola may appear dry and scaly.

- Nipples may have pus or exudate.

- Nipples may be swollen and edematous.

- Nipple tissue may be firm and not graspable by the infant.

- Single, affected nipple pore may be red or white, or have blister with pus or exudate.

- Nipple may blanch with breast-feeding, or during thermal/pressure stimulation.

- Nipple may appear creased or slanted after breast-feeding.

Assessment

- Sore nipples
  - R/O mastitis
  - R/O engorgement
  - R/O inverted nipples
  - R/O *Herpes simplex* virus infection
  - R/O eczema of nipple(s)
  - R/O *Candida albicans* infection
  - R/O normal nipple tenderness (peaking on approximate postpartum day 3)
  - R/O syphilis
  - R/O impetigo
  - R/O maternal varicella infection
  - R/O faulty sucking by infant
  - R/O ankyloglossia (short lingual frenulum) of infant

Plan

Diagnostic Tests

- Culture nipple/areola for suspected herpes simplex virus or *C. albicans*, as indicated

- KOH preparation and microscopy of skin scrapings from nipple/areola (for evidence of candida infection), as indicated.

- VDRL or RPR, as indicated

Treatment/Management

- Infant should be correctly positioned at the breast (Auerbach & Riordan, 1993).

  ▶ Mouth should be wide open with lips flanged, nose and chin should be close to the breast, and cheeks should be full, not dimpling

  ▶ Infant should not be sucking only on the tip of the nipple, but drawing it far into the mouth.

  ▶ Quiet swallows should be heard during feeding, not "clicks" which indicate that the breast is not sufficiently filling the oral cavity

- Maintain correct position of breast. Support as necessary (Woolridge, 1986).

  ▶ Breast support should facilitate grasp of nipple and areolar tissue as well as the ducts behind areola.

  ▶ The nipple should not be pointed upward, which may occur when the mother puts excessive pressure on the skin above the nipple.

- Apply warm, wet compresses to nipples 1 to 5 minutes before and after breast-feeding to increase comfort and assist in healing nipples (Buchko et. al, 1993).

- Express a small amount of breast milk on to nipples after breast-feeding and allow to air dry before covering with clothing. (Chute, 1992)

- Apply a hypoallergenic lanolin cream to nipples after breast-feeding; this may provide soothing comfort and assist in healing if skin is dry.

  NOTE: Lanolin not recommended for individuals with wool allergies (Lawrence, 1994).

- On cracked or open areas, a small amount of 1 percent hydrocortisone ointment may be applied after each feeding. Most of the medication is absorbed, so it does not need to be removed prior to the next feeding (Lawrence, 1994).

- Provide symptomatic relief with analgesics:

  ▶ Acetaminophen 325 mg, one to two tablets every 4 hours, as needed

  ▶ Ibuprofen 200 mg, one to two tablets every 4 to 6 hours, as needed (Lawrence, 1994; Townsend et al., 1984)

  NOTE: Clients with ulcers or clients sensitive to aspirin should not take ibuprofen. Advise clients to take ibuprofen with food.

  ▶ Salicylates (e.g., aspirin 325–500 mg, one to two tablets p.o. every 4 hours, as needed) are acceptable for occasional use, although there is a potential for antiplatelet effect in the infant. It is best to wait 1 or 2 hours after a dose to breast-feed (Anderson, 1991).

  NOTE: These over-the-counter analgesics are absorbed in minimal amounts in milk and generally have no effect on infant except where stated.

- Observe for proper removal of infant from breast. A finger placed in the corner of the infant's mouth breaks the suction and prevents pulling of the nipple.

- Use breast shells to keep clothing away from nipples. Breast shells with air holes may be the most effective.

- Rest nipple(s) by using manual expression or a large electric piston pump for at least 24 hours in the cases of extreme pain unrelieved by other corrective measures.

- Nipple shields have been used in some situations to protect damaged nipples from further damage. Use with caution; shields have been associated with decreased milk supply (Auerbach, 1990).

- In cases of maternal *C. albicans* or thrush in the infant, care for nipples correctly.

  ▶ Rinse nipples after each feeding with water or a mild vinegar-and-water solution (1 tablespoon vinegar in 1 cup of water).

  ▶ Apply clotrimazole, miconazole, *or* nystatin cream to nipples sparingly after feeds; rub in well. Creams are generally well absorbed and need not be removed prior to the next breast-feeding (Auerbach & Riordan, 1993).

  ▶ Treat mother and infant simultaneously.

    – Infant treatment for *C. albicans*/thrush

      * Oral nystatin solution, 1 cc swabbed in mouth q.i.d. several minutes after feeding.

      * Treat any concurrent *Candida* diaper rash.

  ▶ Treat any concurrent maternal vaginal yeast. See Chapter 14.7, *Vaginitis*.

Consultation

- Consult with a physician, as indicated, for suspected herpes or syphilis.

- Refer infant to a pediatrician, as indicated, for suspected herpes or syphilis.

- Refer mother to a dermatologist, as indicated, for unusual exudate or persistent sore nipples.

- Refer mother to a lactation consultant for more extensive breast-feeding education and/or further assessment, as indicated.

Patient Education

- Discuss the importance of continuing to breast-feed or express milk to meet the infant's nutritional requirements and maintain the milk supply.

- Advise regarding good breast hygiene, proper handwashing, use of clean bras, and importance of frequent breast-pad changes.

- Discuss proper breast care, including refraining from using soaps and nonprescribed lotions on the nipples.

- Review information regarding the signs and symptoms of mastitis, including instructions to notify provider should they occur.

- Advise the client that changing breast-feeding positions may allow sore areas to heal.

- Recommend that the client air dry nipples for several minutes after feedings (Chute, 1992).

- Caution the client not to allow infant to breast-feed for long periods without strict attention to the position and suck.

- Advise the client to avoid breast pads with waterproof barriers.

- Instruct the client to avoid engorgement and long intervals between feedings, which may make it more difficult for the infant to grasp the nipple adequately.

- Advise client to begin feeding on the least affected side, so that the suck is not as vigorous on the second breast.

- Inform clients using breast shields that studies have demonstrated significantly lowered milk intake with the use of these devices; in addition it may be difficult for client to discontinue their use (Auerbach, 1990; Woolridge, Baum & Drewett, 1980).

- Provide thrush education.

  ▶ Instruct client to wash hands frequently, especially after contact with nipples or the baby's diaper or mouth.

  ▶ Instruct client to change breast pads frequently and to wear clean bras.

  ▶ Advise client that conditions of moisture, darkness, and warmth favor yeast growth; discuss ways of minimizing them.

  ▶ Instruct client to wash and boil all breast pump parts that come into contact with milk and all rubber nipples and pacifiers daily.

Follow-up

- Observe for mastitis.

- The client is to contact provider if she doesn't experience relief after 24 to 48 hours of treatment.

- Candidiasis resolves more slowly. Instruct the client to return if symptoms persist more than 4 to 5 days after initiation of treatment.

- Nipples that blanch after feeds also take longer to heal, but improvement in symptoms should occur with careful management techniques.

- Document in problem list and progress notes

Suckling Problems

Suckling problems are a major concern for both the breast-feeding mother and the breast-fed infant, because milk transfer is impaired. During suckling the nipple and a portion of the areola are drawn into the infant's mouth, forming a "teat." The tongue then compresses the palate in a wavelike movement that helps to draw milk out of the lactiferous sinuses and into the infant's mouth (Auerbach & Riordan, 1993). If the infant is unable to obtain mother's milk correctly and efficiently, the mother may experience engorgement followed by a reduction in milk supply. She may experience undue pain and trauma to the nipple and areolar tissue as a result of a faulty suckle. The practitioner must be aware of the interplay of the factors involved in milk production, and the importance of identifying problems before either milk supply is impacted or the infant suffers any consequences, such as weight loss or dehydration. When the infant is unable to stimulate the milk supply, the mother must stimulate and sustain the supply expressing the milk by hand or using mechanical means.

Database

Subjective

- The client may complain that the infant is unable to breast-feed, refuses the breast, or will not latch onto the breast.

- Infant will not breast-feed for long periods of time.

- Infant may gag or almost choke on the milk.

- Client may experience pain every time infant breast-feeds. See Sore Nipples section.

Objective

- Infant's weight gain may be below expected normal for age.

- Infant is unable to latch onto the breast

- Infant is unable to sustain suckling.

- Infant is unable to hold breast and nipple in the mouth.

- Few swallows are heard as infant breast-feeds.

- Infant may have signs of insufficient milk intake such as infrequent voiding, infrequent stooling, or unusual sleepiness.

- Infant may have history of perinatal depression (especially those with low Apgar scores), or may have genetic condition that impacts ability to suckle, such as Down syndrome.

- Nipple shape after feeding may reveal sucking obstruction (e.g., compressed flattened nipple).

Assessment

- Suckling problems
  - R/O dehydration, hyperbilirubinemia, or hypoglycemia of infant (Lawrence, 1994)
  - R/O medical illness or condition of infant
  - R/O a breast shape, fullness, or skin type that impairs infant grasp
  - R/O common abnormalities of infant's mouth structure, such as cleft lip or palate, small jaw, or short lingual frenulum
  - R/O nipple trauma affecting latch
  - R/O medication or drug side effects (e.g., medications used during labor or postpartum)
  - R/O excessive pacifier use
  - R/O position-caused sucking difficulties

Plan

Diagnostic Tests

- For suspected infant dehydration, hypoglycemia, or hyperbilirubinemia, infant serum sodium, glucose, and bilirubin levels may be abnormal.

Treatment/Management

- Observe breast-feeding.
  - ▶ Watch infant at the breast.
  - ▶ Look for adequate grasp of nipple and evidence of milk ejection reflex followed by swallows.
  - ▶ Look for strength and coordination of suck at breast.
  - ▶ Correct position, if necessary.
  - ▶ Position the infant facing the mother tummy-to-tummy.
  - ▶ Position mother's hand on breast with thumb on top and four fingers below for support, if needed.
- Assess type of breast pump, if one is in use.
  - ▶ Large hospital-grade breast pumps are much more efficient than small, hand-held battery or electric pumps.
  - ▶ Mothers with large breasts may require additional consultation regarding adequate type of breast pump (Auerbach & Riordan, 1993).
- Supplement the infant with expressed breast milk or formula, as needed.
- Develop a plan to include infant suckle improvement (e.g., using supplemental nursing system, dropper feeds, suck training, etc.) (Auerbach & Riordan, 1993; Marmet & Shell, 1984)
- Treat sore nipples/engorgement. See the appropriate guidelines in this chapter.
- See also Patient Education section.

Consultation

- Consult with/refer to a pediatrician, as indicated, if an infant health problem is suspected.
- Refer infants suspected of dehydration, hypoglycemia, sepsis, or those unable to obtain adequate milk intake for immediate care.
- Refer to a lactation consultant, as indicated, for assistance with milk supply maintenance, techniques to establish breast-feeding for infant, techniques to improve infant's suckle, and follow-up.

Patient Education

- Explain the position of the lactiferous sinuses and the importance of the infant's ability to empty them efficiently during breast-feeding.

- Instruct the client in alternate massage to aid in response of milk ejection reflex during feedings (Auerbach & Riordan, 1994; Bowles, Stutte, & Hensley, 1988):

  ▶ Massage the base of the breast when infant begins rapid, shallow suckling movements without swallows.

  ▶ Stop the massage when the infant begins the slower suckle with swallows.

- Instruct client to hand express milk or use large effective pump after feedings to augment milk supply.

- Explain that milk supply problems combined with suckling problems may take days to weeks to correct, but that if corrective measures are continued, the client may be successful.

Follow-up

- Monitor closely infants with slow weight gain.

- Follow client until suckling problems are resolved; this may take days to weeks.

- Document in problem list and progress notes.

Figure 16.1

Schematic Diagram of Breast

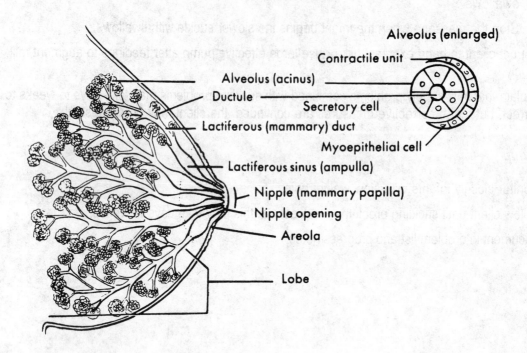

Alveolus (enlarged)

Contractile unit

Alveolus (acinus)

Ductule

Secretory cell

Lactiferous (mammary) duct

Myoepithelial cell

Lactiferous sinus (ampulla)

Nipple (mammary papilla)

Nipple opening

Areola

Lobe

Source: Auerbach, K., & Riordan, J. (1993). Breastfeeding and human lactation. Copyright 1993. Boston: Jones and Bartlett Publishers. Reprinted with permission.

REFERENCES

Alexander, J., Grant, A., & Campbell, M. (1992). Randomized controlled trial of breast shells and Hoffman's exercises for inverted and non-protractile nipples. *British Medical Journal, 304*, 1030–1032.

Anderson, A. (1982). Suppressed prolactin but normal neurophysin levels in cigarette smoking breastfeeding women. *Clinical Endocrinology, 17*, 363–368.

Anderson, P. (1991). Drug use during breast-feeding. *Clinical Pharmacology, 10*, 594–624.

Anderson, P., & Valdéz, V. (1993). Increasing breast milk supply. *Clinical Pharmacy, 12*, 479–480.

Auerbach, K. (1990). The effect of nipple shields on maternal milk volume. *Journal of Gynecological and Neonatal Nursing, 19*(5), 419–427.

Auerbach, K., & Riordan, J. (1993). *Breast-feeding and human lactation.* Boston, MA: Jones and Bartlett.

Bowlew, B., Stutte, P., & Hensley, J. (1988). Alternate massage in breast-feeding. *Genesis, 9*, 5–9.

Buchko, B.L., Pugh, L.C., Bishop, B.A., Cochran, J.F., Smith, L.R., & Lerew, D.J. (1994). Comfort measures in breast-feeding, primiparous women. *Journal of Obstetrical, Gynecological and Neonatal Nursing, 23*(1), 46–52.

Budd, S., Erdman, S. & Long, D. (1993). Improved lactation with metoclopramide. *Clinical Pediatrics, 32*, 53–56.

Cadwell, K. (1981). Improving nipple graspability and success at breast-feeding. *Journal of Gynecological Neonatal Nursing, 4*, 277–279.

Chute, G. (1992). Promoting breast-feeding success: An overview of basic management. *NAACOG's Clinical Issues in Perinatal and Women's Health Nursing, 3*(4), 570–582.

Daly. S., & Hartman, P. (1995). Infant demand and milk supply. Part two: The short term control of milk synthesis in lactating women. *Journal of Human Lactation, II* (1), 27–37.

Evans, K., Evans, R., & Simmer, K. (1995). Effect of the method of breast-feeding on breast engorgement, mastitis, and infantile colic. *Acta Paediatrica, 84*, 849–52

Hale, T., (1997). *Medications and mother's milk.* Amarillo, TX: Pharmasoft Medical Publishing.

Hauben, D., & Mahler, D. (1983). A simple method for the correction of the inverted nipple. *Plastic Reconstructive Surgery, 7*, 556.

Hoffman, J. (1953) A suggested treatment for inverted nipples. *American Journal of Obstetrics and Gynecology. 66*(2), 346–348.

Hopkinson, J., Schanler, R., Fraley, J., & Garza, C. (1992). Milk production by mothers of premature infants: influence of cigarette smoking. *Pediatrics 90*, 934–938.

Lawrence, R. (1994). *Breast-feeding: A guide for the medical profession* (4th ed.). St. Louis, MO: Mosby.

Marmet, C., & Shell, E. (1984). Training neonates to suck correctly. *Maternal-Child Nursing, 9*, 401–405.

Marmet, C., Shell, E., & Marmet, R. (1990). Neonatal frenotomy may be necessary to correct breast-feeding problems. *Journal of Human Lactation, 6*, 117–121.

Marmet, C. (1992). *Manual expression of breast milk.* Encino, CA: The Lactation Institute.

Multicentre Randomised Controlled Trial of Alternative Treatments for Inverted and Non-Protractile Nipples in Pregnancy Trial Collaborative Group (MAIN) (1994). Preparing for breast-feeding: The treatment of inverted and non-protractile nipples in pregnancy. *Midwifery, 10*, 200–221

Neifert, M., McDonough S., and Neville, M. (1981). Failure of lactogenesis associated with placental retention. *American Journal of Obstetrics and Gynecology, 140*, 477–478.

Neifert, M., Seacat, J., & Jobe, W. (1985). Lactation failure due to insufficient glandular development of the breast. *Pediatrics, 76*(5), 823–827.

Thomsen, A. C., Espersen, T., & Maigaard, S. (1983). Course and treatment of milk stasis, noninfectious inflammation of the breast, and infectious mastitis in nursing women. *American Journal of Obstetrics and Gynecology, 149*(5), 492–495.

Townsend, R. J., Benedetti, T. J., Erickson, S. H., Cengis, C., Gillespie, W. R., Gshwend, J., & Albert, K. S. (1984). Excretion of ibuprofen into breast milk. *American Journal of Obstetrics and Gynecology, 149*(2), 184–186.

Woolridge, M. (1986). Aetiology of sore nipples. *Midwifery 2*, 172–176.

Woolridge, M., Baum, J., & Drewett, R. (1980). Effect of a traditional and of a new nipple shield on sucking patterns and milk flow. *Early Human Development, 4*, 357–364.

Woolridge, M, Ingram, J., & Baum, J . (1990). Do changes in pattern of breast usage alter the baby's nutrient intake?. *Lancet, 336*(8712), 395–397.

World Health Organization. (1998). *Protecting, promoting, and supporting breast-feeding: The special role of maternity services.* (a joint WHO/UNICEF statement). Geneva, Switzerland: World Health Organization.

SECTION 17

INFANT HEALTH SUPERVISION

Section 17

INFANT HEALTH SUPERVISION

(Birth to 2 Months of Age)

Maureen T. Shannon

Newborn care involves evaluation of the physical health of the infant, as well as an assessment of the dynamics of the newly constituted family. The work of preparing and adapting to a new infant begins long before birth. During prenatal visits expectant parents should have been asked about how they expect their lives to change after the birth of the infant. In addition, assessment of the parents' ability to provide basic care for the infant (e.g., food, shelter, clothing), their previous experiences with caring for an infant or children, plans they have for resuming their usual life activities, available support systems, and any specific concerns they may have should have been conducted. They should have been provided information about infant safety (e.g., infant car seats), and issues that are pertinent to the infant's care during the first few hours and days after birth (e.g., method of feeding, circumcision) should have been discussed. In addition, ongoing evaluations of the stability of the couple's relationship, as well as the possibility of domestic violence, should have occurred.

This chapter is intended to familiarize the reader with the routine assessment of term, appropriate for gestation (AGA) infants during the first few weeks of life, and will focus on three time periods: the newborn evaluation performed within 24 hours after birth, the first out-of-hospital visit (usually scheduled between 2 and 10 days after birth), and the first routine child health supervision visit (usually scheduled between 1 to 2 months of age). For a more in-depth presentation of pediatric health care, the reader is referred to *Rudolph's Fundamentals of Pediatrics* (1994) edited by A. M. Rudolph and R. K. Kamei, available from Appleton and Lange publishers.

Newborn Evaluation

The immediate newborn period is a transition phase from intrauterine to extrauterine life. It requires adaptations in the neonate's pulmonary, circulatory, thermoregulatory, gastrointestinal, and endocrine systems. Prenatal factors and intrapartum events can effect this adaptation if significant perinatal or medical complications have occurred. A complete physical examination of the neonate is essential to determine his/her adaptation to extrauterine life, the presence of any existing problems, and the appropriate follow-up evaluations indicated (e.g., routine scheduling of out-of-hospital visits, additional laboratory evaluations, public health nurse [PHN] home visits).

Another essential component of the initial evaluation of the neonate is the review of the mother's medical record and an interview with the mother or both parents. In general, the mother will have been through the physically exhausting process of childbirth, which should be considered when interpreting her interactions with her infant. Ideally, questions should be posed in an open ended manner to elicit perceptions about the birth experience and the neonate by the parents, as well as provide an opportunity for addressing specific questions about the neonate they may have.

Database

Subjective

The following areas should be assessed during the initial interview. See also Chapter 4.3, *The Postpartum Visit.*

- Intrapartum experience
  - ▶ Assessment of the actual labor and delivery experience of the mother/couple compared to expectations
  - ▶ Level of fatigue of mother/couple
  - ▶ Level of physical discomfort of mother at this time
  - ▶ Medication(s) she has received for discomfort (e.g., narcotic analgesic)
  - ▶ Time interval between birth of neonate and the mother's or couple's physical contact with the neonate
  - ▶ Mother's/couple's expectation of infant's appearance and behavior compared to actual experience once infant seen
- Infant feeding
  - ▶ What type of feeding is the mother planning?
  - ▶ If breast-feeding is planned, does she understand techniques and the nutritional requirements for breast-feeding?
  - ▶ If bottle-feeding is planned, has a formula been chosen? Is the preparation of the formula clearly understood? Does she have access to refrigeration, clean running water, bottles and nipples?
  - ▶ Is the mother/couple comfortable holding and feeding the infant?
  - ▶ What type of feeding schedule do they anticipate?
- Physical environment
  - ▶ Is the home set up to receive the infant (room or space for infant, crib or bassinet, clothing, diapers)?
  - ▶ What type of transportation is planned for returning home, and getting the infant to scheduled medical visits and emergency visits. If transportation is by car, is an infant car safety seat available for use? Are the parents familiar with the proper location of this in the car (i.e., not in the front passenger seat) and how to secure it?
- Support systems
  - ▶ Anticipated help with household tasks at home
  - ▶ Previous experience with infant care; if limited, person(s) available to the mother or couple to help with infant care or to answer their questions
  - ▶ If other children, perception of these children's needs and plans to address these needs; person(s) available to help with child care, if needed (e.g., transportation to school)
  - ▶ Emotional support system(s)

- Infant health care
  - ▶ Planned access to the health care system for routine questions and for emergencies
  - ▶ Designated primary pediatric clinician for infant; planned date of first office visit
  - ▶ Understanding of routine infant care (e.g., cord care, sleeping cycles, frequency of feeding, normal elimination, immunizations, symptoms of problems, taking temperature and reading a thermometer, etc.)

Objective

- Direct observation of parent-infant interaction is as important as the physical examination of the infant. Observe the way the infant is held and cuddled. Note parental responses to the infant's needs. The infant's ability to attach and suck appropriately when feeding as well as the mother's feeding technique (whether breast-feeding or bottle-feeding) is important to observe. Note the infant's various states (i.e., sleeping, crying, active alert, quiet alert) and parental responses to these states. Finally, observe the mother's interactions with her partner as a means of evaluating their support of each other.

- If possible, perform the physical examination in the presence of both parents after the infant's temperature has stabilized and vital signs have been obtained. It should proceed in a manner that will minimize disturbing the infant so that accurate assessments can be made. Generally, the examination of the oropharynx, extremities, and reflexes, components of the examination that may elicit crying, should be done after completing assessment of the head (i.e., fontanels), heart, and lungs.

  - ▶ In general, note the infant's state (active alert, quiet alert, sleeping, crying), spontaneous activity, respirations, and presence of abnormal signs (e.g., respiratory retractions or grunting, generalized cyanosis, irritability, etc.).

  - ▶ Observe vital signs. The following are the normal ranges observed in a neonate:
    - Temperature within the first 24 hours is 36° to 37.5° C (96° to 99.5° F).
    - Pulse rate is between 95 to 180 beats per minute (bpm) and varies with the neonate's activity.
    - Respirations are usually irregular with a rate between 40 to 60 per minute (Sola, Bull, Durlat, Partridge, & Rogido, 1994).

  - ▶ Length, weight, and head circumference should be plotted on standard growth charts for full term and premature infants (available from Ross Products, Division of Abbott Laboratories, Columbus, OH 43215-1724) (see Figures 17.1, 17.2, 17.3, and 17.4 for examples of standard growth charts for term male and female infants). These parameters should be within two standard deviations of the mean value for the neonate's gestational age at birth.

  - ▶ Assess skin for color (e.g., pink, acrocyanosis, cutis marmorata, pallor, jaundice, meconium staining) and turgor, presence of birth marks (e.g., Mongolian spots, nevus simplex, nevus flammeus, cavernous hemangiomas), lanugo, vernix caseosa, scaling, and rashes (e.g., milia, erythema toxicum).

  NOTE: The presence of pallor may indicate chronic anemia, asphyxia, or shock. Jaundice within the first 24 hours of age is considered abnormal. Acrocyanosis (cyanosis of the hands and feet) and cutis marmorata (mottling of the skin) are commonly observed and are a result of the unstable vasomotor response in newborns. Central or generalized cyanosis is an abnormal physical finding (Sola et al., 1994).

▶ Assess head for the presence of cranial molding, cephalohematoma, caput succedaneum, craniotabes, and abrasions (due to scalp electrode placement or trauma during birth [e.g., improperly placed forceps]). Palpate the cranial sutures, the anterior and posterior fontanels.

NOTE: The anterior fontanel, located between the coronal and sagittal sutures, is diamond shaped, flat, and measures approximately 2 cm by 2 cm. Inability to palpate the anterior fontanel may be a result of overriding of the sutures (during the birth process) or an abnormal fusion of the sutures (e.g., craniosynostosis). The posterior fontanel, located between the sagittal and lamboidal sutures, is triangular in shape and is barely palpable at birth (Sola et al., 1994).

▶ Assess face for symmetry of movement, dysmorphic features, and edema or ecchymosis (usually observed with face presentations or if there was a tight nuchal cord during delivery).

▶ Assess eyes for subconjunctival hemorrhages (as a result of rupture of scleral capillaries during the birth process), scleral icterus, discharge, eyelid edema, epicanthal folds, hypertelorism, slanted palpebral fissures, nystagmus, and fixed strabismus. Pupillary reaction to light should be elicited and be symmetrical. Evaluate for the presence of the retinal red reflex (if a white reflex is observed this indicates an abnormality such as corneal opacification, retinoblastoma, chorioretinitis).

▶ Assess ears for patency of external auditory canals, evidence of low-set ears (can be indicative of genetic syndromes), and presence of auricular tags or sinuses. Evaluate the infant's hearing by making a sudden noise and observing the infant for a response (e.g., Moro reflex).

▶ Assess nose for patency of nares (to rule out unilateral or bilateral choanal atresia). Note evidence of dislocation of the septum or possibly dysmorphic features (e.g., beaked nose, flat, broad nasal bridge)

▶ Assess mouth with the infant at rest and when crying. Observe for evidence of clefts of the soft or hard palate, micrognathia, retrognathia, glossoptosis, and macroglossia (these may occur as isolated findings or in association with congenital anomalies or syndromes). The presence of small mucoid cysts (e.g., Epstein's pearls) are a normal variant. Observe the infant's cry, which should be strong and without stridor.

▶ Assess neck for symmetry, masses, webbing, and edema. Palpate both clavicles to rule out the presence of fractures.

▶ Assess chest for the presence of breast buds, engorgement, accessory nipples, and secretion. Note respiratory rate and rhythm, presence of expiratory grunting, sternal or intercostal retractions, cyanosis, asymmetrical chest wall movement, pectus excavatum, and pectus carinatum. Auscultation of the lungs should reveal bilateral breath sounds; crackles should not be noted 2 to 4 hours after birth.

▶ Assess heart rate and rhythm; the rate will vary between 95 to 180 beats per minute (bpm) depending upon the infant's activity. A heart rate exceeding 200 bpm at rest or less than 80 beats per minute (bpm) requires further evaluation (e.g., electrocardiogram [ECG]). Auscultation of the heart will reveal a loud second heart sound (S_2) without splitting during the first 3 hours after birth. Within 48 hours the majority of infants will demonstrate a split S_2. A systolic murmur may be evident during the first 2 days of life, but will usually resolve after that time. Peripheral pulses should be palpated in all four extremities.

NOTE: Blood pressure readings are not usually obtained in neonates unless symptoms of congenital heart disease or heart failure are observed. When blood pressure readings are indicated they should be obtained in all four extremities to rule out the possibility of coarctation of the aorta (Sola et al., 1994).

▶ Assess abdomen. Inspect the cord for the presence and number of vessels (two arteries, one vein). Assess for peristaltic movements, evidence of abnormal abdominal masses, omphalitis, hernias, and persistent urachus.

NOTE: Observation of the abdomen will usually reveal the normal distention that is a result of poor abdominal muscle tone, diaphragmatic movements associated with respirations, and the enlarged neonatal liver. Lack of this distention is often noted in small-for-gestational-age infants, but may signify the presence of a diaphragmatic hernia or esophageal atresia. The neonatal liver edge is usually palpated below the right costal margin. The kidneys may be felt as small midabdominal masses.

▶ Assess the genitalia.

– For term females, assessment normally reveals the labia majora covering the labia minora and clitoris, a hymenal appendix may be observed at the vaginal orifice, and a milky white vaginal discharge may be evident (as a result of withdrawal of maternal hormones after delivery). Abnormal findings include hypertrophied clitoris (associated with virilizing adrenal hyperplasia), ambiguous genitalia, or hydrometrocolpos (due to an imperforate hymen).

– For term males, assessment normally reveals the testes in the scrotum, a tight prepuce (which should not be retracted), and a small penis with the urethral meatus at the end of the penis. Abnormal findings include scrotal swelling (e.g., hydrocele, testicular torsion), undescended testes, epispadias, hypospadias, hydrocoele(s), hernia(s), and ambiguous genitalia.

▶ Assess anus for patency (e.g., passage of meconium).

NOTE: Meconium stool is passed within the first 24 hours after birth in 90 percent of infants and by 48 hours in 99 percent of infants (Sola et al., 1994). Failure to pass meconium by 24 to 48 hours requires further evaluation to rule out the possibility of imperforate anus.

▶ Assess extremities for muscle tone, symmetry of movements, and number of fingers and toes. Note evidence of hip dislocation or dysplasia (e.g., hip click when legs are abducted), syndactyly, polydactyly, rudimentary digits, or foot abnormalities.

▶ Assess spine for dimpling, presence of hair tufts, nevus, and lipomas in the lumbar-sacral area (can be associated with spina bifida) and evidence of a pilonidal dimple in the sacrococcygeal area (may indicate a sinus tract).

▶ Neurological assessment includes observation of the neonate's states of alertness, variations in states, ability to fix and follow a human face, response to sound, head control, spontaneous motor activity (symmetry, intensity, tremors, jerks, convulsions), and presence of primitive reflexes (see Table 17.1, Neurological/Developmental Assessment of Infants).

Assessment

- Normal, AGA term neonate
- Maternal/parental attachment established and appropriate
- Breast-feeding/bottle-feeding adequate
- Normal circumcision site (if appropriate)
- Immunizations—Hepatitis B series initiated
- List other diagnosis, as indicated (e.g., jaundice, anemia, hypospadias)

Plan

Diagnostic Tests

- Screening tests during the neonatal period are mandated by state laws and may include
  - ▶ Metabolic tests, specifically thyroid (i.e., thyroxine [T4], thyroid stimulating hormone [TSH], phenylketonuria, galactosemia, biotinidase deficiency, congenital adrenal hyperplasia, maple syrup urine disease, homocystinuria, tyrosinemia, and cystic fibrosis testing
  - ▶ Hemoglobinathy screening
  - ▶ Toxoplasmosis testing
  - ▶ Syphilis serology testing of cord blood
- Other tests should be ordered as indicated by physical examination findings (e.g., complete blood count [CBC], total bilirubin, Coombs testing, toxicology screening, etc.).
- If not already obtained during pregnancy, human immunodeficiency virus (HIV) antibody testing should be offered to the mother. This is especially important for women with unknown HIV status who are nursing their infants, since HIV can be transmitted from nursing women to their infants. Women who decline HIV antibody testing for themselves, but consent to the testing of their infants should be educated regarding the implications of this test in terms of their own HIV status. Specifically, a positive HIV antibody test in an infant less than 18 months of age reflects maternal infection and *risk* of HIV infection in the infant and the need for further viral testing of the infant (see Chapter 14.5, *Human Immunodeficiency Virus*).

Consultation

- Consult with a physician for any abnormal physical finding or any disturbance in observed parent-infant interactions.

- Consult with social worker and/or social services department for dysfunctional parent-infant interaction.

Treatment/Management

- Vitamin K, 1.0 mg IM or subcutaneously is routinely given shortly after birth to prevent hemorrhagic disease of the newborn.

  NOTE: Infants weighing less than 1500 grams receive a 0.5 mg dose.

- Erythromycin ophthalmic drops (one drop in each eye) is administered to prevent gonococcal conjunctivitis.

- Currently, the initiation of hepatitis B virus (HBV) vaccine series within 4 weeks after birth in neonates born to hepatitis B antigen negative women is now recommended (Centers for Disease Control & Prevention [CDC], 1998). In many states this series is initiated prior to the neonate's discharge from the hospital with subsequent immunizations required at 1 and 6 months of age (see Figure 17.5, Recommended Childhood Vaccination Schedule—United States, January–December, 1998). There are two vaccine preparations available for administration as follows:

  ▶ Recombivax HB® 2.5 µg (0.25 mL) IM

  ▶ Engerix-B®10 µg (0.5 mL) IM

- Infants should remain in the hospital until the following have been observed:

  ▶ Vital signs are stable for a minimum of 12 hours.

  ▶ Both urination and passage of meconium have been documented.

  ▶ There is no evidence of bleeding from a circumcision site for a minimum of 2 hours.

  ▶ The infant is able to successfully breast-feed or bottle-feed.

  ▶ Maternal laboratory data are complete and there are no indications for further infant treatment (e.g., ABO incompatibility, sepsis, etc.).

  ▶ Maternal/parental ability to care for infant and recognize signs and symptoms of an emergency is demonstrated.

  ▶ An appropriate home environment for the infant is available.

  ▶ A pediatric clinician responsible for the primary care of the infant is identified and a follow-up outpatient visit has been scheduled as indicated.

Patient Education

- Nutrition

  ▶ For breast-feeding, review the need for maternal rest, adequate nutrition and fluid intake, nipple care, methods to relieve breast engorgement (e.g., tight, supportive bra, cool compresses, etc.), frequency of feedings (i.e., every 2 to 3 hours for a minimum of 10 minutes on each breast), techniques to help infant latch onto the breast and release suction, and need for vitamin D 400 IU per day supplementation in areas where significant sun deprivation (e.g., Alaska) (see also Section 16, *Lactation*).

▶ For bottle-feeding, review type of commercial formula to be used (e.g., cow's milk formulas, soy-based formulas), proper preparation of formula (e.g., powder, concentrate, or ready-to-use), adequate caloric intake (e.g., 3 ounces per pound per day, 100 kilocalories per kilogram per day), importance of avoidance of hot spots due to the use of a microwave to warm formula, positioning of bottle for feedings (do not prop), and frequency of feeding (e.g., every 2 to 3 hours) (American Academy of Pediatrics, 1993; Jaskiewicz, 1996; Overby, 1994).

- Injury/illness prevention

  ▶ Infant car seat should be properly secured, not placed in an front air-bag seat.

  ▶ Crib slats must be less than 2 $^3/_8$ inches apart, firm mattress, no pillows.

  ▶ Infant should sleep only on back (to reduce possibility of sudden infant death syndrome [SIDS]).

  ▶ Do not shake the infant.

  ▶ Hot water heater thermostat should be set below 120° F (48.8°C).

  ▶ Never leave infant unattended, especially on soft surfaces or in tub of water. Always keep one hand on the baby.

  ▶ No smoking in environments in which infant is staying.

  ▶ Do not drink hot liquids while holding the infant.

  ▶ Review how to take temperature, read a thermometer, and define a fever that requires notification of a pediatric clinician (i.e., temperature greater than 38° C/100.4° F) .

  ▶ Parental recognition of symptoms that should prompt medical contact: fever, jaundice, diarrhea, dehydration, irritability, lethargy, seizures, apnea, and failure to nurse/bottle-feed.

  ▶ Understanding of what to do in emergency, telephone numbers to call if an emergency occurs (e.g., emergency room, pediatric clinician's number, local poison control center).

- Infant care

  The following aspects of normal infant care should be reviewed (Jaskiewicz, 1996).

  ▶ Sleep patterns—may sleep a total of 20 hours a day, awakening every 2 to 4 hours to nurse/bottle-feed.

  ▶ Nursing/bottle-feeding—every 2 to 4 hours. Bottle-fed term AGA infants will consume approximately 2 to 3 ounces per feeding. A newborn infant should not be permitted to go more than 5 hours between feedings (Overby, 1994).

  ▶ Cord care—alcohol swabbing of cord stump after each diaper change until the cord falls off.

  ▶ Circumcision care—petroleum jelly to prevent freshly scabbing areas from adhering to diaper and to protect the penis from irritation by urine.

  ▶ Variations in crying patterns (e.g., hunger, discomfort, etc.). Total crying time normally observed in newborns is 2 to 3 hours per day (Baker, 1996).

▶ Change from meconium stools (dark greenish-black, pasty consistency) to transitional stools (bright yellow, seedy consistency).

▶ Vaginal discharge/bleeding—small amount is normal and may continue for up to 2 weeks after birth. Discharge can be wiped away with warm water in a front-to-back motion (i.e., prepuce to perineum).

▶ Prior to the administration of the hepatitis B immunization, the mother/parents should receive written information about the vaccination, and give consent for its administration (Siegal, 1996).

● Family care

▶ The mother needs adequate rest, nutrition and opportunities to maintain her own health in order to care for her infant.

▶ Discuss the role of her partner in terms of the mother's support and infant care.

▶ Discuss potential outside sources of support for the mother and her partner.

▶ Discuss ways to integrate time for other children, and ways to explore their reactions/involvement with the infant.

▶ Review previous successful coping strategies of the mother, couple, and family.

▶ If history of or suspicion regarding domestic violence, review cyclic nature of episodes, possibility for escalation of violence because of new infant, and safety measures.

▶ Recommend educational materials about infant care.

NOTE: A good resource is *Taking Care of Your Child: A Parent's Guide to Complete Medical Care* by R.H. Pantell, J.F. Fries, and D.M. Vickery (1999), Perseus Publishing Company. This is an easy-to-read guide for parents or child care givers regarding normal growth and development of children (infancy through adolescence) that also provides information about one hundred pediatric problems. It includes decision-making charts for each pediatric problem so adults can readily follow recommended interventions.

Follow-up

● Since breast milk often does not come in for 2 to 3 days and jaundice often peaks around the third day of life, all infants should be evaluated within 48 to 72 hours after an early discharge (e.g., discharge within 24 hours after delivery). This assessment should occur either in the home or pediatric clinician's office.

● An appointment for a routine evaluation by a pediatric clinician 1 to 2 weeks after birth should have been made, depending upon the needs of the infant.

● Document any identified problem or condition and receipt of hepatitis B vaccine in the progress notes and problem list.

First Posthospital Visit Evaluation

Early discharge of mothers and infants from the hospital is increasing nationally. Despite legislation mandating 48 hours of insurance coverage if requested by physicians, it seems highly likely that many newborns will continue to be at home within 24 hours after birth and most will be discharged well before 48 hours. Follow-up evaluations in these situations is essential. For infants sent home before 24 hours, a telephone call the next day is essential, as well as a scheduled visit with a health provider within 3 days. For those infants who stay in the hospital for more than 48 hours, a repeat health visit should occur within 4 to 7 days after discharge depending on the parents' level of skills and previous experiences with infant care, and the individual needs of the infant. For example, a jaundiced infant with a positive Coombs test will need closer monitoring after discharge than a normal-term infant without evidence of jaundice.

In addition, the first week can be a time of substantial stress for the family since the woman is recuperating from delivery and everyone is adapting to a new schedule that may include little time for sleep. Considerable parental anxiety may also occur in response to the physical adjustments being made by the newborn. Assuming appropriate education occurred before and immediately after birth, subsequent office visits offer opportunities to review, reinforce, and clarify issues of importance about the newborn and the family. Whenever possible, a copy of the infant's and mother's discharge summaries should be obtained and reviewed prior to the visit.

Database

Subjective

- Begin the visit by posing questions to the mother/couple that will address the adjustment of the family to the newborn and elicit special concerns of either parent. Questions should specifically address the following issues about the infant:

  ▶ Consolability

  ▶ Sleep patterns

  ▶ Temperament (e.g., quiet, active, irritable, etc.)

  ▶ Feeding type (formula v. nursing), frequency, success, and any problems (e.g., sore nipples, confusion about formula preparation)

  ▶ Bladder and bowel function

  ▶ Parental tasks, rest, coping strategies, available respite care

  ▶ Maternal fatigue, symptoms of depression or postpartum complications

  ▶ Responses of other children to the infant

Objective

- Try to observe the following parent-infant interactions:

  ▶ Couple's interactions with each other

  ▶ Responsiveness to infant's cues (e.g., comforting of infant)

  ▶ Accomplishment of infant care tasks (e.g., diapering, feeding, burping, etc.)

- The infant examination may include all of the components listed under the Objective section for the Newborn Evaluation with the following areas specifically targeted during this visit:

  ▶ Observe the infant's general state (e.g., active alert, quiet alert, sleeping, crying), spontaneous activity, respiratory effort, and presence of abnormal signs (e.g., irritability).

  ▶ Asses vital signs

  - Loss of up to 10 percent of birth weight is normal during the first few days of life. The infant may not regain birthweight until 7 to 10 days after birth (Overby, 1994). However, any drop below two standard deviations of the mean on the growth chart warrants close monitoring to assure infant does not become dehydrated (see Figures 17.1 and 17.3).

  - The length and head circumference will be similar to initial measurements observed during the newborn examination. Plot these on standard growth charts (should be within two standard deviations of the mean value for the infant's gestational age at birth—see Figure 17.1, 17.2, 17.3, and 17.4).

  - Temperature should be within normal limits (WNL).

  - Respirations should occur at a rate between 30 to 60 per minute without evidence of nasal flaring, grunting or retractions; the respirations may be irregular with very brief periods of apnea.

  - Pulse rate should be between 95 and 180 bpm depending upon the infant's activity.

  ▶ Assess skin for color (especially the presence of pallor, cyanosis, jaundice) and turgor.

  NOTE: The presence of pallor may indicate chronic anemia. Jaundice is commonly observed in term newborns during the first several days of life. However, jaundice that increases in amount, persists beyond 7 days of life, or is associated with a complication (e.g., ABO incompatibility) requires further evaluation and consultation with a physician (McHenry, 1996).

  ▶ Assess head for the resolution of any previously noted cranial molding, cephalohematoma, caput succedaneum, abrasions, and/or overriding cranial sutures. Palpate the anterior and posterior fontanels (which should be flat, not depressed or bulging) (Sola et al., 1994).

  ▶ Assess face for resolution of previously noted edema or ecchymosis.

  ▶ Assess eyes for resolution of previously noted subconjunctival hemorrhages, discharge, or eyelid edema. Observe for nystagmus, pupillary reaction to light, and the presence of the retinal red reflex.

  ▶ Assess the ears and evaluate the infant's hearing by making a sudden noise and observing the infant for a response.

  ▶ Assess nose for patency of nares

  ▶ Assess mouth and observe the infant's cry, which should be strong and without stridor.

  ▶ Assess chest for the presence of breast buds, engorgement, accessory nipples, secretion. Note the respiratory rate and rhythm, presence of expiratory grunting, sternal or intercostal retractions, or cyanosis.

  ▶ Auscultation of the lungs should reveal bilateral breath sounds; crackles should not be noted.

  ▶ Assess the heart rate and rhythm; the rate will vary between 95 to 180 bpm depending upon the infant's activity. A heart rate exceeding 200 bpm at rest or less than 80 bpm requires further evaluation. Auscultation of the heart will reveal a split S_2 within 48 hours after birth in the majority of infants. A systolic murmur previously documented during the first 2 days of life will usually resolve by this visit. Peripheral pulses should be palpated in all four extremities.

▶ Assess the abdomen. Inspect the umbilicus for evidence of infection. Assess for peristaltic movements, evidence of abnormal abdominal masses, hernias, or persistent urachus.

▶ Assess the genitalia and diaper area.

  – For term females, assess for vaginal discharge, labial adhesions, or evidence of a rash

  – For term males, assess for the presence of undescended testes, hydrocele, or hernias. If the infant has been circumcised, evaluate the site for any evidence of an infection.

▶ Musculoskeletal evaluation includes assessment of the spine for deviation, extremities for muscle tone, symmetry of movements, and evidence of hip dislocation or dysplasia.

▶ Neurological assessment includes observation of the neonate's states of alertness, variations in states, ability to fix and follow a human face, response to sound, head control, spontaneous motor activity (symmetry, intensity, tremors, jerks, convulsions) and presence and symmetry of reflexes.

Assessment

- Normal ___ day old infant
- Maternal/parental attachment established and appropriate
- Breast-feeding/bottle-feeding adequate
- Circumcision site healing
- Immunizations, as indicated (e.g., Hepatitis B vaccine #1)
- List other diagnosis, as indicated (e.g., hyperbilirubinemia, anemia)

Plan

Diagnostic Tests

- If available, review the results of any screening tests done prior to discharge (e.g., metabolic tests, hemoglobinopathy screening, etc.). If screening tests were not obtained prior to hospital discharge, discuss these tests with the mother or both parents and obtain them at this visit.

- Obtain other laboratory tests as indicated by physical examination findings or based on the discharge plan of care (e.g., total bilirubin, CBC, etc.).

Consultation

- Consult with a physician for any abnormal physical examination findings, laboratory results, or disturbance in parent-infant interaction.

- Consult with a social worker or social service department for dysfunctional parent-infant interaction, as indicated.

Treatment/Management

- If a hepatitis B immunization series was not initiated prior to discharge from the hospital, it should be considered for administration at this time (see Treatment section of Newborn Evaluation for types of hepatitis vaccines and dosages).

- Consult with a physician and/or institution-specific protocols for the appropriate plan of care indicated for identified conditions, including psychosocial problems.

Patient Education

- See the Patient Education section for Newborn Evaluation

- Discuss and provide written information about the recommended schedule for immunizations of children (see Figure 17.5, Recommended Childhood Vaccination Schedule—United States, January– June 1996).

Follow-up

- All families should be evaluated until the infant's physical health and growth has stabilized and the parents' adjustment is satisfactory. Specific problems (e.g., jaundice) may require daily monitoring until resolved.

- A routine office visit should be scheduled for between 4 to 8 weeks.

- Document any identified problems or conditions and the receipt of hepatitis B vaccine (if given during this visit) in the progress notes and problem list.

One- to Two-Month Evaluation

Current recommendations call for routine infant visits between 1 and 2 months after birth. By the time the infant is 1 month of age, parents have gained considerable experience in caring for their infant and, hopefully, are adapting. There should be a sense of what is needed to feed and comfort their infant. During the first month, colic often emerges. This intense crying, often inconsolable, characteristically occurs in late afternoon and spontaneously resolves by about 3 months. Sleep patterns are still irregular and most infants still wake at night for a feeding. Parent's fatigue levels should be assessed. Although the Family Medical Leave Act grants parents 12 weeks of unpaid leave, many parents return to work by 6 weeks, so child care arrangements should be discussed.

Database

Subjective

- In addition to the areas listed under the Subjective section of the First Posthospital Evaluation, the following should be addressed:

  ▶ Problems and strategies for dealing with fussiness and crying

  ▶ Infant's eye contact, fixing on, following of objects

  ▶ Mother's/parents' adjustment to returning to work

Objective

- Perform direct observation of parental interactions with the infant and between each other, and perform a complete physical exam (Melman, 1996; Overby, 1994):

- Note the infant's general state (e.g., active alert, quiet alert, sleeping, crying), spontaneous activity, respiratory effort, and presence of abnormal signs (e.g., irritability).

- Asses vital signs (optional if infant not clinically ill).

- Plot height, weight, head circumference on growth chart (see Figures 17.1 through 17.4).

  NOTE: The infant's weight should be following the percentile line established at birth. A falloff of more than two percentiles requires consultation to evaluate for dehydration/malnutrition. An increase of more than two percentiles on head circumference requires consultation to evaluate for hydrocephalus.

- Evaluate skin for color and turgor. Jaundice as a result of breast-feeding should have resolved by this age.

- Assess head and note complete resolution of birth associated cephalohematoma, caput succedaneum, and abrasions. The anterior fontanel is palpable measuring 2 cm by 2 cm, but should be flat. The posterior fontanel is not palpable at 2 months.

  ▶ Eye examination should reveal a red reflex. Note esotropia, exotropia fixed strabismus, or discharges.

  ▶ Assess nose for patency of nares, discharge.

  ▶ Assess mouth for evidence of thrush.

  ▶ Evaluate neck for masses.

  ▶ Lymph nodes are normally not palpated at this age.

- Assess chest.

  ▶ Breast buds may still be evident. Note respiratory rate and rhythm. Auscultation of the lungs should reveal bilateral breath sounds; crackles should not be noted.

  ▶ Note heart rate and rhythm and assess for first and second heart sounds, presence of and/or changes in previously noted murmurs. Peripheral pulses should be palpated in all four extremities.

- Assess the abdomen. Inspect the umbilicus for evidence of infection. Assess for peristaltic movements, evidence of abnormal abdominal masses, hernias, or persistent urachus.

- Musculoskeletal evaluation includes assessment of the spine for deviation, extremities for muscle tone, range of motion, symmetry of movements, and evidence of hip dislocation or dysplasia

- Assess the genitalia and diaper area.

  ▶ For term females, assess for vaginal discharge, labial adhesions, or evidence of a rash.

  ▶ For term males, assess for the presence of undescended testes, hydrocele, hernias, or a rash. The circumcision site should be healed by 6 to 8 weeks.

- Neurological includes evaluation of the infant's attention to voices, ability to smile and coo responsively (by 6 weeks), and ability to lift head, neck, and upper chest when lying prone (by 2 months of age). Primitive reflexes may still be present and should be symmetrical.

Assessment

- Normal ___ week old infant
- Maternal/parental attachment established and appropriate
- Breast-feeding/bottle-feeding adequate
- Routine immunizations administered
- List other diagnosis as indicated

Plan

Diagnostic Tests

- No diagnostic tests are indicated unless an abnormal condition is documented or suspected.

Consultation

- Consult with a physician for any abnormal physical examination findings, laboratory results, or significant disturbance in parent-infant interaction.

- Consult with a social worker or social service department if dysfunctional parent-infant interaction, as indicated.

Treatment/Management

- Provide parents with written information, and counsel them about the risks, benefits, and common side effects of each of the immunizations recommended for administration at this visit. Once parental consent is obtained, the following immunizations may be administered (see also Figure 17.5):

  ▶ Administer hepatitis B virus immunization #1 at 1 month of age, if not previously given (see Treatment section of Newborn Evaluation for doses of different preparations).

  ▶ Administer hepatitis B virus immunization #2 at 6 to 8 weeks.

  ▶ The Hemophilus influenza type B (Hib) immunization #1 dose is 0.5 mL IM. Various preparations of Hib vaccines are available, including a preparation in combination with DPT. Once a preparation is initiated, all subsequent immunizations should be with the same preparation. All preparations require the administration of the same dose (i.e., 0.5 mL IM).

  ▶ The diphtheria, tetanus, pertussis (DTP) immunization #1 dose is 0.5 mL IM administered at 6 to 8 weeks of age.

    NOTE: Diphtheria, tetanus, acellular pertussis (DTaP) vaccine is now the recommended vaccine, but is not yet available in a preparation combined with Hib. Whole cell DTP is an acceptable alternative to the acellular vaccine and available in combination with Hib as one vaccine.

▶ Administer polio vaccine #1 at 6 to 8 weeks of age.

NOTE: Oral polio virus (OPV) vaccine (an individual single oral preparation) or inactivated polio virus (IPV) 0.5 mL IM may be administered. Annually, six to ten cases of oral-vaccine-acquired polio (often occurring in immunocompromised patients or the elderly) have been reported (Rosaf, 1995). IPV may be given as an alternative to OPV; however, IPV must be given intramuscularly. IPV administration is recommended for any infant with an immune deficiency disorder, perinatally exposed to HIV, or who has a family member with an immune deficiency (CDC, 1998).

NOTE: The majority of immunizations are not associated with significant side effects or adverse events. However, whole cell pertussis (DPT) has been observed to cause fretfulness, fever (> 37.8 ° C/100° F), erythema/induration/pain at the site of the injection, and drowsiness (Siegal, 1996). Parents should be aware of these symptoms and advised to contact the pediatric clinician if the infant develops any possible adverse events (specifically encephalopathy, convulsions, persistent/inconsolable crying, high-pitched crying, a shocklike state, or an immediate allergic reaction) within 7 days after the administration of a DPT (Siegal, 1996). An infant experiencing a reported adverse event after administration of a DPT should not receive future immunizations containing whole cell pertussis.

● Consider the administration of acetaminophen liquid 10 mg/kg orally just prior to immunizing with DPT to reduce the incidence of fever and discomfort (Rosaf, 1995). Subsequent administration of acetaminophen liquid 10 mg/kg orally every 4 to 6 hours may be indicated to control fever.

Patient Education

See Patient Education sections of the Newborn and First Posthospital Visit evaluations. In addition to the information provided in those sections, the following should be discussed:

● Nutrition (Cavallo & Alfaro, 1996)

▶ Formula-fed infants should receive iron-fortified formula.

▶ Solid foods are not recommended until the infant is 4 to 6 months of age.

▶ Do not add solids (e.g., cereals) to bottles.

▶ Do not give honey during the first year of life due to the possibility of botulism.

▶ Diluted fruit juice (half strength) may be given after 4 weeks of age to infants if they have demonstrated adequate weight gain for their size and age.

▶ At this age, vitamin and fluoride supplementations are not needed for a bottle-fed infant or breast-fed infant whose mother maintains an adequate lactation diet.

● Infant care

▶ Discuss ways to promote normal sleep patterns, including beginning a sensible bed time routine.

▶ Review infant crying patterns and ways to soothe the infant.

▶ Discuss anticipated development of infant during next few weeks/months (e.g., increased cooing, repetition of pleasant sounds, prolonged attention to sounds, responds to familiar voices, blowing bubbles, head control continuing to strengthen).

- Injury prevention
  - ▶ Instruct the parents to always test the water temperature before bathing the infant.
  - ▶ Discuss safe toys, avoiding toys with small parts.
  - ▶ Review proper placement of car seat.
  - ▶ Review recognition of signs and symptoms of illness and procedures to contact health professionals.
  - ▶ Refer parents (and baby-sitters) to infant CPR classes.
  - ▶ Recommend that a list of emergency procedures and telephone numbers be prepared for baby-sitters.
- Family care
  - ▶ Encourage parents to spend time taking care of themselves and socializing with other adults, if possible.
  - ▶ If there are other children in the family, advise parents to allocate, whenever possible, a special time and/or activity with each child during this time.

Follow Up

- The next office visit after this evaluation should be in 2 months for a normally growing and developing infant with parents and family demonstrating adequate caretaking and coping skills.
- Document any identified problems and receipt of immunizations in the progress notes and problem list.

Table 17.1

Neurological/Developmental Assessment of Infants

Activity	Infant's Response	Age Absent (weeks)
Primitive reflexes		
Moro	Present at birth	12
Asymmetric tonic neck	Present at birth	12
Palmar grasp	Present at birth	12
Stepping	Present at birth	8
Postural Reflexes		
Pull to sit		
– Complete head lag	Present at birth	8
– Slight head lag	Present by 12 weeks	20
Body lying prone		
– Head lies in line with body	Present at birth	4–8
– Head turns to one side	Present by 4 weeks	
Ventral suspension		
– Head drops below body	Present at birth	6
– Briefly holds head in plane of body	Present by 6 weeks	
– Head sustained in plane of body	Present by 6 weeks	
Responsiveness		
Sound		
– Startles to noise	Present at birth	4
– Alerts or quiets to noise	Present at birth–8 weeks	
– Responds to human voice	Present by 2–4 weeks	
– Sustained attention to sound	Present by 8–16 weeks	
– Responds to familiar voice	Present by 8–16 weeks	
Eye gaze		
– Follows dangling object from midline to < 45 degrees	Present at birth–4 weeks	
– Follows dangling object from midline to 90 degrees	Present by 4 weeks	
Social smile	Present by 4–8 weeks	
Cooing	Present by 8 weeks	

Sources: Overby, K. J. 1994. Pediatric Health Supervision. In *Rudolph's fundamentals of pediatrics*, eds. A. M. Rudolph & R. K. Kamei, pp. 1–44. East Norwalk, CT: Appleton & Lange; Schmidt, R. E., & Oppenheimer, S. 1996. Normal Motor and Cognitive Development. In *Handbook of pediatric primary care*, ed. R. C. Baker, pp. 71–78. Boston: Little, Brown & Company.

Figure 17.1

Growth Record for Boys Ages Birth to 36 Months: Head Circumference and Weight

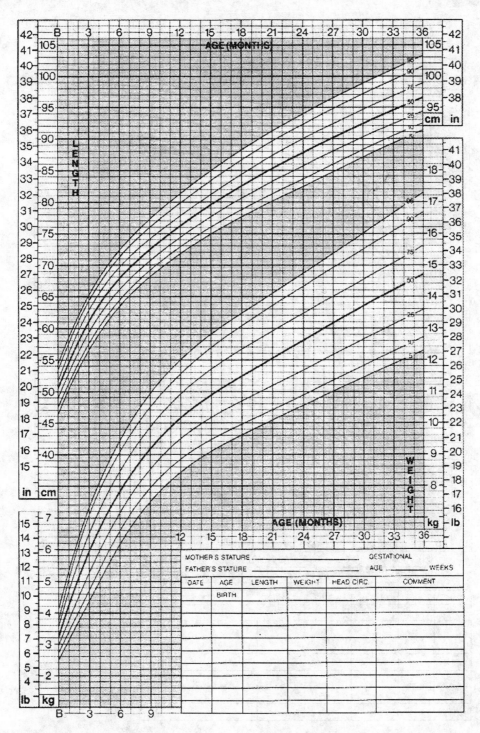

Figure 17.2

Growth Record for Boys Ages Birth to 36 Months: Length and Weight

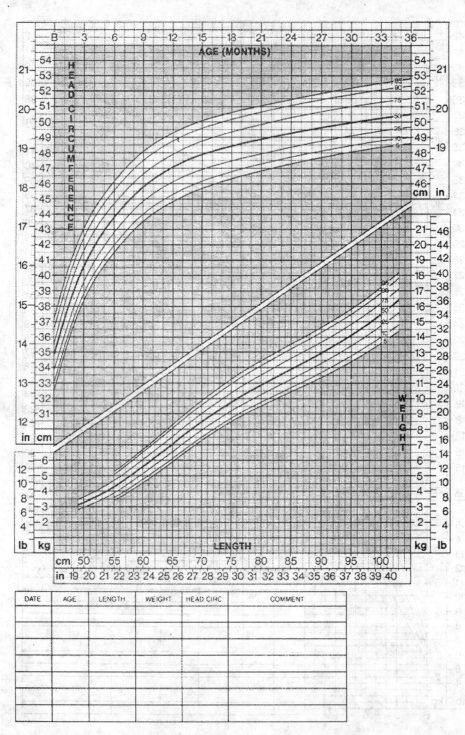

DATE	AGE	LENGTH	WEIGHT	HEAD CIRC	COMMENT

Source: Reprinted with permission from Ross Laboratories copyright © 1982 . Adapted from Hamill, P.V., Drizd, T.A., Johnson, C.L., Reed, R.B., Foche, A.R., & Moore, W.M. 1979. Physical Growth: National Center for Health Statistics Percentiles. *American Journal of Clinical Nutrition, 32*, p.607–629.

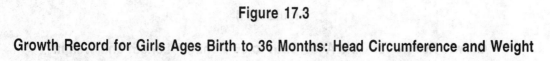

Figure 17.3

Growth Record for Girls Ages Birth to 36 Months: Head Circumference and Weight

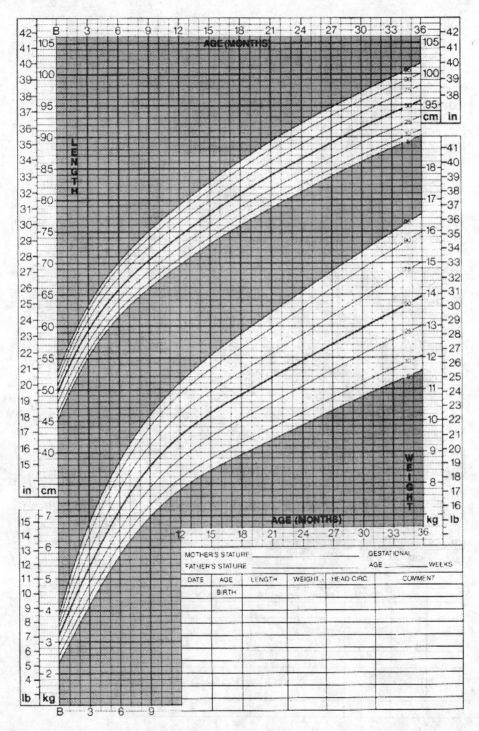

Source: Reprinted with permission from Ross Laboratories copyright © 1982 . Adapted from Hamill, P.V., Drizd, T.A., Johnson, C.L., Reed, R.B., Foche, A.R., & Moore, W.M. 1979. Physical Growth: National Center for Health Statistics Percentiles. *American Journal of Clinical Nutrition, 32,* p.607–629.

Figure 17.4

Growth Record for Girls Ages Birth to 36 Months: Length and Weight

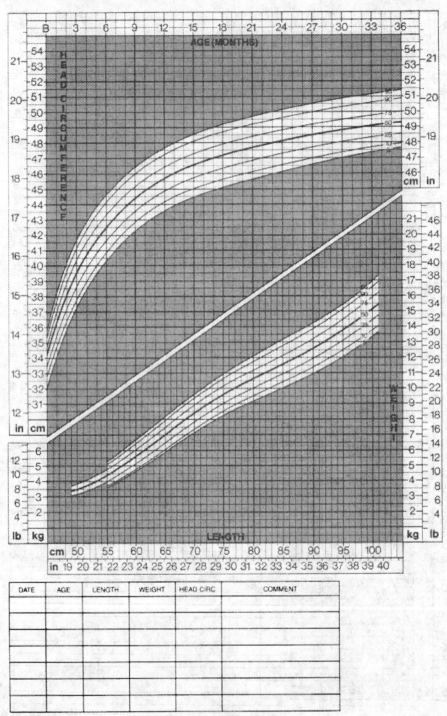

DATE	AGE	LENGTH	WEIGHT	HEAD CIRC	COMMENT

Source: Reprinted with permission from Ross Laboratories copyright © 1982 . Adapted from Hamill, P.V., Drizd, T.A., Johnson, C.L., Reed, R.B., Foche, A.R., & Moore, W.M. 1979. Physical Growth: National Center for Health Statistics Percentiles. *American Journal of Clinical Nutrition, 32*, p.607–629.

Figure 17.5

Recommended Childhood Immunization Schedule—United States, January–June 1998

Vaccines are listed under the routinely recommended ages.

| Light Shaded Bars | indicate range of acceptable ages for vaccination |
| Darker Shaded Bars | indicate vaccines to be assessed and given if necessary during the early adolescent visit |

Age ▸ Vaccine ▾	Birth	1 mos	2 mos	4 mos	6 mos	12 mos	15 mos	18 mos	4-6 years	11-12 years	14-16 years
Hepatitis B[1,2]	Hepatitis B-1		Hep B-2		Hep B-3					Hep B[2]	
Diphtheria, Tetanus, Pertussis[3]			DTaP or DTP	DTaP or DTP	DTaP or DTP		DtaP or DTP[3]		DTaP or DTP	Td	
H.influenzae type b[4]			Hib	Hib	Hib	Hib					
Polio[5]			Polio[5]	Polio[5]	Polio[5]				Polio[5]		
Measles, Mumps, Rubella[6]						MMR			MMR[6]	MMR[6]	
Varicella Virus Vaccine[7]						Var				Var Vaccine[7]	

This schedule indicates the recommended age for routine administration of currently licensed vaccines. Some combination vaccines are available and may be used whenever administration of all components of the vaccine is indicated. Providers should consult the manufacturers' package inserts for detailed recommendations. Vaccines are listed under the routinely recommended ages. Bars indicate range of acceptable ages for vaccination. Shaded bars indicate catch-up vaccination: at 11-12 years, hepatitis B vaccine should be administered to children not previously vaccinated, and varicella virus vaccine should be administered to unvaccinated children who lack a reliable history of chicken pox.

Infant Health Supervision

1. **Infants born to hepatitis B surface antigen (HbsAg)-negative mothers** should receive 2.5 mg of Merck vaccine (Recombivax HB) or 10 mg of SmithKline Beecham (SB) vaccine (Energix-B. The second dose should be administered>1 month after the first dose. The third dose should be given at least 2 months after the second, but not before 6 months of age.

    Infants born to HbsAg-positive mothers should receive 0.5 ml hepatitis B immune globulin (HBIG) within 12 hours of birth and either 5 mg of Merck vaccine (Recombivax HB) or 10 mg of SB vaccine (Energix-B) at a separate site. The second dose is recommended at age 1 month and the third dose at age 6 months.

    Infants born to mothers whose HbsAg status is unknown should receive either 5 mg of Merck vaccine (Recombivax HB) or 10 mg of SB vaccine (Energix-B) within 12 hours of birth. The second dose of vaccine is recommended at age 1 month and the third dose at age 6 months. Blood should be drawn at the time of delivery to determine the mother's HbsAg status; if it is positive, the infant should receive HBIG as soon as possible (no later than age 1 week). The dosage and timing of subsequent vaccines doses should be based on the mother's HbsAg status.

2. Children and adolescents who have not been vaccinated against hepatitis B during infancy may begin the series during any childhood visit. Those who have not previously received three doses of hepatitis B vaccine should initiate or complete the series at age 11-12 years, and older adolescents should be vaccinated whenever possible. The second dose should be administered at least 1 month after the first dose, and the third dose should be administered at least 4 months after the first dose and at least 2 months after the second dose.

3. Diphtheria and tetanus toxoids and acellular pertussis vaccine (DTaP) is the preferred vaccine for all doses in the vaccination series, including completion of the series in children who have received one or more doses of whole-cell diphtheria and tetanus and toxins and pertussis vaccine (DTP). Whole-cell DTP is an acceptable alternative to DTaP. The fourth dose of DTaP may be administered as early as 12 months of age, provided 6 months have elapsed since the third dose and if the child is considered unlikely to return at age 15-18 months. Tetanus and diphtheria toxoids (Td), absorbed, for adult use, is recommended age 11-12 years if at least 5 years have elapsed since the last dose of DTP, DTaP, or diphtheria and tetanus toxoids. Subsequent routine Td boosters are recommended every 10-years.

4. Three H.influenza type b(Hib) conjugate vaccines are listed for infant use. If PRP-OMP (PedavaxHIB [Merck]) is administered at ages 2 and 4 months, a dose at age 6 months is not required.

5. Two poliovirus vaccines are currently licensed in the United States: inactivated poliovirus (IPV) and oral poliovirus (OPV). The following schedules are all acceptable by ACIP, AAP, and AAFP, and parents and providers may choose among them:

    a) IPV at ages 2 and 4 months and OPV at age 12-18 months and at age 4-6 years

    b) IPV at ages 2, 4, and 12-18 months and at age 4-6 years

    c) OPV at ages 2, 4, and 6-18 months and at age 4-6 years.

    ACIP routinely recommends Schedule (a). IPV is the only poliovirus vaccine recommended for immunocompromised persons and their household contacts.

6. The second dose of measles-mumps-rubella vaccine is routinely recommended at 4-6 years of age, or at age 11-12 years, but may be administered during any visit provided at least 1 month has elapsed since receipt of the first dose and that both doses are administered at or after age 12 months. Those who have not previously received the second dose should complete the schedule no later than the 11 to 12-year visit.

7. Susceptible children may receive varicella vaccine (Var) during any visit after the first birthday, and unvaccinated persons who lack a reliable history of chicken pox should be vaccinated at age 11-12 years. Susceptible persons ≥ 13 years should receive two doses at least 1 month apart.

Use of trade names and commercial sources is for identification only and does not imply endorsement by the Public Health Service or the U.S. Department of Health and Human Services.

Source: Reprinted with permission. Centers for Disease Control and Prevention (CDC) 1998. Recommended Childhood Immunization Schedule—United States, 1998. *Morbidity and Mortality Weekly Reports*, 47 (1),8-12.

References

American Academy of Pediatrics (AAP) (1993). *Pediatric nutrition handbook.* Elk Grove Village, IL: Author.

Baker, R.C. (1996). Infantile colic. In R.C. Baker (Ed.), *Handbook of pediatric primary care* (pp. 145–147). Boston: Little, Brown, & Company.

Centers for Disease Control and Prevention (CDC) (1998). Recommended childhood immunization schedule—United States, 1998. *Morbidity and Mortality Weekly Reports, 47*(1), 8–12.

Cavallo A. & Alfaro, M.P. (1996). Nutrition. In R.C. Baker (Ed.), *Handbook of pediatric primary care* (pp. 33–40). Boston: Little, Brown, & Company.

Hamill, P.V., Drizd, T.A., Johnson, C.L., Reed, R.B., Foche, A.R., & Moore, W.M. (1979). Physical growth: National Center for Health Statistics percentiles. *American Journal of Clinical Nutrition, 32,* 607–629.

Jaskiewicz, J. (1996). Anticipatory guidance. In R.C. Baker (Ed.), *Handbook of pediatric primary care* (pp. 41–60). Boston: Little, Brown, & Company.

McHenry, C.L. (1996). Hyperbilirubinemia in the term infant. In R. C. Baker (Ed.), *Handbook of pediatric primary care* (pp. 142–144). Boston: Little, Brown, & Company.

Melman, S.T. (1996). The physical examination. In M.W. Schwartz (Ed.), *Clinical handbook of pediatrics* (pp. 5–27). Baltimore, MD: Williams & Wilkins.

Overby, K.M. (1994). Pediatric health supervision. In A. M. Rudolph & R. K. Kamei (Eds.), *Rudolph's fundamentals of pediatrics* (pp. 1–44). East Norwalk, CT: Appleton & Lange.

Rosaf, E. (1995). Immunizations. In M. W. Schwartz (Ed.), *Clinical handbook of pediatrics* (pp. 48–55). Baltimore, MD: Williams & Wilkins.

Rudolph, A.M., & Kamei, R.K. (Eds.). (1994). *Rudolph's Fundamentals of Pediatrics.* East Norwalk, CT: Appleton & Lange.

Schmidt, R.E. & Oppenheimer, S. (1996). Normal motor and cognitive development. In R.C. Baker (Ed.), *Handbook of pediatric primary care* (pp. 71–78). Boston: Little, Brown, & Company.

Schwartz, M. W. (1996). Outline of history and physical examination. In M.W. Schwartz (Ed.) *Clinical handbook of pediatrics* (pp. 1–5). Baltimore, MD: Williams & Wilkins.

Siegal, R.M. (1996). Immunizations. In R.C. Baker (ED.), *Handbook of pediatric primary care* (PP. 24–40). Boston: Little, Brown, & Company.

Sola, A., Bull, D., Durlat, I., Partridge, J.C., & Rogido, M. (1994). The perinatal period. In A.M. Rudolph & R.K. Kamei (Eds.), *Rudolph's fundamentals of pediatrics* (pp. 85–138). East Norwalk, CT: Appleton & Lange.

SECTION 18

NUTRITION

SECTION 18

NUTRITION

Yolanda M. Gutierrez

Nutrition knowledge in the care of pregnant and lactating women continues to expand. Health professionals need skills to identify nutritional needs and factors that place the client in a special category of nutritional risk. The purpose of this chapter is to provide guidelines for health professionals so they can offer meaningful diet counseling to pregnant women and their families, taking into consideration nutritional, economic, social, and ethnic variables. This will enable them to participate in the process of nutritional assessment during client care.

The various health care delivery systems in existence today are creating multidimensional roles for health professionals, including those of teachers, consultants, interdisciplinary team builders, resource managers, and allocators. At the same time, many uncertainties in nutritional knowledge still exist, making the field of nutritional science especially controversial and demanding of clinical judgment. To identify the relationship of food intake and nutritive quality to the kind of health problem reported, a series of minimum skills should be mastered. These skills include

- Knowledge of and rationale for the increased nutritional needs during pregnancy and lactation
- Knowledge of the nutritive value of foods and the major food sources of nutrients that are likely to be deficient in American diets
- Knowledge of food groups and recommended servings of these foods according to the client's needs
- Ability to take an adequate diet history
- Ability to assess dietary needs
- Ability to use clinical judgment for the recommendation of vitamin and mineral supplements other than routine prenatal vitamins
- Ability to plan nutritional care based on medical and nutritional aspects of care
- Ability to implement and follow up on a client's nutritional care plan
- Ability to prepare adequately for instruction (i.e., with educational handouts, referrals, and audiovisual materials)
- Ability to present information clearly and effectively
- Assertiveness in contacting and competence in discussing nutritional care with the physician/nutritionist or other health personnel (the health team approach)
- Ability to evaluate effectiveness of teaching (e.g., client's intended behavior for improvement or changes in diet)
- Ability to document nutrition intervention in medical records.

To assist in acquiring these skills, the practitioner should have access to at least seven major publications pertinent to maternal nutrition.

- Institute of Medicine (IOM), National Academy of Sciences, Food and Nutrition Board. (1990). *Nutrition during pregnancy Part I: Weight gain, Part II: Nutrient supplements*. Washington, DC: National Academy Press.

- National Academy of Sciences, National Research Council. (1998). *Recommended dietary allowances* (11th ed.). Washington, DC: National Academy Press.

- California Department of Health Services, (1990). *Nutrition during pregnancy and the post-partum period: A manual for health care professionals*. Sacramento, CA. (The manual can be ordered from: California Department of Health Services, Maternal and Child Health Branch ATTN: Administrative Management Section 714 P Street, Room 740 Sacramento, CA 95814.)

- Gutierrez, Y. (1990a). Maternal and infant nutrition in the fourth trimester. In K.A. May (Ed.), *Comprehensive maternity nursing*. Philadelphia, PA: J.B. Lippincott Co.

- Gutierrez, Y.M. (1990b). Nutritional aspects of pregnancy. In K.A. May (Ed.), *Comprehensive maternity nursing*. Philadelphia, PA: J.B. Lippincott Co.

- Gutierrez, Y.M. (1994). *Nutrition in health maintenance & health promotion for primary care providers*. University of California, San Francisco, School of Nursing. (Available through UCSF Nursing Press, School of Nursing, Room N535C, 521 Parnassus Avenue, Box 0608, San Francisco, San Francisco, CA. 94143-0604).

- California Department of Health Services, Maternal and Child Health Branch. (1992). *Sweet Success: Guidelines for Care*.

Preconception Nutrition Counseling

Maternal health, including healthy nutrition, begins before conception. The mother brings to the gestation her past history, including her previous diet and nutritional status. A healthy, well-nourished woman whose nutritional status was good prior to becoming pregnant has a very good chance of delivering a healthy full-term baby of normal birth weight. A well-nourished body usually has a small surplus of all essential nutrients. This surplus can be crucial in the first trimester of pregnancy, when the ability to eat is impaired by the hormonal shifts and the tissues and organs of the embryo are being differentiated. This is the time when adequate nutrition is believed to help protect against some birth defects.

Need for Preconception Nutritional Counseling

Two problems, low birth weight and congenital anomalies, have proved particularly resistant to current obstetric care. Part of the problem is that those who provide obstetric care are generally asked to enter the race to deliver a healthy baby only after the race has begun; all too often, they are placed in the uncomfortable position of practicing prenatal catch-up rather than primary prevention. (Cefalo, & Moos, 1995). However, other risk factors contribute to low birth weight and congenital anomalies. The Institute of Medicine (1985 & 1990) clustered risk factors for low birth weight into five groups:

- Demographic risks, including age, race, marital status, and education
- Medical risks predating pregnancy

- Medical risks in the current pregnancy, including poor weight gain, short interpregnancy interval, selected infections, first to second trimester bleeding and anemia

- Behavioral risks, such as smoking and alcohol use

- Health care risks, such as inadequate prenatal care

Many of these risks factors for low birth weight, such as smoking, can be identified before conception. It is becoming increasingly clear that the mother's preconceptional weight status is an important determinant of pregnancy outcome. Obese clients should reduce their weight before pregnancy, since weight reduction during pregnancy is not recommended. Because a rapid prepregnancy weight loss may deplete the body of essential nutrients, the client should stabilize her weight for 2 to 3 months before conception. At the time of conception, the client should be on a diet of 1,800 to 2,000 kcal/day in combination with an exercise program.

Cefalo and Moos, (1995) clustered the possible causes for the rising rates of congenital malformations into four groups:

- The increasing number of women who are giving birth either at younger or older ages

- The current prevalence of alcohol abuse in women of childbearing age

- The increasing risk of chemical exposure

- Medical advances to allow women who had previously been unlikely to give birth because of chronic disease, such as phenylketonuria and diabetes mellitus, to carry a pregnancy to term.

Minimum Preconceptional Screening for Nutritional Risk

The goal of preconceptional nutritional counseling is to

- Identify nutritional excesses and deficiencies

- Educate clients about importance of nutrition before and during pregnancy and it's relation to pregnancy outcome

The special physiology of the female creates more variable nutrient requirements during different stages of the life cycle than for that of the male (Gutierrez, 1994). Undernutrition is more apt to occur in women than men because their total daily food intake is lower. Women today are also influenced by cultural pressures that promote dieting and limit their intake of essential nutrients, which can compromise nutritional status.

The minimum nutritional screening should include the following assessments:

- Does the client practice vegetarianism?

- Does the client practice pica?

- Does the client have a history of bulimia or anorexia?

- Does the client follow a special diet now or did she have a special diet prescribed as a child?

- Does the client supplement her diet with vitamins and/or minerals?

- Does the client use medications that affect nutrient balance?

- Does the client have an intolerance for milk and/or other food allergies?

- Does the client have a history of tobacco, drug and alcohol abuse?

- Is the client's weight appropriate for height and the hematocrit.

Two of the preconception nutritional risk factors will be specifically discussed, eating disorders (anorexia and bulimia) and the use of supplements. In view of the fact that the incidence of eating disorders is prevalent and still growing among females and the recommendations for supplementations are constantly changing, these areas will be focused on.

Eating Disorders

Bulimia and anorexia nervosa are chronic conditions whose identifications and interventions are best undertaken in the preconceptional period. Anorexia is characterized by low self-esteem, unrealistic goals, and a delusional denial of the appearance of thinness. Because anorexics engage in extreme fasting, anorexia nervosa is usually associated with amenorrhea. Therefore, if an anorectic client should become pregnant, her risks are similar to those of a woman who conceives under famine conditions. Bulimia, or food gorging and emesis, may occur independently of a diagnosis of anorexia nervosa. It is characterized by repeated episodes of binge eating followed by inappropriate compensatory behaviors such as self-induced vomiting; misuse of laxatives, diuretics, or other medications; fasting; or excessive exercise. A distorted perception of body shape and weight is an essential feature of both anorexia nervosa and bulimia nervosa.

Eating disorders are complex disorders involving two sets of issues and behaviors: those directly relating to food and weight and those involving the relationships with oneself and with others. Therefore, only registered dietitians with additional training and experience in the treatment of eating disorders are qualified to carry out the nutrition interventions. It is the position of the American Dietetic Association (ADA) that nutrition education and intervention be integrated into the team treatment of clients with anorexia nervosa, bulimia nervosa, and binge eating during the assessment and treatment phases of outpatient and/or inpatient therapy (ADA, 1994). Ideally, the preconception team should include professionals who specialize in the treatment of persons with eating disorders and who can address the medical, psychiatric, dental, psychological, and nutritional needs of the client. The approach for nutritional intervention could be called "psychonutritional" because the counseling skills of the dietitian are under constant supervision and communication with the psychotherapist and the other members of the health team (ADA, 1994).

Anorexia Nervosa

Diagnostic Criteria (Diagnostic and Statistical Manual of Mental Disorders [DSM-IV], [994])

- Body Weight less than 85% of expected or refusal to maintain weight

- Intense fear of weight gain or becoming fat, though underweight

- Disturbance in experience of weight/shape, weight/shape has undue influence on self-evaluation, or denial of seriousness of current low body weight

- Amenorrhea for 3 consecutive menstrual cycles in postmenarcheal females

Restricting Type: Currently not engaged in binge-eating or purging behavior

Binge-Eating/Purging Type: Regularly engaged in binge-eating or purging

Nutrition Management (Outpatient)

- Restore nutritional adequacy and hydration.
  - ▶ Multivitamin and mineral supplement, 100% RDA
  - ▶ Assure minimum nutrient intake especially protein, iron, zinc and calcium
  - ▶ Adequate fluid intake
- Plan food intake for gradual weight gain.
  - ▶ Interim target weight, optimum weight gain is 0.25 to 0.75 pounds/week at first; 1 to 2 pounds/week later
  - ▶ Recommend calorie intake to achieve 85% relative body weight or 10th percentile body mass index (BMI)
  - ▶ Put client in charge of eating enough to improve health parameters; weight goals used clinically (only for health care team to assess progress)
- Adopt more normal eating and exercise pattern.
  - ▶ Smaller, frequent feedings
  - ▶ Mealtime with family or friends
  - ▶ Restrict physical activity until stable; gradually increase
  - ▶ No caffeine, diet foods, laxatives
  - ▶ Able to eat with others
- Agree on the role of parent(s).
  - ▶ Provide appropriate foods, snacks, and meals at home; regular family meals
  - ▶ Refrain from commenting on client's weight, food intake, appearance, etc.
  - ▶ Take inappropriate products out of the house: diet pills, laxatives, diet foods
- Provide nutrition counseling.
  - ▶ Discuss body image.
  - ▶ Assess attitudes towards food.
  - ▶ Discuss cultural issues.
  - ▶ Assess ability to choose own foods.
  - ▶ Dispel myths about foods and about fasting.

Bulimia Nervosa

Diagnostic Criteria (DSM-IV)

- Recurrent episodes of binge eating
- Eating a large amount of food in a discrete period of time
- Lack of control over eating during binge
- Recurrent compensatory behavior to prevent weight gain (vomiting, laxatives, diuretics, other medications, fasting, or excessive exercise)
- Binge eating and compensatory behaviors occur at least twice a week for 3 months
- Self-evaluation unduly influenced by body shape and weight
- Disturbance does not occur exclusively during episodes of anorexia nervosa

Purging Type: Currently engaged in self-induced vomiting or laxative, diuretic, or enema misuse

Nonpurging Type: Currently engaged in compensatory behaviors other than purging behaviors to prevent weight gain, such as fasting or excessive exercise

Nutrition Management (Outpatient)

- Restore nutritional adequacy and hydration.
  - ▶ Multivitamin and mineral supplement, 100% RDA
  - ▶ Adequate fluid intake
- Adopt more normal eating and exercise patterns.
  - ▶ Eat at least three times a day (no meal skipping)
  - ▶ Do not restrict carbohydrate-containing foods
  - ▶ Pre-plan meals and snacks, especially eating out
  - ▶ Avoid foods associated with binge
  - ▶ At first, use foods that are pre-portioned (roll, bagel, potato, yogurt)
  - ▶ Include high fiber foods (salad, vegetables, fruit, whole grains)
  - ▶ Eat meals and snacks sitting down, preferably with others
  - ▶ No laxatives, fasting, restrictive eating, caffeine abuse, ipecac
  - ▶ Regular aerobic exercise three to five times a week
- Obtain nutrition counseling.
  - ▶ Increase appropriate expectation for body weight/shape.
  - ▶ Explore cultural issues.
  - ▶ Increase awareness of triggers for bingeing and purging episodes.
  - ▶ Explore alternate coping strategies.

▶ Develop appropriate goals:

    – Decrease number of bingeing and purging episodes.

    – Decrease guilt associated with bingeing.

    – Break bingeing and purging cycle (binge without purging).

    – Decrease extent of binge.

    – Develop ability to eat "forbidden" foods.

Binge-eating Disorder

<u>Diagnostic Criteria (DSM-IV)</u>

- Recurrent episodes of binge eating

    ▶ Eating a large amount of food in a discrete period of time

AND

    ▶ Lack of control over eating during binge

- Binge eating episodes are associated with three *or more* of the following:

    ▶ Eating more rapidly than normal

    ▶ Eating until feeling uncomfortably full

    ▶ Eating large amounts of food when not feeling physically hungry

    ▶ Eating alone because of being embarrassed by how much one is eating

    ▶ Feeling disgusted with oneself, depressed, or very guilty after overeating

- Marked distress regarding binge eating

- The binge eating occurs, on average, at least 2 days a week for 6 months

  Note: The method of determining frequency differs from that used for bulimia nervosa.

- The binge eating is not associated with the regular use of inappropriate compensatory behaviors (e.g., purging, fasting, excessive exercise) and does not occur exclusively during the course of anorexia nervosa or bulimia nervosa.

<u>Preconceptional Supplements</u>

Folic Acid

Recent studies have suggested that preconceptional supplementation of folic acid reduces the risk of neural tube defects(NTDs). The preconception period denotes the time from 1 to 3 months before conception to week 6 of gestation. (Rayburn, Stanley, and Garrett, 1996).

Folic acid is one of the nutrients most likely to be deficient in a nonpregnant and pregnant woman's diet. It is found in foods such as liver, spinach, asparagus, broccoli, and most grains. Folic acid is needed for the rapid division of cells, normal protein metabolism, and erythropoiesis. Currently, the

National Research Council encourages a recommended dietary allowance (RDA) for women over 14 years of age to be 400 micrograms of folic acid, and the RDA during pregnancy is 600 micrograms (National Academy of Sciences,1998).

Food folates are easily oxidized and may be destroyed by lengthy cooking. Cigarette smoking, alcohol, and some diseases and drugs may also affect folate status. Studies showed that smokers require an average folate intake of 658 mcg/day to achieve a plasma folic acid level comparable with that of a nonsmoker consuming 200 mcg/day. In addition, early studies showed that oral contraceptive agents depress folic acid status. (IOM,1990; Rayburn et al., 1996).

In 1992, the Centers for Disease Control and Prevention recommended that all women of childbearing age increase folic acid intake. There are three options to achieve this goal: 1) increase dietary folic acid intake, 2) folate supplementation or 3) fortification of food with folate.

Dietary Folic Acid Intake

Foods that are high in folic acid include the following:

- Fortified breakfast cereals
- Dried beans and peas
- Liver/meats
- Spinach and other leafy greens
- Oranges and grapefruits
- Peanuts and sunflower seeds

The best sources of dietary folic acid within these food groups are listed in Table 18.1. Dairy products and breads are poor sources of folic acid. Dairy products range from 22 mcg to 10 mcg (yogurt 1 cup and cheddar cheese $1/2$ cup). Breads range from 29 mcg to 8 mcg (hard roll enriched and white bread).

Two sample menus are presented in Table 18.2 to assist health care providers in guiding preconceptional women to increase their consumption of folic acid. The total number of kilocalories in the sample menus are not presented because energy requirements of women vary with age, body size, activity, and body build, and the aim of the sample menus is to meet the recommendation of folic acid by diet.

Folic Acid Supplementation

The public and health care providers have been exposed to an overwhelming number of dietary recommendations for folic acid. The percent daily value for folate used on food labels is based on 400 mcg, the Reference Daily Intake (RDI). Equivalent units, such as 0.4 mg, are also used.

There was a twofold difference in recommended folic acid intake between the 1989 Recommended Dietary Allowances (RDA) (180 mcg/day for adult women) and the RDIs (400 mcg/day). Another point of confusion is the persistence of the no-longer-acceptable term, folacin. In general, folic acid supplementation is recommended at the level of 400 to 800 micrograms (0.4 to 0.8 milligrams) per day to decrease the chance of having a baby with neural tube defects. This dose is low enough to prevent the masking of neurological manifestations of pernicious anemia due to B_{12} deficiency.

The Committee on Obstetrics: Maternal and Fetal Medicine of the American College of Obstetricians/Gynecologists (ACOG) recommended in 1993 that patients at risk of having an infant with a NTD defect, including

- Couples with a close relative with NTD,
- Women with insulin dependent diabetes, and
- Women with seizure disorders

should be offered treatment with 4 mg of folic acid daily. Regardless whether treatment is directed toward reducing an occurrence or recurrence, the committee recommends that additional folic acid should be started 1 month before becoming pregnant and continued throughout the first 6 weeks of a well-dated pregnancy or 3 months of a less well-dated pregnancy. The committee also recommends that maternal serum alpha-fetoprotein screening at 15 to 18 weeks should be offered routinely, since folate therapy alone does not guarantee the abolition of these major birth defects. (Rayburn et al., 1996).

Fortification of Foods with Folate

In the first major change in food fortification in more than 50 years, the US Food and Drug Administration (FDA) implemented a program to increase dietary folate intake by the American public. On February 29, 1996, Dr. David Kessler, FDA Commissioner, announced plans to begin fortification of enriched flour with 140 mcg folic acid per 100 grams of flour. The amount of folate in the enriched flour will be nearly four times that in whole-grain flour. Compliance is now in effect as of January 1, 1998. The FDA's goal is to increase the folate intake of women in their childbearing years while preventing excessive intake by other population groups.

Nutritional Risk Factors

The following risk factors are California Department of Health Services (1990) standards appropriate to determine eligibility for public health programs such as WIC, as they identify individuals who may be predisposed to poor nutritional status and will benefit from nutritional education. Other states may have other guidelines.

Anthropometric

- Moderately overweight
  Greater than 120 percent of desirable pregravid weight for height.

  ▶ Body mass index (BMI) of greater than 26.0 to 29.0 (see the Body Mass Index section below)

- Very overweight
  Greater than 135 percent of desirable pregravid weight for height

  ▶ BMI of greater than 29.0

- Underweight

  ▶ Less than 90 percent of desirable pregravid weight for height

  ▶ BMI of less than 19.8

- Inadequate weight gain (during pregnancy) during trimesters 2 and 3

  ▶ Less than 1 pound (.05 kg) per month for very overweight women

  ▶ Less than 2 pound (1 kg) per month for all other women

- Excessive weight gain (during pregnancy)

  ▶ More than 6.5 lb. (3 kg) per month

Biochemical (Laboratory)

- Anemia

  ▶ Nonpregnant, 12 through 14 years

    – Hemoglobin (Hb) below 11.8 g/dL (or 118 g/L)

    – Hematocrit (Hct) below 35.5 vol % (or 0.35)

  ▶ Nonpregnant, 15 years or older

    – Hb below 12.0 g/dL (or 120 g/L)

    – Hct below 36.0 vol % (or 0.36)

  ▶ Pregnant, weeks 1 through 13

    – Hb below 11.0 g/dL (or 110 g/L)

    – Hct below 33.0 vol % (or 0.33)

  ▶ Pregnant, weeks 14 through 28

    – Hb below 10.5 g/dL (or 105 g/L)

    – Hct below 32.0 vol % (or 0.32)

  ▶ Pregnant, weeks 29+

    – Hb below 11.0 g/dL (or 110 g/L)

    – Hct below 33.0 vol % (or 0.33)

- Hypovolemia (inadequate plasma volume expansion during pregnancy)

  ▶ Between 24 and 34 weeks

    – Hb above 13.9 g/dL (or 139 g/L)

    – Hct above 41.9 vol % (or 0.419)

- Abnormal glucose levels
  - ▶ 1-hour glucose loading test
    - – Venous plasma glucose above 140 g/dL (7.8 mmol/L) 1 hour after 50-gm oral glucose load
  - ▶ 3-hour 100-gm oral glucose tolerance test—two or more of the following venous plasma concentrations must be met or exceeded (California Department of Health Sciences, 1998):
    - – Fasting, 95 mg/dL
    - – 1-hour, 180 mg/dL
    - – 2-hour, 155 mg/dL
    - – 3-hour, 140 mg/dL

Clinical Physical / Medical / Obstetrical

- Previous obstetrical complications
  - ▶ Hyperemesis gravidarum
  - ▶ Gestational diabetes
  - ▶ Preeclampsia
  - ▶ Anemia
  - ▶ Preterm labor
  - ▶ Inadequate weight gain
  - ▶ Neonatal death (death within first 28 days after birth)
  - ▶ Stillbirth (greater than 20 weeks gestation)
  - ▶ Fetal loss (less than 20 weeks gestation
  - ▶ Premature delivery (less than 37 weeks gestation)
  - ▶ Low-birth-weight infant (less than 2,500 g)
  - ▶ Small-for-gestational-age infant
  - ▶ High-birth-weight infant (more than 4,000 g)
  - ▶ Congenital anomaly
  - ▶ Postpartum hemorrhage
- Adolescence
  - ▶ Less than 18 years at last menstrual period
  - ▶ Less than reproductive biologic year 3 (biologic age is the chronologic age minus the menarcheal age)
- High parity
  - ▶ 5 or more previous deliveries at greater than 20 weeks gestation

- Short interpregnancy interval
  - ▶ 12 months or less between delivery (or termination of pregnancy) and conception
- Breastfeeding
  - ▶ Breastfeeding during current pregnancy
  - ▶ Inadequate milk supply
- Current medical/obstetrical complications
  - ▶ Diabetes (insulin-dependent, non-insulin-dependent, or gestational)
  - ▶ Hypertension (chronic or associated with preeclampsia)
  - ▶ Chronic renal disease
  - ▶ Chronic liver disease
  - ▶ Cancer
  - ▶ Cardiopulmonary disease:
    - – Functional heart disease (New York Heart Association class 2 or higher)
    - – Organic disease (e.g., tuberculosis, pneumonia)
    - – Asthma requiring treatment
  - ▶ Thyroid disease
  - ▶ Gastrointestinal disease (including parasites, malabsorption more severe than lactase deficiency)
  - ▶ Use of prescribed drugs known to affect or suspected of affecting the fetus (e.g., dilantin or phenobarbital for epilepsy)
  - ▶ Multiple Pregnancy
  - ▶ Intrauterine growth restriction (IGUR)
  - ▶ Severe infection (e.g., pyelonephritis, hepatitis, toxoplasmosis, listeriosis, HIV infection)
  - ▶ Venereal disease (positive VDRL, genital herpes, chlamydia, trichomoniasis)
  - ▶ Anesthesia/surgery/trauma shortly before or during the perinatal period
  - ▶ Systemic evidence of nutritional deficiency

Socioeconomic

- Low income
  - ▶ Eligible for local, state, or federal assistance programs
- Substance abuse
  - ▶ Alcohol
    - – Average daily intake of more than 1 oz absolute alcohol (1 oz absolute alcohol = 2 mixed drinks or 2 cans of beer or 2, 6 oz glasses of wine)
    - – Binge drinking

▶ Cigarettes

   – More than 10 cigarettes/day

▶ Recreational /street drugs

   – Use of narcotics, cocaine, hallucinogens, marijuana, amphetamines, and/or other recreational/street drugs

▶ Over-the-counter (OTC) medications and herbal remedies

   – Chronic use of laxatives, antacids or other OTC drugs know to affect nutritional status

   – Use of herbal remedies known or suspected to cause toxic side effects

▶ Vitamin and mineral supplements

   – Excessive use of nutrient supplements (over toxicity limits)

Vitamin A	> 25,000 IU daily
Vitamin D	> 400 IU daily
Vitamin C	> 2,000 mg daily
Vitamin B_6	> 100 mg daily
Iodine	> 11 mg daily

▶ Caffeine

   – Excessive intake of caffeine (more than 300 mg/day). This amount of caffeine is found in about 3 cups coffee, 4 cups tea, or 6 cans of cola

● Pica

   ▶ Eating of nonfood substances

● Psychological problems

   ▶ Depression influencing appetite or eating

   ▶ Current or past history of eating disorders (e.g., anorexia nervosa, bulimia)

   ▶ Mental retardation

   ▶ Mental illness

Diet

● Poor diet/inappropriate food consumption

   ▶ Less than minimum recommended servings from each group in the Daily Food Guide for Women (see Table 18.3, Daily Food Guide)

   ▶ Excessive intake of fat, sugar or salt

Pregnancy Nutritional Guidelines

During pregnancy, the mother must meet her own nutritional needs, in addition to the needs of the growing fetus. Although this growth process means that requirements for all nutrients are increased during pregnancy, some nutrients are of particular importance in pregnancy.

Calories

Additional calories are needed during pregnancy to support increased tissue synthesis by the mother and fetus and the additional metabolic cost incurred by this new tissue. Adequate intake of calories for energy is necessary for optimal protein utilization and tissue growth. The generally accepted figure for the total energy cost of pregnancy is 80,000 kcal. When this figure is divided over the length of pregnancy, it averages out to an additional 300 calories per day above nonpregnant needs. Because caloric requirements are difficult to predict and vary widely among pregnant women, factors such as maternal age, activity, height, preconception weight, health, and stage of pregnancy must be considered. Because of differences in these parameters, individual caloric needs should be calculated by allowing a minimum of 36 kcal per kilogram of pregnant body weight. The pregnant adolescent's energy needs may be as high as 50 kcal/kg/day, depending on her daily activity levels and growth rate (National Academy of Sciences, National Research Council, 1998).

Protein

Additional protein is needed in increased amounts during pregnancy to provide sufficient amino acids for fetal development, blood volume expansion, and growth of maternal breast and uterine tissues. The current recommended dietary allowances (RDA) for protein intake is an additional 10 grams protein per day over nonpregnant needs. It is important to remember that adequate protein intake without adequate calories should be avoided: If caloric intake is below the required amount, protein will be used for maternal energy needs rather than for its primary function of tissue building and maintenance.

Vitamins

Generally, requirements for all vitamins are increased during pregnancy. The only exception is vitamin A for which no increment of vitamin A intake is necessary during pregnancy. The accelerated energy and protein metabolisms require increased amounts of vitamins for tissue synthesis and energy production. Vitamins requiring special attention in pregnancy are iron and folic acid (folate). The recommendations to pregnant women about these vitamins should stress that the needs during pregnancy are increased and the intake in most diets is low.

The 1990 MCH Daily Food Guide (see Table 18.3) has been developed to ensure an intake of at least 80 percent of the RDA for pregnant and lactating women of average height (64 inches) and average weight (120 pounds preconception). The current MCH Daily Food Guide is based on computerized analyses of sample menus. Consequently, the recommended number of servings from each group are actually considered to be the minimum during pregnancy and lactation. If the guide is followed, and if it is recognized that each food group has more nourishing and less nourishing choices within it, using it will ensure an intake of at least 80 percent of the RDAs. This tool is the most practical and best available for the health care provider in evaluating the adequacy of the pregnant or lactating woman's diet. After the 24-hour food consumption recall has been completed, the food intake reported by the woman is then compared to the recommended servings of the Daily Food Guide for the pregnant/lactating woman. If the woman is postpartum and nonlactating, the column in the guide labeled Postpartum/Nonlactating can be used.

Consider the following factors when comparing a patient's diet to the Daily Food Guide.

Calories. Depending on the choice of foods within each group, the calorie intake based on the Daily

Food Guide can range from 2,000 to 3,000 calories for the pregnant and lactating woman. Therefore, to consume adequate calories (most pregnant women need at least 2,300), increase the servings of the food groups. But if foods not listed are eaten or methods of food preparation increase the calories from fats, encourage the client to make nutritious selections.

Protein. Each serving recommended on the Daily Food Guide supplies approximately 7 grams of protein, 1.2 mg of iron (supplementation needed), and 0.9 mg of zinc. However, light poultry, meat, fish, and tofu are lower in zinc than other foods in this group. In general, the Daily Food Guide provides about 150 percent of the RDA for protein. It is important to understand that the RDA level of protein must be exceeded in order to insure an adequate intake of B_6, iron, and zinc in the diet.

Calcium. Each serving of the milk group supplies approximately 275 to 300 mg of calcium. Milk is also a good source of vitamin D. For some women, this food group serves as the primary source of protein in the diet. If the recommended number of servings from this group is inadequate, the calcium intake is likely to be inadequate. Current RDA during pregnancy is 1,300 mg.

Folic Acid. Each serving of dark green vegetables contributes significant amounts of folic acid and magnesium; average is 75 μg/serving of folic acid and 30 mg/serving of magnesium.

Vitamin C–rich Foods. Each serving supplies about 60 mg of vitamin C. In addition, most foods from this group are good sources of folic acid and vitamin A. Those foods that are particularly rich in vitamin A provide more than 2,750 IU per serving. They include such foods as cantaloupe, mango, papaya, greens, bok choy, and spinach.

Breads and Cereals. This group is divided into two parts: whole grains and enriched products. Whole grain breads, cereals, and pastas provide significantly more magnesium, zinc, vitamins E, B_6, and folic acid, and fiber than enriched products. It is recommended that at least half of the bread and cereal servings eaten daily be made from whole grains (California Department of Health Services, 1990).

Screening Indices for Nutritional Status

Height

Recommended weight gain during pregnancy varies depending on pregravid weight status. It must be remembered that desirable body weight is an abstract rather than an absolute concept. Height/weight tables may not be representative for some segments of the population (such as lower socioeconomic groups and specific ethnic groups); they ignore other risk factors (such as smoking), they do not measure degree of fatness or fat distribution, and they have relied on an ill-defined concept of "frame size." Nutrition is a multifaceted issue, as is client assessment, especially in the area of weight management. Health care professionals should use height/weight tables with caution and in conjunction with other parameters to assist in assessment of nutritional status.

Desirable Body Weight (DBW) Calculations

For women, 5 feet = 100 lbs. Add 5 lbs per inch (e.g., 5 ft 4 in = 120 lbs ± 10 lbs for individual variations)

See Table 18.4, *Desirable Weight for Height: For Women 25 Years or Older.*

Calculations to Determine Percentage of Standard Weight

To determine the percentage of standard weight, let us use the example of a woman who is 5 ft 4 in and weighs 100 pounds (5 ft 4 in = 120 lbs DBW). She is 83 percent of desirable body weight.

$$\frac{100 \text{ lbs (actual weight)}}{120 \text{ lbs (desired weight or DBW)}} \times 100 = 83\%$$

If she were 150 pounds instead of 100 pounds she would be 125 percent DBW.

$$\frac{150 \text{ lbs (actual weight)}}{120 \text{ lbs (desired weight or DBW)}} \times 100 = 125\%$$

Body Mass Index (Quetelet Index)

The body mass index (BMI) or Quetelet Index accounts for differences in body composition by defining the level of adiposity according to the relationship of weight to height and eliminates dependence on frame size. The formula is as follows:

$$BMI = \frac{\text{weight (in kilograms)}}{\text{height in meters}^2}$$

or

$$BMI = \frac{\text{weight (in pounds)}}{\text{height in inches}^2} \times 700$$

For example, if a woman weighs 135 pounds and is 5 feet 4 inches and the metric BMI is used she has a BMI of 23, her " ideal" or "normal" weight.

$$\frac{135 \text{ pounds}}{2.2 \text{ pounds/kg}} = 61.36 \text{ kg}$$

5 ft 4 in = 64 inches

$$\frac{64 \text{ inches}}{2.54 \text{ centimeters/inch}} = 162.5 \text{ centimeters } or \text{ 1.63 meters}$$

$$1.63^2 = 2.66$$

$$\text{Therefore the BMI} = \frac{61.36 \text{ kg}}{2.66} = 23$$

The Food and Nutrition Board of the Institute of Medicine's Committee on Nutritional Status during Pregnancy and Lactation; National Academy of Sciences issued its report in 1990. The committee agreed on the following weight-for-height categories for women:

- Underweight: BMI <19.8

- Normal weight: BMI 19.8 to 26.0
- Overweight: BMI >26.0 to 29.0
- Obese: BMI >29.0

The cut-off points generally correspond to 90, 120, and 135 percent of the Metropolitan Life Insurance Company weight-for-height standards. See Table 18.5.

At the present time the definition of obesity and its assessment with regard to health is being reconsidered. A consensus has emerged classifying overweight and obesity on the basis of BMI. The National Institutes of Health (NIH) Expert Panel on the Identification, Evaluation, and Treatment of Overweight and Obesity in Adults defines overweight as a BMI from 25 to 29.9, obesity as a BMI from 30 to 39.9, and extreme obesity as a BMI $\geq$ 40. (Rippe, 1998). This information is important to assist clinicians to determine the best range weight gain during pregnancy.

Weight Gain During Pregnancy

Desirable weight gain recommendations during pregnancy are based on pregravid weight. The California Department of Health Services (1990) classifies pregravid weight-for-height as follows:

- Underweight: $\leq$ 90% DBW
- Desirable: 91–120% DBW
- Moderately overweight: 121–135% DBW
- Very overweight: > 135% DBW

Recommendations for total weight gain in relation to pregravid weight is as follows (California Department of Health Services, 1990):

- Underweight: 28–36 lbs
- Desirable: 24–32 lbs
- Moderately overweight: 24–32 lbs
- Very overweight: 20–24 lbs (individualize)
- Twins: 40 lbs or more

In 1993, the American College of Obstetrics and Gynecology (ACOG, 1993) adapted the recommendations of weight gain during pregnancy from the Institute of Medicine (1990), proposing the following ranges:

- Underweight   28–40 lbs
- Normal weight   25–35 lbs
- Overweight   15–25 lbs
- Obese   15 lbs
- Twin gestation   35–45 lbs

Note that modifications in weight gain may be needed for special risk categories, such as women who smoke, teens, multiple gestation, etc. For twin pregnancies, these are general guidelines only. The optimal weight gain for these individuals will depend on a variety of factors. Therefore individualized nutrition counseling is important to interpret the significance of weight gain patterns.

Prenatal Weight Gain Grid

The recommended rate of weight gain is depicted on the grid (see Table 18.6, Prenatal Weight Gain Grid). This grid provides a visual comparison of the woman's actual weight gain to the recommended pattern, which will differ according to her pregravid weight.

The upper line of the grid corresponds to the upper end of the recommended range of weight gain for underweight women; the middle line is the midpoint of the recommended range for normal or overweight women; and the lower line represents the lower end of the recommended range for very overweight women. The weight gain pattern in the table may vary for adolescents, smokers, women with multiple pregnancies, or women with poor weight gain in early pregnancy.

Optimum prenatal care includes routine use of the Prenatal Weight Gain Grid, which is not only an effective tool for patient education but for clinical evaluation as well.

Initiation of the Individualized Plan of Care

Based on the client's subjective and objective data obtained to establish a nutritional assessment, the health care provider proceeds to initiate the individualized plan of care for the client.

Diagnostic Tests

- Hemoglobin and hematocrit
- Serum iron/TIBC
- Red blood cell count
- Serum ferritin
- Glucose screen
- Urinalysis
- Additional lab(s) as indicated

Treatment/Management

- Monitor weight (pre-pregnant and interval weight gain); record patient's height, and calculate DBW
- Complete 24-hour diet recall
- Review patient's medical, OB, and social history
- Review medication intake
- Review laboratory results

Consultation

Medical nutrition therapy (MNT) is required if the pregnant women experience any of the obstetrical complications listed in Nutritional Risk Factors section, under Current Medical/Obstetrical Complications.

Patient Education

- Provide the client with a weight-gain rationale (desirable pattern of gain and components of weight gain during pregnancy).
- Instruct client regarding use of Daily Food Guide (see Table 18.3).
- Recommend modifications, if appropriate.
  - ▶ Dietary modifications for nutritionally-related health problems (e.g., hypertension)
  - ▶ Physical activity
  - ▶ Recommendations regarding ingestion of coffee, alcohol, drugs and cigarettes
- Review educational materials.
- Assess the need for special considerations.
  - ▶ Use of vitamin/mineral supplements including iron
  - ▶ Pica
  - ▶ Lactose intolerance
  - ▶ Vegetarian diets
  - ▶ Religious/cultural influences
  - ▶ Food allergies
  - ▶ Remedies for nausea, vomiting, heartburn, constipation
  - ▶ Preparation for breastfeeding
  - ▶ Infant nutrition guidelines
  - ▶ Food assistance programs
  - ▶ Eating disorders (e.g., anorexia, bulimia)

Follow-up

- Document in progress notes
  - ▶ Content of the counseling session
  - ▶ The type of nutrition education received (for example, basic nutrition and review of food groups, or high-risk patient receiving more aggressive nutritional intervention, such as diet modification)
  - ▶ The specific behavioral objectives for the patient
  - ▶ Materials used or given

- ▶ Patient's response to counseling
- ▶ The inability or refusal of the patient to attend or participate in nutrition counseling and education
- ▶ Progress of the patient and future plans
- Evaluation of client's success
  - ▶ Demonstrated improvements in physiological or biochemical indicators of health
  - ▶ Behavior intentions; answers to the following questions:
    - – What does the patient intend to eat tomorrow for breakfast?
    - – What snacks does she think she will have tomorrow?
    - – Does she intend to buy special foods tomorrow?
    - – What foods does she intend to add for lunch/dinner, and why is she choosing these foods?
    - – Does she intend to walk or exercise tomorrow?

Dietary Modifications for Nutritionally Related Health Problems

Hypertension

The dietary factors that have been implicated with varying degrees of certainty in the pathogenesis of hypertension include

- Excessive sodium
- Energy balance (obesity)
- Inadequate intakes of magnesium
- Inadequate intakes of calcium
- Excessive alcohol
- Inadequate intake of polyunsaturated fats

A large body of evidence suggests that dietary sodium plays a particularly important role in the development of hypertension. There is, however, also evidence to suggest that sodium is not very important. The truth probably falls somewhere in between; that is, for some people sodium may be very important while for others it is not.

Data on the role of other dietary factors is suggestive, but at best preliminary. Obesity clearly is a risk factor for hypertension. Few would argue that weight loss is an effective treatment modality for most obese hypertensive patients. **There should be no weight loss for pregnant women.**

Current indications for the treatment of mild hypertension remain controversial. The present recommendations on the dietary treatment of hypertension include

- Decrease dietary sodium (processed foods and added salt, only moderate during pregnancy).

- Monitor weight for pregnant obese women (avoid excessive gains, follow adequate recommendations, increase exercise, modify behavior).

- Increase potassium (increase fruits, vegetables and juices).

- Increase dietary fiber (increase whole grains, fruits and vegetables).

- Increase proportion of unsaturated fat (decrease animal fat).

- Recommend no alcohol intake during pregnancy.

Gestational Diabetes Mellitus

In the United States, 90,000 women are diagnosed with gestational diabetes mellitus (GDM) annually, amounting to 1 to 5 percent of the pregnant population. Risk factors include obesity (more than 120 percent of DBW), glucosuria (greater than 2+), age more than 25 years, family history of diabetes, previous birth of a macrosomic neonate, previous history of GDM, and previous fetal death of unknown etiology. However, 50 percent of all patients with GDM, do not have the above risk factors. A number of studies reveal a higher prevalence of GDM, among Asian, African-American, Native American, and Hispanic women.

GDM is a carbohydrate intolerance of variable severity with onset or first recognition during pregnancy. Various physiologic changes during pregnancy, including elevated levels of hormones, contribute to a natural rise in blood glucose and decrease in overall glucose tolerance during the second half of pregnancy. Maternal metabolism usually compensates for this altered state by secreting extra insulin; however, women with GDM decompensate from a euglycemic state to a hyperglycemic state. (Pesicka, Riley, & Thomson, 1996).

Women with GDM typically have normal carbohydrate tolerance before pregnancy, and their carbohydrate tolerance returns to normal after delivery. Unfortunately, approximately 50 percent of women who experience GDM go on to develop Type II diabetes mellitus later in life.

Maternal complications of GDM include spontaneous abortion, premature labor and/or delivery, polyhydramnios, preeclampsia and cesarean delivery secondary to macrosomia. The most common neonatal complications include macrosomia, hyperbilirubinemia and hypoglycemia. If undetected or untreated, GDM can cause intrauterine fetal demise due to ketoacidosis, hypoxia and/or respiratory distress syndrome. A normal perinatal mortality rate can be achieved when GDM is diagnosed and treated.

Screening Criteria

- Glucose measurement in plasma

- 50 gm oral glucose load – administered between the 24th and 28th weeks of pregnancy and without regard to time of day or time of last meal — to all pregnant women who have not been identified as having glucose intolerance before the 24th week

- Venous plasma glucose measured 1 hour later

- A value greater than or equal to 140 mg/dL in venous plasma (indicates the need for a full diagnostic glucose tolerance test)

Diagnostic Criteria

- 100 gm oral glucose load-administered in the morning after overnight fast for at least 8 hours but not more than 14 hours, and after at least 3 days or unrestricted diet (greater or equal to 150 gm carbohydrate) and physical activity.

- Venous plasma glucose measured fasting and at 1-, 2-, and 3- hours post-glucose load administration. Subject should remain seated and not smoke throughout the test.

- Two or more of the following venous plasma glucose concentrations must be met or exceeded for positive diagnosis (California Department of Health Services, 1998):

  ▶ Fasting, 95 mg/dL

  ▶ 1-hour post-glucose load, 180 mg/dL

  ▶ 2-hours post-glucose load, 155 mg/dL

  ▶ 3-hours post-glucose load, 140 mg/dL

General Dietary Recommendations

- Common treatment for GDM includes diet, exercise and insulin.

- Nutrition is the first-line management strategy. Up to 80 percent of women can be managed through diet alone.

- The American Dietetic Association (ADA) advises that all women with GDM receive nutrition counseling by a registered dietitian. This is a condition that requires medical nutrition therapy (MNT), defined as the use of specific nutrition services to treat an illness, injury or condition.

- Most studies confirm that the key to successfully managing women with GDM involves individualized counseling regarding each woman's dietary habits, lifestyles demands, and cultural influences. This strategy leads to the supportive environment needed to maintain strict restrictions on dietary intake.

- There are different degrees of glucose intolerance. Some women are more sensitive than others to certain types of carbohydrates. One woman may be able to tolerate milk at breakfast, while another may not.

- Recommendations for daily blood glucose self-monitoring and maintenance of the recommended diet and activity pattern, aim to create a partnership in care between health care provider and patient.

Modifications of Meal Patterns

The following provides some general information about the modifications in meal patterns and food selections necessary for gestational diabetes. This nutrition information can be reinforced by the health team.

Eating Pattern

- Plan six small meals a day or three meals and three snacks.

- Space meals and snacks at regular intervals, about 2 to 3 hours apart.

- Schedule meals and snacks at approximately the *same time* each day. Skipping meals or snacks is discouraged because it may result in weight loss, urinary ketone excretion or overeating later in the day.

- Recommend inclusion of a protein-rich food at each meal and a bedtime snack such as cheese, meat, fish, eggs or poultry.

Morning Meal

During the morning blood glucose levels are more difficult to maintain within the normal values. Hormonal and overnight fasting are contributing factors; therefore, the composition of the morning meal is particularly important.

- Eat a relatively small meal, lower in carbohydrate content (15-30 grams).

- Exclude foods containing primarily simple sugars such as fruit, fruit juice, and milk.

- Exclude highly processed dry breakfast cereals.

- Recommend whole grain breads, tortillas, or hot cereals, such as old-fashioned oatmeal or instant oat bran.

- Recommend a protein-rich food for the morning meal, such as cheese, meat, eggs, poultry, or dried beans.

- Add milk to other meals or snacks. Blood glucose values 1 hour after meal (post prandial or post meal peak) are normal at 100-130 mg/dL. (California Department of Health Services, 1990 and 1998)

Types of Foods to Recommend

- High-fiber and complex carbohydrate-rich foods such as whole grain breads, corn tortillas, and whole grain pasta are helpful.

- Other high-fiber foods such as hot cereals (oatmeal and oat bran) and dried beans and legumes are particularly good choices because of the soluble fiber content that slows the blood glucose rise.

- Fresh fruits and vegetables are nutrient rich. Frozen varieties may also be used. Canned fruits and vegetables are less desirable because of possible added sugar, losses in nutrient content, and lower fiber content.

- Encourage patients to read labels carefully on all packaged or canned foods for hidden simple sugars: dextrose, sucrose, honey, molasses, fructose, corn syrup, brown sugar, maple syrup, modified food starch.

- Counsel patients to consume as much of the following "free" foods as desired: lettuce, mustard greens, herbs, mushrooms, chilies, lemon juice, radish, garlic, broth, vinegar, and herb tea.

<u>Foods Not Recommended</u>

- Convenience foods generally result in a more rapid rise in blood glucose than fresh or less processed foods. Encourage patients to avoid the following products:

  ▶ Canned soups

  ▶ Instant potatoes

  ▶ Instant noodles or cereals

  ▶ Frozen dinners or entrees

  ▶ Packaged stuffing mix or fast foods, such as hamburgers or pizza.

  NOTE: These foods are also usually high in fat and sodium, which can contribute to excess weight gain or unexplained rises in blood sugar levels.

- Beverages such as fruit juices, juice drinks, soft drinks, and nectars should not be used. Flavored mineral waters and sodas with added juice may also contain added sugars.

- Desserts and other sweets such as cookies, cakes, candy, pies, chocolate, table sugar, jams, and jellies should not be eaten.

- Foods with hidden sugars, such as chocolate milk, granola, soy milk, applesauce, yogurt, commercially prepared spaghetti sauce, teriyaki sauce, and canned fruits, are not good choices.

<u>Strategies to Avoid Excess Weight Gain</u>

- Food Preparation: Remove all visible fat. For example, cut off the fat from beef and the skin from poultry.

- Cooking Methods: Bake, broil, steam, boil, or barbecue foods to reduce the fat used in cooking. Frying foods in large amounts of oil is not recommended. Less fat may be used by cooking with nonstick pans or PAM® instead of oil, margarine, or butter.

- Types of Foods: Use lean cuts of meat, such as roast beef, turkey, ham, or chicken more often; use luncheon meat, sausage, or hot dogs less often. Kilocalories can be decreased easily by using nonfat or low-fat dairy products, such as skim milk cheeses (mozzarella, ricotta, cottage cheese) and low-fat plain yogurt or milk.

- Added Fats: Identify sources of added fat in the diet and moderate their use (e.g., butter, margarine, mayonnaise, salad dressings, cream, sour cream, cream cheese, bacon, olives, nuts, avocados, etc.

Exercise Recommendations

Unrestricted Activity

- Blood glucose control may be improved with regular exercise. Recommend <u>walking</u> at least 10 to 15 minutes after each meal. Pregnant women should check with their health care provider about the types of exercise and the amount allowed.

Restricted Activity

Health professionals must be sensitive about eating difficulties when the patient must restrict her activity during pregnancy. Some women not only have a normal appetite, but the combination of less activity and boredom of lying in bed all day can increase food cravings and intake so that too much weight gain occurs. Others find that the combination of constant bed rest along with anxiety ("Will my baby be all right?") decreases appetite and weight gain. Many find that inactivity can cause constipation which is uncomfortable and may also make eating seem less appealing.

<u>Preventing Excessive Appetite and High Weight Gain</u>

- Eat at regular times.

- Eat more low-caloric, high-nutrient foods, such as raw vegetables, fruit, low or nonfat milk, low-fat yogurt, and diluted juices.

- Write down what is eaten. Try to identify when and what could be deleted throughout the day (e.g., cookies).

- Include the intake of low-caloric but nutritious snacks, such as plain yogurt/fruit, hard-boiled eggs, celery, fruit juice popsicles, unbuttered popcorn, and mineral water.

- Refer to the nutritionist for advice on diet.

<u>Preventing Poor Appetite/Low Weight Gain</u>

- Eat small, frequent meals and do not go too long (3 hours or more) without food.

- Eat at regular times.

- Choose foods that give the most nutrition for the calories (e.g., milk, hard-boiled eggs, milk shake, yogurt).

- Drink fluids between, rather than during, meals.

- Write down what is eaten. Identify when and what could be added throughout the day (e.g., peanuts, trail mix, milkshake).

- Schedule visitors at mealtime for company.

- Refer to the nutritionist for advice on diet.

- Include the intake of high-caloric but nutritious snacks.

<u>Preventing Constipation</u>

- See Chapter 5.2, *Constipation*.

- Because of the need for restricted activity, no regular exercise is advised.

- May be helpful to try 2 to 3 tablespoons/day of unprocessed bran; it can be used on cereals, as coating for baked chicken, sprinkled on soups, etc.

- If dietary measures are not producing results, a stool softener may be recommended.

<u>Food Preparation and Availability</u>

- Plan a list of foods that require little or no preparation. Some examples are eggs (hard boiled), cheese or cottage cheese, yogurt, whole grain breads, and peanut butter. Others are canned fruits, fresh peaches and pears, nuts, mandarin oranges, and small cans of fruit juice.

- Keep a pitcher of water or fluids by the bed. Advise the woman to drink at least 4 to 6 cups of liquids per day.

- Keep a thermos by the bed and use it for soups, milks, or shakes.

- Refer the client to counseling services, as indicated, to help her maintain a positive attitude. Remind the client that what she eats is especially important now. These are critical growing periods for the baby and essential nutrients are needed now especially if the baby comes early.

Vitamin/Mineral Supplements

Although the need for vitamins and minerals is increased during pregnancy, a well-balanced diet based on the Daily Food Guide can provide all the nutrients for optimal maternal and fetal health with the exception of iron and possibly folic acid. However, vitamin and mineral supplementation is a common self-care practice.

The California Department of Health Services and the National Academy of Sciences, who have established the Recommended Dietary Allowances (RDA), recommend that all pregnant women receive daily supplements of 30 mg elemental iron. (See the Folic Acid section under Preconceptional Supplements.) Most prenatal supplements contain a variety of vitamins and minerals in addition to the recommended levels of folic acid and iron. Certain nutrient interactions, as well as other factors, need to be considered when choosing an appropriate prenatal supplement.

Prenatal Supplement Characteristics

First, there is no ideal supplement available. There are more than 40 essential nutrients that must come from food because the body is not able to synthesize them. Nutritional supplements should complement a healthy diet (see Table 18.7, Dietary Sources of Iron; Table 18.1, Best Sources of Folic Acid; and Table 18.8, Dietary Sources of Calcium).

- Recommendations for supplementation of a specific nutrient are still inconclusive. For example, there is insufficient evidence upon which to base a recommendation for routine zinc supplementation during pregnancy. However, zinc supplementation is recommended during pregnancy when the pregnant woman is being given more than 30 mg of supplemental iron per day. According to the Institute of Medicine report of 1990, the level of zinc supplementation that is safe for pregnant women has not been clearly established. Doses used in zinc supplementation studies in pregnant women ranged from 15 to 45 mg/day. Daily zinc intakes of 50 mg are sufficient to impair copper and iron metabolism. (IOM, 1990).

- The recommended folic acid content of a prenatal supplement should be at least at the level of 300 mcg per daily dose (see Folic Acid in the Preconceptional Supplements section regarding different recommendations).

- The recommended iron content of a prenatal supplement should be at the level of 30 mg per daily dose; see Chapter 9.3, *Anemia—Iron, Folate, and Vitamin B$_{12}$ Deficiency*.

- The recommended content of a prenatal vitamin/mineral supplement is presented in Table 18.10. In general prenatal supplements should not contain high levels of calcium and magnesium and the calcium should not be in the form of calcium phosphate (because of nutrient interactions). A high level of supplementation of any nutrient may be defined, in general, as an intake at least ten times the RDA level.

- The recommended prenatal supplement should contain vitamin E and zinc at, or near, the Recommended Dietary Allowance levels (15 IU and 20 mg, respectively) and should contain 2 mg of vitamin B_6 per daily dose.

- Vitamin/mineral supplements should be reasonably priced and readily available.

NOTE: There is *no* recommendation to include Vitamin A in the prenatal vitamin/mineral supplements. The National Research Council's Committee on Dietary Allowances (1998) recommends 800 µg retinol equivalents (µg RE) per day for nonpregnant women of childbearing age; and does not recommend an increase during pregnancy. This 800 µg RE is equivalent to 2,700 IU of vitamin A. Toxicity has been reported at levels of at least 25,000 to 50,000 IU daily.

Calcium Supplements

Calcium supplements may be recommended during pregnancy for women unwilling or unable to ingest sufficient calcium from milk products or other nondairy calcium-rich foods. The amount of calcium required from supplements depends on the diet. If more than 250 to 300 mg of supplemental calcium is required daily, it is recommended that the dosage be split into 250 to 300 mg increments and that each be taken with a meal or snack to enhance absorption. Daily supplementation with more than a gram (1,000 mg) of calcium is *not* recommended because it may inhibit iron and zinc absorption.

The amount of elemental calcium in common calcium supplements is shown in Table 18.9.

Some calcium supplements list contents only in grains. A grain equals approximately 65 mg; thus a 10-grain tablet supplies 650 mg. If the 10-grain tablet contains calcium lactate, which is 14 percent elemental calcium, each tablet would provide approximately 91 mg of elemental calcium (14 percent of 650 mg equals 91 mg) (California Department of Health Services, 1990). The forms of calcium listed in Table 18.9 are recommended because they are more easily absorbed. Calcium phosphate is *not* recommended because this form of calcium is poorly absorbed and also interferes with iron absorption. Because stomach acidity normally decreases somewhat in pregnancy, it has been demonstrated that calcium citrate is far better absorbed.

Fewer studies are available regarding the calcium absorption of other suggested calcium sources such as brand-name antacids, or oyster shell.

Tums®, for example, is used primarily for its antacid properties; nutrition scientists also know that for calcium to be absorbed properly it requires an acid medium. Therefore, to rely on Tums to meet calcium needs is questionable; although it may help, it is not known how much.

Management of Women Requiring Calcium Supplementation

Lactase deficiency may make milk products unacceptable to some women. Symptoms of lactase deficiency include gas, intestinal pain, cramps, and possibly vomiting or diarrhea after ingesting lactose from milk products. Two thirds of the world's population experiences some degree of lactase deficiency after early childhood. Most Hispanics, African-Americans, Asians, and Native Americans are lactase deficient to some degree, but may still be able to digest limited amounts of lactose. There is evidence for a physiological "adaptation" in pregnancy to improve the efficiency of lactose absorption. Therefore, a woman can be encouraged to consume small amounts of milk ($1/_2$ cup) or other milk products several times a day rather than a large amount at any one time. It has also been found that milk products are better tolerated by lactase-deficient individuals when eaten in combination with other foods.

Women unable to tolerate any quantity of milk can substitute naturally aged hard cheeses or fermented milk products, such as yogurt. These foods have negligible lactose content and, thus, may be better tolerated. Yogurt also has the advantage of containing lactase, which can help digest lactose from the other foods ingested at the same meal. Various other products are available for use by lactase-deficient persons. For example, milk containing predigested lactose (such as Lactaid®) may be tolerated very well. The enzyme lactase is also sold commercially and can be added to regular milk to predigest the lactose.

Because calcium requirements increase during pregnancy and lactation, lactase deficiency may not present a significant problem if nonmilk products are tolerated. All women consuming less than the recommended number of servings of milk products should substitute foods from the nondairy, calcium-rich foods, such as sardines, tofu, broccoli, turnip greens, kale, or mustard greens. Clients also may have to increase intake of foods from the protein food group to compensate for the protein and other nutrients usually contributed by milk products. In cases where too few servings of milk products or nondairy calcium-rich foods are consumed, supplementation with calcium and possibly vitamin D may be necessary.

Postpartum Nutritional Guidelines

The nutritional quality of a woman's diet remains very important during the postpartum period, regardless of whether she chooses to breast-feed or bottle-feed her baby. In either case, she is recovering from the physiologic stresses of pregnancy and delivery, as well as coping with the additional work and demands of the new baby. Dietary modifications begun during pregnancy can be extended into the interconceptional period, and should focus on maintaining health and reducing the risk of chronic disease. Consequently, encourage the postpartum woman to continue the following:

- Continue to follow dietary guidelines.

- Gradually lose the weight gained during pregnancy.

- Minimize use of harmful substances (alcohol, cigarettes, drugs), particularly if breastfeeding.

- Drink when thirsty (approximately 2 to 3 quarts of liquids daily if breastfeeding).

Constipation may be a problem for a few weeks after delivery. Encourage women to drink plenty of fluids (at least six 8-ounce glasses daily) and eat foods rich in fiber, such as whole grains, legumes, vegetables, and fruits. Exercise, such as walking, will also be helpful. Excessive flatulence is common after a cesarean section. It can be lessened by decreasing the intake of known offenders, which vary among individuals. The most common offenders are legumes, onions, cabbage, and wheat. Eating small, frequent meals, and taking frequent walks may also be helpful.

Breastfeeding

Breastfeeding is currently favored over formula feeding in the United States. Advances in the field of infant feeding and nutrition have revealed that breastfeeding has many advantages, both nutritional and immunologic.

Maternal Nutrition During Lactation

The breastfeeding woman must produce an adequate volume of milk that meets her baby's nutritional needs. A woman's caloric, fluid, protein, vitamin, and mineral requirements increase during the breastfeeding period. Lactating women produce an average of 600 to 800 mL of milk daily, but it takes several weeks for most mother-infant pairs to reach this quantity. Therefore, an extra 300 to 500 calories per day above the usual intake will be needed during lactation (National Academy of Sciences, 1990). Further caloric increases are indicated for women in whom gestation weight gain is subnormal, weight during lactation falls below standards for height and age, lactation continues for longer than 3 to 4 months, or more than one infant is being nursed.

Protein requirements increase during lactation to 65 grams per day during the first 6 months and decrease slightly 62 grams during the second 6 months of lactation. See Table 18.3, Daily Food Guide, for recommended servings of the different food groups.

Maternal Fluid Requirements

The breastfeeding mother should drink to satisfy thirst (approximately 2 to 3 quarts of liquid daily). This fluid is essential to provide the liquid volume for the breast milk and to meet the mother's normal needs. There are no data to support the assumption that increasing fluid beyond the recommended intake will increase milk volume. In order to insure an adequate fluid intake, breastfeeding mothers can be encouraged to drink a beverage (preferably water, juice, or milk) each time they nurse the baby.

It is best to avoid excessive coffee, tea, and caffeine-containing soft drinks because the caffeine in these beverages has a diuretic effect. Although only a small amount (1%) of the caffeine a mother ingests passes into her milk, caffeine does reach the infant and it can accumulate over time.

Tips for Feeding a Baby

- Breast milk or formula is sufficient for the first 4 to 6 months of life for most babies.

- Many babies show signs of readiness for solid food by the age of 6 months. When the baby is ready for baby food

  ▶ Introduce the simplest foods first.

    - At first, offer small amounts (1 tablespoon or less) of food from a spoon. Make the food thin and smooth by mixing it with a little breast milk or formula.

  ▶ Add only one new food at a time (no mixtures) and wait 5 to 7 days to see how the baby adjusts to that food. If the baby shows an allergic reaction, discontinue that food and discuss the reaction with the baby's health care provider.

- Allergy symptoms are vomiting, diarrhea, colic, skin rash, eczema, wheezing, and runny nose. Usually symptoms occur 2 to 3 days after introduction of the food.

- Foods most likely to cause allergies are cow's milk, egg white, wheat, peanuts, corn, soybeans, citrus, strawberries, tomatoes, chocolate, and fish.

• As the baby grows older, vary the textures of the foods provided. A 6-month-old needs strained (very thin) food. By 8 months most babies do well with mashed, lumpy foods. By 10 months give the baby bits of tender, well-cooked foods to feed himself or herself.

• For homemade baby food, the client will need some inexpensive kitchen equipment. Refer her to a nutritionist for information on making baby food. Store-bought baby food is nutritious if you follow these suggestions:

  ▶ Buy only preparations of single foods (there is as much protein in one jar of strained chicken as in four jars of chicken and noodles).

  ▶ Read labels and avoid sugars, salt, and starches.

  ▶ Check the date on the top of the jar for freshness, and make sure the vacuum poptop has not been broken.

  ▶ Do not feed the baby directly from the jar unless she or he can eat the entire portion in one sitting; refrigerated leftovers eaten later can cause food poisoning.

• Bottle feeding is for water, formula, or breast milk **only.**

  ▶ No solids (cereals, etc.) should be put in bottles; feed solids with a spoon.

  ▶ Kool-aid®, sodas, and even juices can give a baby cavities when fed from a bottle. Juices should be given from a cup. Avoid Kool-aid and sodas because they provide only empty calories.

  ▶ Always hold the baby when giving a bottle. Propping the bottle can cause problems such as choking, cavities, and ear infections.

• Never force the baby to finish food or milk she or he doesn't want. Overfeeding can lead to weight problems.

• Do not give the baby the following foods during the first year or two of life: nuts, raw carrots, popcorn, seeds or other foods that might cause choking, or honey in any form (honey can cause food poisoning).

Food Assistance Programs

Women, Infants and Children (WIC) is a food assistance program funded by USDA and administered by each state's Department of Health. First, it provides food assistance and nutrition education for pregnant and postpartum women and infants. Secondly, it involves ongoing health care because all applicants must be screened by a health care provider. Low-income women, infants and children (varies according to funding levels) who have been identified as being at nutritional risk are eligible. Participants receive a monthly coupon book that may be redeemed at any grocery store for the approved items (infant formula, juice, eggs, milk, cereal, cheese).

The Commodity Supplemental Food Program is administered in different states by different state entities (in California it operates under the Economic Opportunity Council but in other states it may be under the WIC program or EFNEP). Low-income women (pregnant and one-year postpartum), infants and children (up to 72 months) are eligible. Participants receive a monthly package including a combination of the following: iron-fortified formula, juice, cereal, eggs, milk, vegetables, meat, beans, mashed potatoes, and peanut butter. Applicants may be enrolled by the nutritionist or community health worker.

The Extended Food and Nutrition Education Program (EFNEP) is a nutrition education program administered by the USDA. Community aides trained in nutrition visit families with children to educate them about nutritious low-cost foods.

Table 18.1

Best Sources of Folic Acid Within Six Food Groups.

FOOD	AMOUNT	MCG FOLIC ACID
CEREALS (fortified)		
Total	1 cup	466
Product 19	1 cup	466
Just Right	1 cup	466
Grape Nuts	1 cup	402
Raisin Bran	1 cup	400
BEANS (cooked)		
Lentils	1 cup	358
Black beans	1 cup	256
Small white beans	1 cup	246
Black eye peas	1 cup	225
Refried beans	1 cup	211
LIVER/MEATS		
Chicken liver	1/2 cup	538
Beef liver	1/4 pound	162
Roast beef	1 slice	11
Hamburger	3 ounces	8
Eggs	1 large	20
SPINACH/LEAFY GREENS		
Spinach (cooked)	1/2 cup	120
Spinach (raw, chopped)	1 cup	108
Asparagus (frozen, boiled)	1/2 cup	121
Turnip greens (fresh, boiled)	1/2 cup	85
Lettuce (romaine)	1 cup	76
ORANGES/FRUITS		
Orange (fresh)	1	40
Cantaloupe	1 cup	27
Grapefruit	1	22
Banana	1	21
Tangerine	1	17
PEANUTS/SUNFLOWER SEEDS		
Spanish peanuts	1/2 cup	175
Sunflower seeds	1/2 cup	163
Mixed nuts	1/2 cup	59
Pecans	1/2 cup	20
Peanut butter	1 tbs.	12

SOURCE: California Department of Health Services, (1990). Nutrition during pregnancy and the post-partum period: A manual for health care professionals. Sacramento, CA: Author.

Table 18.2

Sample Menus

Sample Menu #1	Folic Acid (mcg)	Sample Menu #2	Folic Acid (mcg)
FOOD		**FOOD**	
Breakfast		**Breakfast**	
1 breakfast taco made with:		1 1/2 cup Kelloggs Bran Flakes	207
1 flour tortilla	4	1 cup low-fat milk	12
1 scrambled egg	18	6 oz orange juice, frozen, diluted	72
1.4 cup cooked potatoes	4		
6 ounces canned orange juice	30		
Snack			
1 banana	21		
Lunch		**Lunch**	
2 burritos made with:		Vegetable soup made with:	
2 flour tortillas	8	1/2 cup lima beans	20
1 cup refried beans	211	6 saltine crackers	3
1/3 cup grated cheese	7	cheese sandwich made with:	
Salad made with:		2 ounces American cheese	4
1 cup iceberg lettuce	30	2 slices whole wheat bread	31
1/2 tomato	9	1 cup cantaloupe	27
Dinner		**Dinner**	
1 cup carne guisada	6	3 ounces pork chop	4
1 cup Mexican rice	6	1/2 cup white rice	3
2 corn tortillas	10	1/2 cup fresh turnip green, boiled	85
1/2 cup canned sweet corn	40	1/2 cup winter squash	29
1/2 cup boiled zucchini squash	15	1 slice whole wheat bread	15
1 cup flan	10	1 serving apple crisp	
TOTAL	429	**TOTAL**	512

Source: Adapted from Women Infant and Children (WIC) Program. (1996). *Women: Get folic acid from your food.* Department of Health, Maternal and Child Health.

Table 18.3

Daily Food Guide for Pregnant/Breastfeeding Women (all ages)

FOOD GROUPS	SERVINGS NEEDED	FOODS	SERVING SIZES
Fruits and Vegetables **Vitamin A Rich** 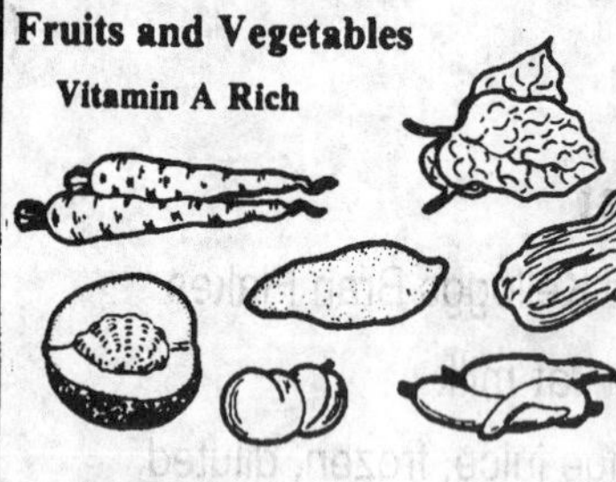	1	cantaloupe or mango	¼ medium
		papaya	½ medium
		apricots	3 medium
		tomato	2 medium
		bok choy, carrots, greens, spinach, sweet potato, or winter squash	½ cup cooked or 1 cup raw
		chili peppers	2 tbsp raw or cooked
Vitamin C Rich 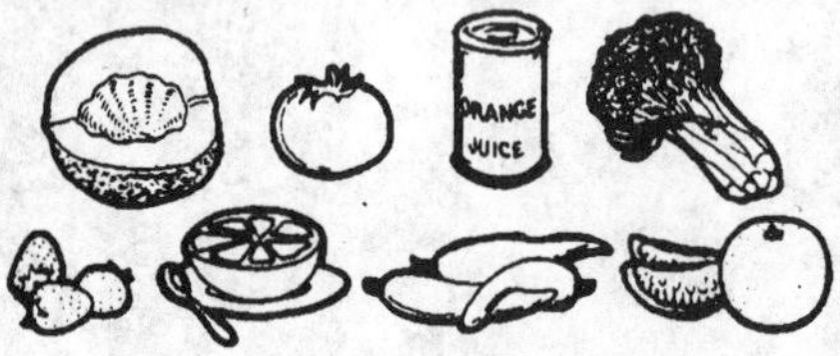	1	juices: orange, grapefruit, or juice with added Vitamin C	6 ounces
		cantaloupe or papaya	¼ medium
		grapefruit	½ medium
		orange, lemon, or kiwi	1 medium
		tangerine or tomato	2 medium
		chili peppers	2 tbsp raw
		broccoli, Brussels sprouts, strawberries, cauliflower, or green pepper	½ cup cooked or raw
		cabbage	½ cup cooked or 1 cup raw
Other 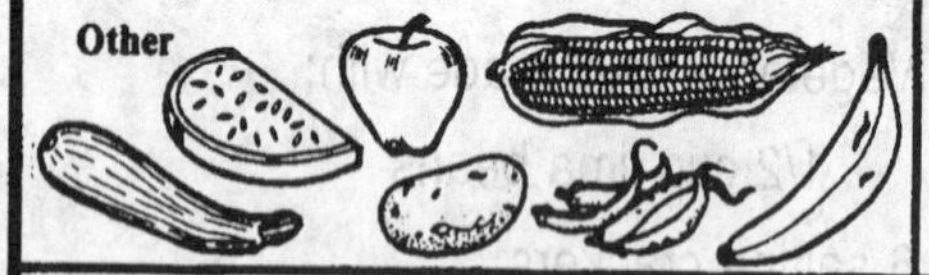	3	raisins	¼ cup
		grapes or watermelon	½ cup
		apple, banana, nectarine, peach, or pear	1 medium
		asparagus, green beans, potato, peas, yellowneck squash, zucchini, or corn	½ cup cooked or raw
		lettuce	1 cup raw
Breads, Grains and Cereals 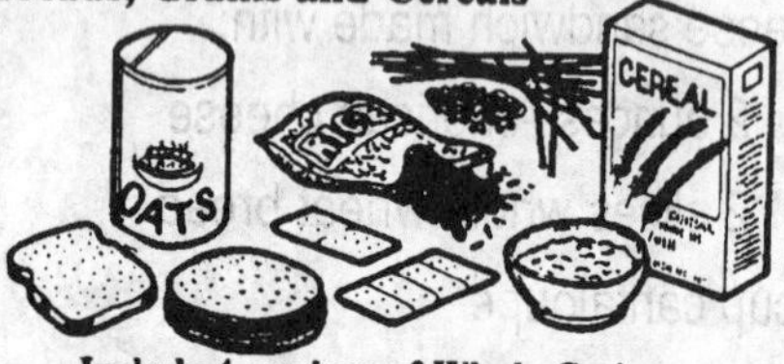 **Include 4 servings of Whole Grains**	7	bread	1 slice
		tortilla	1 small
		cold cereal	¾ cup
		hot cereal	½ cup
		cooked macaroni, noodles, or spaghetti	½ cup
		cooked rice	½ cup
		hot dog or hamburger bun	½
		biscuit, roll, or muffin	1 small
		crackers	8
		pancake	1 medium
Milk Products 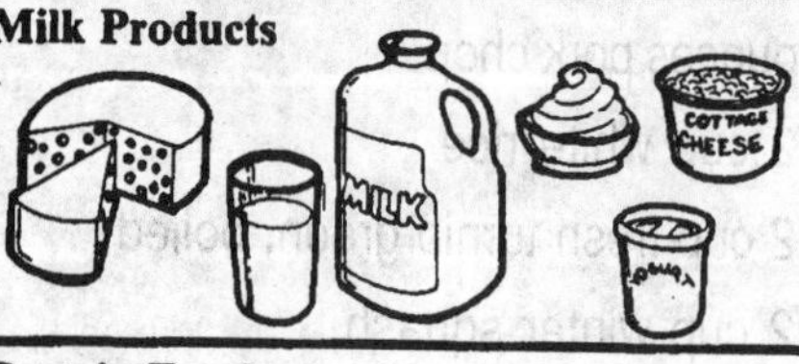	3	milk, yogurt, pudding, or custard	1 cup
		cheese	1½ ounces
		cottage cheese	2 cups
		frozen yogurt, ice milk, or ice cream	1½ cups
Protein Foods 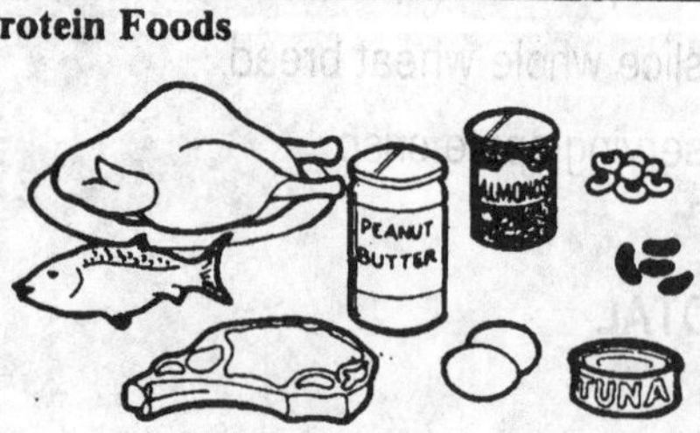	1	cooked dry beans or peas	½ cup
		peanut butter	2 tablespoons
		nuts or seeds	¼ cup
		tofu	3 ounces
	2	cooked beef, chicken, turkey, fish, pork, or lamb (Common Serving Size is 2 to 3 ounces)	1 piece
		Substitute for 1 ounce meat, poultry, fish:	
		eggs 1	
		canned tuna or other canned fish ⅛ cup	

Source: California Department of Health Services. (1990). *Nutrition during pregnancy and the post-partum period: A manual for health care professionals.* Sacramento, CA: Author.

Table 18.4

Desirable Weight for Height: For Women 25 Years or Older*

Height (in)	Desirable Weight Range (lbs)	Midpoint of Desirable Weight Range (lbs)	<90% of Midpoint of Desirable Weight Range (lbs)	>120% of Midpoint of Desirable Weight Range (lbs)	>135% of Midpoint of Desirable Weight Range (lbs)
58	92-121	106	94	128	144
59	95-124	109	97	132	148
60	98-127	112	100	136	152
61	101-130	115	102	139	156
62	104-134	119	106	144	162
63	107-138	122	109	148	166
64	110-142	126	112	152	171
65	114-146	130	116	157	177
66	118-150	134	119	162	182
67	122-154	138	123	167	188
68	126-159	142	126	172	193
69	130-164	147	131	178	200
70	134-169	151	134	183	205

*Height without shoes; weight without clothes

Source: Adapted from California Department of Health Services (1990). *Nutrition during pregnancy and the post-partum period: A manual for health care professionals.* Sacramento, CA: Author.

Table 18.5

BMI Standards

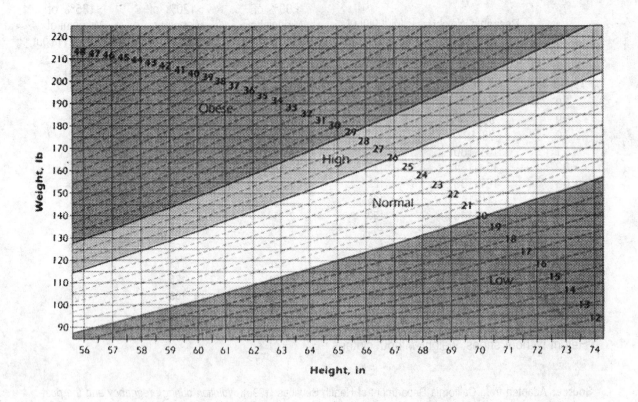

Directions: To find BMI category (e.g., obese), find the point where the woman's height and weight intersect. To estimate BMI, read the bold number on the dashed line that is closest to this point.

Source: Food and Nutrition Board, Institute of Medicine, 1992

Table 18.6
Prenatal Weight Gain Grid

Getting Started

Select the weight gain chart that uses the units of measurement (pounds or Kilograms) used in your practice. Plot the pregnant woman's weight on this weight gain chart using one of the following methods. Use a colored pen to highlight the dashed line that corresponds to the woman's prepregnancy BMI category.

If Prepregnancy Weight Is Known

1. Write the woman's prepregnancy weight, rounded to the nearest pound or kilogram, on the blank line to the left of the zero on the left-hand side of the grid; then mark an x at 0 gain for 0 weeks.
2. Fill in the rest of the blanks along the left side of the grid, adding the prepregnancy weight to the weight gain shown at each horizontal line. For example, if the woman's prepregnancy weight was 120 lb, 126 lb is the prepregnancy weight plus a 5-lb gain, 131 lb is the prepregnancy weight plus a 10-lb gain, and so on.
3. At each subsequent visit, have the woman plot her current weight at the point corresponding to the number of weeks of gestation.

If Prepregnancy Weight Is Not Known

1. Mark an x on the highlighted dashed line at the point that corresponds to the correct number of weeks.
2. Move horizontally from that point to find the corresponding point on the vertical axis, which shows weight, and write the woman's current weight to the left of that point.
3. If the woman's initial weight does not fall on the horizontal line, estimate the number to write in the blank at the nearest horizontal line (add or subtract up to 2 lb or 1 kg). Then fill in the rest of the blanks up the left side of the grid by adding 5 lb (or 2 kg) for each horizontal line. See example below.

Prenatal Weight Gain Chart

Prepregnancy BMI<19.8 (..............), Prepregnancy BMI 19.8–26.0 (Normal Body Weight) (----------)
Prepregnancy BMI>26.0 (— — —)

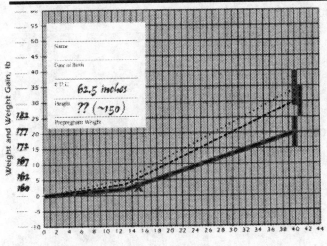
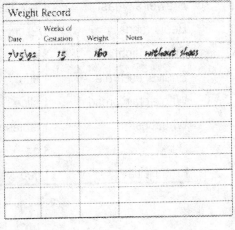

Plotting Weight

- Accurately record weeks of gestation and weight in the "Weight Record" box for future reference.
- Mark an x on the chart at the point that corresponds to that weight and number of weeks of pregnancy.
- See *Nutrition During Pregnancy and Lactation* for tips on interpreting weight gain.
- Consider writing comments (e.g., "ran out of food," "edema 2+," "nausea and vomiting resolved") that will be useful in later interpretation of the weight gain pattern.

Source: California Department of Health Services. (1990). *Nutrition during pregnancy and the post-partum period: A manual for health care professionals.* Sacramento, CA: Author.

Table 18.7

Dietary Sources of Iron

Food	Serving	Mg Iron
Beef liver	3 oz	7.5-12
Sunflower seeds	1/2 cup	5.1
Dried apricots	1/2 cup	3.6
Blackstrap molasses	1 tablespoon	3.2
Almonds	1/2 cup	2.7
Cashews	1/2 cup	2.6
Soybeans	1/2 cup	2.5
Raisins	1/2 cup	2.5
Lentils	1/2 cup	2.1
Turkey, dark	3 oz	2.0
Lima beans	1/2 cup	2.0
haddock or cod fish	6 oz	1.0
Spinach	1 cup	1.7
Brussels sprouts	1 cup	1.7
Peanuts	1/2 cup	1.6
Peas	1/2 cup	1.4
Brewer's yeast	1 tablespoon	1.4
Beet greens	1/2 cup	1.4
Turkey, light	3 oz	1.0
Endive, escarole	1 cup	1.0
Whole grain bread	1 slice	.08
Wheat germ	1 tablespoon	.05
Duck	3 oz	2.0
Prune juice	1 cup	10.5

Source: Adapted from California Department of Health Services. (1990). *Nutrition during pregnancy and the post-partum period: A manual for health care professionals.* Sacramento, CA: Author.

Table 18.8

Dietary Sources of Calcium

Food	Amount	Mg Calcium
Dairy Products		
Milk, whole	1 cup	288
Milk, low-fat (2%)	1 cup	297
Milk, skim	1 cup	298
Buttermilk	1 cup	296
Yogurt (low-fat)	1 cup	270
Nonfat milk powder	1/2 cup	367
Fish		
Fish canned with bones	3 oz	345
Oysters	1 cup	226
Shrimp	1 cup	147
Tofu (soy curd)*	4 oz	150
Sesame Seeds		
Ground or meal	1/2 cup	270
Vegetables **		
Collard greens	1 cup	360
Dandelion greens	1 cup	150
Okra	1 cup	150
Bok choy	1 cup	250
Kale	1 cup	200
Mustard greens	1 cup	180
Broccoli	1 stalk	267
Turnip greens	1 cup	267

* Fortified soy milk, which is acceptable, can offer the same calcium content as milk.
** Vegetables and grains may contain relatively high levels of calcium, but the mineral is bound by oxalates or phytates, and hence not well absorbed. The above vegetables offer unbound calcium.

Source: Adapted from: California Department of Health Services (1990). *Nutrition during pregnancy and the post-partum period: A manual for health care professionals.* Sacramento, CA: Author.

Table 18.9

Amount of Elemental Calcium in Common Supplements

Supplements	Calcium	Required to provide 600 mg Calcium
Calcium carbonate	40%	1500 mg
Calcium citrate	24%	2500 mg
Calcium lactate	14%	4275 mg
Calcium gluconate	9%	6675 mg

Source: California Department of Health Services (1990). Adapted from (IOM, 1990).

Table 18.10

Recommended Contents of a Prenatal Vitamin/Mineral Supplements

NUTRIENT	AMOUNT
Vitamin B$_6$	2 mg
Folate	300 mcg
Vitamin C	50 mg
Vitamin D	200 IU
Calcium	250 mg
Iron	30 mg
Zinc	15 mg
Copper	2 mg

Source: California Department of Health Services (1990). Maternal and Child Health Branch. Nutrition during pregnancy and the post-partum period: A manual of health professionals, June 1990. Adapted from (IOM, 1990)

Table 18.11

Relationships Between Diet and Health

- Obesity increases the risk for coronary heart disease, noninsulin-dependent diabetes, and hypertension. Obesity also increases the risk of gall bladder disease, degenerative joint disease, and some types of cancer (e.g., breast, endometrial).

- Frequent consumption of highly cariogenic foods (those containing fermentable, orally retained carbohydrates), especially between meals, can nullify some of the preventive benefits of adequate fluoride intake and promote dental caries.

- Excessive sodium and inadequate potassium intake have been associated with high blood pressure. A possible role for dietary calcium and magnesium in the regulation of blood pressure has also been suggested.

- Total fat, saturated fat, and cholesterol intake are contributing risk factors for heart disease.

- Low dietary fiber may contribute to the symptoms of chronic constipation, diverticulosis, and some types of irritable bowel syndrome.

- Dietary fat has been associated epidemiologically with some types of cancer (e.g., breast, colon).

- Poor nutritional status may enhance susceptibility or impair response to infections.

- Inadequate intakes of calcium and/or vitamin D may put women at risk for osteoporosis later in life.

- Inadequate intake of iron predisposes premenopausal women to iron-deficiency anemia.

NOTE: In addition to the above relationships between diet and common diseases, some birth control methods may affect nutritional status. Oral contraceptives tend to alter the metabolism of certain nutrients, and the intrauterine device (IUD) may cause greater-than-usual menstrual losses, increasing the need for iron.

To help all preconceptional, pregnant, postpartum, and lactating women achieve optimal nutritional status, nutritional services should be available from health care professionals who are trained to provide the best quality of care, who are well informed, and who keep up-to-date with well-documented publications. Health care professionals should be prepared to alert women to the fact that excessive or inappropriate consumption of some nutrients and food substances contributes to adverse health conditions.

Table 18.12

Dietary Sources of Folacin

Rich Sources	More than 75 mcg per serving
Asparagus	6 stalks or 1/2 cup cooked
Beans: garbanzo, kidney, navy, pinto	1/2 cup cooked
Lentils	1/2 cup cooked
Lettuce: romaine	1 cup raw
Orange juice	6 oz
Spinach	1 cup raw *or* 1/2 cup cooked
Yeast, nutritional	

Good Sources	35 to 75 mcg per serving
Avocado	1/2 medium
Beans: baked, pork and beans	1/2 cup cooked
Bean sprouts	1 cup raw
Beets, fresh	1/2 cup cooked
Broccoli	1/2 cup cooked
Brussels sprouts	1/2 cup cooked
Cabbage	1 cup raw
Collards	1/2 cup cooked
Corn	1/2 cup cooked
Falafel (garbanzo croquettes)	3 patties
Humus (garbanzo-sesame dip)	1/2 cup
Lettuce (Bibb, Boston, endive)	1 cup raw
Liver	1 oz cooked
Mustard greens	1/2 cup cooked
Orange	1 medium
Peanuts	1/4 cup
Peas, green	1/2 cup cooked
Peas, split	1/2 cup cooked
Pineapple juice	6 oz
Sesame butter (tahini)	3 tablespoons
Soybean kernels, roasted	2 $1/2$ tablespoons
Sunflower seeds	1 oz or 1/4 cup
Tomato juice	6 oz
Vegetable juice cocktail	6 oz

Source: Adapted from California Department of Health Services (1990). *Nutrition during pregnancy and the post-partum period: A manual for health care professionals.* Sacramento, CA: Author.

References

American College of Obstetricians and Gynecologists (ACOG). (1993). The Committee on Obstetrics: Maternal and Fetal Medicine.

American Dietetic Association (ADA) Reports. (1994). Position of the American Dietetic Association: Nutrition in the treatment of anorexia nervosa, bulimia nervosa, and binge eating. *Journal of the American dietetic Association. 94*(8):902–907.

American Psychiatric Association. (1994). *Diagnostic and Statistical Manual of Mental Disorders (DSD - IV)* (4th ed.). Washington, DC: Author.

California Department of Health Services, Maternal Child Health Branch. (1998). *Guidelines for Care: California Diabetes and Pregnancy Program.* Sacramento, CA.

California Department of Health Services, (1990). *Nutrition during pregnancy and the post-partum period: A manual for health care professionals.* Sacramento, CA. (The manual can be ordered from the California Department of Health Services, Maternal and Child Health Branch ATTN: Administrative Management Section 714 P Street, Room 740, Sacramento, CA 95814).

Cefalo, R.C. & Moos, M.K. (1995). *Preconceptional Health Care: A Practical Guide* (2nd ed.) St Louis: Mosby.

Gutierrez, Y. (1990a). Maternal and infant nutrition in the fourth trimester. In K.A. May (Ed.), *Comprehensive maternity nursing.* Philadelphia, PA: J.B. Lippincott Co.

Gutierrez, Y.M. (1990b). Nutritional aspects of pregnancy. In K A. May (Ed.), *Comprehensive maternity nursing.* Philadelphia, PA: J. B. Lippincott Co.

Gutierrez, Y. M. (1994). *Nutrition in health maintenance & health promotion for primary care providers.* University of California, San Francisco, School of Nursing. (Available through UCSF Nursing Press, School of Nursing, N535C, University of California San Francisco, San Francisco, CA. 94143–0608).

Institute of Medicine. (1985). *Preventing low birth weight.* Washington, DC: National Academic Press.

Institute of Medicine (IOM), National Academy of Sciences, Food and Nutrition Board. (1990). *Nutrition during Pregnancy Part I: Weight Gain, Part II: Nutrient Supplements.* Washington, DC: National Academy Press.

National Academy of Sciences, National Research Council. (1998). Recommended dietary allowances (11th ed.). Washington, DC: National Academy Press.

Rayburn, W.F.; Stanley, J.R. & Garrett, M.E. (1996). Preconceptional Folate Intake and Neural Tube Defects. *Journal of the American College of Nutrition. 15*(2):121–125.

Rippe, J.M.; Suellyn Crossley, RD; Rhonda Ringer. (1998). Obesity as a chronic disease: Modern medical and lifestyle management. In *The obesity epidemic: A mandate for a multidisciplinary approach.* Supplement to the American Dietetic Association. October 1998. V. 98 Supplement 2. p.59-515.

Texas Department of Health. (1996). *Women Get Folic Acid From Your Food.* Maternal and Child Health, Women Infant and Children (WIC) Program. Houston, TX.

INDEX

Notes for Use of the Index

Patient complaints are the primary way to enter the index. Drug names (both pharmacological and commercial) are indexed under the complaint for which they may be used.

Many acronyms appear here (375+ defined, 70+ undefined). Each defined acronym appears under the full title or phrase in the Index of Text. The page citations at the full listing lead the user to the definition (which is not necessarily the first mention) and to description of the material, if any. The acronym itself, with a *See* reference to the full entry, appears in the separate Index of Acronyms that follows the Index of Text. The index does not include reference to every use of the acronyms or to the undefined ones.

Symptoms of complaints are found in several arrangements. They may be listed in the Clinical Guideline as 'Symptomatology,' as a list of symptoms or just as patient complaints. They are indexed as 'symptomatology' or as 'symptoms' under the applicable disease or condition.

Pathogens

Index of Text

A

INDEX

Vaginitis, 1057-76
  common vulvovaginal irritants, 1072
  contraindication, 1069
  postpartum atrophic, 1059, 1064-67
  prevention strategies, 1073
  symptoms, 1061-62
Vaginosis, bacterial, 1057
Valsalva's maneuver, 488
Varicella, 76-77
  effects on infant, 76
  vaccination, 76
Varicella vaccine (Var), 1158
Varicella virus vaccine, VARIVAX®, 836
Varicella zoster immune globulin (VZIG),
    831
  candidates for, 839
Varicella zoster virus (VZV), 826-40
  acetaminophen, 833
  acyclovir, 833
  amoxicillin, 834
  calamine lotion, 833
  camphor-menthol, 833
  clavulanic acid, 834
  dicloxacillin, 833
  exposure needing VZIG, 838
  exposure/treatment chart, 840
  mupirocin, 833
  preventive measures, 837
  reinfection, 827
  symptoms, 828
  vaccine, 828
Varicosities, 297-99
VDRL in CSF (VDRL-CSF), 1040
Venereal disease research laboratory
    (VDRL), 1038
Venereal warts. See Condylomata
    acuminata
Venous thromboembolic disease, 555-62
  contraindication, 559
  symptomatology, 556-57
Ventilation/perfusion (V/Q), 560
Vertigo, 247-50
  causes, 247
Video display terminal (VDT), 431
Vitamin A, 73
  risk of excess, 7

Vitamin B$_{12}$ deficiency, 650-70
  lack in vegetarian diet, 651, 663
Vitamin/mineral supplements
  calcium, 1189-90
  folic acid, 1188
  iron, 1188
  zinc, 1188
Vomiting, 282-90
  acupuncture for, 288
  alternate remedies, 288
  list of medicines. See Nausea
  self-help, 287

W

Weight gain, grid for prenatal women, 1199
Weight risks, 7
Weight, desired for women, 1197
White blood cells (WBCs), 279
Within normal limits (WNL), 181
Women, Infants, Children (WIC), 25

X Y Z

Yellow fever, 205
  contraindication, 217
  waiver, 216
Zalcitabine (ddC), 1019
Zidovudine (ZDV or AST)
  ACTG protocol, 993, 1012
Zinc, food sources, 662
Zollinger-Ellison syndrome, 622

Index of Acronyms
starts on next page